THOUSANDS OF NEW LISTINGS, THOUSANDS OF NEW CHOICES . . . *GIVE YOURSELF—AND YOUR FAMILY—THE GIFT OF GOOD HEALTH!*

Whether you're trying to maintain a healthy lifestyle or are under a doctor's supervision, you can depend on Corinne T. Netzer, the bestselling expert who sets the standard against which all others are measured with the most accurate and up-to-date information available. *The Complete Book of Food Counts,* now completely revised and updated for the **eighth** edition, helps you make *informed* choices among the foods you love best—from fast-food salads to the most exotic cuisine—with all-new information on a wide variety of new products. Take it to the office . . . keep a copy in the kitchen . . . carry it with you on trips . . . it's quick, easy, and indispensable—the ultimate one-volume reference for today's health-conscious consumer!

Thousands more listings than ever before!

THE COMPLETE BOOK OF FOOD COUNTS
EIGHTH EDITION

CORINNE T. NETZER

P9-BZG-862

Books by Corinne T. Netzer

The Corinne T. Netzer Annual Calorie Counter
The Complete Book of Food Counts
Corinne T. Netzer's Big Book of Miracle Cures
The Corinne T. Netzer Carbohydrate Dieter's Diary
The Complete Book of Vitamin and Mineral Counts
The Corinne T. Netzer Carbohydrate Counter
The Corinne T. Netzer Dieter's Diary
The Corinne T. Netzer Encyclopedia of Food Values
The Corinne T. Netzer Fat Gram Counter
The Corinne T. Netzer Low-Fat Diary
The Dieter's Calorie Counter
The Corinne T. Netzer Dieter's Activity Diary

Available from Dell

Eighth Edition

THE
COMPLETE
BOOK
OF
FOOD COUNTS

Corinne T. Netzer

A DELL BOOK

THE COMPLETE BOOK OF FOOD COUNTS, EIGHTH EDITION
A Dell Book / January 2009

Published by
Bantam Dell
A Division of Random House, Inc.
New York, New York

Dell is a registered trademark of Random House, Inc., and the colophon is a trademark of Random House, Inc.

ISBN 978-0-440-24320-5

Printed in the United States of America
Published simultaneously in Canada

www.bantamdell.com

OPM   10 9 8 7 6 5 4 3 2 1

For
Jack and Chris Healy

Introduction

The eighth edition of *The Complete Book of Food Counts* is the largest compilation of essential food data in this format. It contains data (calories, protein, carbohydrates, fat, cholesterol, sodium, and fiber) for basic generic foods, brand-name foods, and restaurant chains. Whether you are interested in dieting or nutrition—or both—you will find this book unique and invaluable as a reference.

Since this book is alphabetized, you should have no difficulty finding whatever you wish to look up. There are, however, times when you may have to look in more than one place. If you are searching for a particular food and cannot find it immediately, look for it under a category, such as cakes, puddings, cookies, soups. Wherever sensible, I have cross-referenced listings, but the pressure of space has made it impossible to do that for every item.

Compare only foods listed in similar measures. This rule particularly applies to the confusion between measures by capacity and measures by weight. Eight ounces is not necessarily equivalent to eight fluid ounces or one cup. Eight ounces is a measure of how much something weighs; one cup is a measure of how much space it occupies. For instance, a cup of lightweight food, such as puffed rice or popcorn, weighs about one ounce, and eight ounces of the same product would fill many cups. Naturally, you can convert a similar unit of measure into a smaller or larger amount. The following table may be useful in making such conversions.

Equivalents by Capacity
(all measures level)
1 quart = 4 cups
1 cup = 8 fluid ounces
= ½ pint
= 16 tablespoons
2 tablespoons = 1 fluid ounce
1 tablespoon = 3 teaspoons

Equivalents by Weight
1 pound = 16 ounces
3.57 ounces = 100 grams
1 ounce = 28.35 grams

All the material contained in *The Complete Book of Food Counts* is based on information from the U.S. government, from producers and processors of brand-name foods, and from food chains. The data contained herein is the most complete and accurate information available as this book goes to press. Please bear in mind that seasonal and regional differences can affect the nutritional value of foods. Also, the food industry often changes recipes and sizes and may discontinue products or add new ones. In the future I will revise and update this book to keep you completely informed.

Good luck and good dieting.

Corinne T. Netzer

ABBREVIATIONS AND SYMBOLS

cal.	calories
carbo.	carbohydrates
chol.	cholesterol
cont.	container
diam.	diameter
fl.	fluid
gms.	grams
"	inch
<	less than
>	more than
mgs.	milligrams
lb(s).	pound(s)
n.a.	not available
oz.	ounce(s)
pc(s).	piece(s)
pkg.	package
pkt.	packet
prot.	protein
sod.	sodium
sq.	square
tbsp.	tablespoon
tsp.	teaspoon
tr.	trace
w/	with
*	prepared according to basic package directions, except as noted

THE
COMPLETE
BOOK
OF
FOOD COUNTS

A

Food and Measure	cal.	prot. (gms)	carbo. (gms)	fat (gms)	chol. (mgs)	sod. (mgs)	fiber (gms)
Abalone, meat only							
raw, 4 oz.	119	19.4	6.8	.9	96	341	0
Abalone, canned							
(*Roland* Limpets/							
Locos), ⅓ cup	45	9.0	1.0	.5	120	881	0
Abiyuch, ½ cup, 4 oz.	79	1.7	20.1	.1	0	23	6.0
Abruzzese sausage							
(*Boar's Head*), 1 oz.	100	8.0	<1.0	8.0	25	500	0
Acai blackberry drink							
(*Snapple*), 8 fl. oz. .	120	0	30.0	0	0	15	0
Acai juice, 8 fl. oz.:							
(*Bossa Nova* Original)	94	0	23.0	0	0	15	0
berry (*R.W. Knudsen*							
Organic)	100	1.0	24.0	0	0	15	0
Acai juice blends,							
8 fl. oz.:							
blueberry (*Bossa Nova*)	89	0	21.0	0	0	14	0
mango or passion fruit							
(*Bossa Nova*)	89	0	23.0	0	0	14	0
raspberry (*Bossa Nova*)	89	0	23.0	0	0	13	0
Acerola, fresh:							
10 fruits	15	.2	3.7	.1	0	3	.5
peeled, 1 cup	31	.4	7.5	.3	0	7	1.1
Acerola juice, fresh,							
8 fl. oz.	56	1.0	11.6	.7	0	7	.7
Acorn squash:							
raw:							
(*Frieda's*), 3 oz. . . .	35	1.0	9.0	0	0	0	2.0
4" squash, 15.2 oz.	172	3.5	44.9	.4	0	13	6.6
cubed, 1 cup	56	1.1	14.6	.1	0	4	2.1
baked, cubed, ½ cup .	57	1.1	14.9	.1	0	4	4.5
boiled, mashed, ½ cup	42	.8	10.8	.1	0	4	3.2
Adobo fresco, 1 tbsp.	41	.4	3.3	3.8	0	3087	.3

Food and Measure	cal.	prot. (gms)	carbo. (gms)	fat (gms)	chol. (mgs)	sod. (mgs)	fiber (gms)
Adobo sauce (*Doña Maria*), 2 tbsp.	230	2.0	10.0	15.0	0	370	2.0
Adzuki beans:							
dry (*Arrowhead Mills Organic*), ¼ cup ...	130	8.0	26.0	0	0	0	5.0
boiled, ½ cup	147	8.7	28.5	.1	0	9	8.4
Adzuki beans, canned (*Eden* Aduki Organic), ½ cup	110	7.0	19.0	0	0	10	5.0
Agave nectar (*Madhava*), 1 tbsp.	60	0	16.0	0	0	0	1.0
Aioli, see "Mayonnaise, refrigerated"							
Alfredo sauce, in jar, ¼ cup:							
(*Bertolli*)	110	2.0	3.0	10.0	40	460	0
(*Ragú* Classic)	110	1.0	2.0	10.0	30	350	0
cheese, 4 (*Classico*) ..	80	2.0	3.0	7.0	35	350	0
creamy (*Classico*) ...	80	1.0	3.0	7.0	40	490	0
garlic:							
(*Bertolli*)	110	2.0	3.0	10.0	30	360	0
roasted (*Classico*) .	70	1.0	3.0	6.0	30	430	1.0
Parmesan (*Ragú*)	70	2.0	3.0	5.0	25	440	0
red pepper, roasted (*Classico*)	60	1.0	3.0	5.0	35	310	0
tomato:							
Parmesan (*Delallo* Parmigiano)	110	1.0	3.0	10.0	30	400	0
sun-dried (*Classico*)	90	2.0	4.0	7.0	35	430	1.0
Alfredo sauce, refrigerated, ¼ cup:							
(*Buitoni*)	130	4.0	4.0	11.0	35	390	0
(*Buitoni* Light)	90	4.0	5.0	6.0	15	350	0
Alfredo sauce mix, creamy garlic (*McCormick*), 2 tbsp.	90	3.0	4.0	6.0	20	860	0
Allspice, 1 tsp.	5	.1	1.4	.2	0	1	.4
Almond, shelled, 1 oz., except as noted:							
(*Diamond*), ¼ cup, 1.1 oz.	170	6.0	6.0	15.0	0	0	4.0
(*Planters*)	170	6.0	5.0	15.0	0	0	3.0
(*Planters* Nut-rition) ..	170	6.0	6.0	15.0	0	40	3.0

Food and Measure	cal.	prot. (gms)	carbo. (gms)	fat (gms)	chol. (mgs)	sod. (mgs)	fiber (gms)
(*Planters* Salted)	160	6.0	6.0	15.0	0	60	3.0
raw, ¼ cup:							
(*Shiloh Farms*							
Organic), 1.2 oz.	210	7.0	7.0	18.0	0	0	4.0
(*SunRidge Farms*							
Organic), 1.1 oz.	190	8.0	5.0	15.0	0	0	4.0
(*Tree of Life*), 1.1 oz.	180	6.0	6.0	16.0	0	0	3.0
dried	167	5.7	5.8	14.8	0	3	3.1
dry-roasted:							
(*SunRidge Farms*),							
¼ cup, 1.1 oz. ...	180	7.0	6.0	16.0	0	0	4.0
salted	167	4.6	6.9	14.7	0	221	3.9
hickory honey (*Kettle*)	160	6.0	6.0	15.0	0	240	3.0
honey-roasted, 1 oz. .	168	5.2	7.9	14.2	0	37	3.9
oil-roasted, salted ...	176	5.8	4.5	16.4	0	221	3.2
sliced:							
(*Diamond*), 1.1 oz.	180	6.0	6.0	15.0	0	0	3.0
(*Planters*), 1.2 oz. .	200	7.0	6.0	18.0	0	0	4.0
slivered:							
(*Diamond*), ¼ cup,							
1.1 oz.	170	7.0	6.0	15.0	0	0	4.0
(*Planters*), 2 oz. ...	340	12.0	11.0	31.0	0	0	6.0
smoked:							
(*Blue Diamond*							
Smokehouse) ...	170	6.0	5.0	16.0	0	150	3.0
(*Planters* Nut-rition)	170	6.0	6.0	15.0	0	120	3.0
roasted (*New England Natural*),							
1.1 oz.	180	5.0	8.0	15.0	0	300	3.0
tamari:							
(*SunRidge Farms*							
Organic), 1.1 oz.	180	7.0	5.0	15.0	0	75	3.0
raw (*Tree of Life*) ..	170	<5.0	7.0	16.0	0	80	<4.0
tamari, roasted:							
(*Eden* Organic)	160	8.0	8.0	11.0	0	65	4.0
(*SunRidge Farms*),							
¼ cup, 1.1 oz. ..	160	6.0	6.0	14.0	0	100	3.0
toasted	167	5.8	6.5	14.4	0	3	3.2
Almond butter, 1 oz.							
or 2 tbsp.:							
all varieties (*Arrowhead Mills*)	200	7.0	6.0	17.0	0	0	4.0
creamy/crunchy:							
(*Kettle Roaster Fresh*)	180	5.0	6.0	17.0	0	55	2.0

Food and Measure	cal.	prot. (gms)	carbo. (gms)	fat (gms)	chol. (mgs)	sod. (mgs)	fiber (gms)
Almond butter, creamy/crunchy *(cont.)*							
(*Kettle Roaster Fresh Unsalted*)	180	5.0	6.0	17.0	0	0	2.0
(*MaraNatha* Natural/ Organic)	190	7.0	6.0	16.0	0	0	4.0
(*MaraNatha* Natural/ Organic Raw) . . .	195	7.0	6.0	16.0	0	0	4.0
honey (*MaraNatha*) . .	180	6.0	9.0	14.0	0	70	3.0
Almond flour (*Shiloh Farms*), 1 oz.	170	6.0	6.0	15.0	0	0	3.0
Almond meal, 1 oz. . .	116	11.2	8.2	5.2	0	2	n.a.
Amaranth, whole grain:							
(*Arrowhead Mills* Organic), ¼ cup . . .	180	7.0	31.0	3.0	0	10	7.0
(*Shiloh Farms* Organic), ¼ cup	195	7.0	36.0	3.0	0	0	6.0
Amaranth flakes, see "Cereal"							
Amaranth leaves:							
raw, trimmed, ½ cup .	4	.3	.6	<.1	0	3	n.a.
boiled, drained, ½ cup	14	1.4	2.7	.1	0	14	n.a.
Anasazi beans, dry (*Shiloh Farms* Organic), ¼ cup . . .	150	10.0	27.0	.5	0	0	9.0
Anchovy, fresh, European, meat only, raw, 1 oz.	37	5.8	0	1.4	17	29	0
Anchovy, canned, in olive oil, except as noted, drained:							
flat fillets:							
(*Roland*), 6 pcs.	25	4.0	0	1.0	16	860	0
(*Roland* Spanish), 4 pcs.	30	4.0	0	1.5	10	950	0
(*Vigo*), 6 pcs.	25	3.0	0	1.5	15	700	0
mini, soy oil (*Costamar*), 15 pcs. . .	30	3.0	0	2.0	15	1010	0
5 medium, .7 oz. . .	42	5.8	0	1.9	3	734	0
w/garlic and parsley (*Roland* Silverskin), 5 pcs.	25	4.0	0	1.0	15	900	0
pieces, safflower oil (*Alessi*), 2 pcs., .9 oz.	25	4.0	0	1.0	16	860	0

Food and Measure	cal.	prot. (gms)	carbo. (gms)	fat (gms)	chol. (mgs)	sod. (mgs)	fiber (gms)
rolled, w/capers:							
(*Roland*), 6 pcs.	25	4.0	0	1.0	16	860	0
(*Vigo*), 4 pcs.	25	3.0	0	1.5	12	880	0
Anchovy paste							
(*Roland*), 1 tbsp. . .	30	2.0	0	2.5	25	1140	0
Angel-hair pasta:							
dry, see "Pasta"							
refrigerated (*Buitoni*),							
1¼ cups	230	10.0	43.0	2.5	45	20	2.0
Angel-hair pasta							
dish mix, 1 cup*:							
and herbs (*Pasta Roni*)	310	9.0	41.0	13.0	5	820	2.0
Parmesan (*Pasta Roni*)	310	9.0	39.0	14.0	5	870	2.0
primavera (*Pasta Roni*)	310	9.0	37.0	15.0	5	990	2.0
tomato, spicy (*Near East*)	230	8.0	40.0	6.0	0	590	3.0
Angel-hair pasta							
entree, frozen, 1 pkg.:							
marinara, 10 oz.:							
(*Lean Cuisine One Dish Favorites*) . .	260	8.0	48.0	4.0	5	690	4.0
(*Smart Ones*)	200	8.0	37.0	2.0	0	610	4.0
meat sauce (*Michelina's Budget Gourmet*), 8 oz.	290	11.0	48.0	5.0	10	410	4.0
Anise seed, 1 tsp. . . .	7	.4	1.1	.3	0	<1	.3
Antelope, meat only, roasted, 4 oz.	170	33.4	0	3.0	143	51	0
Apple, fresh:							
(*Dole/Dole* Cameo), 5.4-oz. pc.	80	0	22.0	0	0	0	5.0
(*Frieda's* Lady), 5 oz. .	80	0	21.0	.5	0	0	3.0
raw, w/peel:							
2¾" apple	81	.3	21.1	.5	0	1	3.7
sliced, ½ cup	32	.1	8.4	.2	0	0	3.0
raw, peeled:							
2¾" apple	72	.2	19.0	.4	0	<1	2.4
sliced, ½ cup	31	.1	8.2	.2	0	0	1.0
cooked, peeled, sliced, boiled, ½ cup	45	.2	11.7	.3	0	1	2.0
Apple, can/jar (see also "Applesauce"):							
baby, in light syrup (*Roland*), ½ cup . .	50	0	12.0	0	0	20	2.0

Food and Measure	cal.	prot. (gms)	carbo. (gms)	fat (gms)	chol. (mgs)	sod. (mgs)	fiber (gms)
Apple, can/jar *(cont.)*							
baked, sliced, in syrup (*Lucky Leaf/ Musselman's* Dutch), ½ cup	170	0	41.0	0	0	40	3.0
caramel crème parfait (*Dole*), 4.3-oz. cont.	120	0	25.0	2.0	0	10	1.0
fried, ½ cup:							
(*Luck's*)	110	0	29.0	0	0	30	2.0
(*Lucky Leaf*)	170	0	43.0	0	0	20	2.0
(*Musselman's*)	130	0	32.0	0	0	30	2.0
cinnamon (*Luck's*) .	100	0	25.0	0	0	30	2.0
seasoned (*Glory*) ..	80	0	21.0	0	0	170	1.0
rings, spiced (*Lucky Leaf*), 1 ring	35	0	9.0	0	0	5	0
sliced (*Lucky Leaf*), ½ cup	50	0	12.0	0	0	20	1.0
Apple, coated, candy or caramel, w/nuts (*Tastee*), 3-oz. pc. .	160	3.0	26.0	5.0	0	20	4.0
Apple, dried:							
(*Amport Foods*), 11 pcs., 1.4 oz.	100	0	26.0	0	0	160	3.0
(*Sun•Maid*), ¼ cup, 1.4 oz.	120	1.0	29.0	0	0	135	2.0
baked (*Nature Valley* Fruit Crisps), .5-oz. pkg.	50	0	13.0	0	0	75	1.0
rings:							
(*Shiloh Farms* Organic), 8 pcs., 1.4 oz. ..	120	0	23.0	0	0	5	0
(*Tree of Life*), 6 pcs., 1.3 oz.	90	0	25.0	0	0	35	3.0
(*Tree of Life* Organic), 1 oz.	40	0	27.0	0	0	55	0
dehydrated, ½ cup ...	104	.4	28.1	.2	0	74	7.4
sulfured, 1 ring	16	.1	4.2	0	0	6	4.2
sulfured, ½ cup	104	.4	28.3	.1	0	75	7.5
Apple, fried, see "Apple, can/jar"							
Apple, frozen/ refrigerated:							
baked (*Stouffer's* Harvest), 6 oz.	190	0	40.0	3.0	0	5	2.0

Food and Measure	cal.	prot. (gms)	carbo. (gms)	fat (gms)	chol. (mgs)	sod. (mgs)	fiber (gms)
cinnamon (*Shedd's Spread Country Crock*), ½ cup	130	0	26.0	2.5	0	200	1.0
unheated, ½ cup	42	0	10.7	0	0	3	1.6
Apple butter, 1 tbsp.:							
(*Apple Time/Lucky Leaf/Musselman's*) .	30	0	8.0	0	0	0	0
(*Eden* Organic)	20	0	4.0	0	0	0	1.0
(*R.W. Knudsen* Organic)	35	0	9.0	0	0	0	0
(*Shiloh Farms*)	20	0	5.0	0	0	0	0
cherry (*Eden* Organic)	25	0	6.0	0	0	0	<1.0
cider or spiced (*Smucker's*)	45	0	11.0	0	0	10	0
Apple cider, see "Apple juice"							
Apple crisp mix (*Marzetti's*), ⅛ pkg.	120	1.0	27.0	0	0	90	1.0
Apple dip, see "Fruit dip"							
Apple drink:							
(*Lincoln*), 8 fl. oz. ...	130	0	31.0	0	0	10	0
(*R.W. Knudsen Sensible Sipper*), 4.23-oz. box	30	<1.0	8.0	0	0	5	0
(*Snapple*), 8 fl. oz. ...	120	0	30	0	0	10	0
(*Tropicana* Light), 10-fl.-oz. bottle ...	65	0	18.0	0	0	20	0
Apple drink mixer:							
green (*Angostura*), 2 fl. oz.	70	0	17.0	0	0	5	0
sour (*Rose's* Cocktail Infusions), 1.5 fl. oz.	60	0	16.0	0	0	20	0
Apple juice, 8 fl. oz., except as noted:							
(*After the Fall* Organic)	90	0	22.0	0	0	20	0
(*Apple & Eve* Clear) ..	110	1.0	26.0	0	0	5	0
(*Apple & Eve* Natural)	110	1.0	27.0	0	0	10	0
(*Apple Time/Lincoln/ Lucky Leaf*)	120	0	31.0	0	0	25	0
(*Eden* Organic)	90	0	24.0	0	0	0	0
(*Fragile Planet* Organic)	120	0	28.0	0	0	15	0
(*Langers* Cider/Juice/ Harvest)	120	0	28.0	0	0	0	0

Food and Measure	cal.	prot. (gms)	carbo. (gms)	fat (gms)	chol. (mgs)	sod. (mgs)	fiber (gms)
Apple juice (cont.)							
(Martinelli's Gold Medal Juice/Cider/ Unfiltered)	140	1.0	35.0	0	0	0	0
(Minute Maid)	110	0	28.0	0	0	20	0
(Minute Maid), 10-fl.-oz. bottle . . .	140	0	35.0	0	0	25	0
(Mott's Natural)	110	0	27.0	0	0	10	0
(Mott's Original)	120	0	29.0	0	0	10	0
(Nantucket Nectars Organic Cloudy) . . .	120	0	29.0	0	0	30	0
(Nantucket Nectars Pressed)	120	0	30.0	0	0	15	<1.0
(Odwalla)	140	0	34.0	0	0	25	0
(R.W. Knudsen Natural/Organic/ Cider & Spice)	120	<1.0	30.0	0	0	25	0
(Santa Cruz Organic) .	120	<1.0	30.0	0	0	25	0
(Snapple Green Apple), 11.5-oz. can	160	0	41.0	0	0	15	0
(Tree of Life)	120	<1.0	30.0	0	0	25	0
(Tropicana Orchard Style), 12 fl. oz. . . .	170	0	43.0	0	0	20	0
(Veryfine)	110	0	27.0	0	0	35	0
frozen*:							
(Cascadian Farm Organic)	120	0	29.0	0	0	0	0
(Langers)	120	0	28.0	0	0	15	0
(Minute Maid)	110	0	28.0	0	0	0	0
sparkling:							
(Langers Cider) . . .	120	0	28.0	0	0	15	0
(Lucky Leaf/Mussel- man's Cider)	150	0	36.0	0	0	20	0
(Martinelli Cider) . .	140	1.0	35.0	0	0	0	0
(Martinelli Juice), 10-fl.-oz. bottle .	180	1.0	43.0	0	0	0	<1.0
(R.W. Knudsen Crisp/Organic) . .	120	<1.0	30.0	0	0	25	0
Apple juice blend, 8 fl. oz., except as noted:							
berries and cherry (Ceres Secrets of the Valley)	130	0	32.0	0	0	10	0

Food and Measure	cal.	prot. (gms)	carbo. (gms)	fat (gms)	chol. (mgs)	sod. (mgs)	fiber (gms)
grape, white (*Minute Maid*), 6.75 fl. oz.	100	0	25.0	0	0	15	0
pear (*Tropicana* Organic Orchard Medley)	120	0	29.0	0	0	25	0
sparkling, all varieties (*Martinelli*)	110	0	27.0	0	0	4	0
strawberry:							
(*Minute Maid*), 6.75 fl. oz.	100	0	25.0	0	0	15	0
(*Veryfine*)	130	0	31.0	0	0	30	0
Apple juice concentrate (*Eden* Organic), 1 fl. oz.	110	0	28.0	0	0	10	0
Apple pastry, fillo (see also "Turnover"), frozen:							
pocket (*Aunt Trudy's* Organic), 5-oz. pc.	340	5.0	65.0	7.0	0	140	3.0
strudel (*The Fillo Factory* Organic), ⅛ of 22-oz. pkg.	290	3.0	47.0	10.0	0	110	2.0
Applesauce, ½ cup, except as noted:							
unsweetened/natural:							
(*Apple Time*)	50	0	13.0	0	0	10	2.0
(*Eden* Organic)	60	0	13.0	0	0	10	2.0
(*Langers*)	50	0	13.0	0	0	5	2.0
(*Mott's/Mott's* Organic)	50	0	14.0	0	0	0	1.0
(*Santa Cruz Organic*)	60	0	13.0	0	0	20	2.0
cinnamon (*Eden* Organic), 4-oz. cont.	70	0	17.0	0	0	10	2.0
cinnamon (*Santa Cruz Organic*)	90	0	21.0	0	0	25	2.0
Granny Smith (*Mott's Healthy Harvest Sauce*), 3.9-oz. cont.	50	0	13.0	0	0	0	1.0
sweetened:							
(*Lucky Leaf*)	90	0	22.0	0	0	10	2.0
(*Lucky Leaf*), 4-oz. cont.	80	0	20.0	0	0	10	2.0
(*Mott's* Classic/ Organic)	110	0	27.0	0	0	0	1.0

Food and Measure	cal.	prot. (gms)	carbo. (gms)	fat (gms)	chol. (mgs)	sod. (mgs)	fiber (gms)
Applesauce, sweetened *(cont.)*							
(*Mott's* Classic), 4-oz. cont.	100	0	24.0	0	0	0	1.0
(*Mott's* Chunky/ Homestyle)	90	0	23.0	0	0	0	1.0
(*Mott's* Organic), 4-oz. cont.	70	0	18.0	0	0	0	1.0
cinnamon (*Lucky Leaf*)	100	0	25.0	0	0	10	2.0
cinnamon (*Mott's*) .	120	0	29.0	0	0	0	1.0
cinnamon (*Tree of Life* Organic) ...	120	<1.0	20.0	0	0	0	2.0
Applesauce fruit blend, ½ cup, except as noted:							
all varieties:							
(*Mott's Healthy Harvest Sauce*), 3.9-oz. cont.	50	0	13.0	0	0	0	1.0
except blueberry (*Santa Cruz Organic*)	60	0	15.0	0	0	20	2.0
except mixed berry (*Mott's*), 4-oz. cont.	90	0	23.0	0	0	0	1.0
apricot or blackberry (*Santa Cruz Organic*), 4-oz. cont.	70	0	19.0	0	0	17	2.0
berry, mixed (*Mott's*), 4-oz. cont.	100	0	25.0	0	0	0	1.0
blueberry (*Santa Cruz Organic*)	70	0	16.0	0	0	20	2.0
cherry (*Eden* Organic)	70	0	17.0	0	0	10	3.0
cranberry raspberry (*Mott's Plus*), 3.9-oz. cont.......	50	0	13.0	0	0	0	3.0
pomegranate (*Mott's Plus*), 3.9-oz. cont.	50	0	13.0	0	0	0	1.0
raspberry (*Santa Cruz Organic*), 4-oz. cont.	60	0	13.0	0	0	20	2.0
strawberry (*Eden* Organic)	60	0	13.0	0	0	10	2.0
Apricot, fresh:							
(*Dole*), 3 medium, 4 oz.	60	0	11.0	1.0	0	0	1.0

Food and Measure	cal.	prot. (gms)	carbo. (gms)	fat (gms)	chol. (mgs)	sod. (mgs)	fiber (gms)
3 medium, 12 per lb. . .	51	1.5	11.8	.4	0	1	2.5
pitted, halves, ½ cup .	37	1.1	8.6	.3	0	1	1.9
pitted, sliced, ½ cup .	40	1.2	9.2	.3	0	2	2.0
Apricot, can/jar,							
½ cup, halves,							
except as noted:							
in juice, w/liquid	59	.8	15.1	<.1	0	5	2.0
in extra light syrup							
(*Del Monte* Lite) . . .	60	0	16.0	0	0	10	1.0
in light syrup:							
(*Del Monte Orchard*							
Select)	80	<1.0	21.0	0	0	10	1.0
chunks (*S&W* Sun)	90	1.0	22.0	0	0	25	1.0
almond flavor (*Del*							
Monte)	90	0	22.0	0	0	10	1.0
in heavy syrup:							
(*Del Monte*)	100	0	26.0	0	0	10	1.0
whole (*S&W*)	120	<1.0	29.0	0	0	10	1.0
Apricot, dried:							
(*Amport Foods*), 7 pcs.,							
1.4 oz.	100	2.0	24.0	0	0	0	3.0
(*Sun•Maid* California),							
¼ cup, 1.4 oz.	100	1.0	26.0	0	0	0	3.0
(*Sun•Maid* Mediterra-							
nean), 1.4 oz.	100	1.0	23.0	0	0	15	3.0
(*SunRidge Farms* Fancy),							
5 pcs., 1.4 oz.	100	1.0	25.0	0	0	0	3.0
(*SunRidge Farms* Turk-							
ish), 1.4 oz.	110	1.0	25.0	0	0	0	2.0
(*Sunsweet* Mediter-							
ranean), 1.4 oz. . . .	100	1.0	23.0	0	0	25	3.0
diced (*Amport Foods*),							
¼ cup, 1.4 oz.	100	1.0	25.0	0	0	0	3.0
dehydrated, ½ cup . . .	190	2.9	49.3	.4	0	15	n.a.
sulfured, ½ cup	155	2.4	40.1	.3	0	7	5.9
Apricot, frozen,							
sweetened, ½ cup .	119	.9	30.4	.1	0	5	2.1
Apricot juice, 8 fl. oz.:							
(*Ceres*)	130	0	32.0	0	0	15	0
(*R.W. Knudsen* Nectar)	130	<1.0	30.0	0	0	30	0
Apricot kernels (*Shiloh*							
Farms Organic),							
¼ cup	210	7.0	7.0	19.0	0	0	3.0

Food and Measure	cal.	prot. (gms)	carbo. (gms)	fat (gms)	chol. (mgs)	sod. (mgs)	fiber (gms)
Apricot nectar:							
(*Goya*), 8 fl. oz.	130	1.0	31.0	0	0	15	0
(*Goya*), 12 fl. oz.	220	1.0	53.0	0	0	25	1.0
(*Santa Cruz Organic* 100%), 8 fl. oz.	120	0	29.0	0	0	35	<1.0
Arby's:							
breakfast:							
biscuit:							
plain	273	5.0	28.0	15.0	1	786	1.0
bacon	340	9.0	29.0	21.0	13	1028	1.0
bacon/egg/cheese	461	17.0	30.0	28.0	169	1446	1.0
chicken	417	15.0	39.0	23.0	17	1240	1.0
ham	323	14.0	29.0	17.0	15	1315	1.0
ham/egg/cheese ..	444	21.0	31.0	24.0	171	1734	1.0
sausage	436	10.0	28.0	31.0	32	1160	1.0
sausage gravy ..	961	7.0	107.0	68.0	12	3755	1.0
sausage/egg/ cheese	557	18.0	30.0	38.0	187	1579	1.0
croissant:							
bacon/egg	337	11.0	23.0	22.0	187	651	1.0
bacon/egg/cheese	378	14.0	23.0	22.0	198	850	1.0
ham/cheese	274	13.0	22.0	12.0	53	842	1.0
ham/egg/cheese .	441	23.0	25.0	24.0	345	1358	1.0
sausage/egg	433	12.0	23.0	32.0	208	784	1.0
sausage/egg/ cheese	475	15.0	23.0	32.0	216	982	1.0
sourdough:							
bacon/egg/cheese	437	20.0	40.0	16.0	174	1220	2.0
egg/cheese	392	17.0	40.0	12.0	166	1058	2.0
ham/egg/cheese .	442	26.0	41.0	14.0	180	1586	2.0
sausage/egg/ cheese	556	22.0	40.0	28.0	197	1431	2.0
wrap:							
bacon/egg/cheese	515	16.0	50.0	29.0	166	1367	2.0
ham/egg/cheese .	575	25.0	51.0	31.0	185	2005	2.0
sausage/egg/ cheese	689	21.0	50.0	45.0	202	1849	2.0
breakfast items:							
blueberry muffin	320	4.0	49.0	12.0	20	480	1.0
French *Toastix* ..	312	8.0	44.0	13.0	0	492	1.0
syrup	78	0	20.0	0	0	25	0
sandwiches/melts:							
beef, roast:							
Arby's melt	302	16.0	36.0	12.0	30	921	2.0

Food and Measure	cal.	prot. (gms)	carbo. (gms)	fat (gms)	chol. (mgs)	sod. (mgs)	fiber (gms)
bacon/beef/							
cheddar	521	27.0	45.0	27.0	64	1573	2.0
beef/cheddar . . .	445	22.0	44.0	21.0	51	1274	2.0
French dip/Swiss	473	32.0	38.0	18.0	79	1679	3.0
large	547	42.0	41.0	28.0	102	1869	3.0
medium	415	31.0	34.0	21.0	73	1379	2.0
regular	320	21.0	34.0	14.0	44	953	2.0
sourdough melt .	355	18.0	40.0	14.0	30	1047	2.0
super	398	21.0	40.0	19.0	44	1060	2.0
Swiss melt	303	16.0	37.0	12.0	29	919	2.0
fish, fillet	535	21.0	59.0	25.0	55	954	2.0
fish, spicy Cajun . .	595	21.0	59.0	32.0	68	881	3.0
ham sourdough melt	380	19.0	39.0	13.0	31	1280	2.0
ham/Swiss melt . . .	268	17.0	35.0	5.0	25	1042	1.0
Chicken Naturals:							
bacon/Swiss:							
crispy	624	36.0	52.0	29.0	68	1320	2.0
grilled	462	38.0	38.0	17.0	25	1333	2.0
Cordon Bleu:							
crispy	657	41.0	49.0	32.0	76	1624	2.0
grilled	495	43.0	35.0	19.0	34	1637	2.0
fillet, crispy	577	30.0	50.0	30.0	52	902	3.0
fillet, grilled	414	32.0	36.0	17.0	9.0	914	3.0
Market Fresh:							
BLT, ultimate . . .	779	23.0	75.0	45.0	51	1571	6.0
corned beef Reuben	590	32.0	55.0	32.0	77	1685	3.0
pecan chicken							
salad	769	30.0	79.0	39.0	74	1240	9.0
roast beef, Swiss	777	37.0	73.0	41.0	89	1743	5.0
roast ham, Swiss	691	33.0	75.0	31.0	59	1952	5.0
turkey Reuben . .	594	40.0	56.0	30.0	86	1318	3.0
turkey/ranch/bacon	818	46.0	75.0	38.0	102	2146	5.0
turkey/Swiss . . .	708	41.0	74.0	30.0	83	1677	5.0
toasted subs:							
French dip/Swiss	622	37.0	68.0	20.0	79	3397	3.0
Italian, classic . .	787	33.0	67.0	39.0	84	2612	3.0
Philly beef	739	32.0	64.0	37.0	85	1881	3.0
turkey bacon club	619	42.0	65.0	18.0	82	2052	3.0
Market Fresh wraps:							
BLT, ultimate	648	29.0	45.0	44.0	51	1530	5.0
chicken, Southwest	567	36.0	42.0	29.0	88	1481	4.0
corned beef Reuben	560	36.0	42.0	29.0	77	1556	6.0
pecan chicken salad	638	30.0	48.0	38.0	74	1199	8.0

Food and Measure	cal.	prot. (gms)	carbo. (gms)	fat (gms)	chol. (mgs)	sod. (mgs)	fiber (gms)
Arby's Market Fresh wraps *(cont.)*							
turkey Reuben	564	44.0	43.0	27.0	86	1189	6.0
turkey/ranch/bacon	683	45.0	44.0	37.0	102	2103	4.0
Chicken Naturals:							
popcorn, large	531	35.0	39.0	26.0	59	1666	3.0
popcorn, regular ..	365	24.0	27.0	18.0	40	1145	2.0
BBQ sauce	44	0	11.0	0	0	343	0
Buffalo sauce ...	10	0	2.0	1.0	0	790	0
Popcorn Shakers ..	585	36.0	51.0	27.0	59	2795	3.0
Market Fresh salads, no dressing/extras:							
chicken club	426	28.0	26.0	23.0	172	1029	4.0
Martha's Vineyard .	277	26.0	24.0	8.0	72	451	4.0
Santa Fe chicken:							
popcorn	416	25.0	37.0	18.0	46	940	6.0
grilled	283	29.0	21.0	9.0	72	521	6.0
dressing/add-ons:							
almonds, sliced ...	81	4.0	2.0	8.0	0	0	1.0
croutons	77	2.0	7.0	5.0	1	116	0
ranch dressing:							
buttermilk	325	1.0	4.0	34.0	28	657	0
buttermilk, light .	112	1.0	13.0	6.0	0	472	1.0
Santa Fe	296	1.0	4.0	31.0	21	692	0
raspberry vinaigrette	194	0	18.0	14.0	0	387	0
tortilla strips	71	1.0	9.0	3.0	0	25	1.0
sides/*Sidekickers:*							
fries, cheddar	465	6.0	51.0	28.0	2	1311	5.0
fries, curly:							
large	631	8.0	73.0	37.0	0	1476	7.0
medium	397	5.0	46.0	24.0	0	928	4.0
small	338	4.0	39.0	20.0	0	791	4.0
cheddar sauce ..	30	0	2.0	2.0	1	181	0
fries, home style:							
large	566	6.0	82.0	37.0	0	1029	6.0
medium	377	4.0	55.0	25.0	0	686	4.0
small	302	3.0	44.0	20.0	0	549	3.0
Jalapeño Bites:							
large, 10	611	11.0	58.0	43.0	56	1052	4.0
regular, 5	305	5.0	29.0	21.0	28	526	2.0
Loaded Potato Bites:							
large, 10	707	23.0	54.0	44.0	27	1601	5.0
regular, 5	353	11.0	27.0	22.0	13	800	2.0
mozzarella sticks:							
large, 8	849	36.0	75.0	56.0	90	2730	4.0

Food and Measure	cal.	prot. (gms)	carbo. (gms)	fat (gms)	chol. (mgs)	sod. (mgs)	fiber (gms)
regular, 4	426	18.0	38.0	28.0	45	1370	2.0
marinara sauce .	30	1.0	4.0	2.0	0	0	1.0
onion petals:							
large	828	10.0	88.0	57.0	2	831	5.0
regular	331	4.0	35.0	23.0	1	332	2.0
potato cakes, 3 ...	369	3.0	39.0	28.0	0	587	3.0
potato cakes, 2 ...	246	2.0	26.0	18.0	0	391	2.0
sauce/condiments:							
Arby's Sauce	15	0	4.0	0	0	177	0
Bronco Berry Sauce	122	0	30.0	0	0	36	0
cheddar sauce	30	0	2.0	2.0	1	181	0
honey mustard dipping sauce ...	129	0	6.0	12.0	9	151	0
Horsey Sauce	62	0	3.0	5.0	5	173	0
ketchup pkt.	13	0	3.0	0	0	158	0
mayo, .5 oz.	105	0	0	11.0	9	74	0
ranch sour cream dipping sauce ...	158	1.0	2.0	16.0	0	277	0
red ranch sauce ...	72	0	5.0	5.0	0	105	0
Spicy Three Pepper Sauce	22	0	3.0	1.0	0	140	0
Tangy Southwest Sauce	333	1.0	5.0	35.0	29	371	0
shakes, regular size:							
chocolate	507	13.0	83.0	13.0	34	357	0
Jamocha	498	13.0	81.0	13.0	34	393	0
strawberry	498	13.0	81.0	13.0	34	363	0
vanilla	437	13.0	66.0	13.0	34	350	0
desserts:							
chocolate chip cookie	202	2.0	26.0	10.0	15	213	1.0
cinnamon roll, see "*T.J. Cinnamons*"							
turnover:							
apple, iced	377	4.0	65.0	16.0	0	201	2.0
cherry, iced	377	4.0	65.0	15.0	0	201	2.0
chocolate	400	6.0	37.0	25.0	0	190	4.0
Arctic char, raw, meat only, 4 oz.	207	25.0	0	9.1	30	91	0
Arrowhead:							
raw, 1 medium, 2⅝" .	12	.6	2.4	<.1	0	3	<1.0
boiled, drained, 1 medium, .4 oz. ...	9	.5	1.9	<.1	0	2	<1.0
Arrowroot, raw, sliced, ½ cup	36	2.5	8.0	.1	0	16	.8

Food and Measure	cal.	prot. (gms)	carbo. (gms)	fat (gms)	chol. (mgs)	sod. (mgs)	fiber (gms)
Arrowroot flour, 1 cup	457	.4	112.8	.1	0	2	4.4
Artichoke, globe, fresh:							
raw,							
(*Dole*), 1 medium,							
2 oz. edible	25	2.0	6.0	0	0	70	3.0
4.5-oz. choke	60	4.2	13.5	.2	0	120	6.9
5.7-oz. choke	76	5.3	17.0	.2	0	152	8.9
boiled, drained,							
1 medium, 4.2 oz.	60	4.2	13.4	.2	0	114	6.5
hearts, boiled, drained,							
½ cup	42	2.9	9.4	.1	0	80	4.5
Artichoke, can or jar,							
hearts (see also							
"Artichoke, marinated"),							
in water:							
(*Progresso*), 2 pcs.,							
4.6 oz.	30	1.0	7.0	0	0	400	2.0
(*Vigo* Quartered), 8 pcs.	30	2.0	6.0	0	0	240	1.0
all varieties:							
(*Fanci Food*), 4.6 oz.	20	2.0	3.0	0	0	480	2.0
(*Roland*), ½ cup ..	35	2.0	6.0	0	0	420	4.0
Artichoke, frozen,							
hearts:							
(*Birds Eye/C&W*),							
12 pcs., 3 oz.	40	2.0	7.0	1.0	0	55	5.0
9-oz. pkg.	96	6.7	19.8	1.1	0	120	9.9
Artichoke, Jerusalem,							
see "Jerusalem							
artichoke"							
Artichoke, marinated:							
(*Delallo*), 1 oz.	25	.5	2.0	1.5	0	90	.5
(*Progresso*), 1.1 oz. .	60	0	2.0	5.0	0	110	0
quartered (*S&W*),							
2 pcs., 1 oz.	20	0	2.0	2.0	0	80	1.0
salad:							
(*Fanci Food*), 1 oz.	25	1.0	2.0	1.0	0	90	.5
(*Roland*), 2 tbsp. .	60	0	2.0	5.0	0	100	0
whole (*Roland*), 2 pcs.	20	1.0	2.0	1.5	0	130	1.0
Artichoke appetizer:							
canned:							
caponata (*Alessi*),							
⅓ of 7-oz. can ..	130	2.0	7.0	6.0	0	460	3.0
pâté (*Alessi*), 2 tbsp.	118	1.0	1.0	12.5	0	310	3.0

Food and Measure	cal.	prot. (gms)	carbo. (gms)	fat (gms)	chol. (mgs)	sod. (mgs)	fiber (gms)
frozen, and cheese, in mini fillo shells (*Athens*), 2 pcs., 1 oz.	70	2.0	5.0	4.5	10	170	0
Artichoke dip, see "Spinach dip"							
Arugula, fresh:							
10 leaves	5	.5	.7	.1	0	5	.3
½ cup	3	.3	.4	<.1	0	<1	.2
baby (*Fresh Express Organic*), 3 oz. ...	20	2.0	3.0	.5	0	25	1.0
Asparagus, fresh:							
raw, spears, trimmed:							
(*Dole*), 5 pcs., 3.3 oz.	25	2.0	4.0	0	0	0	2.0
4 small, 1.8 oz. ..	14	1.3	2.6	.1	0	1	1.2
purple (*Frieda's*), 3 oz.	20	4.0	4.0	0	0	0	1.0
white (*Frieda's*), 3 oz.	20	2.0	4.0	0	0	0	2.0
boiled, 4 spears, ½"-diam. base	14	1.6	2.5	.2	0	7	1.3
boiled, drained, cuts, ½ cup	22	2.3	3.8	.3	0	10	1.9
Asparagus, can/jar:							
all styles (*Del Monte*), ½ cup	20	2.0	3.0	0	0	365	1.0
spears:							
(*Green Giant*), 4.5 oz., approx. 5 pcs.	20	2.0	3.0	0	0	430	1.0
(*Le Sueur* Extra Large), 4.3 oz., approx. 3 pcs.	20	2.0	3.0	0	0	420	1.0
(*Roland*), ⅔ cup ..	20	2.0	3.0	0	0	450	2.0
(*S&W*), ½ cup	20	2.0	3.0	0	0	365	1.0
marinated (*Vigo*), 3 pcs.	10	1.0	1.0	0	0	75	0
white (*Fanci Food*), ½ cup	20	2.0	3.0	0	0	510	2.0
white (*Roland*), ⅔ cup	20	2.0	3.0	0	0	510	2.0
cuts, ½ cup:							
(*Green Giant*)	20	2.0	3.0	0	0	420	1.0
(*Green Giant* 50% Less Sodium) ...	20	2.0	3.0	0	0	210	1.0
drained, ½ cup	23	2.6	3.0	.8	0	350	2.0

Food and Measure	cal.	prot. (gms)	carbo. (gms)	fat (gms)	chol. (mgs)	sod. (mgs)	fiber (gms)
Asparagus, frozen:							
boiled, drained, 1 cup	50	5.3	8.8	.8	0	7	2.9
spears:							
(*Birds Eye*), 7 pcs.,							
3 oz.	20	2.0	3.0	0	0	0	0
(*C&W*), 7 pcs., 3 oz.	20	2.0	3.0	0	0	5	<1.0
(*Seabrook Farms*),							
7 pcs., 3 oz.	20	3.0	3.0	0	0	5	2.0
4 pcs.	14	1.9	2.4	.1	0	5	1.1
cuts:							
(*Birds Eye*), ¾ cup .	20	2.0	3.0	0	0	0	0
(*Cascadian Farm*							
Organic), ⅔ cup	20	2.0	3.0	0	0	85	<1.0
(*Green Giant Simply*							
Steam), ⅔ cup ..	20	2.0	3.0	0	0	90	<1.0
Asparagus, pickled,							
in jars, white (*Roland*),							
⅔ cup	40	2.0	8.0	0	0	510	2.0
Asparagus bean, see							
"Winged bean"							
Asparagus combina-							
tions, frozen:							
(*Birds Eye* Stir-fry),							
1 cup cooked	80	3.0	15.0	0	0	35	2.0
corn, yellow/white,							
baby carrots							
(*Birds Eye* Steam-							
fresh), ⅔ cup	70	2.0	13.0	.5	0	15	1.0
Atemoya (*Frieda's*),							
3 oz.	80	2.0	20.0	0	0	10	4.0
Au jus gravy, canned							
(*Campbell's*), ¼ cup	5	1.0	0	0	0	230	0
Au jus gravy mix:							
(*Lawry's*), ¼ cup* ...	25	<1.0	4.0	1.0	0	320	0
(*McCormick*), ¼ cup*	5	0	1.0	0	0	310	0
Aubergine, see							
"Eggplant"							
Australian blue squash							
(*Frieda's*), ¾ cup,							
3 oz.	30	1.0	7.0	0	0	0	1.0
Avocado:							
(*Del Monte*),							
⅓ medium, 1.1 oz.	55	1.0	3.0	5.0	0	0	3.0

Food and Measure	cal.	prot. (gms)	carbo. (gms)	fat (gms)	chol. (mgs)	sod. (mgs)	fiber (gms)
all varieties:							
cubed, 1 cup	240	3.0	12.8	22.0	0	11	10.1
pureed, ½ cup	184	2.3	9.8	16.6	0	8	7.7
California:							
pulp from							
1 medium, 6.1 oz.	289	3.4	14.9	26.7	0	14	11.8
pureed, ½ cup	192	2.3	9.9	17.7	0	9	7.8
Florida, pureed, ½ cup	138	2.6	9.0	11.6	0	2	6.4
seedless (*Frieda's*							
Cocktail), 1.4-oz. pc.	60	1.0	3.0	6.0	0	0	2.0
Avocado dip (see also							
"Guacamole")							
(*Litehouse*), 2 tbsp.	140	1.0	2.0	15.0	15	210	0
Avocado sauce							
(*Calavo*), 2 tbsp. ..	15	<1.0	2.0	.5	0	150	1.0

B

Food and Measure	cal.	prot. (gms)	carbo. (gms)	fat (gms)	chol. (mgs)	sod. (mgs)	fiber (gms)
Baba ganoush, see "Eggplant appetizer"							
Bacon, cooked, 2 slices, except as noted:							
(*Applegate Farms*) ...	60	4.0	0	5.0	10	290	0
(*Boar's Head*)	70	4.0	0	6.0	10	190	0
(*Dietz & Watson*)	70	4.0	1.0	6.0	15	250	0
(*Hormel* Micro)	80	5.0	0	7.0	20	300	0
(*Old Smokehouse*) ...	110	7.0	1.0	9.0	20	410	0
(*Oscar Mayer*)	70	4.0	0	6.0	15	290	0
(*Oscar Mayer* Center Cut)	50	4.0	0	4.0	15	270	0
(*Range Brand*)	110	7.0	0	9.0	20	460	0
hickory (*Tyson*)	90	5.0	0	7.0	15	240	0
maple flavor (*Hormel*)	80	5.0	0	7.0	15	270	0
mesquite (*Hormel*) ..	80	5.0	0	7.0	15	330	0
peppercorn, cracked (*Farmer John*)	70	5.0	0	5.0	15	180	0
precooked:							
(*Hormel*), 2½ slices	70	5.0	0	5.0	20	290	0
(*Oscar Mayer*), .5 oz.	70	5.0	0	5.0	15	220	0
hickory (*Tyson*) ...	90	5.0	0	7.0	15	240	0
thick cut, 1 slice:							
(*Oscar Mayer*), .4 oz.	60	4.0	0	5.0	10	250	0
hickory or peppered *Farmland*), .5 oz.	70	3.0	0	6.0	10	230	0
turkey, see "Turkey bacon"							
uncured:							
(*Hormel Natural Choice*)	80	5.0	0	7.0	15	360	0

Food and Measure	cal.	prot. (gms)	carbo. (gms)	fat (gms)	chol. (mgs)	sod. (mgs)	fiber (gms)
(*Hormel Natural Choice* Lower Sodium)	80	5.0	0	7.0	15	180	0
(*Oscar Mayer*)	60	7.0	0	5.0	15	400	0
Bacon, Canadian, 2 oz., except as noted:							
(*Applegate Farms*) . . .	90	12.0	1.0	4.0	35	500	0
(*Boar's Head*)	70	12.0	1.0	2.0	35	570	0
(*Dietz & Watson*)	70	11.0	1.0	2.0	30	490	0
(*Hormel/Red Label*) . .	70	11.0	0	2.5	30	650	0
(*Organic Prairie*), 1 oz.	50	7.0	0	2.5	20	190	0
(*Oscar Mayer*), 1.9 oz.	60	9.0	1.0	2.0	30	480	0
unheated	89	11.7	1.9	4.0	28	799	0
Bacon, Irish, back (*Dawn Irish Gold*), 2 slices, 2 oz.	140	10.0	1.0	10.0	30	570	0
Bacon, Italian (pancetta), 1 oz.:							
(*Applegate Farms*) . . .	90	6.0	0	7.0	25	460	0
(*Dietz & Watson*)	60	8.0	1.0	3.0	22	750	0
"Bacon," vegetarian, frozen, 2 slices, except as noted:							
(*Morningstar Farms* Veggie Strips)	60	2.0	2.0	4.5	0	230	1.0
(*Worthington* Stripples)	60	2.0	2.0	4.5	0	220	<1.0
Canadian (*Yves*), 3 slices, 2 oz.	80	17.0	2.0	.5	0	400	0
Bacon bits, 1 tbsp.:							
(*Oscar Mayer*)	25	3.0	0	1.5	5	220	0
bits (*Hormel*)	25	3.0	0	1.5	5	240	0
pieces (*Hormel*)	25	3.0	0	1.5	10	180	0
"Bacon" bits, imitation, 1½ tbsp.:							
(*Bac'n Pieces*)	30	3.0	2.0	1.5	0	220	0
chips/bits (*Bac-Os*) . .	30	3.0	2.0	1.5	0	120	0
Bacon dip, 2 tbsp.:							
and cheddar (*Kraft*) . .	60	1.0	3.0	5.0	5	170	0
tomato (*Marzetti's*) . .	120	1.0	2.0	12.0	20	190	0
Bagel, 1 pc.: plain:							
(*Cobblestone Mill*) .	280	10.0	57.0	1.0	0	470	2.0

Food and Measure	cal.	prot. (gms)	carbo. (gms)	fat (gms)	chol. (mgs)	sod. (mgs)	fiber (gms)
Bagel, plain *(cont.)*							
(*Pepperidge Farm*) .	260	9.0	54.0	1.0	0	500	3.0
(*Thomas'*)	290	11.0	56.0	2.0	0	540	3.0
plain, onion, poppy, or							
sesame, 2 oz.	157	6.0	30.4	.9	0	304	1.3
blueberry (*Thomas'*) .	300	11.0	60.0	2.5	0	470	3.0
brown sugar							
cinnamon, mini							
(*Pepperidge Farm*) .	120	4.0	24.0	.5	0	150	2.0
cinnamon raisin:							
(*Pepperidge Farm*) .	270	8.0	57.0	1.0	0	450	3.0
swirl (*Thomas'*) . . .	290	10.0	58.0	2.0	0	480	4.0
everything:							
(*David's Deli*)	230	8.0	46.0	1.0	0	360	2.0
(*Pepperidge Farm*) .	260	9.0	53.0	1.5	0	400	2.0
(*Thomas'*)	300	12.0	54.0	4.0	0	510	3.0
maple (*David's Deli*							
French Toast)	230	7.0	48.0	1.5	5	85	<1.0
multigrain:							
(*David's Deli*)	190	8.0	42.0	1.0	<5	290	5.0
(*Cobblestone Mill*) .	280	10.0	58.0	1.5	0	410	3.0
oatmeal and honey							
(*Thomas'*)	290	11.0	58.0	2.0	0	460	3.0
onion (*Thomas'*)	290	11.0	57.0	2.0	0	530	3.0
raisin (*Thomas'*)	270	9.0	55.0	1.0	0	210	2.0
whole wheat:							
(*Pepperidge Farm*) .	250	11.0	49.0	1.5	0	450	6.0
(*Thomas'*)	270	12.0	55.0	2.0	0	440	8.0
mini (*Pepperidge*							
Farm)	100	4.0	20.0	.5	0	180	3.0
Bagel chips/crisps:							
plain, 1 oz.:							
(*New York Style*) . .	140	3.0	17.0	6.0	0	70	1.0
(*Stacy's Simply*							
Naked)	130	3.0	20.0	3.5	0	270	1.0
cinnamon raisin (*New*							
York Style), 1 oz. .	130	2.0	17.0	6.0	0	80	1.0
everything, 1 oz.:							
(*New York Style*) . .	130	3.0	15.0	7.0	0	300	1.0
(*Stacy's*)	130	3.0	19.0	4.0	0	390	2.0
garlic, 1 oz.:							
(*New York Style*) . .	130	3.0	16.0	6.0	0	200	1.0
toasted (*Stacy's*) . . .	130	3.0	20.0	3.5	0	260	2.0

Food and Measure	cal.	prot. (gms)	carbo. (gms)	fat (gms)	chol. (mgs)	sod. (mgs)	fiber (gms)
multigrain (*New York Style*), 1 oz.	130	4.0	17.0	6.0	0	180	2.0
sea salt (*New York Style*), 1 oz.	130	4.0	16.0	6.0	0	310	1.0
sesame (*New York Style*), 1 oz.	140	3.0	15.0	7.0	0	290	1.0
whole wheat, 1 oz.:							
(*New York Style*)	120	4.0	16.0	6.0	0	180	2.0
(*Stacy's*)	130	4.0	19.0	4.0	0	260	2.0
Bagel w/cream cheese (*Philadelphia* To-Go), 3.2 oz.:							
plain cream cheese	240	6.0	34.0	9.0	30	420	2.0
chive and onion	240	6.0	34.0	8.0	30	440	2.0
Baked beans, ½ cup, except as noted:							
(*Allens* Homestyle)	140	6.0	29.0	1.0	0	410	5.0
(*Allens* Original)	150	6.0	29.0	1.0	0	350	8.0
(*B&M* Country)	170	7.0	36.0	1.5	<5	710	7.0
(*B&M* Original, 8 oz.)	180	7.0	31.0	3.0	<5	420	8.0
(*B&M* Original, 16 oz.)	170	7.0	31.0	2.0	<5	400	8.0
(*Bush's* Bold & Spicy)	110	6.0	24.0	1.0	0	560	5.0
(*Bush's* Boston)	150	6.0	31.0	1.0	0	440	5.0
(*Bush's* Country)	160	6.0	33.0	1.0	0	680	5.0
(*Bush's* Homestyle)	140	6.0	29.0	1.0	0	550	5.0
(*Bush's* Original)	140	6.0	29.0	1.0	0	550	5.0
(*Bush's Grillin' Beans* Smokehouse)	170	7.0	34.0	1.0	0	570	5.0
(*Bush's Grillin' Beans* Steakhouse)	180	6.0	39.0	.5	0	510	5.0
(*Ranch Style* Original)	130	5.0	19.0	3.0	0	600	5.0
(*Ranch Style* Texas)	130	6.0	20.0	3.0	0	600	6.0
(*Van Camp's* Homestyle)	170	7.0	33.0	1.0	0	680	6.0
(*Van Camp's* Original)	140	7.0	30.0	1.0	0	540	6.0
bacon, maple cured:							
(*Allens*)	140	6.0	27.0	1.0	0	450	4.0
(*Bush's*)	140	6.0	28.0	1.0	0	620	5.0
(*S&W*)	140	5.0	29.0	.5	0	510	6.0
bacon onion w/brown sugar (*B&M*)	190	8.0	36.0	2.0	<5	450	8.0
barbecue:							
(*Allens*)	150	6.0	29.0	1.0	0	410	5.0
(*B&M*, 16 oz.)	190	8.0	39.0	.5	0	570	9.0

Food and Measure	cal.	prot. (gms)	carbo. (gms)	fat (gms)	chol. (mgs)	sod. (mgs)	fiber (gms)
Baked beans, barbecue *(cont.)*							
(*B&M*, 28 oz.)	190	8.0	38.0	1.0	0	680	9.0
(*Bush's*)	150	6.0	32.0	1.0	0	510	5.0
(*S&W* Country) ...	140	6.0	28.0	.5	0	510	6.0
(*S&W* Ranch)	140	6.0	25.0	1.5	0	640	8.0
Southern pit (*Bush's* Grillin' Beans) ..	170	6.0	35.0	.5	0	550	6.0
bourbon brown sugar (*Bush's Grillin' Beans*)	170	7.0	35.0	.5	0	480	6.0
brown sugar bacon (*Campbell's*)	160	5.0	30.0	2.5	<5	470	8.0
hickory bacon (*Van Camp's*)	150	7.0	32.0	1.0	0	470	5.0
honey (*Bush's*)	160	6.0	32.0	1.0	0	540	6.0
honey mustard (*S&W*)	140	6.0	28.0	.5	0	600	6.0
jalapeño (*Ranch Style*)	120	5.0	19.0	2.5	0	740	6.0
maple flavor (*B&M*) ..	160	7.0	31.0	1.0	0	340	8.0
maple sugar (*S&W*) ..	150	7.0	29.0	0	0	640	6.0
navy beans, w/sorghum and mustard (*Eden Organic*)	150	8.0	27.0	0	0	130	7.0
onion:							
(*Allens*)	140	5.0	25.0	1.5	0	410	4.0
(*Bush's*)	140	6.0	29.0	1.0	0	550	5.0
w/pork:							
(*Campbell's*)	140	6.0	25.0	1.5	5	440	7.0
(*Wagon Master*) ..	130	7.0	23.0	1.0	0	420	9.0
(*Wagon Master*, 1 lb.)	130	7.0	21.0	1.0	0	330	6.0
red kidney (*B&M*) ...	200	8.0	36.0	3.0	<5	460	6.0
vegetarian:							
(*Allens*)	140	6.0	28.0	0	0	460	4.0
(*Amy's Organic*) ...	120	6.0	24.0	.5	0	480	6.0
(*B&M*, 8 oz.)	160	7.0	31.0	1.0	0	380	8.0
(*B&M*, 16 oz.)	160	7.0	28.0	1.0	0	380	8.0
(*B&M*, 28 oz.)	150	8.0	30.0	1.0	0	390	8.0
(*Bush's*)	130	6.0	29.0	0	0	550	5.0
Baking mix (see also "Biscuit mix"):							
(*Arrowhead Mills Organic*), ⅓ cup ...	130	5.0	28.0	1.0	0	390	2.0
(*Hodgson Mill* Multi Purpose), ¼ cup ..	100	4.0	22.0	2.0	0	0	3.0

Food and Measure	cal.	prot. (gms)	carbo. (gms)	fat (gms)	chol. (mgs)	sod. (mgs)	fiber (gms)
("Jiffy"), ¼ cup	130	2.0	21.0	4.5	0	310	<1.0
gluten free (Arrowhead Mills Organic), 1/20 pkg.	110	1.0	21.0	2.0	0	40	<1.0
whole wheat (Hodgson Mill Insta-Bake), ⅓ cup	138	4.0	29.0	1.0	0	290	3.0
Baking powder (Calumet), ¼ tsp.	0	0	0	0	0	100	0
Baking soda, ½ tsp. .	0	0	0	0	0	630	0
Baklava, frozen: (Athens/Apollo), 2 pcs., 2 oz.	230	3.0	30.0	11.0	0	75	1.0
chocolate (The Fillo Factory), 2-oz. pc. .	260	3.0	35.0	10.0	0	85	1.0
maple walnut (Aunt Trudy's Organic), ⅓ of 5-oz. pkg. ...	190	3.0	24.0	10.0	0	45	1.0
oatmeal raisin (Aunt Trudy's Organic), ⅓ of 5.5-oz. pkg. ...	180	3.0	34.0	4.5	0	50	1.0
raspberry (The Fillo Factory), 2-oz. pc. .	270	3.0	35.0	11.0	0	85	0
soy nut (Aunt Trudy's Organic), ⅓ of 5.5-oz. pkg.	190	4.0	29.0	6.0	0	60	2.0
walnut (The Fillo Factory), 2-oz. pc. .	270	3.0	35.0	12.0	5	105	0
Balsam pear: (Frieda's Bittermelon), 1 cup, 3 oz.	15	1.0	3.0	0	0	0	2.0
leafy-tips, ½ cup: raw	7	1.3	.8	.2	0	3	.6
boiled, drained	10	1.0	2.0	.1	0	4	.6
pods, ½" pcs., ½ cup: raw	8	.5	1.7	.1	0	3	1.3
boiled, drained	12	.5	2.7	.1	0	4	1.2
Balsamic glaze (Roland), 1 tbsp. ...	20	0	4.0	0	0	0	0
Bamboo shoots, fresh: raw, slices, ½ cup ...	21	2.0	4.0	.2	0	3	.7
boiled, drained, slices, ½ cup	8	.9	1.2	.1	0	3	<1.0

Food and Measure	cal.	prot. (gms)	carbo. (gms)	fat (gms)	chol. (mgs)	sod. (mgs)	fiber (gms)
Bamboo shoots, canned, ½ cup:							
(*La Choy*)	10	<1.0	2.0	0	0	10	<1.0
drained	13	1.1	2.1	.3	0	5	2.0
Banana (see also "Plantain"), fresh:							
(*Chiquita*), 1 medium, 4.4 oz.	110	1.0	29.0	0	0	0	4.0
(*Frieda's* Baby Nino/ Burro), 3-oz. pc. . .	80	1.0	20.0	0	0	0	1.0
1 medium, 8¾" long .	105	1.2	26.7	.6	0	1	2.7
sliced, ½ cup	69	.8	17.6	.4	0	1	1.8
mashed, ½ cup	104	1.2	26.4	.5	0	1	2.7
red (*Frieda's*), 5 oz. . .	130	1.0	33.0	.5	0	0	2.0
red, 7¼" long	118	1.6	30.7	.3	0	1	n.a.
Banana, dried:							
(*Frieda's*), 1.2 oz.	130	1.0	33.0	.5	0	0	2.0
(*Fruit Additions*), 1.4 oz.	130	2.0	35.0	0	0	0	1.0
chips:							
(*Amport Foods*), ¼ cup, 1.1 oz. . .	150	1.0	20.0	7.0	0	0	0
(*SunRidge Farms*), 35 pcs., 1.4 oz. .	210	1.0	23.0	13.0	0	0	3.0
(*SunRidge Farms* Organic), 1.4 oz.	210	0	17.0	14.0	0	0	1.0
(*Tree of Life*), 1.6 oz.	240	1.0	27.0	15.0	0	0	4.0
dehydrated, ¼ cup . . .	87	1.0	22.1	.5	0	1	1.9
Banana drink (*R.W. Knudsen Sensible Sipper*), 4.23 oz. . .	35	<1.0	9.0	0	0	5	0
Banana drink blend (*After the Fall Banana Casablanca*), 8 fl. oz.	150	1.0	37.0	0	0	20	0
Banana juice blend, mango carrot (*Nantucket Nectars*), 8 fl. oz.	140	0	30.0	0	0	30	0
Banana milk drink, see "Milk, flavored"							
Banana squash (*Frieda's*), 3 oz. . . .	30	1.0	7.0	0	0	0	1.0

Food and Measure	cal.	prot. (gms)	carbo. (gms)	fat (gms)	chol. (mgs)	sod. (mgs)	fiber (gms)
Barbecue sauce (see also "Grilling sauce"), 2 tbsp.:							
(*Annie's Natural* Organic)	45	0	9.0	1.0	0	240	0
(*Bear-Man Black Bear Boogie*)	40	0	8.0	1.0	0	220	0
(*Bear-Man Growlin' Grizzly*)	60	1.0	12.0	1.0	0	290	<1.0
(*Bilardo Brothers* Original)	25	1.0	5.0	0	0	240	1.0
(*Bone Suckin' Sauce*) .	50	0	11.0	0	0	230	0
(*Buccaneer Blends* Sticky Rum)	50	0	13.0	0	0	340	0
(*Bull's-Eye* Original) . .	60	0	13.0	0	0	330	0
(*Consorzio* Organic) . .	45	1.0	11.0	0	0	280	0
(*Cowtown* Kansas City)	45	1.0	11.0	0	0	290	0
(*Emeril's* Kicked Up) .	40	0	11.0	0	0	360	0
(*Hunt's* Original)	60	0	15.0	0	0	280	<1.0
(*Hunt's* Original Bold)	50	0	13.0	0	0	310	<1.0
(*KC Masterpiece* Original)	60	0	15.0	0	0	240	0
(*Kraft* Char-Grill)	50	0	13.0	0	0	450	0
(*Kraft* Original)	50	0	12.0	0	0	440	0
(*Kraft* Original Light) .	20	0	4.0	0	0	330	0
(*Kraft* Thick 'n Spicy) .	50	0	12.0	0	0	430	0
(*Mrs. Renfro's*)	35	<1.0	8.0	0	0	220	0
(*Roland* Char Siu) . . .	75	1.0	15.0	1.0	0	800	1.0
(*Sweet Baby Ray's* Original)	70	0	17.0	0	0	290	0
(*Vienna*)	60	1.0	16.0	0	0	390	0
(*Woody's* Cook-in' Concentrate)	50	<1.0	4.0	4.0	0	490	1.0
all varieties (*Maull's*) .	60	0	13.0	0	0	300	0
apple maple (*Buccaneer Blends*)	60	0	14.0	0	0	200	0
Asian (*San-J*)	35	3.0	7.0	0	0	860	0
brown sugar, spicy (*Kraft* Thick 'n Spicy)	60	0	15.0	0	0	350	0
Chinese style:							
(*Ah-So* Original) . . .	70	0	24.0	0	0	480	0
smoky (*Ah-So*)	100	0	24.0	0	0	480	0

Food and Measure	cal.	prot. (gms)	carbo. (gms)	fat (gms)	chol. (mgs)	sod. (mgs)	fiber (gms)
Barbecue sauce *(cont.)*							
chipotle:							
(*Texas Longhorn*) ..	35	0	8.0	0	0	10	0
hot (*Annie's Naturals* Organic)	50	0	10.0	1.0	0	260	0
garlic:							
(*Pain is Good Garlic-Que*)	30	1.0	8.0	0	0	240	0
honey (*Roland*) ...	100	0	22.0	1.0	0	160	0
honey-roasted (*Kraft*)	50	0	12.0	0	0	350	0
ginger, sweet (*World Harbors* Australian)	70	0	16.0	0	0	540	0
hickory:							
(*Hunt's*)	45	0	11.0	0	0	350	<1.0
brown sugar (*Hunt's*)	70	0	18.0	0	0	390	<1.0
brown sugar (*KC Masterpiece*) ...	60	0	15.0	0	0	320	0
honey (*Hunt's*)	50	0	13.0	0	0	420	<1.0
smoke (*Kraft*)	50	0	12.0	0	0	430	0
smoke (*Kraft* 18 oz.)	40	0	9.0	0	0	420	0
smoke (*Kraft Thick 'n Spicy*)	50	0	12.0	0	0	450	0
smoke, honey (*Kraft*)	60	0	14.0	0	0	360	0
smoke, w/onion bits (*Kraft*)	45	0	11.0	0	0	360	0
honey:							
(*Kraft* Sweet Recipes)	50	0	13.0	0	0	360	0
(*Kraft Thick 'n Spicy*)	60	0	13.0	0	0	340	0
mango (*Buccaneer Blends*)	60	0	13.0	0	0	260	0
mustard (*Hunt's*) ..	50	0	13.0	0	0	330	<1.0
mustard (*Kraft*) ...	50	0	13.0	0	0	280	0
and spice (*Bilardo Brothers*)	30	1.0	7.0	0	0	240	1.0
spicy (*Kraft*)	50	0	14.0	0	0	360	0
hot:							
(*Bone Suckin' Sauce*)	45	0	10.0	0	0	110	0
(*Buccaneer Blends* Fra Diavlo)	45	1.0	11.0	0	0	260	0
(*Cowtown* Night of the Living)	40	0	10.0	0	0	210	0
(*Kraft*)	40	0	9.0	0	0	500	0
jalapeño (*Texas Longhorn* Rodeo) ..	35	0	8.0	0	0	10	0

Food and Measure	cal.	prot. (gms)	carbo. (gms)	fat (gms)	chol. (mgs)	sod. (mgs)	fiber (gms)
jerk, Jamaican (*Pain is Good*)	60	1.0	14.0	0	0	270	0
maple, smoky (*Annie's Naturals* Organic) . .	45	0	9.0	1.0	0	220	0
mesquite:							
(*Buccaneer Blends*)	45	0	11.0	0	0	250	0
smoke (*Kraft*)	40	0	9.0	0	0	420	0
molasses (*Emeril's Sweet 'n Easy*)	50	0	15.0	0	0	400	0
Southern style:							
(*Pain is Good*)	60	1.0	14.0	0	0	270	0
vinegar (*Bilardo Brothers*)	25	1.0	5.0	0	0	145	1.0
spare rib (*Mee Tu*) . . .	80	0	19.0	0	0	260	1.0
sweet (*Emeril's Original*)	45	0	12.0	0	0	390	0
sweet/sour (*Woody's*)	70	0	17.0	0	0	610	1.0
tropical (*Emeril's*)	45	0	12.0	0	0	390	1.0
Barbecue seasoning							
(*Grill Mates*), ¾ tsp.	0	0	0	0	0	200	0
Barley:							
dry, ¼ cup:							
(*Shiloh Farms Organic Hulled/ Hulless/Grits*) . . .	140	5.0	35.0	1.0	0	0	6.0
pearled (*Arrowhead Mills* Organic) . .	160	5.0	32.0	1.0	0	5	8.0
pearled	176	5.0	38.9	.6	0	5	7.8
dry, flakes (*Shiloh Farms* Organic), ½ cup	180	5.0	37.0	1.0	0	5	6.0
cooked, pearled, ½ cup	97	1.8	22.2	.4	0	3	3.0
Barley flour:							
(*Arrowhead Mills* Organic), ⅓ cup . . .	95	3.0	19.0	1.0	0	0	4.0
(*Shiloh Farms* Organic), ¼ cup	75	3.0	19.0	.5	0	0	3.0
Barley malt syrup							
(*Eden* Organic), 1 tbsp.	60	1.0	14.0	0	0	0	0
Basella, see "Vine spinach"							
Basil, fresh:							
1 oz.	8	.7	1.2	.2	0	0	.3

Food and Measure	cal.	prot. (gms)	carbo. (gms)	fat (gms)	chol. (mgs)	sod. (mgs)	fiber (gms)
Basil, fresh *(cont.)*							
5 medium leaves	1	.1	.1	<.1	0	0	.1
chopped, 2 tbsp.	1	.1	.2	<.1	0	0	.2
Basil, dried, ground:							
1 tbsp.	11	.7	2.7	.2	0	2	.5
1 tsp.	.4	.2	.9	.1	0	<1	.2
Basil-garlic seasoning							
(*McCormick* Blends),							
1 tsp.	15	0	2.0	0	0	350	0
***Baskin-Robbins*,**							
4-oz. scoop:							
ice cream:							
butter pecan	280	5.0	24.0	18.0	50	95	1.0
cherries jubilee	240	4.0	30.0	12.0	45	80	1.0
chocolate	260	5.0	33.0	14.0	50	130	0
chocolate *World*							
Class	280	5.0	31.0	16.0	45	95	0
chocolate almond ..	300	7.0	32.0	18.0	45	120	1.0
chocolate chip	270	5.0	28.0	16.0	55	95	1.0
chocolate chip							
cookie dough ...	290	5.0	36.0	15.0	55	130	1.0
chocolate fudge ...	270	4.0	35.0	15.0	50	140	0
cookies 'n cream,							
Oreo	280	5.0	32.0	15.0	50	150	1.0
Gold Medal Ribbon	260	5.0	34.0	13.0	45	150	0
Jamoca	240	5.0	26.0	13.0	55	90	0
Jamoca almond							
fudge	270	6.0	31.0	15.0	40	80	1.0
mint chocolate chip	270	5.0	28.0	16.0	55	95	1.0
nutty coconut	300	6.0	28.0	20.0	45	90	1.0
peanut butter 'n							
chocolate	320	7.0	31.0	20.0	45	180	1.0
peanut butter cup,							
Reese's	300	6.0	31.0	18.0	50	130	0
pistachio almond ..	290	7.0	25.0	19.0	50	85	1.0
pralines 'n cream ..	270	4.0	34.0	14.0	45	170	0
rocky road	290	5.0	36.0	15.0	45	120	1.0
rum raisin	250	4.0	34.0	11.0	45	80	0
strawberry	220	4.0	28.0	11.0	40	70	0
strawberry							
cheesecake	270	5.0	32.0	14.0	55	115	0
toffee, *Heath*	300	5.0	38.0	15.0	45	180	0
vanilla	260	4.0	26.0	16.0	65	70	0
vanilla, French	280	4.0	26.0	18.0	120	85	0

Food and Measure	cal.	prot. (gms)	carbo. (gms)	fat (gms)	chol. (mgs)	sod. (mgs)	fiber (gms)
lighter side:							
ice, lime daiquiri ..	130	0	33.0	0	0	15	0
ice cream, low fat, no sugar added:							
caramel turtle ...	160	5.0	37.0	4.0	10	170	0
chocolate chip ..	150	6.0	31.0	5.0	10	140	1.0
espresso 'n cream	180	5.0	32.0	4.0	10	120	1.0
pineapple coconut	120	5.0	27.0	2.0	10	140	0
sherbet:							
orange	160	1.0	34.0	2.0	10	40	0
rainbow	160	1.0	34.0	2.0	10	40	0
rock 'n pop swirl	190	1.0	37.0	4.0	10	45	0
wild 'n reckless .	160	1.0	33.0	2.0	10	40	0
sorbet, lemon	130	0	33.0	0	0	15	0
yogurt, frozen:							
Strawberry Cheese Louise	190	5.0	35.0	3.5	10	150	1.0
vanilla, nonfat ..	150	6.0	32.0	0	5	105	0
Bass (see also "Sea Bass"), meat only:							
freshwater, 4 oz.:							
raw	129	21.4	0	4.2	77	79	0
baked or broiled ...	166	27.4	0	5.4	99	102	0
striped, 4 oz.:							
raw	110	20.1	0	2.7	91	78	0
baked or broiled ...	141	25.8	0	3.4	117	100	0
Batter/breading mix (see also "Panko crumb coating mix" and specific listings), ¼ cup:							
(*Old Bay Better Batter*)	110	2.0	13.0	.5	0	690	0
(*Old Bay Dip & Crisp*)	110	3.0	15.0	2.0	0	800	0
batter:							
(*Don's Chuck Wagon*)	100	4.0	20.0	0	0	580	1.0
(*Golden Dipt* Fry Easy)	100	2.0	20.0	0	0	770	0
batter, tempura:							
(*Golden Dipt* Fry Easy)	100	1.0	21.0	0	0	150	0
(*Roland*)	100	2.0	24.0	0	0	210	0
breading (*Golden Dipt* Fry Easy)	120	2.0	20.0	1.0	0	750	0
Bay leaf, dried, crumbled, 1 tsp....	5	.1	.3	.1	0	<1	<1.0

Food and Measure	cal.	prot. (gms)	carbo. (gms)	fat (gms)	chol. (mgs)	sod. (mgs)	fiber (gms)
Bean dip, 2 tbsp., except as noted:							
(*Fritos* Original)	40	2.0	5.0	1.0	0	170	1.0
black bean:							
(*Bearito's* Fat Free) .	30	2.0	6.0	0	0	170	1.0
(*Emerald Valley* Organic)	45	2.0	6.0	1.5	0	120	1.0
(*Guiltless Gourmet*)	40	2.0	7.0	0	0	125	2.0
jalapeño (*Fritos* Hot) .	40	2.0	5.0	1.0	0	210	1.0
three-bean (*Emerald Valley* Organic)	35	2.0	6.0	0	0	140	2.0
vegetarian (*Bearito's*) .	30	2.0	6.0	0	0	170	2.0
Bean entree (see also "Rice entree" and specific beans), frozen, Masala, w/rice (*Ethnic Gourmet*), 11-oz. pkg.	400	14.0	67.0	8.0	0	530	1.0
Bean salad, see "Beans, mixed"							
Bean sauce, Asian:							
black bean:							
chili, see "Chili sauce, Asian"							
garlic (*Lee Kum Kee*), 1 tbsp. . . .	30	1.0	4.0	1.0	0	1270	1.0
spicy (*Roland*), 2 tbsp.	60	2.0	9.0	1.5	0	1090	2.0
brown bean, spicy (*House of Tsang*), 1 tbsp.	15	0	3.0	0	0	130	0
Bean sprouts, fresh, see specific listings							
Bean sprouts, canned:							
(*La Choy*), ⅔ cup . . .	15	<1.0	3.0	0	0	60	1.0
(*Roland*), ½ cup	25	3.0	3.0	0	0	270	2.0
Beans, see specific listings							
Beans, baked, see "Baked beans"							
Beans, mixed, can or jar, ½ cup:							
(*Bush's*)	110	7.0	19.0	0	0	500	6.0

Food and Measure	cal.	prot. (gms)	carbo. (gms)	fat (gms)	chol. (mgs)	sod. (mgs)	fiber (gms)
(*S&W* New York Deli Style)	90	4.0	17.0	0	0	670	6.0
(*S&W* San Antonio) ..	90	6.0	20.0	.5	0	670	6.0
(*S&W* Santa Fe)	90	6.0	21.0	.5	0	680	6.0
w/pork (*Luck's*)	130	7.0	21.0	1.5	0	360	7.0
salad (*S&W*)	90	4.0	19.0	0	0	620	6.0
salad, three bean:							
(*Furmano's*)	90	2.0	17.0	1.0	0	250	2.0
(*Green Giant*)	80	3.0	18.0	0	0	470	3.0
seasoned (*Glory* Crock Pot)	130	7.0	25.0	0	0	620	7.0
Beans, snap or string, see "Green bean"							
Beans and franks, canned:							
(*Hormel*), 7.5-oz can .	280	11.0	32.0	12.0	50	1310	5.0
(*Van Camp's Beanee Weenee*), 7.75 oz. .	340	20.0	39.0	11.0	60	1320	11.0
barbecue (*Van Camp's Beanee Weenee*), 7.75 oz.	260	15.0	35.0	8.0	30	940	9.0
w/chili (*Van Camp's Beanee Weenee*), 7.75 oz.	240	14.0	26.0	9.0	45	990	6.0
hickory smoked (*Van Camp's Beanee Weenee*), 7.75 oz. .	290	13.0	43.0	7.0	35	800	14.0
Beans and rice, see "Rice dishes" and "Rice entree"							
Bear, meat only, simmered, 4 oz. ...	294	36.8	0	15.2	111	81	0
Béarnaise sauce, in jars (*Reese*), 2 tbsp.	80	1.0	1.0	8.0	70	360	0
Béarnaise sauce mix (*McCormick*), 1 tsp.	10	0	1.0	0	0	180	0
Beaver, meat only, roasted, 4 oz.	240	39.5	0	7.9	133	67	0
Bee pollen (*Tree of Life*), 1 tsp.	30	.3	3.4	.8	0	30	0
Beechnuts, dried, shelled, 1 oz.	164	1.8	9.5	14.2	0	11	n.a.

Food and Measure	cal.	prot. (gms)	carbo. (gms)	fat (gms)	chol. (mgs)	sod. (mgs)	fiber (gms)
Beef, choice grade, trimmed to ¼" fat, except as noted, meat only, 4 oz.:							
brisket, whole:							
braised, lean w/fat .	437	26.6	0	35.8	107	69	0
braised, lean only . .	274	33.7	0	14.5	105	79	0
chuck, arm pot roast:							
braised, lean w/fat .	395	30.6	0	29.2	112	67	0
braised, lean only . .	255	37.4	0	10.5	115	75	0
chuck, blade roast:							
braised, lean w/fat .	412	29.7	0	31.5	117	73	0
braised, lean only . .	298	35.2	0	16.3	120	81	0
flank steak, trimmed to 0" fat:							
braised, lean only . .	269	31.8	0	14.7	81	82	0
broiled, lean only . .	256	30.0	0	14.2	77	92	0
ground, see "Beef, ground"							
porterhouse steak:							
broiled, lean w/fat .	346	28.2	0	25.1	94	69	0
broiled, lean only . .	247	31.9	0	12.2	91	75	0
rib, whole: roasted,							
lean w/fat	426	25.1	0	35.4	96	71	0
roasted, lean only .	276	30.9	0	15.9	91	82	0
rib, large end (ribs 6-9):							
roasted, lean w/fat .	434	25.3	0	36.2	96	71	0
roasted, lean only .	284	31.2	0	16.7	92	83	0
rib, small end (ribs 10-12):							
broiled, lean w/fat .	376	26.7	0	31.3	95	70	0
broiled, lean only . .	264	31.8	0	14.3	91	78	0
round, bottom:							
braised, lean w/fat .	322	32.5	0	20.3	109	57	0
braised, lean only . .	249	35.8	0	10.7	109	58	0
round, eye of:							
roasted, lean w/fat .	273	30.2	0	16.0	82	67	0
roasted, lean only .	198	32.9	0	6.5	78	70	0
round, full cut: broiled,							
lean w/fat	272	31.0	0	15.4	91	69	0
broiled, lean only . .	217	33.1	0	8.3	88	73	0
round, tip:							
roasted, lean w/fat .	280	30.1	0	16.9	94	70	0
roasted, lean only .	213	32.6	0	8.3	92	74	0

Food and Measure	cal.	prot. (gms)	carbo. (gms)	fat (gms)	chol. (mgs)	sod. (mgs)	fiber (gms)
round, top:							
broiled, lean w/fat .	254	34.2	0	12.0	96	68	0
broiled, lean only ..	214	35.9	0	6.7	95	69	0
fried, lean w/fat ...	314	36.7	0	17.4	110	77	0
fried, lean only	257	39.8	0	9.7	110	81	0
shank, crosscuts:							
braised, lean w/fat .	298	34.8	0	16.6	91	69	0
braised, lean only ..	228	38.2	0	7.2	88	73	0
shortribs:							
braised, lean w/fat .	534	24.5	0	47.6	107	57	0
braised, lean only ..	335	34.9	0	20.6	105	66	0
sirloin, top:							
broiled, lean w/fat .	305	31.3	0	19.0	102	70	0
broiled, lean only ..	229	34.4	0	9.1	101	75	0
fried, lean w/fat ...	370	31.9	0	25.9	111	79	0
fried, lean only	270	36.8	0	12.4	112	87	0
T-bone steak:							
broiled, lean w/fat .	338	28.3	0	24.0	94	69	0
broiled, lean only ..	243	31.9	0	11.8	91	75	0
tenderloin:							
broiled, lean w/fat .	345	28.4	0	24.8	98	67	0
broiled, lean only ..	252	32.0	0	12.7	95	71	0
top loin:							
broiled, lean w/fat .	338	28.8	0	23.8	90	71	0
broiled, lean only ..	243	32.5	0	11.5	86	77	0
Beef, choice grade, trimmed to ⅛" fat, meat only, lean w/fat, 4 oz.:							
brisket, braised:							
whole	375	29.3	0	27.8	105	73	0
flat half	338	32.5	0	22.1	91	52	0
point half	396	27.7	0	30.8	104	78	0
chuck, braised:							
arm	350	34.2	0	22.6	93	56	0
blade	407	29.9	0	30.9	117	73	0
ground, see "Beef, ground"							
rib, whole, broiled ...	399	25.2	0	32.3	81	71	0
rib, whole, roasted ...	414	25.6	0	33.8	95	73	0
rib, large end:							
broiled ...:......	420	23.7	0	35.4	82	71	0
roasted	429	25.5	0	35.5	96	71	0

Food and Measure	cal.	prot. (gms)	carbo. (gms)	fat (gms)	chol. (mgs)	sod. (mgs)	fiber (gms)
Beef *(cont.)*							
rib, small end:							
broiled	345	27.8	0	25.1	132	56	0
roasted	407	25.3	0	33.1	94	71	0
round, full cut, broiled	266	31.2	0	14.7	90	70	0
round, bottom:							
braised	288	37.3	0	14.2	91	48	0
roasted	253	29.5	0	14.1	91	42	0
round, eye, roasted . .	240	32.3	0	11.4	73	42	0
round, tip, roasted . . .	259	30.9	0	14.0	93	71	0
round, top:							
braised	284	38.7	0	13.2	102	51	0
broiled	254	34.8	0	11.6	75	45	0
panfried	302	37.4	0	15.7	110	77	0
sirloin, top:							
broiled	291	30.4	0	17.9	94	61	0
panfried	355	32.6	0	23.9	111	81	0
steak, broiled:							
porterhouse	339	26.4	0	25.1	84	73	0
T-bone	324	27.3	0	20.0	74	75	0
tenderloin:							
broiled	310	30.0	0	20.2	74	59	0
roasted	375	27.1	0	28.8	96	74	0
top loin, broiled	315	29.7	0	20.9	110	59	0
Beef, canned,							
see "Beef entree,							
can/pkg." and							
specific listings							
Beef, corned (see also							
"Beef lunch meat"),							
brisket, cooked, 4 oz.	285	20.6	.5	21.5	111	1286	0
Beef, corned, canned:							
(*Goya*), 2 oz.	120	14.0	0	7.0	50	450	0
(*Hormel*), 2 oz.	120	15.0	0	6.0	20	490	0
(*Libby's/Libby's*							
Hawaiian), 2 oz. . . .	120	14.0	0	7.0	40	490	0
hash, see "Beef hash"							
Beef, dried (see also							
"Beef jerky"):							
(*Dietz & Watson*), 2 oz.	70	16.0	0	2.0	20	740	0
(*Hormel Pillow Pack*),							
10 slices, 1 oz.	50	9.0	0	1.5	30	650	0
cured, 1 oz.	47	8.3	.4	1.1	n.a.	984	0

Food and Measure	cal.	prot. (gms)	carbo. (gms)	fat (gms)	chol. (mgs)	sod. (mgs)	fiber (gms)
Beef, frozen/ refrigerated, raw, 4 oz., except as noted:							
ground (*Organic Prairie*):							
90% lean	250	30.0	0	13.0	95	75	0
85% lean	280	29.0	0	17.0	100	80	0
chub	300	20.0	0	23.0	85	80	0
patty, 5.25 oz.	380	26.0	0	30.0	105	100	0
rib eye steak (*Organic Prairie*), 6.1 oz. ...	470	47.0	0	31.0	160	100	0
sirloin, marinated:							
(*Shady Brook Farms* Tri-Tip Roast Steakhouse Classic) ..	180	20.0	2.0	10.0	50	520	0
garlic Chardonnay (*Shady Brook Farms* Tri-Tip Roast)	180	18.0	4.0	9.0	50	550	0
ginger (*Shady Brook Farms* Tri-Tip Roast Sizzling) ..	210	20.0	9.0	10.0	50	390	0
peppercorn (*Always Tender*)	130	18.0	2.0	5.0	45	450	0
tequila lime (*Always Tender*)	130	18.0	2.0	5.0	45	480	0
teriyaki (*Always Tender*)	130	18.0	4.0	5.0	45	450	0
strip steak:							
(*Organic Prairie* New York), 6.6 oz. ...	450	50.0	0	28.0	150	110	0
garlic pepper (*Always Tender*) .	200	21.0	2.0	12.0	45	340	0
strips, three-pepper (*Always Tender*) ...	210	21.0	2.0	13.0	50	710	0
Beef, frozen/refrigerated, cooked (see also "Beef entree, frozen"), 5 oz., except as noted:							
brisket, barbecued, sliced (*Hormel*) ...	290	18.0	23.0	13.0	65	1170	0
burger (*Applegate Farms* Organic), 3 oz.	195	21.0	0	12.0	70	85	0
cubed, teriyaki (*Simply Simmered*)	100	10.0	10.0	3.0	20	940	1.0

Food and Measure	cal.	prot. (gms)	carbo. (gms)	fat (gms)	chol. (mgs)	sod. (mgs)	fiber (gms)
Beef, frozen/refrigerated, cooked *(cont.)*							
pot roast, in gravy							
(*Tyson*)	170	23.0	2.0	8.0	65	730	0
ribs, center cut,							
w/barbecue sauce							
(*Lloyd's*), 2 ribs							
w/sauce, 7.5 oz.	620	32.0	25.0	43.0	140	1730	0
roast:							
(*Hormel*)	210	28.0	3.0	10.0	80	450	0
in brown gravy							
(*Tyson*)	130	17.0	5.0	4.0	50	600	0
Italian style, au jus							
(*Hormel*)	220	28.0	2.0	11.0	85	240	0
Salisbury steak,							
w/gravy (*Hormel*) .	170	15.0	6.0	10.0	60	890	0
shredded, barbecue							
original sauce w/							
(*Lloyd's*), ¼ cup . . .	90	7.0	11.0	1.5	15	390	<1.0
steak:							
strips, seasoned							
(*Tyson* Bag), 3 oz.	140	18.0	1.0	6.0	55	500	1.0
strips, seasoned							
(*Tyson* Box), 3 oz.	130	18.0	1.0	6.0	55	420	0
tips, in bourbon							
sauce (*Tyson*) . .	180	20.0	12.0	5.0	45	480	0
steak, breaded:							
country fried (*Tyson*),							
3.2-oz. patty	310	10.0	15.0	23.0	25	710	1.0
fingers (*Tyson*),							
2 pcs., 2.5 oz. . .	250	8.0	14.0	18.0	20	650	1.0
Stroganoff (*Hormel*) .	220	22.0	4.0	13.0	75	520	0
tips, w/gravy:							
(*Hormel*)	170	21.0	5.0	8.0	60	700	1.0
in gravy (*Tyson*) . . .	200	17.0	5.0	12.0	55	530	0
Beef, ground (see also "Beef, frozen/refrigerated, raw"), retail cuts, 4 oz.:							
raw:							
95% lean	155	24.3	0	6.0	70	75	0
90% lean	199	22.7	0	11.3	74	75	0
85% lean	244	21.1	0	17.0	77	75	0
80% lean	288	19.5	0	22.7	81	76	0
75% lean	332	17.9	0	28.4	85	76	0

Food and Measure	cal.	prot. (gms)	carbo. (gms)	fat (gms)	chol. (mgs)	sod. (mgs)	fiber (gms)
crumbles, pan-browned:							
95% lean	219	33.1	0	8.6	101	96	0
90% lean	261	32.3	0	13.7	101	99	0
85% lean	290	31.4	0	17.4	102	101	0
80% lean	308	30.6	0	19.7	101	103	0
75% lean	314	30.4	0	20.7	101	105	0
patty, broiled:							
95% lean	202	29.8	0	8.0	86	74	0
90% lean	246	29.6	0	13.3	96	77	0
85% lean	284	29.4	0	17.6	102	82	0
80% lean	307	29.2	0	20.2	103	85	0
75% lean	315	29.0	0	21.3	101	88	0
patty, pan-broiled:							
95% lean	186	29.3	0	7.0	86	81	0
90% lean	231	28.6	0	12.1	93	85	0
85% lean	263	27.9	0	15.9	98	90	0
80% lean	274	27.3	0	18.1	98	94	0
75% lean	281	26.6	0	18.6	94	99	0
"Beef," vegetarian, canned (see also "Burger, vegetarian"):							
(*Worthington Prime Stakes*), 3.2-oz. pc.	120	9.0	7.0	6.0	0	440	1.0
(*Worthington Vegetable Steaks Low Fat*), 2 slices, 2.5 oz. . . .	80	15.0	2.0	1.0	0	300	2.0
"Beef," vegetarian, frozen/refrigerated:							
(*Loma Linda* Swiss Stake), 3.25-oz. pc.	130	9.0	9.0	6.0	0	430	3.0
(*Worthington Stakelets*), 2.5-oz. pc. . . .	150	14.0	7.0	7.0	0	480	2.0
burger, see "Burger patty, vegetarian"							
burger, on wheat bun:							
cheeseburger style (*Nate's Mighty Bites*), 4.5-oz. pc.	330	20.0	33.0	13.0	0	800	5.0
hamburger style (*Nate's Mighty Bites*), 4-oz. pc.	310	16.0	35.0	12.0	0	600	6.0
corned (*Worthington*), 3 slices, 2 oz.	140	10.0	5.0	9.0	0	460	0

Food and Measure	cal.	prot. (gms)	carbo. (gms)	fat (gms)	chol. (mgs)	sod. (mgs)	fiber (gms)
"Beef," vegetarian, frozen/refrigerated *(cont.)*							
ground, ⅓ cup:							
(*Yves* Lettuce Wrap)	60	7.0	8.0	.5	0	350	2.0
(*Yves* Original)	60	10.0	5.0	.5	0	270	2.0
(*Yves* Taco Stuffer)	90	11.0	5.0	2.5	0	300	3.0
lunch meat (*Yves*),							
4 slices, 2.2 oz. . . .	110	15.0	4.0	2.0	0	360	1.0
Philly steak (*Tofurky*)							
5 slices, 1.8 oz. . . .	100	12.0	7.0	3.0	0	370	3.0
skewers (*Yves*), 2.8 oz.	100	14.0	10.0	.5	0	400	3.0
strips, 3 oz.:							
(*Lightlife*)	70	11.0	6.0	0	0	460	4.0
steak (*Morningstar Farms Meal Starters*), 12 pcs.	150	22.0	8.0	3.5	0	530	1.0
steak, natural ingredients (*Morningstar Farms Meal Starters*), 12 pcs.	140	23.0	5.0	3.0	0	720	1.0
Beef appetizer, frozen:							
filet mignon, bacon wrapped (*Original Rangoon*), 4 pcs. . .	280	21.0	0	18.0	55	540	0
steak/cheese wontons (*Original Rangoon Rangoons*), 1 pc. . .	225	11.0	40.0	12.0	40	470	0
Beef dinner, frozen, 1 pkg.:							
boneless rib, barbecue sauce (*Healthy Choice*), 11 oz.	340	20.0	50.0	7.0	50	600	10.0
pot roast (*Healthy Choice*), 11 oz.	310	15.0	45.0	7.0	45	500	5.0
roast (*Healthy Choice*), 11.4 oz.	330	21.0	42.0	7.0	60	550	4.0
Salisbury steak:							
(*Healthy Choice*), 12.5 oz.	360	20.0	46.0	9.0	40	600	7.0
(*Stouffer's*), 16 oz. .	710	41.0	48.0	39.0	100	1820	3.0
(*Swanson Hungry-Man*), 16.25 oz. .	580	31.0	41.0	34.0	90	1250	6.0
steak, bourbon, sweet (*Healthy Choice*), 12.3 oz.	330	21.0	43.0	7.0	40	600	5.0

Food and Measure	cal.	prot. (gms)	carbo. (gms)	fat (gms)	chol. (mgs)	sod. (mgs)	fiber (gms)
steak tips, bourbon (*Stouffer's*), 14 oz. .	570	23.0	65.0	24.0	45	1120	4.0
Stroganoff (*Healthy Choice*), 11 oz.	340	20.0	44.0	9.0	50	460	5.0
tips portobello (*Healthy Choice*), 11.25 oz. .	300	20.0	33.0	8.0	35	600	7.0
"Beef" dinner, vegetarian, frozen, Salisbury steak (*Amy's* Country Dinner), 11-oz. pkg.	390	11.0	60.0	12.0	15	570	8.0
Beef entree, can/pkg. (see also "Beef entree, microwave"):							
chow mein (*La Choy*), 1 cup	90	8.0	11.0	2.0	15	880	2.0
pepper Oriental (*La Choy*), 1 cup	100	9.0	12.0	2.5	20	1110	3.0
roast, w/gravy (*Hormel*), ⅔ cup	180	23.0	8.0	6.0	50	320	0
stew:							
(*Dinty Moore*), 1 cup	210	11.0	19.0	10.0	30	970	2.0
(*Dinty Moore*), 7.5-oz. can	190	10.0	15.0	10.0	30	900	2.0
(*Dinty Moore* Steakhouse), 1 cup . . .	170	14.0	16.0	6.0	45	960	2.0
taco, cheesy (*Betty Crocker Complete Meals*), ⅕ pkg. . . .	250	8.0	43.0	5.0	15	1160	1.0
Beef entree, frozen (see also "Beef, frozen/refrigerated, cooked"), 1 pkg., except as noted:							
Asian style (*Lean Cuisine*), 9.25 oz. . .	200	13.0	29.0	3.0	25	550	3.0
Bolognese (*Contessa*):							
w/sauce, 8 oz.	370	18.0	41.0	15.0	30	660	3.0
w/out sauce, 6.5 oz.	320	17.0	35.0	13.0	30	160	2.0
and broccoli (*Lean Cuisine*), 9 oz.	170	15.0	14.0	6.0	35	520	3.0
broccoli and (*Stouffer's Skillets*), ½ of 12.5-oz. pkg. .	320	19.0	47.0	6.0	35	1140	3.0

Food and Measure	cal.	prot. (gms)	carbo. (gms)	fat (gms)	chol. (mgs)	sod. (mgs)	fiber (gms)
Beef entree, frozen (cont.)							
Burgundy:							
(Michelina's Signature), 8.5 oz.	300	18.0	25.0	14.0	30	1070	2.0
oven-roasted (Lean Cuisine Spa Cuisine), 9.25 oz.	300	17.0	43.0	7.0	35	640	3.0
stew (Contessa), 1¾ cups	240	13.0	22.0	11.0	30	810	3.0
chipped, creamed (Stouffer's), ½ of 11-oz. pkg.	140	9.0	9.0	7.0	35	590	0
fajita, see "Fajita"							
garlic sesame (South Beach Living), 9 oz.	210	15.0	15.0	9.0	25	730	3.0
goulash (Contessa), 1½ cups	250	16.0	34.0	5.0	50	740	4.0
lo mein (Birds Eye Voila!), 1 cup*	230	12.0	37.0	3.0	25	1120	2.0
Merlot (Healthy Choice Café Steamers), 10 oz.	220	17.0	22.0	6.0	25	580	5.0
Mongolian (Contessa):							
w/sauce, 8 oz.	310	13.0	48.0	8.0	25	690	2.0
w/out sauce, 7 oz. .	220	12.0	35.0	3.5	25	140	2.0
orange (South Beach Living), 8.2 oz.	220	15.0	23.0	7.0	35	770	3.0
pepper steak:							
(Smart Ones), 10 oz.	250	15.0	36.0	4.5	25	710	3.0
green (Stouffer's), 10.5 oz.	240	18.0	32.0	4.0	30	910	3.0
and rice (Michelina's Authentico), 8 oz.	270	11.0	47.0	4.0	10	520	2.0
and rice (Michelina's Lean Gourmet), 8 oz.	270	11.0	47.0	4.0	10	710	2.0
and peppers Oriental (Michelina's Yu Sing), 8 oz.	260	10.0	47.0	3.0	10.0	880	2.0
peppercorn (Lean Cuisine), 8.75 oz. . .	220	14.0	25.0	7.0	25	690	3.0
picadillo (Ethnic Gourmet), 10 oz. . .	340	10.0	36.0	13.0	25	650	3.0

Food and Measure	cal.	prot. (gms)	carbo. (gms)	fat (gms)	chol. (mgs)	sod. (mgs)	fiber (gms)
pineapple teriyaki (*Smart Ones Fruit Inspirations*), 9 oz.	260	18.0	38.0	4.5	40	740	0
portobello (*Lean Cuisine*), 9 oz.	220	16.0	25.0	6.0	30	660	2.0
pot roast:							
(*Lean Cuisine*), 9 oz.	200	15.0	21.0	6.0	25	690	3.0
(*Michelina's Signature*), 10 oz.	240	18.0	31.0	6.0	10	930	3.0
(*Smart Ones*), 9 oz.	170	19.0	11.0	5.0	50	740	3.0
(*Stouffer's*), 8.9 oz.	240	16.0	27.0	8.0	35	980	3.0
Yankee (*Stouffer's Skillets*), ½ of 12-oz. pkg.	300	17.0	39.0	8.0	40	1070	3.0
rice, cheesy (*Old El Paso* Complete Skillet Meal), 1 cup*	250	9.0	37.0	8.0	20	720	4.0
roast/roasted:							
(*Smart Ones*), 9 oz.	210	14.0	19.0	9.0	45	550	2.0
oven (*Lean Cuisine*), 9.25 oz.	210	16.0	18.0	8.0	35	690	2.0
portobello gravy (*Smart Ones*), 9 oz.	190	19.0	11.0	8.0	50	680	3.0
Salisbury steak:							
(*Lean Cuisine*), 9.5 oz.	280	24.0	25.0	9.0	50	610	3.0
(*Michelina's Lean Gourmet*), 8 oz.	190	11.0	23.0	6.0	35	760	2.0
(*Smart Ones*), 9 oz.	200	20.0	12.0	8.0	45	820	3.0
(*Smart Ones*), 9.5 oz.	260	23.0	26.0	7.0	40	820	3.0
(*Stouffer's*), 9.63 oz.	410	23.0	30.0	22.0	50	1090	2.0
(*Stouffer's* Homestyle), 16 oz.	710	41.0	48.0	39.0	100	1820	3.0
and garlic mashed potatoes (*Healthy Choice*), 8 oz.	220	14.0	24.0	6.0	15	560	5.0
w/gravy (*Michelina's Authentico*), 8.5 oz.	380	13.0	28.0	22.0	50	1150	2.0
w/gravy, potatoes (*Michelina's Authentico*), 8 oz.	350	12.0	25.0	20.0	45	1080	2.0
savory (*South Beach Living*), 9.4 oz.	220	20.0	16.0	8.0	40	930	3.0
shepherd's pie (*Blake's Organic*), 8 oz.	240	14.0	26.0	9.0	30	520	2.0

Food and Measure	cal.	prot. (gms)	carbo. (gms)	fat (gms)	chol. (mgs)	sod. (mgs)	fiber (gms)
Beef entree, frozen *(cont.)*							
sirloin:							
and Asian vegetables							
(*Smart Ones*), 9 oz.	160	17.0	13.0	4.0	35	680	3.0
roasted (Michelina's							
Lean Gourmet),							
8 oz.	230	13.0	34.0	5.0	15	950	2.0
steak:							
chicken fried							
(*Michelina's*							
Signature), 9 oz.	380	13.0	32.0	22.0	55	1000	2.0
and garlic potato							
(*Birds Eye Voila!*),							
1 cup*	190	9.0	22.0	7.0	15	630	5.0
grilled whiskey							
(*Healthy Choice*							
Café Steamers),							
9.5 oz.	250	18.0	34.0	4.0	30	580	6.0
tips portobello (*Lean*							
Cuisine), 7.5 oz. . .	180	15.0	13.0	7.0	40	460	3.0
steak, teriyaki:							
(*Lean Cuisine*),							
10.5 oz.	280	19.0	37.0	6.0	30	680	3.0
(*Stouffer's Skillets*),							
½ of 11.75-oz. pkg.	310	17.0	49.0	5.0	25	1390	6.0
stir-fry:							
(*Contessa*):							
w/sauce, 8 oz. . .	180	17.0	23.0	3.0	35	700	4.0
w/out sauce, 7 oz.	120	15.0	11.0	3.0	35	260	4.0
(*Contessa* Le Menu):							
w/sauce, 8 oz. . .	170	14.0	24.0	2.5	30	660	4.0
w/out sauce, 7 oz.	120	12.0	12.0	2.5	30	220	4.0
Hunan, w/ (*Lean*							
Cuisine Spa							
Cuisine), 8.5 oz. .	270	15.0	37.0	7.0	20	610	2.0
Stroganoff:							
(*Michelina's*							
Authentico), 8 oz.	400	13.0	38.0	18.0	35	740	2.0
(*Michelina's Lean*							
Gourmet), 8 oz. .	290	15.0	39.0	7.0	20	500	2.0
(*Michelina's*							
Signature), 8.5 oz.	300	19.0	35.0	8.0	30	920	2.0
(*Stouffer's* Homestyle),							
9.75 oz. . , ...	380	22.0	34.0	17.0	70	990	2.0

Food and Measure	cal.	prot. (gms)	carbo. (gms)	fat (gms)	chol. (mgs)	sod. (mgs)	fiber (gms)
tips, Southern (*Lean Cuisine*), 8.75 oz. . . .	250	15.0	36.0	5.0	25	630	3.0
and vegetables:							
(*Stouffer's Skillets* Homestyle), ½ of 12.5-oz. pkg.	300	19.0	32.0	11.0	40	1390	6.0
and rice (*Michelina's Authentico* Oriental), 8 oz. . . .	340	11.0	57.0	6.0	10	890	1.0
Beef entree, microwave, 10-oz. cont., except as noted:							
(*Hormel Compleats*):							
and beans, barbeque sauce	390	29.0	43.0	11.0	55	1100	3.1
homestyle	220	11.0	30.0	6.0	15	600	0
pot roast, w/potato, carrots	270	24.0	29.0	6.0	50	1470	2.0
roast, w/gravy, potato	230	23.0	27.0	3.0	50	1230	2.0
Salisbury steak w/potato, gravy .	280	16.0	30.0	11.0	50	1340	3.0
steak and peppers .	210	20.0	22.0	5.0	50	580	0
steak tips	280	21.0	29.0	9.0	40	950	1.0
stew:							
(*Dinty Moore* Big Bowl), 8.3 oz. . . .	200	10.0	13.0	12.0	40	1040	0
(*Dinty Moore* Micro Bowl), 10 oz. . . .	250	15.0	22.0	11.0	45	1300	2.0
(*Dinty Moore* Micro Cup), 7.5 oz. . . .	150	10.0	15.0	6.0	25	890	2.0
(*Hormel* Micro Cup Meal), 7.5 oz. . . .	150	10.0	15.0	6.0	25	890	2.0
"Beef" entree, vegetarian, frozen:							
(*Yves* Bowl Santa Fe), 10.5-oz. pkg.	360	15.0	57.0	9.0	0	790	5.0
pepper steak (*Hain Vegetarian Classics*), 10-oz. pkg.	310	26.0	41.0	6.0	0	440	9.0
Salisbury steak (*Amy's* Country Dinner), 11-oz. pkg.	390	11.0	60.0	12.0	15	570	8.0

Food and Measure	cal.	prot. (gms)	carbo. (gms)	fat (gms)	chol. (mgs)	sod. (mgs)	fiber (gms)
Beef entree mix, see "Hamburger entree mix"							
Beef gravy, ¼ cup:							
(*Campbell's*)	25	1.0	3.0	1.0	<5	270	0
(*Campbell's* Fat Free) .	15	1.0	3.0	0	0	300	0
(*Campbell's* Micro) ...	25	1.0	3.0	1.0	<5	310	0
(*Franco-American* Slow Roast)	25	1.0	3.0	.5	<5	310	0
(*Franco-American* Slow Roast Nonfat)	20	1.0	3.0	0	<5	300	0
(*Heinz* Home Style Savory)	30	1.0	4.0	1.0	<5	390	0
Beef hash, canned, 1 cup, except as noted:							
corned beef:							
(*Armour*)	440	19.0	23.0	30.0	100	840	2.0
(*Hormel/Mary Kitchen*)	390	21.0	22.0	24.0	80	1000	2.0
(*Hormel/Mary Kitchen*), 7.5-oz. can	350	18.0	20.0	22.0	70	900	2.0
(*Hormel/Mary Kitchen* Less Fat)	290	21.0	24.0	12.0	60	1070	2.0
(*Libby's*)	420	19.0	33.0	24.0	55	1230	3.0
roast beef							
(*Mary Kitchen*)	390	21.0	22.0	24.0	70	790	2.0
Beef jerky, 1 oz., except as noted:							
(*Pemmican* Premium Cut Original)	80	13.0	4.0	1.0	35	610	1.0
(*Pemmican* Premium Cut Steakhouse) ...	80	14.0	1.0	1.5	10	530	0
(*Rustler's*), 1 pc.	35	4.0	0	2.0	10	170	0
(*Slim Jim* Original Canister), 4 pcs....	170	6.0	2.0	15.0	40	490	<1.0
(*Slim Jim* Original Handipack), 5 pcs., 1.4-oz. box	210	8.0	3.0	19.0	50	610	<1.0
all varieties (*Pemmican* Steak Tips)	70	9.0	5.0	1.5	20	510	0
hickory smoke:							
(*Organic Prairie*) ..	75	9.0	5.0	2.0	25	420	0

Food and Measure	cal.	prot. (gms)	carbo. (gms)	fat (gms)	chol. (mgs)	sod. (mgs)	fiber (gms)
(*Pemmican* Tender)	80	12.0	3.0	2.0	35	720	1.0
(*Slim Jim* Natural)	80	12.0	4.0	1.5	30	470	0
mild (*Slim Jim* Canister), 4 pcs.	170	6.0	2.0	15.0	40	490	<1.0
peppered:							
(*Pemmican* Natural)	80	13.0	3.0	1.0	35	670	1.0
(*Pemmican* Premium Cut), 1.8 oz.	140	24.0	5.0	2.0	65	1220	1.0
(*Pemmican* Tender)	80	12.0	3.0	2.0	35	720	1.0
(*Slim Jim* Natural)	80	12.0	4.0	1.5	30	470	0
pepperoni (*Slim Jim* Canister), 4 pcs.	170	6.0	2.0	15.0	40	490	<1.0
shredded:							
hickory smoke or peppered (*Pemmican*)	80	12.0	3.0	2.0	35	720	1.0
teriyaki (*Pemmican*)	80	12.0	3.0	2.0	35	730	1.0
teriyaki (*Pemmican* Natural), 1.8 oz.	140	24.0	5.0	2.0	65	1220	1.0
Beef lunch meat (see also "Bologna" and "Pastrami"), 2 oz., except as noted:							
corned:							
(*Black Bear*)	60	10.0	2.0	1.5	30	550	0
(*Black Bear* Brisket)	90	9.0	2.0	5.0	35	550	0
(*Boar's Head* First Cut Brisket)	80	12.0	0	4.0	40	460	0
(*Boar's Head* Top Round)	80	14.0	0	2.5	30	490	0
(*Di Lusso*)	90	10.0	0	6.0	30	620	0
(*Dietz & Watson* Brisket)	70	12.0	1.0	2.5	30	590	0
(*Dietz & Watson* Extra Lean)	70	12.0	1.0	1.5	30	500	0
(*Healthy Deli*)	80	11.0	2.0	3.0	30	480	0
(*Hebrew National* Brisket)	80	13.0	1.0	3.5	35	520	0
London broil:							
(*Black Bear*)	60	12.0	0	1.5	30	390	0
(*Dietz & Watson*)	70	12.0	0	2.0	30	330	0
peppered eye round:							
(*Applegate Farms*)	80	12.0	0	3.0	30	200	0
(*Boar's Head*)	90	14.0	0	3.0	40	190	0

Food and Measure	cal.	prot. (gms)	carbo. (gms)	fat (gms)	chol. (mgs)	sod. (mgs)	fiber (gms)
Beef lunch meat *(cont.)*							
roast/roasted:							
(*Applegate Farms* Deli Counter) ...	80	12.0	0	3.0	30	200	0
(*Applegate Farms/ Applegate Farms* Organic)	110	19.0	0	3.0	50	230	0
(*Black Bear* Choice)	80	12.0	0	3.5	30	240	0
(*Dietz & Watson*) ..	70	12.0	0	2.0	30	200	0
(*Dietz & Watson* Angus/Trim Tied)	70	12.0	0	2.0	30	190	0
(*Hansel 'n Gretel*) .	70	11.0	2.0	1.5	30	310	0
(*Hatfield Deli Choice*)	80	15.0	0	1.5	35	290	0
(*Healthy Deli*)	70	12.0	1.0	2.0	15	290	0
(*Hormel Natural Choice*)	60	11.0	0	2.0	25	500	0
(*Organic Prairie*) ..	120	16.0	0	5.0	40	270	0
Cajun (*Di Lusso*) ..	80	11.0	0	4.0	30	370	0
eye round (*Black Bear*)	70	12.0	0	2.0	30	390	0
eye round (*Dietz & Watson*)	70	13.0	0	2.0	30	290	0
Italian (*Black Bear*)	60	12.0	0	1.5	30	390	0
Italian (*Boar's Head*)	80	12.0	1.0	2.0	40	370	0
Italian (*Di Lusso*) ..	80	13.0	0	3.0	35	160	0
Italian (*Dietz & Watson*)	70	13.0	0	1.5	30	290	0
seasoned (*Boar's Head Londonport*)	80	14.0	2.0	2.0	40	350	0
seasoned (*Di Lusso*)	80	12.0	0	3.0	30	210	0
seasoned (*Di Lusso* Rare)	80	12.0	0	4.0	35	250	0
seasoned (*Hormel Natural Choice*) .	80	12.0	0	3.0	30	250	0
slow-roasted, shaved (*Oscar Mayer*), ¼ of 7-oz. pkg. ..	60	10.0	0	2.5	30	520	0
top round (*Boar's Head* Low Sodium)	80	15.0	<1.0	2.5	30	80	0
roasted, oven:							
(*Black Bear*)	60	12.0	0	1.5	30	290	0
(*Boar's Head* Top Round No Salt) .	90	14.0	0	3.0	30	40	0
Cajun (*Boar's Head*)	80	14.0	0	2.0	35	260	0

Food and Measure	cal.	prot. (gms)	carbo. (gms)	fat (gms)	chol. (mgs)	sod. (mgs)	fiber (gms)
Beef potato puffs,							
frozen (*Goya*), 1 pc.	140	6.0	18.0	5.0	10	400	3.0
Beef sandwich (see also "Flatbread melts" and "Panini"), frozen:							
w/cheddar (*Oscar Mayer Deli Creations* Steakhouse), 7.2-oz. pc.	450	29.0	50.0	15.0	60	1420	3.0
cheeseburger (*White Castle*), 2 pcs., 3.7 oz.	310	14.0	26.0	17.0	40	610	1.0
hamburger (*White Castle*), 2 pcs., 3.2 oz.	270	12.0	25.0	13.0	30	370	1.0
Beef sausage, see "Sausage" and specific listings							
Beef seasoning mix:							
pot roast:							
(*McCormick* Slow Cookers), 2 tsp. .	15	1.0	2.0	0	0	440	0
(*McCormick Bag 'n Season*), 1 tsp. . . .	10	0	1.0	0	0	390	0
stew:							
(*Lawry's*), 1 tsp. . . .	10	0	2.0	0	0	500	0
(*Lawry's Meal Makers*), 1 tbsp. .	10	0	3.0	0	0	700	0
(*McCormick*), 2 tsp.	15	0	2.0	0	0	510	0
(*McCormick* Slow Cookers), 2 tsp. .	10	0	2.0	0	0	650	0
(*McCormick Bag 'n Season*), 1 tsp. . . .	15	1.0	1.0	0	0	670	0
Stroganoff:							
(*Lawry's*), 1 tbsp. . . .	20	0	5.0	0	0	520	0
(*McCormick*), 2 tsp.	15	0	3.0	0	0	350	0
(*McCormick* Slow Cookers), 1 tsp. .	10	0	2.0	0	0	460	0
Swiss steak (*McCormick Bag 'n Season*), 1 tsp.	15	0	2.0	0	0	430	0
Beef stew, see "Beef entree"							
Beefalo, meat only, roasted, 4 oz.	213	34.8	0	7.2	66	93	0

Food and Measure	cal.	prot. (gms)	carbo. (gms)	fat (gms)	chol. (mgs)	sod. (mgs)	fiber (gms)
Beefsteak leaf, pickled, see "Shiso leaf powder"							
Beer, 12 fl. oz.:							
regular	146	.9	13.2	0	0	19	0
light	100	.7	4.8	0	0	10	0
Beerwurst, pork and beef, 2 oz.	155	7.8	2.4	12.6	35	410	.5
Beet, fresh:							
raw:							
(*Frieda's*), ½ cup, 3 oz.	35	1.0	8.0	0	0	65	2.0
2 medium, 2" diam.	70	2.6	15.6	.3	0	126	4.6
trimmed, sliced, ½ cup	29	1.1	6.5	.1	0	53	1.9
boiled, drained:							
2 medium, 2" diam.	44	1.7	10.0	.2	0	77	1.7
sliced, ½ cup	38	1.4	8.5	.2	0	65	1.4
Beet, can/jar, ½ cup, except as noted:							
whole (*Freshlike*), 3 small, 4.4 oz. ...	40	1.0	9.0	0	0	240	2.0
sliced:							
(*Del Monte*)	35	1.0	8.0	0	0	290	2.0
(*Freshlike* Small) ..	35	1.0	9.0	0	0	230	2.0
(*Veg-All*)	40	<1.0	8.0	0	0	300	1.0
or julienne (*S&W*) .	35	1.0	8.0	0	0	290	2.0
Harvard (*Greenwood Sweet & Tangy*) ...	100	1.0	27.0	0	0	370	1.0
pickled:							
whole (*Roland*) ...	30	2.0	5.0	0	0	650	2.0
whole or sliced (*Greenwood*), 1 oz.	25	0	6.0	0	0	100	0
sliced (*Del Monte*) .	80	1.0	19.0	0	0	380	2.0
sliced (*Freshlike*), 4 pcs., 1 oz.	20	0	4.0	0	0	20	0
sliced (*S&W*), 1 oz.	15	0	4.0	0	0	50	1.0
Beet greens, ½ cup:							
raw, 1" pcs.	4	.4	.8	<.1	0	38	.7
boiled, drained, 1" pcs.	20	1.9	3.9	.1	0	173	2.1
Berliner, pork and beef, 1 oz.	65	4.3	.7	4.9	13	368	0
Berries, mixed, dried (*Welch's* Medley), 1.4 oz.	135	1.0	32.0	0	0	5	1.0

Food and Measure	cal.	prot. (gms)	carbo. (gms)	fat (gms)	chol. (mgs)	sod. (mgs)	fiber (gms)
Berries, mixed, frozen, 1 cup, except as noted:							
(*Cascadian Farm* Organic Harvest) ..	60	1.0	17.0	0	0	0	4.0
(*C&W* Ultimate Medley)	90	2.0	20.0	0	0	0	9.0
(*Dole* Organic/Wildly Nutritious)	70	0	17.0	0	0	0	5.0
(*Tree of Life* Organic), ¾ cup	60	0	16.0	0	0	0	3.0
Berry drink blend, 8 fl. oz., except as noted:							
(*Apple & Eve* Very), 6.75 fl. oz.	100	0	24.0	0	0	15	0
(*Bolthouse Farms* Berry Boost Smoothie) ..	110	1.0	30.0	0	0	0	4.0
(*Bolthouse Farms* Blue Goodness Smoothie)	180	0	45.0	0	0	20	8.0
(*Hi-C Blast Berry Blue*)	120	0	32.0	0	0	15	0
(*Honest Tea* Organic Black Forest)	30	0	8.0	0	0	5	0
(*Minute Maid* Breakfast Blend)	120	0	32.0	0	0	20	0
(*Odwalla* Berries GoMega)	160	3.0	34.0	2.0	0	15	3.0
(*R.W. Knudsen* Sensible Sipper), 4.23-oz. box	35	<1.0	9.0	0	0	5	0
(*SoBe* Black & Blue Berry Brew)	120	0	31.0	0	0	25	0
(*Tropicana* Light), 10-fl.-oz. bottle ...	70	0	18.0	0	0	20	0
(*Tropicana* Smoothie), 11-fl.-oz. bottle ...	220	1.0	54.0	0	0	30	2.0
(*V8 Splash*)	70	0	18.0	0	0	50	0
wild:							
(*Blue Energy*), 8.3 oz.	120	0	29.0	0	0	200	0
(*Hi-C Blast*)	120	0	32.0	0	0	140	0
punch:							
(*Minute Maid*)	120	0	32.0	0	0	15	0
(*Minute Maid* Cooler)	100	0	26.0	0	0	15	0
(*Tropicana*)	130	0	32.0	0	0	15	0
frozen* (*Minute Maid*)	110	0	31.0	0	0	0	0

Food and Measure	cal.	prot. (gms)	carbo. (gms)	fat (gms)	chol. (mgs)	sod. (mgs)	fiber (gms)
Berry juice blend, 8 fl. oz., except as noted:							
(*After the Fall* Oregon)	130	0	32.0	0	0	15	0
(*Dole*)	140	<1.0	35.0	0	0	15	0
(*L&A/Langers*)	120	0	30.0	0	0	15	0
(*Minute Maid*), 10 fl. oz.	150	0	36.0	0	0	25	0
(*Minute Maid*), 11.5 fl. oz.	170	0	42.0	0	0	30	0
(*Santa Cruz Organic* Nectar)	110	<1.0	30.0	0	0	25	0
Biryani paste, see "Curry paste"							
Biscuit, plain or buttermilk, 2 oz. . . .	206	3.5	27.5	9.4	<1	596	.7
Biscuit, frozen/ refrigerated, 1 pc.:							
(*Grands!* Extra Rich) .	210	4.0	26.0	10.0	0	580	<1.0
(*Grands!* Homestyle Original)	190	4.0	24.0	8.0	0	590	<1.0
(*Grands! Butter Tastin'*)	190	4.0	24.0	9.0	0	590	<1.0
(*Grands! Butter Tastin'* Flaky Layers)	190	4.0	24.0	9.0	0	550	<1.0
(*Pillsbury Butter Tastin'* Microwave)	200	4.0	24.0	10.0	0	630	<1.0
(*Pillsbury Butter Tastin'* Oven Baked)	180	4.0	22.0	8.0	0	560	<1.0
(*Pillsbury Butter Tastin'* Golden Homestyle)	100	2.0	14.0	4.0	0	360	0
(*Pillsbury Butter Tastin'* Perfect Portions) . .	190	4.0	23.0	9.0	0	440	<1.0
(*Pillsbury Country*) . .	150	4.0	29.0	2.0	0	570	1.0
buttermilk:							
(*Grands!*)	190	4.0	24.0	8.0	0	600	<1.0
(*Grands!* Flaky Layers)	190	4.0	24.0	9.0	0	550	<1.0
(*Grands!* Reduced Fat)	170	4.0	26.0	6.0	0	590	<1.0
(*Pillsbury*)	150	4.0	29.0	2.0	0	570	1.0
(*Pillsbury* Micro) . .	200	4.0	24.0	10.0	0	630	<1.0
(*Pillsbury Golden Homestyle*)	100	2.0	14.0	4.0	0	360	0
(*Pillsbury Golden Layers*)	110	2.0	14.0	4.5	0	360	0

Food and Measure	cal.	prot. (gms)	carbo. (gms)	fat (gms)	chol. (mgs)	sod. (mgs)	fiber (gms)
cheddar garlic (*Pillsbury* Oven Baked) .	190	4.0	22.0	9.0	0	670	<1.0
flaky:							
(*Grands!* Flaky Layers/Original) .	190	4.0	24.0	9.0	0	550	<1.0
(*Pillsbury* Flaky Layers Oven Baked)	170	4.0	20.0	9.0	0	500	0
(*Pillsbury Golden Layers*)	110	2.0	14.0	4.5	0	360	0
honey butter (*Pillsbury Golden Layers*)	110	2.0	14.0	5.0	0	280	0
sandwich style, extra large (*Pillsbury*) . . .	280	6.0	34.0	13.0	0	840	1.0
shortcake (*Grands!* Homestyle)	190	3.0	26.0	8.0	0	520	<1.0
Southern (*Pillsbury*) .	180	4.0	21.0	9.0	0	560	<1.0
wheat (*Grands!* Golden)	180	4.0	27.0	7.0	0	590	2.0
Biscuit mix (see also "Baking mix"):							
butter (*Martha White* Quick & Easy Homestyle), 1/3 cup	190	3.0	22.0	10.0	20	470	<1.0
buttermilk, 1/3 cup:							
(*Bisquick* Complete)	150	3.0	21.0	6.0	0	370	<1.0
(*"Jiffy"*)	160	3.0	27.0	5.0	<5	420	<1.0
extra rich (*Martha White* Quick & Easy)	190	3.0	22.0	10.0	20	460	<1.0
cheese, three (*Bisquick* Complete), 1/3 cup .	160	3.0	22.0	7.0	0	350	<1.0
cheese garlic, 1/3 cup:							
(*Bisquick* Complete)	160	2.0	22.0	7.0	0	350	<1.0
(*Martha White* Quick & Easy) . .	190	3.0	21.0	10.0	20	410	<1.0
honey butter (*Bisquick* Complete), 1/3 cup .	150	2.0	24.0	5.0	0	290	<1.0
Bison, meat only, 4 oz.:							
roasted	162	32.3	0	2.7	93	65	0
ground, pan-broiled . .	270	27.0	0	17.2	94	83	0
Bitter melon, see "Balsam pear"							
Bitters (*Angostura*), 2 tbsp.	50	0	14.0	0	0	390	0

Food and Measure	cal.	prot. (gms)	carbo. (gms)	fat (gms)	chol. (mgs)	sod. (mgs)	fiber (gms)
Black bean, dried:							
boiled, ½ cup	113	7.6	20.4	.5	0	1	7.5
turtle:							
dry (*Shiloh Farms*							
Organic), ¼ cup .	150	10.0	28.0	<1.0	0	10	9.0
boiled, ½ cup	120	7.5	22.4	.3	0	3	4.9
Black bean, canned							
(see also "Refried							
beans"), ½ cup:							
(*Allens*)	100	6.0	19.0	.5	0	400	8.0
(*Bush's*)	110	8.0	23.0	.5	0	450	7.0
(*Eden* Organic)	110	7.0	18.0	1.0	0	15	6.0
(*Furmano's*)	90	6.0	16.0	0	0	420	5.0
(*Glory* Sensibly							
Seasoned)	100	6.0	18.0	0	0	250	4.0
(*Progresso*)	100	6.0	17.0	.5	0	400	5.0
(*Roland*)	120	8.0	21.0	0	0	430	6.0
(*S&W*)	70	5.0	17.0	0	0	480	6.0
(*S&W* Less Salt)	70	5.0	17.0	0	0	240	6.0
(*Walnut Acres* Organic)	120	8.0	22.0	0	0	85	5.0
(*Westbrae Natural*							
Organic)	100	6.0	19.0	0	0	140	5.0
(*Zapata*)	110	7.0	19.0	1.0	0	100	7.0
Caribbean:							
(*Eden* Organic)	90	7.0	20.0	.5	0	135	7.0
(*S&W*)	90	6.0	18.0	0	0	540	7.0
w/rice (*Glory*)	90	4.0	16.0	1.5	0	450	2.0
seasoned (*Trappey's*) .	120	7.0	20.0	1.5	0	410	7.0
spicy (*Roland*)	110	6.0	17.0	2.0	0	450	5.0
Black bean mix, instant							
(*Fantastic*), ¼ cup .	130	7.0	22.0	1.5	0	260	11.0
Black bean sauce, see							
"Bean sauce"							
Black currant juice,							
8 fl. oz.:							
(*R.W. Knudsen*							
Organic Nectar) . . .	110	0	27.0	0	0	15	<1.0
(*R.W. Knudsen* Just							
Black Currant)	100	1.0	15.0	0	0	5	0
Blackberry, fresh,							
½ cup	37	.5	9.2	.3	0	tr.	3.6
Blackberry, canned,							
in light syrup							
(*Oregon*), ½ cup . .	120	1.0	29.0	0	0	10	6.0

Food and Measure	cal.	prot. (gms)	carbo. (gms)	fat (gms)	chol. (mgs)	sod. (mgs)	fiber (gms)
Blackberry, dried							
(*Frieda's* Marionberry),							
1/3 cup, 1.4 oz. ...	98	0	32.0	.5	0	0	2.0
Blackberry, frozen:							
(*Cascadian Farm*							
Organic), 1 cup ...	80	1.0	22.0	1.0	0	0	7.0
(*Dole*), 1 cup	90	2.0	22.0	0	0	0	7.0
unsweetened, 1/2 cup .	49	.9	11.8	.3	0	1	3.8
Blackberry juice blend							
(*Odwalla Shake*),							
8 fl. oz.	150	2.0	36.0	0	0	10	0
Black-eyed peas (see							
also "Cowpeas"):							
fresh (*Frieda's*), 1/3 cup,							
3 oz.	130	8.0	21.0	1.0	0	250	11.0
dry (*Shiloh Farms*							
Organic), 1/4 cup ...	140	10.0	25.0	.5	0	7	5.0
mature, boiled, 1/2 cup	100	6.7	17.9	.5	0	3	5.6
Black-eyed peas,							
canned, 1/2 cup:							
(*Allens* Dry)	110	7.0	18.0	1.0	0	275	4.0
(*Allens/East Texas Fair*)	120	7.0	21.0	1.0	0	350	6.0
(*Bush's*)	100	5.0	15.0	0	0	480	3.0
(*Eden* Organic)	90	6.0	16.0	1.0	0	25	4.0
(*Glory*)	100	6.0	17.0	.5	0	570	3.0
(*Glory* Sensibly							
Seasoned)	100	7.0	17.0	0	0	250	3.0
(*Luck's*)	120	6.0	20.0	2.0	0	350	4.0
w/bacon:							
(*Allens*)	120	7.0	20.0	1.5	0	390	5.0
(*Bush's*)	95	6.0	17.0	1.5	0	370	3.0
(*Trappey's*)	120	7.0	19.0	2.0	0	350	5.0
jalapeño (*Bush's*) ..	110	6.0	18.0	1.0	5	630	5.0
jalapeño (*Trappey's*)	110	6.0	19.0	2.0	0	470	5.0
pork (*Sunshine*) ...	120	7.0	20.0	1.5	0	390	5.0
w/rice (*Glory*)	90	5.0	17.0	.5	0	680	2.0
w/snaps:							
(*Allens/East Texas*							
Fair)	120	8.0	20.0	1.0	0	420	5.0
(*Bush's*)	110	7.0	17.0	.5	0	550	5.0
Black-eyed peas,							
frozen, 1/2 cup:							
(*McKenzie's*)	110	7.0	21.0	.5	0	10	4.0
boiled, drained	112	7.2	20.2	.6	0	5	4.3

Food and Measure	cal.	prot. (gms)	carbo. (gms)	fat (gms)	chol. (mgs)	sod. (mgs)	fiber (gms)
Blimpie:							
breakfast:							
Bluffin	129	5.0	25.0	1.0	0	242	2.0
bacon/egg/cheese	293	16.0	27.0	14.0	157	973	2.0
egg/cheese	245	13.0	27.0	10.0	149	771	2.0
ham/egg/cheese .	280	18.0	29.0	11.0	164	1049	2.0
sausage/egg/							
cheese	395	19.0	27.0	24.0	179	1081	2.0
biscuit, buttermilk .	224	5.0	31.0	9.0	2	778	1.0
bacon/egg/cheese	387	16.0	33.0	21.0	158	1509	1.0
egg/cheese	339	13.0	33.0	18.0	150	1306	1.0
ham/egg/cheese .	375	18.0	34.0	19.0	166	1585	1.0
sausage/egg/							
cheese	489	19.0	33.0	32.0	180	1616	1.0
croissant	232	5.0	27.0	12.0	3	283	1.0
bacon/egg/cheese	393	16.0	29.0	24.0	160	1011	1.0
egg/cheese	345	12.0	29.0	21.0	152	808	1.0
ham/egg/cheese .	381	17.0	30.0	21.0	167	1087	1.0
sausage/egg/							
cheese	495	18.0	29.0	35.0	182	1118	1.0
panini, 4"	494	26.0	67.0	14.0	181	1480	2.0
panini, 6"	773	43.0	96.0	24.0	360	2368	3.0
cold subs, 6" regular:							
Blimpie Best	420	25.0	49.0	14.0	55	1371	3.0
Buffalo chicken ...	520	31.0	46.0	23.0	67	1525	2.0
club	386	25.0	49.0	10.0	47	1063	3.0
ham and Swiss ...	391	25.0	50.0	10.0	50	1026	3.0
roast beef/cheese ..	408	31.0	47.0	11.0	62	1051	3.0
seafood	333	13.0	56.0	7.0	19	840	4.0
tuna	483	25.0	46.0	21.0	55	776	3.0
turkey/cheese	393	26.0	49.0	10.0	46	1405	3.0
panini grilled, 6" regular:							
beef/turkey/cheese .	609	34.0	58.0	31.0	92	2037	3.0
Cuban	413	29.0	43.0	11.0	65	1628	1.0
pastrami special ...	463	32.0	47.0	14.0	65	1564	3.0
Reuben	571	34.0	54.0	24.0	75	1221	3.0
ultimate club	395	260	43.0	13.0	53	1215	1.0
hot subs, 6" regular:							
BLT	346	15.0	46.0	11.0	17	872	3.0
chicken, Buffalo ...	520	31.0	46.0	23.0	67	1525	2.0
chicken, grilled	334	24.0	46.0	6.0	42	678	3.0
gardenburger	382	14.0	64.0	8.0	0	1006	6.0
meatball	509	24.0	50.0	24.0	45	1297	4.0

Food and Measure	cal.	prot. (gms)	carbo. (gms)	fat (gms)	chol. (mgs)	sod. (mgs)	fiber (gms)
pastrami	454	30.0	48.0	17.0	61	1375	3.0
steak and onion ...	499	26.0	45.0	24.0	72	1233	1.0
wrap, regular:							
beef and cheddar ..	684	32.0	59.0	36.0	85	1928	6.0
BLT, ultimate	703	29.0	60.0	39.0	82	2303	6.0
chicken Caesar	607	30.0	56.0	29.0	61	1586	6.0
Italian, zesty	569	28.0	59.0	26.0	69	1979	6.0
Southwestern	530	23.0	61.0	22.0	54	1771	6.0
steak and onion	774	28.0	62.0	47.0	84	1795	6.0
dressing/condiments:							
dressing, 1.5 oz.:							
blue cheese	230	2.0	2.0	24.0	25	440	0
Caesar, creamy .	210	1.0	2.0	21.0	10	520	0
Dijon honey	180	1.0	8.0	17.0	15	240	0
Italian, fat free ..	25	0	5.0	0	0	390	0
Italian, light	20	0	2.0	1.0	0	770	0
ranch, buttermilk	230	1.0	2.0	24.0	10	380	0
ranch, light	70	1.0	8.0	4.0	0	310	0
Thousand Island	210	0	6.0	20.0	15	350	0
mayo, 1 oz.	202	0	0	22.0	20	202	0
mayo, chipotle or							
horseradish, 1 oz.	100	0	4.0	10.0	20	30	0
sauce, red hot, 1 oz.	10	0	2.0	0	0	760	0
soup, 8.6 oz.:							
bean w/ham	140	8.0	23.0	1.0	0	2250	11.0
beef steak noodle ..	120	8.0	14.0	3.0	30	780	1.0
beef stew	170	17.0	18.0	4.0	45	880	2.0
broccoli cheese ...	190	6.0	15.0	8.0	15	940	3.0
chicken gumbo ...	90	6.0	13.0	2.0	10	1280	2.0
chicken noodle	130	7.0	18.0	4.0	30	1040	2.0
chicken rice	250	14.0	15.0	10.0	30	1030	4.0
chili grande	250	18.0	30.0	9.0	40	1230	18.0
clam chowder	170	7.0	28.0	3.0	25	1060	2.0
corn chowder	210	6.0	29.0	7.0	5	890	4.0
minestrone	90	4.0	14.0	3.0	0	1150	4.0
onion, French	80	2.0	11.0	4.0	0	1020	1.0
potato, cream of ..	190	5.0	24.0	9.0	5	860	3.0
seafood gumbo ...	100	4.0	16.0	2.0	20	850	2.0
tomato basil ravioli	110	4.0	22.0	1.0	10	720	0
turkey vegetable rice	110	4.0	19.0	2.0	20	800	2.0
vegetable, harvest .	100	4.0	19.0	1.0	0	920	3.0
vegetable beef	80	4.0	13.0	1.5	5	1010	2.0
side salads:							
cole slaw	160	1.0	20.0	9.0	5	240	2.0

Food and Measure	cal.	prot. (gms)	carbo. (gms)	fat (gms)	chol. (mgs)	sod. (mgs)	fiber (gms)
Blimpie side salads *(cont.)*							
macaroni	330	5.0	28.0	22.0	15	790	2.0
potato	230	3.0	28.0	12.0	10	490	3.0
potato, Northwest .	260	3.0	22.0	17.0	25	390	3.0
salad, no dressing, regular:							
chef	176	18.0	10.0	7.0	47	805	2.0
chicken Caesar	124	18.0	42.0	3.0	42	420	2.0
seafood	122	6.0	17.0	4.0	19	582	3.0
tuna	272	18.0	7.0	18.0	55	517	2.0
Sicilian	351	19.0	11.0	25.0	59	1081	2.0
Blintz, frozen, 1 pc., 2.2 oz., except as noted:							
apple:							
(*Golden*)	80	3.0	16.0	2.0	10	150	1.0
(*Ratner's*)	100	3.0	21.0	1.0	25	120	0
raisin (*Empire Kosher*)	80	3.0	16.0	2.0	10	150	1.0
blueberry:							
(*Golden*)	90	2.0	18.0	1.0	10	150	1.0
(*Ratner's*)	90	2.0	20.0	1.0	25	100	0
cheese:							
(*Empire Kosher*) ..	80	6.0	13.0	2.0	15	135	2.0
(*Golden*)	80	6.0	13.0	2.0	15	135	2.0
(*Kineret*)	65	2.0	12.0	1.0	0	120	0
(*Old Fashioned Kitchen*), 2.5 oz.	100	8.0	14.0	1.5	5	190	<1.0
vanilla/orange flavor (*Ratner's* Cholov Yisroel)	90	5.0	14.0	1.5	30	160	0
cherry (*Golden*)	100	3.0	18.0	1.0	5	150	2.0
chocolate (*Ratner's*) ..	120	3.0	22.0	3.0	5	130	0
potato:							
(*Empire Kosher*) ..	90	3.0	15.0	4.0	5	170	2.0
(*Golden*)	90	3.0	15.0	4.0	5	170	2.0
(*Kineret*)	70	2.0	12.0	2.0	0	110	0
vegetable (*Golden*) ...	120	3.0	16.0	5.0	15	200	1.0
Blood sausage, 1 oz.	107	4.1	.4	9.8	34	n.a.	0
Bloody Mary drink mixer:							
(*Angostura*), 4 fl. oz. .	20	0	4.0	0	0	560	0
spicy (*Pain is Good* Original/Cajun/ Jamaican), 1 fl. oz.	5	0	1.0	0	0	182	0

Food and Measure	cal.	prot. (gms)	carbo. (gms)	fat (gms)	chol. (mgs)	sod. (mgs)	fiber (gms)
Bloody Mary seasoning							
(*Angostura*), 1 tsp. .	0	0	0	0	0	300	0
Blue squash, see "Australian blue squash"							
Blueberry, fresh:							
(*Del Monte*), 1 cup . . .	100	1.0	27.0	0	0	0	3.0
½ cup	41	.5	10.2	.3	0	5	2.0
Blueberry, canned:							
in light syrup (*Oregon*), ½ cup	110	<1.0	26.0	0	0	5	2.0
in heavy syrup, ½ cup	113	.8	28.2	.4	0	4	1.9
Blueberry, dried, ¼ cup, 1.4 oz.:							
(*Frieda's*)	140	1.0	33.0	0	0	0	4.0
(*Sunsweet*)	140	1.0	33.0	0	0	0	3.0
(*Tree of Life*)	150	4.0	38.0	0	0	0	4.0
wild:							
(*Eden* Organic)	150	<1.0	35.0	0	0	15	5.0
(*Fruit Additions*) . . .	150	1.0	35.0	0	0	30	6.0
(*Hodgson Mill*) . . .	120	1.0	32.0	1.0	0	0	6.0
Blueberry, frozen, 1 cup, except as noted:							
(*Cascadian Farm* Organic)	70	<1.0	17.0	1.0	0	0	4.0
(*C&W* Ultimate), ¾ cup	70	0	16.0	0	0	0	3.0
(*Dole*)	70	0	17.0	1.0	0	0	4.0
(*Dole* Wild)	70	0	16.0	0	0	15	6.0
(*Dole* Wild Organic) . .	70	0	17.0	0	0	0	4.0
(*Tree of Life* Organic) .	80	0	20.0	0	0	0	2.0
unsweetened, ½ cup .	40	.3	9.4	.5	0	1	2.1
sweetened, ½ cup . . .	94	.5	25.2	.2	0	2	2.4
Blueberry glaze:							
(*Litehouse*), 3 tbsp. . .	70	0	17.0	0	0	45	0
(*Marie's*), 2 tbsp.	40	0	10.0	0	0	35	0
(*Marzetti's*), 3 tbsp. . .	60	0	15.0	0	0	65	0
Blueberry juice, 8 fl. oz.:							
(*After the Fall* Maine Coast)	120	0	31.0	0	0	15	0
(*R.W. Knudsen* Nectar)	110	0	28.0	0	0	15	0
(*R.W. Knudsen* Just Blueberry) . . .	100	0	24.0	0	0	10	0

Food and Measure	cal.	prot. (gms)	carbo. (gms)	fat (gms)	chol. (mgs)	sod. (mgs)	fiber (gms)
Blueberry juice *(cont.)*							
(Simply Nutritious							
Vita Blueberry)	120	0	30.0	0	0	10	0
(Walnut Acres)	130	0	28.0	0	0	10	0
smoothie blend							
(Odwalla Blueberry							
B Monster)	140	0	33.0	0	0	10	0
sparkling (*R.W.*							
Knudsen)	110	0	28.0	0	0	15	0
Blueberry juice blend,							
8 fl. oz.:							
banana (*Nantucket*							
Nectars Organic) ..	110	0	28.0	0	0	30	1.0
pomegranate (*R.W.*							
Knudsen Organic) .	130	0	33.0	0	0	10	0
Blueberry juice							
concentrate:							
(*R.W. Knudsen*),							
8 fl. oz.*	100	0	24.0	0	0	10	0
wild (*Tree of Life*),							
8 tsp.	120	0	31.0	0	0	10	0
Bluefish, meat only:							
raw, 4 oz.	141	22.7	0	4.8	67	68	0
baked or broiled, 4 oz.	180	29.1	0	6.2	86	87	0
Boar, wild, meat only,							
roasted, 4 oz.	181	32.1	0	5.0	87	68	0
Bockwurst, raw, 1 oz.	87	3.8	.1	7.8	17	313	0
Bok choy, see							
"Cabbage, Chinese"							
Bologna (see also							
"Ham bologna,"							
etc.), 2 oz., except							
as noted:							
(*Boar's Head* 28%							
Lower Sodium) ...	150	8.0	0	13.0	30	410	0
(*Dietz & Watson*)	170	7.0	3.0	14.0	30	510	0
(*Dietz & Watson* Ring)	150	7.0	2.0	13.0	50	500	0
(*Hansel 'n Gretel*							
Classic)	150	8.0	3.0	12.0	30	670	0
(*Hatfield* Ring)	110	9.0	2.0	11.0	35	420	0
(*Hatfield Deli Choice*) .	160	7.0	2.0	14.0	30	550	0
(*Johnsonville* Ring) ..	170	7.0	1.0	15.0	35	460	0
(*Oscar Mayer*), 1 oz. .	90	3.0	1.0	8.0	30	300	0

Food and Measure	cal.	prot. (gms)	carbo. (gms)	fat (gms)	chol. (mgs)	sod. (mgs)	fiber (gms)
(*Oscar Mayer* Light), 1 oz.	60	3.0	2.0	4.0	20	300	0
beef:							
(*Boar's Head*)	150	7.0	0	13.0	35	520	0
(*Di Lusso*)	170	6.0	1.0	16.0	35	590	0
(*Dietz & Watson*) ..	170	7.0	3.0	14.0	35	510	0
(*Farmland* Black Angus)	180	6.0	2.2	16.6	30	680	0
(*Hansel 'n Gretel*) .	160	7.0	4.0	13.0	30	710	0
(*Hebrew National* Chub)	180	6.0	0	17.0	15	420	0
(*Hebrew National* Lean)	90	8.0	1.0	5.0	20	440	0
(*Johnsonville* Ring)	170	7.0	1.0	15.0	35	460	0
(*Oscar Mayer*), 1 oz.	90	3.0	1.0	8.0	20	310	0
(*Oscar Mayer* Light), 1 oz.	60	3.0	2.0	4.0	15	310	0
w/cheese (*Oscar Mayer*), 1 oz.	90	3.0	1.0	8.0	20	320	0
garlic:							
(*Hatfield* Ring)	120	9.0	3.0	8.0	35	500	0
(*Boar's Head*)	150	7.0	1.0	13.0	35	530	0
German:							
(*Dietz & Watson*) ..	140	7.0	1.0	12.0	30	490	0
(*Hansel 'n Gretel*) .	150	8.0	3.0	12.0	30	670	0
(*Hatfield Deli Choice*)	170	7.0	2.0	14.0	30	560	0
(*Obermeiser*)	180	6.0	6.0	15.0	40	700	0
(*Wunderbar*)	190	6.0	5.0	16.0	20	600	0
garlic (*Black Bear*) .	160	7.0	1.0	14.0	30	450	0
Lebanon (*Boar's Head*)	100	11.0	3.0	5.0	40	680	0
pork and beef:							
(*Boar's Head*)	150	7.0	1.0	13.0	35	530	0
(*Di Lusso*)	150	7.0	2.0	12.0	35	590	0
"Bologna," vegetarian, frozen, slices:							
(*Worthington Bolono*), 3 slices, 2 oz.	80	11.0	3.0	3.0	0	660	2.0
(*Yves*), 4 slices, 2.2 oz.	80	14.0	2.0	2.5	0	480	0
Boniato (*Frieda's*), 3 oz.	100	1.0	24.0	0	0	10	3.0
Bonito, meat only, raw, 4 oz.	146	29.3	.5	2.3	n.a.	50	0
Bonito flakes (*Eden* Organic), 2 tbsp. ...	5	1.0	0	0	1	4	0

Food and Measure	cal.	prot. (gms)	carbo. (gms)	fat (gms)	chol. (mgs)	sod. (mgs)	fiber (gms)
Borage:							
raw, 1" pcs., ½ cup ..	9	.8	1.4	.3	0	35	<1.0
boiled, drained, 4 oz. .	28	2.4	4.0	.9	0	98	<2.0
Bouillon, 1 cube, pkt. or							
tsp., except as noted:							
beef:							
(*Herb-Ox* Cube) ...	5	0	1.0	0	0	910	0
(*Herb-Ox* Instant) ..	5	0	1.0	0	0	900	0
(*Herb-Ox* Instant							
Broth/Seasoning)	5	0	1.0	0	0	1040	0
(*Herb-Ox* Instant							
Broth/Seasoning							
Low Sodium) ...	10	0	2.0	0	0	0	0
(*Maggi*), ½ cube ..	15	0	1.0	1.0	0	1340	0
chicken:							
(*Herb-Ox* Cube) ...	5	0	1.0	0	0	910	0
(*Herb-Ox* Instant) ..	5	0	1.0	0	0	870	0
(*Herb-Ox* Instant							
Broth/Seasoning)	5	0	1.0	0	0	1100	0
(*Herb-Ox* Instant							
Broth/Seasoning							
Low Sodium) ...	10	0	2.0	0	0	0	0
(*Maggi*), ½ cube ..	10	0	1.0	.5	0	1280	0
garlic (*Herb-Ox*) ...	5	0	1.0	0	0	1100	0
garlic herb (*Herb-Ox*							
Instant)	5	0	1.0	0	0	860	0
vegetable (*Herb-Ox*) ..	5	0	1.0	0	0	960	0
Bow-tie pasta dish							
mix, four cheese							
(*Knorr Lipton Italian*							
Sides), ¾ cup	220	8.0	38.0	4.0	10	770	1.0
Bow-tie pasta entree,							
frozen, and chicken							
(*Lean Cuisine*), 9.5 oz.	230	16.0	32.0	4.5	45	660	3.0
Boysenberry, fresh,							
see "Blackberry"							
Boysenberry, canned,							
in light syrup							
(*Oregon*), ½ cup ..	120	<1.0	27.0	0	0	10	3.0
Boysenberry, frozen,							
unsweetened, ½ cup	33	.7	8.1	.1	0	1	2.6
Boysenberry nectar							
(*R.W. Knudsen*),							
8 fl. oz.	130	<1.0	31.0	0	0	20	0

Food and Measure	cal.	prot. (gms)	carbo. (gms)	fat (gms)	chol. (mgs)	sod. (mgs)	fiber (gms)
Brains, 4 oz.:							
beef, fried	222	14.3	0	18.0	2262	179	0
lamb, fried	310	19.2	0	25.2	2840	178	0
pork, braised	156	13.8	0	10.8	2894	103	0
veal, fried	242	16.4	0	19.0	2404	200	0
Bran, see "Cereal" and specific grains							
Bratwurst, cooked, 1 link:							
(*Applegate Farms* Organic), 3 oz.	170	12.0	2.0	12.0	45	660	0
(*Black Bear*), 3.2 oz.	240	11.0	0	22.0	40	670	0
(*Boar's Head*), 4 oz.	300	19.0	0	25.0	75	650	0
(*Dietz & Watson*), 2 oz.	270	13.0	0	21.0	50	550	0
(*Johnsonville* Beer Precooked/Stadium Style), 2.7 oz.	240	9.0	2.0	22.0	50	760	0
(*Johnsonville* Heat & Serve), 2.9 oz.	280	12.0	3.0	24.0	55	980	0
(*Johnsonville* Original/ Beer 'n Bratwurst/ Irish O'Garlic), 3 oz.	270	15.0	2.0	22.0	60	810	0
(*Johnsonville* Stadium Style), 3.6 oz.	330	12.0	2.0	30.0	65	1020	0
(*Organic Prairie*), 3 oz.	210	13.0	1.0	19.0	50	720	0
beef, smoked (*Johnsonville*), 2.7 oz.	240	9.0	2.0	21.0	60	640	0
cheddar (*Johnsonville*), 3 oz.	270	15.0	3.0	22.0	60	890	0
hot and spicy (*Johnsonville*), 3 oz.	280	16.0	3.0	22.0	55	840	0
smoked (*Johnsonville*), 2.7 oz.	240	9.0	2.0	21.0	60	640	0
turkey (*Shady Brook Farms*), 3 oz.	140	14.0	2.0	8.0	50	500	0
turkey, raw, 3.8 oz.:							
(*Jennie-O* Beer 'N Turkey)	230	15.0	4.0	18.0	70	660	0
(*Jennie-O* Original)	170	17.0	2.0	10.0	70	670	0
cheddar (*Jennie-O*)	230	16.0	2.0	20.0	75	780	0
"Bratwurst," vegetarian, frozen, 1 link:							
(*Boca*), 2.5 oz.	140	14.0	6.0	7.0	0	760	1.0
(*Yves* Classic), 3.4 oz.	160	19.0	9.0	5.0	0	840	1.0

Food and Measure	cal.	prot. (gms)	carbo. (gms)	fat (gms)	chol. (mgs)	sod. (mgs)	fiber (gms)
"Bratwurst," vegetarian *(cont.)*							
(*Yves* Zesty Italian), 3.4 oz.	150	19.0	9.0	5.0	0	650	2.0
Bratwurst burger, grilled (*Johnsonville*), 2.5-oz. pc. ..	230	12.0	2.0	19.0	50	630	0
Braunschweiger (see also "Liverwurst"), 2 oz.:							
(*Black Bear*)	180	9.0	2.0	15.0	55	500	0
(*Boar's Head* Lite) ...	120	9.0	1.0	8.0	50	450	0
(*Di Lusso*)	130	8.0	2.0	10.0	100	660	0
(*Dietz & Watson*)	170	8.0	3.0	14.0	100	530	0
(*Hansel 'n Gretel*) ...	170	9.0	4.0	13.0	95	730	0
Brazil nuts:							
(*Diamond*), ¼ cup shelled, 6 pcs. in shell	200	4.0	4.0	20.0	0	0	2.0
shelled, 8 medium or 6 large, 1 oz.	186	4.1	3.6	18.8	0	<1	1.6
Bread, 1 slice, except as noted:							
baguette (*Cobblestone Mill*), ⅓ pc.	170	6.0	34.0	1.5	0	360	2.0
buttermilk, sweet (*Pepperidge Farm* Farmhouse)	120	4.0	23.0	1.5	0	190	1.0
cinnamon swirl							
(*Cobblestone Mill*) .	80	3.0	15.0	1.5	0	140	<1.0
(*Pepperidge Farm*) .	80	2.0	15.0	1.5	0	110	<1.0
(*Pepperidge Farm* Whole Grain) ...	100	4.0	18.0	1.5	0	150	2.0
brown sugar (*Pepperidge Farm*)	110	3.0	21.0	2.0	0	140	<1.0
cinnamon swirl raisin:							
(*Cobblestone Mill*) .	90	2.0	17.0	1.5	0	110	<1.0
(*Pepperidge Farm*) .	80	2.0	15.0	1.5	0	100	<1.0
(*Pepperidge Farm* Whole Grain) ...	100	4.0	18.0	1.5	0	140	3.0
(*Sun•Maid*)	100	3.0	18.0	1.5	5	130	1.0
(*Wonder*)	80	2.0	15.0	1.5	0	110	0
focaccia (*Alessi* Classica), ¼ pkg., 2.2 oz.	150	5.0	28.0	2.5	0	730	2.0

Food and Measure	cal.	prot. (gms)	carbo. (gms)	fat (gms)	chol. (mgs)	sod. (mgs)	fiber (gms)
French (see also "baguette," above):							
(*Cobblestone Mill* Sliced), 2 slices .	130	5.0	26.0	1.0	0	290	1.0
(*Pepperidge Farm* Hot & Crusty Thin), 2 slices ..	150	4.0	30.0	1.5	0	240	1.0
honey flax (*Pepperidge Farm* Natural)	100	5.0	19.0	2.0	0	170	3.0
Italian:							
(*Pepperidge Farm*) .	90	3.0	17.0	1.0	0	190	<1.0
(*Pepperidge Farm* Hot & Crusty), 2" slice	150	5.0	29.0	2.0	0	250	1.0
(*Wonder*)	80	2.0	14.0	1.0	0	170	0
(*Wonder* Light), 2 slices	80	5.0	18.0	.5	0	270	5.0
kamut (*Shiloh Farms* Organic Sprouted) .	90	7.0	16.0	1.0	0	120	2.0
multigrain:							
(*Arnold* Whole Grains Double Protein)	110	6.0	18.0	2.0	0	200	3.0
(*Pepperidge Farm* Whole Grain Golden Harvest) .	110	4.0	20.0	2.0	0	200	4.0
(*Roman Meal* Muesli)	110	5.0	19.0	1.5	0	160	2.0
7 (*Arnold* Whole Grains)	110	4.0	22.0	1.5	0	190	3.0
7 (*Healthy Choice*) .	80	4.0	18.0	1.0	0	170	3.0
7 (*Pepperidge Farm* Light), 3 slices ..	130	7.0	26.0	1.0	0	270	4.0
7 (*Pepperidge Farm* Carb Style)	60	5.0	8.0	1.5	0	150	3.0
7 (*Pepperidge Farm* Farmhouse)	110	4.0	21.0	1.5	0	170	2.0
7 (*Roman Meal*) ..	100	4.0	20.0	1.5	0	200	2.0
7 (*Shiloh Farms* Organic Sprouted)	100	6.0	18.0	0	0	120	3.0
7, honey (*Nature's Own* 20 oz.)	70	3.0	14.0	1.0	0	105	1.0
7, honey (*Nature's Own* 24 oz.)	80	3.0	15.0	1.0	0	115	1.0
8 (*Roman Meal*) ..	90	4.0	17.0	1.0	0	170	1.0

Food and Measure	cal.	prot. (gms)	carbo. (gms)	fat (gms)	chol. (mgs)	sod. (mgs)	fiber (gms)
Bread, multigrain (cont.)							
9 (*Nature's Own*) ..	120	4.0	24.0	1.5	0	190	2.0
9 (*Pepperidge Farm* 100% Natural Whole Grain) ...	100	4.0	20.0	2.0	0	180	3.0
12 (*Arnold* Whole Grains)	110	4.0	21.0	2.0	0	200	3.0
12 (*Nature's Own*) .	90	5.0	20.0	1.0	0	220	3.0
12 (*Pepperidge Farm Farmhouse*)	120	4.0	21.0	2.0	0	180	3.0
12 (*Roman Meal*) .	110	4.0	19.0	2.0	0	190	2.0
15 (*Arnold* Whole Grains)	120	5.0	21.0	2.5	0	190	3.0
15 (*Pepperidge Farm* Whole Grain)	120	4.0	20.0	2.0	0	180	3.0
nan, tandoori:							
(*Kontos*), 2.8 oz. pc.	255	9.0	40.0	6.0	0	510	2.0
garlic (*Fabulous Flats*), 2.2 oz.	160	4.0	28.0	3.0	5	450	1.0
oat:							
crunchy (*Pepperidge Farm Farmhouse*)	120	5.0	21.0	1.5	0	160	2.0
honey (*Pepperidge Farm* Whole Grain Soft)	110	4.0	20.0	2.0	0	170	3.0
nutty (*Pepperidge Farm Farmhouse*)	120	4.0	21.0	2.5	0	170	3.0
oat bran, honey (*Roman Meal*)	110	4.0	20.0	1.5	0	200	2.0
oatmeal:							
(*Pepperidge Farm*) .	70	2.0	12.0	1.0	0	130	1.0
(*Pepperidge Farm* Light), 3 slices ..	140	7.0	27.0	1.0	0	260	2.0
(*Pepperidge Farm* Whole Grain) ...	110	4.0	20.0	2.0	0	170	3.0
soft (*Pepperidge Farm Farmhouse*)	120	4.0	21.0	1.5	0	200	1.0
pita (see also "Pita chips"), 1 pc.:							
(*Aladdin*)	160	6.0	34.0	.5	0	280	1.0
garlic (*Aladdin*) ...	160	6.0	33.0	0	0	270	1.0
onion (*Aladdin*) ...	160	6.0	34.0	.5	0	270	1.0
spelt (*Shiloh Farms*)	150	6.0	29.0	1.0	0	125	4.0

Food and Measure	cal.	prot. (gms)	carbo. (gms)	fat (gms)	chol. (mgs)	sod. (mgs)	fiber (gms)
whole wheat (*Aladdin*)	150	6.0	31.0	.5	0	260	3.0
whole wheat (*Shiloh Farms*)	140	6.0	31.0	0	0	130	3.0
potato:							
(*Cobblestone Mill*) .	80	3.0	15.0	1.0	0	130	<1.0
(*Martin's*)	80	4.0	15.0	1.0	0	120	2.0
(*Wonder* Country) .	90	2.0	17.0	1.0	0	160	<1.0
whole wheat (*Martin's*)	70	6.0	14.0	1.0	0	125	4.0
pumpernickel:							
(*Beefsteak*)	70	2.0	13.0	1.0	0	180	<1.0
(*Cobblestone Mill* German)	80	3.0	15.0	1.0	0	200	1.0
(*Pepperidge Farm* Family)	80	3.0	15.0	1.0	0	190	1.0
(*Pepperidge Farm* Party), 5 slices . .	130	5.0	23.0	1.5	0	320	3.0
(*Rubschlager* Danish/ Westphalian), 1-oz. slice	70	2.0	14.0	.5	0	135	2.0
rye:							
(*Beefsteak* Hearty) .	70	2.0	13.0	1.0	0	200	<1.0
(*Beefsteak* Light), 2 slices	80	4.0	20.0	1.0	0	220	5.0
(*Beefsteak* Soft) . . .	70	2.0	14.0	1.0	0	180	<1.0
(*Cobblestone Mill* Jewish)	80	3.0	15.0	1.0	0	240	1.0
(*Pepperidge Farm* Party), 5 slices . .	130	4.0	25.0	2.0	0	460	2.0
seeded (*Levy's* Real Jewish) . . .	90	2.0	16.0	1.5	0	240	1.0
seeded (*Pepperidge Farm*)	80	3.0	15.0	1.0	0	170	2.0
seedless (*Levy's* Real Jewish) . . .	90	2.0	17.0	1.5	0	240	1.0
seedless (*Pepperidge Farm*) . .	80	3.0	14.0	1.0	0	170	1.0
rye/pumpernickel (*Pepperidge Farm* Deli Swirl)	80	3.0	14.0	1.0	0	180	1.0
sourdough:							
(*Cobblestone Mill* San Francisco) . .	80	3.0	16.0	.5	0	180	<1.0

Food and Measure	cal.	prot. (gms)	carbo. (gms)	fat (gms)	chol. (mgs)	sod. (mgs)	fiber (gms)
Bread, sourdough *(cont.)*							
(*Pepperidge Farm Farmhouse*)	120	4.0	22.0	1.5	0	220	1.0
wheat:							
(*Home Pride*)	70	2.0	13.0	1.0	0	160	1.0
(*Nature's Own Double Fiber*) ...	50	3.0	13.0	.5	0	135	5.0
(*Nature's Own Double Fiber Specialty*)	100	5.0	23.0	1.0	0	210	7.0
(*Nature's Own Light*), 2 slices ..	80	5.0	19.0	1.0	0	200	5.0
(*Nature's Own Wheat 'n Fiber*) .	60	5.0	9.0	1.5	0	150	2.0
(*Nature's Own Whitewheat 20 oz.*), 2 slices .	100	6.0	22.0	2.0	0	230	5.0
(*Nature's Own Whitewheat 24 oz.*), 2 slices .	110	6.0	23.0	2.0	0	250	5.0
(*Pepperidge Farm Light Style Soft*), 3 slices	130	7.0	26.0	1.5	0	280	4.0
(*Wonder Light*), 2 slices	80	4.0	18.0	.5	0	240	5.0
dark (*Pepperidge Farm 100% Natural Whole Grain German*) ..	100	4.0	20.0	1.5	0	210	3.0
honey (*Nature's Own Light*), 2 slices ..	90	5.0	19.0	1.0	0	200	5.0
honey (*Nature's Own Sandwich 20 oz.*)	60	3.0	12.0	.5	0	125	1.0
honey (*Nature's Own Sandwich 24 oz.*)	70	3.0	13.0	.5	0	135	1.0
honey (*Pepperidge Farm Simply Delicious*), 2 slices ..	160	6.0	30.0	2.0	0	260	4.0
honey (*Wonder Whole Grain*), 2 slices	140	6.0	26.0	2.0	0	330	4.0
wheat, whole:							
(*Arnold Whole Grains*)	110	5.0	20.0	1.0	0	210	3.0

Food and Measure	cal.	prot. (gms)	carbo. (gms)	fat (gms)	chol. (mgs)	sod. (mgs)	fiber (gms)
(*Arnold* Whole Grains Double Fiber)	100	4.0	21.0	1.5	0	200	5.0
(*Healthy Choice* Whole Grain) ...	80	3.0	18.0	1.0	0	170	3.0
(*Nature's Own* 20 oz.)	50	4.0	10.0	1.0	0	115	2.0
(*Nature's Own* 24 oz.)	60	4.0	11.0	1.0	0	125	2.0
(*Nature's Own* Specialty)	100	5.0	21.0	1.5	0	240	3.0
(*Nature's Own* Sugar Free Whole Grain)	50	3.0	11.0	1.0	0	110	2.0
(*Pepperidge Farm* 100% Natural Whole Grain) ...	100	4.0	20.0	2.0	0	180	3.0
(*Pepperidge Farm* Simply Delicious), 2 slices	160	7.0	27.0	2.5	0	270	4.0
(*Pepperidge Farm* Thin Sliced)	70	2.0	12.0	1.0	0	90	2.0
(*Pepperidge Farm* Very Thin Sliced), 3 slices	110	4.0	20.0	2.0	0	230	3.0
(*Pepperidge Farm* Whole Grain) ...	110	4.0	20.0	1.5	0	150	3.0
(*Pepperidge Farm* Carb Style)	60	5.0	8.0	1.5	0	170	3.0
(*Pepperidge Farm* Farmhouse)	110	5.0	19.0	2.0	0	150	3.0
(*Roman Meal* 100%)	100	5.0	20.0	1.5	0	180	2.0
(*Roman Meal* Original), 2 slices	130	5.0	25.0	2.0	0	250	2.0
(*Wonder* Whole Grain), 2 slices ..	130	6.0	26.0	1.5	0	320	4.0
w/bran (*Roman Meal* Double Fiber)	100	5.0	19.0	2.0	0	180	5.0
honey (*Pepperidge Farm* Whole Grain Soft)	110	4.0	20.0	2.0	0	170	3.0
stone ground (*Wonder*)	80	4.0	14.0	1.0	0	170	2.0
stone ground (*Pepperidge Farm* Thin)	70	2.0	12.0	1.0	0	90	2.0

Food and Measure	cal.	prot. (gms)	carbo. (gms)	fat (gms)	chol. (mgs)	sod. (mgs)	fiber (gms)
Bread *(cont.)*							
wheat berry, honey:							
(*Nature's Own* Specialty)	110	6.0	22.0	1.0	0	190	3.0
(*Nature's Own* Specialty Organic Flour)	100	4.0	22.0	1.0	0	190	3.0
(*Pepperidge Farm Farmhouse*)	120	4.0	22.0	1.5	0	190	2.0
(*Roman Meal*)	100	5.0	19.0	1.5	0	180	2.0
white:							
(*Arnold* Country) ..	120	4.0	23.0	2.0	0	260	1.0
(*Arnold* Country Whole Grain) ...	110	4.0	21.0	2.0	0	210	2.0
(*Nature's Own* Light), 2 slices	80	5.0	19.0	1.0	0	190	5.0
(*Pepperidge Farm* Canadian)	100	3.0	18.0	1.5	0	180	1.0
(*Pepperidge Farm* Original Thin) ...	70	2.0	13.0	1.0	0	100	1.0
(*Pepperidge Farm* Sandwich), 2 slices	130	4.0	23.0	2.5	0	250	<1.0
(*Pepperidge Farm* Sandwich Family), 2 slices	150	4.0	26.0	3.0	0	300	<1.0
(*Pepperidge Farm* Simply Delicious Whole Grain), 2 slices	160	6.0	28.0	2.0	0	260	4.0
(*Pepperidge Farm* Toasting)	80	3.0	16.0	1.0	0	170	0
(*Pepperidge Farm* Very Thin Sliced), 3 slices	120	4.0	24.0	1.0	0	250	1.0
(*Pepperidge Farm Farmhouse* Country)	120	4.0	22.0	1.5	0	180	2.0
(*Pepperidge Farm Farmhouse* Hearty)	120	4.0	22.0	1.5	0	250	1.0
(*Pepperidge Farm Farmhouse* Whole Grain)	110	4.0	21.0	2.0	0	180	3.0
(*Wonder* 12 oz.), 2 slices	90	3.0	18.0	1.0	0	190	<1.0

Food and Measure	cal.	prot. (gms)	carbo. (gms)	fat (gms)	chol. (mgs)	sod. (mgs)	fiber (gms)
(*Wonder* Light), 2 slices	80	4.0	18.0	.5	0	260	5.0
(*Wonder* Whole Grain), 2 slices ..	130	6.0	25.0	2.0	0	300	4.0
Bread, frozen/ refrigerated:							
baguette, demi (*Pepperidge Farm* Artisan Hearth Fired), 2 slices, ¾"	130	4.0	28.0	.5	0	320	2.0
challah (*Kineret*), 2 oz., ⅛ loaf	140	5.0	27.0	1.0	20	220	<1.0
dough, 1.8 oz.:							
wheat (*Rhodes*) ...	130	6.0	24.0	2.0	0	280	2.0
white (*Rhodes*) ...	140	5.0	24.0	2.0	0	280	2.0
dough, sweet, see "Dough, sweet"							
French, crusty (*Pillsbury*), ⅙ loaf .	120	4.0	24.0	1.5	0	300	<1.0
garlic bread, 2 slices:							
(*Mamma Bella*) ...	150	3.0	17.0	9.0	5	230	1.0
(*Mamma Bella* Cholesterol Free)	150	3.0	16.0	8.0	0	220	1.0
(*New York*), 1" slices	180	5.0	25.0	7.0	0	400	1.0
(*New York* Home-style)	150	3.0	17.0	9.0	<5	230	1.0
(*New York* Less Fat), 1" slices	160	5.0	27.0	3.0	0	370	1.0
(*Pepperidge Farm*), ½" slices	170	4.0	24.0	7.0	0	250	2.0
cheese (*Mamma Bella*)	150	3.0	17.0	8.0	5	230	1.0
5 cheese (*Pepperidge Farm*), ½" slices	190	5.0	24.0	8.0	<5	300	2.0
mozzarella (*Pepperidge Farm*), ¼" slices	160	5.0	22.0	6.0	0	250	2.0
Parmesan (*Pepperidge Farm*), ½" slices	160	5.0	23.0	6.0	0	270	2.0
roasted (*Pepperidge Farm* Premium), ½" slices	170	4.0	21.0	8.0	0	320	2.0

Food and Measure	cal.	prot. (gms)	carbo. (gms)	fat (gms)	chol. (mgs)	sod. (mgs)	fiber (gms)
Bread, frozen/refrigerated *(cont.)*							
garlic bread baguette, buttery (*Alexia Artisan*), 2 pcs., 1.5 oz.	130	4.0	19.0	4.5	10	250	<1.0
Italian, (*Pillsbury Country*), ⅛ loaf . .	110	4.0	21.0	1.5	0	270	<1.0
rosemary olive oil, petite (*Pepperidge Farm* Artisan Hearth Fired), 2" slice	130	4.0	27.0	1.0	0	300	2.0
sourdough, petite (*Pepperidge Farm* Artisan Hearth Fired), 2" slice	130	5.0	27.0	.5	0	330	2.0
toast, 1 slice:							
cheese garlic (*Mamma Bella*) .	150	2.0	13.0	10.0	0	260	0
cracked pepper Parmesan (*Pepperidge Farm*) . . .	150	4.0	21.0	6.0	<5	230	<1.0
garlic (*Mamma Bella Traditional*)	160	2.0	12.0	11.0	0	250	0
garlic, roasted (*Pepperidge Farm*)	150	4.0	18.0	7.0	0	260	1.0
Romano herb (*Pepperidge Farm*)	150	4.0	18.0	7.0	<5	220	1.0
toast, Texas, 1 slice:							
cheese (*New York*) .	180	5.0	20.0	9.0	5	350	1.0
5 cheese (*Mamma Bella*)	180	5.0	20.0	9.0	5	350	1.0
5 cheese (*New York*)	170	5.0	16.0	10.0	5	360	1.0
5 cheese (*Pepperidge Farm*)	150	4.0	18.0	7.0	<5	200	1.0
garlic (*New York*) . .	150	3.0	15.0	9.0	0	260	1.0
garlic (*New York Lite*)	130	2.0	18.0	4.5	0	270	1.0
garlic (*New York 6 Carb*)	120	4.0	8.0	8.0	0	160	2.0
garlic (*Pepperidge Farm*)	150	3.0	18.0	7.0	0	190	2.0
mozzarella Monterey Jack (*Pepperidge Farm*)	160	5.0	20.0	7.0	<5	250	<1.0

Food and Measure	cal.	prot. (gms)	carbo. (gms)	fat (gms)	chol. (mgs)	sod. (mgs)	fiber (gms)
Parmesan (New York)	180	6.0	18.0	10.0	5	370	1.0
Parmesan (Pepperidge Farm) ...	160	4.0	14.0	9.0	20	250	<1.0
whole grain (Pepperidge Farm) ...	150	4.0	14.0	8.0	0	250	2.0
Bread, mix (see also "Bread mix, sweet"), dry mix, ¼ cup: (Watkins Good Tastings)	140	3.0	29.0	0	0	250	1.0
barley, w/soy (Hodgson Mill)	121	5.0	23.0	1.0	0	215	2.0
cheese and herb (Hodgson Mill) ...	130	5.0	21.0	1.0	0	250	<1.0
multigrain: (Arrowhead Mills Organic)	140	6.0	28.0	.5	0	115	3.0
9, w/soy (Hodgson Mill)	120	5.0	22.0	1.5	0	150	3.0
potato, w/soy (Hodgson Mill)	110	5.0	23.0	0	0	170	1.0
rye, caraway, w/soy (Hodgson Mill) ...	110	5.0	22.0	1.0	0	190	3.0
white, w/soy (Hodgson Mill)	120	5.0	22.0	.5	0	170	1.0
whole wheat: (Arrowhead Mills Organic)	140	6.0	27.0	1.0	0	140	4.0
honey, w/soy (Hodgson Mill)	120	5.0	22.0	.5	0	160	2.0
Bread mix, sweet, 1/14 pkg. mix, except as noted:							
apple cinnamon (Pillsbury Quick) ..	130	1.0	26.0	2.0	0	115	<1.0
banana: (Betty Crocker Quick), 1/12 loaf*	170	3.0	25.0	7.0	35	200	0
(Pillsbury Quick) ..	110	2.0	22.0	1.0	0	125	<1.0
blueberry (Pillsbury Quick) ..	120	1.0	24.0	1.5	0	100	<1.0
carrot (Pillsbury Quick), 1/16 pkg. ...	110	2.0	22.0	1.0	0	125	<1.0

Food and Measure	cal.	prot. (gms)	carbo. (gms)	fat (gms)	chol. (mgs)	sod. (mgs)	fiber (gms)
Bread mix, sweet *(cont.)*							
chocolate chip swirl							
(*Pillsbury* Quick) ..	150	1.0	27.0	4.5	0	140	<1.0
cinnamon swirl (*Pillsbury* Quick)	150	1.0	27.0	4.0	0	140	0
cinnamon streusel (*Betty Crocker* Quick), 1/14 loaf*	180	3.0	28.0	7.0	30	160	0
corn, see "Corn bread mix"							
cranberry:							
(*Pillsbury* Quick) ..	120	2.0	26.0	1.5	0	115	<1.0
orange (*Betty Crocker* Quick), 1/12 loaf*	180	3.0	29.0	6.0	35	180	<1.0
date (*Pillsbury* Quick)	130	2.0	28.0	1.5	0	115	1.0
gingerbread, whole wheat (*Hodgson Mill*), ¼ cup	110	2.0	24.0	0	0	260	2.0
lemon poppy seed (*Pillsbury* Quick) ..	130	2.0	25.0	2.5	0	120	<1.0
nut (*Pillsbury* Quick) .	120	2.0	23.0	3.0	0	135	<1.0
pecan swirl (*Pillsbury* Quick)	150	1.0	25.0	5.0	0	140	<1.0
pumpkin (*Pillsbury* Quick), 1/12 pkg. .	130	2.0	27.0	1.5	0	150	1.0
pumpkin spice (*Krusteaz* Quick), 1/10 loaf*	220	3.0	32.0	9.0	45	240	1.0
Bread crumbs (see also "Panko crumbs"), ¼ cup or 1 oz.:							
plain:							
(*Progresso*)	110	4.0	20.0	1.5	0	220	1.0
(*Vigo*)	110	4.0	19.0	1.5	0	200	1.0
garlic herb (*Progresso*)	110	4.0	20.0	1.5	0	540	1.0
Italian:							
(*Contadina*)	100	3.0	19.0	1.5	0	720	1.0
(*Progresso*)	110	4.0	20.0	1.5	0	470	1.0
(*Vigo*)	110	4.0	21.0	1.6	0	490	2.0
Parmesan (*Progresso*)	110	4.0	19.0	1.5	0	870	1.0
Bread stick:							
plain (*Alessi* Thin), 9 pcs., 1 oz.	110	3.0	22.0	1.5	0	280	1.0

Food and Measure	cal.	prot. (gms)	carbo. (gms)	fat (gms)	chol. (mgs)	sod. (mgs)	fiber (gms)
garlic, 5 pcs.:							
(*Alessi*), 1.1 oz. ...	120	4.0	24.0	1.5	0	230	2.0
herb, thin (*Torino* Grissini), .5 oz. .	60	2.0	12.0	.5	0	150	0
pizza (*Torino* Grissini), 5 pcs., .5 oz.	60	2.0	12.0	.5	0	95	0
rosemary (*Alessi*), 9 pcs., 1 oz.	110	3.0	22.0	1.5	0	280	1.0
sesame (*Alessi*), 4 pcs., 1 oz.	110	4.0	22.0	2.0	0	210	4.0
Bread stick, frozen/ refrigerated:							
(*Pillsbury* Soft), 2 pcs.	140	4.0	25.0	2.5	0	370	<1.0
corn bread (*Pillsbury* Twists), 1 pc.	140	3.0	18.0	6.0	0	340	0
garlic:							
(*Mamma Bella/New York*), 1 pc.	170	5.0	24.0	6.0	0	300	1.0
(*Pepperidge Farm*), 1 pc.	160	5.0	25.0	4.5	0	320	1.0
(*Pillsbury*), 2 pcs. .	170	4.0	24.0	7.0	0	570	<1.0
herb (*Pillsbury*), 2 pcs., ½ tsp. spread	170	5.0	24.0	6.0	0	540	<1.0
Parmesan w/garlic (*Pillsbury*), 2 pcs., ½ tsp. spread	170	5.0	24.0	6.0	0	540	<1.0
Breadfruit, raw, ½ cup	113	1.2	29.8	.3	0	2	5.4
Breadfruit seeds:							
raw, 1 oz.	54	2.1	8.3	1.6	0	7	1.5
boiled, shelled, 1 oz. .	48	1.5	9.1	.7	0	7	1.4
roasted, shelled, 1 oz.	59	1.8	11.4	.8	0	8	1.7
Breading mix, see "Batter/breading mix," "Panko crumb coating mix," and specific listings							
Breadnut tree seeds, dried, 1 oz.	104	2.4	22.5	.5	0	15	4.2
Breakfast dish, see "Egg breakfast" and specific listings							

Food and Measure	cal.	prot. (gms)	carbo. (gms)	fat (gms)	chol. (mgs)	sod. (mgs)	fiber (gms)
Breakfast sandwich/ **pastry** (see also "Burrito, breakfast" and "Taquito, breakfast"), frozen, 1 pc.:							
bagel, sausage/egg/ cheese (*Jimmy Dean*)	380	13.0	34.0	21.0	115	770	1.0
biscuit:							
sausage/egg/cheese (*Aunt Jemima*) ..	340	12.0	27.0	21.0	110	830	<1.0
sausage/egg/cheese (*Jimmy Dean*) ..	430	13.0	28.0	30.0	115	830	1.0
cheese/egg, and:							
bacon (*Toaster Scrambles*)	180	4.0	15.0	12.0	25	330	0
bacon (*Toaster Scrambles Reduced Fat*) ...	160	4.0	16.0	9.0	25	340	0
ham (*Toaster Scrambles*)	180	4.0	15.0	11.0	25	340	0
sausage (*Toaster Scrambles*)	180	4.0	15.0	12.0	25	320	0
sausage (*Van's Stuffed*)	330	10.0	29.0	19.0	65	450	1.0
croissant, sausage/egg/ cheese:							
(*Aunt Jemima*)	350	13.0	22.0	23.0	145	680	<1.0
(*Jimmy Dean*)	430	13.0	30.0	29.0	115	740	1.0
egg/cheese, Western (*Van's Stuffed*)	320	10.0	29.0	18.0	75	480	1.0
English muffin:							
ham and cheese (*Smart Ones*) ...	200	13.0	27.0	5.0	15	480	2.0
sausage/egg/cheese (*Jimmy Dean*) ..	230	12.0	27.0	9.0	95	670	1.0
French toast:							
(*Pop•Tarts*)	220	3.0	35.0	8.0	0	180	<1.0
(*Toaster Strudel*) ..	190	3.0	26.0	9.0	10	190	<1.0
sausage/egg/cheese (*Aunt Jemima*) ..	320	14.0	24.0	20.0	200	720	<1.0
griddle cake:							
ham/egg/cheese (*Aunt Jemima*) ..	240	9.0	33.0	8.0	110	870	<1.0

Food and Measure	cal.	prot. (gms)	carbo. (gms)	fat (gms)	chol. (mgs)	sod. (mgs)	fiber (gms)
sausage/egg/cheese (*Aunt Jemima*) . .	360	12.0	30.0	21.0	145	930	<1.0
ham and cheese (*Van's Stuffed*)	330	8.0	31.0	18.0	20	470	<1.0
Southwestern (*Toaster Scramble* Reduced Fat)	160	4.0	15.0	9.0	25	340	<1.0
tofu scramble (*Amy's* Pocket)	180	11.0	23.0	6.0	0	520	<1.0
wrap, 4.6 oz.:							
(*South Beach Living* All American) . . .	230	19.0	22.0	9.0	15	590	6.0
(*South Beach Living* Denver Style) . . .	210	17.0	22.0	8.0	15	630	6.0
Southwestern (*South Beach Living*) . . .	190	16.0	22.0	6.0	10	480	6.0
Southwestern, vegetarian (*Boca*) . . .	200	14.0	25.0	7.0	5	510	6.0
vegetarian (*Boca* Original)	220	16.0	27.0	7.0	5	640	6.0
Broad bean, fresh:							
raw, ½ cup	40	3.1	6.4	.4	0	28	2.3
boiled, drained, 4 oz.	64	5.4	11.5	.6	0	47	<3.0
Broad bean, mature:							
dry:							
(*Shiloh Farms* Organic Fava), ¼ cup	70	7.0	22.0	0	0	20	12.0
peeled (*Frieda's* Habas), ½ cup, 3 oz.	100	6.0	17.0	0	0	5	4.0
boiled, ½ cup	93	6.5	16.7	.3	0	4	4.6
Broad bean, mature, canned, ½ cup:							
(*Progresso* Fava)	100	6.0	17.0	.5	0	250	5.0
w/liquid	91	7.0	15.9	.3	0	580	4.7
Broccoli, fresh:							
raw, 8.7-oz. stalk	42	4.5	7.9	.5	0	40	4.5
raw, chopped, ½ cup .	12	1.3	2.3	.2	0	12	1.3
boiled, drained:							
1 stalk, 6.3 oz.	51	5.4	9.1	.6	0	46	5.2
chopped, ½ cup . . .	22	2.3	3.9	.2	0	20	2.3
Broccoli, Chinese, see "Kale, Chinese"							

Food and Measure	cal.	prot. (gms)	carbo. (gms)	fat (gms)	chol. (mgs)	sod. (mgs)	fiber (gms)
Broccoli, frozen:							
spears:							
(*Birds Eye*), 2 spears, 3.1 oz.	30	2.0	4.0	0	0	25	2.0
(*Green Giant Simply Steam*), 3.5 oz., approx. 3 spears	25	2.0	4.0	0	0	120	2.0
baby (*Birds Eye*), 4 spears, 3 oz. ..	30	1.0	4.0	0	0	20	2.0
10-oz. pkg.	84	8.7	15.2	1.0	0	49	8.5
spears or chopped, boiled, drained, 1 cup	52	5.7	9.8	.2	0	44	5.5
florets:							
(*Birds Eye* Baby/ Steamfresh/C&W), 1 cup	30	1.0	4.0	0	0	20	2.0
(*Cascadian Farm* Organic Bag), ⅔ cup, 3 oz. ...	25	2.0	4.0	0	0	20	2.0
(*Cascadian Farm* Organic Box), 1⅓ cups, 3 oz. ..	20	1.0	3.0	0	0	120	2.0
(*Green Giant Select*), 1⅓ cups	20	1.0	4.0	0	0	20	2.0
cuts:							
(*Birds Eye* Tender/ Steamfresh), 1 cup	30	2.0	4.0	0	0	20	2.0
(*Cascadian Farm* Organic), ⅔ cup	25	2.0	4.0	0	0	20	2.0
(*Green Giant* Bag), ⅔ cup cooked ..	25	1.0	4.0	0	0	20	2.0
(*Green Giant* Box No Sauce), ⅔ cup	25	1.0	4.0	0	0	105	2.0
chopped:							
(*Birds Eye*), ¾ cup .	30	1.0	4.0	0	0	20	2.0
(*Green Giant*), ½ cup cooked ..	25	1.0	4.0	0	0	20	2.0
10-oz. pkg.	75	8.0	13.6	.8	0	68	8.5
in butter sauce, spears (*Green Giant*), 4 oz., approx. 3 pcs.	40	2.0	6.0	1.5	<5	330	2.0
in cheese sauce:							
(*Birds Eye*), ½ cup .	90	3.0	8.0	5.0	5	490	1.0
(*Green Giant*), ⅔ cup	60	2.0	7.0	2.5	0	460	2.0

Food and Measure	cal.	prot. (gms)	carbo. (gms)	fat (gms)	chol. (mgs)	sod. (mgs)	fiber (gms)
(*Green Giant* Zesty), ¾ cup	60	2.0	8.0	2.0	0	470	1.0
(*Green Giant Just for One*), 4.25 oz. ..	60	2.0	7.0	3.0	0	470	2.0
cheddar (*C&W*), 1⅓ cups	70	4.0	7.0	2.5	5	370	2.0
cheddar, white (*Green Giant*), ¾ cup ..	60	2.0	8.0	2.0	<5	470	1.0
three cheese (*Green Giant* Bag), ½ cup cooked	45	2.0	6.0	2.0	5	350	1.0
Broccoli combinations, frozen, 1 cup, except as noted:							
(*Birds Eye* Stir Fry) ..	30	1.0	5.0	0	0	35	2.0
carrots:							
(*Cascadian Farm Purely Steam*), Organic), ¾ cup*	60	2.0	8.0	3.0	0	250	3.0
(*Green Giant Simply Steam*), ¾ cup cooked	60	2.0	8.0	3.0	0	260	3.0
w/garlic, herbs (*Green Giant*), ½ cup cooked ..	40	2.0	7.0	.5	0	200	2.0
carrots, cauliflower, cheese sauce (*Green Giant*), ½ cup cooked	50	2.0	7.0	1.5	<5	370	2.0
carrots, water chestnuts:(*Birds Eye*)	35	1.0	6.0	0	0	35	2.0
sugar snaps (*Birds Eye Steamfresh*), ¾ cup	35	1.0	6.0	0	0	25	2.0
cauliflower:							
(*Birds Eye/Birds Eye Steamfresh*)	25	1.0	4.0	0	0	25	2.0
garlic herb sauce (*Green Giant Select*), ½ cup cooked	50	2.0	6.0	2.0	5	310	2.0
cauliflower, carrots: (*Birds Eye Steamfresh*), ¾ cup	30	1.0	5.0	0	0	30	2.0

Food and Measure	cal.	prot. (gms)	carbo. (gms)	fat (gms)	chol. (mgs)	sod. (mgs)	fiber (gms)
Broccoli combinations, cauliflower, carrots, frozen *(cont.)*							
cheese sauce (*Green Giant*), ⅔ cup ..	60	2.0	8.0	2.5	0	460	2.0
cauliflower, peppers (*Birds Eye*)	25	1.0	3.0	0	0	20	1.0
florets, w/onion, mushrooms, peppers (*Birds Eye*)	30	1.0	4.0	0	0	15	1.0
green beans, onion, pepper (*Birds Eye*) .	30	1.0	5.0	0	0	10	2.0
red pepper, sugar snaps, water chestnuts (*C&W Vegetable Stand Combinations*)	30	1.0	5.0	0	0	10	1.0
Broccoli pot pie, frozen (*Amy's*), 7.5 oz. ...	430	11.0	46.0	22.0	45	630	4.0
Broccoli rabe, fresh:							
(*Andy Boy*), 3 oz. ...	30	3.0	3.0	0	0	45	2.0
(*Frieda's* Rapini), 3 oz.	25	3.0	4.0	0	0	25	0
Broccoli rabe, frozen (*Seabrook Farms*), 1 cup	25	2.0	4.0	0	0	35	2.0
Broccoli snacks, frozen:							
w/cheddar, breaded (*Veggie Patch* Bites), 3 pcs., 2.6 oz.	150	5.0	17.0	8.0	10	380	4.0
and cheese, breaded (*Morningstar Farms* Veggie Bites), 3 pcs., 3 oz.	190	8.0	16.0	10.0	5	550	1.0
Broccolini, fresh (*Mann's*), 8 stalks, 2.9 oz. ...	35	3.0	6.0	0	0	25	1.0
Broccoli-cheese pie, frozen (*The Fillo Factory*), ⅕ of 24-oz. pkg.	280	12.0	26.0	15.0	30	430	2.0
Broccoli-cheese pocket, frozen, 1 pc.:							
(*Amy's*), 4.5 oz.	270	8.0	37.0	10.0	15	560	3.0
cheddar (*Aunt Trudy's*), 5 oz.	320	12.0	34.0	15.0	30	480	3.0
Brown gravy, w/onion, canned (*Campbell's*), ¼ cup	25	0	4.0	1.0	0	330	<1.0

Food and Measure	cal.	prot. (gms)	carbo. (gms)	fat (gms)	chol. (mgs)	sod. (mgs)	fiber (gms)
Brown gravy mix:							
(*McCormick*), ¼ cup*	20	0	3.0	1.0	0	340	0
(*McCormick* Less Sodium), ¼ cup*	20	0	3.0	.5	0	230	0
Brownie, 1 pc., except as noted:							
(*Hershey's*), 1.5 oz.	200	2.0	28.0	9.0	0	30	1.0
(*Reese's*), 1.5 oz.	200	3.0	27.0	9.0	0	45	1.0
caramel (*Awrey's Bursts*), 1.5 oz.	140	1.0	23.0	6.0	10	150	<1.0
chocolate, triple, iced (*Awrey's* Indulgence), 2 oz.	230	2.0	34.0	10.0	25	125	<1.0
fudge:							
nut (*Awrey's* Decadent), 2 oz.	230	2.0	33.0	11.0	25	120	<1.0
w/walnuts (*Little Debby*), 2.2 oz.	290	3.0	40.0	13.0	10	150	1.0
mint (*Awrey's* Brownie Bursts), 1.5 oz.	150	<1.0	24.0	6.0	10	135	<1.0
peanut butter:							
(*Awrey's* Brownie Bursts), 1.5 oz.	150	1.0	22.0	7.0	10	220	<1.0
iced (*Awrey's* Sensation), 2 oz.	250	3.0	32.0	13.0	25	140	<1.0
raspberry filled (*Awrey's* Bursts), 1.5 oz.	170	1.0	29.0	6.0	10	150	1.0
Brownie, microwave, 1 cont.:							
chocolate, hot (*Guiltless Gourmet*), 2 oz.	200	4.0	42.0	3.0	20	190	3.0
fudge:							
hot (*Betty Crocker Warm Delights*), 3.1 oz.	370	5.0	61.0	12.0	0	270	3.0
peanut butter (*Betty Crocker Warm Delights*), 3.3 oz.	400	5.0	63.0	12.0	0	290	7.0
Brownie, mix:							
(*Arrowhead Mills* Organic), 1/20 pkg.	90	1.0	21.0	1.5	0	65	<1.0
(*Arrowhead Mills* Organic Gluten Free), 1/20 pkg.	110	1.0	21.0	2.0	0	40	<1.0

Food and Measure	cal.	prot. (gms)	carbo. (gms)	fat (gms)	chol. (mgs)	sod. (mgs)	fiber (gms)
Brownie mix *(cont.)*							
(*Betty Crocker* Supreme Original), 1/20 pkg.*	160	2.0	27.0	5.0	20	115	1.0
(*Pillsbury* Traditional), 1/12 pkg.	150	2.0	24.0	6.0	0	120	<1.0
caramel swirl (*Pillsbury* Fudge Supreme), 1/12 pkg.	130	1.0	27.0	2.5	0	100	<1.0
cheesecake swirl (*Pillsbury* Fudge Supreme), 1/18 pkg.	100	1.0	20.0	2.5	0	75	<1.0
chocolate: (*Pillsbury* Fudge Supreme Extreme), 1/16 pkg.	120	1.0	22.0	3.0	0	65	1.0
dark (*Betty Crocker*), 1/20 pkg.*	170	2.0	24.0	7.0	20	105	1.0
dark (*Betty Crocker* Supreme), 1/20 pkg.*	170	2.0	25.0	7.0	20	110	0
double (*Pillsbury* Fudge Supreme), 1/16 pkg.	110	1.0	23.0	2.0	0	85	<1.0
frosted (*Pillsbury* Fudge Supreme), 1/16 pkg.	140	1.0	27.0	3.5	0	105	<1.0
milk (*Pillsbury* Fudge Classics), 1/20 pkg.	110	1.0	23.0	2.0	0	70	<1.0
chocolate chunk: (*Betty Crocker/Betty Crocker* Triple Supreme), 1/20 pkg.*	180	2.0	25.0	9.0	20	95	1.0
(*Pillsbury* Fudge Supreme), 1/16 pkg.	120	1.0	22.0	3.5	0	70	<1.0
triple (*Pillsbury*), 1/12 pkg.	160	2.0	24.0	6.0	0	105	<1.0
walnut (*Betty Crocker* Supreme), 1/20 pkg.*	180	2.0	23.0	10.0	20	95	1.0
frosted (*Betty Crocker* Supreme), 1/20 pkg.*	200	2.0	31.0	9.0	20	130	1.0
fudge: (*Betty Crocker*), 1/20 pkg.*	170	2.0	22.0	9.0	20	95	1.0

Food and Measure	cal.	prot. (gms)	carbo. (gms)	fat (gms)	chol. (mgs)	sod. (mgs)	fiber (gms)
(*Betty Crocker* Low Fat), 1/18 pkg.*	130	2.0	27.0	2.5	0	115	1.0
(*Betty Crocker* Pouch), 1/9 pkg.*	190	2.0	27.0	8.0	25	125	1.0
(*Betty Crocker* Ultimate), 1/20 pkg.*	180	2.0	24.0	8.0	20	100	<1.0
(*Dr. Oetker*), 1/6 pkg.	100	1.0	23.0	0	0	60	1.0
(*Dr. Oetker* Organic), 1/9 pkg.	160	1.0	36.0	.5	0	90	1.0
(*"Jiffy"*), 1/8 pkg.	120	1.0	22.0	3.5	0	120	<1.0
(*No Pudge!* Original), 1/12 pkg.	110	2.0	28.0	0	0	100	1.0
(*Pillsbury* Brownie Classics Traditional), 1/16 pkg.	110	1.0	22.0	2.0	0	80	<1.0
fudge toffee (*Pillsbury* Fudge Classics), 1/20 pkg.	110	1.0	23.0	2.5	0	85	<1.0
mint or raspberry fudge (*No Pudge!*), 1/12 pkg.	110	2.0	28.0	0	0	100	1.0
peanut butter:							
(*Betty Crocker* Supreme), 1/20 pkg.*	180	3.0	24.0	9.0	20	105	1.0
swirl (*Pillsbury* Fudge Supreme), 1/16 pkg.	140	2.0	23.0	4.5	0	100	<1.0
turtle (*Betty Crocker* Supreme), 1/20 pkg.*	170	2.0	23.0	9.0	20	100	<1.0
walnut:							
(*Betty Crocker* Supreme), 1/20 pkg.*	180	2.0	22.0	9.0	20	95	0
(*Martha White*), 1/20 pkg.	130	2.0	23.0	3.5	20	120	1.0
(*Pillsbury* Fudge Supreme), 1/12 pkg.	140	2.0	24.0	4.5	0	85	1.0
w/whole wheat flour, flax seeds (*Hodgson Mill*), 3 tbsp.	120	3.0	28.0	.5	0	80	2.0
Browning sauce (*Gravy Master*), ¼ tsp.	0	0	<1.0	0	0	30	0
Bruschetta, frozen, pesto, mozzarella, tomato (*Cedarlane*), 1.25-oz. pc.	100	3.0	10.0	5.0	5	190	.5

Food and Measure	cal.	prot. (gms)	carbo. (gms)	fat (gms)	chol. (mgs)	sod. (mgs)	fiber (gms)
Bruschetta spread/ **topping,** 2 tbsp., except as noted:							
(*Buitoni* Classic)	30	1.0	2.0	2.0	0	140	0
(*Cedar's* Fresh), ½ cup	120	1.0	5.0	9.0	0	350	1.0
all varieties (*Roland*) .	60	<1.0	7.0	1.0	0	0	0
artichoke (*Delallo*) . . .	60	0	1.0	6.0	0	135	1.0
basil and tomato or extra garlic (*Classico*), 1 tbsp.	15	0	1.0	1.0	0	55	0
olive (*Delallo*)	70	0	1.0	8.0	0	140	0
Brussels sprouts, fresh:							
raw (*Dole*), 4 pcs. . . .	40	2.0	6.0	0	0	25	3.0
raw, 1/2 cup	19	1.5	3.9	.1	0	11	1.8
boiled, .7-oz. pc.	8	.5	1.8	.1	0	4	.9
boiled, drained, ½ cup	30	2.0	6.8	.4	0	17	3.4
Brussels sprouts, frozen:							
(*Birds Eye* Box), 10 pcs., 3 oz.	45	3.0	8.0	0	0	15	3.0
(*Birds Eye* Tender), 6 pcs., 3 oz.	45	3.0	8.0	0	0	15	3.0
(*Birds Eye Steamfresh* Baby Premium Select), 10 pcs.	45	3.0	8.0	0	0	15	3.0
(*Birds Eye Steamfresh* Baby Singles), 3.25-oz. bag	50	3.0	9.0	0	0	20	3.0
(*C&W* Petite), 10 pcs., 3 oz.	45	3.0	8.0	0	0	15	3.0
butter sauce, baby, ½ cup cooked:							
(*Green Giant* Bag) .	70	4.0	10.0	1.0	<5	320	3.0
(*Green Giant* Box) .	60	3.0	9.0	1.0	<5	312	3.0
Brussels sprouts combination, **frozen:** cauliflower, carrots							
(*Birds Eye*), 1 cup . .	40	2.0	7.0	0	0	35	2.0
Buckwheat, grain:							
1 oz.	97	3.8	20.3	1.0	0	<1	2.8
1 cup	584	22.5	121.6	5.8	0	1	17.0
Buckwheat flour:							
(*Arrowhead Mills* Organic), ⅓ cup . . .	115	5.0	20.0	1.5	0	0	6.0
(*Hodgson Mill*), <¼ cup	100	2.0	22.0	1.0	0	0	3.0

Food and Measure	cal.	prot. (gms)	carbo. (gms)	fat (gms)	chol. (mgs)	sod. (mgs)	fiber (gms)
(*Shiloh Farms* Organic),							
¼ cup	100	4.0	21.0	1.0	0	0	3.0
1 cup	402	15.1	84.7	3.7	0	13	12.0
Buckwheat groats:							
(*Arrowhead Mills*							
Organic), ¼ cup . . .	150	5.0	31.0	1.0	0	0	4.0
(*Shiloh Farms* Organic),							
¼ cup	140	5.0	30.0	1.0	0	0	3.0
roasted, dry, ¼ cup:							
(*Shiloh Farms*							
Organic Kasha) .	140	5.0	30.0	1.0	0	0	3.0
(*Wolff's* Kasha) . . .	170	6.0	35.0	1.0	0	10	2.0
roasted, cooked, 1 cup	182	6.7	39.5	1.2	0	8	4.5
Buffalo wing sauce,							
see "Wing sauce"							
Buffalo wing seasoning							
(*McCormick*), 1 tbsp.	30	0	5.0	0	0	710	0
Bulgur:							
dry:							
(*Shiloh Farms*),							
¼ cup	140	5.0	30.0	.5	0	0	5.0
(*Shiloh Farms*							
Organic), ⅓ cup .	150	5.0	33.0	.5	0	0	4.0
¼ cup	120	4.3	26.6	.5	0	6	6.4
cooked, 1 cup	152	5.6	33.8	.4	0	9	8.2
Bulgur salad, see							
"Tabouli"							
Bun, see "Roll"							
Bun, sweet, 1 pc.:							
cheese (*Entenmann's*),							
3 oz.	320	6.0	40.0	15.0	55	320	1.0
cherry puffs (*Enten-*							
mann's), 2.8 oz. . . .	310	4.0	35.0	18.0	10	270	1.0
cinnamon swirl							
(*Entenmann's*), 3 oz.	320	5.0	44.0	14.0	45	280	2.0
Bun, sweet, frozen/							
refrigerated, 1 pc.,							
except as noted:							
blueberry (*Sister Schu-*							
bert's), 2 pcs.	190	3.0	33.0	6.0	15	210	1.0
caramel (*Pillsbury*) . .	170	2.0	24.0	7.0	0	320	<1.0
cinnamon (*Sister Schu-*							
bert's), 2 pcs.	220	3.0	37.0	7.0	20	200	1.0

Food and Measure	cal.	prot. (gms)	carbo. (gms)	fat (gms)	chol. (mgs)	sod. (mgs)	fiber (gms)
Bun, sweet, frozen/refrigerated *(cont.)*							
cinnamon, w/icing:							
(*Grands!*)	310	5.0	54.0	9.0	0	640	1.0
(*Pillsbury*)	150	2.0	23.0	5.0	0	340	<1.0
(*Pillsbury* Mini Bites), 3 pcs.	170	2.0	26.0	6.0	0	360	<1.0
(*Pillsbury* Reduced Fat)	140	2.0	24.0	3.5	0	340	<1.0
buttercream icing, rich (*Grands!*) ..	320	5.0	54.0	10.0	0	630	1.0
cream cheese icing (*Grands!*)	310	5.0	54.0	9.0	0	650	1.0
cream cheese icing (*Pillsbury*)	150	2.0	23.0	5.0	0	340	<1.0
knots (*Papa Ciro's*)	111	3.0	20.0	1.7	0	141	2.0
flaky, chocolate iced (*Grands!* Supreme)	380	4.0	47.0	20.0	0	580	1.0
orange (*Sister Schubert's*), 2 pcs.	190	2.0	31.0	6.0	15	200	0
orange, w/icing (*Pillsbury*)	170	2.0	25.0	7.0	0	340	<1.0
Bun, sweet, mix (*Pillsbury* Hot Roll), ¼ cup	110	4.0	21.0	1.5	5	210	<1.0
Burbot, meat only:							
raw, 4 oz.	102	21.9	0	.9	68	110	0
baked or broiled, 4 oz.	130	28.1	0	1.2	87	141	0
Burdock root:							
raw (*Frieda's* Gobo Root), 3 oz.	60	1.0	15.0	0	0	0	3.0
raw, 7.3-oz. pc.	112	1.3	13.6	.1	0	4	5.1
raw, pieces, ½ cup ..	43	.9	10.3	.1	0	3	1.9
boiled, 1" pcs., ½ cup	55	1.3	13.2	.1	0	3	1.1
Burger, vegetarian (see also "Beef," vegetarian"):							
canned:							
(*Linda Redi-Burger*), ⅝" slice, 3 oz. ..	120	18.0	7.0	2.5	0	450	4.0
(*Loma Linda Vege-Burger*), ¼ cup ..	60	12.0	2.0	.5	0	130	2.0
(*Worthington Vegetarian Burger*), ¼ cup ..	70	10.0	3.0	1.5	0	250	1.0
frozen/refrigerated:							
ground (*Boca*), 2 oz.	60	13.0	6.0	.5	0	270	3.0

Food and Measure	cal.	prot. (gms)	carbo. (gms)	fat (gms)	chol. (mgs)	sod. (mgs)	fiber (gms)
ground (*Morningstar Farms Grillers Recipe Crumbles*), ⅔ cup	80	10.0	4.0	2.5	0	240	3.0
ground, sausage style (*Morningstar Farms Recipe Crumbles*), ⅔ cup	90	11.0	5.0	2.5	0	440	1.3.0
patty, see "Burger patty, vegetarian,"							
taco seasoned (*Frieda's SoyTaco*), 1 oz. . .	50	4.0	3.0	3.0	0	180	2.0
mix (*Fantastic* Nature's Burger), ¼ cup ...	170	8.0	29.0	3.0	0	300	4.0
Burger patty, vegetarian, frozen, 1 pc., 2.5 oz., except as noted:							
(*Amy's* Bistro)	90	5.0	13.0	2.5	0	340	2.0
(*Boca* Organic Vegan)	100	13.0	9.0	2.5	0	470	4.0
(*Boca* Original)	70	13.0	6.0	.5	0	280	4.0
(*Garden Gourmet* Veggie Patties), 2.6 oz. ...	90	7.0	6.0	4.0	0	430	4.0
(*Gardenburger*)	100	5.0	14.0	3.5	5	420	5.0
(*Gardenburger* Classic)	110	12.0	8.0	5.0	0	390	4.0
(*Gardenburger* Flame Grilled)	90	11.0	5.0	4.0	0	420	4.0
(*Gardenburger* Garden Vegan)	100	10.0	12.0	1.0	0	230	3.0
(*Morningstar Farms* Classic), 2.25 oz. ..	150	14.0	9.0	6.0	0	280	3.0
(*Morningstar Farms* Vegan)	90	13.0	8.0	1.5	0	460	4.0
(*Morningstar Farms* Garden Veggie Patties), 2.25 oz. ..	110	10.0	9.0	3.5	0	350	3.0
(*Morningstar Farms* Garden Veggie Patties), 3.5 oz. ...	150	18.0	10.0	5.0	0	650	4.0
(*Morningstar Farms* Grillers Original), 2.25 oz.	130	15.0	5.0	6.0	0	260	2.0
(*Morningstar Farms* Grillers Vegan)	100	12.0	7.0	2.5	0	280	4.0
(*Morningstar Farms* Grillers Prime)	170	17.0	4.0	9.0	0	360	2.0

Food and Measure	cal.	prot. (gms)	carbo. (gms)	fat (gms)	chol. (mgs)	sod. (mgs)	fiber (gms)
Burger patty, vegetarian *(cont.)*							
(*Worthington Fri-Pats*),							
2.25 oz.	130	15.0	5.0	6.0	0	320	3.0
(*Yves*), 2.6 oz.	110	14.0	8.0	4.0	0	440	2.0
all American:							
(*Amy's*)	120	10.0	15.0	3.0	0	390	3.0
(*Boca*)	90	14.0	4.0	3.0	5	280	3.0
(*Boca* Organic)	140	15.0	9.0	5.0	5	500	4.0
Asian (*Morningstar*							
Farms), 2.4 oz.	100	7.0	10.0	4.0	0	490	2.0
black bean:							
chipotle (*Garden-*							
burger)	80	5.0	13.0	2.5	0	250	5.0
spicy (*Morningstar*							
Farms), 2.75 oz. .	140	12.0	13.0	4.5	0	410	5.0
California:							
(*Amy's*)	140	6.0	19.0	5.0	0	430	4.0
(*Gardenburger*) . . .	90	3.0	12.0	3.5	0	380	2.0
char-broiled (*Garden*							
Gourmet), 2.6 oz. . .	100	14.0	2.0	4.0	0	440	4.0
cheddar (*Morningstar*							
Farms), 2.25 oz. . . .	150	13.0	10.0	7.0	0	480	3.0
cheeseburger:							
(*Boca*)	100	12.0	5.0	5.0	5	360	3.0
(*Boca* Organic)	120	15.0	7.0	4.5	5	650	3.0
Chicago (*Amy's*)	160	10.0	20.0	5.0	5	390	3.0
"chicken," see "Chicken,"							
vegetarian"							
garlic, roasted:							
(*Boca*)	70	12.0	6.0	1.5	0	370	4.0
(*Boca* Organic)	130	16.0	9.0	3.0	0	470	4.0
herb-crusted cutlet							
(*Gardenburger*) . . .	150	10.0	11.0	9.0	0	460	3.0
mushroom (*Morning-*							
star Farms), 2.25 oz.	110	7.0	8.0	6.0	0	220	<1.0
okara (*Morningstar*							
Farms), 2.25 oz. . . .	120	12.0	6.0	5.0	0	300	3.0
onion, roasted:							
(*Boca*)	70	11.0	7.0	1.0	0	300	4.0
(*Boca* Organic)	130	15.0	10.0	3.0	0	420	4.0
Philly cheese steak							
burger (*Morningstar*							
Farms), 2.25 oz. . . .	120	10.0	6.0	6.0	5	400	3.0

Food and Measure	cal.	prot. (gms)	carbo. (gms)	fat (gms)	chol. (mgs)	sod. (mgs)	fiber (gms)
pizza burger, tomato basil (*Morningstar Farms*), 2.4 oz.	120	10.0	7.0	6.0	10	160	3.0
portobello:							
(*Gardenburger*) . . .	90	5.0	15.0	2.5	5	360	5.0
garlic (*Veggie Patch*)	120	11.0	8.0	6.0	0	320	4.0
Southwest (*Morningstar Farms*), 2.4 oz.	130	6.0	21.0	3.0	5	340	2.0
sun-dried tomato basil (*Gardenburger*) . . .	100	5.0	15.0	3.0	5	310	5.0
Texas (*Amy's*)	120	12.0	14.0	2.5	0	350	3.0
Tex-Mex:							
(*Morningstar Farms Tex-Mex*)	110	9.0	17.0	1.0	0	320	3.0
(*Tofurky*), 3.5 oz. . .	120	12.0	14.0	2.0	0	250	3.0
Thai (*Morningstar Farms*), 2.4 oz.	100	10.0	7.0	3.5	0	400	3.0
tomato basil (*Morningstar Farms*), 2.25 oz.	120	12.0	8.0	4.0	<5	340	2.0
vegetable, w/soy:							
garden (*Boca Organic*)	130	15.0	9.0	3.0	0	400	4.0
grilled (*Boca*)	80	12.0	7.0	1.0	0	300	4.0
veggie medley:							
(*Amy's* Quarter Pound), 4 oz. . . .	220	20.0	25.0	5.0	0	640	6.0
(*Gardenburger*) . . .	90	5.0	15.0	3.0	0	440	5.0
(*Morningstar Farms*), 2.25 oz.	120	11.0	11.0	4.0	0	260	2.0
Burger King:							
breakfast:							
biscuit:							
bacon/egg/cheese	410	16.0	31.0	25.0	150	1320	1.0
ham/egg/cheese .	390	16.0	31.0	22.0	145	1410	1.0
sausage	390	12.0	28.0	26.0	35	1020	1.0
sausage/egg/ cheese	530	20.0	31.0	37.0	175	1490	1.0
Croissan'wich:							
egg/cheese	300	12.0	26.0	17.0	145	740	<1.0
bacon/egg/cheese	340	15.0	26.0	20.0	155	890	<1.0
ham/egg/cheese .	340	18.0	26.0	18.0	160	1230	1.0
sausage/cheese .	370	14.0	23.0	25.0	50	810	<1.0
sausage/egg/ cheese	470	19.0	26.0	32.0	180	1060	<1.0

Food and Measure	cal.	prot. (gms)	carbo. (gms)	fat (gms)	chol. (mgs)	sod. (mgs)	fiber (gms)
Burger King, breakfast *(cont.)*							
Double Croissan'wich:							
double bacon ...	430	21.0	27.0	27.0	175	1250	<1.0
double ham	420	27.0	27.0	23.0	185	2210	1.0
double sausage .	680	29.0	26.0	51.0	220	1590	1.0
ham/bacon	420	24.0	27.0	24.0	180	1600	1.0
ham/sausage ...	550	28.0	27.0	37.0	205	2040	1.0
sausage/bacon ..	550	25.0	27.0	39.0	200	1420	1.0
omelet sandwich:							
enormous	730	37.0	44.0	45.0	330	1940	2.0
ham	290	13.0	33.0	13.0	85	870	1.0
French toast sticks:							
3 pcs.	240	4.0	26.0	13.0	0	260	1.0
5 pcs.	390	7.0	43.0	22.0	0	440	2.0
hash browns:							
large	620	5.0	60.0	40.0	0	1200	6.0
medium	430	4.0	42.0	28.0	0	830	4.0
small	260	2.0	25.0	17.0	0	500	2.0
cini-minis	390	7.0	51.0	18.0	20	560	2.0
vanilla icing ...	110	0	21.0	3.0	0	40	0
jam, grape/strawberry	30	0	7.0	0	0	0	0
syrup	80	0	21.0	0	0	20	0
burgers:							
Angus steak burger	640	33.0	55.0	33.0	185	1260	3.0
BK burger:							
double stacker ...	610	34.0	32.0	39.0	125	1100	1.0
triple stacker ...	800	48.0	33.0	54.0	185	1450	1.0
quad stacker ...	1000	62.0	34.0	68.0	240	1800	1.0
BK Veggie	420	23.0	46.0	16.0	10	1100	7.0
no mayo	340	23.0	46.0	8.0	0	1030	7.0
w/cheese	470	25.0	47.0	20.0	20	1320	7.0
burger bacon, 1 pc.	15	1.0	0	1.0	5	50	0
cheeseburger	330	17.0	31.0	16.0	55	780	1.0
double	500	30.0	31.0	29.0	105	1030	1.0
Double Whopper ..	900	47.0	51.0	57.0	175	1090	3.0
no mayo	740	47.0	51.0	39.0	160	950	3.0
w/cheese	990	52.0	52.0	64.0	195	1520	3.0
w/cheese, no mayo	830	52.0	52.0	47.0	180	1380	3.0
hamburger	290	15.0	30.0	12.0	40	560	1.0
double	410	25.0	30.0	21.0	85	600	1.0
Triple Whopper ...	1130	67.0	51.0	74.0	255	1160	3.0
no mayo	980	66.0	51.0	57.0	240	1020	3.0
w/cheese	1230	71.0	52.0	82.0	275	1590	3.0

Food and Measure	cal.	prot. (gms)	carbo. (gms)	fat (gms)	chol. (mgs)	sod. (mgs)	fiber (gms)
w/cheese, no mayo	1070	71.0	52.0	65.0	260	1450	3.0
Whopper	670	28.0	51.0	39.0	95	1020	3.0
no mayo	510	28.0	51.0	22.0	80	880	3.0
w/cheese	760	33.0	52.0	47.0	115	1450	3.0
w/cheese, no mayo	600	32.0	52.0	30.0	100	1310	3.0
Whopper, Jr.	370	15.0	31.0	21.0	50	570	2.0
no mayo	290	15.0	31.0	12.0	40	490	2.0
w/cheese.......	410	18.0	32.0	24.0	60	780	2.0
w/cheese, no mayo	330	17.0	31.0	16.0	55	710	2.0
sandwiches:							
BK Big Fish	640	24.0	67.0	32.0	65	1450	3.0
no tarter sauce ..	470	23.0	65.0	13.0	50	1240	3.0
chicken, original ...	660	24.0	52.0	40.0	70	1440	4.0
.no mayo	450	23.0	52.0	17.0	50	1250	4.0
Chick'n Crisp	480	15.0	36.0	31.0	45	870	1.0
no mayo	320	15.0	36.0	13.0	30	730	1.0
Tendercrisp chicken	790	33.0	68.0	44.0	70	1640	5.0
Tendergrill chicken	510	37.0	49.0	19.0	75	1180	4.0
no mayo	400	36.0	49.0	7.0	70	1090	4.0
BK chicken fries:							
6 pcs.	260	12.0	18.0	15.0	35	650	2.0
9 pcs.	390	18.0	26.0	23.0	50	980	3.0
12 pcs.	520	25.0	35.0	31.0	65	1300	4.0
Chicken Tenders:							
4 pcs.	170	9.0	11.0	10.0	25	480	0
5 pcs.	210	12.0	13.0	12.0	35	600	0
6 pcs. ....:...	250	14.0	16.0	15.0	40	720	0
8 pcs.	340	19.0	21.0	20.0	55	960	<1.0
dipping sauce, 1 oz.:							
barbecue	40	0	11.0	0	0	310	0
Buffalo	80	0	2.0	8.0	5	350	0
honey mustard	90	0	8.0	6.0	10	180	0
ranch	140	1.0	1.0	15.0	5	95	0
sweet and sour ...	45	0	11.0	0	0	55	0
sides:							
Cheesy Tots:							
6 pcs.	210	7.0	20.0	12.0	20	650	2.0
9 pcs.	320	10.0	30.0	18.0	30	970	2.0
12 pcs.	430	14.0	40.0	24.0	40	1300	3.0

Food and Measure	cal.	prot. (gms)	carbo. (gms)	fat (gms)	chol. (mgs)	sod. (mgs)	fiber (gms)
Burger King, sides *(cont.)*							
fries, salted:							
king	600	6.0	69.0	33.0	0	990	6.0
large	500	5.0	57.0	28.0	0	820	5.0
medium	360	4.0	41.0	20.0	0	590	4.0
small	230	2.0	26.0	13.0	0	380	2.0
fries, no salt added:							
king	600	6.0	69.0	33.0	0	640	6.0
large	500	5.0	57.0	28.0	0	530	5.0
medium	360	4.0	41.0	20.0	0	380	4.0
small	230	2.0	26.0	13.0	0	240	2.0
ketchup, 1 pkt.	10	0	3.0	0	0	125	0
mayo, 1 pkt.	80	0	1.0	9.0	10	75	0
onion rings:							
king	500	7.0	62.0	25.0	0	720	5.0
large	440	6.0	53.0	22.0	0	620	5.0
medium	310	4.0	37.0	15.0	0	440	3.0
small	140	2.0	18.0	7.0	0	210	2.0
onion ring sauce ..	150	0	3.0	15.0	15	210	<1.0
salad, garden, no dressing/extras:							
Tendergrill chicken .	240	33.0	8.0	9.0	80	720	4.0
Tendercrisp chicken	410	29.0	26.0	22.0	70	1080	5.0
no chicken	90	5.0	7.0	5.0	15	125	3.0
side salad	15	1.0	3.0	0	0	0	1.0
salad dressing, 2 oz.:							
Caesar, creamy ...	210	3.0	4.0	21.0	25	610	0
honey mustard	270	1.0	15.0	23.0	20	520	0
Italian, light	120	0	5.0	11.0	0	440	0
ranch	190	1.0	2.0	20.0	20	560	0
ranch, fat free	60	1.0	15.0	0	0	740	2.0
croutons, garlic Parmesan	60	1.0	9.0	2.0	0	120	0
shakes, 16 fl. oz.:							
chocolate	470	8.0	75.0	14.0	55	320	1.0
strawberry	460	7.0	73.0	14.0	55	240	0
vanilla	400	8.0	57.0	15.0	60	240	0
Oreo sundae:							
chocolate	680	9.0	105.0	24.0	55	480	2.0
strawberry	660	9.0	103.0	23.0	55	380	1.0
vanilla	510	9.0	87.0	24.0	60	400	1.0
beverages:							
Icee, cherry or *Coca-Cola*, medium ...	140	0	40.0	0	0	10	0

Food and Measure	cal.	prot. (gms)	carbo. (gms)	fat (gms)	chol. (mgs)	sod. (mgs)	fiber (gms)
Mocha *BK Joe*	380	6.0	66.0	10.0	40	290	1.0
dessert, pie:							
Dutch apple	300	2.0	45.0	13.0	0	270	1.0
Hershey's sundae ..	310	3.0	32.0	19.0	10	220	1.0
Burger sauce, see							
"Sandwich spread"							
Burrito (see also							
"Burrito, breakfast"),							
frozen, 1 pc.:							
bean/cheese:							
(*Amy's*), 6 oz.	300	11.0	43.0	9.0	10	580	6.0
(*Cedarlane Dr. Sears*							
Zone), 6 oz.	350	27.0	37.0	13.0	15	380	8.0
(*El Monterey*), 4 oz.	220	8.0	35.0	6.0	5	490	4.0
(*El Monterey*), 5 oz.	280	10.0	43.0	8.0	5	560	5.0
(*El Monterey* XX							
Large!), 10 oz. ..	570	19.0	87.0	17.0	10	1110	9.0
(*Nate's*), 6 oz.	350	25.0	21.0	18.0	50	560	12.0
w/chicken (*Cedarlane*							
Dr. Sears Zone),							
6.5 oz.	320	24.0	33.0	12.0	40	550	6.0
bean/rice (*Amy's*), 6 oz.	280	9.0	48.0	6.0	0	550	5.0
bean/rice/cheese:							
(*Cedarlane* Low-Fat							
Organic), 6 oz. ..	260	13.0	48.0	1.0	0	490	7.0
(*Nate's*), 6 oz.	330	23.0	23.0	15.0	45	530	12.0
beef/bean:							
(*El Monterey*), 4 oz.	290	8.0	34.0	14.0	15	490	3.0
(*El Monterey*), 5 oz.	370	10.0	42.0	17.0	20	610	4.0
(*El Monterey*), 8 oz.	590	17.0	68.0	27.0	30	980	7.0
(*El Monterey* XX							
Large!), 10 oz. ..	740	21.0	84.0	35.0	40	1230	8.0
mild (*Patio*), 5 oz. .	300	10.0	44.0	10.0	<5	740	5.0
spicy (*El Monterey*							
Red Hot), 5 oz. ...	380	11.0	42.0	18.0	20	700	4.0
spicy (*El Monterey*							
Red Hot), 8 oz. ...	600	17.0	68.0	29.0	35	1120	7.0
spicy (*El Monterey*							
Red Hot XX							
Large!), 10 oz. ...	750	21.0	86.0	36.0	40	1400	9.0
beef/bean, green chili:							
(*El Monterey*), 4 oz.	290	8.0	33.0	13.0	15	490	3.0
(*El Monterey*), 5 oz.	360	10.0	41.0	17.0	20	610	4.0

Food and Measure	cal.	prot. (gms)	carbo. (gms)	fat (gms)	chol. (mgs)	sod. (mgs)	fiber (gms)
Burrito, beef/bean, green chili *(cont.)*							
(*El Monterey* XX Large!), 10 oz. . .	720	20.0	84.0	33.0	40	1220	7.0
beef/bean, red chili:							
(*El Monterey*), 4 oz.	300	8.0	34.0	14.0	15	460	3.0
(*El Monterey* XX Large!), 10 oz. . .	740	21.0	86.0	34.0	40	1140	8.0
(*Patio*), 5 oz.	310	9.0	42.0	11.0	10	730	4.0
beef steak, shredded/ cheese (*El Monterey* Supreme), 8 oz. . . .	450	21.0	58.0	14.0	50	920	2.0
black bean, 6 oz.:							
rice (*Amy's*)	270	9.0	45.0	6.0	5	620	4.0
vegetable (*Amy's*) .	280	9.0	44.0	8.0	0	580	4.0
chicken:							
(*El Monterey*), 4 oz.	210	7.0	31.0	7.0	10	520	1.0
(*José Olé* Monterey), 5 oz.	270	12.0	40.0	6.0	15	700	2.0
(*Patio*), 5 oz.	280	9.0	42.0	8.0	15	740	2.0
and cheese (*El Monterey*), 8 oz.	460	22.0	60.0	15.0	35	1090	3.0
w/chili verde sauce (*Cedarland* Organic), 5 oz.	230	9.0	27.0	10.0	20	540	2.0
w/salsa roja (*Cedarlane*), 5 oz.	220	9.0	27.0	9.0	20	610	2.0
Southwestern (*Amy's*), 5.5 oz.	300	12.0	43.0	10.0	15	680	6.0
steak/cheese:							
(*José Olé*), 5 oz. . . .	300	13.0	39.0	10.0	25	510	2.0
shredded (*El Monterey*), 5 oz.	290	12.0	41.0	9.0	20	590	1.0
taco picante, spicy (*El Monterey*), 4 oz.	280	8.0	32.0	13.0	15	520	2.0
vegetable, roasted, and cheese (*Cedarlane* Organic), 6 oz.	330	14.0	48.0	8.0	15	590	3.0
Burrito, breakfast, frozen, 1 pc.:							
(*Amy's*), 6 oz.	250	9.0	38.0	7.0	0	540	5.0
chorizo/egg/cheese (*El Monterey*), 8 oz.	490	19.0	57.0	22.0	150	960	2.0
egg/bacon/cheese/salsa (*El Monterey*), 8 oz.	440	19.0	58.0	19.0	70	1430	2.0

Food and Measure	cal.	prot. (gms)	carbo. (gms)	fat (gms)	chol. (mgs)	sod. (mgs)	fiber (gms)
egg/cheese/salsa/bacon (*El Monterey* Supreme), 4.5 oz.	290	13.0	36.0	11.0	120	740	1.0
egg/cheese/sausage (*El Monterey* Supreme), 4.5 oz.	300	10.0	34.0	13.0	75	630	1.0
egg/ham/cheese (*José Olé*), 4 oz.	260	10.0	34.0	9.0	95	770	2.0
egg/sausage/cheese: (*José Olé*), 4 oz. . . .	270	10.0	34.0	11.0	95	750	2.0
potato (*El Monterey*), 8 oz.	510	17.0	60.0	22.0	145	1150	2.0
ranchero (*Cedarlane Dr. Sears Zone*), 10 oz.	300	25.0	33.0	11.0	0	770	4.0
Burrito entree, frozen (*Cedarlane* Grande), ½ of 10-oz. pkg.:							
w/chili verde sauce . .	230	9.0	27.0	10.0	20	540	2.0
w/salsa roja	220	9.0	27.0	9.0	20	610	2.0
Burrito seasoning:							
(*Lawry's*), 2 tsp.	20	<1.0	4.0	0	0	390	<1.0
(*McCormick*), 1 tbsp. . .	25	0	5.0	.5	0	500	0
(*Old El Paso*), 2 tsp. . . .	15	0	4.0	0	0	410	0
(*Ortega*), 11/2 tsp.	20	0	3.0	0	0	230	0
Butter, 1 tbsp., except as noted:							
cultured (*Vermont Butter & Cheese*) . .	110	0	0	12.0	30	<5	0
regular, unsalted:							
(*Land O Lakes*) . . .	100	0	0	11.0	30	0	0
(*Land O Lakes Ultra Creamy*) . .	110	0	0	12.0	30	0	0
(*Organic Valley*) . . .	100	0	0	11.0	30	0	0
(*Organic Valley* European Style) .	110	0	0	12.0	35	0	0
1 stick or 4 oz.	813	1.0	0	92.0	248	12	0
1 tbsp.	100	.1	0	11.4	31	1	0
1 tsp.	34	<.1	0	3.8	10	<1	0
regular, salted:							
(*Land O Lakes*) . . .	100	0	0	11.0	30	95	0
(*Land O Lakes* Light)	50	0	0	6.0	15	100	0
(*Land O Lakes* Ultra Creamy*) . .	110	0	0	12.0	30	85	0

Food and Measure	cal.	prot. (gms)	carbo. (gms)	fat (gms)	chol. (mgs)	sod. (mgs)	fiber (gms)
Butter, regular, salted *(cont.)*							
(*Organic Valley*) . . .	110	0	0	12.0	30	40	0
1 stick or 4 oz.	813	1.0	0	92.0	248	937	0
1 tbsp.	100	.1	0	11.4	31	115	0
1 tsp.	34	<.1	0	3.8	10	39	0
whipped, unsalted:							
(*Land O Lakes*) . . .	50	0	0	6.0	15	0	0
½ cup or 1 stick . .	542	.6	<.1	61.3	165	8	0
1 tbsp.	67	.1	tr.	7.6	20	1	0
1 tsp.	23	tr.	tr.	2.6	7	<1	0
whipped, salted:							
(*Land O Lakes*) . . .	50	0	0	6.0	15	50	0
(*Land O Lakes* Light)	45	0	0	5.0	15	85	0
½ cup or 1 stick . .	542	.6	<.1	61.3	165	625	0
1 tbsp.	67	.1	tr.	7.6	20	78	0
1 tsp.	23	tr.	tr.	2.6	7	26	0
Butter, blend, 1 tbsp.:							
(*Parkay 50/50*)	100	0	0	11.0	15	100	0
w/canola oil:							
(*Land O Lakes*) . . .	100	0	0	11.0	20	90	0
(*Land O Lakes* Light)	50	0	0	5.0	5	90	0
(*Shedd's Spread*							
Country Crock) .	80	0	0	9.0	15	65	0
Butter, flavored, 1 tbsp.:							
garlic (*Land O Lakes*) .	90	0	0	10.0	20	110	0
honey:							
(*Downey's*)	60	0	11.0	1.0	<5	10	0
(*Land O Lakes*) . . .	90	0	4.0	8.0	15	40	0
Butter beans (see also "Lima beans"), canned, ½ cup:							
(*Bush's* Speckled) . . .	110	6.0	19.0	.5	0	420	5.0
(*Eden* Organic)	100	5.0	17.0	1.0	0	35	4.0
(*Furmano's*)	90	5.0	16.0	0	0	430	4.0
(*Glory*)	100	6.0	18.0	0	0	570	5.0
(*S&W*)	80	6.0	19.0	0	0	500	5.0
baby:							
(*Allens*)	120	7.0	22.0	.5	0	460	6.0
(*Bush's*)	120	7.0	19.0	.5	0	510	5.0
green (*Sunshine*)	120	7.0	22.0	.5	0	460	6.0
large:							
(*Allens*)	120	7.0	20.0	1.0	0	290	7.0
(*Bush's*)	100	6.0	18.0	.5	0	450	5.0

Food and Measure	cal.	prot. (gms)	carbo. (gms)	fat (gms)	chol. (mgs)	sod. (mgs)	fiber (gms)
white, w/sausage (*Trappey's*)	110	6.0	21.0	1.0	0	300	6.0
Butter beans, frozen, (*McKenzie's*), ½ cup	100	6.0	20.0	0	0	130	4.0
Butter oil, see "Oil"							
Butterbur, fresh:							
raw, .2-oz. stalk	1	<.1	.2	<.1	0	<1	<1.0
boiled, drained, 4 oz. .	9	.3	2.4	<.1	0	5	n.a.
Butterbur, canned,							
chopped, ½ cup ...	2	.1	.2	.1	0	3	n.a.
Buttercup squash (*Frieda's*), 3 oz. ...	30	1.0	7.0	0	0	0	1.0
Butterfish, meat only:							
raw, 4 oz.	166	19.6	0	9.1	74	100	0
baked or broiled, 4 oz.	212	25.1	0	11.7	94	129	0
Buttermilk, see "Milk"							
Butternut, dried:							
in shell, 1 lb.	750	30.5	14.8	69.8	0	1	5.8
shelled, 1 oz.	174	7.1	3.4	16.2	0	<1	1.3
Butternut squash:							
raw (*Frieda's*), 3 oz. ..	30	1.0	7.0	0	0	0	1.0
raw, cubed, ½ cup ...	32	.7	8.1	.1	0	3	1.1
baked, cubed, ½ cup .	41	.9	10.7	.1	0	4	2.9
Butternut squash, frozen, boiled, drained, mashed, ½ cup ...	47	1.5	12.1	.1	0	2	n.a.
Butterscotch baking chips, 1 tbsp., .5 oz.:							
(*Hershey's*)	80	1.0	9.0	4.0	0	35	0
(*Nestlé Toll House*) ..	70	0	9.0	4.0	0	15	0
Butterscotch syrup (*Smucker's Sundae Syrup*), 2 tbsp.	100	1.0	25.0	0	0	110	0
Butterscotch topping, 2 tbsp.:							
(*Hershey's*)	110	<1.0	27.0	0	0	120	0
caramel (*Smucker's Special Recipe*) ...	140	1.0	31.0	1.0	<5	70	<1.0
(*Smucker's Spoonable*)	120	0	30.0	0	0	105	0

C

Food and Measure	cal.	prot. (gms)	carbo. (gms)	fat (gms)	chol. (mgs)	sod. (mgs)	fiber (gms)
Cabbage, fresh:							
raw:							
(*Glory*), 1 cup, 3 oz.	20	1.0	5.0	0	0	15	2.0
5¾" head, 2½ lbs. . .	228	13.1	49.3	2.4	0	164	20.9
shredded, ½ cup . .	9	.5	1.9	.1	0	6	.8
boiled, drained,							
shredded, ½ cup . .	17	.8	3.4	.3	0	6	2.1
Cabbage, can or jar:							
red, sweet/sour (*Green-*							
wood), ½ cup	100	0	24.0	0	0	380	0
seasoned (*Glory*							
Country), ½ cup . .	30	1.0	6.0	0	0	350	1.0
Cabbage, Chinese,							
fresh, ½ cup,							
except as noted:							
bok choy, raw:							
(*Frieda's/Frieda's*							
Baby), 3 oz.	10	1.0	2.0	0	0	55	1.0
shredded	5	.5	.8	.1	0	23	.4
bok choy, boiled,							
drained, shredded .	10	1.3	1.5	.1	0	29	1.4
napa, raw (*Frieda's*),							
1 cup, 3 oz.	15	1.0	3.0	0	0	10	1.0
pe-tsai, shredded,							
boiled, drained	8	.9	1.4	.1	0	6	1.0
Cabbage, frozen, sea-							
soned (*Glory*), ½ cup	45	1.0	7.0	1.5	0	380	2.0
Cabbage, marinated,							
see "Kim chee"							
Cabbage, mustard,							
raw (*Frieda's* Gai							
Choy), 1 cup, 3 oz.	20	2.0	4.0	0	0	20	2.0
Cabbage, napa, see							
"Cabbage, Chinese"							

Food and Measure	cal.	prot. (gms)	carbo. (gms)	fat (gms)	chol. (mgs)	sod. (mgs)	fiber (gms)
Cabbage, red, fresh:							
raw, whole, 1 lb.	100	5.0	22.2	.9	0	38	7.3
raw, shredded, ½ cup	10	.5	2.1	.1	0	4	.7
boiled, drained,							
shredded, ½ cup ..	16	.8	3.5	.2	0	6	1.5
Cabbage, savoy, fresh:							
raw, whole, 1 lb.	100	7.3	22.1	.4	0	102	11.2
raw, shredded, ½ cup	10	.7	2.1	<.1	0	10	1.1
boiled, drained,							
shredded, ½ cup ..	18	1.3	4.0	.1	0	17	n.a.
Cabbage, stuffed,							
frozen, mini (*Empire*							
Kosher), 2 pcs., 4 oz.	90	9.0	9.0	2.0	25	320	1.0
Cabbage, stuffed, entree,							
frozen (*Lean Cuisine*							
One Dish Favorites),							
9.5 oz.	200	11.0	25.0	6.0	15	690	4.0
Cabbage, Tuscan							
(*Frieda's*), 3 oz. ...	20	1.0	5.0	0	0	15	2.0
Cabbage salad, red							
(*Sabra*), 1 oz.	70	0	6.0	4.5	5	160	0
Cactus pads, fresh:							
raw (*Frieda's*), 3 oz. ..	20	1.0	4.0	0	0	5	1.0
raw, sliced, 1 cup	14	1.1	2.9	.1	0	19	2.0
cooked, 1 pad	4	.4	1.0	<.1	0	6	.6
cooked, 1 cup	22	2.0	4.9	.1	0	30	3.0
Cactus pads, can/jar							
(nopalitos):							
(*Goya* Tender), 23 pcs.,							
4.5 oz.	20	<1.0	3.0	0	0	1180	3.0
chopped (*Doña Maria*),							
2 tbsp.	5	0	1.0	0	0	560	0
pickled (*Sabores*							
Aztecas), 2.1 oz. ..	40	2.0	6.0	0	0	240	5.0
sliced (*Embasa*), 2 tbsp.	5	0	1.0	0	0	830	2.0
Cactus pear, see "Prickly							
pear"							
Cajun sauce, see "Seafood							
sauce"							
Cajun seasoning:							
(*Luzianne*), ¼ tsp.	0	0	0	0	0	260	0
(*McCormick*), ¼ tsp. .	0	0	0	0	0	135	0

Food and Measure	cal.	prot. (gms)	carbo. (gms)	fat (gms)	chol. (mgs)	sod. (mgs)	fiber (gms)
Cake, ⅛ cake, except as noted:							
apple, caramel iced (*Awrey's* Ripple), 1/9 cake	310	2.0	40.0	16.0	10	180	0
apple strudel (*Entenmann's*), ¼ cake . .	350	3.0	52.0	15.0	0	260	2.0
banana crunch (*Entenmann's*)	230	2.0	33.0	10.0	30	270	<1.0
banana split (*Awrey's* Ripple), 1/9 cake . .	350	2.0	45.0	19.0	20	190	<1.0
black and white (*Entenmann's*)	300	2.0	41.0	15.0	30	210	<1.0
butter loaf (*Entenmann's*)	220	3.0	31.0	9.0	70	290	0
caramel buttercream (*Awrey's* Ripple), 1/9 cake	290	2.0	39.0	15.0	10	200	0
carrot, iced:							
cream cheese (*Awrey's*)	340	3.0	41.0	18.0	25	210	1.0
pineapple (*Awrey's* Ripple), 1/9 cake	340	2.0	39.0	19.0	25	220	<1.0
cheese, see "Cheesecake"							
chocolate:							
chocolate iced (*Awrey's*)	320	3.0	54.0	12.0	30	370	1.0
chocolate iced (*Awrey's Bill Knapp's* Celebration)	330	3.0	54.0	12.0	20	380	1.0
French, w/buttercream, chocolate iced (*Awrey's* Ripple), 1/9 cake	280	2.0	42.0	16.0	10	180	0
peppermint iced (*Awrey's* Ripple), 1/9 cake	320	2.0	38.0	18.0	10	220	<1.0
chocolate chip crumb loaf (*Entenmann's*) .	240	3.0	33.0	11.0	35	220	<1.0
chocolate fudge (*Entenmann's*)	270	3.0	40.0	11.0	25	230	2.0
chocolate truffle (*Entenmann's*), ⅙ cake . .	400	3.0	55.0	19.0	40	290	2.0

Food and Measure	cal.	prot. (gms)	carbo. (gms)	fat (gms)	chol. (mgs)	sod. (mgs)	fiber (gms)
coffee cake:							
butterscotch walnut (*Awrey's*), 1/12 cake	200	2.0	24.0	10.0	10	170	<1.0
cheese, cherry top (*Awrey's* 8 x 12), 1/24 cake	140	2.0	17.0	7.0	<5	160	0
crumb, cheese (*Entenmann's*), 1/9 cake	200	4.0	25.0	10.0	35	190	<1.0
raspberry almond (*Awrey's*), 1/12 cake	190	3.0	23.0	9.0	0	180	<1.0
crumb cake:							
(*Entenmann's* Ultimate), 1/10 cake	250	2.0	33.0	13.0	25	270	<1.0
all butter (*Entenmann's* French) .	210	2.0	29.0	10.0	50	230	<1.0
Danish cake:							
cheese twist (*Entenmann's*) ..	230	3.0	29.0	12.0	25	210	<1.0
pecan ring (*Entenmann's*) ..	240	3.0	24.0	15.0	20	150	1.0
raspberry twist (*Entenmann's*) ..	220	3.0	29.0	11.0	15	170	<1.0
walnut ring (*Entenmann's*) ..	240	4.0	24.0	14.0	20	150	2.0
devil's food, marshmallow iced (*Entenmann's*)	280	3.0	40.0	13.0	25	250	<1.0
golden, fudge iced (*Entenmann's*)	290	3.0	41.0	13.0	35	210	1.0
lemon, lemon iced:							
(*Awrey's* Ripple), 1/9 cake	340	2.0	43.0	19.0	10	190	0
lemon buttercream (*Awrey's*)	350	2.0	59.0	12.0	30	440	0
lemon coconut (*Entenmann's*)	320	2.0	38.0	18.0	35	240	<1.0
Louisiana crunch (*Entenmann's*)	330	3.0	49.0	14.0	45	300	<1.0
orange, orange iced (*Awrey's* Ripple), 1/9 cake	310	2.0	40.0	17.0	10	180	0

Food and Measure	cal.	prot. (gms)	carbo. (gms)	fat (gms)	chol. (mgs)	sod. (mgs)	fiber (gms)
Cake *(cont.)*							
raisin loaf (*Entenmann's*)	210	2.0	33.0	8.0	35	220	1.0
sour cream loaf (*Entenmann's*)	210	0	24.0	12.0	40	150	0
strawberry, strawberry iced (*Awrey's* Ripple), 1/9 cake	340	2.0	42.0	19.0	10	180	0
yellow, white iced (*Awrey's*)	360	2.0	58.0	14.0	35	470	0
Cake, frozen, ⅛ cake, except as noted:							
carrot, cream cheese iced (*Mrs. Smith's*), ⅙ cake	300	3.0	37.0	16.0	30	320	2.0
cheese, see "Cheesecake"							
chocolate chip (*Kineret*)	200	2.0	27.0	10.0	45	170	0
chocolate, German (*Pepperidge Farm* 3 Layer)	240	2.0	34.0	10.0	15	200	<1.0
chocolate coconut (*Pepperidge Farm* 3 Layer)	240	2.0	33.0	10.0	20	130	<1.0
chocolate fudge: (*Pepperidge Farm* 3 Layer)	230	2.0	33.0	10.0	20	130	1.0
double (*Smart Ones*), 2.7-oz. pc.	220	4.0	35.0	7.0	45	300	3.0
stripe (*Pepperidge Farm* 3 Layer) ..	240	2.0	34.0	10.0	20	150	2.0
coconut layer (*Pepperidge Farm* 3 Layer) .	240	1.0	35.0	10.0	20	120	<1.0
devil's food (*Pepperidge Farm* 3 Layer)	220	2.0	34.0	9.0	20	170	2.0
golden (*Pepperidge Farm* 3 Layer)	230	2.0	34.0	9.0	15	130	1.0
lemon (*Pepperidge Farm* 3 Layer)	240	2.0	34.0	11.0	25	130	<1.0
marble (*Kineret*)	200	2.0	25.0	10.0	45	180	0
peppermint (*Pepperidge Farm* 3 Layer)	230	2.0	31.0	11.0	25	135	2.0

Food and Measure	cal.	prot. (gms)	carbo. (gms)	fat (gms)	chol. (mgs)	sod. (mgs)	fiber (gms)
pound cake (*Sara Lee*), ¼ cake	300	4.0	35.0	16.0	110	250	<1.0
strawberry shortcake (*Smart Ones*), 3.3 oz.	170	4.0	25.0	6.0	40	260	<1.0
tiramisu (*Kozy Shack*), 3-oz. pc.	220	4.0	29.0	10.0	5	5	1.0
vanilla bean (*Pepperidge Farm* 3 Layer)	220	1.0	35.0	9.0	20	120	<1.0
Cake, microwave, 1 cont.:							
bananas Foster (*Guiltless Gourmet*), 2 oz.	200	3.0	42.0	2.0	15	250	<1.0
black velvet (*Guiltless Gourmet*), 2 oz. ...	200	4.0	42.0	2.5	20	190	3.0
caramel, molten (*Betty Crocker Warm Delights*), 3.4 oz.	360	5.0	64.0	10.0	5	490	3.0
chocolate, molten (*Betty Crocker Warm Delights*), 3.4 oz. ..	370	6.0	61.0	12.0	5	490	3.0
cinnamon swirl (*Betty Crocker Warm Delights*), 3.3 oz. ..	390	4.0	72.0	10.0	0	500	1.0
lemon swirl (*Betty Crocker Warm Delights*), 3.6 oz. ..	380	4.0	72.0	9.0	5	410	1.0
Cake, mix, 1/12 cake*, except as noted:							
(*Moist Supreme Funfetti*), 1/12 pkg.	180	1.0	36.0	3.5	0	300	<1.0
angel food:							
(*Betty Crocker*) ...	140	3.0	32.0	0	0	320	0
(*Pillsbury*)	140	3.0	31.0	0	0	360	0
banana (*Moist Supreme*), 1/12 pkg.	170	1.0	35.0	3.5	0	290	<1.0
butter pecan (*SuperMoist*)	240	3.0	34.0	11.0	55	290	0
carrot (*SuperMoist*), 1/10 cake*	320	4.0	41.0	16.0	65	340	0
cherry chip (*SuperMoist*)	300	4.0	40.0	14.0	65	380	<1.0
chocolate:							
butter recipe (*SuperMoist*) ...	260	3.0	35.0	12.0	75	420	2.0

Food and Measure	cal.	prot. (gms)	carbo. (gms)	fat (gms)	chol. (mgs)	sod. (mgs)	fiber (gms)
Cake mix, chocolate (cont.)							
dark (*Moist Supreme*), 1/12 pkg.	170	2.0	33.0	4.0	0	360	1.0
dark (*SuperMoist*) .	280	4.0	36.0	14.0	55	420	1.0
German (*Moist Supreme*), 1/12 pkg.	170	1.0	34.0	3.5	0	280	<1.0
German (*Super-Moist*)	270	3.0	34.0	14.0	55	360	1.0
milk (*SuperMoist*) .	240	4.0	34.0	11.0	55	290	1.0
triple (*Pillsbury Ultimate Dessert Kit*), 1/9 pkg.	210	2.0	37.0	6.0	0	210	<1.0
chocolate caramel (*Pillsbury Ultimate Dessert Kit*), 1/9 pkg. .	190	1.0	38.0	0	8	210	<1.0
chocolate fudge (*SuperMoist*)	270	3.0	34.0	14.0	55	370	1.0
cookies and cream (*Pillsbury Ultimate Dessert Kit*), 1/9 pkg.	210	1.0	39.0	5.0	0	270	1.0
coffee cake (*Aunt Jemima Easy Mix*), 1/8 cake*	180	3.0	28.0	6.0	30	250	1.0
devil's food:							
(*"Jiffy"*), 1/5 pkg.	210	3.0	39.0	5.0	0	450	1.0
(*Moist Supreme*), 1/12 pkg.	160	2.0	35.0	2.5	0	330	1.0
(*SuperMoist*)	270	4.0	34.0	14.0	55	380	1.0
fudge, hot (*Betty Crocker Complete Desserts*), 1/8 cake*	440	5.0	78.0	13.0	5	550	3.0
gingerbread (*Betty Crocker Cake & Cookie*), 1/8 cake* ..	220	3.0	39.0	6.0	25	370	2.0
golden:							
butter recipe (*Moist Supreme*), 1/12 pkg.	170	1.0	35.0	3,5	0	290	<1.0
yellow (*"Jiffy"*), 1/5 pkg.	210	2.0	40.0	4.5	0	340	0
lemon:							
(*Moist Supreme*), 1/12 pkg.	170	1.0	35.0	3.5	0	300	<1.0
(*SuperMoist*)	240	3.0	34.0	11.0	55	290	0

Food and Measure	cal.	prot. (gms)	carbo. (gms)	fat (gms)	chol. (mgs)	sod. (mgs)	fiber (gms)
pineapple:							
(*Moist Supreme*), 1/12 pkg.	170	1.0	35.0	3.5	0	290	<1.0
upside-down (*Betty Crocker*), ⅙ cake*	390	3.0	65.0	13.0	35	330	0
pound (*Betty Crocker*), ⅛ cake*	260	4.0	45.0	8.0	55	210	0
rainbow chip (*Super-Moist*), 1/10 cake*	300	4.0	40.0	14.0	55	370	1.0
pumpkin cream cheese swirl (*Pillsbury Ultimate Dessert Kit*), 1/9 pkg.	260	2.0	51.0	5.0	0	250	2.0
spice (*SuperMoist*) ..	240	3.0	34.0	11.0	55	290	0
strawberry:							
(*Moist Supreme*), 1/12 pkg.	170	1.0	35.0	3.5	0	290	<1.0
(*SuperMoist*)	240	3.0	34.0	11.0	55	290	0
and cream (*Pillsbury Ultimate Dessert Kit*), 1/9 pkg. ...	170	1.0	36.0	3.0	0	200	<1.0
vanilla:							
(*SuperMoist*)	250	3.0	330	11.0	55	300	0
French or golden (*SuperMoist*) ...	240	3.0	34.0	11.0	55	290	0
white:							
(*"Jiffy"*), 1/5 pkg. ...	210	2.0	40.0	4.5	0	340	0
(*Moist Supreme* Classic), 1/12 pkg. ...	170	1.0	35.0	3.5	0	290	1.0
(*SuperMoist*)	230	3.0	330	10.0	0	300	0
yellow:							
(*Moist Supreme* Classic), 1/12 pkg.	170	1.0	35.0	3.5	0	290	<1.0
(*SuperMoist*)	240	3.0	34.0	11.0	55	290	0
butter recipe (*SuperMoist*) ...	250	3.0	35.0	12.0	75	370	0
Cake, snack (see also specific listings), 1 pc., except as noted:							
apple puffs (*Entenmann's*), 3 oz.	290	3.0	39.0	14.0	0	260	1.0
berry, mixed, shortbread (*Awrey's* Fruit Squares), 1.5 oz. ...	170	1.0	29.0	6.0	15	150	<1.0

Food and Measure	cal.	prot. (gms)	carbo. (gms)	fat (gms)	chol. (mgs)	sod. (mgs)	fiber (gms)
Cake, snack *(cont.)*							
butter (*Awrey's* Fruit Squares), 1.5 oz.:							
date nut	180	2.0	28.0	7.0	25	170	<1.0
lemon	160	1.0	30.0	4.5	25	170	<1.0
raspberry	150	1.0	28.0	4.5	25	180	1.0
chocolate, w/crème:							
(*Devil Dogs*), 1.6 oz.	170	2.0	26.0	7.0		150	1.0
(*Ding Dongs*), 2 pcs., 2.8 oz. ..	360	2.0	41.0	19.0	10	230	1.0
(*Hostess Ho-Hos*), 1 oz.	120	1.0	18.0	6.0	10	75	0
(*Oreo Cakesters*), 2 pcs., 2 oz.	250	2.0	36.0	12.0	5	260	1.0
(*Yodels*), 2 pcs., 2.2 oz.	270	2.0	37.0	14.0	10	140	1.0
coffee cake (*Drake's*), 2 pcs., 2.3 oz.	280	3.0	40.0	12.0	15	200	1.0
cupcake:							
chocolate, w/crème (*Hostess*), 1.75 oz.	180	1.0	31.0	6.0	5	290	1.0
chocolate, w/crème (*Yankee Doodles*), 2 pcs., 2 oz.	220	2.0	33.0	9.0	0	250	1.0
golden, w/crème (*Sunny Doodles*), 2 pcs., 2 oz.	220	2.0	33.0	9.0	15.0	220	0
date nut shortbread (*Awrey's* Fruit Squares), 1.5 oz. ..	180	2.0	26.0	8.0	15	140	1.0
golden, w/crème (*Twinkies*), 1.5 oz. .	150	1.0	27.0	4.5	20	220	0
lemon shortbread (*Awrey's* Fruit Squares), 1.5 oz. ..	170	1.0	29.0	6.0	15	160	<1.0
muffins, chocolate chip, mini (*Hostess*), 2-oz. pouch	260	3.0	29.0	15.0	35	150	<1.0
pecan twirls (*Mrs. Freshley's*), 1 oz. ..	100	1.0	16.0	4.0	0	80	0
strawberry shortbread (*Awrey's* Fruit Squares), 1.5 oz. ..	130	0	19.0	6.0	15	150	0

Food and Measure	cal.	prot. (gms)	carbo. (gms)	fat (gms)	chol. (mgs)	sod. (mgs)	fiber (gms)
Calabaza (*Frieda's*), ½ cup, 3 oz.	10	1.0	2.0	0	0	0	1.0
Calamari, fresh, see "Squid"							
Calamari, frozen, raw, rings (*Principe del Mar* Natural), 1 oz. .	6	1.0	0	.1	15	3	0
Calamari dish, frozen, breaded, fried:							
(*Contessa*), 13 pcs.:							
w/sauce	160	5.0	21.0	6.0	55	370	1.0
w/out sauce	130	5.0	17.0	4.5	55	250	1.0
(*Matlaw's*):							
calamari, 2 oz.	200	7.0	25.0	10.0	70	600	2.0
sauce, ½ cup	70	1.0	6.0	5.0	0	800	2.0
rings (*Mrs. Paul's/ Van de Kamp's*), 15 pcs., 4 oz.	270	10.0	26.0	13.0	105	650	1.0
strips (*Margaritaville Captain's*), ⅓ pkg.:							
calamari, 4 oz.	240	9.0	25.0	12.0	75	710	0
sauce, 2 tbsp.	90	0	3.0	8.0	10	20	0
Calzone, frozen (*Smart Ones*), 10 oz.	290	14.0	47.0	6.0	25	620	6.0
Camouflage melon (*Frieda's*), 5 oz. . . .	50	1.0	13.0	0	0	15	1.0
Candy:							
almond, chocolate coated:							
dark (*CocoaVia*), 1-oz. pkg.	140	3.0	12.0	11.0	0	0	3.0
dark (*Dove*), 13 pcs.	210	3.0	19.0	15.0	5	10	3.0
milk (*Dove*), 13 pcs.	220	4.0	19.0	15.0	5	20	2.0
milk, candy (*M&M's*), ¼ cup, 1.5 oz. . .	230	4.0	25.0	13.0	5	20	2.0
almond, coated:							
carob (*Tree of Life* Natural), 1.4 oz. .	220	3.0	20.0	16.0	0	45	1.0
yogurt (*Tree of Life* Natural), 1.4 oz.	220	3.0	20.0	15.0	0	20	2.0
almond caramel clusters (*Pot of Gold*), 3 pcs., 1.6 oz.	240	4.0	24.0	14.0	5	70	1.0
berry flavor (*Ike & Mike* Blast), 1.4 oz.	140	0	36.0	0	0	30	0

Food and Measure	cal.	prot. (gms)	carbo. (gms)	fat (gms)	chol. (mgs)	sod. (mgs)	fiber (gms)
Candy *(cont.)*							
bridge mix (*Brach's*),							
16 pcs., 1.4 oz. . . .	190	2.0	26.0	8.0	5	40	>1.0
candy corn (*Brach's*),							
22 pcs., 1.4 oz. . . .	140	0	36.0	0	0	115	0
caramel:							
(*Brach's Milk Maid*),							
4 pcs., 1.4 oz. . .	160	2.0	27.0	4.5	0	95	0
(*Sugar Babies*),							
30 pcs., 1.6 oz. . .	180	0	41.0	1.5	0	40	0
(*Sugar Daddy*							
Large), 1.7-oz. pc.	200	1.0	43.0	2.5	0	65	0
(*Sugar Mama*),							
7 pcs., 1.4 oz. . .	160	0.0	35.0	2.5	0	45	0
rolls (*Brach's Milk*							
Maid Royals),							
5 pcs., 1.3 oz. . .	140	0	28.0	3.5	0	65	0
caramel, chocolate coated:							
(*Junior* Caramels),							
1.4 oz.	170	1.0	35.0	3.0	0	30	<1.0
(*Milk Duds*), 1.4 oz.	170	1.0	28.0	6.0	0	100	0
(*Rolo*), 1.7-oz. pkg.	230	3.0	33.0	10.0	5	85	0
cookie bar (*Twix*),							
2 bars	280	3.0	37.0	14.0	5	115	1.0
peanut, nougat,							
white chocolate							
(*Zero*), 1.8-oz. bar	230	3.0	37.0	8.0	0	115	<1.0
peanut clusters							
(*Brach's*), 2 pcs. .	180	3.0	20.0	10.0	0	90	<1.0
cashew, chocolate coated:							
(*Planters*), 1.4 oz. .	210	4.0	20.0	14.0	5	15	1.0
(*Planters* Chocolate							
Lovers), 1.5 oz. .	230	5.0	20.0	16.0	5	25	1.0
cherry, chocolate coated, 2 pcs., 1 oz.:							
dark (*Cella's*)	110	1.0	19.0	4.5	0	10	<1.0
milk (*Cella's*)	120	1.0	20.0	4.5	5	20	1.0
cherry flavor:							
(*Twizzlers* Bites),							
17 pcs., 1.4 oz. .	140	1.0	32.0	.5	0	95	0
(*Twizzlers* Nibs),							
2.25-oz. pkg. . . .	220	1.0	50.0	2.0	0	100	0

Food and Measure	cal.	prot. (gms)	carbo. (gms)	fat (gms)	chol. (mgs)	sod. (mgs)	fiber (gms)
(*Twizzlers Pull-n-Peel*), 2 pcs.	160	1.0	36.0	1.0	0	100	0
twists (*Twizzlers*), 4 pcs., 1.6 oz. ..	160	1.0	36.0	1.0	0	105	0
chocolate, dark:							
(*Brach's Stars*), 10 pcs., 1.3 oz. .	180	2.0	26.0	10.0	0	0	3.0
(*Cacao Reserve by Hershey 65%*), 4 blocks, 1.4 oz.	220	3.0	21.0	15.0	n.a.	n.a.	4.0
(*Cadbury Royal Dark*), 10 blocks, 1.4 oz.	210	2.0	24.0	13.0	<5	0	3.0
(*CocoaVia*), .8 oz. .	100	1.0	12.0	6.0	0	0	2.0
(*Dove*), 1.3-oz. bar .	190	2.0	22.0	12.0	5	0	3.0
(*Dove Promise*), 5 pcs., 1.4 oz. ...	210	2.0	24.0	13.0	5	0	3.0
(*Hershey's* Extra Dark Pure), 3 blocks, 1.3 oz.	210	3.0	20.0	13.0	<5	5	4.0
(*Hershey's Kisses Special Dark*), 9 pcs., 1.4 oz. ..	180	2.0	25.0	12.0	<5	15	3.0
(*Hershey's Special Dark*), 1.4-oz. bar	180	2.0	25.0	12.0	<5	15	3.0
(*Tropical Source*), 1.5 oz.	230	2.0	21.0	15.0	0	9	1.0
almond (*Hershey's Kisses Special Dark*), 1.4 oz.	230	3.0	22.0	14.0	<5	0	3.0
almond (*Hershey's Nuggets Special Dark*), 4 pcs.	180	3.0	20.0	13.0	<5	10	3.0
almond, toasted (*Tropical Source*), 1.5 oz.	250	3.0	21.0	17.0	0	15	1.0
candy coated (*M&M's*), 1.7 oz.	240	2.0	33.0	11.0	5	10	2.0
w/chocolate crème (*Dove* Sugar Free), 5 pcs.	190	2.0	22.0	15.0	5	0	3.0
w/crisps, rice (*Tropical Source*), 1.5 oz. .	240	3.0	25.0	14.0	0	16	1.0
crispy (*CocoaVia*), .7-oz. bar	90	2.0	11.0	5.0	0	10	2.0

Food and Measure	cal.	prot. (gms)	carbo. (gms)	fat (gms)	chol. (mgs)	sod. (mgs)	fiber (gms)
Candy, chocolate, dark *(cont.)*							
honey almond nougat (*Toblerone* Bittersweet), 1.2 oz. . .	170	1.0	20.0	9.0	5	5	2.0
w/macadamias, cranberries (*Hershey's* Extra Dark), 1.3 oz.	210	3.0	20.0	13.0	<5	0	4.0
w/mint or raspberry crème (*Dove* Sugar Free), 5 pcs.	190	2.0	22.0	15.0	5	0	3.0
mint crunch (*Tropical Source*), 1.5 oz. .	220	2.0	26.0	13.0	0	17	1.0
mint truffle (*Kisses*), 9 pcs., 1.4 oz. . .	210	2.0	25.0	14.0	<5	35	1.0
orange (*Terry's*), 1.5 oz.	240	1.0	28.0	13.0	5	5	3.0
raspberry (*Tropical Source*), 1.5 oz. .	240	2.0	24.0	15.0	0	17	1.0
truffle (*Hershey's Nuggets Special Dark*), 4 pcs., 1.4 oz. . .	220	2.0	24.0	13.0	5	40	2.0
chocolate, dark milk:							
(*Cacao Reserve by Hershey* Arriba), 4 blocks, 1.4 oz.	230	4.0	18.0	17.0	5	30	2.0
(*Cacao Reserve by Hershey* Java), 4 blocks, 1.4 oz.	220	3.0	21.0	14.0	10	35	1.0
(*Hershey's* Antioxidant), 1.25-oz. bar	180	3.0	21.0	11.0	10	30	1.0
(*Hershey's* Whole Bean), 1.25-oz. bar	180	4.0	18.0	12.0	10	40	6.0
chocolate, milk:							
(*Brach's Stars*), 10 pcs., 1.3 oz. .	200	2.0	24.0	11.0	5	45	0
(*Cadbury Dairy Milk*), 10 blocks, 1.4 oz.	220	3.0	24.0	12.0	10	45	<1.0
(*CocoaVia*), .8 oz. . .	110	1.0	13.0	6.0	5	15	0
(*Dove*), 1.3-oz. bar .	200	2.0	22.0	12.0	5	0	1.0
(*Dove Promise*), 5 pcs., 1.4 oz. . . .	220	2.0	24.0	13.0	5	25	1.0
(*Hershey's*), 1.9-oz. bar	270	4.0	33.0	16.0	15	45	1.0

Food and Measure	cal.	prot. (gms)	carbo. (gms)	fat (gms)	chol. (mgs)	sod. (mgs)	fiber (gms)
(*Hershey's Hugs*), 9 pcs., 1.4 oz. ..	210	3.0	23.0	12.0	10	45	0
(*Hershey's Kisses*), 9 pcs., 1.4 oz. ..	230	3.0	24.0	13.0	10	35	1.0
(*Hershey's Nuggets*), 4 pcs., 1.4 oz. ..	200	3.0	25.0	12.0	10	35	1.0
(*Hershey's* Sticks), .4-oz. pc.	60	<1.0	6.0	3.5	<5	10	0
(*Symphony*), 1.5 oz.	210	3.0	24.0	13.0	10	40	<1.0
almond (*Cadbury Roast Almond*), 10 blocks, 1.4 oz.	220	4.0	21.0	13.0	10	80	1.0
almond (*CocoaVia*), .8-oz. bar	110	2.0	12.0	7.0	5	15	1.0
almond (*Dove*), ⅓ of 3.67-oz. bar	190	3.0	19.0	12.0	5	20	2.0
almond (*Hershey's*), 1.4-oz. bar	210	4.0	21.0	14.0	10	25	2.0
almond (*Hershey's Kisses*) 9 pcs., 1.4 oz.	210	4.0	21.0	14.0	10	30	1.0
almond (*Hershey's Nuggets*), 4 pcs., 1.3 oz.	200	4.0	20.0	13.0	10	25	2.0
almond/toffee (*Symphony*), 1.5 oz. ..	230	4.0	23.0	14.0	10	55	1.0
candy coated (*Hershey's Kissables*), 1.4 oz.	180	1.0	28.0	9.0	5	55	<1.0
candy coated (*M&M's*), 1.7 oz.	240	2.0	34.0	10.0	5	30	1.0
caramel (*Caramello*), 6 blocks, 1.5 oz.	200	3.0	27.0	9.0	10	50	<1.0
caramel (*Hershey's* Extra Creamy), 1.25-oz. bar	180	2.0	22.0	9.0	10	40	<1.0
caramel filled (*Hershey's* Sticks), .4-oz. pc.	60	<1.0	7.0	3.0	<5	10	0
caramel filled (*Hershey's Kisses*), 9 pcs., 1.5 oz. ..	200	3.0	27.0	9.0	10	70	<1.0
caramel miniatures (*Dove*), 5 pcs. ..	200	2.0	24.0	11.0	5	45	1.0

Food and Measure	cal.	prot. (gms)	carbo. (gms)	fat (gms)	chol. (mgs)	sod. (mgs)	fiber (gms)
Candy, chocolate, milk *(cont.)*							
cherry cordial crème (*Hershey's Kisses*), 9 pcs., 1.5 oz. ..	200	2.0	29.0	8.0	5	30	0
coconut crème (*Hershey's Kisses*), 9 pcs., 1.4 oz. ..	220	2.0	23.0	15.0	5	25	1.0
crisps (*Crunch*), 1.55-oz. bar	220	2.0	29.0	12.0	5	15	1.0
crisps (*Krackel*), 1.4-oz. bar	210	2.0	28.0	10.0	<5	50	<1.0
crisps, w/caramel (*Crunch*), 1.52-oz. bar	210	2.0	28.0	12.0	5	40	<1.0
crisps, wafers (*Crunch Crisp*), 1.7-oz. bar	240	3.0	32.0	13.0	0	65	1.0
dulce de leche (*Hershey's Kisses*), 8 pcs., 1.3 oz. ..	180	3.0	24.0	8.0	10	70	<1.0
egg (*Cadbury*), 1.4 oz.	180	2.0	25.0	8.0	5	25	<1.0
egg, caramel (*Cadbury*), 1.2 oz.	170	2.0	21.0	9.0	<5	60	<1.0
egg, crème (*Cadbury*), 1.2 oz.	150	1.0	25.0	8.0	<5	20	<1.0
egg, mini (*Cadbury*), 12 pcs, 1.4 oz. ..	190	2.0	28.0	8.0	5	30	<1.0
fruit/nut (*Cadbury Fruit & Nut*), 10 blocks, 1.4 oz.	200	4.0	24.0	10.0	5	30	1.0
honey almond nougat (*Toblerone*), 1.2 oz.	170	2.0	21.0	9.0	10	15	1.0
honey almond nougat (*Toblerone*), 1.76-oz bar	260	3.0	32.0	13.0	10	25	1.0
macadamia (*Mauna Loa*), 1.4-oz. bar	190	2.0	22.0	15.0	10	10	2.0
mint (*Hershey's Kisses*), 9 pcs., 1.4 oz. ..	230	3.0	24.0	13.0	10	35	1.0
mint, candy coated (*M&M's*), 1.5 oz.	210	2.0	29.0	10.0	5	40	2.0
orange (*Terry's*), 1.5 oz.	230	3.0	27.0	12.0	10	30	1.0

Food and Measure	cal.	prot. (gms)	carbo. (gms)	fat (gms)	chol. (mgs)	sod. (mgs)	fiber (gms)
peanut butter filled (*Hershey's*), 4 blocks, 1.5 oz.	220	4.0	22.0	15.0	5	90	1.0
peanut butter filled (*Hershey's Kisses*), 9 pcs., 1.4 oz. . .	230	4.0	21.0	15.0	5	110	1.0
raisins/almonds (*Hershey's Nuggets*), 4 pcs., 1.4 oz. . .	190	3.0	23.0	11.0	10	30	1.0
toffee/almonds (*Hershey's Nuggets*), 4 pcs., 1.3 oz. . .	200	3.0	21.0	13.0	10	60	<1.0
truffle (*Hershey's Kisses*), 9 pcs., 1.5 oz. . .	210	2.0	25.0	14.0	<5	45	2.0
truffle (*Hershey's Nuggets*), 4 pcs., 1.4 oz. . .	210	3.0	23.0	12.0	5	55	<1.0
chocolate, white:							
cookies and cream (*Hershey's*), .6 oz.	90	1.0	11.0	4.5	<5	45	0
honey almond nougat (*Toblerone*), 1.2 oz.	180	2.0	20.0	10.0	5	30	0
chocolate chews (*Tootsie Roll*), 1.4 oz.	140	1.0	28.0	3.0	0	15	0
chocolate thins (*Andes*), 8 pcs., 1.3 oz.:							
cherry jubilee	200	2.0	22.0	13.0	0	20	1.0
crème de menthe . .	200	2.0	22.0	13.0	0	20	<1.0
mint parfait	210	2.0	22.0	13.0	0	20	0
toffee crunch	200	2.0	24.0	11.0	0	45	0
chocolate twists (*Twizzlers*), 4 pcs., 1.6 oz.	160	2.0	33.0	2.5	0	85	<1.0
cinnamon:							
hard (*Brach's* Disks), 3 pcs., .6 oz. . . .	70	0	17.0	0	0	10	0
hot (*Hot Tamales*), 20 pcs., 1.4 oz. .	150	0	36.0	0	0	15	0
circus peanuts (*Brach's*), 6 pcs. . . .	160	<1.0	39.0	0	0	0	0
coconut, Neapolitan (*Brach's* Sundaes), 3 pcs., 1.3 oz.	160	1.0	28.0	5.0	0	75	1.0
coconut bar, chocolate:							
(*Mounds*), 1.7 oz. .	230	2.0	29.0	13.0	0	55	3.0
(*SunSpire*), 1.75 oz.	260	2.0	27.0	15.0	0	40	0

Food and Measure	cal.	prot. (gms)	carbo. (gms)	fat (gms)	chol. (mgs)	sod. (mgs)	fiber (gms)
Candy, coconut bar, chocolate *(cont.)*							
almond (*Almond Joy*), 1.6 oz.	220	2.0	26.0	13.0	0	70	2.0
almond (*SunSpire*), 1.75 oz.	260	3.0	25.0	16.0	5	40	3.0
coffee beans, dark chocolate coated (*SunSpire* Organic), 1.18-oz. bag	170	2.0	20.0	9.0	0	0	2.0
cotton candy (*Charms Fluffy Stuff*), .6-oz. bag . .	70	0	17.0	0	0	0	0
cranberry, dark chocolate coated (*SunSpire* Organic), 1.8-oz. bag .	160	1.0	24.0	6.0	0	0	2.0
fruit flavor, assorted:							
(*Brach's* Jube Jels), 12 pcs., 1.4 oz. . .	140	0	34.0	0	0	40	0
(*Brach's Fruitos* All Natural), .9 oz. . .	80	1.0	19.0	0	0	30	0
(*Hawaiian Punch*), .8-oz. pkg.	70	1.0	16.0	0	0	25	0
(*Jolly Rancher Stix*), .6-oz. pkg.	70	0	17.0	0	0	10	0
(*Mott's* All Natural), .8-oz. pkg.	70	1.0	16.0	0	0	5	0
(*Swedish Fish*), 1.5 oz.	140	0	36.0	0	0	30	0
all varieties (*Dots*), 12 pcs., 1.5 oz. .	140	0	35.0	0	0	10	0
all varieties, except sours (*Skittles*), 2.2-oz. pkg.	250	0	56.0	3.0	0	10	0
fruit flavor, chews:							
(*Brach's*), 5 pcs., 1.3 oz.	150	0	32.0	2.5	0	50	0
(*Ike & Mike*), 23 pcs., 1.4 oz.	140	0	36.0	0	0	25	0
(*Starburst*), 2.1 oz.	240	0	48.0	5.0	0	0	0
(*Tootsie Roll*), 1.4 oz.	140	1.0	28.0	3.0	0	15	0
sour (*Starburst*), 2.1-oz. pkg.	240	0	47.0	5.0	0	0	0
sour (*Twizzlers Sourz*), 1.8 oz. . .	180	1.0	40.0	1.5	0	370	<1.0

Food and Measure	cal.	prot. (gms)	carbo. (gms)	fat (gms)	chol. (mgs)	sod. (mgs)	fiber (gms)
fruit flavor, gummy:							
(*Dots*), 1.5 oz.	140	0	35.0	0	0	10	0
(*Jolly Rancher*), 9 pcs., 1.4 oz. . .	120	2.0	28.0	0	0	35	0
(*Jujubes*), 55 pcs., 1.4 oz.	110	0	28.0	0	0	5	0
(*Orchard Fruit*), 1.4 oz.	130	2.0	29.0	0	0	15	0
fruit flavor, hard:							
(*Charms* Square), 2 pcs., .2 oz. . . .	20	0	6.0	0	0	0	0
(*Jolly Rancher*), 3 pcs., .6 oz. . . .	70	0	17.0	0	0	10	0
(*Jolly Rancher* Sugar Free*), .6 oz.	35	0	13.0	0	0	0	0
(*Life Savers*), 2 pcs.	20	0	5.0	0	0	0	0
sour balls (*Charms*), .2-oz. pc.	20	0	5.0	0	0	0	0
fruit/ginger (*Tree of Life* Bears), 1 oz. . .	90	<1.0	22.0	0	0	10	0
ginger chews (*The Ginger People*), 2 pcs., .4 oz.	40	0	10.0	0	0	0	0
gum, chewing, 1 pc., except as noted:							
(*Abra Cabubble*) . . .	45	0	10.0	0	0	0	0
(*Bubblicious*)	25	0	6.0	0	0	0	0
(*Bubblicious Burst*)	20	0	5.0	0	0	0	0
(*Big Red/Juicy Fruit/ Wrigley's Spear- mint/Doublemint/ Winterfresh*)	10	0	2.0	0	0	0	0
all varieties, except wild strawberry (*Bubble Yum*) . . .	25	0	6.0	0	0	0	0
wild strawberry (*Bubble Yum*) . . .	10	0	3.0	0	0	0	0
jelly beans:							
(*Brach's*), 14 pcs., 1.4 oz.	150	0	37.0	0	0	5	0
(*Jelly Belly*), 35 pcs., 1.4 oz.	140	0	37.0	0	0	10	0
(*Jolly Rancher*), 30 pcs., 1.4 oz. . .	120	0	30.0	0	0	60	0

Food and Measure	cal.	prot. (gms)	carbo. (gms)	fat (gms)	chol. (mgs)	sod. (mgs)	fiber (gms)
Candy, jelly beans *(cont.)*							
(*Orchard Fruit*),							
25 pcs., 1.4 oz. . .	140	0	35.0	0	0	10	0
(*Starburst* Original),							
¼ cup, 1.5 oz. . . .	160	0	39.0	0	0	15	0
sour (*Starburst*),							
¼ cup, 1.5 oz. . . .	160	0	38.0	0	0	15	0
tropical (*Starburst*),							
¼ cup, 1.5 oz. . . .	150	0	37.0	0	0	20	0
licorice:							
(*Crows*), 12 pcs.,							
1.5 oz.	140	0	35.0	0	0	10	0
(*Twizzlers*), 4 pcs.,							
1.6 oz.	150	1.0	35.0	1.0	0	210	0
(*Twizzlers* Bites),							
17 pcs., 1.4 oz. . .	130	1.0	31.0	.5	0	180	0
(*Twizzlers* Nibs),							
29 pcs., 1.4 oz. . .	140	1.0	31.0	1.0	0	180	0
candy coated (*Good & Plenty*),							
33 pcs., 1.4 oz. . .	140	<1.0	35.0	0	0	120	0
soft (*Lucky Country*),							
4 pcs., 1.4 oz. . . .	120	1.0	28.0	.5	0	40	0
wheels (*Haribo*),							
3 pcs., 1.7 oz. . . .	130	3.0	30.0	0	0	230	0
lollipop, 1 pop, except as noted:							
(*Charms* Sweet/ Sour), .6 oz.	70	0	17.0	0	0	0	0
(*Charms* Sweet/Sour Junior), .5 oz. . .	50	0	14.0	0	0	0	0
(*Charms Blow Pop*), .6 oz.	60	0	16.0	0	0	0	0
(*Charms Blow Pop* Junior), .5 oz. . .	50	0	14.0	0	0	0	0
(*Charms Blow Pop* Super), 1.3 oz. . .	130	0	35.0	0	0	0	0
(*Dum Dum Pops*), 2 pcs., .5 oz. . . .	70	0	13.0	0	0	0	0
(*Jolly Rancher* As- sorted), .6 oz. . .	60	0	16.0	0	0	15	0
(*Jolly Rancher* Filled), .6 oz. . . .	60	0	15.0	0	0	15	0

Food and Measure	cal.	prot. (gms)	carbo. (gms)	fat (gms)	chol. (mgs)	sod. (mgs)	fiber (gms)
(*Tootsie Caramel Apple Pops*), .6 oz.	60	0	15.0	0	0	15	0
(*Tootsie Pops*), .6 oz.	60	0	15.0	0	0	0	0
(*Tootsie Pops* Mini), 3 pcs., .5 oz. . . .	50	0	13.0	0	0	0	0
(*Tootsie Pops* Mini Sugar Free), 3 pcs., .5 oz.	40	0	14.0	0	0	0	0
macadamias, coated:							
butter candy glaze (*Mauna Loa*), 1 oz.	160	1.0	10.0	13	<5	65	2.0
candy (*Mauna Loa*), 1.4 oz.	210	2.0	22.0	13.0	5	20	1.0
chocolate, dark (*Mauna Loa*), 1.5 oz.	220	3.0	22.0	17.0	<5	120	3.0
chocolate, milk (*Mauna Loa*), 1.5 oz.	240	4.0	21.0	17.0	10	135	2.0
chocolate, milk (*Mauna Loa Mountains*), 4 pcs., 1.5 oz. . .	230	3.0	22.0	16.0	10	35	1.0
chocolate, milk, toffee (*Mauna Loa*), 1.4 oz.	220	3.0	20.0	16.0	10	45	1.0
chocolate trio (*Mauna Loa*), 1.3 oz.	220	3.0	18.0	15.0	<5	25	1.0
malt balls, coated:							
carob (*Tree of Life Natural*), 1.4 oz. . .	200	0	28.0	10.0	0	80	0
chocolate (*Brach's Malts*), 1.4 oz. . .	190	2.0	30.0	7.0	10	25	<1.0
chocolate (*Whoppers*), 18 pcs., 1.4 oz. .	180	1.0	31.0	7.0	0	115	0
marshmallow:							
(*Kraft Jet-Puffed*), 1.1 oz.	100	1.0	24.0	0	0	25	0
all flavors (*Kraft Fun-Mallows*), 1.1 oz.	100	1.0	24.0	0	0	20	0
chocolate (*Kraft Jet-Puffed Choco-Mallows*), 1.1 oz.	100	1.0	25.0	0	0	30	0

Food and Measure	cal.	prot. (gms)	carbo. (gms)	fat (gms)	chol. (mgs)	sod. (mgs)	fiber (gms)
Candy, marshmallow *(cont.)*							
mini (*Kraft Jet-Puffed*), 1 oz. . . .	90	1.0	23.0	0	0	30	0
strawberry (*Kraft Jet-Puffed*), 1.1 oz.	100	1.0	24.0	0	0	25	0
toasted coconut (*Kraft Jet-Puffed*), 1.6 oz.	170	1.0	31.0	4.5	0	60	0
marzipan (*Biermann*), .42-oz. pc.	50	1.0	10.0	1.0	0	5	1.0
mint:							
(*Brach's* Kentucky), 7 pcs., .6 oz. . . .	60	0	16.0	0	0	0	0
(*Brach's Ice Blue Mint Coolers*), 3 pcs., .6 oz. . . .	70	0	17.0	0	0	10	0
(*Hot Tamales Ice*), 20 pcs., 1.4 oz. . . .	140	0	36.0	0	0	20	0
(*Star Brites*), 3 pcs., .5 oz.	60	0	15.0	0	0	10	0
mint, chocolate coated:							
(*Junior* Mints), 16 pcs., 1.4 oz. . .	170	1.0	35.0	3.0	0	30	<1.0
(*SunSpire*), 1.3 oz. .	170	0	29.0	5.0	5	20	1.0
(*York* Peppermint Pattie), 1.4-oz. pc.	140	<1.0	31.0	2.5	0	10	<1.0
nonpareils:							
(*Brach's Sprinkles*), 17 pcs., 1.4 oz. .	200	2.0	29.0	9.0	15	35	<1.0
(*Brimfield's* 70% Dark), 1.4 oz.	210	2.0	25.0	12.0	0	0	3.0
(*Pearls*), 21 pcs., 1.5 oz.	200	1.0	28.0	11.0	0	0	2.0
nougat, w/chocolate:							
(*Milky Way* Classic), 2-oz. bar	260	2.0	41.0	10.0	5	95	1.0
(*Milky Way Midnight*), 1.76-oz. bar	220	2.0	36.0	8.0	5	90	1.0
(*Milky Way 2 To Go*), 1.8-oz. bar	230	2.0	36.0	9.0	5	85	1.0
(*3 Musketeers*), 2.13-oz. bar	260	2.0	46.0	8.0	5	110	1.0
(*3 Musketeers* 2 To Go), 1.7-oz. bar .	200	1.0	35.0	6.0	5	85	1.0

Food and Measure	cal.	prot. (gms)	carbo. (gms)	fat (gms)	chol. (mgs)	sod. (mgs)	fiber (gms)
chocolate (*Charleston Chew*), 1.9 oz. . .	230	2.0	43.0	6.0	0	30	1.0
mint (*3 Musketeers*), 2 pcs., 1.25 oz. .	150	1.0	26.0	5.0	0	65	1.0
strawberry (*Charleston Chew*), 1.9 oz. . .	230	2.0	43.0	6.0	0	30	0
vanilla (*Charleston Chew*), 1.9 oz. . . ·	230	2.0	44.0	6.0	0	30	0
nougat, jelly (*Brach's*), 3 pcs., 1.3 oz.	150	0	32.0	2.5	0	50	0
orange slices (*Brach's*), 3 pcs., 1.5 oz.	150	0	38.0	0	0	10	0
peanut, butter toffee:							
(*Fisher*), 1 oz.	130	3.0	17.0	6.0	0	150	1.0
(*Old Dominion*), 1 oz.	140	4.0	16.0	7.0	0	20	2.0
fudge (*Brach's*), 7 pcs., 1.5 oz. . .	190	3.0	28.0	8.0	0	75	1.0
maple (*Brach's*), 7 pcs., 1.5 oz. . .	200	3.0	30.0	8.0	0	70	1.0
peanut, chocolate coated:							
(*Brach's* Clusters), 3 pcs., 1.4 oz. . .	210	4.0	21.0	13.0	5	65	2.0
(*Brach's* Double Dippers), 1.4 oz.	210	4.0	23.0	12.0	10	65	2.0
(*Chewets Peanut Chews*), 3 pcs. . . .	170	3.0	22.0	9.0	0	55	2.0
(*Mr. Goodbar*), 1.7 oz.	260	5.0	26.0	17.0	<5	60	2.0
(*Planters*), 1.4 oz. .	220	5.0	19.0	14.0	5	15	2.0
cocoa (*Hershey's Really Nuts!*), 2.5-oz. pkg.	350	8.0	36.0	23.0	5	200	3.0
dark, candy (*M&M's*), 1.5 oz.	220	4.0	25.0	12.0	0	10	2.0
milk, candy (*M&M's*), 1.74 oz.	250	5.0	30.0	13.0	5	25	2.0
peanut, coated:							
carob (*Tree of Life Natural*), 1.4 oz. .	220	3.0	20.0	16.0	0	45	<1.0
French burnt (*Brach's*), 31 pcs., 1.4 oz.	170	3.0	29.0	6.0	0	0	1.0
yogurt (*Tree of Life Natural*), 1.4 oz. .	220	4.0	19.0	15.0	0	20	<1.0

Food and Measure	cal.	prot. (gms)	carbo. (gms)	fat (gms)	chol. (mgs)	sod. (mgs)	fiber (gms)
Candy (cont.)							
peanut bar:							
(*Munch*), 1.4 oz. . .	220	6.0	18.0	15.0	10	140	2.0
(*Planters*), 1.6 oz. .	230	7.0	22.0	14.0	0	10	2.0
caramel chocolate (*Planters* Carb Well), 1.35 oz. . . .	180	6.0	17.0	13.0	0	140	2.0
chocolate (*Chew-ets/ Peanut Chews*), 3 pcs., 1 oz.	140	3.0	17.0	6.0	0	30	<1.0
peanut butter crunch (*Planters* Carb Well), 1.35 oz.	160	6.0	16.0	12.0	0	140	2.0
peanut brittle:							
(*Cayten's* Gourmet), 3 pcs., 1.6 oz. . .	200	4.0	28.0	9.0	5	15	1.0
(*Palmer's*), .5 oz. . .	60	1.0	11.0	2.0	0	55	0
peanut butter, w/chocolate:							
(*Brach's* Clusters), 2 pcs., 1.3 oz. . .	200	4.0	17.0	13.0	5	45	1.0
(*5th Avenue*), 2 oz.	280	4.0	35.0	14.0	0	140	2.0
(*Reese's NutRageous*), 2 oz.	260	6.0	28.0	16.0	<5	75	2.0
(*Reese's Peanut Butter Cups*), 1.8 oz. . .	260	6.0	29.0	15.0	<5	180	2.0
(*Reese's Peanut Butter Cups Big Cup*), 1.4 oz.	210	4.0	22.0	12.0	<5	150	1.0
(*Reese's Pieces*), 1.5 oz.	210	5.0	26.0	10.0	0	85	1.0
(*Reese's Whipps*), 1.9 oz.	230	4.0	36.0	9.0	0	130	<1.0
coconut (*Zagnut*), 1.5 oz.	200	3.0	31.0	8.0	0	90	1.0
cookie bar (*Twix*), 2 bars	280	5.0	28.0	17.0	5	120	2.0
crispy crunchy (*Reese's*), 1.7 oz. .	230	5.0	26.0	14.0	<5	115	2.0
nougat (*Reese's Fast Break*), 2 oz.	260	5.0	35.0	13.0	<5	200	2.0
wafer bar (*Reese-Sticks*), 1.5 oz. . .	230	4.0	23.0	13.0	0	135	1.0

Food and Measure	cal.	prot. (gms)	carbo. (gms)	fat (gms)	chol. (mgs)	sod. (mgs)	fiber (gms)
white (*Reese's Peanut Butter Cups*), 1.8 oz.	260	2.0	29.0	15.0	<5	180	2.0
white (*Reese's Peanut Butter Cups Big Cup*), 1.4 oz.	200	5.0	20.0	12.0	<5	170	1.0
peanut caramel bar:							
(*Baby Ruth*), 2.1-oz.	280	4.0	39.0	14.0	0	130	1.0
(*PayDay*), 1.8 oz. ..	240	7.0	27.0	13.0	0	120	2.0
(*PayDay* Avalanche), 1.8 oz.	260	5.0	29.0	14.0	0	105	2.0
(*PayDay* Pro Trail Mix), 1.8 oz.	220	15.0	22.0	8.0	0	135	1.0
(*Snickers*) 2.1 oz. ...	280	4.0	35.0	14.0	5	140	1.0
(*Snickers* Dark), 1.8 oz.	250	4.0	30.0	13.0	5	125	2.0
(*Snickers Charged*), 1.8-oz. bar	250	4.0	31.0	13.0	5	120	1.0
(*Whatchamacallit*), 1.6-oz. bar	240	3.0	28.0	13.0	<5	150	<1.0
almond (*Snickers*), 1.76-oz. bar	240	3.0	32.0	11.0	5	80	1.0
pecan caramel clusters (*Pot of Gold*), 3 pcs., 1.6 oz.	250	3.0	24.0	16.0	5	65	1.0
pretzel, caramel, peanut, chocolate (*Take 5*), 1.5-oz. bar	210	4.0	25.0	11.0	<5	180	1.0
pretzel, coated (*Snyder's Hershey's Dips*), 1 oz.:							
dark chocolate	140	2.0	22.0	4.5	<5	130	2.0
milk chocolate	140	2.0	19.0	6.0	<5	100	<1.0
white chocolate ...	140	3.0	19.0	6.0	<5	110	0
pretzel, yogurt coated (*Tree of Life*), 1.4 oz.	190	2.0	28.0	9.0	0	75	0
raisins, coated:							
carob (*Tree of Life Natural*), 1.4 oz. ..	180	1.0	28.0	9.0	0	45	<1.0
chocolate (*Brach's California*), 35 pcs., 1.4 oz.	170	1.0	28.0	6.0	10	10	1.0
chocolate (*CocoaVia*), 1.2-oz. pkg.	150	2.0	22.0	6.0	5	15	1.0

Food and Measure	cal.	prot. (gms)	carbo. (gms)	fat (gms)	chol. (mgs)	sod. (mgs)	fiber (gms)
Candy, raisins, coated *(cont.)*							
chocolate, dark (*Sun-Spire* Organic), 1.18-oz. bag	160	1.0	23.0	7.0	0	0	2.0
chocolate, milk (*Sun•Maid*), 1.1 oz.	170	2.0	26.0	6.0	5	20	1.0
raisins, yogurt coated:							
(*Tree of Life*), 1.4 oz.	180	1.0	27.0	8.0	0	20	<1.0
chocolate (*Sun•Maid*), 1 oz.	120	1.0	22.0	4.0	0	20	1.0
vanilla (*Sun•Maid*), 1 oz.	130	1.0	21.0	5.0	0	20	1.0
root beer (*Brach's* Barrels), 3 pcs., .6 oz. .	70	0	17.0	0	0	5	0
soy nuts, chocolate coated (*GeniSoy*), 1 oz.	140	5.0	15.0	8.0	0	20	1.0
spearmint (*Brach's* Leaves), 1.4 oz. ...	130	0	34.0	0	0	15	0
spice drops (*Brach's*), 12 pcs., 1.4 oz. ...	130	0	33.0	0	0	15	0
strawberry filled, hard (*Brach's*), 2 pcs.	50	0	13.0	0	0	15	0
strawberry flavor:							
(*Twizzlers Strawz*), 1.6-oz. pkg.	150	1.0	35.0	1.0	0	150	0
twists (*Twizzlers*), 4 pcs., 1.6 oz. ..	160	1.0	36.0	1.0	0	95	0
taffy (*Brach's* Salt Water), 5 pcs.	170	0	36.0	2.5	00	35	0
toffee bar, chocolate:							
(*Heath*), 1.4 oz. ...	210	1.0	24.0	13.0	5	135	<1.0
(*Skor*), 1.4 oz.	210	1.0	24.0	12.0	15	120	<1.0
crunch (*SunSpire*), 1.75 oz.	280	3.0	24.0	19.0	40	130	0
truffles, chocolate:							
(*Truffelettes*), 4 pcs., 1.1 oz.	189	1.6	14.0	14.0	0	18	1.4
dark (*Cacao Reserve by Hershey*), 1.8 oz.	260	4.0	23.0	22.0	15	20	4.0
milk (*Cacao Reserve by Hershey*), 1.8 oz.	290	3.0	25.0	22.0	15	45	1.0
wafer, w/chocolate:							
(*KitKat*), 1.5-oz. bar	210	3.0	28.0	11.0	<5	30	<1.0

Food and Measure	cal.	prot. (gms)	carbo. (gms)	fat (gms)	chol. (mgs)	sod. (mgs)	fiber (gms)
caramel (*KitKat*), 1.4-oz. bar	200	3.0	26.0	11.0	5	35	<1.0
extra crispy (*KitKat*), 1.6-oz. bar	230	3.0	29.0	12.0	<5	35	<1.0
Cane juice, dehydrated (*Tree of Life Organic*), 1 level tsp.	15	0	3.0	0	0	10	0
Cane syrup:							
(*Mrs. Renfro's*), ¼ cup	250	0	63.0	0	0	15	0
1 tbsp.	52	0	13.4	0	0	<1	0
Cannellini beans, see "Kidney beans"							
Cannelloni entree, frozen, four cheese (*Lean Cuisine One Dish Favorites*), 9⅛-oz. pkg.	240	17.0	30.0	6.0	20	690	3.0
Cantaloupe:							
(*Dole*), ¼ medium ...	50	1.0	12.0	0	0	25	1.0
½ of 5" melon	94	2.3	22.3	.7	0	23	2.1
cubed, 1 cup	56	1.4	13.4	.5	0	14	1.3
Caper berries:							
(*Roland*), 2 tbsp.	0	0	1.0	0	0	410	0
in balsamic vinegar (*Alessi*), 2 pcs. ...	0	0	0	0	0	120	0
Capers, 1 tbsp., except as noted:							
(*Costamar*)	0	0	0	0	0	315	0
(*Crosse & Blackwell*) .	5	0	1.0	0	0	350	0
(*Roland* Capote/Nonpareille/Surfines)	0	0	0	0	0	85	0
(*Roland* Organic)	0	0	1.0	0	0	315	0
(*Vigo*), 1 tsp.	0	0	0	0	0	140	0
in salt (*Roland*)	5	0	0	0	0	70	0
in sherry wine vinegar (*Roland*)	5	0	1.0	0	0	315	0
Capicola, see "Ham lunch meat"							
Capon, see "Chicken"							
Caponata, see "Artichoke appetizer" and "Eggplant appetizer"							
Cappuccino, see "Coffee"							

Food and Measure	cal.	prot. (gms)	carbo. (gms)	fat (gms)	chol. (mgs)	sod. (mgs)	fiber (gms)
Carambola, fresh:							
(*Frieda's* Starfruit),							
5 oz.	45	1.0	11.0	0	0	0	4.0
1 medium, 4.7 oz. . . .	42	.7	9.9	.4	0	2	3.4
sliced, ½ cup	18	.3	1.0	.2	0	1	1.5
Carambola, dried							
(*Frieda's* Starfruit),							
1.4 oz.	120	2.0	29.0	0	0	5	1.0
Caramel dip, see							
"Fruit dip"							
Caramel syrup, 2 tbsp.:							
(*Hershey's Classic*							
Caramel Sundae) . .	100	0	25.0	0	0	100	0
(*Santa Cruz Organic*) .	120	0	29.0	0	0	20	0
(*Smucker's Sundae*							
Syrup)	100	1.0	25.0	0	0	110	0
Caramel topping (see							
also "Butterscotch							
topping"), 2 tbsp.:							
(*Smucker's*)	120	0	29.0	0	0	110	0
(*Smucker's* Sugar Free)	90	0	24.0	0	0	65	0
(*Smucker's Magic*							
Shell)	220	2.0	14.0	17.0	5	30	0
dulce de leche:							
(*Hershey's*)	110	<1.0	28.0	0	0	135	0
(*Smucker's*)	150	1.0	26.0	4.5	5	60	0
hot (*Smucker's*)	140	1.0	27.0	3.5	0	55	0
Caraway seed, 1 tsp. . .	7	.4	1.1	.3	0	<1	<1.0
Cardamom, ground,							
1 tsp.	6	.2	1.4	.1	0	<1	.5
Cardoon:							
raw (*Frieda's*), 3 oz. . . .	15	1.0	4.0	0	0	140	1.0
raw, shredded, ½ cup	18	.6	4.4	.1	0	151	1.4
boiled, drained, 4 oz. .	25	.9	6.0	.1	0	200	n.a.
Caribou, meat only,							
roasted, 4 oz.	189	33.8	0	5.0	123	68	0
Carissa, sliced, ½ cup	46	.4	10.2	1.0	0	2	n.a.
Carnival squash							
(*Frieda's*), 3 oz. . . .	30	1.0	7.0	0	0	0	1.0
Carob chips, baking:							
(*Sunspire*), 2 tbsp. . . .	70	1.0	10.0	3.5	0	0	1.0
malt sweetened (*Tree*							
of Life), 15 pcs. . . .	70	1.0	9.0	4.0	0	5	1.0

Food and Measure	cal.	prot. (gms)	carbo. (gms)	fat (gms)	chol. (mgs)	sod. (mgs)	fiber (gms)
unsweetened (*SunSpire*), 2 tbsp.	70	2.0	8.0	3.5	0	50	2.0
Carob drink mix, powder, 3 tsp.	45	.2	11.2	tr.	0	12	<1.0
Carob flour, ¼ cup . .	99	1.2	22.9	.2	0	9	10.2
Carob powder (*Shiloh Farms*), 1 tbsp. . . .	45	0	11.0	0	0	12	1.0
Carp, meat only:							
raw, 4 oz.	144	20.2	0	6.4	75	58	0
baked or broiled, 4 oz.	184	25.9	0	8.1	95	71	0
Carrot, fresh:							
raw:							
(*Dole*), 7" long, 1¼" diam.	35	1.0	8.0	0	0	40	2.0
(*Frieda's Gold*), 3 oz.	35	1.0	9.0	0	0	30	3.0
whole, 7½", 2.8 oz.	31	.7	7.3	.1	0	25	2.2
shredded (*Dole Fresh Favorites*), 3 oz.	40	1.0	9.0	0	0	45	2.0
shredded, ½ cup . .	24	.6	5.6	.1	0	19	1.7
raw, baby:							
(*Mann's*), 3 oz.	38	1.0	9.0	0	0	44	2.0
1 medium, 2¾" long	4	.1	.8	.1	0	3	.2
peeled mini (*Dole*), 3 oz., ¾ cup	40	1.0	9.0	–	0	45	2.0
boiled, drained, sliced, ½ cup	35	.9	8.2	.1	0	52	2.6
Carrot, can/jar, ½ cup:							
baby, whole:							
(*Roland* Can)	35	1.0	7.0	.5	0	400	3.0
(*Roland* Jar)	35	1.0	11.0	0	0	400	2.0
(*S&W*)	35	0	8.0	0	0	300	3.0
crinkle (*Freshlike*) . . .	45	1.0	11.0	0	0	180	3.0
julienne (*S&W*)	35	0	8.0	0	0	300	3.0
sliced:							
(*Allens* Tiny)	35	0	8.0	0	0	40	3.0
(*Del Monte*)	35	0	8.0	0	0	300	3.0
w/liquid	28	.8	6.2	.2	0	297	1.1
drained	17	.5	4.0	.1	0	176	1.1
honey:							
(*Glory*)	50	0	12.0	0	0	220	2.0
glazed (*Del Monte Savory Sides*) . .	70	1.0	18.0	0	0	440	1.0

Food and Measure	cal.	prot. (gms)	carbo. (gms)	fat (gms)	chol. (mgs)	sod. (mgs)	fiber (gms)
Carrot, frozen, ⅔ cup, except as noted:							
(*C&W* Parisienne) ...	35	1.0	7.0	0	0	15	3.0
baby (*C&W*)	35	1.0	7.0	0	0	60	2.0
sliced:							
(*Birds Eye*)	35	0	7.0	0	0	55	2.0
boiled, drained, ½ cup	26	.9	6.0	.1	0	43	2.6
honey glazed (*Green Giant*), 1 cup	90	1.0	15.0	3.0	0	190	3.0
Carrot chips (*Hain*), 1 oz.	150	2.0	15.0	9.0	0	170	1.0
Carrot drink blend, orange mango (*Nantucket Nectars*), 8 fl. oz.	120	0	28.0	0	0	30	0
Carrot juice, 8 fl. oz.:							
(*Bolthouse Farms*) ...	70	2.0	14.0	0	0	150	>1.0
(*Earthbound Farm Organic*)	70	2.0	14.0	0	0	150	<1.0
(*Odwalla*)	70	2.0	15.0	0	0	160	1.0
Carrot juice blend (see also "Orange juice blend"), 8 fl. oz.:							
orange (*After the Fall 24 Karrot*)	120	1.0	28.0	0	0	55	0
orange apple (*Odwalla*)	100	1.0	23.0	0	0	65	0
Carrot-celery dip (*Marzetti's*), 1.5 oz.	230	1.0	2.0	24.0	10	390	0
Casaba melon:							
⅒ of 7¾" melon	43	1.5	10.2	.2	0	20	1.3
cubed, 1 cup	44	1.5	10.5	.2	0	10	1.4
Cashew, 1 oz., except as noted:							
(*Beer Nuts*)	170	5.0	8.0	13.0	0	80	1.0
(*Fisher* Jumbo)	170	5.0	8.0	15.0	0	140	1.0
(*Frito-Lay* Whole), 3 tbsp.	180	4.0	4.0	15.0	0	120	1.0
(*Kettle*)	160	5.0	8.0	14.0	0	85	1.0
(*Planters* Salted), 2-oz. pkg.	330	10.0	16.0	28.0	0	320	3.0
(*Planters* Whole/ Jumbo/Salted)	170	5.0	8.0	14.0	0	115	1.0
(*Planters* Whole Lightly Salted)	170	5.0	8.0	14.0	0	60	1.0

Food and Measure	cal.	prot. (gms)	carbo. (gms)	fat (gms)	chol. (mgs)	sod. (mgs)	fiber (gms)
(*Really Nuts! Mauna Loa*), 1.5-oz. pkg...	250	8.0	11.0	21.0	0	130	1.0
(*SunRidge Farms* Organic), 1.1 oz.	170	5.0	10.0	13.0	0	95	<1.0
(*SunRidge Farms* Roasted Jumbo), 1.1 oz. ...	180	5.0	8.0	15.0	0	105	<1.0
raw, ¼ cup:							
pieces (*SunRidge Farms*)	170	5.0	9.0	14.0	0	105	<1.0
whole (*Shiloh Farms*)	190	5.0	11.0	15.0	0	5	1.0
dry-roasted:							
(*Planters*), .7 oz. ..	160	5.0	9.0	12.0	0	140	1.0
18 medium, 1 oz. ...	163	4.4	9.3	13.2	0	4	.9
whole or halves, 1 cup	787	21.0	44.8	63.5	0	21	4.1
halves and pieces:							
(*Planters*)	170	5.0	8.0	14.0	0	115	1.0
(*Planters* 11.1 oz.) .	170	6.0	7.0	14.0	0	120	1.0
(*Planters* Lightly Salted	170	5.0	8.0	14.0	0	55	1.0
honey-roasted, 1 pkg.:							
(*Frito-Lay*)	280	6.0	14.0	22.0	0	110	1.0
(*Planters*), 2 oz. ...	310	9.0	23.0	24.0	0	170	3.0
oil-roasted:							
18 medium, 1 oz. ...	163	4.6	8.1	13.7	0	5	1.1
whole/halves, 1 cup .	748	21.0	37.1	62.7	0	22	4.9
Cashew butter, 2 tbsp.:							
(*MaraNatha* Natural Roasted)	190	5.0	10.0	15.0	0	0	2.0
(*Tree of Life*)	180	4.0	9.0	15.0	0	0	1.0
all varieties (*Arrowhead Mills*)	160	4.0	9.0	13.0	0	0	<1.0
creamy (*Kettle Roaster Fresh*)	160	5.0	8.0	14.0	0	0	1.0
Cassava (see also "Yuca root"), raw:							
14.4-oz. root	653	5.6	155.2	1.1	0	57	7.3
1 cup	330	2.8	78.4	.6	0	29	3.7
Catfish, channel, meat only:							
farmed, 4 oz.:							
raw	153	17.7	0	8.6	15	60	0
baked or broiled ...	172	21.2	0	9.1	73	91	0

Food and Measure	cal.	prot. (gms)	carbo. (gms)	fat (gms)	chol. (mgs)	sod. (mgs)	fiber (gms)
Catfish *(cont.)*							
wild, 4 oz.:							
raw	108	18.6	0	3.2	66	49	0
baked or broiled . . .	119	20.9	0	3.2	82	57	0
Catfish entree, frozen:							
cornmeal breaded (*Mrs.*							
Paul's), 4-oz. fillet .	230	11.0	26.0	10.0	25	780	1.0
strips, fried (*Delta*							
Pride Country Crisp),							
4 oz.	240	10.0	20.0	12.0	25	450	0
Catjang, boiled, ½ cup	100	7.0	17.5	.6	0	16	3.1
Cauliflower, fresh:							
raw:							
(*Dole*), ⅙ medium							
head, 3.5 oz. . . .	25	2.0	5.0	0	0	30	2.0
florets, 3 pcs.	14	1.1	2.9	.1	0	17	1.4
1" pcs., ½ cup	13	1.0	2.6	.1	0	15	1.3
boiled, drained, 1" pcs.,							
½ cup	14	1.1	2.6	.3	0	9	1.7
green:							
raw, ⅕ head	28	2.7	5.7	.3	0	22	3.0
raw, 1" pcs., ½ cup	16	1.5	3.0	.2	0	12	1.6
boiled, drained,							
1" pcs., ½ cup . .	20	1.9	3.9	.2	0	14	2.0
Cauliflower, frozen:							
florets (*Birds Eye/C&W*),							
4 pcs., 3 oz.	25	1.0	4.0	0	0	25	1.0
boiled, drained, 1" pcs.,							
½ cup	17	1.5	3.4	.2	0	16	2.0
cheese sauce:							
(*Green Giant* Box),							
½ cup	50	2.0	6.0	2.5	0	410	1.0
3 cheese (*Green*							
Giant Bag), ½ cup							
cooked	45	2.0	6.0	2.0	5	350	1.0
garlic (*Birds Eye*							
Steamfresh), 1 cup	40	1.0	5.0	1.5	0	330	1.0
Cauliflower combination,							
frozen, w/carrots,							
snow peas (*Birds Eye*),							
1 cup	30	1.0	6.0	0	0	35	2.0
Cavatelli pasta entree,							
frozen (*Celentano*),							
1 cup	240	9.0	46.0	1.5	10	15	3.0

Food and Measure	cal.	prot. (gms)	carbo. (gms)	fat (gms)	chol. (mgs)	sod. (mgs)	fiber (gms)
Caviar (see also "Roe"), 1 tbsp.:							
lumpfish, black or red:							
(*Roland*)	15	2.0	0	.5	50	420	0
(*Romanoff*)	15	1.0	0	1.0	50	380	0
salmon (*Romanoff*) ..	35	0	0	1.5	55	310	0
whitefish, black							
(*Romanoff*)	25	1.0	1.0	1.5	45	300	0
Cayenne, see "Pepper"							
Ceci bean, see "Garbanzo bean"							
Celeriac, fresh, raw:							
(*Frieda's* Celery Root),							
¾ cup, 3 oz.	35	1.0	8.0	0	0	85	2.0
trimmed, 4 oz.	44	1.7	10.4	.3	0	113	2.0
trimmed, ½ cup	31	1.2	7.2	.2	0	78	1.4
Celery:							
raw:							
(*Del Monte*), 2 stalks,							
3.9 oz.	20	1.0	2.0	0	0	100	2.0
7½"-stalk, 1.6 oz. ..	6	.3	1.5	.1	0	35	.7
diced, 1/2 cup	10	.5	2.2	.1	0	52	1.0
boiled, drained, diced,							
½ cup	13	.6	3.0	.1	0	68	1.2
Celery, canned, hearts							
(*Roland*), ½ cup ..	15	1.0	2.0	0	0	360	1.0
Celery, Chinese							
(*Frieda's* Kahn							
Choy), 1 cup, 3 oz.	15	1.0	3.0	0	0	75	1.0
Celery, dried, flake/							
seed (*Tone's*), 1 tsp.	9	.4	.9	.5	0	4	.3
Celery root, see "Celeriac"							
Celery salt (*McCormick*),							
¼ tsp.	0	0	0	0	0	250	0
Celtus, raw, trimmed:							
1 oz.	6	.2	1.0	.1	0	3	.3
.3-oz. leaf	1	<.1	.3	0	0	1	.1
Cereal, ready-to-eat							
(see also specific grains),							
1 cup, except as noted:							
amaranth flakes:							
(*Arrowhead Mills*							
Organic)	140	4.0	26.0	2.0	0	0	3.0

Food and Measure	cal.	prot. (gms)	carbo. (gms)	fat (gms)	chol. (mgs)	sod. (mgs)	fiber (gms)
Cereal, ready-to-eat, amaranth flakes *(cont.)*							
(*Health Valley* Organic), ¾ cup ...	100	3.0	24.0	0	0	90	4.0
bran:							
(*All-Bran*), ½ cup ..	80	4.0	23.0	1.0	0	80	10.0
(*All-Bran* Extra Fiber), ½ cup	50	3.0	20.0	1.0	0	120	13.0
(*All-Bran Bran Buds*), ⅓ cup	70	2.0	24.0	1.0	0	200	13.0
(*Fiber One*), ½ cup	60	2.0	25.0	1.0	0	105	14.0
(*Post 100%*), ⅓ cup	80	4.0	22.0	1.0	0	125	9.0
flakes (*Kellogg's Complete*), ¾ cup	90	3.0	23.0	.5	0	210	5.0
flakes (*Post*), ¾ cup	100	3.0	24.0	.5	0	220	5.0
w/yogurt bites (*All Bran*), 1¼ cups .	190	6.0	44.0	3.0	0	240	10.0
bran, raisin:							
(*Cascadian Farm Organic*)	180	5.0	43.0	1.5	0	340	6.0
(*Erewhon* Organic) .	170	5.0	40.0	1.0	0	100	6.0
(*Fiber One Clusters*)	170	4.0	45.0	1.0	0	260	11.0
(*Health Valley* Organic), 1¼ cups .	190	5.0	47.0	0	0	90	6.0
(*Kellogg's Raisin Bran*)	190	5.0	45.0	1.5	0	350	7.0
(*Kellogg's Raisin Bran* Organic) ...	190	5.0	46.0	1.0	0	380	8.0
(*Kellogg's Raisin Bran Crunch*) ...	190	3.0	45.0	1.0	0	210	4.0
(*Para su Familia*), 1¼ cups	170	4.0	41.0	1.0	0	300	6.0
(*Post*)	190	4.0	46.0	1.0	0	300	8.0
(*Total*)	160	3.0	40.0	1.0	0	250	5.0
buckwheat flakes, maple (*Arrowhead Mills* Organic)	170	4.0	35.0	1.0	0	190	1.0
corn:							
(*Barbara's Puffins* Original), ¾ cup .	90	2.0	23.0	1.0	0	190	5.0
(*Chex Corn*)	120	2.0	26.0	.5	0	290	1.0
(*Cocoa Puffs*), ¾ cup	110	1.0	23.0	1.5	0	150	1.0
(*Corn Pops*)	120	1.0	28.0	0	0	120	<1.0
(*Health Valley* Crunch-Ems!*) ...	110	4.0	27.0	0	0	160	2.0

Food and Measure	cal.	prot. (gms)	carbo. (gms)	fat (gms)	chol. (mgs)	sod. (mgs)	fiber (gms)
(*Kix*), 1¼ cups	110	2.0	25.0	1.0	0	210	3.0
(*Malt-O-Meal Colossal Crunch*), ¾ cup	120	1.0	26.0	1.5	0	230	0
(*Malt-O-Meal Corn Bursts*)	120	1.0	28.0	0	0	270	0
(*Trix*)	120	1.0	28.0	1.5	0	180	1.0
berry (*Lucky Charms*)	110	1.0	26.0	1.0	0	190	1.0
cinnamon (*Barbara's Puffins*), ⅔ cup .	100	2.0	26.0	1.0	0	150	6.0
honey nut (*Chex*), ¾ cup	120	2.0	28.0	.5	0	230	1.0
peanut butter (*Barbara's Puffins*), ¾ cup	110	3.0	23.0	2.0	0	230	2.0
puffed (*Arrowhead Mills*)	60	2.0	12.0	1.0	0	5	2.0
corn flakes:							
(*Arrowhead Mills Organic*)	120	2.0	27.0	0	0	70	2.0
(*Barbara's Organic*)	110	2.0	25.0	1.0	0	140	1.0
(*Erewhon Organic*), 1¼ cups	210	5.0	45.0	2.5	0	100	3.0
(*General Mills Country*)	120	2.0	28.0	.5	0	300	1.0
(*Kellogg's Corn Flakes*)	100	2.0	24.0	0	0	200	1.0
(*Kellogg's Frosted Flakes*), ¾ cup ..	110	1.0	27.0	0	0	140	1.0
(*La Lechera*), ¾ cup	100	1.0	24.0	.5	0	170	1.0
blue (*Health Valley Organic*), ¾ cup .	100	3.0	24.0	0	0	10	3.0
frosted (*Malt-O-Meal*), ¾ cup	120	2.0	28.0	0	0	180	1.0
corn and amaranth (*Erewhon Aztec Organic*)	110	2.0	26.0	0	0	70	1.0
corn and oat, ¾ cup:							
(*Cap'n Crunch*)	110	1.0	23.0	1.5	0	200	1.0
(*Health Valley Cranberry Crunch*) ..	200	5.0	41.0	3.0	0	30	4.0
corn and rice:							
(*Caramel Nut Crunch*)	210	3.0	41.0	3.5	0	310	1.0
(*Crispix*)	110	2.0	25.0	0	0	210	<1.0

Food and Measure	cal.	prot. (gms)	carbo. (gms)	fat (gms)	chol. (mgs)	sod. (mgs)	fiber (gms)
Cereal, ready-to-eat *(cont.)*							
corn and wheat, ¾ cup:							
(*Malt-O-Meal Coco-Roos*)	120	1.0	26.0	1.5	0	135	1.0
(*Malt-O-Meal Honey Graham Squares*)	130	1.0	25.0	3.0	0	270	1.0
granola, ½ cup, except as noted:							
(*Almond Raisin Crisp Granola*) . .	220	7.0	36.0	9.0	0	50	6.0
(*Apple Raisin Walnut Granola Organic*)	230	6.0	33.0	8.0	0	0	4.0
(*Banana Crunch Granola Organic*)	190	6.0	35.0	3.0	0	10	4.0
(*Cascadian Farm Oats & Honey Organic*), ⅔ cup	230	5.0	42.0	6.0	0	120	3.0
(*Cape Cod Cranberry Granola*) . .	200	5.0	41.0	2.5	0	35	3.0
(*Goji Berry Crunch Granola*)	200	5.0	32.0	7.0	0	90	3.0
(*Granola Crisp*) . . .	230	6.0	34.0	8.0	0	55	4.0
(*Hemp and Flax Granola Organic*)	230	6.0	34.0	9.0	0	60	4.0
(*Honey Crunch Granola*)	280	8.0	37.0	13.0	0	20	4.0
(*Kashi Mountain Medley*)	220	6.0	37.0	7.0	0	110	6.0
(*Kashi Orchard Spice*)	220	6.0	37.0	7.0	0	130	6.0
(*Magical Maple Granola*)	220	6.0	34.0	8.0	0	20	3.0
(*SunRidge Farms Organic Magic Muesli*)	210	6.0	35.0	6.0	0	30	5.0
all varieties (*Health Valley* Low-Fat), ⅔ cup	180	5.0	43.0	1.0	0	90	6.0
almonds/raisins (*Breadshop SuperNatural*) . . .	220	5.0	34.0	8.0	0	0	4.0
ancient grains flakes (*Breadshop*)	200	4.0	38.0	4.0	0	180	4.0

Food and Measure	cal.	prot. (gms)	carbo. (gms)	fat (gms)	chol. (mgs)	sod. (mgs)	fiber (gms)
berry crunch, triple (*Breadshop*)	210	5.0	34.0	8.0	0	65	4.0
cinnamon raisin (*Breadshop Organic*)	220	4.0	39.0	7.0	0	65	4.0
cinnamon raisin (*Cascadian Farm Organic*), ⅔ cup	210	5.0	42.0	3.0	0	200	3.0
cranberry pecan (*Earthbound Farm Organic*)	220	4.0	36.0	8.0	0	0	5.0
honey nut (*Breadshop*)	240	6.0	33.0	10.0	0	0	4.0
maple (*Breadshop Organic Vermont*)	220	5.0	34.0	7.0	0	85	4.0
maple almond (*Earthbound Farm Organic*)	260	6.0	31.0	14.0	0	0	4.0
mocha almond crunch (*Breadshop*)	210	5.0	33.0	8.0	0	40	4.0
oat honey (*Mother's*)	210	5.0	35.0	6.0	0	20	3.0
praline/cream (*Breadshop Organic*) ..	210	5.0	32.0	8.0	0	45	4.0
w/raisins (*Kellogg's Low Fat*), ⅔ cup	230	4.0	49.0	3.0	0	150	3.0
w/out raisins (*Kellogg's Low Fat*) .	190	4.0	40.0	2.5	0	110	3.0
raspberry crunch (*SunRidge Farms Organic*)	220	6.0	38.0	6.0	0	5	4.0
spelt, apple cinnamon (*VitaSpelt Organic*)	220	5.0	33.0	8.0	0	15	3.0
spelt and kamut (*Shiloh Flaky*) ...	220	7.0	45.0	1.5	0	0	4.0
kamut, puffed (*Arrowhead Mills Puffed Kamut Organic*) ...	50	3.0	11.0	0	0	0	2.0
kamut flakes: (*Arrowhead Mills Organic*) ..	120	4.0	25.0	1.0	0	70	2.0
(*Erewhon Organic*), ⅔ cup	110	5.0	25.0	0	0	75	4.0

Food and Measure	cal.	prot. (gms)	carbo. (gms)	fat (gms)	chol. (mgs)	sod. (mgs)	fiber (gms)
Cereal, ready-to-eat, kamut flakes *(cont.)*							
w/cranberries (*Arrowhead Mills* Organic)	170	5.0	36.0	1.0	0	90	3.0
millet, puffed (*Arrowhead Mills*)	60	2.0	11.0	.5	0	0	1.0
millet rice flakes (*Nature's Path* Organic), ¾ cup	110	3.0	21.0	1.5	0	90	3.0
multigrain (see also "granola," above):							
(*Annie's Cinna Bunnies*), ¾ cup	120	2.0	28.0	.5	0	210	1.0
(*Apple Jacks*)	120	1.0	28.0	.5	0	150	1.0
(*Barbara's* Organic GrainShop), ½ cup	80	3.0	24.0	1.0	0	120	8.0
(*Barbara's* Honey Crunch'n Oats), ⅔ cup	110	2.0	25.0	1.5	0	105	3.0
(*Basic 4*)	200	4.0	43.0	3.0	0	320	3.0
(*Cascadian Farm* Organic Squares), ¾ cup	110	3.0	25.0	1.0	0	115	2.0
(*Cascadian Farm* Hearty Morning Organic), ¾ cup .	200	5.0	43.0	3.0	0	360	8.0
(*Cheerios*)	110	2.0	23.0	1.0	0	200	3.0
(*Chex* Multi-Bran), ¾ cup	160	3.0	39.0	1.5	0	310	6.0
(*Fiber One Honey Cluster*)	160	5.0	42.0	1.5	0	280	13.0
(*Froot Loops*)	120	1.0	26.0	1.0	0	140	1.0
(*Fruit-e-O's* Organic)	120	3.0	25.0	1.5	0	85	2.0
(*GoLean*)	140	130	30.0	1.0	0	85	10.0
(*GoLean Crunch!* Original)	190	9.0	36.0	3.0	0	95	8.0
(*Good Friends*)	170	5.0	43.0	2.0	0	130	12.0
(*Grape-Nuts*), ½ cup	200	6.0	48.0	1.0	0	290	7.0
(*Grape-Nuts* Organic), ½ cup . .	210	8.0	45.0	1.0	0	290	7.0
(*Grape-Nuts O's*) . .	120	2.0	28.0	0	0	140	2.0
(*Health Valley* Empower)	200	5.0	42.0	3.0	0	170	6.0

Food and Measure	cal.	prot. (gms)	carbo. (gms)	fat (gms)	chol. (mgs)	sod. (mgs)	fiber (gms)
(*Health Valley* Heart Wise)	200	11.0	37.0	3.0	0	140	5.0
(*Health Valley* Organic Golden Flax), ¾ cup	190	6.0	38.0	3.0	0	80	6.0
(*Kellogg's Müeslix*), ⅔ cup	200	5.0	40.0	3.0	0	170	4.0
(*Kellogg's Toasted Honey Crunch*), 1¼ cups	220	3.0	50.0	1.5	0	320	2.0
(*Malt-O-Meal Apple Zings*)	130	1.0	30.0	1.0	0	150	1.0
(*Malt-O-Meal Honey Buzzers*), 1⅓ cups	110	1.0	26.0	.5	0	220	1.0
(*Malt-O-Meal Honey & Oat Blenders*), ¾ cup	120	2.0	25.0	1.5	0	150	1.0
(*Nature's Path* Organic Mesa Sunrise), ¾ cup	120	3.0	24.0	1.5	0	130	3.0
(*Nature's Path* Heritage Organic), ¾ cup	110	4.0	23.0	1.0	0	135	6.0
(*New England Natural* Muesli Organic), ½ cup .	220	8.0	40.0	5.0	0	40	8.0
(*Product 19*)	100	2.0	25.0	0	0	210	1.0
(*Vive*), 1¼ cups ...	170	4.0	43.0	2.5	0	100	12.0
almond (*Honey Bunches of Oats*), ¾ cup .	130	3.0	25.0	2.5	0	150	2.0
berry, mixed (*Post LiveAction Crunch*)	190	4.0	43.0	1.5	0	250	7.0
berry, red (*Nature's Path Flax Plus Organic*), ¾ cup .	220	6.0	41.0	4.5	0	170	7.0
cinnamon or oats and honey (*Nature Valley*) ..	230	4.0	48.0	3.0	0	220	4.0
cinnamon clusters (*Honey Bunches of Oats*), ¾ cup .	120	2.0	25.0	1.5	0	150	2.0
dates/raisins/walnuts (*Post Fruit & Bran*)	200	4.0	42.0	3.0	0	260	6.0

Food and Measure	cal.	prot. (gms)	carbo. (gms)	fat (gms)	chol. (mgs)	sod. (mgs)	fiber (gms)
Cereal, ready-to-eat, multigrain (cont.)							
flakes (*Arrowhead Mills* Organic) ..	170	5.0	33.0	2.0	0	180	3.0
flakes (*Grape-Nuts*), ¾ cup	110	3.0	24.0	1.0	0	120	3.0
flakes (*Health Valley* Organic Healthy Fiber), ¾ cup ...	100	3.0	23.0	0	0	15	4.0
flakes (*Kashi*)	180	6.0	41.0	1.0	0	150	6.0
flakes (*Nature's Path* Organic), ¾ cup .	110	4.0	24.0	1.0	0	110	5.0
flakes (*Smart Start* Antioxidants) ...	190	3.0	43.0	.5	0	280	3.0
honey almond flax (*GoLean Crunch!*)	200	9.0	34.0	5.0	0	140	8.0
honey nut (*Clusters*)	210	4.0	49.0	1.0	0	290	3.0
honey-roasted (*Honey Bunches of Oats*), ¾ cup .	120	2.0	25.0	1.5	0	150	2.0
nuggets (*Kashi*), ½ cup	210	7.0	47.0	1.5	0	260	7.0
nut (*Post LiveAction Harvest Crunch*) .	210	5.0	38.0	7.0	0	300	8.0
peach (*Honey Bunches of Oats*), ¾ cup	120	2.0	26.0	2.0	0	135	2.0
peach/raisins/almond (*Post Fruit & Bran*)	190	4.0	42.0	3.0	0	260	6.0
pecans, crunchy (*Post Selects Great Grains*), ½ cup	220	5.0	38.0	6.0	0	150	4.0
puffed (*Kashi* Puffs)	70	2.0	15.0	.5	0	0	1.0
puffed, honey (*Kashi* Puffs)	120	3.0	25.0	1.0	0	6	2.0
raisins/dates/ pecans (*Post Selects Great Grains*), ½ cup ..	210	4.0	40.0	4.5	0	130	4.0
shredded (*Barbara's Spoonfuls*), ¾ cup	120	4.0	24.0	1.5	0	200	4.0
strawberry (*Honey Bunches of Oats*), ¾ cup	120	2.0	26.0	1.5	0	140	2.0

Food and Measure	cal.	prot. (gms)	carbo. (gms)	fat (gms)	chol. (mgs)	sod. (mgs)	fiber (gms)
vanilla almond crunch (*Cascadian Farm Organic*), ¾ cup .	200	4.0	41.0	3.0	0	210	3.0
oat/oats:							
(*Alpha Bits*)	120	3.0	27.0	1.0	0	125	2.0
(*Barbara's* Organic Breakfast O's) ...	120	4.0	22.0	2.0	0	125	3.0
(*Cascadian Farm Purely O's Organic*)	110	3.0	22.0	2.0	0	280	3.0
(*Cheerios*)	100	3.0	20.0	2.0	0	190	3.0
(*Life*), ¾ cup	120	3.0	25.0	1.5	0	160	2.0
(*Lucky Charms*), ¾ cup	110	2.0	22.0	1.0	0	190	1.0
(*Oatios* Original Organic)	110	5.0	22.0	2.0	0	125	3.0
almond, crunchy (*Oatmeal Crisp*) .	240	6.0	46.0	5.0	0	115	4.0
apple cinnamon (*Barbara's* Organic O's), ¾ cup	120	3.0	24.0	1.5	0	85	2.0
apple cinnamon (*Cheerios*), ¾ cup	120	2.0	25.0	1.5	0	120	1.0
apple cinnamon (*Oatios* Organic) .	120	3.0	18.0	1.0	0	60	2.0
brown sugar (*Quaker* Oatmeal Squares)	210	6.0	44.0	2.5	0	250	5.0
cinnamon (*Life*), ¾ cup	120	3.0	25.0	1.5	0	150	2.0
cinnamon (*Quaker* Oatmeal Squares)	230	6.0	48.0	2.5	0	260	5.0
cinnamon crunch (*Mother's*)	230	6.0	48.0	3.0	0	250	5.0
flakes, wild blueberry clusters (*Heart to Heart*) .	200	6.0	42.0	2.5	0	130	4.0
frosted (*Cheerios*), ¾ cup	110	2.0	23.0	1.0	0	170	2.0
w/fruit juice (Fruity *Cheerios*), ¾ cup	100	1.0	23.0	1.0	0	135	2.0
honey almond (*Oatios* Organic) .	120	3.0	17.0	1.0	0	50	2.0
honey graham (*Life*), ¾ cup	230	3.0	25.0	1.5	0	160	2.0

Food and Measure	cal.	prot. (gms)	carbo. (gms)	fat (gms)	chol. (mgs)	sod. (mgs)	fiber (gms)
Cereal, ready-to-eat, oat/oats *(cont.)*							
honey nut (*Barbara's* Organic O's), ¾ cup	120	3.0	24.0	2.0	0	80	2.0
honey nut (*Cascadian Farm* O's Organic)	120	3.0	24.0	2.0	0	250	2.0
honey nut (*Cheerios*), ¾ cup	110	3.0	22.0	1.5	0	190	2.0
honey nut (*Malt-O-Meal Scooters*)	110	2.0	24.0	1.5	0	210	2.0
honey toasted (*Heart to Heart*), ¾ cup	110	4.0	25.0	1.5	0	90	5.0
maple brown sugar (*Oatmeal Crisp*)	220	5.0	48.0	2.5	0	125	4.0
raisin (*Oatmeal Crisp*)	230	5.0	51.0	2.5	0	110	4.0
shredded (*Barbara's* Bite Size), 1¼ cups	220	6.0	46.0	2.5	0	260	5.0
shredded, vanilla almond (*Barbara's* Bite Size)	220	7.0	42.0	3.0	0	210	4.0
oat bran: (*Cracklin' Oat Bran*), ¾ cup	200	4.0	35.0	7.0	0	150	6.0
(*Health Valley Organic Oat Bran O's*), ¾ cup	100	3.0	23.0	0	0	90	3.0
almond crunch (*Health Valley*), ½ cup	200	6.0	34.0	3.0	0	90	5.0
toasted (*Mother's*), ¾ cup	120	4.0	24.0	1.5	0	200	3.0
oat bran flakes: (*Arrowhead Mills* Organic)	140	5.0	24.0	2.5	0	80	4.0
(*Kellogg's Complete*), ¾ cup	110	3.0	23.0	1.0	0	210	4.0
(*Health Valley* Organic), ¾ cup	100	3.0	24.0	0	0	90	4.0
(*Smart Start* Original), 1¼ cups	230	7.0	46.0	3.0	0	140	5.0
cinnamon raisin (*Smart Start*)	190	6.0	38.0	2.5	0	115	5.0

Food and Measure	cal.	prot. (gms)	carbo. (gms)	fat (gms)	chol. (mgs)	sod. (mgs)	fiber (gms)
maple brown sugar (*Smart Start*), 1¼ cups	230	7.0	46.0	3.0	0	140	5.0
raisins (*Health Valley* Organic), ¾ cup	110	3.0	26.0	0	0	90	4.0
oats and rice (*Arrowhead Mills* Organic Nature O's)	130	4.0	25.0	2.0	0	0	2.0
rice:							
(*Berry Krispies*) ...	120	2.0	27.0	0	0	220	0
(*Chex* Rice)	100	2.0	23.0	.5	0	240	0
(*Frosted Krispies*), ¾ cup	110	1.0	27.0	0	0	220	0
(*Health Valley* Rice Crunch-Ems!) ..	110	4.0	26.0	0	0	150	2.0
(*Rice Krispies*), 1¼ cups	120	2.0	29.0	0	0	320	0
(*Rice Krispies Treats*), ¾ cup ..	120	1.0	26.0	1.5	0	170	0
(*Special K*)	120	7.0	22.0	.5	0	220	<1.0
brown (*Barbara's* Organic Crisps) .	120	2.0	25.0	1.0	0	125	1.0
brown, crispy (*Erewhon* Organic) ..	110	2.0	25.0	0	0	180	1.0
brown, crispy, w/berries (*Erewhon*)	120	2.0	27.0	.5	0	100	1.0
brown, crispy, frosted (*New Morning* Cocoa Crisp Rice), ¾ cup	120	2.0	26.0	.5	0	100	1.0
brown, crispy/puffs (*Erewhon Rice Twice*), ¾ cup ..	120	2.0	26.0	0	0	60	0
crispy (*Malt-O-Meal*), 1¼ cups	130	2.0	29.0	0	0	300	0
flakes (*Arrowhead Mills* Organic Sweetened)	180	3.0	40.0	1.0	0	190	1.0
honey (*Barbara's* Puffins), ¾ cup .	120	2.0	25.0	1.5	0	125	2.0
puffed (*Arrowhead Mills*)	60	1.0	14.0	0	0	0	<1.0

Food and Measure	cal.	prot. (gms)	carbo. (gms)	fat (gms)	chol. (mgs)	sod. (mgs)	fiber (gms)
Cereal, ready-to-eat, rice *(cont.)*							
puffed (*Malt-O-Meal*)	60	1.0	13.0	0	0	0	0
w/strawberries (*Rice Krispies*)	110	1.0	26.0	0	0	220	0
rice and wheat:							
(*Organic Promise Strawberry Fields*)	120	2.0	28.0	0	0	200	1.0
flakes, chocolate or cinnamon pecan (*Special K*), ¾ cup	120	2.0	25.0	2.0	0	180	1.0
flakes, fruit/yogurt (*Special K*), ¾ cup	120	2.0	27.0	1.0	0	135	1.0
flakes, red berries (*Special K*)	110	3.0	25.0	0	0	220	1.0
flakes, vanilla almond (*Special K*), ¾ cup	110	2.0	25.0	1.5	0	160	1.0
vanilla almond (*Kellogg's Special K*), ¾ cup	110	2.0	25.0	1.5	0	160	1.0
spelt flakes:							
(*Arrowhead Mills Organic*)	120	4.0	24.0	1.0	0	100	3.0
(*Nature's Path Organic*), ¾ cup . . .	80	3.0	20.0	.5	0	150	3.0
and cranberries (*Arrowhead Mills Organic*)	170	5.0	35.0	1.0	0	120	4.0
wheat:							
(*Barbara's* Organic Crispy), ¾ cup . .	110	3.0	25.0	.5	0	180	3.0
(*Chex* Wheat), ¾ cup	160	5.0	38.0	1.0	0	340	5.0
(*Golden Grahams*), ¾ cup	120	2.0	26.0	1.0	0	270	1.0
(*Malt-O-Meal Blueberry Muffin Tops*), ¾ cup . . .	130	1.0	24.0	3.5	0	140	1.0
(*Malt-O-Meal Cinnamon Toasters*), ¾ cup	130	1.0	24.0	3.5	0	140	1.0
(*Malt-O-Meal Golden Puffs*), ¾ cup . . .	110	2.0	24.0	0	0	65	0
(*Total*), ¾ cup	100	2.0	23.0	.5	0	190	3.0
(*Total Honey Clusters*), ¾ cup	170	3.0	38.0	1.5	0	250	3.0

Food and Measure	cal.	prot. (gms)	carbo. (gms)	fat (gms)	chol. (mgs)	sod. (mgs)	fiber (gms)
(*Weetabix* Organic), 2 pcs.	120	4.0	28.0	1.0	0	130	4.0
(*Weetabix* Organic Crispy Flakes), ¾ cup	110	3.0	24.0	.5	0	180	4.0
(*Weetabix* Organic Crispy Flakes & Fiber), 1¼ cups .	170	6.0	44.0	1.5	0	320	6.0
(*Wheaties*), ¾ cup .	100	3.0	22.0	.5	0	190	3.0
cranberry crunch (*Total*), 1¼ cups	190	4.0	44.0	1.5	0	280	4.0
whole (*Cascadian Farm Great Measure* Organic) . . .	190	9.0	43.0	2.0	0	150	9.0
whole, caramel (*Fiber One* Delight)	180	3.0	41.0	3.0	0	260	9.0
whole, cinnamon toast (*Eggo*)	100	2.0	26.0	3.0	0	130	2.0
whole, maple syrup (*Eggo*)	120	2.0	27.0	1.5	0	160	2.0
wheat, puffed:							
(*Arrowhead Mills*) .	60	3.0	12.0	0	0	0	2.0
(*Barbara's Organic Wild Puffs*)	100	2.0	23.0	.5	0	40	<1.0
(*Malt-O-Meal*)	60	2.0	11.0	0	0	0	1.0
wheat, shredded:							
(*Arrowhead Mills* Organic)	190	6.0	38.0	1.0	0	5	6.0
(*Barbara's*), 2 pcs. .	140	4.0	31.0	0	0	0	5.0
(*Kellogg's Mini-Wheats*), approx. 30 pcs., 2.1 oz.	200	6.0	46.0	1.5	0	10	6.0
(*Malt-O-Meal Frosted Mini Spooners*)	190	5.0	45.0	1.0	0	10	6.0
(*Organic Promise Autumn Wheat*) .	190	5.0	45.0	1.0	0	0	6.0
(*Post Shredded Wheat* Original), ⅙ of 10-oz. pkg.	160	5.0	37.0	1.0	0	0	6.0
(*Post Shredded Wheat 'N Bran Spoon Size*), 1¼ cups	200	6.0	49.0	1.0	0	0	8.0

Food and Measure	cal.	prot. (gms)	carbo. (gms)	fat (gms)	chol. (mgs)	sod. (mgs)	fiber (gms)
Cereal, ready-to-eat, wheat, shredded *(cont.)*							
(*Post Shredded Wheat Spoon Size*)	170	6.0	40.0	1.0	0	0	6.0
cinnamon brown sugar (*Post Shredded Wheat Spoon Size*)	210	4.0	47.0	1.5	0	65	6.0
frosted (*Kellogg's Mini-Wheats*), 24 pcs., 1.9 oz. .	190	4.0	44.0	1.0	0	0	5.0
frosted (*Kellogg's Mini-Wheats* Big Bite), 5 pcs., 1.8 oz. .	180	5.0	41.0	1.0	0	5	5.0
frosted (*Post Shredded Wheat Spoon Size*)	180	4.0	43.0	1.0	0	0	5.0
frosted, cinnamon streusel (*Kellogg's Mini-Wheats*), 24 pcs., 1.8 oz. .	180	4.0	44.0	1.0	0	0	5.0
frosted, maple brown sugar (*Kellogg's Mini-Wheats*), 24 pcs., 1.8 oz. .	190	4.0	44.0	1.0	0	0	5.0
frosted, strawberry or vanilla crème (*Kellogg's Mini-Wheats*), 24 pcs., 1.8 oz. .	180	4.0	43.0	1.0	0	0	5.0
honey nut (*Post Shredded Wheat Spoon Size*)	190	4.0	44.0	1.5	0	70	5.0
maple brown sugar (*Malt-O-Meal Mini Spooners*)	190	5.0	46.0	1.0	0	10	6.0
strawberry or vanilla cream (*Malt-O-Meal Mini Spooners*) .	190	5.0	45.0	1.0	0	10	6.0
wheat and rice, ¾ cup: (*Cinnamon Toast Crunch*)	130	1.0	25.0	3.0	0	220	1.0
(*Cinnamon Toast Crunch* Reduced Sugar)	110	2.0	23.0	2.5	0	170	3.0
and soy, flakes (*Kellogg's Special K* Low Carb)	100	10.0	14.0	3.0	0	110	5.0

Food and Measure	cal.	prot. (gms)	carbo. (gms)	fat (gms)	chol. (mgs)	sod. (mgs)	fiber (gms)
Cereal, cooking/hot							
(see also specific grains), uncooked, ¼ cup, except as noted:							
barley (*Erewhon Barley Plus* Organic)	170	5.0	37.0	1.0	0	0	4.0
bulgur:							
(*Arrowhead Mills* Organic)	150	5.0	34.0	.5	0	0	4.0
w/soy (*Hodgson Mill*)	115	10.0	22.0	1.0	0	0	3.0
farina, see "wheat," below							
grits, see "Corn grits"							
multigrain:							
(*Country Choice* Organic), ½ cup .	130	5.0	29.0	1.0	0	0	5.0
(*Kashi* Pilaf), ½ cup*	170	6.0	30.0	3.0	0	15	6.0
(*Red River* Original)	154	5.5	27.0	2.5	0	4	5.7
(*Red River* Ready to Serve), 1 pkt. . . .	136	4.9	24.0	2.2	0	0	5.3
4 (*Arrowhead Mills* Organic Plus Flax)	140	5.0	28.0	1.5	0	0	9.0
7 (*Arrowhead Mills* Organic), ⅓ cup .	140	8.0	28.0	1.0	0	0	6.0
7 (*Arrowhead Mills* Organic Wheat Free)	150	5.0	30.0	2.5	0	0	3.0
apple cinnamon (*Quaker Simple Harvest*), 1 pkt. .	150	4.0	32.0	1.5	0	90	4.0
w/flax, soy (*Hodgson Mill*), ⅓ cup	160	7.0	25.0	3.0	0	0	6.0
honey cinnamon (*GoLean*), 1 pkt. .	150	8.0	26.0	2.0	0	100	5.0
maple brown sugar (*Red River* Ready to Serve), 1 pkt. .	153	4.6	29.0	1.8	0	0	4.5
maple brown sugar pecan (*Quaker Simple Harvest*), 1 pkt. .	160	4.0	30.0	3.5	0	75	4.0
vanilla, almond, honey (*Quaker Simple Harvest*), 1 pkt. .	160	4.0	31.0	3.0	0	75	4.0

Food and Measure	cal.	prot. (gms)	carbo. (gms)	fat (gms)	chol. (mgs)	sod. (mgs)	fiber (gms)
Cereal, cooking/hot *(cont.)*							
oat/oats:							
(*Country Choice* Organic Old Fashioned/ Quick), ½ cup ..	150	5.0	27.0	3.0	0	0	4.0
(*Quaker* Old Fashioned/ Quick), ½ cup ..	150	5.0	27.0	3.0	0	0	4.0
flakes (*Arrowhead Mills* Organic), ⅓ cup	130	5.0	23.0	2.0	0	0	4.0
rolled (*Mother's*), ½ cup	150	5.0	27.0	3.0	0	0	4.0
rolled, creamy vanilla (*GoLean*), 1 pkt.	150	9.0	25.0	2.0	0	100	7.0
steel cut (*Arrowhead Mills* Organic) ..	160	6.0	27.0	3.0	0	0	8.0
steel cut (*Country Choice* Organic) .	150	5.0	27.0	3.0	0	0	4.0
steel cut (*Hodgson Mill*)	150	5.0	27.0	2.5	0	0	4.0
steel cut (*Quaker*) .	150	5.0	27.0	2.5	0	0	4.0
oat bran:							
(*Arrowhead Mills* Organic), ⅓ cup .	130	6.0	21.0	2.5	0	0	4.0
(*Hodgson Mill*) ...	120	6.0	23.0	3.0	0	3	6.0
(*Mother's*), ½ cup .	150	7.0	25.0	3.0	0	0	6.0
oatmeal:							
(*Arrowhead Mills* Organic Old Fashioned), ⅓ cup ..	130	5.0	23.0	2.0	0	0	4.0
w/flax (*Arrowhead Mills* Organic), 1 pkt. ..	140	5.0	24.0	3.0	0	70	4.0
maple apple spice (*Arrowhead Mills* Organic), 1 pkt. ..	140	4.0	26.0	2.0	0	45	3.0
oatmeal, instant, 1 pkt.:							
(*Arrowhead Mills* Organic Original)	110	4.0	19.0	2.0	0	0	2.0
(*Country Choice* Organic Original)	110	4.0	19.0	2.0	0	0	3.0
(*Mother's*), ½ cup .	150	5.0	27.0	3.0	0	0	4.0
(*Nature's Path* Organic Original)	210	7.0	37.0	3.5	0	160	63.0

Food and Measure	cal.	prot. (gms)	carbo. (gms)	fat (gms)	chol. (mgs)	sod. (mgs)	fiber (gms)
(*Nature's Path Hemp Plus* Organic) ...	160	5.0	30.0	2.5	0	105	4.0
(*Quaker*)	100	4.0	19.0	2.0	0	80	3.0
(*Quaker* Organic) ..	100	4.0	19.0	2.0	0	0	3.0
w/added oat bran (*Erewhon* Organic)	130	6.0	25.0	2.5	0	0	4.0
apple, baked (*Quaker Oatmeal Express*)	200	4.0	42.0	2.5	0	320	4.0
apple cinnamon (*Erewhon* Organic)	130	5.0	24.0	2.0	0	100	3.0
apple cinnamon (*Heart to Heart*) .	160	4.0	33.0	2.0	0	110	5.0
apple cinnamon (*Nature's Path* Organic)	210	5.0	40.0	2.5	0	100	4.0
apple cinnamon (*Quaker*)	130	3.0	27.0	1.5	0	170	3.0
apple cinnamon (*Quaker* Crunch)	190	4.0	39.0	2.5	0	170	4.0
brown sugar (*Quaker Oatmeal Express*)	200	5.0	42.0	2.5	0	290	3.0
cinnamon, raisin (*Erewhon* Organic)	130	4.0	24.0	2.5	0	100	4.0
cinnamon pecan (*Quaker*)	180	4.0	33.0	4.0	0	290	3.0
cinnamon roll (*Quaker*)	160	4.0	33.0	2.0	0	240	3.0
cinnamon roll (*Quaker Oatmeal Express*)	200	5.0	41.0	2.5	0	250	4.0
cinnamon spice (*Quaker*)	170	4.0	35.0	2.0	0	250	3.0
w/flax (*Nature's Path FlaxPlus* Organic)	210	6.0	38.0	3.0	0	140	5.0
w/flax (*Uncle Sam*)	130	5.0	24.0	3.0	0	20	5.0
honey nut (*Quaker*)	170	4.0	31.0	3.5	0	240	3.0
maple (*Country Choice* Organic) .	170	4.0	32.0	2.0	0	60	3.0
maple, golden brown (*Heart to Heart*) .	160	4.0	33.0	2.0	0	100	5.0
maple brown sugar (*Quaker*)	160	4.0	33.0	2.0	0	270	3.0

Food and Measure	cal.	prot. (gms)	carbo. (gms)	fat (gms)	chol. (mgs)	sod. (mgs)	fiber (gms)
Cereal, cooking/hot, oatmeal, instant *(cont.)*							
maple brown sugar (*Quaker* Crunch)	190	4.0	39.0	2.5	0	220	3.0
maple brown sugar (*Quaker* Organic)	150	4.0	31.0	2.0	0	95	3.0
maple spice (*Erewhon* Organic) ..	130	5.0	25.0	2.0	0	100	3.0
raisin, date, walnuts (*Quaker*)	140	3.0	27.0	2.5	0	240	3.0
raisin spice (*Heart to Heart*)	150	3.0	33.0	2.0	0	100	4.0
raisin spice (*Quaker*)	150	3.0	33.0	2.0	0	240	3.0
rice, brown:							
(*Arrowhead Mills* Organic)	150	3.0	32.0	1.0	0	0	2.0
(*Lundberg* Purely Organic)	150	3.0	32.0	1.5	0	0	3.0
almond, sweet (*Lundberg*), ⅓ cup	200	3.0	40.0	3.5	0	0	4.0
cream (*Erewhon* Organic)	170	5.0	36.0	1.0	0	30	1.0
rye (*Roman Meal Cream of Rye*), ⅓ cup	130	6.0	27.0	1.0	0	0	6.0
wheat:							
(*Arrowhead Mills* Bear Mush)	150	5.0	32.0	1.0	0	0	2.0
(*Cream of Wheat* 2½ Minute), 3 tbsp.	120	4.0	23.0	0	0	85	1.0
(*Cream of Wheat* Instant), 1 pkt. ...	100	3.0	19.0	0	0	160	1.0
(*Farina* Original), 3 tbsp.	120	3.0	22.0	0	0	0	<1.0
(*Malt-O-Meal* Original), 3 tbsp.	130	5.0	27.0	.5	0	0	1.0
chocolate or creamy hot (*Malt-O-Meal*), 3 tbsp.	130	4.0	27.0	0	0	0	1.0
cracked (*Hodgson Mill*)	110	5.0	25.0	1.0	0	0	5.0
maple brown sugar (*Malt-O-Meal*) ..	170	4.0	37.0	.0	0	0	1.0

Food and Measure	cal.	prot. (gms)	carbo. (gms)	fat (gms)	chol. (mgs)	sod. (mgs)	fiber (gms)
Cereal, frozen (*Amy's* Organic), 9-oz. pkg.:							
cream of rice	170	2.0	39.0	1.0	0	220	2.0
rolled oats	220	6.0	42.0	3.5	0	220	5.0
steel cut oats	220	6.0	42.0	3.5	0	190	4.0
Cereal bar, see "Granola/cereal bar"							
Cervelat, see "Summer sausage"							
Chayote:							
raw:							
1 medium, 7.2 oz. .	49	1.8	11.0	.6	0	8	6.1
1" pcs., ½ cup	16	.6	3.6	.2	0	3	2.0
boiled, drained:							
(*Dole*), ½ cup	17	1.0	4.0	0	0	3	2.0
1" pcs., ½ cup	19	.5	4.1	.4	0	1	2.3
Cheddarwurst:							
(*Black Bear*), 3.2-oz. link	270	12.0	4.0	23.0	40	750	0
(*Dietz & Watson*), 2 oz.	270	14.0	1.0	23.0	65	800	0
Cheese (see also "Cheese food" and "Cheese spread"), 1 oz., except as noted:							
American, white or yellow, except as noted:							
(*Alpine Lace*)	90	7.0	1.0	7.0	20	300	0
(*Boar's Head*)	100	6.0	1.0	9.0	25	380	0
(*Boar's Head* Lower Sodium/Fat)	90	6.0	1.0	6.0	20	300	0
(*Kraft* Singles Organic), ⅔ oz. ...	60	4.0	1.0	4.0	10	230	0
(*Kraft* Singles Select), ⅔ oz.	70	4.0	1.0	6.0	20	310	0
(*Kraft Deli Deluxe* 8 oz.)	100	5.0	1.0	9.0	30	460	0
(*Land O Lakes*) ...	110	5.0	2.0	9.0	25	480	0
(*Land O Lakes* Light)	70	7.0	1.0	4.5	15	390	0
(*Land O Lakes* Singles), ¾ oz. ...	70	4.0	2.0	5.0	15	300	0
(*Sargento Burger-Cheese*), ⅔ oz. .	70	4.0	<1.0	6.0	20	240	0

Food and Measure	cal.	prot. (gms)	carbo. (gms)	fat (gms)	chol. (mgs)	sod. (mgs)	fiber (gms)
Cheese, American *(cont.)*							
sharp (*Land O Lakes*)	110	6.0	1.0	9.0	25	400	0
white (*Di Lusso*) ..	100	5.0	2.0	9.0	25	480	0
white (*Kraft* Singles),							
⅔ oz.	60	4.0	1.0	4.5	15	250	0
yellow (*Di Lusso*) ..	110	6.0	1.0	9.0	20	360	0
yellow (*Kraft* Singles),							
⅔ oz.	60	3.0	1.0	4.5	15	250	0
asiago (*BelGioioso*) ..	100	7.0	0	8.0	25	340	0
(*Auribella*)	110	7.0	0	9.0	30	265	0
blue/bleu:							
(*Athenos*)	100	6.0	<1.0	8.0	30	390	0
(*Boar's Head*)	90	6.0	0	8.0	30	280	0
blue, crumbled:							
(*Athenos*), 3 tbsp. ..	110	7.0	2.0	9.0	30	430	<1.0
(*Litehouse* Idaho),							
¼ cup, 1.1 oz. ..	100	5.0	2.0	8.0	35	400	0
(*Organic Valley*) ...	100	6.0	1.0	8.0	25	380	0
(*Sargento*), ¼ cup .	100.	6.0	1.0	8.0	25	380	0
brick (*Land O Lakes*) .	110	7.0	1.0	8.0	25	170	0
Brie	95	5.9	.1	7.9	20	229	0
butterKäse (*Boar's Head*)	100	6.0	0	9.0	30	180	0
Camembert	85	5.6	.1	6.9	20	239	0
caraway	107	7.1	.9	8.3	2.6	196	0
Chedarella (*Land O Lakes*)	110	7.0	0	9.0	25	190	0
cheddar:							
(*Alpine Lace*)	90	7.0	0	7.0	20	180	0
(*Boar's Head*)	110	7.0	0	10.0	30	180	0
(*Cabot* Classic Vermont/Old School/ Vintage/Private Stock/Wheel) ...	110	7.0	<1.0	9.0	30	180	0
(*Cabot* Light 50% Reduced Fat) ...	70	8.0	<1.0	4.5	15	170	0
(*Kraft* Organic)	120	7.0	0	10.0	30	190	0
(*Sargento* Slices) ..	80	5.0	0	6.0	20	140	0
all styles (*Di Lusso*)	110	7.0	1.0	9.0	30	180	0
all styles (*Land O Lakes*)	110	7.0	0	9.0	30	190	0
medium (*Kraft*) ...	120	6.0	0	10.0	30	180	0
medium (*Kraft* 8 oz.)	110	7.0	1.0	9.0	30	180	0
mild (*Cabot*)	110	7.0	<1.0	9.0	30	180	0

Food and Measure	cal.	prot. (gms)	carbo. (gms)	fat (gms)	chol. (mgs)	sod. (mgs)	fiber (gms)
mild (*Cracker Barrel Cracker Cuts*) ...	120	6.0	0	10.0	30	180	0
mild (*Kraft* Longhorn)	110	7.0	0	9.0	30	180	0
mild (*Kraft Deli Deluxe* Slices), .8 oz.	90	5.0	0	8.0	25	160	0
mild (*Organic Valley*)	110	7.0	0	9.0	30	170	0
mild (*Sargento* Cube), 7 pcs., 1.1 oz. ..	120	7.0	<1.0	10.0	30	190	0
mild or sharp (*Kraft*)	120	6.0	0	10.0	30	180	0
mild or extra sharp (*Kraft* Sticks) ...	120	6.0	0	10.0	30	180	0
raw, mild or sharp (*Organic Valley*) .	110	7.0	0	9.0	30	170	0
sharp (*Boar's Head*)	110	7.0	<1.0	9.0	30	190	0
sharp (*Cabot* Extra/ Seriously)	110	7.0	<1.0	9.0	30	180	0
sharp (*Cracker Barrel Cracker Cuts*) ...	120	6.0	0	10.0	30	190	0
sharp (*Cracker Barrel/ Kraft* Sticks Reduced Fat)	90	7.0	1.0	6.0	20	240	0
sharp (*Kraft Deli Deluxe* Slices) ..	110	6.0	1.0	9.0	30	440	0
sharp, extra (*Adams Reserve*)	110	7.0	1.0	9.0	30	180	0
sharp, extra (*Cracker Barrel/Kraft*)	120	6.0	0	10.0	30	180	0
sharp, extra (*Cracker Barrel* Reduced Fat) ...	90	7.0	1.0	6.0	20	240	0
sharp, white (*Cracker Barrel* Vermont/ Cracker Cuts*) ...	110	7.0	0	9.0	30	180	0
stick (*Organic Valley* Stringles)	110	7.0	0	9.0	30	170	0
stick (*Sargento*) ...	110	7.0	1.0	9.0	30	180	0
cheddar, flavored:							
all varieties (*Dietz & Watson*)	110	6.0	<1.0	9.0	28	270	0
bacon (*Kraft*)	90	5.0	2.0	7.0	20	480	0
chipotle (*Sargento*), ¾-oz. slice	80	5.0	1.0	6.0	10	150	0

Food and Measure	cal.	prot. (gms)	carbo. (gms)	fat (gms)	chol. (mgs)	sod. (mgs)	fiber (gms)
Cheese, cheddar, flavored *(cont.)*							
chipotle, habanero, or sun-dried tomato basil *(Cabot)*	110	7.0	<1.0	9.0	30	180	0
garlic, roasted *(Kraft)*	80	5.0	1.0	2.0	25	380	0
horseradish *(Boar's Head)*	110	6.0	2.0	9.0	30	190	0
horseradish *(Cabot)*	110	6.0	1.0	9.0	30	270	0
jalapeño *(Cabot Reduced Fat)*	70	8.0	<1.0	4.5	15	170	0
cheddar, shredded, ¼ cup or 1 oz.:							
(Cabot)	110	7.0	<1.0	9.0	30	180	0
(Kraft Fat Free)	45	9.0	1.0	0	5	280	0
(Kraft Organic)	120	6.0	1.0	10.0	30	180	0
(Organic Valley)	110	7.0	1.0	9.0	30	180	0
double *(Sargento Artisan Blends)*	110	7.0	1.0	9.0	30	190	0
mild *(Kraft)*	100	6.0	1.0	8.0	30	170	0
mild *(Sargento Reduced Fat)*	80	7.0	<1.0	6.0	20	180	0
mild or sharp *(Sargento Chef-Style/Classic)*	110	7.0	1.0	9.0	30	190	0
mild or sharp *(Kraft 2% Fat)*	80	7.0	1.0	6.0	20	230	0
mild or sharp, fine *(Kraft)*	110	6.0	1.0	9.0	25	180	0
sharp, extra *(Cracker Barrel)*	80	7.0	1.0	6.0	20	240	0
cheddar, smoked *(Dietz & Watson)*	110	6.0	<1.0	9.0	28	270	0
cheddar blend, shredded ¼ cup:							
w/bacon *(Sargento Bistro)*	110	7.0	2.0	9.0	25	190	0
chipotle *(Sargento Bistro)*	100	6.0	1.0	8.0	15	190	0
Jack *(Kraft Mexican)*	110	6.0	1.0	9.0	25	190	0
Jack *(Sargento)*	110	7.0	1.0	9.0	30	180	0
Jack, w/jalapeño *(Kraft Mexican)*	110	6.0	1.0	9.0	25	190	0

Food and Measure	cal.	prot. (gms)	carbo. (gms)	fat (gms)	chol. (mgs)	sod. (mgs)	fiber (gms)
Monterey Jack							
(*Kraft*)	100	6.0	1.0	8.0	25	170	0
mozzarella (*Cabot*							
Fancy)	100	7.0	1.0	7.0	20	180	0
cheddar Monterey Jack:							
cubes (*Kraft*)	120	7.0	1.0	10.0	30	200	0
cubes (*Kraft* 2%							
Milk)	90	8.0	1.0	6.0	20	270	0
marbled (*Kraft*) ...	110	7.0	1.0	9.0	30	200	0
Cheshire	110	6.6	1.4	8.7	29	198	0
Colby:							
(*Boar's Head*)	110	7.0	<1.0	9.0	30	170	0
(*Cracker Barrel*							
Slices), ¾ oz. ...	80	5.0	0	7.0	20	135	0
(*Kraft*)	110	6.0	1.0	9.0	30	180	0
(*Kraft* 2% Milk) ...	80	7.0	0	6.0	20	220	0
(*Land O Lakes*) ...	110	7.0	1.0	9.0	25	190	0
(*Organic Valley*) ...	110	7.0	<1.0	9.0	25	170	0
(*Sargento*), ¾ oz. ...	80	5.0	<1.0	7.0	20	140	0
Colby Jack:							
(*Boar's Head*)	110	6.0	0	9.0	25	180	0
(*Di Lusso*)	110	6.0	1.0	9.0	30	200	0
(*Land O Lakes Co-*							
Jack)	110	7.0	0	9.0	25	190	0
(*Sargento*), ⅔ oz. .	70	4.0	0	6.0	15	125	0
marbled (*Cracker*							
Barrel Cracker							
Cuts/Kraft)	110	7.0	1.0	9.0	30	180	0
stick (*Organic Valley*							
Stringles)	110	7.0	0	9.0	30	200	0
stick (*Sargento*) ...	110	6.0	<1.0	9.0	25	190	0
Colby Jack, shredded,							
¼ cup or 1 oz.:							
(*Kraft*)	100	6.0	1.0	8.0	25	190	0
(*Kraft* 2% Milk) ...	80	7.0	1.0	5.0	15	230	0
(*Sargento* Classic) .	110	6.0	1.0	9.0	30	190	0
fine (*Kraft*)	100	6.0	1.0	8.0	25	190	0
cottage, 4%, ½ cup:							
(*Breakstone's*)	120	12.0	6.0	5.0	25	430	0
(*Friendship*)	110	15.0	3.0	5.0	20	380	0
(*Land O Lakes*) ...	110	11.0	5.0	4.5	20	410	0
(*Organic Valley*) ...	110	14.0	5.0	5.0	15	450	0
cottage, 2%, ½ cup:							
(*Breakstone's*)	90	12.0	6.0	2.5	15	400	0

Food and Measure	cal.	prot. (gms)	carbo. (gms)	fat (gms)	chol. (mgs)	sod. (mgs)	fiber (gms)
Cheese, cottage, 2% *(cont.)*							
(*Knudsen* Low Fat) .	100	13.0	6.0	2.5	15	440	0
(*Land O Lakes*) ...	100	13.0	5.0	2.5	15	480	0
(*Organic Valley*) ...	100	15.0	4.0	2.0	10	450	0
pot (*Friendship*) ...	90	15.0	3.0	2.5	10	400	0
cottage, 1%, ½ cup:							
(*Land O Lakes*) ...	90	13.0	5.0	1.5	10	460	0
(*Light n' Lively*) ...	80	12.0	6.0	1.5	10	420	0
cottage, low fat, 4 oz.:							
(*Breakstone's Live-Action*)	90	10.0	8.0	2.0	15	380	3.0
mixed berry (*Breakstone's Live-Action*)	110	8.0	18.0	1.5	10	310	3.0
mixed berry (*Knudsen LiveActon*) ..	120	8.0	18.0	1.5	10	310	3.0
pineapple (*Breakstone's/Knudsen LiveAction*)	110	8.0	17.0	1.5	10	310	3.0
cottage, low fat, w/topping, 5.5-oz. cont.:							
apple cinnamon (*Breakstone's Cottage Doubles*) ...	140	11.0	18.0	2.5	15	390	0
apple cinnamon (*Knudsen Cottage Doubles*)	140	11.0	18.0	2.0	15	400	0
blueberry (*Breakstone's/Knudsen Cottage Doubles*)	140	11.0	18.0	2.5	15	400	1.0
peach (*Knudsen Cottage Doubles*) ...	140	11.0	17.0	2.5	15	390	1.0
peach or pineapple (*Breakstone's Cottage Doubles*) ...	130	11.0	16.0	2.0	15	400	0
pineapple (*Knudsen Cottage Doubles*)	130	11.0	17.0	2.5	15	390	0
raspberry (*Breakstone's Cottage Doubles*)	140	11.0	17.0	2.5	15	400	1.0
raspberry (*Knudsen Cottage Doubles*)	150	11.0	20.0	2.5	15	400	1.0
strawberry (*Breakstone's Cottage Doubles*)	130	11.0	17.0	2.0	15	400	0

Food and Measure	cal.	prot. (gms)	carbo. (gms)	fat (gms)	chol. (mgs)	sod. (mgs)	fiber (gms)
strawberry (*Knudsen Cottage Doubles*)	140	11.0	19.0	2.5	15	400	0
cottage, nonfat, ½ cup:							
(*Breakstone's*)	80	12.0	8.0	0	10	450	0
(*Cabot*)	70	13.0	5.0	0	5	410	0
(*Knudsen*)	80	13.0	7.0	0	5	430	0
(*Land O Lakes*) ...	80	14.0	6.0	0	5	380	0
(*Light n' Lively*) ...	80	12.0	8.0	0	10	460	0
peach (*Friendship*) .	110	12.0	15.0	0	<5	300	0
pineapple (*Hood*) ..	100	10.0	16.0	0	5	240	0
cream cheese, 2 tbsp.:							
(*Boar's Head*)	100	2.0	2.0	10.0	30	100	0
(*Organic Valley* Bar)	100	2.0	2.0	10.0	30	100	0
(*Organic Valley* Tub)	90	1.0	2.0	9.0	25	140	0
(*Philadelphia* Bar) .	100	2.0	1.0	10.0	30	90	0
(*Philadelphia* Bar Fat Free)	30	4.0	2.0	0	5	200	0
(*Philadelphia* Light)	60	3.0	2.0	4.5	15	150	0
(*Philadelphia* Tub) .	90	2.0	2.0	9.0	35	130	0
(*Smart Balance*) ...	90	3.0	2.0	6.0	15	105	0
blueberry (*Philadel- phia*)	90	1.0	5.0	7.0	30	110	0
chive/onion (*Phila- delphia* Light) ...	60	2.0	3.0	4.5	15	170	0
garlic, roasted (*Phila- delphia* Light) ...	60	3.0	3.0	4.5	15	180	0
honey nut (*Philadel- phia*)	90	1.0	4.0	8.0	30	125	0
peaches and cream (*Philadelphia Cream Swirls*)	90	1.0	5.0	7.0	30	110	0
pineapple (*Philadel- phia*)	90	1.0	4.0	7.0	30	115	0
salmon (*Philadelphia*)	90	2.0	1.0	8.0	30	220	0
strawberry (*Phila- delphia*)	90	1.0	5.0	8.0	30	120	0
strawberry (*Phila- delphia* Light) ...	70	2.0	6.0	4.0	15	120	0
vegetable, garden (*Philadelphia*) ...	90	1.0	2.0	8.0	35	160	0
cream cheese, whipped, 2 tbsp.:							
(*Philadelphia*)	60	1.0	1.0	6.0	20	90	0

Food and Measure	cal.	prot. (gms)	carbo. (gms)	fat (gms)	chol. (mgs)	sod. (mgs)	fiber (gms)
Cheese, cream, whipped *(cont.)*							
berry, mixed (*Philadelphia*)	70	1.0	1.0	5.0	15	55	0
chive (*Philadelphia*)	60	1.0	1.0	6.0	15	130	0
cinnamon brown sugar (*Philadelphia*)	70	1.0	3.0	6.0	20	55	0
garlic herb (*Philadelphia*)	60	1.0	1.0	6.0	20	100	0
ranch (*Philadelphia*)	60	1.0	1.0	6.0	15	150	0
crescenza-stracchino (*BelGioioso*)	80	4.0	0	6.0	20	140	0
Edam (*Boar's Head*) . .	90	7.0	0	7.0	20	280	0
farmer:							
(*Friendship*)	50	5.0	0	2.5	10	120	0
kefir (*Lifeway*), 2 tbsp.	40	3.0	4.0	1.5	6	10	0
feta:							
(*Athenos* Mild)	80	5.0	<1.0	6.0	20	190	0
(*Athenos* Traditional/ in Brine)	80	6.0	<1.0	6.0	20	330	0
(*Boar's Head*)	60	5.0	1.0	4.0	10	370	0
(*Fage* Greek)	70	5.0	0	6.0	15	180	0
(*Organic Valley*) . . .	60	5.0	<1.0	4.0	10	430	0
basil tomato (*Athenos*)	80	6.0	1.0	6.0	20	320	1.0
garlic herb (*Athenos*)	80	5.0	1.0	6.0	20	320	0
peppercorn (*Athenos*)	80	5.0	<1.0	6.0	20	330	1.0
feta, crumbled, ¼ cup:							
(*Athenos* Mild)	90	6.0	1.0	7.0	20	220	<1.0
(*Athenos* Traditional)	90	7.0	2.0	7.0	20	390	<1.0
(*Athenos* Traditional Reduced Fat) . . .	70	7.0	1.0	4.5	10	470	<1.0
(*Kraft Crumbles*) . .	90	7.0	2.0	7.0	25	390	1.0
basil tomato, garlic herb or lemon garlic, oregano (*Athenos*)	90	7.0	2.0	7.0	25	380	<1.0
peppercorn (*Athenos*)	90	6.0	2.0	7.0	25	390	<1.0
roasted pepper, garlic (*Athenos*)	90	6.0	3.0	7.0	25	370	<1.0
(*Finlandia Lappi*)	100	7.0	<1.0	8.0	25	160	0
fontina:							
(*BelGioioso*)	100	6.0	0	8.0	25	170	0
(*Denmark's Finest*)	90	7.0	0	7.0	15	160	0

Food and Measure	cal.	prot. (gms)	carbo. (gms)	fat (gms)	chol. (mgs)	sod. (mgs)	fiber (gms)
gjetost:							
(*Ekté*)	120	3.0	11.0	8.0	35	85	1.0
(*Ski Queen*)	130	3.0	11.0	9.0	30	90	0
Gloucester, double							
(*Boar's Head*)	110	7.0	0	10.0	35	200	0
goat:							
(*Vermont Butter &*							
Cheese Chèvre) .	80	5.0	1.0	6.0	20	45	0
(*Woolwich Dairy*							
Castile)	90	5.0	1.0	7.0	30	30	0
ash log (*Woolwich*							
Dairy Tre Fratello)	80	5.0	1.0	6.0	25	135	0
creamy (*Vermont*							
Butter & Cheese)	50	3.0	1.0	4.5	20	70	0
log, crumbles, or							
rounds (*Woolwich*							
Dairy)	70	5.0	1.0	6.0	25	100	0
log or disc (*Woolwich*							
Dairy Capella) . .	80	5.0	1.0	6.0	25	140	0
hard type	128	8.7	.6	10.1	30	98	0
semisoft type	103	6.1	.7	8.5	22	146	0
soft type	76	5.3	.3	6.0	·13	104	0
goat, brie (*Woolwich*							
Dairy)	90	6.0	1.0	7.0	30	180	0
goat, cheddar, raw							
(*Shiloh Farms*):							
mild or no salt	120	8.0	<1.0	9.0	20	81	0
sharp	110	7.0	<1.0	8.0	30	120	0
goat, feta:							
(*Shiloh Farms*)	110	6.0	0	9.0	15	150	0
(*Vermont Butter &*							
Cheese)	70	4.0	1.0	6.0	25	310	0
goat, Jack:							
(*Shiloh Farms* Just							
Jack)	110	7.0	<1.0	9.0	20	130	0
chive or tomato basil							
(*Shiloh Farms*) . .	100	7.0	0	8.0	20	110	0
goat, mozzarella							
(*Shiloh Farms*)	105	7.0	<1.0	8.5	25	238	0
gorgonzola:							
(*BelGioioso Creamy*							
Gorg)	100	6.0	0	8.0	30	280	0
crumbled (*Athenos*),							
3 tbsp.	110	7.0	2.0	9.0	30	400	<1.0

Food and Measure	cal.	prot. (gms)	carbo. (gms)	fat (gms)	chol. (mgs)	sod. (mgs)	fiber (gms)
Cheese *(cont.)*							
Gouda:							
(*Boar's Head*)	110	6.0	0	9.0	30	280	0
(*Finlandia* Stick) . . .	100	7.0	0	8.0	19	168	0
smoked (*Dietz & Watson*)	100	6.0	<1.0	8.0	25	270	0
(*Grana* American)	110	10.0	0	7.0	25	260	0
Gruyère	117	8.5	.1	9.2	31	95	0
havarti:							
(*Applegate Farms*), 1.5 oz.	180	7.0	0	15.0	37	225	0
(*Finlandia* Stick) . . .	109	7.0	<1.0	9.0	23	168	0
(*Land O Lakes*) . . .	110	6.0	0	9.0	25	180	0
cream, all varieties (*Boar's Head*) . . .	110	6.0	0	10.0	35	210	0
Italian, shredded, ¼ cup:							
4 cheese (*Organic Valley*)	90	7.0	1.0	7.0	20	220	0
4 cheese (*Sargento* Reduced Fat)	80	8.0	1.0	4.5	15	220	0
5 cheese (*Kraft*)	90	7.0	1.0	6.0	20	240	0
6 cheese (*Sargento* Classic)	90	7.0	1.0	7.0	20	200	0
(*Italico*)	100	6.0	0	8.0	30	280	0
Jack style, raw milk (*Organic Valley*) . . .	100	7.0	0	8.0	25	170	0
jalapeño Jack (*Land O Lakes*)	90	5.0	1.0	8.0	20	420	0
(*Jarlsberg*):							
loaf	100	7.0	0	8.0	25	130	0
loaf, lite	70	9.0	0	5.0	10	130	0
thin sliced	70	5.0	0	6.0	15	100	0
thin sliced, lite	50	7.0	0	2.5	10	100	0
wheel	100	7.0	0	8.0	20	180	0
Kasseri (*BelGioioso*) .	110	7.0	0	9.0	30	270	0
Limburger	93	5.7	.1	7.7	26	227	0
mascarpone:							
(*BelGioioso*)	120	2.0	0	13.0	35	15	0
(*BelGioioso* Tiramisu)	130	2.0	0	13.0	35	15	0
(*Sorrento*)	130	2.0	2.0	13.0	45	15	0
Mediterranean style (*Kraft Crumbles*) . .	90	7.0	1.0	7.0	20	280	0
Mexican (*Kraft Crumbles* Reduced Fat)	80	7.0	1.0	5.0	15	250	0

Food and Measure	cal.	prot. (gms)	carbo. (gms)	fat (gms)	chol. (mgs)	sod. (mgs)	fiber (gms)
Mexican, shredded, ¼ cup:							
(*Organic Valley*) ...	110	7.0	1.0	9.0	30	170	0
4 cheese (*Kraft*) ...	100	6.0	1.0	9.0	25	190	0
4 cheese (*Kraft* 2%)	80	7.0	1.0	5.0	15	240	0
4 cheese (*Sargento* Classic)	110	6.0	1.0	9.0	25	200	0
4 cheese (*Sargento* Reduced Fat) ...	80	8.0	<1.0	6.0	20	200	0
Monterey Jack:							
(*Boar's Head*)	100	6.0	0	9.0	25	180	0
(*Dietz & Watson*) ..	90	7.0	<1.0	9.0	25	180	0
(*Kraft* 8 oz.)	100	6.0	0	9.0	30	190	0
(*Kraft* 16 oz.)	110	6.0	0	9.0	30	190	0
(*Land O Lakes*) ...	110	7.0	0	9.0	25	190	0
(*Organic Valley*) ...	100	7.0	0	9.0	30	170	0
(*Sargento*), ¾ oz. ..	80	5.0	0	6.0	20	135	0
hot pepper or jalapeño (*Land O Lakes*) .	110	6.0	1.0	9.0	25	190	0
jalapeño (*Boar's Head*)	100	6.0	0	9.0	25	170	0
Monterey Jack, shredded, ¼ cup:							
(*Colby*)	110	7.0	1.0	9.0	30	170	0
(*Kraft*)	100	6.0	1.0	8.0	25	190	0
(*Sargento* Classic) .	110	7.0	1.0	9.0	30	190	0
Morbier (*Montboisse*)	99	6.5	.7	7.0	23	220	0
mozzarella:							
(*Alpine Lace*)	70	6.0	1.0	5.0	20	200	0
(*Boar's Head*)	90	6.0	1.0	7.0	20	150	0
(*Di Lusso*)	90	6.0	0	7.0	15	150	0
(*Dietz & Watson*) ..	90	6.0	<1.0	7.0	20	200	0
(*Kraft* Singles), ¾ oz.	50	4.0	1.0	3.0	10	290	0
(*Kraft* Deli Deluxe Slices), ¾ oz. ...	60	6.0	0	5.0	10	150	0
(*Kraft* String-ums) .	80	7.0	1.0	6.0	20	220	1.0
(*Kraft* String-ums Organic)	80	7.0	1.0	6.0	15	200	1.0
(*Land O Lakes*) ...	90	7.0	1.0	6.0	15	190	0
(*Organic Valley*) ...	80	7.0	<1.0	6.0	20	190	0
(*Sargento*), ¾ oz. ..	60	5.0	1.0	4.0	10	140	0
whole (*Polly-O*) ...	80	6.0	1.0	6.0	20	200	0
part skim (*Kraft*) ..	80	7.0	1.0	6.0	20	220	0
part skim (*Polly-O*) .	70	6.0	1.0	5.0	15	200	0
nonfat (*Polly-O*) ...	35	7.0	1.0	0	5	220	0

Food and Measure	cal.	prot. (gms)	carbo. (gms)	fat (gms)	chol. (mgs)	sod. (mgs)	fiber (gms)
Cheese (cont.)							
mozzarella, fresh:							
(BelGioioso)	80	5.0	0	6.0	20	40	0
(Polly-O)	80	5.0	0	7.0	20	15	0
cream filled (Bel-							
Gioioso Burrata) .	90	5.0	0	7.0	20	85	0
mozzarella, shredded,							
¼ cup:							
(Cabot)	80	8.0	1.0	6.0	15	170	0
(Kraft)	80	6.0	1.0	5.0	20	220	0
(Kraft Organic)	80	7.0	1.0	5.0	15	200	0
(Kraft 2% Milk) ...	70	8.0	1.0	4.0	15	200	0
(Organic Valley) ...	90	7.0	1.0	6.0	20	190	0
(Sargento ChefStyle/							
Classic)	80	7.0	1.0	6.0	15	190	0
whole (Polly-O) ...	90	6.0	1.0	7.0	20	190	0
whole (Sargento							
Artisan Blends) .	90	7.0	1.0	7.0	25	190	0
part skim (Polly-O)	80	7.0	1.0	5.0	15	200	0
nonfat (Kraft)	45	8.0	2.0	0	5	340	0
nonfat (Polly-O) ...	40	8.0	1.0	0	5	240	0
mozzarella blend,							
shredded, ¼ cup:							
asiago, roasted garlic							
(Sargento Bistro)	80	7.0	2.0	5.0	15	270	0
Parmesan, fine							
(Polly-O)	90	6.0	1.0	7.0	20	210	0
provolone (Sargento							
Artisan Blends) .	90	6.0	0	7.0	20	170	0
sun-dried tomato							
(Sargento Bistro)	90	7.0	1.0	6.0	20	220	0
Muenster:							
(Alpine Lace)	100	7.0	0	9.0	20	85	0
(Boar's Head)	100	6.0	0	8.0	25	180	0
(Di Lusso)	100	6.0	0	8.0	30	190	0
(Finlandia)	110	7.0	0	10.0	25	150	0
(Land O Lakes) ...	100	7.0	0	8.0	25	180	0
(Organic Valley) ...	100	7.0	0	8.0	25	180	0
(Sargento), ¾ oz. ...	80	5.0	0	6.0	20	135	0
baby (Finlandia							
Oltermanni)	100	7.0	0	8.0	20	160	0
nacho taco, shredded							
(Sargento Bistro),							
¼ cup	110	7.0	1.0	9.0	30	200	0

Food and Measure	cal.	prot. (gms)	carbo. (gms)	fat (gms)	chol. (mgs)	sod. (mgs)	fiber (gms)
Neufchâtel:							
(*Organic Valley* Bar), 2 tbsp., 1.1 oz. . . .	80	2.0	1.0	6.0	20	115	0
(*Organic Valley* Tub), 2 tbsp., 1.1 oz. . . .	70	2.0	2.0	6.0	20	140	0
(*Philadelphia*)	70	2.0	1.0	6.0	20	120	0
Parmesan (*BelGioioso/ BelGioioso* Vegetarian)	110	10.0	0	7.0	25	260	0
Parmesan, grated, 2 tsp.:							
(*Kraft*)	20	2.0	0	1.5	5	85	0
(*Kraft* Reduced Fat)	20	1.0	2.0	1.0	5	80	0
(*Polly-O*)	20	2.0	0	1.5	5	85	0
(*Sargento*)	25	2.0	0	1.5	5	80	0
Romano (*Kraft*) . . .	20	2.0	0	1.5	5	85	0
Romano (*Polly-O*) .	20	2.0	0	1.5	5	85	0
Parmesan, shredded:							
(*Buitoni*), 1 tbsp. . . .	20	2.0	0	1.5	5	60	0
(*Kraft*), ¼ cup	110	9.0	1.0	8.0	25	400	0
(*Organic Valley*), ¼ cup	110	10.0	0	7.0	20	350	0
(*Sargento Artisan Blends*), 2 tsp. . . .	20	2.0	0	1.5	<5	55	0
Romano and asiago (*Kraft*), ¼ cup . .	110	9.0	1.0	8.0	25	370	0
pepato (*BelGioioso*) . .	100	7.0	0	8.0	25	340	0
pepper, hot:							
(*Alpine Lace*)	90	7.0	1.0	7.0	20	300	0
(*BelGioioso Peperoncino*) . . .	100	7.0	0	8.0	25	340	0
pepper Jack:							
(*Di Lusso*)	100	7.0	1.0	8.0	30	170	0
(*Kraft*)	110	6.0	1.0	9.0	30	170	0
(*Kraft Deli Deluxe* Slices), .8 oz. . . .	90	5.0	0	7.0	25	150	0
(*Land O Lakes*) . . .	110	6.0	1.0	9.0	25	190	0
(*Organic Valley*) . . .	100	6.0	0	8.0	25	220	0
(*Sargento*), ¾ oz. . .	80	4.0	0	6.0	20	140	0
pepperoni:							
(*Black Bear*)	90	5.0	2.0	7.0	20	480	0
(*Dietz & Watson*) . .	110	6.0	<1.0	9.0	28	270	0
pizza, shredded, ¼ cup:							
(*Sargento Double Cheese*)	90	7.0	1.0	6.0	20	190	0

Food and Measure	cal.	prot. (gms)	carbo. (gms)	fat (gms)	chol. (mgs)	sod. (mgs)	fiber (gms)
Cheese, pizza, shredded *(cont.)*							
4 cheese (*Kraft*) . . .	90	6.0	1.0	7.0	20	220	0
mozzarella/cheddar							
(*Kraft*)	90	6.0	1.0	7.0	20	200	0
mozzarella/provolone/							
Parmesan (*Polly-O*)	90	7.0	1.0	7.0	20	230	0
Port du Salut	100	6.7	.2	8.0	35	151	0
provolone:							
(*Boar's Head* Lower							
Sodium)	100	7.0	1.0	8.0	20	140	0
(*Boar's Head* Picante)	100	7.0	1.0	8.0	25	250	0
(*Di Lusso*)	100	7.0	1.0	8.0	20	240	0
(*Kraft Deli Deluxe*) .	100	7.0	0	8.0	25	230	0
(*Organic Valley*) . . .	100	7.0	1.0	8.0	20	250	0
medium (*BelGioioso*)	100	7.0	0	8.0	30	320	0
mild (*BelGioioso*) . .	100	7.0	0	8.0	25	120	0
sharp (*BelGioioso*) .	110	7.0	0	9.0	30	320	0
smoke flavor							
(*Land O Lakes*) .	100	7.0	1.0	8.0	20	250	0
quark (*Vermont Butter*							
& Cheese), 2 oz. . .	80	5.0	2.0	6.0	15	80	0
ricotta, ¼ cup:							
(*Polly-O* Lite)	70	8.0	3.0	3.0	10	80	0
(*Polly-O* Original) . .	110	7.0	2.0	8.0	25	65	0
(*Sargento* Light) . . .	60	5.0	3.0	2.5	15	55	0
whole (*BelGioioso*							
Ricotta con Latte)	100	8.0	0	7.0	25	100	0
whole (*Organic*							
Valley)	100	6.0	3.0	7.0	20	100	0
whole (*Sargento*) . .	90	7.0	3.0	6.0	25	75	0
part skim (*Polly-O*)	90	8.0	2.0	6.0	20	65	0
part skim (*Sargento*)	70	6.0	3.0	4.5	25	85	0
nonfat (*Polly-O*) . . .	45	8.0	3.0	0	5	80	0
nonfat (*Sargento*) . .	50	5.0	5.0	0	10	65	0
Romano (*BelGioioso*) .	100	9.0	0	7.0	25	330	0
Romano, grated:							
(*Alessi* Pecorino/							
Pepato), 1 tbsp. . .	25	2.0	0	2.0	5	120	0
(*Kraft*), 2 tsp.	20	2.0	0	1.5	5	85	0
Romano, shredded							
(*Buitoni*), 1 tbsp. . . .	20	2.0	0	1.5	5	50	0
Roquefort	105	6.1	.6	8.7	26	513	0
(*Snorfrisk*)	70	2.0	2.0	8.0	15	170	0

Food and Measure	cal.	prot. (gms)	carbo. (gms)	fat (gms)	chol. (mgs)	sod. (mgs)	fiber (gms)
string cheese:							
(*Polly-O String-Ums*)	80	7.0	1.0	6.0	20	220	0
(*Sargento*)	80	8.0	<1.0	6.0	15	240	0
(*Sargento* 5 oz.), .8-oz. pc.	70	6.0	<1.0	4.5	15	200	0
Swiss:							
(*Applegate Farms*), ⅔-oz. slice	80	5.0	0	6.0	15	35	0
(*Boar's Head* Gold Label Import) . . .	110	8.0	<1.0	8.0	20	70	0
(*Boar's Head* Lacey)	90	9.0	0	6.0	15	35	0
(*Boar's Head* Natural No Salt)	110	8.0	1.0	8.0	25	10	0
(*Cracker Barrel* Emmentaler Slices), ¾ oz.	80	6.0	0	7.0	20	35	0
(*Di Lusso*)	100	8.0	1.0	8.0	25	60	0
(*Finlandia*)	110	8.0	0	8.0	20	80	0
(*Finlandia* Black Label)	110	8.0	0	8.0	20	170	0
(*Finlandia* Heavenly Light)	70	9.0	0	4.0	10	130	0
(*Finlandia* Presliced), .8 oz.	86	6.0	0	7.0	16	62	0
(*Finlandia* Thin Sliced), .5 oz.	55	4.0	0	4.0	10	39	0
(*Kraft* Singles), ¾ oz.	60	4.0	2.0	4.5	15	280	0
(*Kraft* Singles 2% Milk), ¾ oz.	50	4.0	2.0	2.5	10	310	0
(*Kraft* Singles Fat Free), ¾ oz.	30	5.0	2.0	0	5	280	0
(*Kraft Deli Deluxe* Natural Slices), ¾ oz.	80	6.0	0	7.0	20	35	0
(*Kraft Deli Deluxe* Slices 8 oz.)	90	6.0	1.0	7.0	25	340	0
(*Kraft Deli Deluxe* Slices 16 oz.) . . .	110	8.0	0	9.0	30	50	0
(*Kraft Deli Deluxe* Slices), ¾ oz. . . .	80	6.0	0	7.0	20	35	0
(*Kraft Deli Deluxe* 2% Milk), ¾ oz.	70	6.0	0	4.5	15	50	0
(*Land O Lakes*) . . .	110	8.0	1.0	8.0	25	115	0

Food and Measure	cal.	prot. (gms)	carbo. (gms)	fat (gms)	chol. (mgs)	sod. (mgs)	fiber (gms)
Cheese, Swiss *(cont.)*							
(*Sargento* Aged/Thin),							
⅔-oz. slice	70	5.0	0	5.0	20	40	0
(*Sargento* Reduced							
Fat), ¾-oz. slice .	60	7.0	1.0	4.0	10	30	0
(*Sargento* Thick) . .	110	8.0	1.0	8.0	25	60	0
Swiss, baby:							
(*Boar's Head*)	110	7.0	<1.0	9.0	25	135	0
(*Cracker Barrel*) . . .	110	7.0	0	9.0	25	110	0
(*Di Lusso*)	110	7.0	1.0	9.0	30	75	0
(*Land O Lakes*) . . .	110	8.0	1.0	8.0	25	115	0
(*Organic Valley*) . . .	110	7.0	0	9.0	25	125	0
(*Sargento*), ⅔ oz. . .	70	5.0	0	5.0	15	40	0
Swiss, shredded:							
(*Kraft*), ¼ cup	110	7.0	1.0	8.0	25	60	0
(*Sargento* Artisan							
Blends), ¼ cup .	110	8.0	<1.0	8.0	25	60	0
Swiss and cheddar,							
smoky (*Kraft*)	100	5.0	1.0	8.0	25	380	0
taco, shredded, ¼ cup:							
(*Kraft* Mexican) . . .	120	7.0	1.0	10.0	30	240	0
(*Sargento* Bistro) . .	110	7.0	1.0	9.0	30	200	0
Cheese appetizer/snack,							
frozen:							
in fillo shell (*The Fillo*							
Factory Tyropita),							
3 pcs., 3 oz.	230	7.0	19.0	14.0	40	310	0
mozzarella sticks,							
breaded (*Alexia*							
Mozzarella Stix),							
2 pcs., 1.3 oz.	120	5.0	13.0	7.0	15	220	<1.0
three cheese, 2 pcs.:							
(*Athens/Apollo*							
Tyropita), 2 oz. . .	180	6.0	14.0	11.0	25	310	0
mini, tomato fillo							
(*Athens*), 1 oz. . .	70	3.0	7.0	3.5	5	270	0
Cheese bun, see "Bun,							
sweet"							
Cheese w/crackers,							
see "Cheese dip kit"							
Cheese dip, 2 tbsp.:							
(*Cheez Whiz* Light) . . .	80	6.0	6.0	3.5	20	500	0
(*Cheez Whiz* Original)	90	3.0	4.0	7.0	30	490	0
(*Fritos*)	45	1.0	3.0	3.0	<5	310	0

Food and Measure	cal.	prot. (gms)	carbo. (gms)	fat (gms)	chol. (mgs)	sod. (mgs)	fiber (gms)
blue cheese:							
(*Marzetti's*)	140	1.0	1.0	15.0	25	250	0
peppercorn (*Marie's*)	100	2.0	2.0	10.0	15	220	0
cheddar:							
jalapeño (*Fritos*) ...	50	1.0	4.0	4.0	5	300	0
mild (*Fritos*)	60	1.0	3.0	4.0	5	330	0
chili (*Fritos*)	45	1.0	3.0	3.0	<5	310	0
cream cheese, see "Fruit dip"							
Monterey Jack (*Tostitos* Queso) ..	40	1.0	4.0	2.5	<5	210	0
nacho:							
(*Bravo*)	50	1.0	3.0	4.5	0	250	0
(*Mrs. Renfro's*) ...	30	1.0	4.0	1.5	0	150	0
salsa con queso:							
(*Cheez Whiz*)	90	3.0	4.0	7.0	30	500	0
(*Chi-Chi's*)	45	1.0	4.0	3.0	0	280	0
(*Chi-Chi's* Mild) ...	90	2.0	3.0	8.0	10	520	0
(*Tostitos*)	40	<1.0	5.0	2.5	<5	280	<1.0
bean (*Taco Bell* Home Originals) .	35	1.0	2.0	2.0	0	300	1.0
chili (*Taco Bell* Home Originals) .	40	2.0	3.0	2.0	5	470	0
mild or medium (*Old El Paso* Cheese n' Salsa)	40	<1.0	3.0	3.0	0	280	0
mild or medium (*Taco Bell* Home Originals)	25	1.0	1.0	2.0	0	220	0
medium (*Old El Paso* Cheese n' Salsa Low Fat) ..	30	<1.0	4.0	1.5	0	280	0
Cheese dip kit:							
cheddar (*Sargento Cheese Dips!*):							
w/bagel chips, 3 oz.	280	9.0	24.0	17.0	15	1130	<1.0
w/pretzels, 3.75 oz.	360	9.0	47.0	16.0	15.0	1430	2.0
w/tortilla chips, 3 oz.	320	7.0	26.0	21.0	15	860	1.0
w/cheddar sticks (*Sargento*), 1 oz. ..	100	2.0	11.0	6.0	<5	360	0
w/crackers:							
(*Sargento*), 1 oz. ..	100	2.0	10.0	5.0	5	360	0
Colby Jack (*Kraft To Go!*), 1.5 oz. .	170	8.0	10.0	11.0	30	280	1.0

Food and Measure	cal.	prot. (gms)	carbo. (gms)	fat (gms)	chol. (mgs)	sod. (mgs)	fiber (gms)
Cheese dip kit, with crackers *(cont.)*							
cheddar (*Kraft To Go!*), 1.5 oz. .	190	7.0	10.0	13.0	30	310	0
w/pretzels (*Sargento*), . .9 oz.	90	2.0	13.0	3.0	<5	260	<1.0
w/sticks (*Sargento*), 1 oz.	100	2.0	12.0	5.0	<5	290	0
Cheese dish, pkg. (*Tasty Bite* Paneer Makhani), 5 oz. . . .	120	6.0	10.0	8.0	10	440	2.0
Cheese food (see also "Cheese spread"), 1 oz., except as noted:							
(*Velveeta* Loaf)	80	5.0	3.0	6.0	25	410	0
(*Velveeta* 2% Milk) . . .	60	5.0	4.0	3.0	15	410	0
(*Velveeta* Slices 12 oz.), ¾ oz.	60	4.0	2.0	4.0	15	270	0
(*Velveeta* Slices 16 oz.), .8 oz.	60	4.0	2.0	4.5	15	300	0
(*Velveeta* Slices Extra Thick), 1.2 oz.	100	5.0	3.0	7.0	30	410	0
w/hot pepper (*Land O Lakes*)	100	5.0	2.0	8.0	25	420	0
w/jalapeño (*Land O Lakes* Presliced) . . .	90	5.0	2.0	7.0	20	450	0
Mexican:							
hot (*Velveeta*)	90	5.0	3.0	6.0	25	430	0
mild (*Velveeta*)	80	5.0	3.0	6.0	25	400	0
w/onion (*Land O Lakes*)	90	5.0	2.0	7.0	20	420	0
pepper Jack (*Velveeta*)	80	5.0	3.0	6.0	25	430	0
w/pepperoni (*Land O Lakes*)	90	5.0	2.0	7.0	25	430	0
shredded (*Velveeta*), ¼ cup, 1.3 oz.	130	8.0	3.0	9.0	30	500	0
Cheese powder (*Cabot Cheddar Shake!*), 2 tsp.	25	1.0	1.0	1.5	5	220	0
Cheese sauce, chipotle or jalapeño con queso (*Pain is Good*), 1 oz.	168	5.0	4.0	11.0	0	240	2.0
Cheese sauce, cooking, can/jar, ¼ cup:							
cheddar, double (*Ragú*)	100	2.0	3.0	9.0	25	510	0

Food and Measure	cal.	prot. (gms)	carbo. (gms)	fat (gms)	chol. (mgs)	sod. (mgs)	fiber (gms)
mild (*Zapata*)	60	2.0	7.0	2.5	10	490	0
nacho (*Mrs. Renfro's*)	60	1.0	7.0	3.5	0	310	0
spicy, jalapeño (*Zapata*)	50	2.0	4.0	3.5	15	260	0
Cheese sauce mix, four (*McCormick*), 1⅓ tbsp.	40	1.0	5.0	1.5	5	600	0
Cheese seasoning (*Molly McButter* Natural), 1 tsp.	5	0	1.0	0	0	125	0
Cheese spread (see also "Cheese"), 1 oz. or 2 tbsp., except as noted:							
(*Boursin*):							
Apple, Cranberry & Cinnamon	120	2.0	3.0	12.0	30	90	0
Fig, Raisin & Nut ..	120	2.0	.2	12.0	35	90	0
Garlic & Fine Herbs	120	2.0	1.0	13.0	35	180	0
pepper	120	2.0	1.0	13.0	35	200	0
Shallot & Chive ...	120	2.0	1.0	13.0	35	180	0
(*Finlandia Viola*)	87	3.0	1.0	8.0	19	280	0
all varieties, except Swiss (*Kaukauna* Log)	90	6.0	4.0	6.0	15	230	1.0
American (*Kraft Easy Cheese*)	90	5.0	2.0	6.0	20	410	0
bacon:							
(*Kraft*)	90	5.0	1.0	8.0	25	570	0
cheddar (*Hans' All Natural*)	100	3.0	6.0	7.0	20	200	0
smoky (*Kaukauna/ WisPride* Ball) ...	90	6.0	4.0	6.0	15	230	1.0
beef and onion (*Kaukauna* Ball) ...	120	2.0	5.0	10.0	30	180	1.0
blue cheese:							
(*Kraft Roka*)	80	3.0	2.0	7.0	20	340	0
almond (*Hans' All Natural*)	100	4.0	5.0	7.0	20	370	0
cheddar:							
(*Cheez-It*)	90	4.0	3.0	6.0	15	510	0
(*Kraft Easy Cheese*)	90	5.0	2.0	6.0	20	410	0
and bacon (*Kraft Easy Cheese*) ...	90	5.0	2.0	6.0	20	410	0

Food and Measure	cal.	prot. (gms)	carbo. (gms)	fat (gms)	chol. (mgs)	sod. (mgs)	fiber (gms)
Cheese spread *(cont.)*							
cheddar, sharp:							
(*Hans' All Natural*) .	100	4.0	4.0	7.0	26	200	0
(*Kaukauna* Ball/Log)	90	6.0	4.0	6.0	15	230	1.0
(*Kraft Easy Cheese*)	80	4.0	2.0	6.0	10	450	0
extra (*Kaukauna/ WisPride* Ball) ..	100	6.0	4.0	7.0	15	230	0
extra (*Kaukauna/ Wispride* Lite) ..	70	5.0	5.0	3.5	15	190	0
extra or smoky (*Kaukauna/ WisPride*)	90	5.0	3.0	7.0	20	190	0
cheddar, white:							
(*Cheez-It*)	90	4.0	3.0	6.0	15	540	0
(*Kaukauna/WisPride* Extremely Creamy Vermont)	100	3.0	3.0	8.0	20	170	0
w/roasted red pepper (*Philadelphia* Cracker Spreads)	80	2.0	1.0	8.0	25	105	0
cheddar and cream cheese (*Kaukauna/ WisPride* Ball)	100	6.0	3.0	7.0	20	190	1.0
cheddar/Swiss, double, all varieties (*Wis-Pride* Log)	90	6.0	4.0	6.0	15	230	1.0
cheese, three, Italian (*Kaukauna* Extremely Creamy)	100	4.0	3.0	8.0	25	190	0
chipotle (*Kaukauna* Extremely Creamy) .	100	4.0	3.0	8.0	20	180	0
cream cheese, see "Cheese"							
garlic herb:							
(*Kaukauna/WisPride*)	90	2.0	2.0	8.0	30	180	0
(*Kaukauna/ WisPride* Ball) ..	120	2.0	5.0	10.0	30	180	1.0
horseradish:							
(*Kaukauna/WisPride*)	90	5.0	3.0	7.0	20	210	0
(*Kaukauna/WisPride* Ball)	90	6.0	4.0	6.0	15	230	1.0
(*Kaukauna/WisPride* Extremely Creamy)	100	3.0	3.0	8.0	20	170	0

Food and Measure	cal.	prot. (gms)	carbo. (gms)	fat (gms)	chol. (mgs)	sod. (mgs)	fiber (gms)
cheddar (*Hans' All Natural*)	90	3.0	5.0	5.0	20	190	0
jalapeño cheddar (*Hans' All Natural*) .	90	3.0	6.0	5.0	20	230	0
mozzarella garlic (*Kaukauna/WisPride* Extremely Creamy) .	90	2.0	1.0	9.0	20	220	0
onion, Vidalia (*Kaukauna* Ball) ...	100	5.0	3.0	7.0	20	190	0
Parmesan:							
w/garlic, herbs (*Philadelphia* Cracker Spreads)	90	2.0	1.0	9.0	25	130	0
ranch (*Kaukauna*) ..	90	5.0	3.0	6.0	20	240	0
pepper Jack, w/jalapeño (*Philadelphia* Cracker Spreads) ..	90	2.0	1.0	8.0	25	160	0
pesto (*Kaukauna* Extremely Creamy) ..	100	4.0	3.0	8.0	25	200	0
pimento (*Kraft*)	80	2.0	3.0	6.0	20	170	0
pineapple (*Kraft*)	70	2.0	4.0	5.0	15	120	0
port wine:							
(*Kaukauna/WisPride*)	90	5.0	4.0	7.0	20	190	0
(*Kaukauna/WisPride* Lite)	70	5.0	5.0	3.5	15	190	0
(*Kaukauna/WisPride* Ball)	90	6.0	4.0	6.0	15	230	1.0
ranch cream cheese (*Kaukauna/WisPride* Ball)	120	2.0	6.0	10.0	30	180	1.0
sharp (*Kraft Old English*)	90	5.0	1.0	8.0	25	520	0
Swiss:							
(*Kaukauna/WisPride* Ball/Log)	80	6.0	2.0	6.0	20	420	0
almond (*Hans' All Natural*)	100	5.0	4.0	8.0	20	240	0
almond (*Kaukauna*)	90	5.0	3.0	7.0	20	140	0
vegetable, garden:							
(*Kaukauna/WisPride*)	90	2.0	2.0	8.0	25	190	0
(*Kaukauna/WisPride* Ball)	120	2.0	5.0	10.0	30	180	1.0
Cheeseburger, see "Beef sandwich"							

Food and Measure	cal.	prot. (gms)	carbo. (gms)	fat (gms)	chol. (mgs)	sod. (mgs)	fiber (gms)
Cheesecake, French style (*Entenmann's* Deluxe), ⅙ cake . . .	390	6.0	39.0	24.0	40	400	<1.0
Cheesecake, frozen:							
(*Baby Watson*), ¼ cake	370	6.0	31.0	25.0	55	230	0
(*Sara Lee* Original), ¼ cake	330	8.0	35.0	17.0	70	260	<1.0
New York style:							
(*Sara Lee*), ⅙ cake	480	7.0	47.0	30.0	135	490	1.0
(*Smart Ones*), 2.5-oz. pc.	150	5.0	21.0	5.0	15	140	<1.0
Cheesecake mix, dry:							
(*Jell-O* No Bake Homestyle), ⅙ pkg.	220	2.0	44.0	4.5	0	400	1.0
(*Jell-O* No Bake Real), ⅙ pkg.	220	2.0	42.0	5.0	0	380	1.0
cherry (*Eagle Brand Cherry Cheesecake Treasures*), ⅙ pkg. .	380	6.0	72.0	8.0	15	400	1.0
Cheesecake snack:							
bars, 1.5-oz. pc.:							
(*Philadelphia* Classic)	190	2.0	20.0	11.0	15	85	0
marble brownie (*Philadelphia.*) . .	170	3.0	20.0	9.0	25	110	1.0
strawberry (*Philadelphia* Snack Bars)	180	2.0	22.0	9.0	10	80	0
bites, 1-oz. pc.:							
strawberry, chocolate covered (*Philadelphia* Snack Bites)	130	1.0	15.0	7.0	10	55	0
turtle (*Philadelphia* Snack Bites)	130	2.0	14.0	7.0	10	70	0
petite, assorted (*Atlanta Cheesecake Co.*), 5 pcs., 2.5 oz.	220	4.0	24.0	13.0	65	170	1.0
Cherimoya (see also "Custard apple"):							
(*Frieda's*), 5 oz.	120	2.0	34.0	.5	0	0	3.0
1 medium, 1.9 lb. . . .	515	7.1	131.3	2.2	0	n.a.	13.1
Cherry, fresh:							
(*Dole*), 1 cup, 4.9 oz. .	90	2.0	22.0	.5	0	0	3.0
sour, red, ½ cup:							
w/pits	26	.5	6.3	.2	0	2	.6
red, pitted	39	.8	9.4	.2	0	3	.9

Food and Measure	cal.	prot. (gms)	carbo. (gms)	fat (gms)	chol. (mgs)	sod. (mgs)	fiber (gms)
sweet, w/pits, ½ cup .	52	.9	12.0	.7	0	1	1.7
sweet, 10 medium ...	49	.8	11.3	.7	0	<1	1.6
Cherry, can/jar, pitted, ½ cup, except as noted:							
dark, sweet:							
in light syrup (*Trader Joe's* Morello)	110	1.0	27.0	0	0	10	1.0
in heavy syrup (*Oregon* Bing) ..	110	1.0	26.0	0	0	10	1.0
in heavy syrup (*Del Monte*)	100	<1.0	24.0	0	0	10	<1.0
in extra heavy syrup (*S&W*)	140	1.0	34.0	0	0	10	1.0
light, sweet, in heavy syrup (*Oregon* Royal Anne)	110	1.0	26.0	0	0	10	1.0
red, tart, in water (*Oregon*), ⅔ cup ..	60	1.0	14.0	0	0	10	2.0
sour, pitted:							
in light syrup	95	.9	24.3	.1	0	9	1.0
in heavy syrup	116	.9	29.8	.1	0	9	1.0
sweet, w/liquid:							
in juice	68	1.1	17.3	<.1	0	4	1.9
in light syrup	84	.8	21.8	.2	0	4	1.9
Cherry, dried:							
(*Roland*), ⅓ cup	140	1.0	34.0	0	0	10	2.0
(*Sunsweet*), ¼ cup, 1.4 oz.	100	1.0	30.0	0	0	5	2.0
bing (*Frieda's*), ¼ cup, 1.4 oz.	120	2.0	26.0	0	0	5	3.0
sour/tart:							
(*Eden* Montmorency), ¼ cup, 1.6 oz. ..	140	0	36.0	0	0	15	3.0
(*Frieda's*), ⅓ cup, 1.4 oz.	150	2.0	33.0	0	0	0	2.0
(*Shiloh Farms*), ⅓ cup, 1.4 oz. ..	135	3.0	31.0	0	0	7	4.0
Cherry, flavored, 1 pc.:							
lemon, lime, passion fruit, or wild berry (*Roland*)	10	0	2.0	0	0	0	0
maraschino (*Roland*) .	10	0	2.0	0	0	0	0

Food and Measure	cal.	prot. (gms)	carbo. (gms)	fat (gms)	chol. (mgs)	sod. (mgs)	fiber (gms)
Cherry, frozen:							
dark sweet (*Dole*), 1 cup	90	2.0	22.0	0	0	0	3.0
sweet (*Cascadian Farm* Organic), 1 cup ...	90	1.0	22.0	0	0	0	3.0
unsweetened, ½ cup .	36	7.1	8.5	.3	0	1	1.2
sweetened, ½ cup ...	116	1.5	29.0	.2	0	1	2.7
Cherry, maraschino, see "Cherry, flavored"							
Cherry, West Indian, see "Acerola"							
Cherry butter, tart (*Eden* Organic Montmorency), 1 tbsp. .	35	0	9.0	0	0	0	1.0
Cherry drink, 8 fl. oz.:							
citrus (*SoBe Courage*)	110	0	30.0	0	0	25	0
wild (*Capri Sun*)	100	0	28.0	0	0	15	0
sparkling (*R.W. Knudsen* 80%)	120	<1.0	31.0	0	0	20	0
Cherry juice, 8 fl. oz., except as noted:							
all varieties (*Cherrish*), 11.5 fl. oz.	142	2.0	35.0	0	0	38	0
(*Walnut Acres* Organic)	140	0	34.0	0	0	15	0
black:							
(*L&A*)	180	0	45.0	0	0	10	0
(*R.W. Knudsen Just Black Cherry*) ...	160	2.0	37.0	0	0	10	0
cider (*R.W. Knudsen*) .	130	<1.0	33.0	0	0	40	0
tart:							
(*Eden* Organic Montmorency) ..	140	1.0	33.0	1.0	0	30	0
(*R.W. Knudsen Just Tart Cherry*)	130	1.0	32.0	0	0	20	0
red (*Santa Cruz* Organic)	120	0	30.0	0	0	25	0
Cherry juice concentrate:							
(*Eden* Organic), 1 fl. oz.	119	1,0	26.0	0	0	20	0
black:							
(*R.W. Knudsen*), 8 fl. oz.*	200	2.0	47.0	0	0	10	0
(*Tree of Life*), 8 tsp.	110	0	28.0	0	0	0	0
Chervil, dried, 1 tsp. .	1	.1	.3	<.1	0	<1	.1

Food and Measure	cal.	prot. (gms)	carbo. (gms)	fat (gms)	chol. (mgs)	sod. (mgs)	fiber (gms)
Chestnut, Chinese, shelled, 1 oz.:							
dried	103	1.9	22.7	.5	0	2	<1.0
boiled or steamed ...	44	.8	9.6	.2	0	1	<1.0
roasted	68	1.3	14.9	.3	0	1	<1.0
Chestnut, European:							
raw, in shell, 1 lb. ...	714	8.1	152.8	7.6	0	9	27.2
raw, shelled, w/peel, 1 cup, 13 pcs.	308	3.5	66.0	3.3	0	4	11.7
dried, peeled, 1 oz. ..	105	1.4	23.3	1.1	0	11	<2.0
boiled, 1 oz.	37	.8	7.9	.4	0	8	<1.0
roasted, peeled:							
1 oz.	70	.9	15.0	.6	0	1	3.3
1 cup, 17 kernels ..	350	4.3	75.7	3.2	0	3	16.7
Chestnuts, European, can/jar:							
(*Minerve*), 4 pcs.	40	<1.0	9.0	0	0	0	2.0
(*Roland*), 4 pcs.	50	<1.0	11.0	.5	0	0	2.0
cream (*Roland* Crème de Marrons), 2 tbsp.	80	<1.0	18.0	0	0	0	0
puree (*Roland*), 2 tbsp.	25	<1.0	6.0	0	0	0	1.0
in water (*Roland*), 4 pcs.	30	<1.0	7.0	0	0	180	1.0
Chia seeds, dried:							
(*Shiloh Farms*), 3 tbsp.	140	5.0	13.0	7.0	0	15	10.0
1 oz.	139	4.4	12.4	10.8	8	5	10.7
Chicken, fresh, 4 oz., except as noted:							
broiler-fryer, roasted:							
w/skin, ½ chicken, 10.5 oz. (15.8 oz. w/bone)	715	81.6	0	40.7	263	244	0
w/skin	271	31.0	0	15.4	100	93	0
meat only	215	32.8	0	8.4	101	98	0
meat only, chopped or diced, 1 cup ..	266	40.5	0	10.4	125	120	0
skin only, 1 oz.	129	5.8	0	11.5	24	18	0
dark meat only	232	31.0	0	11.0	105	105	0
light meat only	196	35.1	0	5.1	96	87	0
breast, w/skin, ½ breast, 3½ oz. (8½ oz. w/bone)	193	29.2	0	7.6	83	69	0
drumstick, w/skin, 1.8 oz. (2.9 oz. w/bone)	112	14.1	0	5.8	48	47	0

Food and Measure	cal.	prot. (gms)	carbo. (gms)	fat (gms)	chol. (mgs)	sod. (mgs)	fiber (gms)
Chicken, fresh *(cont.)*							
leg, w/skin (5.7 oz. w/bone)	265	29.6	0	15.4	105	99	0
thigh, w/skin, 2.2 oz. (2.9 oz. w/bone) .	153	15.5	0	9.6	58	52	0
wing, w/skin, 1.2 oz. (2.3 oz. w/bone) .	99	9.1	0	6.6	29	28	0
capon, roasted, w/skin:							
½ capon, 1.4 lbs. (2 lbs. w/bone) .	1457	184.5	0	74.2	549	313	0
w/skin	260	32.8	0	13.2	98	56	0
ground, see "Chicken, ground"							
roaster, roasted:							
w/skin, ½ chicken, 1 lb. (1½ lbs. w/bone)	1071	115.0	0	64.3	365	349	0
meat w/skin	253	27.2	0	15.2	86	83	0
stewing, stewed:							
w/skin, ½ chicken, 9.2 oz. (13½ oz. w/bone)	744	70.2	0	49.2	205	190	0
meat w/skin	323	30.5	0	21.4	90	83	0
meat only	269	34.5	0	13.5	94	88	0
meat only, chopped or diced, 1 cup ..	332	42.6	0	16.6	117	109	0
Chicken, canned,							
chunk, 2 oz.:							
(*Tyson*)	60	10.0	0	2.5	30	200	0
(*Swanson* Mixin')	100	8.0	1.0	7.0	40	210	<1.0
white (*Valley Fresh*) ..	70	15.0	0	1.0	25	180	0
breast:							
(*Swanson*)	50	9.0	1.0	1.0	25	300	0
(*Tyson*)	60	13.0	0	.5	30	200	0
(*Tyson* Pouch)	70	14.0	0	1.5	45	210	0
white and dark:							
(*Swanson*)	60	10.0	1.0	2.0	30	250	0
(*Valley Fresh*)	80	15.0	0	2.0	50	130	0
Chicken, frozen/ refrigerated, raw, 4 oz., except as noted:							
whole, edible portion:							
(*Empire Kosher* Broiler Fresh) ...	240	21.0	0	17.0	85	220	0

Food and Measure	cal.	prot. (gms)	carbo. (gms)	fat (gms)	chol. (mgs)	sod. (mgs)	fiber (gms)
(*Empire Kosher* Roaster Frozen) .	220	19.0	0	15.0	75	440	0
(*Organic Prairie*) ..	260	21.0	0	17.0	100	80	0
(*Tyson* Roaster)	210	19.0	0	15.0	90	150	0
(*Tyson* Young)	250	19.0	0	19.0	65	70	0
seasoned (*Perdue Oven Ready Roaster*)	200	19.0	1.0	12.0	105	630	0
breast, bone-in (*Perdue Oven Stuffer*) .	150	21.0	0	8.0	70	40	0
breast, bone-in, split: (*Empire Kosher* Fresh)	160	19.0	0	9.0	70	220	0
(*Empire Kosher* Frozen)	160	21.0	0	9.0	65	480	0
(*Perdue Tender & Tasty*)	130	20.0	1.0	4.5	70	390	0
(*Tyson*)	170	21.0	0	10.0	65	160	0
skinless (*Perdue Tender & Tasty*) .	100	21.0	1.0	1.5	80	460	0
skinless (*Tyson*) ...	130	23.0	0	4.0	60	160	0
breast, bone-/ skinless: (*Empire Kosher* Frozen)	100	23.0	0	1.0	60	470	0
(*Organic Prairie*) ..	120	26.0	0	1.5	65	75	0
(*Perdue Fit & Easy*)	110	26.0	0	1.0	75	45	0
(*Perdue Perfect Portions*), 4.8-oz. pc.	130	29.0	0	1.5	80	350	0
(*Perdue Perfect Portions* All Natural), 4.8-oz. pc.	140	32.0	0	1.5	90	60	0
(*Perdue Tender & Tasty*)	120	22.0	1.0	2.5	70	350	0
(*Tyson*)	110	23.0	0	2.5	65	180	0
(*Tyson* Trimmed & Ready)	110	24.0	0	1.5	55	110	0
thin (*Perdue Fit & Easy*), 2.8-oz. pc.	80	17.0	0	1.0	50	30	0
thin (*Tyson* Thin & Fancy Fillet)	120	28.0	0	1.0	60	30	0
thin (*Tyson* Trimmed & Ready)	110	23.0	0	2.5	65	180	0

Food and Measure	cal.	prot. (gms)	carbo. (gms)	fat (gms)	chol. (mgs)	sod. (mgs)	fiber (gms)
Chicken, frozen/refrigerated, raw *(cont.)*							
breast, bone-/skinless, marinated (*Foster Farms Savory Selections*), ½ pc., 3.6 oz.:							
lemon herb	110	20.0	4.0	1.5	65	360	0
peppercorn bacon .	100	21.0	2.0	1.5	30	660	0
teriyaki	120	21.0	7.0	1.5	35	410	0
breast, bone-/skinless, marinated (*Perdue Perfect Portions*), 4.8-oz. pc.:							
garlic, white wine . .	140	29.0	1.0	3.0	75	520	0
herb and pepper Italian	130	27.0	2.0	1.5	105	480	0
teriyaki	160	28.0	7.0	1.5	65	640	0
tomato basil	140	26.0	3.0	1.5	65	690	0
breast, breaded, 1 pc.:							
(*Bell & Evans*), 5.25 oz.	240	27.0	15.0	7.0	60	570	<1.0
(*Bell & Evans* Gluten Free), 5.25 oz. . .	270	27.0	19.0	9.0	55	530	3.0
(*Empire Kosher* Continental), 6.25 oz.	380	27.0	30.0	16.0	70	550	<1.0
garlic Parmesan (*Bell & Evans*) . .	230	27.0	11.0	8.0	65	620	<1.0
garlic Parmesan (*Bell & Evans* Gluten Free)	280	28.0	15.0	12.0	70	600	2.0
Kiev (*Empire Kosher*), 6.25 oz.	590	27.0	24.0	43.0	70	850	0
portobello (*Empire Kosher*), 6.25 oz.	370	27.0	27.0	17.0	70	640	<1.0
breast tenderloin:							
(*Perdue Fit & Easy*)	120	26.0	0	1.0	75	45	0
(*Perdue Tender & Tasty*)	110	22.0	1.0	2.0	85	340	0
(*Tyson Individually Fresh Frozen*) . . .	100	22.0	0	.5	70	110	0
breast tenders (*Tyson*)	100	22.0	0	.5	70	110	0
breast tenders, breaded:							
(*Bell & Evans*)	190	20.0	13.0	6.0	45	440	1.0

Food and Measure	cal.	prot. (gms)	carbo. (gms)	fat (gms)	chol. (mgs)	sod. (mgs)	fiber (gms)
(*Empire Kosher*), 3 pcs., 3 oz.	220	21.0	26.0	3.0	35	490	<1.0
coconut (*Bell & Evans*)	180	18.0	16.0	5.0	45	370	<1.0
drumstick:							
(*Empire Kosher*) ..	160	19.0	0	9.0	80	380	0
(*Perdue*), 2.2-oz. pc.	110	14.0	0	6.0	80	65	0
(*Perdue Oven Stuffer*), 3.6-oz. pc.	190	25.0	0	11.0	125	85	0
(*Perdue Tender & Tasty*)	140	20.0	0	6.0	110	340	0
(*Tyson*)	150	18.0	0	9.0	95	180	0
drumstick, skinless:							
(*Perdue*), 2 pcs., 3.5 oz.	150	24.0	0	5.0	120	100	0
(*Tyson*)	110	19.0	0	4.5	100	180	0
ground, see "Chicken, ground"							
leg, whole (*Perdue*), 5.6-oz. pc.	370	33.0	0	27.0	200	105	0
leg quarters:							
(*Empire Kosher*) ..	210	20.0	0	14.0	90	225	0
(*Perdue Tender & Tasty*)	210	15.0	2.0	17.0	105	410	0
(*Tyson*)	190	18.0	0	13.0	85	180	0
nuggets:							
(*Bell & Evans*)	190	20.0	13.0	6.0	45	440	1.0
(*Bell & Evans* Gluten Free)	180	19.0	12.0	6.0	45	440	1.0
(*Empire Kosher*), 5 pcs., 2.9 oz. ..	230	16.0	2.0	7.0	25	610	0
patties, breaded:							
(*Bell & Evans*)	240	19.0	11.0	14.0	60	300	1.0
(*Bell & Evans* Gluten Free)	230	19.0	13.0	12.0	55	390	2.0
Italian style (*Bell & Evans* Gluten Free)	270	18.0	15.0	16.0	55	610	2.0
w/mozzarella (*Bell & Evans*)	270	18.0	14.0	16.0	55	540	1.0
tenderloin or tenders, see "breast" above							
thigh:							
(*Empire Kosher* Fresh)	220	19.0	0	16.0	95	220	0

Food and Measure	cal.	prot. (gms)	carbo. (gms)	fat (gms)	chol. (mgs)	sod. (mgs)	fiber (gms)
Chicken, frozen/refrigerated, raw, thigh *(cont.)*							
(*Empire Kosher* Quick Frozen)	200	17.0	0	14.0	85	420	0
(*Perdue Tender & Tasty*)	230	17.0	0	18.0	100	310	0
(*Tyson*)	220	16.0	0	17.0	90	170	0
thigh, bone-/skinless:							
(*Perdue Fit & Easy*)	140	22.0	0	6.0	110	80	0
(*Perdue Tender & Tasty*)	140	17.0	0	8.0	105	450	0
(*Perdue Tender & Tasty Individually Frozen*)	160	18.0	0	12.0	105	370	0
(*Tyson Individually Fresh Frozen*)	170	17.0	0	11.0	70	270	0
cutlet (*Tyson*)	130	18.0	0	7.0	90	160	0
thigh, skinless:							
(*Perdue*), 2.7-oz. pc.	160	18.0	0	10.0	100	60	0
(*Tyson*)	130	18.0	0	7.0	90	160	0
wings:							
(*Perdue Tender & Tasty*)	190	17.0	2.0	13.0	100	370	0
(*Perdue Tender & Tasty Individually Frozen*)	210	18.0	0	15.0	105	310	0
(*Tyson*)	220	17.0	0	17.0	105	190	0
Chicken, frozen/ refrigerated, cooked (see also "Chicken entree, frozen"):							
whole, roasted, 3 oz.:							
(*Tyson*)	160	16.0	1.0	11.0	75	490	1.0
dark (*Perdue*)	210	17.0	0	16.0	110	55	0
dark (*Perdue Oven Stuffer*)	210	18.0	0	15.0	100	60	0
white (*Perdue*)	170	21.0	0	10.0	85	45	0
white (*Perdue Oven Stuffer*)	170	21.0	0	9.0	80	50	0
Alfredo (*Bell & Evans*), 4 oz.	200	18.0	3.0	14.0	75	360	
barbecue (*Empire Kosher*), 5 oz.	225	22.0	8.0	12.0	85	780	0
barbecue sauce w/shredded, ¼ cup:							

Food and Measure	cal.	prot. (gms)	carbo. (gms)	fat (gms)	chol. (mgs)	sod. (mgs)	fiber (gms)
honey hickory sauce (*Lloyd's*)	90	6.0	12.0	2.0	20	490	0
original (*Lloyd's*) . .	90	6.0	11.0	2.0	20	440	<1.0
bites, breaded (*Tyson Any'tizers*), 4 pcs., 3.2 oz.:							
cheddar bacon	240	16.0	12.0	14.0	40	600	0
cheddar jalapeno . .	200	13.0	13.0	11.0	35	450	3.0
bites, breaded, mini (*Tyson Any'tizers*), 13 pcs., 3 oz.	270	13.0	15.0	18.0	40	400	1.0
breast, bone-in, half, roasted, 1 pc.:							
(*Tyson*), 6.3 oz. . . .	320	42.0	2.0	16.0	135	830	0
barbecue (*Tyson*), 6.7 oz.	300	36.0	14.0	12.0	135	1050	0
breast, bone-/skinless, roasted (*Tyson*), 4.5-oz. pc.	160	31.0	1.0	3.0	85	720	0
breast, carved (*Perdue Short Cuts*), ½ cup:							
grilled	90	16.0	1.0	2.5	60	470	0
grilled, Italian	100	17.0	2.0	2.0	75	480	0
honey-roasted	90	17.0	2.0	2.0	55	480	0
roasted	90	16.0	0	2.0	80	450	0
Southwest	90	17.0	2.0	2.0	55	520	0
breast, carved, w/sauce (*Perdue Mealtime Starters*), ½ cup:							
Alfredo	150	19.0	5.0	7.0	90	890	0
marinara	130	18.0	8.0	3.0	80	710	0
roast, w/gravy	120	16.0	5.0	4.0	75	700	0
breast, diced, 3 oz.:							
(*Tyson*)	90	20.0	0	1.0	45	250	0
roasted (*Tyson*) . . .	110	19.0	2.0	2.5	60	370	1.0
breast, stuffed, 1 pc.:							
apple cherry (*Hans' All Natural*), 4 oz.	220	18.0	18.0	8.0	55	160	2.0
broccoli (*Empire Kosher*), 5 oz. . .	190	18.0	10.0	9.0	50	670	1.0
broccoli cheese (*Hans' All Natural*), 4 oz.	190	21.0	1.0	11.0	55	300	1.0

Food and Measure	cal.	prot. (gms)	carbo. (gms)	fat (gms)	chol. (mgs)	sod. (mgs)	fiber (gms)
Chicken, frozen/refrigerated, cooked, breast, stuffed *(cont.)*							
pesto (*Hans' All Natural*), 4 oz. . . .	170	21.0	1.0	9.0	50	280	<1.0
smoked turkey and cheese (*Hans' All Natural*), 4 oz. . . .	190	23.0	4.0	9.0	55	200	<1.0
spinach/feta (*Hans' All Natural*), 4 oz.	170	21.0	1.0	9.0	50	280	<1.0
vegetables (*Empire Kosher*), 5 oz. . . .	190	18.0	11.0	9.0	50	670	1.0
breast chunks, breaded, glazed (*Perdue*), 3 oz.:							
barbecue (26 oz.) . .	190	11.0	17.0	8.0	25	630	0
barbecue (48 oz.) . .	170	11.0	17.0	6.0	25	630	0
bourbon	180	12.0	17.0	8.0	25	360	0
Buffalo	180	13.0	14.0	8.0	35	650	0
General Tso's	190	12.0	16.0	8.0	25	610	0
honey barbecue . . .	180	12.0	17.0	8.0	55	520	0
honey Dijon	220	13.0	15.0	13.0	35	510	0
honey mustard	140	11.0	19.0	3.0	25	630	0
breast cutlet, breaded, baked, 3-oz. pc.:							
(*Perdue*)	160	12.0	12.0	7.0	50	470	0
Italian (*Perdue*) . . .	160	13.0	10.0	8.0	35	520	0
breast fillet:							
breaded (*Empire Kosher*), 3 oz. . .	250	19.0	26.0	7.0	35	580	<1.0
breaded (*Tyson*), 4.6-oz. pc.	240	19.0	20.0	9.0	30	680	0
w/gravy (*Hormel*), 5.7 oz.	120	20.0	4.0	3.0	55	1070	0
mesquite (*Tyson*), 3 oz.	130	17.0	1.0	7.0	45	540	0
teriyaki (*Tyson*), 3.1 oz.	170	20.0	7.0	7.0	55	620	0
breast fillet, grilled:							
(*Bell & Evans*), 2.75 oz.	80	18.0	1.0	.5	50	260	0
Buffalo style (*Bell & Evans*), 3 oz. . . .	110	24.0	0	1.0	65	340	0
honey barbecue (*Bell & Evans*), 3.25 oz.	120	22.0	6.0	1.0	55	170	0
breast tenderloin, see "tenderloin," below							

Food and Measure	cal.	prot. (gms)	carbo. (gms)	fat (gms)	chol. (mgs)	sod. (mgs)	fiber (gms)
Buffalo, in crust (*Michelina's Lean Gourmet*), 11 pcs., 3 oz.	190	10.0	23.0	7.0	10	480	1.0
chunks w/sauce (*Simply Simmered*), 5 oz.:							
garlic	140	16.0	10.0	4.0	15	750	3.0
sesame	180	15.0	26.0	2.5	10	750	5.0
sweet and sour . . .	180	15.0	26.0	2.5	10	750	5.0
Szechuan	180	19.0	16.0	4.5	10	810	5.0
teriyaki	190	16.0	23.0	3.5	20	950	1.0
drumstick, roasted (*Tyson*), 2.4 oz. . . .	130	18.0	1.0	6.0	95	500	0
drumsticks and thighs, breaded (*Empire Kosher*), 3 oz.	260	17.0	26.0	9.0	45	520	<1.0
finger, breaded (*Barber Foods*), 3.3-oz. pc.:							
All American	190	16.0	15.0	8.0	35	460	<1.0
Buffalo	160	15.0	18.0	3.5	35	380	<1.0
Italian	190	15.0	15.0	8.0	35	560	<1.0
fries, breaded, 7 pcs.:							
(*Tyson Any'tizers* Homestyle), 3.2 oz.	230	13.0	19.0	11.0	25	590	1.0
ranch (*Tyson Any'tizers*), 3.2 oz.	230	14.0	14.0	13.0	40	560	1.0
ground, see "Chicken, ground"							
medallions, w/sauce (*Tyson*), 5 oz.:							
Italian herb	120	18.0	7.0	2.0	40	640	0
sesame teriyaki . . .	190	18.0	22.0	3.0	50	740	0
white wine/garlic . .	140	19.0	3.0	6.0	45	500	1.0
nuggets:							
(*Applegate Farms*), 7 pcs., 3.1 oz. . .	180	13.0	13.0	10.0	35	230	0
(*Barber Foods*), 4 pcs., 3 oz.	150	14.0	12.0	12.0	35	340	0
(*Empire Kosher*), 5 pcs., 2.9 oz. . .	230	16.0	26.0	7.0	25	610	2.0
(*Foster Farms* Breast), 4 pcs., 2.8 oz. . .	160	13.0	9.0	9.0	25	360	1.0
(*Perdue* Breast Fresh), 5 pcs., 3 oz.	200	10.0	14.0	12.0	50	490	0

Food and Measure	cal.	prot. (gms)	carbo. (gms)	fat (gms)	chol. (mgs)	sod. (mgs)	fiber (gms)
Chicken, frozen/refrigerated, cooked, nuggets *(cont.)*							
(*Perdue* Breast Frozen), 5 pcs., 3.4 oz.	230	12.0	14.0	14.0	60	550	0
(*Tyson*), 5 pcs., 3.2 oz.	280	14.0	16.0	18.0	40	480	0
(*Tyson* Breast), 5 pcs., 3.2 oz. ..	280	13.0	21.0	16.0	50	430	0
baked, whole grain (*Perdue*), 4 pcs., 2.8 oz.	160	12.0	12.0	7.0	50	470	0
w/broccoli, cheddar (*Alexia Chicken Nuggets*), 6 pcs.	200	11.0	13.0	12.0	30	420	>1.0
w/cheese (*Perdue Fresh*), 5 pcs., 3 oz.	210	11.0	12.0	13.0	50	480	0
w/cheese (*Perdue* Frozen), 6 pcs., 3 oz.	220	11.0	13.0	13.0	40	470	0
honey crunch (*Barber Foods*), 5 pcs.	300	15.0	20.0	18.0	45	460	<1.0
Southern style (*Tyson*), 6 pcs., 3 oz.	270	10.0	11.0	21.0	45	570	1.0
spinach, feta (*Alexia Chicken Nuggets*), 6 pcs., 3 oz.	200	11.0	13.0	12.0	30	330	2.0
nuggets, stuffed (*Barber Foods*), 3 pcs.:							
artichoke Parmesan	220	13.0	9.0	15.0	40	480	<1.0
cheddar and bacon	240	14.0	8.0	17.0	45	520	<1.0
cheese, four	230	14.0	9.0	16.0	45	570	<1.0
ham and cheese ...	220	21.0	11.0	15.0	40	510	<1.0
onion, caramelized .	220	13.0	9.0	15.0	45	580	<1.0
patties, breast, breaded, 1 pc.:							
(*Foster Farms*), 4 oz.	240	16.0	18.0	12.0	40	490	0
(*Tyson*), 2.6 oz. ...	180	10.0	12.0	11.0	25	300	1.0
baked (*Perdue*), 4 oz.	230	18.0	14.0	12.0	75	750	0
Southern style (*Tyson*), 2.6 oz. .	240	9.0	10.0	18.0	40	490	1.0
pesto (*Bell & Evans*), 4 oz.	260	16.0	3.0	21.0	60	350	0
popcorn, breaded: (*Perdue* 26 oz.), 3 oz.	220	12.0	19.0	11.0	50	610	0

Food and Measure	cal.	prot. (gms)	carbo. (gms)	fat (gms)	chol. (mgs)	sod. (mgs)	fiber (gms)
(*Perdue* 44 oz.), 3 oz.	200	12.0	19.0	9.0	50	610	0
(*Tyson Any'tizers*), 6 pcs., 2.8 oz. . .	220	12.0	19.0	10.0	25	670	1.0
(*Tyson Popcorn Chicken Bites*), 6 pcs., 2.9 oz. . .	250	14.0	22.0	12.0	30	760	2.0
Buffalo (*Tyson*), 5 pcs., 2.9 oz. . .	170	14.0	11.0	8.0	35	870	1.0
strips, breaded:							
(*Barber Foods* Homestyle), 3 pcs.	260	16.0	26.0	11.0	30	1160	<1.0
(*Louis Rich/Oscar Mayer* Restaurant Style), 3 oz.	170	15.0	14.0	6.0	30	800	0
(*Perdue* Homestyle), 2 pcs., 3 oz.	230	15.0	21.0	9.0	35	593	0
Buffalo (*Perdue*), 2 pcs. 3 oz.	180	14.0	14.0	7.0	35	690	0
Buffalo (*Tyson*), 2 pcs., 3.5 oz. . .	230	14.0	21.0	10.0	45	1250	1.0
crispy (*Tyson*), 2 pcs., 3.3 oz. . .	200	16.0	13.0	10.0	30	520	1.0
strips, breast, 3 oz.:							
(*Tyson*)	120	21.0	1.0	3.5	60	500	0
Buffalo (*Tyson*) . . .	110	21.0	2.0	1.5	65	450	1.0
fajita (*Tyson*)	110	19.0	3.0	2.0	60	450	0
grilled (*Foster Farms*)	100	19.0	2.0	1.5	25	550	0
grilled (*Perdue*) . . .	100	18.0	1.0	2.0	45	470	0
grilled (*Tyson*)	110	19.0	2.0	3.0	50	480	0
grilled, Italian or Southwest (*Louis Rich/Oscar Mayer*)	110	19.0	1.0	3.0	55	770	0
honey-roasted (*Louis Rich/Oscar Mayer*)	130	22.0	3.0	2.5	60	780	0
oven-roasted (*Louis Rich/Oscar Mayer*)	130	22.0	1.0	2.5	60	790	0
Southwest (*Tyson*) .	110	18.0	2.0	3.0	40	400	0
Southwest (*Tyson* Refrigerated) . . .	120	22.0	2.0	2.5	60	250	0
strips, fajita (*Tyson*), 3 oz.	110	17.0	1.0	4.0	55	540	0
tenderloin, breaded:							
(*Foster Farms*), 2 pcs., 3.9 oz. . .	220	17.0	20.0	9.0	35	460	0

Food and Measure	cal.	prot. (gms)	carbo. (gms)	fat (gms)	chol. (mgs)	sod. (mgs)	fiber (gms)
Chicken, frozen/refrigerated, cooked, tenderloin, breaded *(cont.)*							
(*Tyson*), 2.4-oz. pc.	150	10.0	12.0	7.0	20	370	1.0
baked (*Perdue*), 3 oz.	170	12.0	15.0	7.0	50	490	0
Southern (*Tyson*), 2.4-oz. pc.	150	10.0	9.0	7.0	20	360	1.0
spicy (*Tyson*), 2.4-oz. pc.	160	11.0	13.0	7.0	20	620	0
tenders, breaded:							
(*Perdue*), 3 pcs., 3 oz.	180	12.0	13.0	9.0	50	400	0
(*Tyson*), 5 pcs., 3 oz.	240	12.0	15.0	14.0	35	330	0
(*Tyson* Breast), 3 oz.	220	13.0	14.0	12.0	30	350	1.0
honey batter (*Tyson*), 5 pcs., 3 oz.	220	13.0	13.0	13.0	35	250	2.0
thigh, roasted, 1 pc.:							
(*Perdue*), 3.2 oz. . .	240	17.0	0	19.0	115	65	0
(*Tyson*), 3.5 oz. . . .	260	19.0	1.0	20.0	110	620	0
wings, 4 pcs., except as noted:							
barbecue (*Tyson* Any'tizers*), 3 pcs.	200	15.0	7.0	13.0	110	380	0
Buffalo, hot (*Tyson*)	220	20.0	1.0	15.0	110	560	1.0
chipotle (*Foster Farms*)	190	15.0	1.0	14.0	80	430	0
honey barbecue (*Bell & Evans*), 3 pcs.	160	17.0	6.0	8.0	80	240	0
honey barbecue (*Foster Farms*) . .	170	13.0	5.0	10.0	50	390	0
honey barbecue (*Tyson*)	220	15.0	9.0	14.0	95	450	0
hot/spicy (*Foster Farms*)	170	14.0	1.0	13.0	55	460	0
hot/spicy (*Tyson*) . .	220	20.0	1.0	15.0	110	560	0
tequila lime (*Tyson*)	200	20.0	2.0	13.0	125	690	0
teriyaki (*Tyson*) . . .	200	19.0	4.0	12.0	110	390	0
wings, breaded:							
Buffalo (*Perdue*), 2 pcs.	180	14.0	4.0	12.0	80	720	0
Buffalo (*Tyson* Wyngs*), 3 pcs. . . .	130	12.0	7.0	6.0	25	670	0
Buffalo (*Tyson* Any'tizers* Wyngs), 3 pcs.	150	12.0	8.0	7.0	30	680	0

Food and Measure	cal.	prot. (gms)	carbo. (gms)	fat (gms)	chol. (mgs)	sod. (mgs)	fiber (gms)
honey barbecue (*Tyson Any'tizers* Wyngs), 3 pcs. . . .	200	11.0	20.0	8.0	25	450	0
smoky barbecue (*Tyson* Wyngs), 3 pcs.	190	13.0	16.0	8.0	20	530	0
teriyaki (*Tyson* Wyngs), 3 pcs. . . .	220	13.0	21.0	10.0	15	590	0
wings, roasted, hot and spicy (*Tyson*), 3 pcs., 3 oz.	180	16.0	1.0	12.0	80	780	0
Chicken, ground:							
raw, 4 oz.:							
(*Empire Kosher*) . .	150	18.0	1.0	9.0	65	500	0
(*Organic Prairie*) . .	200	21.0	1.0	12.0	95	90	0
(*Perdue*)	180	19.0	0	12.0	135	75	0
breast (*Perdue Fit & Easy*)	100	24.0	0	.5	65	75	0
burgers (*Bell & Evans*)	160	22.0	0	7.0	90	240	0
patties (*Perdue*) . . .	170	19.0	0	11.0	130	75	0
cooked, 3 oz.:							
(*Perdue*)	170	18.0	0	11.0	125	50	0
breast (*Perdue Fit & Easy*)	80	19.0	0	.5	55	60	0
patties (*Perdue*) . . .	170	19.0	0	11.0	130	75	0
"Chicken," vegetarian, canned:							
(*Worthington FriChik*), 2 pcs., 3.2 oz.	140	12.0	3.0	8.0	0	430	1.0
diced, drained (*Worthington* Chik), ¼ cup	50	9.0	2.0	0	0	220	1.0
"Chicken," vegetarian, frozen/refrigerated (see also " 'Chicken' entree, vegetarian"):							
cutlet (*Veggie Patch* Chick'n), 2.5 oz. . . .	140	10.0	15.0	6.0	0	380	3.0
drumstick (*Garden Gourmet*), 1.8 oz. .	90	7.0	10.0	4.0	0	400	2.0
fried w/gravy (*Loma Linda*), 2 pcs., 2.9 oz.	150	12.0	5.0	10.0	0	430	2.0

Food and Measure	cal.	prot. (gms)	carbo. (gms)	fat (gms)	chol. (mgs)	sod. (mgs)	fiber (gms)
"Chicken," vegetarian, frozen/refrigerated *(cont.)*							
nuggets, 3 oz.:							
(*Boca* Chik'n)	180	14.0	17.0	7.0	0	500	3.0
(*Morningstar Farms* Chik'n), 4 pcs. . .	190	12.0	18.0	7.0	0	490	2.0
(*Veggie Patch* Chick'n), 4 pcs. .	190	10.0	22.0	8.0	0	480	3.0
patties, 1 pc., 2.5 oz., except as noted:							
(*Boca* Chik'n)	160	11.0	15.0	6.0	0	430	2.0
(*Gardenburger* Chik'n Grill)	100	13.0	5.0	2.5	0	360	5.0
(*Morningstar Farms Chik Patties*)	150	9.0	16.0	6.0	0	540	2.0
(*Yves* Burger), 2.6 oz.	100	15.0	5.0	3.0	0	420	2.0
breaded (*Gardenburger* Chick'n) .	140	7.0	10.0	9.0	0	400	3.0
Parmesan ranch (*Morningstar Farms Chik Patties*)	170	10.0	17.0	7.0	0	680	2.0
roasted herb, w/organic soy (*Morningstar Farms*), 2.25 oz. .	110	12.0	9.0	2.5	0	340	2.0
spicy (*Boca* Chik'n)	160	11.0	15.0	6.0	0	560	2.0
roll (*Worthington* Meatless), 3/8" slice, 2 oz.	90	9.0	2.0	4.5	0	240	1.0
skewers (*Yves*), 2.8 oz.	100	15.0	7.0	1.0	0	450	4.0
slices:							
(*Worthington* Meatless), 3 pcs.	90	9.0	2.0	4.5	0	250	1.0
smoked (*Yves*), 4 pcs.	100	16.0	5.0	1.5	0	480	0
strips (*Morningstar Farms Meal Starters*), 12 pcs., 3 oz.	140	23.0	6.0	3.5	0	510	1.0
tenders (*Morningstar Farms* Chik'n), 2 pcs., 2.9 oz.	190	12.0	20.0	7.0	0	580	3.0
wings, Buffalo, 3 oz.:							
(*Boca* Chik'n Hot & Spicy)	160	14.0	14.0	7.0	0	700	3.0
(*Morningstar Farms*)	200	11.0	19.0	9.0	0	790	3.0
Chicken bologna (*Foster Farms*), 1-oz. slice	60	4.0	<1.0	5.0	25	280	0

Food and Measure	cal.	prot. (gms)	carbo. (gms)	fat (gms)	chol. (mgs)	sod. (mgs)	fiber (gms)
Chicken coating mix (see also "Batter/breading mix"), seasoned:							
(*Don's Chuck Wagon* Bake & Fry), ¼ cup	95	3.0	21.0	0	0	665	1.0
(*Golden Dipt* Fry Easy Extra Crispy), 1½ tbsp.	60	1.0	9.0	0	0	310	0
(*Golden Dipt* Fry Easy Homestyle), 2 tbsp.	50	0	9.0	0	0	660	0
(*McCormick* Season 'n Fry), 1 tbsp.	35	0	6.0	0	0	760	0
(*McCormick Bag 'n Season*), 1 tbsp.	20	0	3.0	0	0	460	0
(*Oven Fry* Extra Crispy), ⅛ pkg.	60	2.0	10.0	1.0	0	420	0
(*Oven Fry* Homestyle Flour), 1/8 pkg. . . .	40	1.0	7.0	1.0	0	470	0
(*Shake 'n Bake* w/Bag), 1 tbsp.	40	1.0	7.0	1.0	0	220	0
barbecue glaze (*Shake 'n Bake*), 1 tbsp.	45	0	9.0	1.0	0	410	0
Cajun (*Luzianne*), 2 tbsp.	100	3.0	20.0	1.0	0	1260	1.0
country (*McCormick Bag 'n Season*), 2 tsp.	25	0	3.0	1.0	0	880	0
garlic herb (*Shake 'n Bake*), 1 tbsp.	35	1.0	7.0	0	0	190	0
herbs/spice (*Golden Dipt* Fry Easy), 2 tbsp.	70	0	13.0	0	0	490	0
hot and spicy (*Golden Dipt* Fry Easy), 2 tbsp.	50	0	9.0	0	0	430	0
hot and spicy (*Shake 'n Bake*), 1 tbsp.	35	1.0	7.0	1.0	0	170	0
Italian (*Shake 'n Bake*), 1 tbsp.	35	1.0	7.0	.5	0	280	0
Parmesan crust (*Shake 'n Bake* Chicken/ Pork), 1 tbsp.	35	1.0	7.0	.5	0	290	0
ranch and herb crust (*Shake 'n Bake* Chicken/Pork), 1 tbsp.	35	1.0	7.0	0	0	300	0

Food and Measure	cal.	prot. (gms)	carbo. (gms)	fat (gms)	chol. (mgs)	sod. (mgs)	fiber (gms)
Chicken dinner, frozen, 1 pkg.:							
asiago, portobello (*Healthy Choice*), 12.5 oz.	310	21.0	43.0	5.0	30	580	7.0
blackened (*Healthy Choice*), 11 oz.	310	16.0	46.0	6.0	15	600	6.0
boneless (*Swanson Hungry-Man*), 1 lb.	860	32.0	86.0	44.0	110	1300	6.0
breaded, country (*Healthy Choice*), 10.6 oz.	370	15.0	53.0	9.0	25	560	6.0
broccoli Alfredo (*Healthy Choice*), 11.5 oz.	300	17.0	46.0	5.0	25	430	8.0
carbonara w/noodles (*Stouffer's*), 15 oz. .	670	40.0	56.0	32.0	85	1150	6.0
fettuccine Alfredo (*Stouffer's*), 16.75 oz.	620	33.0	69.0	24.0	50	1360	7.0
fiesta (*Healthy Choice*), 12.25 oz.	370	20.0	62.0	4.0	35	450	7.0
grilled (*Healthy Choice*):							
barbecue, 10.5 oz. .	270	15.0	43.0	3.0	30	430	7.0
w/barbecue sauce, smokehouse, 12 oz.	370	17.0	63.0	5.0	30	600	7.0
honey balsamic, 12 oz.	350	13.0	58.0	6.0	25	460	4.0
Monterey, 11oz. . . .	300	17.0	40.0	7.0	30	570	5.0
herb, country (*Healthy Choice*), 11.35 oz. .	240	15.0	34.0	5.0	30	600	5.0
honey glazed (*Healthy Choice*), 11 oz.	280	15.0	39.0	6.0	30	590	7.0
Monterey (*Stouffer's*), 14.25 oz.	530	31.0	54.0	21.0	80	1300	5.0
parmigiana (*Healthy Choice*), 11.6 oz. . .	370	16.0	56.0	9.0	15	500	6.0
roast (*Healthy Choice*), 11.4 oz.	290	16.0	39.0	7.0	25	600	10.0
sesame, w/noodles (*Stouffer's*), 15 oz. .	590	25.0	87.0	16.0	95	1210	6.0
sweet/sour (*Healthy Choice*), 12 oz.	430	16.0	69.0	9.0	20	600	5.0

Food and Measure	cal.	prot. (gms)	carbo. (gms)	fat (gms)	chol. (mgs)	sod. (mgs)	fiber (gms)
teriyaki (*Healthy Choice*), 11 oz.	280	15.0	44.0	4.0	25	550	8.0
Chicken entree, can/ pkg. (see also "Chicken entree, microwave"):							
à la king (*Swanson*), 10.5-oz. can	270	14.0	12.0	18.0	20	1370	2.0
Alfredo, cheesy (*Banquet Homestyle Bakes*), ¾ cup filling, ½ cup pasta	400	14.0	36.0	22.0	45	970	2.0
and biscuits, ⅕ pkg.:							
(*Banquet Homestyle Bakes* Country) .	250	7.0	31.0	11.0	10	930	2.0
buttermilk (*Betty Crocker Complete Meals*)	280	9.0	37.0	11.0	15	950	2.0
creamy (*Banquet Homestyle Bakes*)	350	11.0	39.0	18.0	15	1050	6.0
breast, 4-oz. pouch:							
w/barbecue sauce (*Bumble Bee Prime Fillet*)	170	29.0	10.0	1.5	80	740	0
garlic herb (*Bumble Bee Prime Fillet*)	110	24.0	1.0	1.5	75	490	0
Southwest (*Bumble Bee Prime Fillet*)	120	26.0	<1.0	1.0	80	580	0
cheese, three (*Betty Crocker Complete Meals*), ⅕ pkg.	240	8.0	35.0	7.0	10	870	1.0
chow mein (*La Choy*), 1 cup	100	8.0	10.0	3.0	20	1210	2.0
and dumplings:							
(*Banquet Homestyle Bakes*), ¼ pkg. . . .	230	14.0	33.0	4.5	30	1560	3.0
(*Betty Crocker Complete Meals* Homestyle), ⅕ pkg. . . .	240	8.0	34.0	9.0	15	870	2.0
(*Dinty Moore*), 1 cup	230	12.0	28.0	8.0	35	900	1.0
(*Dinty Moore*), 7.5-oz. can	190	11.0	24.0	6.0	25	890	1.0
(*Luck's*), 1 cup	170	12.0	21.0	4.5	29	1030	2.0
(*Swanson*), 1 cup .	230	11.0	24.0	10.0	35	990	2.0

Food and Measure	cal.	prot. (gms)	carbo. (gms)	fat (gms)	chol. (mgs)	sod. (mgs)	fiber (gms)
Chicken entree, can/pkg. *(cont.)*							
fettuccine (*Betty Crocker Complete Meals*), ⅕ pkg.	240	10.0	31.0	9.0	20	880	1.0
w/pasta, ⅙ pkg.:							
cheesy (*Campbell's Supper Bakes*) . .	170	6.0	28.0	4.0	5	840	1.0
garlic (*Campbell's Supper Bakes*) . .	220	9.0	42.0	1.5	<5	760	2.0
w/rice, ⅙ pkg.:							
herb (*Campbell's Supper Bakes*) . .	180	4.0	38.0	1.5	<5	780	1.0
lemon, herb (*Campbell's Supper Bakes*)	190	4.0	39.0	1.5	<5	780	1.0
roast, w/stuffing (*Campbell's Supper Bakes* Traditional), ⅙ pkg.	160	5.0	29.0	3.0	<5	740	2.0
stew (*Dinty Moore*), 1 cup	220	12.0	17.0	11.0	35	1020	2.0
teriyaki (*La Choy* Bi-Pack), 1 cup	120	7.0	16.0	3.5	20	1370	3.0
Chicken entree, frozen (see also "Chicken, frozen/refrigerated, cooked"), 1 pkg., except as noted:							
à la king (*Stouffer's*), 11.5 oz.	360	18.0	44.0	12.0	35	800	0
Alfredo:							
(*Birds Eye Voila!*), 1 cup*	320	14.0	26.0	17.0	60	480	2.0
(*Birds Eye Voila! Family Skillets*), 1 cup*	250	14.0	35.0	6.0	5	830	3.0
(*Contessa*):							
w/out sauce, 6 oz.	190	15.0	26.0	1.5	30	180	1.0
w/sauce, 9 oz. . .	290	20.0	28.0	10.0	50	700	1.0
(*Green Giant* Complete Skillet Meal), 1¼ cups*	270	17.0	39.0	6.0	30	760	3.0
(*Stouffer's Skillets*), ½ of 25-oz. pkg.	410	28.0	49.0	11.0	60	1080	2.0

Food and Measure	cal.	prot. (gms)	carbo. (gms)	fat (gms)	chol. (mgs)	sod. (mgs)	fiber (gms)
blackened (*Zatarain's* New Orleans), 10.5 oz.	500	23.0	46.0	25.0	110	1320	2.0
w/broccoli (*Lean Cuisine One Dish Favorites*), 10 oz.	260	17.0	34.0	6.0	35	660	3.0
Florentine (*Michelina's Lean Gourmet*), 8 oz. .	250	12.0	34.0	7.0	40	690	2.0
grilled, w/broccoli (*Michelina's Signature*), 10 oz.	410	21.0	39.0	17.0	75	740	2.0
spinach (*Organic Classics*), 9.5 oz.	360	14.0	36.0	12.0	55	570	2.0
w/almonds (*Lean Cuisine*), 8.5 oz.	260	17.0	34.0	6.0	30	490	3.0
arrabiata, penne (*Ethnic Gourmet*), 10 oz. . .	340	28.0	37.0	9.0	60	900	5.0
arroz con pollo (*Jeff Nathan Creations*), 10 oz.	340	26.0	40.0	26.0	65	1220	4.0
baked:							
(*Lean Cuisine*), 8.625 oz.	240	15.0	34.0	4.5	25	650	3.0
breast (*Stouffer's*), 8.9 oz.	250	20.0	20.0	10.0	60	730	1.0
balsamic glazed (*Lean Cuisine Dinnertime Selects*), 12 oz. . . .	350	24.0	43.0	9.0	40	810	6.0
basil:							
cream sauce (*Lean Cuisine*), 8.5 oz. .	280	18.0	35.0	7.0	35	470	2.0
creamy (*Lean Cuisine*), 10.5 oz. . .	290	22.0	34.0	7.0	35	640	2.0
barbecue:							
(*Banquet* BBQ), 10 oz.	250	13.0	31.0	6.0	25	890	5.0
honey mango (*Smart Ones Fruit Inspirations*), 9 oz.	240	9.0	34.0	3.5	30	490	0
biryani (*Ethnic Gourmet*), 10 oz. . .	390	16.0	54.0	12.0	20	1080	4.0
blackened, yellow rice (*Zatarain's* New Orleans), 10.5 oz. .	460	19.0	67.0	13.0	30	1250	2.0

Food and Measure	cal.	prot. (gms)	carbo. (gms)	fat (gms)	chol. (mgs)	sod. (mgs)	fiber (gms)
Chicken entree, frozen *(cont.)*							
breast, strips, breaded, w/potato (*Healthy Choice*), 8 oz.	200	11.0	31.0	3.0	25	600	5.0
breast, stuffed, 6-oz. pc., except as noted: (*Barber Foods Homestyle*)	280	21.0	24.0	11.0	45	860	<2.0
asparagus cheese (*Barber Foods*) . .	320	26.0	17.0	17.0	70	400	<1.0
broccoli cheese (*Barber Foods*) . .	290	23.0	16.0	15.0	65	510	<2.0
broccoli cheese (*Barber Foods* Reduced Fat), 5.5 oz.	250	25.0	11.0	13.0	55	610	<2.0
broccoli cheese (*Tyson*)	310	17.0	23.0	16.0	50	590	2.0
broccoli, cheese, ham (*Barber Foods*), 5 oz. . . .	240	22.0	16.0	10.0	45	520	<2.0
Cordon Bleu (*Barber Foods*)	320	29.0	15.0	16.0	75	640	<1.0
Cordon Bleu (*Barber Foods* Reduced Fat), 5.5 oz.	260	27.0	11.0	13.0	75	700	0
Cordon Bleu (*Tyson*)	380	22.0	20.0	24.0	80	790	1.0
crème brie and apple (*Barber Foods*) . .	340	25.0	23.0	16.0	70	710	<1.0
Kiev (*Barber Foods*)	380	26.0	15.0	24.0	95	390	<1.0
Kiev (*Tyson*)	480	17.0	19.0	37.0	150	420	1.0
Parmesan (*Barber Foods*), 5 oz. . . .	250	19.0	17.0	12.0	45	440	<1.0
scallop and lobster (*Barber Foods*) . .	340	25.0	22.0	17.0	70	520	<1.0
Caesar, grilled (*Lean Cuisine*), 9 oz.	230	19.0	24.0	6.0	30	690	3.0
cacciatore: (*Contessa*), 1½ cups	240	16.0	28.0	7.0	40	870	3.0
w/penne (*Organic Classics*), 10 oz. . .	270	20.0	37.0	4.0	40	390	3.0
Cajun style, w/shrimp (*Healthy Choice Café Steamers*), 10.4 oz.	250	18.0	36.0	3.0	40	600	3.0

Food and Measure	cal.	prot. (gms)	carbo. (gms)	fat (gms)	chol. (mgs)	sod. (mgs)	fiber (gms)
carbonara:							
(*Lean Cuisine*), 9 oz.	270	19.0	33.0	7.0	30	620	2.0
(*Smart Ones*), 9.5 oz.	250	20.0	32.0	4.5	40	660	2.0
cashew (*Contessa*):							
w/sauce, 8 oz.	260	14.0	39.0	5.0	25	730	3.0
w/out sauce, 7 oz. .	200	13.0	27.0	5.0	25	120	3.0
cheese, three:							
(*Birds Eye Voila!*),							
1 cup*	210	13.0	21.0	8.0	30	940	2.0
(*Lean Cuisine*), 8 oz.	220	21.0	14.0	9.0	45	520	2.0
(*Michelina's Lean*							
Gourmet), 8 oz. .	300	14.0	41.0	8.0	40	750	1.0
cheesy (*Birds Eye*							
Voila!), 1 cup*	250	14.0	35.0	6.0	5	830	3.0
chicken fried (*Miche-*							
lina's Signature), 9 oz.	290	15.0	35.0	10.0	125	610	3.0
w/cilantro salsa (*Em-*							
pire Kosher), 10 oz.	260	24.0	27.0	6.0	50	810	2.0
citrus (*Contessa*):							
w/sauce, 8 oz.	220	13.0	26.0	1.5	30	590	4.0
w/out sauce, 6 oz. .	160	10.0	16.0	1.5	30	180	3.0
chow mein, w/rice:							
(*Contessa*):							
w/sauce, 8 oz. ..	340	20.0	53.0	4.0	30	640	54.0
w/out sauce, 7 oz.	280	19.0	40.0	4.0	30	280	5.0
(*Lean Cuisine One*							
Dish Favorites),							
9 oz.	260	14.0	41.0	4.0	25	550	3.0
curry, w/rice:							
(*Contessa*):							
w/sauce, 8 oz. ..	230	12.0	30.0	6.0	25	520	3.0
w/out sauce, 6 oz.	160	12.0	25.0	1.5	25	150	2.0
coconut, w/vege-							
tables (*Ethnic*							
Gourmet Kaeng							
Kary Kai), 10 oz.	390	20.0	54.0	11.0	35	770	2.0
Malay (*Ethnic Gour-*							
met), 10 oz.	410	18.0	59.0	11.0	35	530	3.0
Thai style (*Organic*							
Classics), 10 oz. .	420	19.0	50.0	17.0	40	510	3.0
and dumplings:							
(*Glory* Savory), 11 oz.	290	16.0	40.0	8.0	75.0	1400	6.0
(*Glory* Savory Family							
Size), 1 cup	250	14.0	34.0	7.0	65	1200	5.0

Food and Measure	cal.	prot. (gms)	carbo. (gms)	fat (gms)	chol. (mgs)	sod. (mgs)	fiber (gms)
Chicken entree, frozen (cont.)							
(Stouffer's Skillets),							
¼ of 24-oz. pkg.	370	23.0	41.0	13.0	60	1120	5.0
dumplings, vegetables and (C&W Ultimate Stir Fry Feast):							
1½ cups w/sauce ..	190	11.0	25.0	5.0	30	1350	3.0
1½ cups w/out sauce	160	10.0	20.0	5.0	30	410	2.0
enchilada or fajita, see "Enchilada entree" and "Fajita entree"							
escalloped, and noodles:							
(Stouffer's Family),							
⅕ of 45-oz. pkg. ...	330	14.0	28.0	18.0	35	910	2.0
w/feta, rice (Ethnic Gourmet Kotopoulo Domato), 10 oz.	340	20.0	41.0	11.0	40	410	5.0
fettuccine:							
(Lean Cuisine Dinnertime Selects), 12 oz.	400	33.0	48.0	8.0	50	850	6.0
(Lean Cuisine One Dish Favorites), 9.25 oz.	270	22.0	33.0	6.0	40	690	1.0
(Michelina's Authentico), 8.5 oz.	330	14.0	40.0	12.0	40	650	2.0
(Smart Ones), 10 oz.	340	26.0	42.0	8.0	50	620	4.0
fettuccine Alfredo:							
(Healthy Choice), 8.5 oz.	210	16.0	23.0	5.0	25	570	5.0
(South Beach Living), 9.3 oz.	240	16.0	20.0	7.0	65	690	7.0
w/chicken, broccoli (Michelina's Authentico), 8.5 oz.	310	15.0	36.0	11.0	45	680	2.0
Florentine:							
(Kashi), 10 oz.	290	22.0	31.0	9.0	45	550	5.0
(Lean Cuisine), 8 oz.	200	18.0	14.0	8.0	40	660	3.0
(Lean Cuisine Dinnertime Selects), 13.25 oz.	390	28.0	52.0	8.0	45	840	6.0
fried:							
breast (Stouffer's), 8.9 oz.	360	20.0	30.0	18.0	45	880	2.0

Food and Measure	cal.	prot. (gms)	carbo. (gms)	fat (gms)	chol. (mgs)	sod. (mgs)	fiber (gms)
w/gravy, potatoes (*Michelina's Authentico*), 8 oz. . . .	290	11.0	29.0	15.0	35	930	2.0
garlic:							
(*Birds Eye Voila!*), 1 cup*	240	11.0	21.0	8.0	30	940	3.0
(*Birds Eye Voila! Family Skillets*), 1 cup*	240	11.0	29.0	8.0	20	540	3.0
herb (*South Beach Living*), 8.2 oz. . . .	240	23.0	10.0	10.0	70	550	3.0
Parmesan (*South Beach Living*), 10.1 oz.	270	26.0	22.0	10.0	55	700	8.0
roasted (*Lean Cuisine*), 8⅞ oz. . .	180	21.0	9.0	7.0	40	680	1.0
General Tso's spicy (*Healthy Choice Café Steamers*), 10.8 oz.	430	17.0	66.0	9.0	15	600	5.0
ginger garlic stir-fry (*Lean Cuisine Spa Cuisine*), 9.825 oz. . .	290	17.0	46.0	4.0	30	640	4.0
glazed:							
(*Lean Cuisine*), 8.5 oz.	220	21.0	25.0	3.5	40	500	1.0
(*Michelina's Lean Gourmet*), 8 oz. .	250	10.0	46.0	3.0	20	470	1.0
country (*Healthy Choice*), 8.5 oz. .	210	12.0	30.0	4.0	15	600	3.0
w/green beans, rice (*Michelina's Authentico*), 8 oz. . . .	250	11.0	45.0	3.5	20	850	2.0
grilled:							
(*Lean Cuisine* Fiesta), 8.5 oz.	250	19.0	31.0	5.0	40	560	2.0
barbecue sauce (*Michelina's Lean Gourmet*), 8 oz. . .	260	11.0	36.0	9.0	35	780	3.0
barbecue sauce (*Michelina's Signature*), 9 oz. . . .	290	22.0	40.0	4.5	50	920	3.0
basil (*Healthy Choice Café Steamers*), 10.6 oz.	290	20.0	37.0	6.0	25	580	5.0

Food and Measure	cal.	prot. (gms)	carbo. (gms)	fat (gms)	chol. (mgs)	sod. (mgs)	fiber (gms)
Chicken entree, frozen, grilled *(cont.)*							
herb (*Stouffer's*), 9 oz.	250	19.0	29.0	6.0	35	740	3.0
garlic herb sauce (*Smart Ones*), 9 oz.	180	19.0	10.0	8.0	50	490	2.0
lemon pepper (*Stouffer's*), 9 oz.	240	19.0	24.0	8.0	40	670	4.0
marinara (*Healthy Choice Café Steamers*), 10 oz.	250	20.0	32.0	4.0	30	550	5.0
and pasta (*Healthy Choice*), 8.5 oz. . .	210	15.0	25.0	5.0	25	480	5.0
portobello (*Stouffer's*), 9 oz.	220	18.0	23.0	6.0	35	960	3.0
w/potato (*Healthy Choice*), 8.5 oz. . .	160	11.0	18.0	3.5	25	530	3.0
primavera (*Lean Cuisine Spa Cuisine*), 9.375 oz.	220	18.0	24.0	5.0	25	610	5.0
teriyaki (*Stouffer's*), 9.38 oz.	300	21.0	45.0	3.5	40	880	3.0
teriyaki glaze (*Lean Cuisine*), 10 oz. . .	280	17.0	46.0	3.0	30	500	3.0
white meat, roasted red pepper Alfredo (*Healthy Choice Café Steamers*), 10.3 oz.	240	22.0	23.0	5.0	25	600	4.0
herb, garden (*Birds Eye Voila!*), 1 cup*	280	14.0	30.0	11.0	35	600	3.0
honey Dijon: (*Smart Ones*), 8.5 oz.	220	11.0	38.0	3.5	30	460	2.0
grilled (*Lean Cuisine*), 8 oz.	220	17.0	22.0	7.0	50	640	2.0
honey mustard (*Lean Cuisine*), 8 oz.	250	17.0	37.0	4.0	30	650	1.0
Italiano (*Contessa*):							
w/sauce, 8 oz.	340	20.0	36.0	13.0	65	720	3.0
w/out sauce, 6 oz. .	210	19.0	29.0	2.0	35	210	3.0
jerk, Jamaican style (*Organic Classics*), 9.5 oz.	270	16.0	37.0	7.0	40	620	4.0
korma (*Ethnic Gourmet*), 10 oz. . .	340	21.0	44.0	9.0	40	720	3.0

Food and Measure	cal.	prot. (gms)	carbo. (gms)	fat (gms)	chol. (mgs)	sod. (mgs)	fiber (gms)
kung pao, w/rice:							
(*Ethnic Gourmet*), 11 oz.	370	16.0	53.0	9.0	25	900	3.0
(*South Beach Living*), 8.3 oz.	250	25.0	14.0	9.0	70	630	4.0
lemon:							
(*Lean Cuisine Spa Cuisine*), 9 oz. ..	300	15.0	40.0	9.0	25	570	3.0
piccata (*Organic Classics*), 9.5 oz.	320	14.0	49.0	8.0	35	650	3.0
rosemary (*Kashi*), 10 oz.	330	17.0	45.0	9.0	15	640	5.0
lemongrass:							
(*Lean Cuisine Spa Cuisine*), 9.375 oz.	250	18.0	30.0	6.0	30	610	4.0
coconut (*Kashi*), 10 oz.	300	18.0	38.0	8.0	10	680	7.0
and basil (*Ethnic Gourmet*), 10 oz.	380	20.0	56.0	9.0	30	310	5.0
lime, w/ancho chile sauce (*Ethnic Gourmet*), 10 oz. ..	340	26.0	25.0	15.0	80	730	3.0
linguine, Alfredo sauce (*Michelina's Authentico* Tuscan-Inspired), 8 oz.	300	13.0	44.0	8.0	35	760	2.0
lo mein:							
(*Green Giant Complete Skillet Meal*), 1 cup* ...	190	12.0	31.0	2.0	20	740	3.0
(*Michelina's Yu Sing*), 8.5 oz.	230	13.0	37.0	2.5	25	1280	2.0
mandarin:							
(*Healthy Choice*), 9.1 oz.	240	13.0	39.0	2.5	15	510	5.0
(*Lean Cuisine One Dish Favorites*), 9 oz.	270	14.0	46.0	3.5	30	690	2.0
(*Michelina's Lean Gourmet*), 8 oz. ..	260	9.0	46.0	3.0	15	650	2.0
Margherita (*Healthy Choice Café Steamers*), 10 oz. ...	340	23.0	43.0	8.0	30	550	4.0

Food and Measure	cal.	prot. (gms)	carbo. (gms)	fat (gms)	chol. (mgs)	sod. (mgs)	fiber (gms)
Chicken entree, frozen *(cont.)*							
w/marinara cheese sauce (*South Beach Living Caprese Style*), 9.4 oz.	240	30.0	10.0	8.0	90	650	3.0
Marsala:							
(*Lean Cuisine*), 8⅛ oz.	140	14.0	12.0	4.0	35	620	3.0
(*Organic Classics*), 9.5 oz.	330	14.0	31.0	16.0	60	530	3.0
w/broccoli (*Smart Ones*), 9 oz.	180	20.0	10.0	7.0	50	530	2.0
w/garlic potatoes (*Michelina's Signature*), 8.5 oz. . . .	270	11.0	25.0	14.0	40	1170	2.0
pasta (*Smart Ones Mirabella*), 9.2 oz.	200	12.0	33.0	2.0	15	550	3.0
Mediterranean (*Lean Cuisine Spa Cuisine*), 10.5 oz.	240	19.0	32.0	4.0	40	590	6.0
orange:							
(*Contessa*):							
w/sauce, 9 oz. . .	350	18.0	48.0	9.0	40	710	3.0
w/out sauce, 7 oz.	280	15.0	37.0	9.0	40	210	3.0
à l'orange (*Lean Cuisine*), 9 oz. . .	260	18.0	39.0	3.0	30	580	2.0
glazed (*Michelina's Authentico*), 8.5 oz.	400	13.0	54.0	3.0	25.0	590	1.0
peel (*Lean Cuisine Dinnertime Selects*), 12 oz. .	390	15.0	63.0	9.0	25	850	3.0
sesame (*Smart Ones Fruit Inspirations*), 9 oz. . . .	320	14.0	48.0	8.0	20	680	2.0
Oriental (*Smart Ones*), 9 oz.	230	12.0	39.0	2.5	35	640	2.0
pad Thai, see "Noodle entree"							
Parmesan:							
(*Birds Eye Voila!*), 1 cup*	240	10.0	31.0	8.0	10	580	2.0
(*Boston Market*), 16 oz.	620	33.0	69.0	24.0	50	1580	7.0
(*Lean Cuisine*), 10.875 oz.	260	23.0	31.0	5.0	35	580	4.0

Food and Measure	cal.	prot. (gms)	carbo. (gms)	fat (gms)	chol. (mgs)	sod. (mgs)	fiber (gms)
(*Michelina's Lean Gourmet*), 8 oz. .	250	13.0	37.0	4.5	30	580	2.0
(*Smart Ones*), 11 oz.	290	26.0	35.0	5.0	40	630	4.0
creamy (*Smart Ones*), 9 oz.	210	23.0	12.0	8.0	70	700	3.0
parmigiana (*Stouffer's*), 12 oz.	410	23.0	47.0	14.0	40	900	4.0
pasta and/and pasta:							
(*Kashi* Pomodoro), 10 oz.	280	19.0	38.0	6.0	25	470	6.0
(*Michelina's Authentico* Castellina), 8 oz.	290	14.0	40.0	8.0	40	530	3.0
(*Stouffer's Skillets*), ½ of 25-oz. pkg.	340	28.0	42.0	7.0	40	410	6.0
broccoli bake (*Stouffer's* Family), ⅕ of 45-oz. pkg.	300	19.0	24.0	14.0	45	990	1.0
cheesy (*Green Giant* Complete Skillet Meal), 1¼ cups*	270	17.0	41.0	6.0	35	760	4.0
Cordon Bleu (*Stouffer's* Family), ¼ of 37-oz. pkg.	330	20.0	28.0	15.0	35	920	2.0
cream sauce (*Michelina's Authentico*), 8.5 oz.	380	16.0	43.0	15.0	45	830	2.0
cream sauce (*Michelina's Budget Gourmet*), 8 oz. .	290	12.0	38.0	10.0	35	800	2.0
garlic (*Green Giant* Complete Skillet Meal), 1 cup* . . .	230	13.0	33.0	6.0	30	840	4.0
garlic (*Stouffer's Corner Bistro*), 12 oz.	330	25.0	37.0	9.0	40	890	5.0
garlic (*Stouffer's Skillets*), ½ of 23-oz. pkg.	320	24.0	42.0	6.0	40	1440	6.0
peas/carrots (*Michelina's Authentico*), 8 oz.	280	15.0	35.0	10.0	45	690	2.0
pesto primavera (*Kashi*), 10 oz. . . .	290	11.0	37.0	11.0	5	750	7.0

Food and Measure	cal.	prot. (gms)	carbo. (gms)	fat (gms)	chol. (mgs)	sod. (mgs)	fiber (gms)
Chicken entree, frozen, pasta *(cont.)*							
picante (*Smart Ones*), 9 oz.	260	23.0	32.0	4.0	25	480	4.0
white sauce, noodles (*Michelina's Zap'ems*), 8 oz. .	290	12.0	38.0	10.0	35	800	2.0
peanut sauce (*Lean Cuisine Spa Cuisine*), 9 oz.	280	22.0	30.0	8.0	25	560	5.0
pecan (*Lean Cuisine Spa Cuisine*), 9 oz. .	260	19.0	32.0	6.0	30	690	4.0
penne:							
(*Lean Cuisine Dinner-time Selects*), 12 oz.	330	20.0	52.0	4.5	40	580	5.0
(*Smart Ones* Penne Pollo), 10 oz. . . .	270	14.0	43.0	6.0	45	510	3.0
garlic (*Michelina's Authentico* Tuscan-Inspired), 8 oz. . .	330	16.0	47.0	9.0	40	570	2.0
primavera (*Birds Eye Voila!*), 1 cup*	260	15.0	32.0	7.0	35	660	2.0
red pepper sauce (*South Beach Living*), 9.4 oz. . .	280	22.0	25.0	12.0	50	690	7.0
wine/mushroom sauce (*Michelina's Lean Gourmet*), 8.5 oz.	290	12.0	46.0	6.0	10	550	3.0
pesto primavera (*Birds Eye Voila!*), 1 cup*	210	12.0	24.0	7.0	20	590	2.0
piccata:							
(*Jeff Nathan Crea-tions*), 12 oz. . . .	290	27.0	24.0	6.0	65	1240	6.0
lemon herb (*Smart Ones*), 9 oz.	230	12.0	41.0	1.5	25	540	2.0
pie/pot pie:							
(*Applegate Farms*), 8 oz.	470	14.0	50.0	24.0	30	760	2.0
(*Bell & Evans*), ½ of 16-oz. pkg.	520	16.0	48.0	29.0	80	630	2.0
(*Blake's Natural*), 8 oz.	370	15.0	40.0	17.0	25	380	3.0
(*Blake's Organic*), 8 oz.	340	15.0	34.0	17.0	30	470	5.0
(*Empire Kosher*), 8 oz.	460	21.0	43.0	23.0	25	820	10.0

Food and Measure	cal.	prot. (gms)	carbo. (gms)	fat (gms)	chol. (mgs)	sod. (mgs)	fiber (gms)
(*Stouffer's*) 8 oz. ...	560	20.0	55.0	32.0	55	860	2.0
(*Swanson*), 7 oz. ...	380	10.0	34.0	22.0	35	770	2.0
Alfredo, and broccoli (*Pepperidge Farm*), 1 cup ...	500	13.0	40.0	32.0	35	870	2.0
no vegetables (*Blake's Natural*), 8 oz. ..	360	16.0	34.0	18.0	25	380	1.0
no vegetables (*Blake's* Organic), 8 oz.	290	18.0	25.0	13.0	45	650	3.0
roasted white meat (*Pepperidge Farm*), 1 cup	510	13.0	43.0	32.0	30	870	3.0
portobello (*Lean Cuisine Dinnertime Selects*), 12 oz. ...	390	32.0	48.0	8.0	55	560	2.0
pot stickers, vegetables and (*C&W Pot Sticker Stir Fry Feast*):							
2 cups w/sauce ...	200	10.0	30.0	4.0	15	1200	4.0
2 cups w/out sauce	160	9.0	23.0	4.0	15	230	4.0
primavera w/spirals (*Michelina's Authentico*), 8 oz.	260	13.0	37.0	6.0	30	690	2.0
ranchero sauce, spicy (*Smart Ones* Fiesta), 8.5 oz.	250	12.0	45.0	2.0	25	460	2.0
w/rice:							
and beans (*South Beach Living* Santa Fe), 9 oz. .	340	22.0	35.0	12.0	80	750	4.0
cheesy (*Healthy Choice*), 8.6 oz. .	220	15.0	24.0	6.0	30	600	5.0
confetti pilaf, honey barbecue sauce (*Organic Classics*), 9.5 oz.	320	23.0	49.0	3.5	50	270	2.0
rice, fried, see "Rice entree, frozen"							
roast/roasted:							
Chardonnay (*Healthy Choice Café Steamers*), 10.6 oz.	270	22.0	30.0	6.0	30	550	4.0

Food and Measure	cal.	prot. (gms)	carbo. (gms)	fat (gms)	chol. (mgs)	sod. (mgs)	fiber (gms)
Chicken entree, frozen, roast/roasted (cont.)							
herb (Lean Cuisine), 8 oz.	180	18.0	20.0	3.5	35	590	3.0
w/lemon pepper fettuccine (Lean Cuisine One Dish Favorites), 8⅛ oz. . . .	230	16.0	28.0	6.0	30	580	2.0
Marsala (Healthy Choice Café Steamers), 10.4 oz. . . .	250	38.0	28.0	6.0	30	550	4.0
w/mashed potato (Smart Ones), 9.5 oz.	180	17.0	20.0	4.0	40	820	2.0
w/stuffing (Stouffer's), 9.63 oz.	460	26.0	34.0	24.0	80	990	5.0
rosemary (Lean Cuisine Spa Cuisine), 8.25 oz.	210	17.0	27.0	4.0	35	580	3.0
sesame:							
(Contessa):							
w/sauce, 8 oz. . .	260	14.0	43.0	4.0	25	730	4.0
w/out sauce, 7 oz.	190	13.0	29.0	3.0	25	135	4.0
(Healthy Choice), 8.5 oz.	230	13.0	34.0	4.5	15	600	5.0
(Lean Cuisine), 9 oz.	330	16.0	47.0	9.0	25	650	2.0
(Michelina's Lean Gourmet), 8 oz. .	270	11.0	51.0	2.0	15	660	2.0
(Michelina's Signature), 9 oz.	400	21.0	67.0	4.0	35	600	2.0
stir-fry (Lean Cuisine Spa Cuisine), 9.825 oz.	300	20.0	41.0	6.0	40	680	5.0
smoked sausage, rice:							
(Glory Savory Family Size Casserole), 1 cup	320	14.0	36.0	13.0	45	1030	1.0
(Glory Savory Singles Casserole), 11 oz.	440	18.0	49.0	18.0	60	1390	1.0
Southwest:							
(Birds Eye Voila!), 1 cup*	310	17.0	49.0	5.0	25	1590	3.0
(Kashi), 10 oz.	240	16.0	32.0	5.0	30	680	6.0
stir-fry:							
(Birds Eye Voila!), 1 cup*	200	11.0	31.0	2.5	15	1040	2.0

Food and Measure	cal.	prot. (gms)	carbo. (gms)	fat (gms)	chol. (mgs)	sod. (mgs)	fiber (gms)
(*Contessa*):							
w/sauce, 8 oz. ..	180	14.0	26.0	1.5	30	590	3.0
w/out sauce, 7 oz.	120	13.0	11.0	1.5	30	210	3.0
(*Contessa* le Menu):							
w/sauce, 8 oz. ..	170	12.0	27.0	1.5	25	550	4.0
w/out sauce, 7 oz.	110	11.0	12.0	1.5	25	170	4.0
(*Tyson* Meal Kit),							
2¾ cups*	430	24.0	73.0	4.5	45	1700	5.0
sweet and sour:							
(*Kashi*), 10 oz.	320	18.0	55.0	3.5	35	380	6.0
(*Lean Cuisine*), 10 oz.	300	18.0	51.0	3.0	30	560	2.0
(*Michelina's Lean Gourmet*), 8 oz. .	330	10.0	65.0	3.0	15	640	1.0
(*Michelina's Yu Sing*), 8.5 oz.	350	11.0	68.0	3.0	20	760	1.0
(*Smart Ones*), 9 oz.	140	16.0	13.0	3.0	45	660	2.0
tandoori:							
(*Contessa*):							
w/sauce, 8 oz. ..	200	14.0	27.0	3.5	35	450	3.0
w/out sauce, 7 oz.	190	15.0	25.0	3.0	30	150	2.0
w/spinach (*Ethnic Gourmet*), 10 oz.	170	14.0	19.0	4.5	30	840	3.0
tenderloins (*Stouffer's*), 10 oz.	430	26.0	37.0	20.0	70	1230	3.0
tenders, breaded, fried (*Michelina's Authentico* Littles), 5.5 oz.	310	12.0	33.0	14.0	30	780	3.0
teriyaki:							
(*Birds Eye Voila!*), 1 cup*	200	12.0	34.0	1.5	20	890	2.0
(*Green Giant* Complete Skillet Meal), 1½ cups*	240	13.0	46.0	1.0	20	780	3.0
(*Stouffer's Skillets*), ½ of 25-oz. pkg.	310	23.0	44.0	4.5	50	1130	6.0
stir-fry (*Lean Cuisine One Dish Favorites*), 10 oz.	300	17.0	49.0	4.5	30	690	3.0
and vegetables (*Smart Ones*), 9 oz.	230	14.0	39.0	2.5	25	710	3.0
tetrazzini, Cajun style (*Organic Classics*), 10 oz.	370	25.0	43.0	10.0	55	490	3.0

Food and Measure	cal.	prot. (gms)	carbo. (gms)	fat (gms)	chol. (mgs)	sod. (mgs)	fiber (gms)
Chicken entree, frozen *(cont.)*							
Thai:							
w/rice noodles (*Smart Ones*), 9 oz.	260	14.0	43.0	4.0	25	570	2.0
style (*Lean Cuisine*), 9 oz.	220	17.0	30.0	4.0	30	610	2.0
tikka masala (*Ethnic Gourmet*), 10 oz. . .	260	19.0	32.0	6.0	45	680	3.0
Tuscan/Tuscany:							
(*Healthy Choice Café Steamers*), 10.6 oz.	300	21.0	34.0	8.0	25	560	5.0
(*Lean Cuisine Dinner-time Selects*), 12 oz.	280	22.0	34.0	6.0	40	780	5.0
creamy, w/zucchini (*Smart Ones*), 9 oz.	190	17.0	11.0	9.0	60	620	2.0
vegetables and:							
(*Smart Ones* Home-style), 9 oz.	230	25.0	12.0	9.0	90	660	4.0
Chinese style (*Miche-lina's Budget Gourmet*), 8 oz. .	310	8.0	57.0	5.0	5	670	2.0
fire-grilled (*Smart Ones*), 10 oz. . .	290	18.0	47.0	3.0	45	730	2.0
Italian style (*Miche-lina's Budget Gourmet*), 8 oz. .	270	11.0	44.0	5.0	10	540	4.0
spicy Szechuan (*Smart Ones*), 9 oz.	240	11.0	36.0	5.0	5	900	4.0
Szechuan style (*Mi-chelina's Budget Gourmet*), 8 oz. . .	280	10.0	51.0	2.5	5	880	2.0
and vegetables:							
(*Lean Cuisine*), 10.5 oz.	230	20.0	27.0	5.0	30	640	3.0
(*Smart Ones* Santa Fe), 9 oz.	140	20.0	11.0	2.5	30	800	4.0
grilled (*Stouffer's Skillets*), ½ of 25-oz. pkg.	360	27.0	43.0	9.0	50	870	3.0
pasta, ginger (*Cedar-lane Dr. Sears Zone*), 10 oz. . . .	340	24.0	35.0	12.0	140	650	3.0

Food and Measure	cal.	prot. (gms)	carbo. (gms)	fat (gms)	chol. (mgs)	sod. (mgs)	fiber (gms)
rice bake (*Stouffer's* Grandma's), ¼ of 36-oz. pkg.	360	19.0	37.0	15.0	70	880	1.0
zesty, w/garlic potatoes (*Ethnic Gourmet*), 10 oz.	320	23.0	26.0	13.0	60	720	5.0
Chicken entree, micro-wave, 1 cont.:							
(*Hormel Compleats* Santa Fe), 10 oz. . . .	280	20.0	41.0	4.0	40	550	0
blackened, yellow rice (*Zatarain's* Micro), 6.5 oz.	300	12.0	52.0	4.5	15	1330	1.0
breast w/gravy, 10 oz.:							
w/dressing (*Hormel Compleats*)	280	23.0	35.0	5.0	50	860	1.0
w/potato (*Hormel Compleats*)	210	21.0	24.0	3.0	35	780	2.0
and dumplings:							
(*Dinty Moore* Big Bowl)	220	11.0	29.0	7.0	35	950	.8
(*Dinty Moore* Micro Cup), 7.5 oz. . . .	200	10.0	26.0	6.0	25	890	1.0
(*Hormel Compleats*), 10 oz.	260	13.0	34.0	8.0	50	1140	2.0
(*Luck's* Micro)	160	12.0	21.0	3.5	20	1320	2.0
and noodles (*Hormel Compleats*), 10 oz. .	240	15.0	27.0	8.0	60	1400	2.0
noodles and: (*Dinty Moore* Micro Cup), 7.5 oz.	190	8.0	20.0	9.0	35	1100	1.0
w/penne, Alfredo sauce (*Hormel Compleats*), 10 oz.	360	16.0	28.0	20.0	45	1300	.7
and rice (*Hormel Compleats*), 10 oz. . .	280	11.0	34.0	11.0	40	1170	3.0
sesame (*Hormel Compleats*), 10 oz. . .	320	22.0	41.0	8.0	50	600	0
stew, Southwest (*Dinty Moore* Big Bowl), 1 cup	170	4.0	23.0	4.0	25	700	0
teriyaki, w/rice (*Hormel Compleats*), 10 oz.	270	14.0	51.0	1.5	40	1220	2.0

Food and Measure	cal.	prot. (gms)	carbo. (gms)	fat (gms)	chol. (mgs)	sod. (mgs)	fiber (gms)
"Chicken" entree, vegetarian, frozen, 1 pkg.:							
teriyaki (*Seeds of Change* Hanalei Organic), 10 oz.	300	19.0	47.0	3.5	0	770	4.0
Thai lemongrass (*Yves* Bowl), 10.5 oz.	330	16.0	49.0	9.0	0	910	4.0
Chicken entree mix, 1 cup*:							
cheddar herb (*Annie's* Organic Skillet Meals)	310	31.0	30.0	7.0	75	460	1.0
cheese, four (*Chicken Helper*)	300	24.0	26.0	12.0	55	770	1.0
enchilada, cheesy (*Chicken Helper*)	330	25.0	42.0	7.0	60	830	<1.0
fettuccine Alfredo (*Chicken Helper*)	280	25.0	27.0	8.0	55	790	1.0
fried rice (*Chicken Helper*)	260	22.0	25.0	9.0	125	720	<1.0
jambalaya (*Chicken Helper*)	280	24.0	27.0	8.0	55	810	1.0
teriyaki (*Chicken Helper*)	290	24.0	36.0	6.0	65	900	<1.0
Chicken fat, rendered (*Empire Kosher*), 1 tbsp.	120	0	<1.0	13.0	10	0	0
Chicken giblets, simmered, chopped, 1 cup	228	37.5	1.4	6.9	570	85	0
Chicken gravy, can/jar, ¼ cup:							
(*Campbell's*)	40	0	3.0	3.0	5	260	0
(*Campbell's* Nonfat)	15	1.0	3.0	0	<5	310	0
(*Franco-American* Slow Roast)	20	1.0	3.0	.5	<5	240	0
(*Franco-American* Slow Roast Nonfat)	20	<1.0	4.0	0	<5	250	0
(*Heinz* Home Style Classic)	30	0	3.0	2.0	<5	250	0
(*Pacific* Natural)	25	1.0	4.0	.5	0	270	0
cream of (*Heinz* Home Style)	35	0	4.0	2.0	<5	320	0
Chicken gravy mix (*McCormick*), ¼ cup*	20	0	4.0	0	0	330	0

Food and Measure	cal.	prot. (gms)	carbo. (gms)	fat (gms)	chol. (mgs)	sod. (mgs)	fiber (gms)
Chicken lunch meat, breast, 2 oz., except as noted:							
(*Black Bear*)	70	11.0	1.0	2.0	30	400	0
(*Dietz & Watson*)	70	11.0	1.0	2.0	30	400	0
barbecue:							
(*Black Bear*)	70	11.0	1.0	2.0	30	400	0
(*Boar's Head Bar BQ Basted*)	60	11.0	3.0	.5	30	490	0
(*Jennie-O*)	60	12.0	2.0	1.0	30	420	0
Buffalo style:							
(*Black Bear*)	70	11.0	1.0	2.0	30	420	0
(*Boar's Head Blazing Buffalo*)	60	13.0	0	1.0	35	390	0
(*Di Lusso*)	60	12.0	0	1.0	30	400	0
(*Dietz & Watson*) . .	70	11.0	1.0	2.0	30	420	0
(*Jennie-O*)	60	12.0	0	1.0	30	400	0
grilled or oven-roasted (*Hormel Natural Choice* Carved) . . .	60	12.0	0	1.0	35	230	0
honey barbecue (*Dietz & Watson*) . .	50	12.0	2.0	2.0	30	400	0
mesquite style (*Di Lusso*)	60	12.0	0	1.0	30	450	0
oven-roasted:							
(*Applegate Farms*) .	60	12.0	1.0	1.0	30	290	0
(*Boar's Head Golden Classic*)	60	13.0	0	1.0	35	350	0
(*Di Lusso*)	50	10.0	0	1.5	20	420	0
(*Jennie-O*)	50	11.0	0	0	20	420	0
(*Louis Rich/Oscar Mayer*), 1 oz. . . .	35	5.0	1.0	1.5	15	330	0
(*Oscar Mayer*), ¼ of 10-oz. pkg.	70	11.0	1.0	2.0	35	810	0
(*Oscar Mayer* Thin Sliced)	60	10.0	1.0	1.5	30	710	0
(*Tyson*), 2 slices, 1.6 oz.	40	8.0	1.0	.5	20	530	0
shaved (*Tyson*) . . .	60	10.0	2.0	1.0	25	640	0
roasted:							
(*Applegate Farms* Organic)	60	10.0	1.0	1.5	30	580	0
(*Boar's Head Lemon Pepper*)	60	13.0	1.0	1.0	35	360	0

Food and Measure	cal.	prot. (gms)	carbo. (gms)	fat (gms)	chol. (mgs)	sod. (mgs)	fiber (gms)
Chicken lunch meat *(cont.)*							
rotisserie style:							
(*Black Bear*)	70	11.0	1.0	2.0	30	400	0
(*Dietz & Watson*) . .	70	11.0	1.0	2.0	30	400	0
shaved (*Tyson*) . . .	60	10.0	2.0	1.0	20	640	0
seasoned (*Boar's Head Aroastica*)	60	13.0	0	1.0	35	400	0
smoked:							
(*Applegate Farms*) .	70	12.0	1.0	2.0	30	360	0
(*Applegate Farms Organic*)	70	12.0	1.0	2.0	30	580	0
(*Tyson*), 2 slices, 1.6 oz.	45	9.0	1.0	.5	20	530	0
hickory (*Boar's Head*)	60	13.0	0	.5	35	360	0
mesquite (*Jennie-O*)	50	12.0	0	0	25	420	0
Thai style (*Jennie-O*) .	60	11.0	1.0	1.0	30	490	0
Chicken pie, see "Chicken entree, frozen"							
Chicken salad:							
fresh, see "Salad bowl" and "Salad entree kit"							
refrigerated, ⅓ cup:							
(*Wampler*)	200	9.0	9.0	14.0	30	420	1.0
(*Wampler* Low Fat)	90	8.0	9.0	1.5	20	440	0
Chicken salad kit,							
w/crackers:							
(*Bumble Bee*):							
2.9-oz can salad . . .	140	8.0	10.0	8.0	25	410	0
6 crackers, .6 oz. . .	90	2.0	12.0	4.5	0	180	0
(*Bumble Bee Lunch on the Run*), total kit, 8.2 oz.	470	11.0	62.0	19.5	35	735	1.0
(*Tyson* Salad Kit), 3.8-oz. pkg.	210	18.0	15.0	9.0	50	640	1.0
Chicken sandwich, see "Panini," and "Wrap, filled"							
Chicken sausage, see "Sausage" and specific listings							
Chicken seasoning, (see also "Chicken coating mix" and "Rubs"):							
(*Grill Mates* Montreal), ¼ tsp.	0	0	0	0	0	90	0

Food and Measure	cal.	prot. (gms)	carbo. (gms)	fat (gms)	chol. (mgs)	sod. (mgs)	fiber (gms)
(*McCormick* Original/ Rotisserie), ¼ tsp. . .	0	0	0	0	0	130	0
herb, Italian (*McCormick* Slow Cookers), 2 tsp.	15	0	3.0	0	0	400	0
Chicken wontons, Buffalo, frozen (*Original Rangoon Rangoons*), 3 pcs. . .	220	12.0	29.0	5.0	25	580	<1.0
Chickpeas, see "Garbanzo beans"							
Chicory, witloof:							
(*Frieda's* Endive), 2 cups, 3 oz.	15	1.0	3.0	0	0	20	3.0
5-7" head, 1.9 oz.	9	.5	2.1	.1	0	1	1.6
½ cup	8	.4	1.8	<.1	0	1	1.4
Chicory greens:							
trimmed, 1 oz.	7	.5	1.3	.1	0	13	1.1
chopped, ½ cup	21	1.5	4.2	.3	0	41	3.6
Chicory root:							
1 medium, 2.6 oz. . . .	44	.8	10.5	.1	0	30	n.a.
1" pcs., ½ cup	33	.6	7.9	.1	0	23	n.a.
Chili, canned, 1 cup, except as noted:							
w/beans:							
(*Bush's* Chunky) . . .	260	15.0	28.0	10.0	15	1250	8.0
(*Bush's* Original/ Homestyle)	250	14.0	26.0	10.0	15	1250	7.0
(*Campbell's* Chunky Firehouse/Road-house)	230	15.0	25.0	8.0	30	870	8.0
(*Campbell's* Chunky Grilled Steak) . . .	200	16.0	27.0	3.0	15	870	7.0
(*Dennison's*)	360	20.0	38.0	14.0	40	1030	11.0
(*Dennison's* Chunky)	300	20.0	32.0	10.0	40	1020	9.0
(*Hormel*)	260	16.0	33.0	7.0	30	1200	3.5
(*Hormel* Chunky) . .	260	17.0	32.0	7.0	30	1160	7.0
(*Hormel* Homestyle)	350	16.0	28.0	19.0	40	1020	5.0
(*Hormel* Less Salt) .	260	16.0	33.0	7.0	30	880	7.0
(*Hormel/Hormel* Hot), 7.5-oz. can	230	14.0	29.0	6.0	30	1070	6.0
(*Stagg* Chunkero) . .	320	16.0	28.0	16.0	40	850	6.0
(*Stagg* Classic)	330	17.0	28.0	17.0	45	820	5.0
(*Stagg* Country) . . .	320	15.0	29.0	16.0	45	1130	5.0
(*Stagg* Fiesta Grill)	250	15.0	25.0	10.0	40	950	6.0

Food and Measure	cal.	prot. (gms)	carbo. (gms)	fat (gms)	chol. (mgs)	sod. (mgs)	fiber (gms)
Chili, canned, w/beans *(cont.)*							
(*Stagg Laredo*)	320	18.0	27.0	15.0	45	1150	6.0
(*Stagg Silverado*) . .	250	17.0	30.0	7.0	30	860	6.0
(*Wolf*)	370	21.0	31.0	19.0	40	1020	7.0
hot (*Bush's*)	250	14.0	26.0	10.0	15	1260	7.0
hot (*Dennison's*) . .	350	21.0	11.0	14.0	40	980	2.0
hot (*Dennison's* Chunky)	300	20.0	32.0	10.0	40	930	9.0
hot (*Hormel*)	260	16.0	33.0	7.0	30	1190	7.0
hot (*Stagg Dynamite Hot*)	340	17.0	30.0	17.0	40	800	8.0
hot/spicy (*Hormel*)	260	16.0	33.0	7.0	25	1300	7.0
lean beef (*Wolf*) . . .	220	26.0	15.0	8.0	40	970	8.0
w/out beans:							
(*Bush's* No Bean) . .	240	13.0	16.0	14.0	25	1380	3.0
(*Campbell's Chunky* Hold the Beans) .	240	18.0	20.0	10.0	35	770	5.0
(*Hormel*)	220	16.0	18.0	9.0	40	970	3.0
(*Hormel* Chunky) . .	210	16.0	19.0	8.0	40	1130	4.0
(*Hormel* Less Salt) .	220	16.0	18.0	9.0	40	710	3.0
(*Stagg Steak House*)	320	17.0	14.0	22.0	65	1080	2.0
(*Wolf*)	410	23.0	20.0	28.0	55	1020	7.0
hot (*Hormel*)	220	16.0	18.0	9.0	40	970	3.0
hot (*Wolf*)	400	21.0	20.0	26.0	55	960	5.0
hot/spicy (*Hormel*)	220	16.0	19.0	9.0	40	1030	3.0
mild (*Wolf*)	410	23.0	17.0	29.0	60	1060	5.0
chicken, w/beans:							
(*Stagg* Santa Fe) . .	200	15.0	25.0	4.0	25	900	6.0
(*Stagg* White)	260	17.0	20.0	12.0	70	1010	4.0
(*Stagg* Ranch House)	240	17.0	26.0	8.0	55	780	7.0
turkey, w/beans:							
(*Dennison's*)	210	16.0	29.0	3.0	45	850	7.0
(*Hormel*)	210	17.0	28.0	3.0	45	1250	6.0
(*Stagg Ranchero*) . .	240	22.0	31.0	3.0	35	850	6.0
(*Wolf*)	160	22.0	16.0	2.5	25	1340	8.0
turkey, w/out beans (*Hormel*)	190	23.0	16.0	3.0	80	1230	3.0
vegetable/vegetarian:							
(*Dennison's*)	190	9.0	34.0	1.5	0	800	9.0
(*Hormel*)	190	11.0	35.0	1.0	0	780	11.0
(*Stagg Vegetable Garden*)	200	10.0	37.0	1.0	0	890	8.0
(*Worthington*)	280	24.0	25.0	10.0	0	1130	8.0

Food and Measure	cal.	prot. (gms)	carbo. (gms)	fat (gms)	chol. (mgs)	sod. (mgs)	fiber (gms)
black bean (*Amy's* Organic)	200	13.0	31.0	2.0	0	680	15.0
black bean, mild or spicy (*Health Valley* Organic) . .	150	10.0	32.0	1.0	0	480	8.0
medium (*Amy's* Organic)	250	13.0	30.0	9.0	0	680	7.0
medium (*Amy's* Organic Light Sodium)	250	13.0	20.0	9.0	0	340	7.0
medium, w/vegetables (*Amy's* Organic) .	190	13.0	30.0	6.0	0	680	8.0
spicy (*Amy's* Organic)	250	8.0	26.0	9.0	0	590	7.0
spicy (*Amy's* Organic Light Sodium)	250	13.0	30.0	9.0	0	340	7.0
spicy (*Health Valley* Chunky Organic)	150	9.0	31.0	1.0	0	480	10.0
three bean (*Health Valley* Chunky Organic)	150	10.0	32.0	1.0	0	480	10.0
Chili, frozen (see also "Chili entree, frozen"), 1 cup:							
(*Organic Classics* Our Favorite)	220	14.0	31.0	5.0	15	450	9.0
two bean (*Moosewood* Organic Texas)	200	9.0	34.0	4.0	0	840	8.0
Chili, mix, vegetarian: (*Fantastic*), ¼ cup .	200	16.0	32.0	2.0	0	1160	7.0
Chili beans (see also "Chili starter" and "Mexican beans"), canned, ½ cup:							
(*Bush's*)	120	6.0	20.0	1.0	0	480	6.0
(*Westbrae Natural* Organic)	100	7.0	19.0	0	0	150	5.0
chili sauce (*Bush's*) . .	100	6.0	22.0	.5	0	480	7.0
w/chipotle (*S&W* Santa Fe)	90	7.0	21.0	0	0	570	6.0
w/jalapeño/red pepper (*Eden* Organic)	130	9.0	21.0	0	0	250	7.0
tomato sauce (*S&W*) .	110	7.0	23.0	1.0	0	580	6.0

Food and Measure	cal.	prot. (gms)	carbo. (gms)	fat (gms)	chol. (mgs)	sod. (mgs)	fiber (gms)
Chili entree, frozen, 1 pkg., except as noted:							
bean, three (*Lean Cuisine One Dish Favorites*), 10 oz.	270	9.0	42.0	7.0	10	620	8.0
w/macaroni (*Michelina's Zap'ems Chili-Mac*), 8 oz.	320	13.0	38.0	11.0	25	820	3.0
pot pie, w/corn bread (*Pepperidge Farm*), 1 cup	360	11.0	40.0	17.0	20	890	3.0
w/vegetables:							
and corn bread (*Amy's*), 10.5 oz.	340	11.0	59.0	6.0	10	680	10.0
and tofu (*Helen's Kitchen* Comfort Food), 10 oz.	210	12.0	29.0	4.0	0	380	7.0
vegetarian:							
(*Boca* Meatless), 9.5 oz.	150	20.0	25.0	1.0	0	650	12.0
(*Yves Bowl*), 10.5 oz.	240	21.0	37.0	1.0	0	850	14.0
chipotle (*Ethnic Gourmet*), 10 oz.	260	15.0	29.0	11.0	0	940	5.0
Chili entree, microwave, 1 cont.:							
(*Hormel* Chili'n Mac), 10 oz.	260	17.0	34.0	6.0	30	950	0
(*Hormel* Chili'n Penne), 10 oz.	330	20.0	32.0	13.0	55	990	0
(*Hormel* Chili'n Spuds), 10 oz.	250	14.0	33.0	7.0	20	760	0
w/beans (*Hormel/ Hormel* Hot)	220	13.0	27.0	6.0	20	1010	6.0
w/out beans (*Hormel*)	190	14.0	16.0	8.0	35	860	2.0
Chili pepper, see "Pepper, chili"							
Chili pepper paste, see "Thai sauce"							
Chili pocket sandwich, frozen, vegetable 3-bean (*Aunt Trudy's* Organic), 5-oz. pc.	260	8.0	42.0	7.0	0	300	5.0
Chili powder:							
(*McCormick*), ¼ tsp.	0	0	0	0	0	20	0

Food and Measure	cal.	prot. (gms)	carbo. (gms)	fat (gms)	chol. (mgs)	sod. (mgs)	fiber (gms)
1 tbsp.	24	.9	4.1	1.3	0	76	2.6
1 tsp.	8	.3	1.4	.4	0	26	.9
Chili relish, Indian							
(*Patak's*), 1 tbsp. . .	50	0	0	5.0	0	510	0
Chili sauce, Asian (see							
also specific listings):							
(*Heaven and Earth*							
Dragon Fire), 1 tbsp.	25	0	6.0	0	0	50	0
(*Roland* Srichacha),							
1 tsp.	5	0	1.0	0	0	60	0
black bean (*Heaven*							
and Earth), 1 tbsp. .	30	1.0	4.0	1.5	0	400	0
garlic:							
(*Roland*), 1 tbsp. . . .	10	0	3.0	0	0	540	0
pepper (*A Taste of*							
Thai), 1 tsp.	10	0	2.0	0	0	230	0
ginger (*Roland*), 2 tbsp.	35	0	8.0	0	0	210	0
mango (*Roland*),							
2 tbsp.	45	0	11.0	0	0	220	0
pineapple (*Roland*),							
2 tbsp.	40	0	9.0	0	0	200	0
sweet, 1 tsp.:							
(*Roland*)	10	0	3.0	0	0	60	0
red (*A Taste of Thai*)	10	0	2.0	0	0	40	0
Chili sauce, hot, see							
"Chili sauce, Asian,"							
"Hot sauce" and							
"Thai sauce"							
Chili sauce, tomato:							
(*Del Monte*), 1 tbsp. . .	20	0	5.0	0	0	480	0
(*Heinz*), 1 tbsp.	20	0	4.0	0	0	230	0
(*Wolf* Hot Dog), 2 tbsp.	25	1.0	4.0	1.0	0	120	1.0
Chili seasoning mix:							
(*Carroll Shelby's*							
Texas), 2 tbsp.	60	2.0	12.0	1.0	0	1320	0
(*Lawry's*). 1 tsp.	10	0	2.0	0	0	500	0
(*Lawry's Meal*							
Makers), 1 tbsp.	30	<1.0	5.0	.5	0	270	<1.0
(*McCormick*), 1⅓ tbsp.	30	1.0	5.0	.5	0	310	0
(*McCormick* Less							
Sodium), 1 tbsp. . .	30	1.0	5.0	.5	0	210	0
(*McCormick* Slow							
Cookers), 2 tsp. . . .	15	0	2.0	0	0	420	0
(*Old El Paso*), 2 tsp. . .	15	0	3.0	.5	0	550	1.0

Food and Measure	cal.	prot. (gms)	carbo. (gms)	fat (gms)	chol. (mgs)	sod. (mgs)	fiber (gms)
Chili seasoning mix *(cont.)*							
(*Wick Fowler's* Texas One-Step), ¼ pkg. . .	25	1.0	5.0	1.0	0	360	2.0
hot:							
(*McCormick* Mexican), 1⅓ tbsp. . . .	35	1.0	4.0	1.0	0	340	0
(*Wick Fowler's* 2-Alarm Kit), 3 tbsp.	60	2.0	10.0	2.0	0	980	0
w/lime (*McCormick*), ¼ tsp.	0	0	0	0	0	230	0
mild:							
(*McCormick*), 1⅓ tbsp.	30	1.0	5.0	0	0	400	0
(*Wick Fowler's* False-Alarm Kit), 2 tbsp.	50	2.0	9.0	2.0	0	980	0
Tex-Mex (*McCormick*), 1⅓ tbsp.	35	0	4.0	1.0	0	360	0
white, chicken (*McCormick*), 1 tbsp. . . .	30	0	5.0	.5	0	450	0
Chili starter, canned:							
(*Bush's Chili Magic*),							
Texas, ½ cup	120	5.0	20.0	2.0	0	1130	5.0
Texas, 1 cup*	230	22.0	15.0	9.0	55	880	4.0
traditional, ½ cup .	110	5.0	19.0	1.0	0	890	5.0
traditional, 1 cup* .	220	22.0	15.0	8.0	55	770	3.0
(*S&W* Chili Makin's):							
black bean, ½ cup .	80	6.0	19.0	0	0	750	6.0
homestyle, ½ cup .	80	7.0	19.0	0	0	630	6.0
original, ½ cup . . .	80	5.0	20.0	.5	0	820	5.0
Chimichanga, frozen, 1 pc., except as noted:							
beef/bean:							
(*El Monterey*), 4 oz.	310	8.0	34.0	15.0	15	480	3.0
spicy (*El Monterey* Red Hot XX Large!), 10 oz.	900	21.0	81.0	55.0	35	1100	8.0
chicken/cheese:							
(*José Olé*), 5 oz. . . .	330	11.0	44.0	12.0	20	550	2.0
Monterey Jack (*El Monterey* Supreme), 5 oz. . . .	280	12.0	37.0	10.0	20	640	2.0
steak/cheese:							
(*José Olé*), 5 oz. . . .	340	12.0	40.0	15.0	20	650	2.0
cheddar (*José Olé* Minis), 3 pcs., 3 oz.	250	8.0	29.0	12.0	20	530	3.0

Food and Measure	cal.	prot. (gms)	carbo. (gms)	fat (gms)	chol. (mgs)	sod. (mgs)	fiber (gms)
shredded (*El Monterey* Monterey), 5 oz. . .	330	12.0	35.0	15.0	30	350	1.0
Chimichurri sauce, see "Marinade"							
Chipotle, see "Pepper, chipotle"							
Chipotle dip (*Bison*), 2 tbsp.	50	1.0	2.0	4.5	20	190	0
Chipotle oil (*Watkins* Liquid Spice), 1 tsp.	40	0	0	4.5	0	0	0
Chipotle sauce, 2 tbsp.:							
(*La Morena*)	25	<1.0	6.0	0	0	680	0
three berry (*Fiesta*) . .	20	4.0	3.0	1.0	0	220	6.0
Chipotle seasoning (*Ortega*), 1 tbsp. . .	20	0	4.0	0	0	350	0
Chitterlings, pork, simmered, 4 oz. . . .	344	11.6	0	32.6	162	44	0
Chives:							
fresh, 1 oz.	9	.9	1.2	.2	0	1	.9
fresh, chopped, 1 tbsp. .	1	.1	.1	<.1	0	<1	.1
freeze-dried, 1 tbsp. . . .	1	.<.1	.1	<.1	0	6	<1.0
Chocolate, see "Candy"							
Chocolate, baking, ½ oz., except as noted:							
(*Nestlé Choco Bake*) .	80	1.0	4.0	8.0	0	0	2.0
bars:							
bittersweet (*Baker's*)	70	1.0	7.0	6.0	0	0	1.0
dark (*Hershey's Special Dark*) . . .	70	1.0	9.0	4.5	0	5	<1.0
semisweet (*Baker's*)	70	1.0	8.0	4.5	0	0	1.0
semisweet (*Nestlé Toll House*)	70	<1.0	9.0	4.0	0	0	<1.0
sweet (*German's*) . .	60	1.0	8.0	3.5	0	0	1.0
white (*Baker's*)	80	1.0	8.0	4.5	5	15	0
white (*Nestlé Toll House*)	70	<1.0	9.0	4.0	0	10	0
bars, unsweetened:							
(*Baker's*)	70	2.0	4.0	7.0	0	0	2.0
(*Hershey's*)	80	2.0	4.0	7.0	0	0	2.0
(*Nestlé Toll House*)	70	1.0	4.0	7.0	0	0	2.0
chips or morsels:							
(*SunSpire* Grain Sweetened)	70	1.0	9.0	4.0	0	0	1.0

Chocolate, baking, chips or morsels *(cont.)*

Food and Measure	cal.	prot. (gms)	carbo. (gms)	fat (gms)	chol. (mgs)	sod. (mgs)	fiber (gms)
candy coated, dark (*M&M's* Mini) ...	70	1.0	9.0	3.5	0	0	1.0
candy coated, milk (*M&M's* Mini) ...	70	1.0	10.0	3.5	5	10	0
dark (*Hershey's Special Dark*) ...	70	<1.0	9.0	4.5	0	0	1.0
milk (*Hershey's*) ...	80	1.0	9.0	4.5	<5	10	<1.0
milk (*Hershey's Kisses*), 9 pcs., 1.4 oz.	230	3.0	24.0	13.0	10	35	1.0
milk (*Hershey's Mini Kisses*), 2.7-oz. bag	420	7.0	440	24.0	20	75	2.0
milk (*Nestlé Toll House*)	70	<1.0	9.0	4.0	<5	5	0
milk, caramel swirl (*Nestlé Toll House*)	70	<1.0	9.0	4.0	<5	10	0
mint (*Hershey's*) ..	70	<1.0	10.0	4.5	0	0	<1.0
semisweet (*Hershey's*)	80	<1.0	10.0	4.5	0	0	<1.0
semisweet (*Nestlé Toll House Morsels*)	70	<1.0	9.0	4.0	0	0	<1.0
semisweet (*SunSpire Organic*)	70	1.0	10.0	4.0	0	0	1.0
semisweet, mini (*Nestlé Toll House*)	70	<1.0	9.0	4.0	0	0	<1.0
semisweet, nondairy (*SunSpire Tropical Source*)	70	.5	9.0	4.0	0	1	1.0
semisweet and white swirled (*Nestlé Toll House*)	70	<1.0	9.0	4.0	0	5	0
white (*Hershey's*) ..	80	1.0	9.0	4.0	0	30	0
white (*Nestlé Toll House Morsels*) .	70	0	9.0	4.0	0	15	0
white (*SunSpire*) ..	80	1.0	10.0	4.0	0	0	0
chunks or pieces:							
dark or white, w/macadamias (*Hershey's Special Dark*) ...	90	<1.0	7.0	7.0	0	0	1.0
semisweet (*Nestlé Toll House*), .4 oz.	60	<1.0	8.0	3.5	0	0	<1.0
semisweet (*Baker's*)	70	1.0	9.0	4.5	0	5	1.0

Food and Measure	cal.	prot. (gms)	carbo. (gms)	fat (gms)	chol. (mgs)	sod. (mgs)	fiber (gms)
Chocolate dip, see "Fruit dip"							
Chocolate drink mix (see also "Cocoa mix"):							
(*GoLean* Shake), 2 scoops	220	21.0	32.0	1.0	0	120	7.0
(*Hershey's* Milk Mix), 3 tbsp.	90	0	23.0	0	0	60	<1.0
(*Nesquik*), 2 tbsp. . . .	60	<1.0	14.0	.5	0	30	<1.0
Chocolate milk, see "Milk, flavored"							
Chocolate syrup, 2 tbsp.:							
(*Fox's U-Bet*)	120	1.0	29.0	0	0	35	0
(*Hershey's*)	100	<1.0	24.0	0	0	15	1.0
(*Hershey's* Calcium) . .	90	<1.0	230	0	0	15	1.0
(*Hershey's* Lite)	45	0	11.0	0	0	55	<1.0
(*Hershey's* Sugar Free)	15	0	5.0	0	0	50	0
(*Kahlua* Sauce)	124	0	29.0	0	0	0	0
(*Nesquik*)	100	0	25.0	0	0	55	<1.0
(*Santa Cruz Organic*) .	110	1.0	27.0	3.5	0	0	0
(*Smucker's* Sundae Syrup)	110	1.0	26.0	0	0	20	1.0
dark (*Hershey's* Special Dark)	90	<1.0	24.0	0	0	30	1.0
double (*Hershey's* Sundae)	100	<1.0	24.0	0	0	15	1.0
malt (*Hershey's* Whoppers)	100	0	25.0	0	0	45	<1.0
Chocolate topping, 2 tbsp.:							
(*Hershey's* Shell)	220	<1.0	16.0	18.0	0	15	1.0
(*Smucker's* Magic Shell)	210	1.0	17.0	16.0	0	30	1.0
w/chips, cookie bits, sprinkles (*Hershey's* Triple)	90	1.0	12.0	4.0	0	50	<.10
dark chocolate:							
(*Smucker's Dove*) .	130	<1.0	23.0	4.5	0	25	1.0
w/mint (*Smucker's*)	110	1.0	24.0	1.5	0	50	1.0
fudge:							
(*Smucker's* Micro/ Spoonable)	130	0	28.0	1.5	0	60	1.0

Food and Measure	cal.	prot. (gms)	carbo. (gms)	fat (gms)	chol. (mgs)	sod. (mgs)	fiber (gms)
Chocolate topping, fudge *(cont.)*							
(*Smucker's Magic Shell*)	210	1.0	17.0	16.0	0	45	<1.0
fudge, hot:							
(*Hershey's*)	120	2.0	20.0	4.0	0	90	<1.0
(*Smucker's*)	130	2.0	22.0	4.5	0	45	<1.0
(*Smucker's* Light) .	90	2.0	23.0	0	0	90	2.0
(*Smucker's* Micro) .	120	2.0	22.0	3.5	0	45	<1.0
(*Smucker's* Special Recipe)	130	2.0	20.0	4.5	0	55	<1.0
(*Smucker's* Sugar Free)	90	1.0	24.0	0	0	35	1.0
milk chocolate:							
(*Hershey's Bar in a Jar*)	120	1.0	19.0	5.0	0	40	0
(*Smucker's Dove*) .	130	2.0	21.0	4.0	0	75	<1.0
mocha (*Smucker's*) . .	110	1.0	28.0	0	0	100	<1.0
Chorizo:							
(*Carando*), 1 oz.	100	6.0	1.0	8.0	25	450	0
(*Daniele* Cantimpalo), 1 oz.	80	8.0	<1.0	5.0	17	540	0
(*Del Oro* Mexican Style), 2 oz.	160	8.0	0	14.0	40	360	0
(*Farmer John* Original/ Spicy Hot), 2.5 oz. . .	220	10.0	2.0	19.0	40	390	0
(*Farmer John* Traditional), 2.5 oz.	190	11.0	2.0	15.0	80	680	0
pork and beef, 2 oz. . .	255	13.5	1.0	21.4	49	692	0
turkey and chicken (*Aidells*), 3.5 oz. . . .	180	16.0	2.0	12.0	90	560	0
Chorizo, vegetarian (*Soyrizo*), 4 tbsp., 1.9 oz.	120	7.0	5.0	9.0	0	440	12.0
Chow chow pickle:							
(*Crosse & Blackwell*), 1 tbsp.	10	0	1.0	0	0	200	<1.0
hot or mild (*Mrs. Renfro's*), 1 tbsp. . . .	10	0	3.0	0	0	45	0
sweet, w/cauliflower, ¼ cup	74	.9	16.5	.5	0	321	.9
Chrysanthemum garland, 1" pcs.:							
raw, ½ cup	2	.2	.5	<.1	0	7	.4
boiled, drained, ½ cup	10	.8	2.2	.1	0	27	1.2

Food and Measure	cal.	prot. (gms)	carbo. (gms)	fat (gms)	chol. (mgs)	sod. (mgs)	fiber (gms)
Chutney, 1 tbsp., except as noted:							
apple curry (*Crosse & Blackwell*)	25	0	7.0	0	0	25	0
apricot Chardonnay (*Crosse & Blackwell*)	25	0	6.0	0	0	20	0
cilantro (*Maya Kaimal*), 2 tbsp.	40	1.0	1.0	4.0	0	240	0
coconut (*Maya Kaimal*), 2 tbsp.	40	1.0	1.0	4.0	0	240	0
cranberry (*Crosse & Blackwell*)	40	0	10.0	0	0	0	0
fig (*Maya Kaimal*), 2 tbsp.	25	0	4.0	1.5	0	80	0
ginger (*India Select*) .	46	<1.0	7.0	2.0	0	450	1.0
ginger pineapple (*Neera's*)	31	0	7.0	0	0	54	0
lime chili, w/turmeric (*Fanci Food*)	50	0	13.0	0	0	440	<1.0
mango:							
(*Crosse & Blackwell* Hot/Major Grey) .	60	0	14.0	0	0	170	0
(*Fanci Food*)	60	0	14.0	0	0	105	0
(*Maya Kaimal*), 2 tbsp.	30	0	3.0	2.0	0	90	0
(*Neera's*)	20	0	5.0	0	0	26	0
(*Patak's* Major Grey)	60	0	14.0	0	0	290	0
(*Roland* Major Grey), 2 tbsp.	60	0	14.0	0	0	170	0
(*Taj Gourmet*)	20	0	5.0	0	0	80	0
hot (*Patak's*)	60	0	14.0	0	0	300	0
sweet (*Patak's*)	60	0	14.0	.5	0	310	0
mango pomegranate, w/turmeric (*Fanci Food*)	50	0	13.0	0	0	100	0
mango raisin, w/red chili (*Fanci Food*) ..	60	0	14.0	0	0	100	0
peach:							
(*Crosse & Blackwell* Zinfandel)	25	0	6.0	0	0	20	0
(*Neera's*)	22	0	6.0	0	0	30	0
(*Roland*), 2 tbsp. ...	60	0	16.0	0	0	95	0
pear cardamom:							
(*Crosse & Blackwell*)	25	5	6.0	0	0	10	0
(*Neera's*)	30	0	7.0	0	0	23	1.0

Food and Measure	cal.	prot. (gms)	carbo. (gms)	fat (gms)	chol. (mgs)	sod. (mgs)	fiber (gms)
Chutney (cont.)							
pineapple, w/turmeric							
(*Fanci Food*)	60	0	16.0	0	0	115	0
tomato:							
(*Roland*), 2 tbsp. ...	70	0	17.0	0	0	105	0
mint (*Neera's*)	30	1.0	5.0	2.0	0	54	1.0
roasted (*Prairie*							
Thyme), 2 tbsp. .	40	0	10.0	0	0	75	0
vegetable, hot (*Neera's*)	21	0	2.0	2.0	0	49	0
Cilantro, see							
"Coriander"							
Cinnamon, ground,							
1 tsp.	6	.1	2.1	.1	0	1	1.4
Cinnamon baking							
chips (*Hershey's*),							
1 tbsp., .5 oz.	80	1.0	9.0	4.0	0	45	0
Cinnamon sugar (*Mc-*							
Cormick), 1 tsp. ...	15	0	3.0	0	0	0	0
Cisco, meat only:							
raw, 4 oz.	112	21.5	0	2.2	57	62	0
smoked, 4 oz.	201	18.6	0	13.5	36	545	0
Citronella root, see							
"Lemongrass"							
Citrus drink, 8 fl. oz.,							
except as noted:							
(*Five Alive*)	120	2.0	30.0	0	0	15	0
(*Minute Maid* Breakfast							
Blends)	120	0	30.0	0	0	15	0
(*Minute Maid* Punch) .	120	0	32.0	0	0	15	0
(*Odwalla Citrus C*							
Monster)	150	2.0	36.0	0	0	15	0
(*SoBe Energy*)	110	0	27.0	0	0	15	0
frozen* (*Five Alive*) ..	110	0	29.0	0	0	0	0
Clam, meat only:							
raw:							
4 oz.	84	14.5	2.9	1.1	39	64	0
9 large or 20 small,							
6.3 oz.	133	23.0	4.6	1.8	60	100	0
boiled, poached, or							
steamed, 4 oz.	168	29.0	5.8	2.2	76	127	0
Clam, can or pouch,							
2 oz. or ¼ cup,							
except as noted:							
whole:							

Food and Measure	cal.	prot. (gms)	carbo. (gms)	fat (gms)	chol. (mgs)	sod. (mgs)	fiber (gms)
(*Roland* Pacific), ⅓ cup	45	4.0	6.0	1.0	20	260	0
pink (*Roland*), ½ cup	70	13.0	1.0	1.5	70	450	0
razor (*Roland*), ½ cup	60	12.0	1.0	1.0	50	340	1.0
whole, baby:							
(*Bumble Bee*)	50	9.0	2.0	1.0	40	270	0
(*Chicken of the Sea* Pouch), 2.5 oz.	40	7.0	1.0	.5	15	360	0
(*Roland*), ½ cup ..	50	10.0	2.0	0	48	280	0
chopped or minced:							
(*Bumble Bee*)	25	4.0	2.0	0	10	320	0
(*Chicken of the Sea*)	30	5.0	2.0	0	12	370	0
(*Roland*), ⅓ cup ..	45	10.0	0	0	15	310	0
ocean (*Chincoteague*)	30	6.0	1.0	0	10	290	0
sea (*Chincoteague*)	25	6.0	0	0	15	260	0
Clam, smoked, canned in oil, drained:							
(*Bumble Bee*), 2 oz. ..	130	11.0	1.0	9.0	40	460	0
baby:							
(*Roland*), ⅓ cup ..	90	10.0	2.0	5.0	45	330	2.0
(*Yankee Clipper* 3 oz.), 2.3 oz.	140	14.0	2.0	5.0	45	330	2.0
Clam chowder, see "Soup"							
Clam dish, frozen:							
fried, breaded:							
(*Cape Cod* Premium), 4 oz.	334	11.0	32.0	16.0	13	720	3.0
(*Cape Cod/Chincoteague*), 3 oz.	265	6.0	24.0	16.0	5	527	1.0
(*Mrs. Paul's*), 3 oz.	270	9.0	29.0	13.0	20	690	1.0
strips, breaded (*Schooner*), 7 pcs., 3 oz.	260	6.0	36.0	10.0	0	370	1.0
stuffed, in shell:							
(*Matlaw's* Gourmet), 5-oz. pc.	250	13.0	23.0	12.0	10	950	3.0
(*Matlaw's* New England), 2 pcs., 3.1 oz.	180	8.0	20.0	8.0	0	640	2.0
(*Matlaw's* Tray Pack), 2.2-oz. pc.	110	5.0	12.0	4.5	0	390	1.0

Food and Measure	cal.	prot. (gms)	carbo. (gms)	fat (gms)	chol. (mgs)	sod. (mgs)	fiber (gms)
Clam dish, frozen, stuffed (cont.)							
casino (*Matlaw's*),							
2 pcs., 1.3 oz. . .	60	3.0	7.0	3.0	0	230	<1.0
oreganata (*Matlaw's*),							
2 pcs., 1.2 oz. . .	80	3.0	6.0	5.0	0	125	0
Clam juice:							
(*Roland*), 1 tbsp.	0	1.0	0	0	0	100	0
(*Roland* Can), 1 tbsp. .	0	1.0	0	0	0	130	0
ocean (*Chincoteague*),							
½ cup	10	2.0	1.0	0	0	1490	0
sea (*Chincoteague*),							
½ cup	15	1.0	0	0	0	590	0
Clam sauce, canned:							
red, ½ cup:							
(*Chincoteague*)	100	5.0	8.0	5.0	10	550	<1.0
(*Progresso*)	60	3.0	6.0	1.0	5	430	2.0
white, ½ cup:							
(*Chincoteague*)	120	4.0	9.0	8.0	10	490	0
(*Progresso*)	130	6.0	5.0	10.0	10	750	0
(*Progresso* Deluxe)	150	9.0	5.0	10.0	20	710	0
Cloves, ground:							
1 tbsp.	21	.4	4.0	1.3	0	16	<1.0
1 tsp.	7	.1	1.3	.4	0	5	.2
Cobbler, frozen:							
apple, w/raisins (*Jeff Nathan Creations*),							
½ of 8.5-oz. pkg. . .	310	3.0	47.0	13.0	0	25	2.0
berry (*Marie Callender's*), ¼ pkg.	300	3.0	36.0	15.0	0	180	3.0
Cocktail mixers, see specific listings							
Cocktail sauce, see "Seafood sauce"							
Cocoa, 1 tbsp.:							
(*Nestlé Toll House*) . .	15	1.0	3.0	.5	0	0	1.0
(*Shiloh Farms* Organic)	15	0	2.0	1.0	0	35	1.0
Dutch or unsweetened (*Hershey's*)	20	1.0	3.0	.5	0	95	1.0
Cocoa mix, 1 pkt., except as noted:							
(*Cacao Reserve by Hershey* Classic Mayan Blend)	140	5.0	26.0	2.0	<5	150	2.0

Food and Measure	cal.	prot. (gms)	carbo. (gms)	fat (gms)	chol. (mgs)	sod. (mgs)	fiber (gms)
(*Cacao Reserve by Hershey* Spiced Aztec Blend)	130	5.0	26.0	2.0	<5	150	2.0
(*Hershey's Goodnight Hugs*)	140	3.0	27.0	2.5	<5	190	0
(*Hershey's Goodnight Kisses*)	140	3.0	27.0	3.0	<5	140	<1.0
(*Swiss Miss* Cocoa & Cream)	150	2.0	26.0	4.5	5	170	1.0
(*Swiss Miss* Fat Free)	50	3.0	10.0	0	0	200	<1.0
(*Swiss Miss* No Sugar)	60	2.0	10.0	1.0	0	170	1.0
(*Swiss Miss* Rich & Creamy)	110	2.0	22.0	2.0	<5	170	<1.0
caramel (*Swiss Miss*)	120	1.0	22.0	2.5	0	160	<1.0
chocolate:							
(*Swiss Miss* Rich) .	110	2.0	24.0	1.5	0	160	1.0
Dutch (*Hershey's*) .	200	3.0	41.0	3.0	0	300	2.0
milk (*Swiss Miss*) .	120	1.0	23.0	2.5	0	170	1.0
milk (*Swiss Miss* . Canister), ¼ cup	140	2.0	28.0	3.0	0	210	1.0
milk, w/marshmallows (*Swiss Miss*) ...	120	1.0	24.0	2.0	0	150	1.0
w/marshmallows:							
(*Swiss Miss*)	120	1.0	24.0	2.0	0	150	1.0
(*Swiss Miss* Canister), ¼ cup	140	1.0	29.0	2.5	0	180	1.0
(*Swiss Miss* Marsh-mallow Lovers Fat Free)	70	3.0	13.0	0	0	180	<1.0
mini (*Swiss Miss*) .	120	1.0	24.0	2.0	0	150	1.0
vanilla, French:							
(*Hershey's*)	140	4.0	28.0	1.5	<5	140	0
(*Swiss Miss*)	110	2.0	24.0	2.0	0	160	<1.0
Coconut, fresh, shelled:							
(*Dole*), 1.75 oz.	180	2.0	8.0	17.0	0	10	5.0
(*Frieda's* White/Young), 1.4 oz.	140	1.0	6.0	13.0	0	10	4.0
1 oz.	100	.9	4.3	9.5	0	6	2.6
shredded or grated, 1 cup not packed ..	283	2.7	12.2	26.8	0	16	7.2
Coconut, cream of:							
(*Costamar*), 1 oz.	110	0	19.0	3.0	0	10	0
(*Roland*), 1 oz.	130	0	21.0	5.0	0	20	<1.0
(*Vigo*), 2 tbsp.	110	0	17.0	10.0	0	15	0

Food and Measure	cal.	prot. (gms)	carbo. (gms)	fat (gms)	chol. (mgs)	sod. (mgs)	fiber (gms)
Coconut, dried:							
flaked, sweetened:							
(*Baker's Angel Flake*),							
2 tbsp.	70	1.0	6.0	5.0	0	40	1.0
(*Mounds*), 2 tbsp. .	70	<1.0	6.0	4.5	0	35	1.0
⅓ cup	117	.8	11.8	7.9	0	63	1.1
shredded:							
(*Shiloh Farms* Or-							
ganic), 3 tbsp. ...	100	1.0	4.0	9.0	0	5	2.0
(*Tree of Life* Organic							
Macaroon), 1 oz.	180	2.0	7.0	18.0	0	10	5.0
toasted, 1 oz.	168	1.5	12.6	13.4	0	11	1.0
Coconut, grated, in							
syrup, canned (*Vigo*),							
1 oz.	80	0	16.0	2.5	0	0	1.0
Coconut milk:							
(*Roland*), 2 tbsp.	80	0	3.0	8.0	0	5	1.0
(*Roland* Lite), 2 tbsp. .	25	0	1.0	2.0	0	25	0
(*A Taste of Thai*),							
⅓ cup	140	1.0	2.0	11.0	0	25	0
(*A Taste of Thai* Lite),							
⅓ cup	50	1.0	2.0	4.5	0	15	0
(*Vigo*), ¼ cup	120	0	2.0	12.0	0	10	0
Coconut nectar (*R.W.*							
Knudsen), 8 fl. oz. ..	140	1.0	27.0	5.0	0	55	3.0
Coconut water (*Roland*),							
12 fl. oz.	130	0	29.0	1.5	0	55	0
Cod, meat only:							
Atlantic, 4 oz.:							
raw	93	20.2	0	.8	49	62	0
baked or broiled ...	119	25.9	0	1.0	62	88	0
Pacific, 4 oz.:							
raw	93	20.3	0	.7	42	81	0
baked or broiled ...	119	26.0	0	.9	53	103	0
Cod, canned, Atlantic,							
w/liquid, 4 oz.	119	25.8	0	1.0	62	247	0
Cod, dried, Atlantic,							
salted, 1 oz.	81	17.6	0	.7	42	1968	0
Cod, smoked, Alaskan							
black, see "Sablefish,							
smoked"							
Cod entree, frozen:							
fillet, breaded (*Mrs.*							
Paul's), 4-oz. pc. ..	220	12.0	17.0	121.0	40	430	1.0

Food and Measure	cal.	prot. (gms)	carbo. (gms)	fat (gms)	chol. (mgs)	sod. (mgs)	fiber (gms)
stuffed (*Oven Poppers*), 5-oz. pc.:							
cheese, au gratin ..	220	24.0	5.0	11.0	75	450	1.0
broccoli, cheese ...	150	20.0	4.0	6.0	55	330	1.0
Cod liver, smoked, canned (*Roland*),							
⅓ cup	290	3.0	0	30.0	120	320	0
Cod liver oil, see "Oil"							
Coffee:							
brewed, 6 fl. oz.	4	.1	.8	0	0	4	0
instant, regular,							
1 rounded tsp.	4	.2	.7	tr.	0	1	0
Coffee, flavored, mix (*General Foods International Coffees*), 1⅓ tbsp. or 1 pkt.:							
café Français	60	0	8.0	3.0	0	90	0
café Vienna:							
regular	70	0	12.0	2.0	0	110	0
sugar free	30	0	2.0	2.0	0	60	0
cappuccino:							
Italian	50	0	10.0	1.5	0	45	0
orange	70	0	12.0	2.0	0	100	0
chocolate:							
dark Mayan, café Français	50	0	11.0	1.5	0	30	0
white, Swiss	70	0	12.0	2.5	0	30	0
Viennese	50	0	11.0	1.5	0	25	0
crème caramel	60	0	12.0	2.0	0	50	0
hazelnut Belgian café .	70	0	12.0	2.0	0	55	0
pumpkin spice, café Français	70	1.0	12.0	2.5	0	80	0
Suisse mocha:							
decaf	60	1.0	9.0	2.0	0	35	0
regular	60	0	10.0	2.0	0	40	0
sugar free	30	0	2.0	2.0	0	30	0
vanilla, French:							
decaf	60	0	10.0	2.0	0	55	0
regular or vanilla nut	60	0	10.0	2.5	0	55	0
sugar free	30	0	2.0	2.5	0	50	0
Coffee, iced:							
cappuccino:							
(*AriZona Kahlua* Shake), 10.5 fl. oz.	130	5.0	24.0	2.0	7	130	.5

Food and Measure	cal.	prot. (gms)	carbo. (gms)	fat (gms)	chol. (mgs)	sod. (mgs)	fiber (gms)
Coffee, iced, cappuccino *(cont.)*							
chocolatey, rich (*AriZona* Shake), 10.5 fl. oz.	180	4.0	36.0	2.0	9	150	.5
double-roasted (*AriZona* Shake), 10.5 fl. oz.	180	4.0	36.0	3.5	9	150	.5
mocha (*Bolthouse Farms Perfectly Protein*), 8 fl. oz.	178	10.0	29.0	2.5	13	106	0
caramel (*Frappuccino*), 9.5 fl. oz.	200	6.0	36.0	3.0	15	100	0
coffee:							
(*Frappuccino*), 9.5 fl. oz.	200	6.0	36.0	3.0	15	100	0
(*Starbucks*), 11.5 fl. oz.	100	2.0	23.0	1.0	5	25	0
espresso and cream, 6.5 fl. oz.:							
(*Starbucks Double Shot*)	140	4.0	18.0	6.0	20	70	0
(*Starbucks Double Shot* Light)	70	3.0	6.0	4.0	15	50	0
latte, hazelnut (*Bolthouse Farms Perfectly Protein*), 8 fl. oz. ..	199	10.0	34.0	2.5	13	115	0
mocha, 9.5 fl. oz.:							
(*Frappuccino*)	180	7.0	33.0	3.0	15	95	0
(*Frappuccino* Lite) .	100	6.0	12.0	3.0	15	95	0
Coffee, iced, mix (*General Foods International Coffees Cappuccino Coolers*), 1 pkt.:							
hazelnut	60	0	15.0	0	0	0	1.0
vanilla, French	60	0	15.0	0	0	0	0
Coffee creamer, see "Creamer"							
Coffee substitute (*Kaffree Roma*), 1 tsp.	10	0	0	0	0	0	0
Cold cuts, see "Lunch meat" and specific listings							

Food and Measure	cal.	prot. (gms)	carbo. (gms)	fat (gms)	chol. (mgs)	sod. (mgs)	fiber (gms)
Coleslaw, see "Salad blend kit"							
Coleslaw dressing, see "Salad dressing"							
Coleslaw seasoning (*Watkins*), ½ tsp. . . .	5	0	1.0	0	0	190	0
Collard greens, fresh:							
raw:							
(*Glory*), 2 cups . . .	25	2.0	5.0	0	0	15	3.0
chopped (*Del Monte*), 2 cups	25	1.0	5.0	0	0	30	1.0
chopped, ½ cup . . .	6	.3	1.3	<.1	0	4	.7
trimmed, 1 oz.	9	.4	2.0	.1	0	6	1.0
boiled, drained, chopped, ½ cup . . .	17	.9	3.9	.1	0	10	1.3
Collard greens, canned, ½ cup:							
chopped (*Bush's*)	30	2.0	4.0	0	0	410	2.0
seasoned:							
(*Glory* Sensibly) . . .	20	2.0	4.0	0	0	240	2.0
(*Glory* Southern) . .	35	2.0	5.0	0	0	490	2.0
turkey flavor (*Glory*) .	25	2.0	5.0	0	0	580	2.0
Collard greens, frozen, chopped, ½ cup:							
(*Seabrook Farms*) . . .	30	2.0	2.0	0	0	20	2.0
boiled, drained	31	2.5	6.1	.4	0	42	n.a.
seasoned (*Glory* Savory Accents)	60	2.0	10.0	0	0	630	2.0
Conch, fresh, baked or broiled, 4 oz.	147	29.8	1.9	1.4	74	174	0
Conch, canned, whole baby, in water (*Roland*), ½ cup . .	60	13.0	1.0	.5	100	320	0
Cookie:							
(*Gamesa Marias*), 8 pcs., 1 oz.	120	2.0	24.0	1.5	0	160	<1.0
(*Murray* Big 'Uns), 2 pcs., 1.1 oz.	150	2.0	23.0	5.0	0	120	<1.0
(*Peek Freans* Nice), 1.2 oz.	160	2.0	25.0	6.0	0	100	1.0
(*Pepperidge Farm Bordeaux*), 4 pcs., .9 oz.	130	2.0	19.0	5.0	10	95	<1.0
(*Social Tea* Biscuit 11 oz.), 1.1 oz.	140	2.0	24.0	4.0	0	125	1.0

Food and Measure	cal.	prot. (gms)	carbo. (gms)	fat (gms)	chol. (mgs)	sod. (mgs)	fiber (gms)
Cookie (cont.)							
(*TLC* Happy Trail Mix), 1.1-oz. pc.	130	2.0	21.0	5.0	0	80	4.0
almond:							
(*Alessi* Cantuccini), 5 pcs., 1 oz.	115	3.0	19.0	3.0	12	60	0
butter, toasted (*Tree of Life* Fat Free), .8-oz. pc.	70	2.0	16.0	0	0	35	1.0
thins (*Jules Destrooper*), 8 pcs., 1 oz.	140	2.0	22.0	4.5	15	170	<1.0
amaretti (*Roland*), 10 pcs., 1 oz.	130	2.0	24.0	2.0	0	20	1.0
animal:							
(*Animalitos*), 14 pcs., 1.1 oz.	110	2.0	25.0	.5	0	160	<1.0
(*Austin SeAnimals*), 1-oz. pkg.	130	2.0	20.0	4.5	0	90	<1.0
(*Austin Zoo*), 1 oz. .	130	2.0	25.0	2.0	0	90	<1.0
(*Barbara's Snackimals* Snickerdoodle), 10 pcs., 1.1 oz.	120	2.0	19.0	4.0	0	65	0
(*Barnum's Animals*), 1 oz.	120	2.0	22.0	3.5	0	140	1.0
(*Famous Amos* Safari), 10 pcs., 1 oz.	130	2.0	21.0	4.5	0	115	<1.0
(*Murray* Original), 2-oz. pkg.	250	3.0	43.0	8.0	0	250	<1.0
chocolate chip (*Barbara's Snackimals*), 10 pcs., 1.1 oz. .	120	1.0	19.0	4.0	0	80	0
frosted (*Keebler*), 8 pcs., 1.1 oz. ..	150	1.0	22.0	7.0	0	80	<1.0
iced (*Murray*), 2-oz. pkg.	250	3.0	43.0	7.0	0	240	<1.0
oatmeal (*Barbara's Snackimals*), 10 pcs., 1.1 oz. .	120	1.0	17.0	5.0	0	130	1.0
vanilla (*Barbara's Snackimals*), 10 pcs., 1.1 oz. .	110	2.0	17.0	4.0	0	65	0

Food and Measure	cal.	prot. (gms)	carbo. (gms)	fat (gms)	chol. (mgs)	sod. (mgs)	fiber (gms)
apricot raspberry (*Pepperidge Farm Verona*), 3 pcs., .9 oz.	140	2.0	22.0	5.0	10	100	<1.0
arrowroot (*Nabisco*), .2-oz. pc.	20	0	4.0	.5	0	15	0
assortment (*Murray*), 5 pcs., 1 oz.	130	2.0	19.0	5.0	0	130	<1.0
banana crème (*Murray*), 3 pcs., 1 oz.	140	1.0	21.0	5.0	0	90	<1.0
biscotti:							
almond or chocolate (*New York Style*), 3 pcs., 1 oz.	130	3.0	20.0	4.5	25	35	1.0
chocolate, chocolate dipped (*Nonni's Decadence*), .85-oz. pc.	100	2.0	16.0	4.0	20	70	1.0
butter:							
(*Murray Cookie Jar Classics*), 8 pcs., 1.1 oz.	140	2.0	22.0	5.0	0	130	<1.0
(*Pepperidge Farm Chessmen*), 3 pcs., .9 oz.	120	2.0	18.0	5.0	20.0	80	<1.0
Danish, 4 pcs., 1.1 oz.	160	2.0	19.0	8.0	20	80	1.0
caramel chip, w/fudge strips (*Chips Deluxe*), .7-oz. pc.	100	1.0	13.0	6.0	0	60	<1.0
carob (*Tree of Life Wheat Free California*), .8-oz. pc.	110	1.0	14.0	5.0	0	75	6.0
chocolate:							
(*Barbara's Organic Mini*), .9-oz. pkg.	100	1.0	18.0	2.0	5	150	0
w/almonds, chocolate coated (*Hershey's*), 2 pcs., 1 oz.	150	2.0	16.0	9.0	<5	65	<1.0
cappuccino or toffee (*Pepperidge Farm Marbella*), 3 pcs.	180	2.0	21.0	10.0	5	90	2.0

Food and Measure	cal.	prot. (gms)	carbo. (gms)	fat (gms)	chol. (mgs)	sod. (mgs)	fiber (gms)
Cookie, chocolate *(cont.)*							
w/caramel, chocolate coated (*Hershey's*), 2 pcs., 1 oz.	130	1.0	19.0	6.0	<5	80	<1.0
double, mini (*Hershey Kisses*), .9-oz. pkg.	120	2.0	17.0	5.0	0	55	<1.0
double, mini (*Hershey Kisses*), 24 pcs., 1.1 oz. .	140	2.0	20.0	6.0	0	65	1.0
mini (*Hershey Kisses*), .9-oz. pkg.	130	2.0	16.0	6.0	5	45	<1.0
mint, chocolate coated (*Dove Mint Chocolate Serenade*), 3 pcs., 1.1 oz. . .	160	2.0	19.0	8.0	0	70	1.0
mint, chocolate coated (*York*), 2 pcs., 1 oz.	130	2.0	17.0	8.0	0	50	1.0
w/peanut butter, chocolate coated (*Reese's*), 1 oz. .	150	2.0	17.0	8.0	0	90	<1.0
top (*Pepperidge Farm Geneva*), 3 pcs., 1.1 oz. . .	160	2.0	19.0	9.0	0	95	1.0
wafer (*Famous*), 5 pcs., 1.1 oz. . .	140	2.0	24.0	4.0	5	230	1.0
chocolate cake, Black Forest or mint (*SnackWell's*), .6-oz. pc.	50	1.0	12.0	.5	0	40	0
chocolate chip/chunk:							
(*Chips Ahoy!*), 3 pcs., 1.1 oz. . .	160	2.0	21.0	8.0	0	105	1.0
(*Chips Ahoy! 16 oz.*), 3 pcs., 1.2 oz. . .	160	2.0	22.0	8.0	0	110	1.0
(*Chips Ahoy! Candy Blasts*), .6-oz. pc.	90	1.0	11.0	4.5	0	55	0
(*Chips Ahoy! Chewy* .9-oz. pc.	120	1.0	18.0	6.0	0	80	1.0
(*Chips Ahoy! Chunky*), .6-oz. pc.	80	1.0	11.0	4.5	0	55	1.0
(*Chips Ahoy! Mini*), 5 pcs., 1.1 oz. . .	150	2.0	21.0	8.0	0	100	1.0
(*Chips Deluxe Chocolate Lovers*), .6-oz. pc.	80	<1.0	10.0	4.5	0	65	0

Food and Measure	cal.	prot. (gms)	carbo. (gms)	fat (gms)	chol. (mgs)	sod. (mgs)	fiber (gms)
(*Chips Deluxe* Original), 2-oz. pkg. . . .	300	3.0	37.0	16.0	0	180	1.0
(*Chips Deluxe* Soft 'n Chewy), .6-oz. pc.	80	<1.0	11.0	3.5	0	55	<1.0
(*Chips Deluxe Gripz*), .9-oz. pkg.	120	1.0	18.0	5.0	0	95	<1.0
(*Chips Deluxe Rite Bites*), .75-oz. pkg.	100	1.0	17.0	3.0	0	95	<1.0
(*Country Choice* Organic), 4 pcs., 1 oz.	130	1.0	20.0	5.0	0	140	<1.0
(*Dare* Breaktime), 4 pcs., 1.1 oz. . .	140	1.0	22.0	5.0	0	200	0
(*Dove* Beyond), .75-oz. pc.	110	1.0	13.0	5.0	10	100	1.0
(*Famous Amos*), 4 pcs., 1 oz.	150	1.0	20.0	7.0	<5	105	<1.0
(*Grandma's* Homestyle Big), 1.4-oz. pc.	190	2.0	25.0	9.0	0	105	<1.0
(*Grandma's* Rich 'n Chewy), 1 pkg. . . .	270	2.0	38.0	12.0	10	105	2.0
(*Health Valley* Chunk), .9-oz. pc.	120	1.0	15.0	7.0	10	150	1.0
(*Health Valley* Mini), 4 pcs., 1 oz.	120	1.0	16.0	6.0	5	125	1.0
(*Keebler Soft Batch*), .6-oz. pc.	80	<1.0	11.0	3.5	0	55	<1.0
(*Keebler Soft Batch*), 2.25-oz. pkg. . . .	310	2.0	42.0	14.0	0	220	1.0
(*Murray* Sugar Free), 3 pcs., 1.1 oz. . .	160	2.0	20.0	9.0	<5	130	1.0
(*Murray Cookie Jar Classics*), 8 pcs., 1.1 oz.	140	2.0	22.0	5.0	0	130	<1.0
(*Pepperidge Farm* Sugar Free), 3 pcs.	170	<1.0	22.0	9.0	15	85	1.0
(*Southern Kitchen*), 2 pcs., 1 oz.	140	2.0	19.0	7.0	0	140	<1.0
chocolate (*Health Valley* Mini), 4 pcs., 1 oz.	130	1.0	16.0	7.0	5	110	1.0
chocolate peanut butter (*Chips Deluxe*), .6-oz. pc.	80	1.0	10.0	4.5	0	65	<1.0

Food and Measure	cal.	prot. (gms)	carbo. (gms)	fat (gms)	chol. (mgs)	sod. (mgs)	fiber (gms)
Cookie, chocolate chip/chunk *(cont.)*							
chocolate walnut, dipped (*Dove Oasis*), .75-oz. pc.	110	1.0	13.0	6.0	5	90	1.0
coconut (*Chips Deluxe*), 2 pcs., 1.1 oz.	160	2.0	18.0	9.0	0	90	1.0
dark (*Pepperidge Farm Nantucket*), .9-oz. pc.	140	2.0	16.0	7.0	10	80	0
dark (*Pepperidge Farm Nantucket* Soft), 1.1-oz. pc.	150	2.0	20.0	8.0	10	95	0
dark, brownie (*Pepperidge Farm Captiva* Soft), 1 pc. .	140	1.0	22.0	5.0	<5	65	1.0
dark, double (*Pepperidge Farm Nantucket*), .9-oz. pc.	140	2.0	18.0	7.0	10	80	1.0
dark, pecans (*Pepperidge Farm Chesapeake*), .9-oz. pc.	140	2.0	15.0	8.0	10	80	0
double (*Chips Deluxe Gripz*), 1 pouch .	130	2.0	17.0	5.0	0	115	<1.0
double (*Health Valley* Chunk), .9-oz. pc.	120	1.0	15.0	7.0	5	140	1.0
double (*Health Valley Healthy Chips* Low Fat), 3 pcs., 1.2 oz.	120	2.0	23.0	3.0	0	70	2.0
fudge (*Grandma's* Homestyle Big), 1.4-oz. pc.	170	2.0	27.0	7.0	10	150	1.0
w/fudge stripes (*Chips Deluxe*), .7-oz. pc.	110	1.0	12.0	6.0	0	55	<1.0
macadamia (*Mauna Loa*), 4 pcs., 1 oz.	150	2.0	17.0	9.0	0	80	<1.0
milk (*Pepperidge Farm* Soft), 1 pc.	150	1.0	21.0	7.0	5	70	<1.0
milk, caramel (*Pepperidge Farm* Soft), 1-oz. pc.	140	1.0	21.0	6.0	5	75	<1.0
milk, cashew (*Pepperidge Farm Stowe*), 1 pc. . . .	130	2.0	17.0	6.0	10	75	1.0

Food and Measure	cal.	prot. (gms)	carbo. (gms)	fat (gms)	chol. (mgs)	sod. (mgs)	fiber (gms)
milk, macadamia (*Pepperidge Farm Sausalito*), .9-oz. pc.	140	2.0	16.0	8.0	10	80	0
milk, macadamia (*Pepperidge Farm Sausalito* Mini), 4 pcs. 1 oz.	150	2.0	17.0	8.0	10	90	0
milk, macadamia (*Pepperidge Farm Sausalito* Soft), 1 pc.	160	2.0	19.0	8.0	10	85	0
peanut butter cups (*Chips Deluxe*), .6-oz. pc.	90	1.0	10.0	4.5	0	50	<1.0
pecan (*Famous Amos*), 4 pcs., 1 oz.	150	2.0	18.0	8.0	0	95	1.0
pecan (*Murray* Sugar Free), 3 pcs., 1.1 oz. ..	160	2.0	19.0	10.0	<5	125	2.0
powdered sugar (*Keebler* Danish Wedding), 4 pcs., .9 oz.	130	1.0	18.0	6.0	0	70	<1.0
walnut (*Dove* Rendez-vous), .75-oz. pc.	110	1.0	13.0	6.0	10	100	1.0
white (*Health Valley* Chunk), .9-oz. pc.	140	1.0	17.0	7.0	5	150	0
white, macadamia (*Mauna Loa*), 4 pcs., 1 oz.	150	2.0	17.0	8.0	0	90	<1.0
white, macadamia (*Pepperidge Farm Tahoe*), .9-oz. pc.	130	1.0	17.0	6.0	<5	85	<1.0
white fudge, chunky (*Chips Ahoy!*), .6-oz. pc.	80	1.0	11.0	4.5	0	60	0
chocolate sandwich: (*Country Choice* Organic Cremes), 2 pcs., 1 oz.	130	1.0	19.0	5.0	0	100	<1.0
(*Dipping Delights*), .6-oz. pc.	90	<1.0	13.0	4.0	0	50	<1.0

Food and Measure	cal.	prot. (gms)	carbo. (gms)	fat (gms)	chol. (mgs)	sod. (mgs)	fiber (gms)
Cookie, chocolate sandwich *(cont.)*							
(*Emperador*), 2 pcs., .9 oz.	120	1.0	19.0	4.0	0	105	<1.0
(*Famous Amos* Cremes), 3 pcs., 1.2 oz.	170	2.0	25.0	7.0	0	150	1.0
(*Heath*), 2 pcs., 1 oz.	130	1.0	18.0	7.0	<5	85	<1.0
(*Hershey's*), 2 pcs., 1 oz.	130	1.0	19.0	6.0	0	85	<1.0
(*Murray* Sugar Free), 3 pcs., 1 oz.	130	1.0	19.0	7.0	0	55	1.0
(*Oreo*), 3 pcs., 1.2 oz.	160	2.0	25.0	7.0	0	190	1.0
(*Oreo* Mini Bite Size), 9 pcs., 1 oz.	140	1.0	21.0	6.0	0	160	1.0
(*Oreo* Reduced Fat), 3 pcs., 1.2 oz. . .	150	1.0	27.0	4.5	0	180	1.0
(*Oreo Double Stuf*), 2 pcs., 1 oz.	140	1.0	21.0	7.0	0	120	1.0
(*Pepperidge Farm Brussels*), 3 pcs., 1.1 oz.	150	2.0	20.0	7.0	5	65	1.0
(*Pepperidge Farm Brussels* Mini), 8 pcs., 1 oz.	150	2.0	19.0	7.0	5	65	1.0
(*Pepperidge Farm Lido*), 1 pc.	90	<1.0	10.0	5.0	<5	40	0
(*Pepperidge Farm Milano*), 3 pcs., 1.2 oz.	180	2.0	21.0	10.0	10	80	<1.0
(*Pepperidge Farm Milano* Mini), 6 pcs., 1 oz.	160	2.0	18.0	8.0	10	70	<1.0
(*Pepperidge Farm Milano* Sugar Free), 3 pcs.	170	2.0	21.0	9.0	5	65	<1.0
(*Reese's*), 2 pcs., 1 oz.	140	2.0	18.0	7.0	0	95	<1.0
all varieties (*Health Valley Cookie Cremes*), 2 pcs., .9 oz.	120	1.0	19.0	5.0	0	100	0
amaretto (*Pepperidge Farm Milano*), 2 pcs.	130	1.0	16.0	7.0	<5	65	<1.0

Food and Measure	cal.	prot. (gms)	carbo. (gms)	fat (gms)	chol. (mgs)	sod. (mgs)	fiber (gms)
black and white (*Pepperidge Farm Milano*), 3 pcs. . . .	180	2.0	21.0	10.0	<5	85	1.0
cheesecake (*Dipping Delights*), .6-oz. pc.	90	<1.0	13.0	4.0	0	50	0
chocolate coated (*Oreo*), 1.3 oz. . .	180	2.0	25.0	9.0	0	120	1.0
chocolate crème (*Country Choice Organic*), 2 pcs., 1 oz.	130	1.0	19.0	5.0	0	100	<1.0
chocolate crème (*Murray*), 3 pcs., 1 oz.	140	1.0	21.0	6.0	0	140	0
chocolate crème (*Oreo Double Stuf*), 3 pcs., 1.1 oz. . .	150	1.0	21.0	7.0	0	130	1.0
chocolate crème, mini (*Oreo*), 9 pcs., 1 oz.	140	1.0	21.0	6.0	0	160	1.0
coconut (*Pepperidge Farm Tahiti*), 2 pcs.	170	2.0	17.0	10.0	5	40	2.0
double (*Pepperidge Farm Milano*), 2 pcs., 1 oz. . . . :	180	2.0	21.0	10.0	10	80	<1.0
fudge coated (*Oreo*), .7-oz. pc.	100	1.0	13.0	5.0	0	70	1.0
fudge coated, white (*Oreo*), .7-oz. pc.	100	1.0	13.0	5.0	0	65	0
milk (*Pepperidge Farm Milano*), 3 pcs.	170	2.0	21.0	9.0	10	110	<1.0
mint/crème (*Oreo Double Delight*), 1 oz.	140	1.0	20.0	7.0	0	120	1.0
mint (*Pepperidge Farm Brussels*), 3 pcs., 1.1 oz. . .	190	2.0	22.0	10.0	0	100	1.0
mint (*Pepperidge Farm Milano*), 2 pcs., .9 oz. . . .	130	1.0	16.0	7.0	<5	65	<1.0
mint (*Pepperidge Farm Milano* Mini), 6 pcs., 1 oz.	170	2.0	20.0	9.0	5	85	1.0

Food and Measure	cal.	prot. (gms)	carbo. (gms)	fat (gms)	chol. (mgs)	sod. (mgs)	fiber (gms)
Cookie, chocolate sandwich *(cont.)*							
mint, chocolate coated (*Oreo*), 1.3 oz.	180	2.0	25.0	9.0	0	120	1.0
orange or vanilla (*Pepperidge Farm Milano*), 2 pcs., .9 oz.	130	1.0	16.0	7.0	<5	65	<1.0
raspberry (*Pepperidge Farm Milano*), 2 pcs., .9 oz. ...	130	1.0	16.0	7.0	<5	40	<1.0
and vanilla (*Country Choice* Organic Duplex Crèmes), 2 pcs., 1 oz.	130	1.0	19.0	5.0	0	110	<1.0
and vanilla (*Oreo* Duo), 1.25 oz. ..	170	2.0	25.0	7.0	0	130	1.0
cinnamon (*Gamesa Roscas*), 3 pcs., 1 oz.	130	2.0	22.0	4.0	0	130	1.0
coconut:							
(*Arcoiris*), 6 pcs. ..	220	3.0	44.0	3.5	0	130	1.0
(*Dare* Breaktime), 4 pcs., 1.1 oz. ..	140	2.0	22.0	5.0	0	105	<1.0
(*Gamesa* Barras de Coco), 5 pcs., 1 oz.	120	2.0	21.0	3.5	0	130	<1.0
(*Hawaianas*), 3 pcs., 1 oz.	130	2.0	22.0	3.5	0	115	<1.0
(*Southern Kitchen*), 2 pcs., 1 oz.	150	2.0	19.0	7.0	<5	80	<1.0
w/almonds, chocolate coated (*Almond Joy*), 2 pcs., 1 oz.	140	2.0	17.0	8.0	0	60	<1.0
bars (*Famous Amos*), 4 pcs., 1 oz.	130	2.0	20.0	5.0	0	120	1.0
bars (*Murray Cookie Jar Classics*), 6 pcs., 1.1 oz. ..	150	2.0	24.0	5.0	0	160	<1.0
crème sandwich (*Dare*), .7-oz. pc.	100	<1.0	13.0	5.0	0	75	<1.0
crèmes:							
(*Murray* Duplex), 3 pcs., 1 oz.	130	1.0	21.0	5.0	0	110	0
assorted (*Murray*), 3 pcs., 1 oz.	140	1.0	21.0	5.0	0	105	<1.0

Food and Measure	cal.	prot. (gms)	carbo. (gms)	fat (gms)	chol. (mgs)	sod. (mgs)	fiber (gms)
assorted (*Peek Freans*), 1 oz.	140	1.0	19.0	6.0	0	50	0
devil's food (*Snack-Well's Fat Free*), .6-oz. pc.	50	1.0	12.0	0	0	25	0
fig filled/bar:							
(*Barbara's* Traditional), ⅔-oz. pc.	60	0	14.0	.5	0	20	0
(*Barbara's* Wheat Free), ⅔-oz. pc. .	60	0	13.0	0	0	25	1.0
(*Newtons*), 2 pcs., 1.1 oz.	110	1.0	22.0	2.0	0	125	1.0
(*Newtons* Bars), 1.3-oz. pc.	130	1.0	26.0	2.5	0	140	2.0
(*Newtons* Fat Free 12 oz.), 1 oz. ..	90	1.0	22.0	0	0	125	1.0
(*Newtons* Whole Grain), 1.1 oz. ..	110	1.0	21.0	2.0	0	115	2.0
(*Newtons* Whole Grain Bars), 1.3-oz. pc.	130	1.0	26.0	2.5	0	135	3.0
apple cinnamon (*Barbara's*), ⅔-oz. pc.	60	1.0	14.0	0	0	25	1.0
blueberry (*Barbara's*), ⅔-oz. pc.	70	.0	15.0	.5	0	20	0
raspberry (*Barbara's*), ⅔-oz. pc.	60	0	14.0	0	0	25	1.0
whole wheat (*Barbara's*), ⅔-oz. pc.	60	1.0	13.0	0	0	25	1.0
fudge:							
caramel filled (*Fudge Shoppe*), 2 pcs., 1.1 oz.	160	1.0	20.0	8.0	0	40	0
double (*Murray Sugar Free*), 3 pcs., 1.2 oz. ..	160	2.0	21.0	8.0	<5	95	1.0
sticks (*Fudge Shoppe*), 3 pcs., 1 oz.	150	1.0	20.0	8.0	0	30	0
stripes (*Fudge Shoppe*), 3 pcs., .75 oz. ..	150	1.0	21.0	7.0	0	110	<1.0
stripes (*Fudge Shoppe Rite Bites*), .75-oz. pkg.	100	1.0	16.0	3.5	0	70	<1.0

Food and Measure	cal.	prot. (gms)	carbo. (gms)	fat (gms)	chol. (mgs)	sod. (mgs)	fiber (gms)
Cookie (cont.)							
fudge crème sandwich:							
(*E.L. Fudge* Original),							
.6-oz. pc.	90	1.0	13.0	3.5	<5	50	<1.0
(*E.L. Fudge* Double							
Stuffed), 2 pcs.,							
1.2 oz.	180	2.0	24.0	9.0	<5	95	1.0
chocolate (*Dare*),							
.7-oz. pc.	100	1.0	13.0	5.0	0	75	0
ginger:							
(*Barbara's* Organic							
Mini), .9-oz. pkg.	100	1.0	19.0	2.0	5	150	0
(*Dare* Breaktime),							
4 pcs. 1.1 oz. . . .	130	2.0	23.0	3.5	0	100	0
(*Pepperidge Farm*							
Ginger Family),							
4 pcs.	160	2.0	26.0	5.0	<5	135	1,9
(*Pepperidge Farm*							
Ginger Man),							
4 pcs., .9 oz. . . .	130	2.0	21.0	4.0	10	100	<1.0
thins (*Anna's*), 6 pcs.,							
1 oz.	140	2.0	19.0	7.0	0	150	2.0
ginger snaps:							
(*Country Choice*							
Organic), 5 pcs.,							
1.1 oz.	140	1.0	22.0	5.0	0	85	0
(*Earthbound Farm*							
Organic), 2 pcs.,							
1.1 oz.	120	2.0	18.0	6.0	20	70	0
(*Murray* Old Fashion),							
5 pcs., 1.1 oz. . .	140	2.0	22.0	5.0	0	160	<1.0
(*Murray* Sugar Free),							
7 pcs., 1.1 oz. . .	130	2.0	23.0	5.0	0	115	2.0
(*Nabisco*), 4 pcs.,							
1 oz.	120	1.0	23.0	2.5	0	190	1.0
iced (*Famous Amos*),							
1.75-oz. pkg. . . .	200	3.0	40.0	3.0	0	170	1.0
iced (*Murray* Old							
Fashion), 5 pcs.,							
1.2 oz.	150	2.0	25.0	5.0	0	160	<1.0
ginger lemon sandwich,							
2 pcs., 1 oz.:							
(*Carr's*)	130	1.0	20.0	5.0	0	95	0

Food and Measure	cal.	prot. (gms)	carbo. (gms)	fat (gms)	chol. (mgs)	sod. (mgs)	fiber (gms)
(*Country Choice* Organic Cremes)	130	1.0	19.0	5.0	0	120	<1.0
graham cracker:							
(*Keebler* Original), 8 pcs., 1 oz.	130	2.0	22.0	3.5	0	160	<1.0
amaranth or oat bran (*Health Valley*), 6 pcs., 1 oz.	120	3.0	22.0	3.0	0	80	3.0
oatmeal (*Teddy Grahams*), 1.1 oz.	130	2.0	23.0	3.5	0	125	1.0
rice (*Health Valley*), 6 pcs., 1 oz.	110	3.0	19.0	3.0	0	70	3.0
graham, chocolate:							
(*Annie's Bunny Grahams*), 1.1 oz.	130	2.0	22.0	3.5	0	90	<1.0
(*Honey Maid*), 1.1 oz.	130	2.0	24.0	3.0	0	190	1.0
(*Honey Maid* Sticks), 1.1 oz.	130	2.0	25.0	3.0	0	170	1.0
(*New Morning* Mini Bites), .75 oz.	90	1.0	15.0	2.5	0	100	1.0
(*Teddy Grahams*), 24 pcs., 1.1 oz. . .	130	2.0	22.0	4.5	0	160	1.0
chip (*Annie's Bunny Grahams*), 1.1 oz.	140	2.0	22.0	4.5	0	125	<1.0
chip (*Teddy Grahams*), 24 pcs., 1.1 oz. .	130	1.0	23.0	4.5	0	170	1.0
chip, mini (*Teddy Grahams*), 1.1 oz.	140	2.0	22.0	4.5	0	170	1.0
sticks (*Honey Maid*), 1.1 oz.	130	2.0	24.0	3.0	0	170	1.0
graham, cinnamon:							
(*Honey Maid*), 1.1 oz.	130	2.0	25.0	2.5	0	160	1.0
(*Honey Maid* Low Fat), 1.1 oz.	120	2.0	26.0	1.5	0	170	1.0
(*Honey Maid* Sticks), 1.1 oz.	130	2.0	25.0	3.0	0	170	1.0
(*Honey Maid* Sticks Packs 2 Go), 1 oz.	120	2.0	23.0	2.5	0	160	1.0
(*Keebler*), 8 pcs., 1.1 oz.	130	2.0	23.0	3.5	0	140	1.0
(*Keebler* Low Fat), 8 pcs., 1.1 oz. . .	110	2.0	23.0	1.5	0	140	1.0
(*Murray*), 8 pcs., 1.1 oz.	130	2.0	23.0	3.5	0	140	1.0

Food and Measure	cal.	prot. (gms)	carbo. (gms)	fat (gms)	chol. (mgs)	sod. (mgs)	fiber (gms)
Cookie, graham, cinnamon *(cont.)*							
(*New Morning* Organic), 2 pcs., 1.1 oz.	130	3.0	24.0	3.0	0	170	<1.0
(*Ricanelas*), 8 pcs., 1.1 oz.	140	2.0	24.0	4.0	0	180	2.0
(*Teddy Grahams*), 1.1 oz.	130	2.0	23.0	4.0	0	150	1.0
(*Teddy Grahams* 10 oz.), 1.1 oz. . . .	130	2.0	23.0	4.0	0	140	1.0
shapes (*Keebler* Bug Bites), 1.1 oz.	130	2.0	22.0	4.0	0	125	<1.0
graham, honey:							
(*Annie's Bunny Grahams*), 1.1 oz.	130	2.0	22.0	4.0	0	170	<1.0
(*Honey Maid*), 1.1 oz.	130	2.0	24.0	3.5	0	180	1.0
(*Honey Maid* Bees), 1.1 oz.	130	2.0	22.0	4.0	0	160	1.0
(*Honey Maid* Low Fat), 1.1 oz.	120	2.0	25.0	2.0	0	190	1.0
(*Honey Maid* Sticks), 1.1 oz.	130	2.0	25.0	2.5	0	160	1.0
(*Keebler*), 8 pcs., 1.1 oz.	140	2.0	23.0	4.0	0	150	<1.0
(*Keebler* Low Fat), 8 pcs., 1 oz.	110	2.0	22.0	1.5	0	150	<1.0
(*Murray*), 8 pcs., 1.1 oz.	140	2.0	23.0	4.0	0	150	<1.0
(*New Morning* Organic), 2 pcs., 1.1 oz.	130	3.0	24.0	3.0	0	180	1.0
(*New Morning* Mini Bites), .75 oz. . . .	90	1.0	15.0	2.5	0	110	1.0
(*Teddy Grahams*), 24 pcs., 1.1 oz. .	130	2.0	23.0	4.0	0	150	1.0
graham w/fudge:							
(*Fudge Shoppe*), 3 pcs., 1 oz.	140	1.0	17.0	7.0	0	70	<1.0
(*Murray* Sugar Free), 4 pcs., 1.1 oz. . .	150	2.0	19.0	8.0	0	80	1.0
graham sandwich, s'mores (*Ritz Bits*), 1.1 oz.	150	1.0	22.0	6.0	0	130	1.0

Food and Measure	cal.	prot. (gms)	carbo. (gms)	fat (gms)	chol. (mgs)	sod. (mgs)	fiber (gms)
ladyfingers:							
(*Alessi* Biscotti Savoiardi), 4 pcs., 1 oz.	110	2.0	23.0	1.0	30	80	1.0
(*Roland* Champagne), 6 pcs.	120	2.0	27.0	1.0	30	10	0
(*Roland* Italian), 4 pcs.	110	3.0	22.0	1.0	45	75	0
(*Specialty Brands*), 12 pcs., 3 oz. . . .	310	8.0	59.0	4.5	180	600	1.0
(*Torino*), 4 pcs., 1.2 oz.	120	3.0	25.0	1.0	25	50	<1.0
lemon:							
(*Famous Amos*), 5 pcs., 1.1 oz. . .	140	2.0	22.0	5.0	0	125	<1.0
(*Jackson's* Jumble), 3 pcs., 1.1 oz. . .	150	2.0	23.0	8.0	0	105	0
bars (*Murray Cookie Jar Classics*), 6 pcs., 1.1 oz. . .	150	2.0	24.0	5.0	0	170	<1.0
iced (*Grandma's* Big), 1.4-oz. pkg.	190	3.0	31.0	9.0	0	150	1.0
iced (*Murray* Low Fat), 7 pcs., 1.1 oz.	120	2.0	25.0	1.5	0	110	<1.0
snaps (*Earthbound Farm* Organic), 2 pcs., 1.1 oz. . .	120	2.0	16.0	6.0	25	115	0
wafers (*Murray* Sugar Free), 4 pcs., 1 oz.	130	<1.0	19.0	8.0	0	20	4.0
lemon sandwich:							
(*Austin Lemon Ohs!*), 1.2-oz. pkg.	170	1.0	24.0	7.0	0	95	<1.0
(*Dare* Creme), .7-oz. pc.	100	<1.0	14.0	4.0	0	70	0
(*Emperador*), 6 pcs.	270	3.0	45.0	8.0	0	260	1.0
(*Murray* Cremes), 3 pcs., 1 oz.	150	1.0	22.0	6.0	0	95	0
(*Murray* Sugar Free), 3 pcs., 1 oz.	130	1.0	19.0	7.0	0	55	<1.0
(*SnackWell's* Creme Sugar Free), 3 pcs., 1.1 oz. . .	130	1.0	23.0	6.0	0	135	2.0
macadamia toffee crunch (*Mauna Loa*), 4 pcs., 1 oz.	140	1.0	17.0	8.0	0	100	<1.0

Food and Measure	cal.	prot. (gms)	carbo. (gms)	fat (gms)	chol. (mgs)	sod. (mgs)	fiber (gms)
Cookie *(cont.)*							
maple leaf crème sandwich (*Dare*), .6-oz. pc.	80	<1.0	12.0	3.5	0	60	0
marshmallow, w/chocolate, 2 pcs.:							
(*Arcoiris*), 1 oz. . . .	120	1.0	18.0	5.0	0	50	<1.0
(*Dare* Whippet Original),1.1 oz.	130	1.0	21.0	4.5	0	45	1.0
(*Mallomars*), .9 oz.	120	1.0	18.0	5.0	0	40	1.0
raspberry (*Dare* Whippet), 1.1 oz.	130	1.0	22.0	4.5	0	45	1.0
marshmallow sandwich (*Arcoiris*), 6 pcs. . .	200	3.0	43.0	2.5	0	170	1.0
mint, fudge coated:							
(*Fudge Shoppe* Grasshopper), 4 pcs., 1 oz.	140	1.0	19.0	7.0	0	75	<1.0
(*Fudge Shoppe Rite Bites* Grasshopper), .75-oz. pkg.	100	2.0	14.0	3.5	0	70	1.0
(*Murray* Sugar Free), 4 pcs., .9 oz. . . .	130	1.0	16.0	7.0	0	65	1.0
mint crème (*Fudge Shoppe*), 3 pcs., 1.1 oz.	160	<1.0	20.0	9.0	0	65	<1.0
mint sandwich (*Country Choice* Organic Cremes), 2 pcs., 1 oz.	130	1.0	19.0	5.0	0	100	<1.0
molasses:							
(*Pepperidge Farm* Soft), 1 pc.	130	1.0	22.0	3.5	5	120	0
spiced (*Grandma's* Big), 1 pc.	160	2.0	28.0	4.5	<5	220	1.0
oatmeal:							
(*Barbara's* Organic Mini), .9-oz. pkg.	100	1.0	19.0	2.0	5	140	0
(*Dare* Breaktime), 4 pcs., 1.1 oz. . .	130	2.0	22.0	4.0	0	190	<1.0
(*Murray* Sugar Free), 3 pcs., 1.1 oz. . .	140	2.0	21.0	7.0	0	130	3.0

Food and Measure	cal.	prot. (gms)	carbo. (gms)	fat (gms)	chol. (mgs)	sod. (mgs)	fiber (gms)
(*Pepperidge Farm* Soft), .9-oz. pc. .	140	2.0	22.0	5.0	10	120	1.0
(*Southern Kitchen*), 2 pcs., 1 oz.	140	2.0	20.0	6.0	0	95	1.0
chocolate, dark (*TLC*), 1.1-oz. pc.	130	2.0	21.0	5.0	0	70	3.0
chocolate chip (*Chips Ahoy!* Chewy), 1 oz. . . .	120	1.0	18.0	6.0	0	80ˈ	1.0
chocolate chip (*Country Choice* Organic), .8-oz. pc.	100	2.0	15.0	4.0	5	60	1.0
chocolate chip (*Health Valley* Wheat Free), .8-oz. pc.	100	2.0	14.0	4.0	0	50	1.0
chocolate chip walnut (*Famous Amos*), 4 pcs., 1 oz.	140	1.0	18.0	7.0	<5	110	1.0
iced (*Country Choice* Organic), 4 pcs., 1 oz.	120	1.0	21.0	4.0	0	120	<1.0
iced (*Murray* Low Fat), 7 pcs., 1.1 oz.	120	2.0	25.0	1.5	0	100	<1.0
iced (*Murray* Old Fashion), 5 pcs., 1.2 oz	150	2.0	24.0	6.0	0	200	<1.0
iced (*Southern Kitchen*), 2 pcs., 1 oz.	140	2.0	20.0	5.0	0	85	1.0
peanut crunch (*Health Valley* Wheat Free), .8-oz. pc.	100	2.0	14.0	4.0	0	60	1.0
oatmeal cranberry (*Pepperidge Farm* Soft), .9-oz. pc. . . .	130	2.0	22.0	4.0	5	110	<1.0
oatmeal macaroon sandwich (*Famous Amos*), 3 pcs., 1.2 oz.	170	2.0	24.0	7.0	0	65	<1.0
oatmeal raisin:							
(*Country Choice* Organic), .8-oz. pc.	100	1.0	16.0	3.0	5	65	1.0
(*Grandma's* Homestyle Big), 1.4-oz. pc. .	180	2.0	30.0	6.0	10	240	1.0

Food and Measure	cal.	prot. (gms)	carbo. (gms)	fat (gms)	chol. (mgs)	sod. (mgs)	fiber (gms)
Cookie, oatmeal raisin *(cont.)*							
(*Health Valley* Low Fat), 3 pcs., 1.2 oz.	110	2.0	23.0	1.5	0	105	1.0
(*Health Valley* Wheat Free), .8-oz. pc.	90	2.0	14.0	3.5	0	50	1.0
(*Keebler* Country Style), 2 pcs., 1 oz.	130	2.0	18.0	6.0	0	115	1.0
(*Pepperidge Farm Santa Cruz* Soft), .9-oz. pc.	130	2.0	23.0	4.5	<5	90	2.0
flax (*TLC*), 1.1 oz.	130	2.0	20.0	5.0	0	75	4.0
peanut butter:							
(*Famous Amos*), 4 pcs., 1.1 oz.	150	3.0	17.0	8.0	<5	70	<1.0
(*Grandma's* Home-style Big), 1.4-oz. pc.	200	4.0	24.0	10.0	10	200	1.0
(*Health Valley* Mini), 4 pcs., 1 oz.	120	3.0	16.0	5.0	10	180	0
(*Keebler Soft Batch*), .6-oz. pc.	80	<1.0	10.0	3.5	0	50	0
(*Murray* Sugar Free), 3 pcs., 1.1 oz.	150	3.0	16.0	9.0	<5	130	1.0
(*Southern Kitchen*), 2 pcs., 1 oz.	150	2.0	18.0	8.0	0	110	<1.0
chocolate chip (*Chips Ahoy!* Chunky), .6-oz. pc.	90	1.0	10.0	5.0	0	85	0
fudge coated (*Fudge Shoppe*), 3 pcs., 1.1 oz.	170	3.0	16.0	10.0	0	100	<1.0
peanut butter sandwich:							
(*Famous Amos*), 3 pcs., 1.2 oz.	160	3.0	22.0	7.0	0	65	1.0
(*Murray* Cremes), 3 pcs., 1 oz.	150	2.0	21.0	6.0	0	85	0
(*Nutter Butter*), 1 oz.	130	2.0	19.0	6.0	0	110	1.0
(*Nutter Butter* Bites), 10 pcs., 1.1 oz.	140	2.0	21.0	6.0	0	115	1.0
(*Nutter Butter* Bites), 1.25-oz. pkg.	170	3.0	24.0	7.0	0	135	1.0
(*Nutter Butter* Packs 2 Go), 1.9 oz.	260	4.0	37.0	11.0	5.0	220	1.0

Food and Measure	cal.	prot. (gms)	carbo. (gms)	fat (gms)	chol. (mgs)	sod. (mgs)	fiber (gms)
chocolate coated (*Nutter Butter*), .6-oz. pc.	90	1.0	12.0	4.5	0	45	0
graham, chocolate (*New Morning Graham-Wiches*), 2 pcs., 1 oz.	120	2.0	18.0	5.0	0	95	0
graham, honey (*New Morning Graham-Wiches*), 2 pcs., 1 oz.	130	2.0	18.0	5.0	0	120	0
peanut butter wafer, chocolate coated (*ChocoStix Nutter Butter*), 1 oz.	140	1.0	18.0	8.0	0	50	1.0
puff pastry, glazed (*Alessi Sfogliatine*), 3 pcs., 1 oz.	150	2.0	18.0	8.0	7	75	1.0
rainbow chips: (*Rainbow Chips Deluxe*), .6-oz. pc.	80	1.0	10.0	4.0	0	55	<1.0
mini (*Rainbow Chips Deluxe*), 1.4-oz. pkg.	200	1.0	27.0	10.0	0	125	<1.0
raspberry: (*Newtons*), 2 pcs., 1 oz.	100	1.0	21.0	1.5	0	110	1.0
(*Pepperidge Farm Chantilly*), 2 pcs., .9 oz.	120	1.0	23.0	3.0	0	115	<1.0
shortbread: (*Lorna Doone*), 4 pcs., 1 oz.	140	1.0	20.0	7.0	0	150	0
(*Murray* Sugar Free), 8 pcs., 1.1 oz.	130	2.0	21.0	5.0	0	140	2.0
(*Pepperidge Farm*), 2 pcs., .9 oz. . . .	140	2.0	16.0	7.0	10	105	<1.0
(*Sandies* Simply Shortbread), .6-oz. pc.	80	<1.0	10.0	4.5	5	65	0
(*Sandies Rite Bites*), .75-oz. pkg.	100	1.0	17.0	3.0	0	90	<1.0
(*SnackWell's* Sugar Free), 3 pcs., 1.1 oz.	130	2.0	21.0	6.0	5	140	2.0

Food and Measure	cal.	prot. (gms)	carbo. (gms)	fat (gms)	chol. (mgs)	sod. (mgs)	fiber (gms)
Cookie, shortbread *(cont.)*							
butter pecan or fudge drops (*Sandies*), 4 pcs., 1 oz.	140	1.0	18.0	7.0	0	60	<1.0
fudge dipped (*Murray* Sugar Free), 5 pcs., 1 oz.	150	2.0	21.0	8.0	0	80	1.0
pecan (*Sandies*), .6-oz. pc.	80	1.0	9.0	5.0	<5	50	0
pecan (*Sandies* Reduced Fat), .6-oz. pc.	80	<1.0	11.0	3.5	0	65	0
pecan (*Murray* Sugar Free), 3 pcs., 1.1 oz.	170	2.0	18.0	11.0	<5	110	1.0
pecan chocolate chip (*Sandies*), .6-oz. pc.	80	<1.0	9.0	5.0	0	50	0
spice (*Pepperidge Farm* Snickerdoodle), 1 pc.	140	2.0	22.0	5.0	10	95	<1.0
strawberry:							
(*Newtons*), 2 pcs., 1 oz.	100	1.0	21.0	1.5	0	110	1.0
(*Pepperidge Farm Verona*), 3 pcs., .9 oz.	140	2.0	22.0	5.0	10	100	<1.0
crèmes (*Murray*), 3 pcs., 1 oz.	150	1.0	21.0	5.0	0	90	<1.0
mini (*Newtons* Whole Grain), 1.3-oz. pkg.	130	2.0	27.0	3.0	0	140	2.0
sugar:							
(*Grandma's* Big), 1.4-oz. pc.	190	3.0	22.0	9.0	0	150	1.0
(*Pepperidge Farm* Homestyle), 3 pcs., 1.1 oz. . .	140	2.0	20.0	6.0	15	90	<1.0
(*Pepperidge Farm* Soft), 1 pc.	140	2.0	22.0	5.0	10	90	0
sugar wafer:							
(*Murray*), 5 pcs., 1 oz.	150	1.0	20.0	7.0	0	25	<1.0
(*Murray* Duplex), 5 pcs., 1.1 oz. . .	160	1.0	22.0	7.0	0	30	0
chocolate (*Gamesa*), 3 pcs., 1.2 oz. . .	160	1.0	23.0	7.0	0	30	0

Food and Measure	cal.	prot. (gms)	carbo. (gms)	fat (gms)	chol. (mgs)	sod. (mgs)	fiber (gms)
peanut butter (*Murray*), 5 pcs., 1.1 oz.	160	3.0	17.0	9.0	0	50	<1.0
strawberry (*Gamesa*), 3 pcs., 1.2 oz. . .	160	1.0	24.0	6.0	0	25	0
strawberry (*Murray*), 5 pcs., 1.1 oz. . .	160	1.0	22.0	7.0	0	30	0
vanilla (*Gamesa*), 3 pcs., 1.2 oz. . .	160	1.0	25.0	7.0	0	25	0
vanilla (*Murray* Sugar Free), 4 pcs., 1 oz.	140	1.0	20.0	8.0	0	20	5.0
vanilla, w/chocolate:							
(*Dove Milk Chocolate Moment*), 3 pcs., 1.1 oz. . .	160	2.0	20.0	9.0	5	45	1.0
toffee (*Dove Toffee Chocolate Thrill*), 3 pcs., 1.1 oz. . .	160	2.0	20.0	8.0	5	50	1.0
vanilla sandwich:							
(*Austin* Cremes), 1.2-oz. pkg.	170	1.0	24.0	7.0	0	85	<1.0
(*Cameo*), 1 oz.	130	1.0	21.0	5.0	0	105	0
(*Country Choice* Organic Cremes), 2 pcs., 1 oz.	130	1.0	19.0	5.0	0	120	0
(*Emperador*), 2 pcs., .9 oz.	120	2.0	19.0	3.5	0	75	0
(*Famous Amos*), 3 pcs., 1.2 oz. . .	170	2.0	25.0	7.0	0	100	1.0
(*Grandma's* Mini Bites), 9 pcs., 1.1 oz.	150	2.0	22.0	7.0	<5	80	<1.0
(*Grandma's* Sandwich Cremes), 5 pcs., 1.5 oz. . .	210	2.0	30.0	9.0	0	90	1.0
(*Health Valley* Cookie Cremes), 2 pcs., .9 oz.	120	1.0	19.0	5.0	0	125	0
(*Murray* Cremes), 3 pcs., 1 oz.	140	1.0	22.0	5.0	0	85	0
(*Murray* Sugar Free Cremes), 3 pcs., 1 oz.	130	1.0	20.0	6.0	0	55	<1.0

Food and Measure	cal.	prot. (gms)	carbo. (gms)	fat (gms)	chol. (mgs)	sod. (mgs)	fiber (gms)
Cookie, vanilla sandwich (cont.)							
(*Oreo* Golden), 3 pcs., 1.25 oz.	170	1.0	25.0	7.0	0	120	0
(*Oreo* Golden Mini Bite Size), 1 oz. . .	140	1.0	21.0	6.0	0	105	0
(*SnackWell's* Creme), 1.7-oz. pkg.	210	2.0	38.0	5.0	0	230	1.0
(*Vienna Fingers*), 2 pcs., 1.1 oz. . .	150	1.0	22.0	7.0	0	95	<1.0
(*Vienna Fingers* Reduced Fat), 2 pcs., 1.1 oz. . .	140	1.0	24.0	4.5	0	115	<1.0
w/chocolate crème (*Oreo Uh-Oh*), 1.25 oz.	170	2.0	25.0	7.0	0	135	1.0
vanilla wafer:							
(*Country Choice* Organic), 7 pcs., 1.1 oz.	140	1.0	22.0	5.0	5	100	0
(*Jackson's*), 8 pcs., 1.1 oz.	140	2.0	23.0	4.5	<5	120	<1.0
(*Keebler*), 8 pcs., 1.1 oz.	140	1.0	21.0	6.0	0	120	<1.0
(*Murray*), 8 pcs., 1.1 oz.	150	1.0	22.0	6.0	0	120	<1.0
(*Murray* Sugar Free), 9 pcs., 1.1 oz. . .	130	2.0	24.0	5.0	0	90	2.0
(*Nilla*), 8 pcs., 1.1 oz.	140	1.0	21.0	6.0	5	115	0
(*Nilla* Reduced Fat), 8 pcs., 1 oz.	110	1.0	24.0	2.0	0	110	0
fudge dipped (*Murray* Sugar Free), 4 pcs., 1.1 oz.	150	1.0	19.0	10.0	0	20	4.0
mini (*Keebler*), 18 pcs., 1.1 oz. . .	140	1.0	21.0	6.0	0	120	<1.0
mini (*Nilla*), 1.1 oz.	140	1.0	21.0	6.0	5	115	0
wafer (*Roland* Gaufrettes Eventails), 4 pcs., .9 oz.	110	2.0	6.0	2.0	25	95	0
wafer, w/chocolate (*Bahlsen* Afrika), 8 pcs., 1.1 oz.	170	2.0	17.0	10.0	5	20	2.0

Food and Measure	cal.	prot. (gms)	carbo. (gms)	fat (gms)	chol. (mgs)	sod. (mgs)	fiber (gms)
wafer, rolled, crème filled (*Pepperidge Farm Pirouette*), 2 pcs., .9 oz.:							
cappuccino	120	1.0	18.0	5.0	<5	40	0
chocolate fudge . . .	120	2.0	18.0	4.0	0	30	1.0
chocolate hazelnut .	120	1.0	19.0	5.0	5	40	1.0
mint chocolate	120	1.0	18.0	4.5	<5	40	<1.0
vanilla	120	1.0	18.0	7.0	<5	65	0
Cookie, frozen/ refrigerated, ready-to-bake, 1 pc., except as noted:							
chocolate, triple:							
(*Nestlé Ultimates*) .	170	2.0	23.0	8.0	20	180	1.0
(*Pillsbury Big Deluxe Classics*)	200	2.0	25.0	10.0	10	115	1.0
chocolate candy, w/chips (*Pillsbury*)	100	1.0	13.0	4.5	5	60	0
chocolate chip:							
(*Kineret*)	130	1.0	17.0	7.0	10	85	0
(*Nestlé Toll House*), 1 oz.	130	1.0	18.0	6.0	10	70	<1.0
(*Nestlé Toll House Bar*), .9 oz.	120	1.0	15.0	6.0	15	90	<1.0
(*Nestlé Toll House Jumbo*), 1.5 oz. .	200	2.0	26.0	10.0	20	160	1.0
(*Nestlé Toll House Mini*), 2 pcs., .9 oz.	120	1.0	15.0	6.0	15	90	<1.0
(*Nestlé Ultimates*) .	180	2.0	23.0	9.0	15	150	1.0
(*Pillsbury*)	100	1.0	13.0	5.0	<5	70	0
(*Pillsbury Big Deluxe Classics*)	200	2.0	25.0	10.0	10	140	<1.0
(*Pillsbury Create 'n Bake*), 1½" ball of dough	120	1.0	18.0	5.0	5	90	<1.0
w/walnuts (*Pillsbury*)	100	1.0	12.0	5.0	<5	65	0
chocolate chunk:							
(*Nestlé Toll House*)	120	1.0	15.0	6.0	15	100	<1.0
and chip (*Pillsbury*)	100	1.0	13.0	5.0	<5	70	0
gingerbread (*Pillsbury Create 'n Bake*), 2 balls dough, 1" . .	140	1.0	18.0	7.0	10	105	0

Food and Measure	cal.	prot. (gms)	carbo. (gms)	fat (gms)	chol. (mgs)	sod. (mgs)	fiber (gms)
Cookie, frozen/refrigerated *(cont.)*							
oatmeal:							
chocolate chip (*Pillsbury*)	100	1.0	13.0	4.5	<5	55	<1.0
chocolate chip (*Pillsbury Create 'n Bake*), 1½" ball of dough	130	1.0	17.0	6.0	5	100	<1.0
raisin (*Pillsbury Big Deluxe Classics*) .	170	2.0	26.0	7.0	10	115	1.0
peanut butter:							
(*Nestlé Ultimates*) .	170	2.0	23.0	8.0	15	190	1.0
(*Pillsbury Blossoms*)	130	2.0	17.0	6.0	5	100	0
(*Pillsbury Create 'n Bake*), 1½" ball of dough	130	2.0	16.0	6.0	5	135	0
(*Pillsbury Reese's Pieces*)	100	1.0	13.0	4.5	<5	75	0
chocolate chunk bars (*Pillsbury* Simply Bake), 1/10 pkg. .	180	2.0	23.0	9.0	5	125	0
cup (*Pillsbury Big Deluxe Classics*) .	190	3.0	24.0	9.0	5	160	<1.0
s'mores (*Pillsbury*) . .	100	1.0	13.0	4.5	<5	60	0
sugar:							
(*Nestlé Toll House*)	130	1.0	18.0	6.0	10	100	<1.0
(*Pillsbury*)	100	<1.0	12.0	5.0	5	55	0
(*Pillsbury Create 'n Bake*), ½" slice, 1/16 pkg.	130	1.0	18.0	6.0	10	80	0
turtle:							
(*Nestlé Ultimates*) .	180	1.0	23.0	9.0	15	140	1.0
(*Pillsbury Big Deluxe Classics*)	200	2.0	26.0	10.0	5	105	<1.0
bars (*Pillsbury* Simply Bake), 1/10 pkg. .	180	2.0	23.0	9.0	5	100	<1.0
white chunk macadamia (*Pillsbury Big Deluxe Classics*) . . .	200	2.0	24.0	11.0	10	110	1.0
Cookie, mix:							
bars, 1/20 pkg.:							
(*Eagle Brand Magic*)	110	2.0	15.0	5.0	5	50	1.0
(*Eagle Brand Turtle Temptations*) . . .	140	2.0	19.0	6.0	<5	15	2.0

Food and Measure	cal.	prot. (gms)	carbo. (gms)	fat (gms)	chol. (mgs)	sod. (mgs)	fiber (gms)
chocolate chip:							
(*Arrowhead Mills* Organic), 1 pc.*	90	1.0	16.0	3.0	15	105	0
(*Arrowhead Mills* Organic Gluten Free), 1 pc.*	90	1.0	17.0	3.0	15	125	0
(*Betty Crocker*), 2 pcs.*	170	2.0	21.0	8.0	25	115	0
(*Dr. Oetker* Organic), 1/12 pkg.	120	1.0	24.0	2.0	0	110	0
fudgy (*Betty Crocker* Warm Delights Micro), 1 bowl	340	4.0	58.0	11.0	0	290	2.0
walnut (*Betty Crocker* Warm Delights Micro), 2 pcs.*	170	2.0	21.0	9.0	25	140	1.0
chocolate chunk, double (*Betty Crocker*), 2 pcs.*	150	2.0	21.0	6.0	10	105	0
coconut bar, w/chocolate (*Betty Crocker Almond Joy*), 1/12 pkg.*	200	2.0	21.0	12.0	15	95	2.0
fudge bar (*Eagle Brand Decadent*), 1/11 pkg.	190	3.0	23.0	17.0	5	20	2.0
gingerbread (*Pillsbury*), 1/8 pkg.	210	2.0	39.0	5.0	0	350	0
lemon bar:							
(*Betty Crocker Sunkist*), 1/16 pkg.*	140	2.0	24.0	4.0	40	90	0
(*Eagle Brand Creamy Lemon Delights*), 1/20 pkg.	100	1.0	21.0	1.0	0	200	0
lime bar (*Eagle Brand Key Lime Treasures*), 1/16 pkg.	330	6.0	59.0	9.0	20	220	1.0
oatmeal (*Dr. Oetker* Organic), 1/12 pkg.	110	1.0	24.0	.5	0	110	0
oatmeal chocolate chip (*Betty Crocker*), 2 pcs.*	160	2.0	21.0	8.0	25	120	0
oatmeal raisin:							
(*Arrowhead Mills* Organic), 1 pc.*	90	2.0	16.0	2.0	15	90	<1.0
(*Sun•Maid*), ¼ cup	170	2.0	35.0	2.0	0	120	1.0

Food and Measure	cal.	prot. (gms)	carbo. (gms)	fat (gms)	chol. (mgs)	sod. (mgs)	fiber (gms)
Cookie, mix *(cont.)*							
peanut butter (*Betty Crocker*), 2 pcs.* ..	150	3.0	20.0	6.0	10	150	0
peanut butter bar:							
(*Betty Crocker Reese's*), 1/15 pkg.*	180	2.0	20.0	10.0	10	150	1.0
(*Eagle Brand* Passion), 1/20 pkg.	170	4.0	20.0	8.0	<5	90	1.0
rainbow chocolate candy (*Betty Crocker*), 2 pcs.*	160	2.0	22.0	7.0	25	140	0
sugar (*Betty Crocker*), 2 pcs.*	170	2.0	22.0	6.0	25	105	0
toffee bar:							
(*Betty Crocker Heath* Bits), 1/12 pkg.*	190	1.0	27.0	9.0	15	160	1.0
(*Eagle Brand* Dream), 1/20 pkg.	110	1.0	20.0	3.5	0	65	0
Cookie crumbs:							
(*Oreo*), 2 tbsp.	90	1.0	13.0	4.0	0	95	1.0
graham cracker (*Keebler*), 3 tbsp. ...	70	1.0	13.0	1.5	0	140	1.0
Cookie pie crust, see "Pie crust"							
Coquito nut (*Frieda's*), 11 pcs., 1 oz.	110	1.0	5.0	10.0	0	5	3.0
Coriander, fresh, ¼ cup	1	.1	.1	<.1	0	1	.1
Coriander, dried:							
leaf, 1 tsp.	2	.1	.3	<.1	0	1	.1
seed, 1 tsp.	5	.2	1.0	.3	0	1	.5
Corkscrew pasta dish mix, four cheese (*Pasta-Roni*), 1 cup*	370	11.0	49.0	16.0	10	890	2.0
Corn, fresh:							
baby, .28-oz. ear	9	.3	2.0	.1	0	1	.2
golden or white:							
raw (*Del Monte*), 3.2-oz. ear	80	3.0	18.0	1.0	0	0	3.0
raw, 5-oz. ear	123	4.6	27.2	1.7	0	21	3.9
kernels, boiled, drained, ½ cup .	89	2.7	20.6	1.1	0	14	2.3
white, boiled, drained, 2.72-oz. ear	83	2.6	19.3	1.0	0	13	2.1

Food and Measure	cal.	prot. (gms)	carbo. (gms)	fat (gms)	chol. (mgs)	sod. (mgs)	fiber (gms)
Corn, canned, ½ cup, except as noted:							
baby, whole or cut (*Roland*)	25	2.0	4.0	0	0	280	2.0
kernel, golden:							
(*Del Monte*)	90	2.0	18.0	1.0	0	360	3.0
(*Del Monte* Summer Crisp Vac Pac) . .	70	2.0	13.0	1.0	0	270	3.0
(*Freshlike*)	80	3.0	17.0	1.5	0	310	2.0
(*Furmano's*)	100	2.0	20.0	1.0	0	340	1.0
(*Green Giant* Whole Kernel Sweet) . . .	60	2.0	11.0	.5	0	370	2.0
(*Green Giant* Whole Kernel Sweet Less Sodium)	80	2.0	16.0	.5	0	180	2.0
(*Green Giant Niblets* Extra Sweet), ⅓ cup	50	2.0	10.0	.5	0	200	1.0
(*Green Giant Niblets* Vac Pac), ⅓ cup	80	2.0	16.0	.5	0	230	1.0
(*S&W*)	60	2.0	11.0	1.0	0	360	3.0
(*S&W* Sweet 'n Crisp)	70	2.0	13.0	1.0	0	270	3.0
kernel, golden/white:							
(*Del Monte*)	80	2.0	18.0	.5	0	360	2.0
(*Green Giant* Super Sweet), ⅓ cup . .	60	2.0	12.0	.5	0	200	1.0
kernel, white:							
(*Del Monte*)	60	2.0	11.0	1.0	0	360	3.0
(*Green Giant* Shoe-peg), ⅓ cup	80	2.0	16.0	.5	0	220	1.0
(*Roland* Organic) . .	110	2.0	23.0	1.0	0	145	4.0
cream style:							
(*Del Monte*)	90	2.0	20.0	.5	0	360	2.0
(*Freshlike/Veg-All*), ⅓ cup	100	2.0	21.0	1.0	0	280	2.0
(*Green Giant*)	90	2.0	19.0	.5	0	400	1.0
(*S&W*)	60	1.0	14.0	.5	0	360	2.0
seasoned (*Glory* Skillet Corn)	80	2.0	19.0	.5	0	490	2.0
white (*Del Monte*) .	100	2.0	21.0	1.0	0	360	2.0
in butter sauce (*Del Monte Savory Sides*)	90	2.0	14.0	2.5	5	530	<1.0

Food and Measure	cal.	prot. (gms)	carbo. (gms)	fat (gms)	chol. (mgs)	sod. (mgs)	fiber (gms)
Corn, canned (cont.)							
w/diced pepper:							
(*Freshlike* Selects) .	80	2.0	16.0	1.0	0	240	1.0
(*Green Giant Mexi-corn*), ⅓ cup ...	70	2.0	14.0	.5	0	250	1.0
seasoned (*Del Monte* Fiesta)	50	2.0	12.0	1.0	0	310	2.0
w/tomato, black beans (*Del Monte Savory Sides* Santa Fe) ...	70	3.0	16.0	1.0	0	510	1.0
Corn, frozen, ⅔ cup, except as noted:							
on cob:							
(*Green Giant* Extra Sweet), ½ ear, 2.2 oz.	60	2.0	11.0	1.0	0	0	1.0
(*Green Giant Nibblers* Halves), ½ ear, 2.2 oz.	70	2.0	14.0	.5	0	5	1.0
mini (*Birds Eye Steamfresh* Sweet), 3-oz. ear	90	3.0	19.0	1.0	0	0	1.0
kernel, golden:							
(*Birds Eye* Sweet) .	100	3.0	21.0	1.0	0	0	1.0
(*Birds Eye/Birds Eye Steamfresh* Super Sweet)	70	3.0	14.0	1.0	0	0	2.0
(*Cascadian Farm* Organic Super Sweet), ¾ cup ..	70	2.0	16.0	1.0	0	90	2.0
(*Cascadian Farm* Organic Sweet Bag), ¾ cup	70	3.0	18.0	1.0	0	0	2.0
(*Cascadian Farm* Organic Sweet Box), ¾ cup	90	3.0	19.0	1.0	0	0	2.0
(*C&W* Petite)	100	3.0	21.0	1.0	0	0	1.0
(*C&W Early Harvest* Supersweet)	70	3.0	14.0	1.0	0	0	2.0
(*Green Giant Niblets*), ½ cup cooked ..	80	2.0	17.0	.5	0	5	2.0
(*Green Giant Niblets* Extra Sweet), ½ cup cooked ..	70	2.0	13.0	1.0	0	0	2.0

Food and Measure	cal.	prot. (gms)	carbo. (gms)	fat (gms)	chol. (mgs)	sod. (mgs)	fiber (gms)
(*Green Giant Niblets Simply Steam*), ½ cup cooked ..	80	2.0	18.0	.5	0	60	2.0
kernel, golden/white:							
(*C&W* Petite)	100	3.0	21.0	1.0	0	0	1.0
baby (*Birds Eye*) ..	100	3.0	20.0	1.0	0	0	2.0
kernel, white:							
(*C&W* Petite)	100	3.0	21.0	1.0	0	0	1.0
(*Green Giant Select* Shoepeg), ¾ cup	100	2.0	21.0	1.5	0	0	2.0
(*Green Giant Simply Steam* Shoepeg), ½ cup	70	2.0	15.0	1.0	0	45	2.0
(*McKenzie's* Southern), ½ cup	80	3.0	19.0	1.0	0	10	1.0
baby (*Birds Eye*) ..	90	3.0	18.0	1.0	0	0	3.0
in butter sauce:							
(*Birds Eye*), ½ cup .	150	3.0	28.0	3.0	0	260	2.0
(*Green Giant Niblets*), ⅔ cup cooked ..	110	3.0	21.0	2.0	<5	370	2.0
(*Green Giant Niblets Family Bag*), ½ cup cooked ..	100	3.0	19.0	1.5	<5	280	1.0
(*Green Giant Niblets Just for One*), 4.25-oz tray	120	3.0	24.0	2.0	5	330	2.0
white (*Green Giant* Shoepeg), ¾ cup	110	2.0	22.0	2.0	<5	340	2.0
cheddar bacon (*C&W*), ½ cup	130	4.0	18.0	4.5	10	210	3.0
cheese sauce, bacon (*Birds Eye*), ½ cup .	150	5.0	26.0	4.0	5	470	1.0
cream style (*Green Giant*), ½ cup	110	2.0	24.0	1.0	0	320	2.0
fried (*Glory* Savory Accents), ½ cup ..	110	3.0	24.0	1.5	0	470	2.0
seasoned (*Birds Eye Steamfresh* Southwestern)	90	2.0	16.0	2.0	0	260	1.0
Corn, pickled, baby (*Roland*), ¼ cup ..	10	1.0	2.0	0	0	65	0
Corn, whole-grain:							
1 oz.	103	2.7	21.1	1.3	0	10	2.1
1 cup	605	15.6	123.3	7.9	0	58	12.2

Food and Measure	cal.	prot. (gms)	carbo. (gms)	fat (gms)	chol. (mgs)	sod. (mgs)	fiber (gms)
Corn bran, crude,							
1 cup	170	6.4	65.1	.7	0	5	64.3
Corn cake mix, sweet, dry, ½ cup:							
(*Chi-Chi's*)	100	1.0	23.0	0	0	130	0
(*El Torito*)	100	1.0	22.0	.5	0	120	0
Corn chips, see "Corn crisps/chips"							
Corn combinations, frozen:							
baby corn and:							
green beans, peas (*Birds Eye*), ¾ cup .	70	2.0	13.0	0	0	0	2.0
vegetable blend (*Birds Eye*), ⅔ cup	50	2.0	9.0	1.0	0	10	3.0
black beans:							
onions (*Green Giant* Southwestern), ½ cup cooked . .	90	4.0	18.0	1.0	0	190	4.0
tomatoes (*C&W Salsa Corn*), 1 cup	90	3.0	17.0	.5	0	250	3.0
broccoli florets, red peppers (*C&W Vegetable Stand Combinations*), ⅔ cup	50	2.0	8.0	.5 ·	0	10	2.0
peas, herb butter sauce (*Green Giant*), ¾ cup	80	4.0	14.0	1.5	<5	320	3.0
red peppers, roasted, Southwestern (*Green Giant*), ¾ cup	80	2.0	17.0	.5	0	125	2.0
Corn crisps/chips (see also "Snack chips"), 1 oz., except as noted:							
(*Baja Express* Churritos), 1.1 oz.	160	2.0	18.0	9.0	0	260	2.0
(*Bugles*), 1.1 oz.	160	1.0	18.0	9.0	0	310	<1.0
(*Chipitos* Jumbo)	150	1.0	18.0	8.0	0	170	2.0
(*Corn Nuts*)	120	3.0	20.0	4.5	0	180	2.0
(*Dipsy Doodles*)	160	1.0	16.0	10.0	0	180	1.0
(*Fritos* Original)	160	2.0	15.0	10.0	0	170	1.0
(*Fritos Scoops!*)	160	2.0	16.0	10.0	0	110	1.0
(*Herr's*), 1.1 oz.	160	2.0	17.0	7.0	0	400	1.0
(*Wise/Moore's*)	160	1.0	16.0	10.0	0	180	1.0

Food and Measure	cal.	prot. (gms)	carbo. (gms)	fat (gms)	chol. (mgs)	sod. (mgs)	fiber (gms)
barbecue:							
(*Chipitos*)	150	2.0	16.0	8.0	0	260	2.0
(*Corn Nuts*)	130	2.0	20.0	4.5	0	170	2.0
(*Dipsy Doodles/ Moore's*)	160	1.0	16.0	10.0	0	250	1.0
(*Fritos*)	150	2.0	16.0	10.0	0	280	1.0
honey (*Fritos Flavor Twists*)	160	2.0	16.0	10.0	0	210	1.0
(*Wise*)	160	1.0	16.0	10.0	0	210	1.0
cheddar, white:							
(*Barbara's* Cheesee Puff Bakes)	160	2.0	13.0	11.0	0	190	0
(*Cheetos* Puffs) ...	150	2.0	16.0	9.0	0	290	<1.0
(*Cheez Doodles* Puffed)	150	2.0	15.0	9.0	<5	290	0
cheddar jalapeño (*Cheetos* Crunchy) .	170	2.0	15.0	11.0	<5	250	<1.0
cheese:							
(*Barbara's* Cheese Puffs)	150	2.0	16.0	10.0	0	130	0
(*Barbara's* Cheese Puff Bakes)	160	2.0	13.0	11.0	0	190	0
(*Cheetos* Crunchy) .	160	2.0	15.0	10.0	<5	290	<1.0
(*Cheetos* Crunchy Baked!)	130	2.0	19.0	5.0	0	240	0
(*Cheetos* Puffs) ...	160	2.0	15.0	10.0	0	370	<1.0
(*Cheetos* Puffs Jumbo)	160	2.0	13.0	10.0	<5	350	0
(*Cheetos* Twisted) .	160	2.0	13.0	10.0	0	350	0
(*Cheetos* Flamin' Hot Jumbo Puffs) ...	150	1.0	14.0	10.0	0	300	1.0
(*Cheetos* Mix & More)	160	2.0	14.0	11.0	<5	300	<1.0
(*Cheez Doodles* Crunchy)	150	1.0	17.0	9.0	0	220	0
(*Cheez Doodles* Puffed)	150	2.0	16.0	8.0	0	320	0
(*Cheez Doodles* Reduced Fat) ...	130	2.0	20.0	5.0	<5	220	<1.0
(*Doodle O's*)	160	2.0	14.0	11.0	<5	310	0
(*Herr's* Crunchy Sticks)	150	1.0	17.0	9.0	0	150	<1.0
(*Herr's* Curls)	150	2.0	16.0	8.0	0	350	1.0

Food and Measure	cal.	prot. (gms)	carbo. (gms)	fat (gms)	chol. (mgs)	sod. (mgs)	fiber (gms)
Corn, crisps/chips, cheese *(cont.)*							
(*Jax* Baked Twists/ Curls)	140	2.0	18.0	7.0	<5	360	<1.0
(*Jax* Crunchy), 1.1 oz.	170	2.0	15.0	11.0	<5	210	0
(*Snyder's* Twists) . .	140	2.0	15.0	8.0	<5	230	0
honey or hot (*Herr's* Curls)	150	2.0	16.0	8.0	0	350	1.0
hot (*Cheetos Flamin' Hot*)	170	2.0	15.0	11.0	0	250	<1.0
hot (*Cheetos Flamin' Hot* Baked!)	130	3.0	19.0	5.0	0	240	<1.0
hot (*Cheetos Flamin' Hot* Limón)	160	1.0	15.0	11.0	0	190	<1.0
jalapeño (*Barbara's* Cheese Puffs) . . .	150	2.0	16.0	10.0	0	130	0
nacho (*Bugles*), 1.1 oz.	160	1.0	18.0	9.0	0	330	0
nacho (*Corn Nuts*) .	130	3.0	19.0	5.0	0	240	2.0
nacho (*Wise Nacho Twisters*)	160	2.0	14.0	11.0	0	250	1.0
chili cheese:							
(*Bugles*), 1.1 oz. . .	160	2.0	18.0	9.0	0	310	0
(*Fritos*)	160	2.0	15.0	10.0	0	260	1.0
chili picante (*Corn Nuts*)	130	2.0	19.0	4.5	0	290	2.0
hot (*Fritos Flamin' Hot*)	160	2.0	15.0	10.0	0	160	1.0
onion:							
(*Funyuns*)	140	2.0	18.0	7.0	0	270	<1.0
(*Herr's* Rings)	140	1.0	17.0	7.0	0	400	1.0
(*Wise* Rings)	140	0	20.0	6.0	0	420	0
ranch:							
(*Bugles* Southwest), 1.1 oz.	170	1.0	18.0	10.0	0	310	0
(*Corn Nuts*)	130	3.0	19.0	5.0	0	240	2.0
salsa:							
(*Bugles*), 1.1 oz. . .	160	2.0	18.0	9.0	0	320	<1.0
(*Corn Nuts* Jalisco)	130	3.0	20.0	4.5	0	150	2.0
shrimp chips (*Maui Style*)	140	<1.0	19.0	8.0	0	220	<1.0
tortilla:							
(*Bearito's*)	140	2.0	18.0	7.0	0	80	3.0
(*Bravos* Restaurant/ Round White) . . .	150	2.0	18.0	8.0	0	80	1.0
(*Cape Cod* White Corn)	140	2.0	19.0	7.0	0	110	2.0

Food and Measure	cal.	prot. (gms)	carbo. (gms)	fat (gms)	chol. (mgs)	sod. (mgs)	fiber (gms)
(*Chipitos*)	140	2.0	21.0	6.0	0	200	2.0
(*Chipitos* Restaurant)	130	2.0	18.0	6.0	0	100	1.0
(*Doritos* Toasted) . .	140	2.0	18.0	7.0	0	120	1.0
(*Garden of Eatin'* White Chips) . . .	140	2.0	19.0	6.0	0	70	2.0
(*Snyder's* Restaurant)	130	2.0	20.0	5.0	0	120	4.0
(*Snyder's* White) . .	140	2.0	23.0	4.5	0	110	2.0
(*Santitas*)	130	2.0	19.0	6.0	0	110	1.0
(*Tostitos* Flour) . . .	140	2.0	19.0	7.0	0	95	1.0
(*Tostitos* Restaurant)	140	2.0	19.0	7.0	0	120	1.0
(*Tostitos* Restaurant Light)	90	2.0	20.0	1.0	0	105	1.0
(*Tostitos* Rounds) .	140	2.0	18.0	7.0	0	120	1.0
(*Tostitos* Scoops!) .	140	2.0	18.0	7.0	0	120	1.0
(*Tostitos* Scoops! Baked!)	120	2.0	22.0	3.0	0	150	2.0
bite size (*Herr's*) . . .	140	3.0	18.0	6.0	0	90	2.0
bite size (*Tostitos* Gold)	140	2.0	19.0	7.0	0	110	1.0
bite size (*Tostitos* Rounds)	140	2.0	18.0	8.0	0	110	1.0
black bean (*Kettle*) .	140	3.0	18.0	7.0	0	170	2.0
black bean salsa (*Chipitos*)	140	3.0	18.0	7.0	0	160	3.0
cheddar barbecue (*Doritos* Smokin')	150	2.0	17.0	8.0	0	170	1.0
cheese (*Doritos* Spicy Nacho!) . .	140	2.0	18.0	7.0	0	210	1.0
cheese (*Doritos* Nacho Cheese) . .	140	2.0	17.0	8.0	0	180	1.0
cheese (*Doritos* Nacho Cheese Baked!)	120	2.0	21.0	3.5	0	20	2.0
cheese (*Herr's* Nachitas)	140	2.0	18.0	6.0	0	230	2.0
cheese, nacho (*Bravos*)	150	2.0	17.0	8.0	0	180	1.0
cheese, nacho (*Chipitos*)	140	2.0	19.0	6.0	0	125	2.0
cheese, nacho (*Garden of Eatin'*)	140	2.0	18.0	6.0	0	140	2.0
cheese, nacho (*Guiltless Gourmet*) . .	120	2.0	22.0	3.0	0	250	2.0

Food and Measure	cal.	prot. (gms)	carbo. (gms)	fat (gms)	chol. (mgs)	sod. (mgs)	fiber (gms)
Corn, crisps/chips, tortilla *(cont.)*							
cheese, white nacho (*Doritos* Natural)	150	2.0	17.0	8.0	0	190	1.0
chili lime (*Chipitos*)	140	2.0	18.0	7.0	0	180	2.0
chili lime (*Garden of Eatin'*)	140	2.0	18.0	7.0	0	125	2.0
chili lime (*Kettle*) ..	140	3.0	18.0	7.0	0	140	2.0
chocolate (*Food Should Taste Good*)	140	2.0	19.0	7.0	0	80	3.0
guacamole (*Garden of Eatin'*)	140	2.0	19.0	6.0	0	170	2.0
hot (*Doritos* Fiery Habanero)	130	2.0	16.0	7.0	0	240	<1.0
lime, hint (*Tostitos*)	150	2.0	18.0	8.0	0	160	1.0
Montery Jack/green chili (*Herr's*)	160	2.0	18.0	7.0	0	300	2.0
multigrain (*Herr's*) .	140	2.0	18.0	7.0	0	180	2.5
multigrain (*Kettle*) .	140	3.0	18.0	7.0	0	100	2.0
multigrain (*Tostitos*)	150	2.0	18.0	8.0	0	135	2.0
mini strips or rounds (*Garden of Eatin'*)	140	2.0	19.0	6.0	0	60	2.0
olive (*Food Should Taste Good*)	140	2.0	18.0	7.0	0	80	3.0
peppercorn ranch (*Bravos*)	140	2.0	18.0	7.0	0	220	2.0
pico de gallo (*Garden of Eatin'*)	140	2.0	18.0	7.0	0	150	3.0
ranch (*Doritos Cool Ranch*)	140	2.0	18.0	7.0	0	170	1.0
salsa verde (*Doritos*)	140	2.0	19.0	7.0	0	210	1.0
sweet pepper (*Bravos*)	140	2.0	18.0	7.0	0	180	2.0
taco (*Doritos*)	140	2.0	18.0	7.0	0	170	1.0
tamari (*Garden of Eatin'*)	140	2.0	18.0	7.0	0	160	3.0
tortilla, blue corn:							
(*Bearito's*)	140	2.0	18.0	7.0	0	60	2.0
(*Cape Cod*)	140	2.0	19.0	6.0	0	110	2.0
(*Garden of Eatin'*) .	140	2.0	18.0	7.0	0	60	2.0
(*Garden of Eatin' Little Soy Blues*) .	140	3.0	17.0	7.0	0	70	2.0
(*Garden of Eatin' Red Hot Blues*) ..	140	2.0	18.0	7.0	0	150	2.0

Food and Measure	cal.	prot. (gms)	carbo. (gms)	fat (gms)	chol. (mgs)	sod. (mgs)	fiber (gms)
(*Garden of Eatin' Sesame Blues*) ..	150	3.0	16.0	8.0	0	90	2.0
(*Garden of Eatin' Sunny Blues*) ...	150	2.0	17.0	8.0	0	70	2.0
(*Guiltless Gourmet*)	120	3.0	23.0	3.0	0	250	2.0
(*Kettle*)	140	3.0	18.0	6.0	0	80	2.0
(*Tostitos* Natural) ..	140	2.0	19.0	6.0	0	80	1.0
black bean, spicy (*Guiltless Gourmet*)	120	2.0	19.0	3.0	0	250	2.0
tortilla, red corn: (*Garden of Eatin'*) .	140	2.0	18.0	7.0	0	70	1.0
(*Garden of Eatin' Salsa Reds*)	140	2.0	18.0	7.0	0	170	3.0
tortilla, yellow corn: (*Bearito's*)	140	2.0	19.0	6.0	0	55	1.0
(*Garden of Eatin'*) .	140	2.0	18.0	7.0	0	70	2.0
(*Garden of Eatin' Mini Rounds*) ...	140	2.0	18.0	7.0	0	60	2.0
(*Guiltless Gourmet*)	120	2.0	19.0	3.0	0	250	2.0
(*Kettle*)	140	3.0	18.0	7.0	0	100	2.0
(*Tostitos* Natural) ..	140	2.0	19.0	6.0	0	100	1.0
black bean (*Garden of Eatin'*)	140	3.0	18.0	7.0	0	70	4.0
black bean chili (*Garden of Eatin'*)	140	3.0	17.0	7.0	0	130	4.0
chili lime (*Guiltless Gourmet*)	120	2.0	19.0	3.0	0	250	2.0
chili verde or chipotle (*Guiltless Gourmet*)	120	2.0	22.0	3.0	0	250	2.0
Corn dog, see "Frankfurter, wrapped"							
Corn dog, vegetarian, frozen:							
(*Morningstar Farms* Original), 2.5-oz. pc.	150	7.0	22.0	4.0	0	500	3.0
mini (*Morningstar Farms*), 4 pcs., 2.7 oz.	170	11.0	21.0	4.5	0	580	1.0
Corn dog entree, frozen, w/fries (*Michelina's Authentico*), 5.5 oz.	290	8.0	40.0	10.0	10	950	3.0
Corn flake crumbs (*Kellogg's*), 6 tbsp..	120	2.0	29.0	9.0	9	240	<1.0

Food and Measure	cal.	prot. (gms)	carbo. (gms)	fat (gms)	chol. (mgs)	sod. (mgs)	fiber (gms)
Corn flour:							
(*Shiloh Farms* Organic),							
¼ cup	130	2.4	27.0	1.4	0	0	5.0
wholegrain, 1 oz.	102	2.0	21.8	1.1	0	1	3.8
wholegrain, 1 cup ...	422	8.1	89.9	4.5	0	6	15.7
masa, 1 oz.	103	2.6	21.6	1.1	0	1	2.7
masa, 1 cup	416	10.7	87.0	4.3	0	6	10.9
Corn fritters, frozen:							
(*Delta Pride*), 3 pcs. ...	160	2.0	19.0	9.0	0	85	0
(*Lupita's Texas*),							
1.3-oz. pc.	100	2.0	14.0	4.0	10	200	1.0
Corn grits, ¼ cup,							
except as noted:							
(*Albers* Quick)	140	3.0	31.0	.5	0	0	1.0
(*Quaker/Aunt Jemima*							
Old Fashioned)	150	4.0	32.0	.5	0	0	1.0
(*Quaker/Aunt Jemima*							
Quick)	130	3.0	29.0	.5	0	0	2.0
instant (*Quaker* Original),							
1-oz. pkt.	100	2.0	22.0	0	0	310	1.0
white (*Arrowhead*							
Mills)	150	3.0	33.0	0	0	0	1.0
yellow (*Arrowhead*							
Mills Organic)	130	3.0	30.0	0	0	0	1.0
Corn grits, flavored,							
(*Quaker* Instant),							
1-oz. pkt.:							
bacon, country, flavor	100	3.0	21.0	.5	0	430	1.0
butter flavor	100	2.0	21.0	1.5	0	370	1.0
cheese flavor:							
American	100	2.0	21.0	1.5	0	420	1.0
cheddar	100	3.0	20.0	1.5	0	470	1.0
cheddar blend	100	2.0	20.0	1.0	0	480	1.0
three cheese	100	3.0	20.0	1.0	0	480	1.0
gravy, red-eye, and							
country ham	100	3.0	21.0	.5	0	490	1.0
ham and cheese	100	3.0	20.0	1.5	0	540	1.0
Corn relish, 1 tbsp.:							
(*Mrs. Renfro's*)	15	0	4.0	0	0	45	0
(*Nance's*)	20	0	5.0	0	0	75	0
Corn soufflé, frozen							
(*Stouffer's*), ½ of							
12-oz. pkg.	150	5.0	22.0	5.0	65	490	2.0

Food and Measure	cal.	prot. (gms)	carbo. (gms)	fat (gms)	chol. (mgs)	sod. (mgs)	fiber (gms)
Corn syrup, 2 tbsp.:							
dark (*Karo*)	120	0	31.0	0	0	45	0
light (*Karo*)	120	0	31.0	0	0	35	0
Corn-mozzarella bites, frozen, breaded (*Veggie Patch*), 3 pcs., 2.6 oz.	150	5.0	22.0	7.0	5	380	4.0
Corn bread mix:							
(*Arrowhead Mills* Organic), ¼ cup . . .	120	4.0	25.0	1.0	0	290	2.0
(*Aunt Jemima* Easy Mix), ⅛ pkg.*	160	8.0	37.0	8.0	75	800	1.0
(*Betty Crocker* Cornbread & Muffin), ⅙ pkg.*	160	3.0	25.0	6.0	45	290	<1.0
(*Glory* Homestyle), 1.2-oz. square* . . .	160	2.0	24.0	4.5	35	480	2.0
(*Hodgson Mill*), ¼ cup	130	4.0	27.0	.5	0	240	3.0
(*Kentucky Kernel* Sweet), ¼ cup	120	2.0	24.0	1.5	0	310	0
(*Martha White Cotton Country*), ⅕ pkg. . .	130	2.0	23.0	3.0	20	440	1.0
buttermilk (*Martha White*), ⅕ pkg.	130	2.0	23.0	3.0	20	430	1.0
honey (*Krusteaz*), 2" pc.*	120	3.0	21.0	3.0	15	210	<1.0
honey (*Krusteaz* Fat Free), ¼ cup	120	2.0	27.0	0	0	410	1.0
jalapeno (*Hodgson Mill*), ¼ cup	100	4.0	21.0	.5	0	310	1.0
Mexican (*Martha White*), ⅙ pkg.	110	2.0	18.0	3.0	20	400	<1.0
white (*Martha White Family*), ⅟₁₈ pkg. . . .	110	2.0	21.0	2.0	20	500	1.0
yellow:							
(*Martha White*), ⅕ pkg.	130	3.0	25.0	2.0	20	460	1.0
sweet (*Martha White*), ⅙ pkg. . . .	130	2.0	24.0	3.0	20	250	<1.0
sweet honey (*Martha White*), ⅙ pkg. . . .	130	2.0	24.0	3.5	20	250	2.0
Cornichon, see "Pickle"							
Cornish hen, roasted:							
meat w/skin, 4 oz. . . .	295	25.3	0	20.7	149	73	0
meat only, 4 oz.	152	26.4	0	4.4	120	71	0

Food and Measure	cal.	prot. (gms)	carbo. (gms)	fat (gms)	chol. (mgs)	sod. (mgs)	fiber (gms)
Cornish hen, frozen/ refrigerated:							
whole, raw, 4 oz.:							
(*Empire Kosher* Rock Broiler) ...	165	19.0	0	10.0	85	220	0
w/out giblets (*Tyson*)	200	19.0	0	14.0	130	65	0
whole, roasted, 3 oz.:							
dark (*Perdue*)	200	17.0	0	14.0	125	55	0
light (*Perdue*)	160	21.0	0	8.0	100	40	0
Cornmeal (see also "Corn flour" and "Polenta"):							
blue (*Arrowhead Mills* Organic), ⅓ cup ...	130	3.0	25.0	1.5	0	0	5.0
buttermilk. self-rising (*Martha White*), 3 tbsp.	110	2.0	22.0	1.0	20	450	2.0
white, 3 tbsp.:							
regular (*Martha White*)	110	2.0	22.0	1.0	20	450	2.0
self-rising (*Martha White*)	100	2.0	22.0	1.0	20	440	2.0
white or yellow:							
(*Albers*), 3 tbsp.	110	2.0	24.0	0	0	0	<1.0
(*Hodgson Mill*), <¼ cup	100	3.0	22.0	1.0	0	0	3.0
yellow:							
(*Arrowhead Mills* Organic), ⅓ cup .	120	3.0	27.0	1.0	0	0	3.0
(*Hodgson Mill* Organic), <¼ cup	100	3.0	23.0	1.0	0	0	3.0
(*Shiloh Farms* Organic), ¼ cup ...	210	7.0	43.0	0	0	5	3.0
self-rising (*Hodgson Mill*), <¼ cup ...	90	3.0	21.0	1.0	0	260	3.0
self-rising (*Martha White*), 3 tbsp. ...	110	2.0	22.0	1.0	20	460	2.0
whole grain, ½ cup	221	5.0	46.9	2.2	0	21	4.5
Cornstarch (*Argo*), 1 tbsp.	30	0	7.0	0	0	0	0
Cosmopolitan drink mixer, bottled:							
(*Daily*), 4 fl. oz.	160	0	40.0	0	0	75	0
(*Master of Mixes*), 3 fl. oz.	87	0	18.0	0	0	5	0

Food and Measure	cal.	prot. (gms)	carbo. (gms)	fat (gms)	chol. (mgs)	sod. (mgs)	fiber (gms)
Cottonseed flour, partially defatted, 1 cup	337	38.5	38.1	5.8	8	33	2.8
Cottonseed kernels, roasted, 1 tbsp. . . .	51	3.3	2.2	3.6	0	3	.6
Cottonseed meal, partially defatted, 1 oz.	104	13.9	10.9	1.4	0	10	<1.0
Couscous, dry, ¼ cup, except as noted:							
(*Casbah* Original Organic), ⅓ cup	200	7.0	43.0	1.0	0	5	2.0
(*Casbah* Original Toasted), ⅓ cup . . .	170	5.0	36.0	0	0	0	2.0
(*Fantastic* Organic) . . .	150	6.0	33.0	.5	0	0	1.0
(*Marrakesh Express*), 2 oz.	220	8.0	45.0	0	0	10	1.0
(*Near East*), ⅓ cup . .	220	8.0	46.0	1.0	0	5	2.0
(*Roland*), ⅓ cup	200	6.0	42.0	1.0	0	1	3.0
(*Vigo*), ⅓ cup	190	7.0	41.0	0	0	10	1.0
spinach (*RiceSelect*) .	144	5.0	30.0	1.0	0	4	1.0
toasted (*Marrakesh Express* Grande), 3 scoops	270	10.0	57.0	0	0	10	2.0
tomato (*RiceSelect*) . .	145	5.0	30.0	1.0	0	11	1.0
tri-color (*RiceSelect*) .	150	5.0	31.0	0	0	0	2.0
whole wheat:							
(*Casbah* Organic), ⅓ cup	190	7.0	43.0	1.0	0	5	7.0
(*Fantastic*)	170	7.0	37.0	.5	0	0	6.0
(*Hodgson Mill*) . . .	210	8.0	47.0	1.0	0	0	5.0
(*RiceSelect* Organic)	210	8.0	45.0	1.0	0	0	7.0
whole wheat, w/flax and soy (*Hodgson Mill*), ⅓ cup	230	10.0	48.0	2.0	0	0	6.0
Couscous dish, mix, 2 oz. mix, except as noted:							
broccoli and cheese (*Near East*)	190	8.0	40.0	1.0	0	670	3.0
chicken:							
herbed (*Near East*)	190	8.0	40.0	1.0	0	510	3.0
w/vegetables (*Marrakesh Express*) . .	190	8.0	39.0	0	0	700	2.0

Food and Measure	cal.	prot. (gms)	carbo. (gms)	fat (gms)	chol. (mgs)	sod. (mgs)	fiber (gms)
Couscous dish, mix *(cont.)*							
curry:							
(*Marrakesh Express*)	190	8.0	39.0	0	0	530	2.0
(*Near East* Mediter-							
ranean)	190	8.0	40.0	1.0	0	550	3.0
garlic/olive oil:							
(*Casbah* Organic),							
¼ cup	160	6.0	33.0	1.0	0	420	2.0
(*Near East*)	200	8.0	39.0	2.0	0	570	2.0
lemon spinach (*Casbah*							
Organic), ½ cup . . .	160	6.0	33.0	1.0	0	400	2.0
mango salsa (*Marra-							
kesh Express*)	190	7.0	38.0	0	0	390	1.0
Mediterranean (*Roland*),							
⅓ cup	200	7.0	42.0	1.5	0	550	3.0
mushroom, wild:							
(*Casbah* Organic),							
⅓ cup	160	6.0	33.0	1.0	0	350	2.0
(*Casbah* Toasted),							
⅓ cup	170	6.0	34.0	.5	0	480	2.0
(*Marrakesh Express*)	190	8.0	39.0	.5	0	600	1.0
and herb (*Near East*)	190	8.0	40.0	1.0	0	580	3.0
nutted, w/currants,							
spice (*Casbah* Or-							
ganic), ¼ cup	160	6.0	32.0	2.0	0	420	2.0
Parmesan:							
(*Marrakesh Express*)	200	8.0	39.0	1.0	0	800	1.0
(*Near East*)	200	8.0	39.0	2.0	5	580	2.0
pilaf (*Casbah*), ¼ cup	160	6.0	34.0	1.0	0	400	2.0
pine nut, toasted (*Near							
East*)	200	8.0	38.0	3.0	0	510	2.0
spicy (*Roland*), ⅓ cup	200	7.0	42.0	1.0	0	580	3.0
sun-dried tomato							
(*Marrakesh Express*)	190	8.0	39.0	0	0	600	2.0
tomato lentil:							
(*Near East*)	190	8.0	40.0	1.0	0	670	3.0
(*Roland*), ⅓ cup . .	200	7.0	45.0	1.0	0	460	3.0
vegetable, garden							
(*Roland*), ⅓ cup . .	200	7.0	42.0	1.0	0	420	3.0
whole wheat, w/flax							
and soy (*Hodgson							
Mill*), ⅓ cup:							
chicken and herb . .	250	11.0	52.0	1.0	0	223	6.0
garlic basil	235	10.0	50.0	2.0	0	625	6.0

Food and Measure	cal.	prot. (gms)	carbo. (gms)	fat (gms)	chol. (mgs)	sod. (mgs)	fiber (gms)
mushroom, wild ...	246	11.0	52.0	1.0	0	362	6.0
Parmesan cheese ..	240	10.0	50.0	2.5	10	482	6.0
Couscous stew, frozen (*Moosewood* Organic Moroccan), 10-oz. pkg.	150	5.0	29.0	3.0	0	400	5.0
Cowpeas (see also "Black-eyed peas"), fresh, ½ cup:							
raw:							
immature seeds ...	65	2.1	13.7	.3	0	3	3.6
leafy tips, chopped .	5	.7	.9	<.1	0	1	n.a.
pods, w/seeds	21	1.6	4.5	.1	0	2	n.a.
boiled, drained:							
immature seeds ...	80	2.6	16.8	.3	0	3	4.1
leafy tips, chopped .	6	1.2	.7	0	0	2	n.a.
pods, w/seeds	16	1.2	3.3	.1	0	1	n.a.
Cowpeas, canned or frozen, see "Black-eyed peas"							
Cowpeas, catjang, see "Catjang"							
Crab, meat only:							
Alaska king, 4 oz.:							
raw	95	20.8	0	.7	47	948	0
boiled, poached, or steamed	110	21.9	0	1.7	60	1216	0
blue, 4 oz.:							
raw	99	20.5	.1	1.2	89	332	0
boiled, poached, or steamed	116	22.9	0	2.0	113	316	0
Dungeness, 4 oz.:							
raw	98	19.8	.8	1.1	67	335	0
boiled, poached, or steamed	125	25.3	1.1	1.4	86	429	0
queen, 4 oz.:							
raw	102	21.0	0	1.4	62	611	0
boiled, poached, or steamed	130	26.9	0	1.7	81	784	0
Crab, can or pouch, 2 oz., except as noted: (*Chicken of the Sea* Fancy)	40	7.0	2.0	0	50	400	0

Food and Measure	cal.	prot. (gms)	carbo. (gms)	fat (gms)	chol. (mgs)	sod. (mgs)	fiber (gms)
Crab, can or pouch *(cont.)*							
(*Chicken of the Sea* Premium 3.53-oz. Pouch), 2.5 oz. ...	40	9.0	1.0	0	60	500	0
(*Consul*), ½ cup	45	10.0	0	0	55	370	0
all styles (*Yankee Clipper*)	40	7.0	2.0	0	40	400	0
Dungeness (*SeaBear*)	50	13.0	0	1.0	45	210	0
leg meat (*King Roland*), ½ cup	45	10.0	0	0	55	370	0
lump or jumbo lump (*Chicken of the Sea*)	35	7.0	1.0	.5	50	400	0
pink (*Bumble Bee*) ...	35	7.0	0	.5	50	300	0
white:							
(*Roland*), ½ cup ..	35	8.0	0	0	60	230	0
or lump (*Bumble Bee*)	40	8.0	0	1.0	50	300	0
or pink (*Chicken of the Sea*)	30	7.0	1.0	0	50	400	0
"Crab," imitation, ½ cup, 3 oz., except as noted:							
(*Chicken of the Sea* Premium 3.53-oz. pouch), 2.5 oz.	40	3.0	6.0	0	9	360	1.0
(*Matlaw's*)	80	9.0	10.0	1.0	10	660	0
chunk, flake, or leg style (*Louis Kemp Crab Delights*)	70	7.0	10.0	0	5	460	1.0
shredded (*Louis Kemp Crab Delights* Easy Shreds)	80	7.0	12.0	0	5	720	1.0
Crab apple, fresh:							
(*Frieda's*), 5 oz.	110	1.0	28.0	0	0	0	1.0
sliced, ½ cup	42	.2	11.0	.2	0	1	.6
Crab cake, frozen:							
(*Margaritaville* Coral Reef), ⅙ pkg.:							
crab cake, 3 oz. ...	150	17.0	2.0	8.0	65	480	0
sauce, 1 tbsp.	50	0	2.0	4.0	5	10	0
(*Matlaw's*), 2 oz.	80	5.0	14.0	2.0	5	230	0
deviled, breaded (*Mrs. Paul's*), 3 oz.	220	20.0	12.0	12.0	60	320	3.0

Food and Measure	cal.	prot. (gms)	carbo. (gms)	fat (gms)	chol. (mgs)	sod. (mgs)	fiber (gms)
Crab cake mix (*Old Bay Crab Cake Classic*), 1 tbsp. . . .	25	1.0	3.0	.5	25	240	0
Crab dip seasoning (*Watkins*), 1 tsp. . .	10	0	2.0	0	0	140	0
Crab wontons, frozen, w/cream cheese (*Original Rangoon Rangoons*), 3 pcs. .	220	12.0	29.0	5.0	25	580	<1.0
Cracker (see also "Snack chips" and specific listings):							
(*Barbara's Rite Lite Rounds* Original), 5 pcs., .5 oz.	60	1.0	11.0	2.0	0	200	0
(*Bremner* Cracker), 7 pcs., .5 oz.	60	1.0	10.0	1.0	0	130	0
(*Bremner* Wafer), 7 pcs. .5 oz.	70	2.0	11.0	1.5	0	105	0
(*Breton* Original), 3 pcs., .5 oz.	60	1.0	8.0	2.5	0	110	0
(*Goldfish* Original), 55 pcs., 1.1 oz. . . .	150	3.0	20.0	6.0	0	230	<1.0
(*Health Valley* Organic Mediterranean Stix), 8 pcs., .5 oz.	70	1.0	9.0	3.0	0	210	<1.0
(*Lavosh-Hawaii* Classic/ Bite Size/Mini-Bite), 1 oz.	120	3.0	19.0	3.0	21	290	1.0
(*Ritz* Simply Socials), .5 oz.	70	1.0	10.0	3.0	0	140	1.0
(*Sabrosas*), 11 pcs., 1.1 oz.	150	2.0	20.0	6.0	0	190	0
(*Sociables*), 7 pcs., .5 oz.	70	1.0	9.0	3.5	0	140	0
almond and rice (*Nut Thins*), 16 pcs.:							
original	130	3.0	23.0	2.5	0	115	1.0
cheddar	130	3.0	22.0	4.0	0	250	<1.0
ranch, country	130	3.0	22.0	3.5	0	220	<1.0
smokehouse	130	3.0	23.0	3.0	0	160	<1.0
bruschetta: (*TLC* Mediterranean), 4 pcs., 1 oz.	120	3.0	18.0	4.0	0	140	3.0

Food and Measure	cal.	prot. (gms)	carbo. (gms)	fat (gms)	chol. (mgs)	sod. (mgs)	fiber (gms)
Cracker, bruschetta (cont.)							
vegetable (*Health Valley* Organic), 4 pcs., .6 oz. ...	70	1.0	10.0	3.0	0	210	0
butter/butter flavor:							
(*Cabaret*), 3 pcs., .5 oz.	70	<1.0	9.0	3.5	0	70	0
(*Hain*), 11 pcs., 1.1 oz.	130	3.0	21.0	4.5	0	370	0
(*Keebler Club*), 4 pcs., .5 oz.	70	1.0	9.0	3.0	0	150	<1.0
(*Keebler Club* Reduced Fat), 5 pcs., .6 oz.	70	1.0	12.0	2.5	0	190	<1.0
(*Keebler Club* Snack Sticks), 12 pcs., 1 oz.	130	1.0	19.0	6.0	0	320	<1.0
(*Murray Social Hits*), 9 pcs., 1.1 oz. ..	150	2.0	18.0	8.0	0	230	<1.0
(*Pepperidge Farm* Golden Butter), 4 pcs., .5 oz. ...	70	1.0	11.0	2.5	<5	100	0
(*Ritz* Original), 5 pcs., .6 oz.	80	1.0	10.0	4.0	0	135	0
(*Ritz* Reduced Fat), 5 pcs., .5 oz. ...	70	1.0	11.0	2.0	0	160	0
(*Toasteds* Buttercrisp), 5 pcs., .6 oz. ...	80	1.0	10.0	3.5	0	150	<1.0
(*Town House* Original), 5 pcs., .6 oz. ...	80	<1.0	10.0	4.5	0	160	<1.0
(*Town House* Reduced Fat), 6 pcs., .6 oz.	60	<1.0	11.0	1.5	0	160	<1.0
(*Town House* Toppers), 3 pcs., .5 oz.	70	1.0	9.0	3.0	0	135	0
(*Tree of Life* Golden Classic), 5 pcs., .5 oz.	60	1.0	12.0	<1.0	0	220	0
herb (*Keebler Club* Snack Sticks), 12 pcs., 1 oz. ...	130	1.0	19.0	6.0	0	320	<1.0
honey (*Ritz*), .6 oz.	80	1.0	10.0	4.0	0	70	0
puffed (*Keebler Club*), 24 pcs., 1.1 oz. .	140	2.0	20.0	6.0	0	310	1.0
caraway (*Bremner* Wafer), 7 pcs., .5 oz.	70	2.0	11.0	1.5	0	105	1.0

Food and Measure	cal.	prot. (gms)	carbo. (gms)	fat (gms)	chol. (mgs)	sod. (mgs)	fiber (gms)
caraway rye (*Lavosh-Hawaii*), 1 oz.	115	3.0	20.0	3.0	21	300	1.0
cheddar:							
(*Annie's* Original Bunnies), 50 pcs., 1.1 oz.	150	3.0	19.0	7.0	<5	250	1.0
(*Better Cheddars*), 22 pcs., 1.1 oz. .	160	3.0	18.0	8.0	5	360	1.0
(*Cheese Nips*), 1.1 oz.	150	3.0	19.0	6.0	0	340	1.0
(*Cheese Nips*), 1.25-oz. pkg. . . .	170	3.0	22.0	7.0	0	410	1.0
(*Cheese Nips* Mini Go Pack), 1.1 oz.	150	3.0	19.0	6.0	0	340	1.0
(*Cheez-It Crisps* Crunch), 36 pcs., 1.1 oz.	150	3.0	18.0	8.0	0	280	1.0
(*Cheez-It Stix*), 35 pcs., 1.1 oz. .	150	3.0	18.0	7.0	0	280	<1.0
(*Cheez-It Twisterz*), 17 pcs., 1.1 oz. .	140	2.0	19.0	6.0	0	270	<1.0
(*Combos*), 1 oz. . . .	140	2.0	18.0	6.0	0	290	0
(*Goldfish*), 55 pcs., 1.1 oz.	140	4.0	20.0	5.0	<5	250	<1.0
(*Goldfish* Baby), 89 pcs., 1.1 oz. .	140	4.0	20.0	5.0	<5	250	<1.0
(*Goldfish* Calcium), 55 pcs., 1.1 oz. .	130	3.0	19.0	4.5	<5	250	<1.0
(*Goldfish* Flavor Blasted Xtra), 51 pcs., 1.1 oz. .	140	4.0	18.0	6.0	<5	310	<1.0
(*TLC* Cquntry), 18 pcs., 1.1 oz. .	130	3.0	20.0	4.5	0	220	<1.0
Jack (*Cheez-It*), 25 pcs., 1.1 oz. .	160	3.0	18.0	8.0	0	250	0
ranch, cool (*Cheez-It Twisterz*), 17 pcs., 1.1 oz.	140	2.0	20.0	6.0	0	280	<1.0
sour cream/onion (*Annie's* Bunnies), 55 pcs., 1.1 oz. .	140	3.0	18.0	6.0	0	250	<1.0
white (*Annie's* Bunnies), 55 pcs., 1.1 oz. .	140	3.0	18.0	6.0	0	160	<1.0
white (*Cheez-It*), 25 pcs., 1.1 oz. .	150	2.0	18.0	8.0	0	280	<1.0

Food and Measure	cal.	prot. (gms)	carbo. (gms)	fat (gms)	chol. (mgs)	sod. (mgs)	fiber (gms)
Cracker, cheddar *(cont.)*							
white (*Cheez-It Stix*),							
35 pcs., 1.1 oz. .	150	3.0	18.0	7.0	0	280	<1.0
whole grain (*Goldfish*),							
55 pcs., 1.1 oz. . .	140	4.0	19.0	5.0	<5	250	2.0
whole wheat (*Annie's*							
Bunnies), 50 pcs.,							
1.1 oz.	130	3.0	17.0	6.0	0	250	3.0
cheese:							
(*Carr's* Cheese Melts),							
3 pcs., .5 oz. . . .	60	2.0	7.0	3.0	5	150	<1.0
(*Cheez-It* Big),							
13 pcs., 1.1 oz. .	160	4.0	18.0	8.0	0	250	<1.0
(*Cheez-It* Original),							
27 pcs., 1.1 oz. .	160	3.0	18.0	8.0	0	250	<1.0
(*Cheez-It* Reduced							
Fat), 29 pcs.,							
1.1 oz.	130	4.0	20.0	4.0	0	360	<1.0
(*Cheez-It Gripz*),							
.9-oz. pkg.	130	3.0	16.0	6.0	0	260	<1.0
(*Goldfish* Colors),							
55 pcs., 1.1 oz. .	140	4.0	20.0	5.0	5	260	<1.0
(*Ritz* Real Cheese),							
1.38-oz. pkg. . . .	200	3.0	22.0	11.0	5	400	1.0
(*Ritz* Real Cheese							
Packs to Go),							
1.38-oz. pkg. . . .	200	2.0	22.0	12.0	5	460	1.0
(*Ritz* Handi-Snacks),							
1.1 oz.	110	3.0	13.0	4.5	10	340	0
4 (*Cheese Nips*),							
1.1 oz.	150	3.0	18.0	7.0	0	310	1.0
4 (*Cheez-It Crisps*),							
36 pcs., 1.1 oz. .	150	3.0	18.0	7.0	0	240	<1.0
3 (*Pepperidge Farm*							
Snack Sticks),							
11 pcs., 1.1 oz. .	130	4.0	21.0	3.5	<5	380	<1.0
artisan (*Pepperidge*							
Farm Snack Sticks),							
11 pcs., 1.1 oz. .	130	4.0	20.0	4.0	5	400	1.0
Buffalo flavor (*Gold-*							
fish Flavor Blasted							
Blazin'), 51 pcs.							
1.1 oz.	140	4.0	19.0	6.0	<5	310	<1.0

Food and Measure	cal.	prot. (gms)	carbo. (gms)	fat (gms)	chol. (mgs)	sod. (mgs)	fiber (gms)
chili queso (*Cheez-It Fiesta*), 25 pcs., 1.1 oz.	160	3.0	18.0	8.0	0	270	<1.0
hot/spicy (*Cheez-It*), 26 pcs., 1.1 oz. . .	150	2.0	18.0	8.0	0	280	<1.0
jalapeño (*Goldfish Sabor Explosivo*), 51 pcs., 1.1 oz. . .	150	3.0	17.0	7.0	<5	310	1.0
nacho (*Cheez-It Fiesta*), 25 pcs., 1.1 oz.	160	3.0	18.0	8.0	0	260	1.0
nacho (*Cheez-It Gripz*), .9-oz. pkg.	120	3.0	16.0	5.0	<5	220	<1.0
nacho (*Goldfish Flavor Blasted* Nothin' But), 51 pcs., 1.1 oz. . .	150	3.0	17.0	7.0	<5	250	<1.0
sour cream/onion (*Cheez-It*), 25 pcs., 1.1 oz. . .	160	3.0	19.0	8.0	0	250	<1.0
cheese sandwich:							
(*Cheese Waffies*), 1 oz.	140	2.0	15.0	8.0	<5	380	0
(*Ritz Bits*), 1.5 oz. . .	220	3.0	24.0	13.0	5	480	1.0
(*Ritz Bits* Cheese Now!), 1 oz.	150	2.0	16.0	9.0	5	260	0
bacon cheddar, (*Cheetos*), 1 pkg.	190	3.0	24.0	10.0	0	330	1.0
chedder (*Keebler Club*), 1.3-oz. pkg.	190	4.0	23.0	10.0	0	360	<1.0
cheddar, toast (*Cheetos*), 1 pkg.	200	3.0	23.0	11.0	<5	410	1.0
jalapeño cheddar (*Ritz Bits*), 1.1 oz.	160	2.0	17.0	10.0	5	340	0
jalapeño cheese, toast (*Doritos*), 1 pkg.	200	3.0	23.0	11.0	0	340	1.0
nacho cheese, toast (*Doritos*), 1 pkg.	210	3.0	22.0	12.0	<5	280	1.0
chicken flavor (*Chicken in a Bisket*), 12 pcs., 1.1 oz.	160	2.0	19.0	8.0	0	300	1.0
corn bread (*Town House Bistro*), 2 pcs., .6 oz.	80	1.0	11.0	5.0	5	100	<1.0

Food and Measure	cal.	prot. (gms)	carbo. (gms)	fat (gms)	chol. (mgs)	sod. (mgs)	fiber (gms)
Cracker *(cont.)*							
crispbread wafer							
(*Water Wheel* Original), 16 pcs., .4 oz.	40	1.1	7.3	.2	0	134	.5
flaky (*Carr's Croissant*), 3 pcs., .5 oz.	70	1.0	11.0	2.5	5	100	0
flatbread:							
herb, Italian (*JJ Flats*), .5-oz. pc. .	60	2.0	10.0	2.0	0	95	<1.0
onion (*JJ Flats*), .5-oz. pc.	60	2.0	10.0	2.0	0	140	<1.0
poppy (*JJ Flats*), .5-oz. pc.	60	2.0	10.0	2.0	<5	125	<1.0
seeds and spice (*New York Style Crispini*), 6 pcs., 1 oz.	120	4.0	19.0	3.5	0	190	<1.0
sesame (*New York Style Crispini*), 6 pcs., 1 oz.	120	4.0	20.0	2.5	0	190	1.0
sesame garlic (*New York Style Crispini*), 6 pcs., 1 oz.	120	4.0	19.0	3.0	0	190	<1.0
garlic herb:							
(*All-Bran*), 18 pcs., 1.1 oz.	120	3.0	19.0	6.0	0	330	5.0
(*Town House Toppers*), 3 pcs., .5 oz. ...	70	1.0	9.0	3.0	0	135	0
graham cracker, see "Cookie"							
grain, whole, and seeds (*Dare grainsfirst*), 4 pcs., .6 oz.	90	2.0	12.0	3.0	0	125	2.0
hazelnut/rice (*Nut-Thins*), 16 pcs.	130	2.0	23.0	3.0	0	115	<1.0
herb, garden (*Health Valley* Organic), 4 pcs., .5 oz.	70	1.0	10.0	3.0	0	170	0
herb and garlic (*Tree of Life* Organic), 10 pcs., 1.1 oz. ...	120	2.0	22.0	2.5	0	220	1.0
matzo, 1.1-oz. pc.:							
(*Manischewitz*)	120	3.0	27.0	0	0	0	1.0
(*Streit's*)	110	3.0	25.0	0	0	0	1.0

Food and Measure	cal.	prot. (gms)	carbo. (gms)	fat (gms)	chol. (mgs)	sod. (mgs)	fiber (gms)
multigrain:							
(All-Bran), 18 pcs., 1.1 oz.	130	2.0	19.0	6.0	0	210	5.0
(Breton), 3 pcs., .6 oz.	80	2.0	10.0	3.5	0	160	1.0
(Jacob's Choice Grain), 2 pcs., .5 oz. ...	60	1.0	10.0	2.0	0	135	1.0
(Keebler Club), 4 pcs., .5 oz.	70	1.0	10.0	3.0	0	150	<1.0
(Town House Bistro), 2 pcs., .6 oz. ...	80	1.0	11.0	3.0	0	130	<1.0
(Vinta), .5 oz.	70	1.0	8.0	3.0	0	110	0
(Wheat Thins), 17 pcs., 1.1 oz. .	130	2.0	22.0	4.5	0	230	2.0
(Wheatables), 17 pcs., 1.1 oz. .	140	2.0	20.0	6.0	0	300	1.0
5 grain crunch (Wheat Thins), 1.1 oz.	130	3.0	23.0	4.0	0	230	2.0
7 grain (TLC), 15 pcs., 1.1 oz. .	130	3.0	22.0	3.0	0	160	2.0
7 grain (TLC Stone-ground), 4 pcs., 1 oz.	130	3.0	17.0	5.0	0	140	3.0
10 grain (Lavosh-Hawaii), 1 oz.	110	4.0	19.0	3.0	0	300	3.0
garlic, roasted, thyme (TLC), 4 pcs., 1 oz.	130	3.0	18.0	4.5	0	140	3.0
honey sesame (TLC), 15 pcs., 1.1 oz. .	130	3.0	22.0	3.0	0	160	2.0
puffed (Keebler Club), 24 pcs., 1.1 oz. .	140	2.0	21.0	6.0	0	310	1.0
ranch (TLC Natural), 15 pcs., 1.1 oz. .	130	3.0	22.0	3.0	0	200	2.0
vegetable, fire-roasted (TLC), 15 pcs., 1.1 oz. .	130	3.0	21.0	3.5	0	210	2.0
onion:							
(Toasteds), 5 pcs., .6 oz.	80	1.0	11.0	3.5	0	160	<1.0
slightly (Lavosh-Hawaii), 1 oz.	120	3.0	19.0	3.0	21	300	1.0

Food and Measure	cal.	prot. (gms)	carbo. (gms)	fat (gms)	chol. (mgs)	sod. (mgs)	fiber (gms)
Cracker, onion *(cont.)*							
roasted (*Haute Cuisine*), 10 pcs., 1 oz. . . .	130	2.0	22.0	3.0	0	210	<1.0
toasted (*Tree of Life Organic*), 10 pcs., 1.1 oz.	120	2.0	22.0	2.5	0	210	1.0
Parmesan:							
(*Goldfish*), 60 pcs., 1.1 oz.	130	4.0	20.0	4.0	0	280	<1.0
garlic (*Cheez-It*), 25 pcs., 1.1 oz. .	150	3.0	19.0	7.0	0	270	0
peanut butter sandwich, 1.4-oz. pkg., except as noted:							
(*Ritz Bits*), 1.25 oz.	170	4.0	20.0	10.0	0	280	1.0
(*Ritz Bits 9.5 oz.*), 1 oz.	140	3.0	16.0	8.0	0	240	1.0
cheese crackers (*Austin*)	200	1.0	23.0	10.0	0	400	1.0
cheese crackers (*Austin* Mega Stuffed), 1.7 oz. .	240	6.0	25.0	13.0	0	490	2.0
cheese crackers (*Frito-Lay*)	190	5.0	23.0	9.0	0	370	2.0
chocolatey (*Austin*)	200	3.0	25.0	10.0	0	220	<1.0
and jelly (*Austin*) . .	200	3.0	24.0	10.0	0	300	<1.0
and jelly (*Ritz Bits*), 1 oz.	140	3.0	16.0	7.0	0	230	1.0
toast (*Austin* Toasty)	200	4.0	23.0	10.0	0	410	1.0
toast (*Frito-Lay*) . . .	200	4.0	23.0	10.0	0	310	2.0
pecan/rice (*Nut-Thins*), 16 pcs.	130	2.0	23.0	3.5	0	130	<1.0
pepper, cracked (*Tree of Life* Organic), 10 pcs., 1.1 oz. . . .	120	3.0	23.0	2.0	0	135	<1.0
peppercorn (*Lavosh-Hawaii*), 1 oz.	115	3.0	20.0	3.0	21	300	1.0
pepperoni (*Combos*), 1 oz.	140	2.0	18.0	6.0	0	280	0
pizza flavor, 1.1 oz.:							
(*Goldfish*), 55 pcs. .	140	3.0	20.0	5.0	0	230	<1.0
(*Goldfish Flavor Blasted* Xplosive), 51 pcs.	140	3.0	19.0	6.0	0	280	1.0

Food and Measure	cal.	prot. (gms)	carbo. (gms)	fat (gms)	chol. (mgs)	sod. (mgs)	fiber (gms)
poppy seed, savory (*Barbara's Rite Lite Rounds*), 5 pcs., .5 oz.	60	1.0	11.0	2.0	0	200	0
pretzel cracker:							
(*Goldfish*), 43 pcs., 1.1 oz.	130	3.0	24.0	2.5	0	430	<1.0
(*New York Style Pretzel Flatz* Original), 12 pcs., 1 oz.	110	3.0	23.0	1.0	0	250	1.0
(*Pepperidge Farm* Pretzel Thins), 11 pcs., 1 oz.	110	2.0	21.0	0	0	340	1.0
(*Snyder's* Original), 1.1 oz.	120	2.0	23.0	2.5	0	200	2.0
butter sesame (*Snyder's*), 1.1 oz.	120	3.0	23.0	2.5	0	290	1.0
cheddar, savory (*Pepperidge Farm* Thins), 11 pcs., 1.1 oz.	140	0	26.0	3.0	0	600	1.0
everything (*New York Style Pretzel Flatz*), 12 pcs., 1 oz.	110	3.0	21.0	2.0	0	440	1.0
pumpernickel onion (*Snyder's*), 1 oz.	120	3.0	22.0	2.5	0	230	3.0
pumpernickel (*Pepperidge Farm* Snack Sticks), 15 pcs., 1 oz.	120	3.0	24.0	1.5	0	410	2.0
rice:							
all varieties, except maki rolls (*Roland*), 1.1 oz.	110	2.0	25.0	0	0	280	2.0
maki rolls (*Roland*), 1.1 oz.	110	2.0	25.0	0	0	190	2.0
onion/garlic (*Cedar's*), 16 pcs., 1 oz.	120	2.0	24.0	1.5	0	80	0
rice, brown:							
(*Eden* Organic), 8 pcs., 1.1 oz.	120	3.0	22.0	2.0	0	230	2.0
nori maki (*Eden* Organic), 15 pcs., 1.1 oz.	110	3.0	24.0	0	0	160	2.0
sesame (*San-J*), 5 pcs., 1 oz.	140	4.0	17.0	6.0	0	180	1.0

Food and Measure	cal.	prot. (gms)	carbo. (gms)	fat (gms)	chol. (mgs)	sod. (mgs)	fiber (gms)
Cracker, rice, brown *(cont.)*							
sesame, black *(San-J)*, 5 pcs., 1 oz.	140	4.0	17.0	6.0	0	130	2.0
tamari *(San-J)*, 6 pcs., 1.1 oz.	120	3.0	27.0	0	0	170	<1.0
rice bran *(Health Valley)*, 6 pcs., 1 oz.	110	3.0	19.0	3.0	0	70	3.0
rosemary, 1 oz.:							
(Carr's), 7 pcs.	130	2.0	19.0	5.0	0	230	<1.0
garlic *(Lavosh-Hawaii)*	125	3.0	19.0	3.0	21	230	1.0
rye *(Triscuit)*, 1 oz. . .	120	3.0	19.0	4.5	0	150	3.0
saltines, 5 pcs., .5 oz., except as noted:							
(Murray)	60	1.0	11.0	1.5	0	200	<1.0
(Murray Unsalted Tops)	60	1.0	12.0	1.5	0	90	<1.0
(Premium Fat Free)	60	1.0	12.0	0	0	170	0
(Premium Low Sodium)	60	1.0	11.0	1.5	0	25	0
(Premium Original)	60	1.0	11.0	1.5	0	190	0
(Premium Original 8 oz.)	70	1.0	11.0	1.5	0	220	0
(Premium Unsalted Top)	60	1.0	11.0	1.5	0	130	0
(Zesta Fat Free) . . .	60	1.0	13.0	0	0	280	<1.0
(Zesta Original) . . .	60	1.0	11.0	1.5	0	200	<1.0
multigrain *(Premium)*	60	1.0	10.0	1.5	0	170	0
onion, toasted *(Premium)*	60	1.0	11.0	1.5	0	190	1.0
whole wheat *(Wheat-ines* Original), 4 pcs., .5 oz. . . .	60	1.0	11.0	1.0	0	80	<1.0
whole wheat *(Zesta)*	60	1.0	11.0	1.5	0	230	<1.0
whole wheat, cracked pepper *(Wheatines)*, 4 pcs., .5 oz. . . .	50	1.0	11.0	1.0	0	120	1.0
saltines, mini *(Prem-ium)*, .5 oz.	70	1.0	10.0	2.5	0	140	0
sesame:							
(Bremner Wafer), 7 pcs., .5 oz. . . .	70	2.0	11.0	2.0	0	105	0

Food and Measure	cal.	prot. (gms)	carbo. (gms)	fat (gms)	chol. (mgs)	sod. (mgs)	fiber (gms)
(*Breton*), 3 pcs., .5 oz.	70	2.0	8.0	3.0	0	100	0
(*Health Valley* Organic), 4 pcs., .6 oz. . . .	70	1.0	10.0	3.0	0	200	<1.0
(*Toasteds*), 5 pcs., .6 oz.	80	1.0	10.0	3.5	0	140	<1.0
and flax seed (*Tree of Life* Organic), 10 pcs., 1.1 oz. .	140	3.0	23.0	4.0	0	230	1.0
tamari (*Barbara's Rite Lite Rounds*), 5 pcs., .5 oz. . . .	70	1.0	10.0	2.0	0	200	0
toasted (*Pepperidge Farm* Snack Sticks), 12 pcs., 1.1 oz. .	130	3.0	19.0	5.0	0	290	2.0
soda/water:							
(*Carr's Table Water*), 4 pcs., .5 oz. . . .	60	1.5	12.0	1.0	0	40	0
(*Courtney's* English), 4 pcs., .5 oz. . . .	60	1.0	10.0	1.0	0	140	0
(*Jacob's* Biscuits for Cheese), 3 pcs., .5 oz.	70	1.0	10.0	2.5	0	110	<1.0
(*Jacob's* Cream), 2 pcs., .5 oz. . . .	70	2.0	11.0	2.5	0	80	0
(*Keebler* Export Soda), 3 pcs., .5 oz. . . .	60	1.0	10.0	1.5	0	85	<1.0
(*Pepperidge Farm* Classic), 4 pcs., .5 oz.	60	0	12.0	1.0	0	90	<1.0
(*Tree of Life* Organic Water), 4 pcs., .5 oz.	60	<2.0	12.0	1.0	0	75	0
(*Wellington* Traditional), 4 pcs., .5 oz.	60	2.0	12.0	1.0	0	75	0
all varieties (*Dare* Water Cracker), 5 pcs., .6 oz. . . .	60	1.5	11.0	1.5	0	120	0
assorted (*Carr's* Biscuits for Cheese), 2 pcs., .4 oz. . . .	50	1.0	8.0	2.0	<5	85	<1.0
cheese (*Carr's* Melts), 3 pcs., .5 oz. . . .	60	2.0	7.0	3.0	5	150	<1.0

Food and Measure	cal.	prot. (gms)	carbo. (gms)	fat (gms)	chol. (mgs)	sod. (mgs)	fiber (gms)
Cracker, soda/water *(cont.)*							
cracked pepper (*Carr's Table Water*), 5 pcs., .6 oz.	70	2.0	13.0	1.5	0	100	<1.0
cracked pepper (*Tree of Life* Organic Water), 4 pcs., .5 oz.	60	<2.0	11.0	1.0	0	75	0
garlic, roasted (*Carr's Table Water*), 5 pcs., .6 oz.	70	2.0	12.0	1.5	0	140	<1.0
poppy/sesame (*Carr's*), 4 pcs., .6 oz.	80	2.0	9.0	5.0	<5	135	<1.0
sesame (*Tree of Life* Organic Water), 4 pcs., .5 oz.	70	<2.0	11.0	1.5	0	70	0
sesame, toasted (*Carr's Table Water*), 5 pcs., .6 oz.	70	2.0	12.0	1.5	0	100	<1.0
soup/oyster, .5 oz.:							
(*Bremner* Oyster), 50 pcs.	60	1.0	10.0	1.0	0	130	0
(*Bremner* Soup & Chili), 50 pcs.	60	2.0	11.0	1.5	0	110	0
(*Hain* Oyster), 52 pcs.	60	2.0	12.0	1.0	0	140	0
(*Premium*), 23 pcs.	60	1.0	11.0	1.5	0	170	0
spelt (*Skinny Dippers* Organic), 2 pcs., .6 oz.	50	1.0	10.0	.5	0	100	1.0
toasts, 2 pcs., .6 oz.:							
(*Alessi*)	50	2.0	8.0	0	0	70	0
(*New York Style Panetini*)	80	2.0	10.0	4.0	0	90	0
cheese, 3 (*New York Style Pantini*)	80	2.0	9.0	4.5	0	150	0
garlic (*New York Style Pantini*)	80	2.0	10.0	4.0	0	190	0
garlic Parmesan (*New York Style Pantini*)	80	2.0	9.0	4.5	0	150	0
whole wheat (*Alessi*)	70	2.0	13.0	0	0	70	1.0
vegetable:							
(*Vegetable Thins*), 14 pcs., 1.1 oz.	150	2.0	20.0	7.0	0	330	1.0

Food and Measure	cal.	prot. (gms)	carbo. (gms)	fat (gms)	chol. (mgs)	sod. (mgs)	fiber (gms)
(*Vivant*), 3 pcs., .5 oz.	60	1.0	9.0	2.5	0	120	0
(*Wheat Thins* Harvest), 1.1 oz.	130	2.0	23.0	3.5	0	230	1.0
garden (*Breton*), 3 pcs., .5 oz.	60	1.0	9.0	2.5	0	105	0
garden (*Breton* Minis), 13 pcs., .5 oz.	70	1.0	10.0	3.0	0	170	0
garden (*Tree of Life* Organic), 10 pcs., 1.1 oz.	120	3.0	22.0	2.5	0	250	<1.0
roasted (*Ritz*), .6 oz.	80	1.0	10.0	3.5	0	150	0
wheat:							
(*Hain Wheatettes*), 16 pcs., 1.1 oz.	130	3.0	21.0	3.5	0	270	2.0
(*Pepperidge Farm* Harvest), 3 pcs., .5 oz.	80	1.0	11.0	3.5	0	125	<1.0
(*Toasteds*), 5 pcs., .6 oz.	80	1.0	10.0	3.5	0	160	<1.0
(*Toasteds* Harvest Organic), 5 pcs., 1 oz.	130	2.0	20.0	6.0	0	260	1.0
(*Town House*), 5 pcs., .6 oz.	80	1.0	10.0	4.0	0	140	<1.0
(*Wheat Thins* Big), 11 pcs., 1.1 oz.	150	2.0	21.0	6.0	0	270	1.0
(*Wheat Thins* Low Sodium), 16 pcs., 1.1 oz.	150	2.0	22.0	6.0	0	80	1.0
(*Wheat Thins* Original), 16 pcs., 1.1 oz.	150	2.0	21.0	6.0	0	260	1.0
(*Wheat Thins* Original 4 oz.), 1.1 oz.	150	3.0	21.0	6.0	0	280	1.0
(*Wheatables* Original Golden Wheat), 17 pcs., 1.1 oz.	140	2.0	20.0	6.0	0	340	1.0
(*Wheatables* Reduced Fat), 19 pcs., 1.1 oz.	140	2.0	22.0	4.0	0	320	1.0
(*Wheatsworth*), 5 pcs., .6 oz.	80	2.0	10.0	3.5	0	180	1.0
cracked (*Bremner* Wafer), 7 pcs., .5 oz.	70	2.0	11.0	1.5	0	100	0

Food and Measure	cal.	prot. (gms)	carbo. (gms)	fat (gms)	chol. (mgs)	sod. (mgs)	fiber (gms)
Cracker, wheat *(cont.)*							
honey (*Keebler Club Snack Sticks*), 12 pcs., 1 oz. . . .	130	1.0	19.0	6.0	0	260	<1.0
honey, toasted (*Wheatables*), 17 pcs., 1.1 oz. .	140	2.0	20.0	6.0	0	310	1.0
Parmesan basil (*Wheat Thins*), 1.1 oz.	140	2.0	21.0	5.0	0	290	1.0
ranch (*Wheat Thins*), 1 oz.	130	2.0	20.0	6.0	0	250	1.0
salsa (*Pepperidge Farm Crisps*), 16 pcs., 1.1 oz. .	140	2.0	21.0	6.0	0	270	2.0
stoned (*Archer Farms*), 3 pcs., .5 oz.	60	2.0	11.0	1.5	0	160	<1.0
stoned (*Health Valley Organic*), 4 pcs., .6 oz.	70	1.0	10.0	3.0	0	170	<1.0
stoned (*Red Oval Farms*), 2 pcs., .5 oz. . . .	60	1.0	10.0	1.5	0	210	1.0
stoned (*Red Oval Farms Lower Sodium*), 2 pcs., .5 oz. . . .	60	1.0	11.0	1.5	0	70	1.0
stoned, mini (*Red Oval Farms*), 1.1 oz.	130	3.0	22.0	3.0	0	430	1.0
toasted (*Pepperidge Farm Crisps*), 17 pcs., 1.1 oz. .	140	2.0	21.0	5.0	0	240	2.0
tomato, sun-dried, basil (*Wheat Thins*), 1.1 oz. . . .	140	2.0	20.0	6.0	0	240	1.0
wheat, whole:							
(*Carr's*), 2 pcs., .6 oz.	80	1.0	11.0	3.5	0	100	1.0
(*Health Valley Organic*), 4 pcs., .5 oz. . . .	70	2.0	9.0	3.0	0	170	1.0
(*Ritz*), 5 pcs., .5 oz.	70	1.0	11.0	2.5	0	120	1.0
(*Ritz Simply Social*), .5 oz.	70	1.0	10.0	3.0	0	150	1.0
(*Triscuit Original*), 1 oz.	120	3.0	19.0	4.5	0	180	3.0

Food and Measure	cal.	prot. (gms)	carbo. (gms)	fat (gms)	chol. (mgs)	sod. (mgs)	fiber (gms)
(*Triscuit* Reduced Fat), 1 oz.	120	3.0	21.0	3.0	0	160	3.0
(*Triscuit Thin Crisps*), 15 pcs., 1.1 oz.	130	3.0	21.0	5.0	0	180	3.0
(*Wheat Thins 100%*), 1.1 oz.	140	2.0	21.0	6.0	0	290	2.0
cheddar (*Triscuit*), 1 oz.	120	3.0	19.0	4.5	0	220	3.0
cracked pepper/olive oil (*Triscuit*), 1 oz.	120	3.0	20.0	4.0	0	140	3.0
garlic, roasted (*Triscuit*), 1 oz.	120	3.0	20.0	4.5	0	140	3.0
herb, garden (*Triscuit*), 1 oz.	120	3.0	20.0	4.0	0	125	3.0
rosemary/olive oil (*Triscuit*), 1 oz.	120	3.0	20.0	4.0	0	135	3.0
tomato, fire-roasted (*Triscuit*), 1 oz.	120	3.0	20.0	4.0	0	150	3.0
zwieback (*Nabisco*), .3-oz. pc.	35	1.0	6.0	1.0	0	10	0
Cracker meal, ¼ cup:							
(*Nabisco*)	110	3.0	22.0	0	0	15	1.0
(*Vigo*)	120	3.0	24.0	.5	0	120	1.0
matzo (*Manischewitz*)	130	3.0	23.0	0	0	0	1.0
Cranberry, fresh:							
(*Ocean Spray*), 2 oz.	30	0	7.0	0	0	35	2.0
whole, ½ cup	23	.2	6.0	.1	0	1	2.0
chopped, ½ cup	27	.2	7.0	.1	0	1	2.3
Cranberry, canned, see "Cranberry sauce"							
Cranberry, dried, ⅓ cup, 1.4 oz., except as noted:							
(*Amport Foods*), ¼ cup	150	0	36.0	0	0	5	3.0
(*Craisins*)	130	0	33.0	0	0	0	2.0
(*Earthbound Farm* Organic)	130	0	34.0	0	0	2	2.0
(*Eden* Organic)	140	0	33.0	.5	0	20	2.0
(*Frieda's*), 1 oz.	90	0	23.0	1.0	0	3	1.0
(*Sun•Maid* Cape Cod)	130	0	33.0	0	0	0	2.0
(*SunRidge Farms*), ¼ cup	120	0	33.0	.5	0	0	2.0
(*Sunsweet*)	140	0	35.0	0	0	0	2.0
(*Tree of Life*)	129	0	35.0	0	0	0	3.5

Food and Measure	cal.	prot. (gms)	carbo. (gms)	fat (gms)	chol. (mgs)	sod. (mgs)	fiber (gms)
Cranberry, dried *(cont.)*							
(*Tree of Life* Organic),							
1 oz.	120	0	23.0	0	0	1	<2.0
Cranberry bean:							
boiled, ½ cup	120	8.2	21.5	.4	0	1	3.0
canned, ½ cup	108	7.2	19.7	.4	0	431	n.a.
Cranberry drink,							
8 fl. oz.:							
(*Apple & Eve* Light) . .	40	0	9.0	0	0	10	0
(*Langers*)	140	0	35.0	0	0	10	0
cocktail:							
(*Nantucket Nectars*)	130	0	33.0	0	0	25	0
(*Ocean Spray*)	130	0	33.0	0	0	35	0
(*Ocean Spray*							
Calcium)	150	0	37.0	0	0	35	0
(*Tropicana*)	140	0	34.0	0	0	35	0
nectar (*Santa Cruz*							
Organic)	110	<1.0	27.0	0	0	25	0
white (*Langers*)	120	0	28.0	0	0	10	0
Cranberry drink blend,							
8 fl. oz., except as noted:							
all varieties (*Langers*							
Diet/Low Carb)	30	0	8.0	0	0	10	0
apple (*Cranapple*)	140	0	35.0	0	0	80	0
apple raspberry							
(*Minute Maid*)	120	0	33.0	0	0	25	0
berry (*Langers*)	135	0	34.0	0	0	10	0
cherry (*Cran•Cherry*) .	130	0	32.0	0	0	35	0
grape:							
(*Apple & Eve* Light)	40	0	9.0	0	0	5	0
(*Cran•Grape*)	140	0	35.0	0	0	80	0
(*Langers*)	165	0	41.0	0	0	10	0
(*Minute Maid*)	150	0	39.0	0	0	20	0
frozen* (*Langers*) .	150	0	37.0	0	0	10	0
grapefruit (*SoBe*							
Elixir 3C)	100	0	28.0	0	0	10	0
w/lime (*Langers*)	140	0	35.0	0	0	10	0
lime raspberry							
(*Odwalla B Barrier*)	120	0	30	0	0	15	0
raspberry:							
(*Apple & Eve* Light)	40	0	9.0	0	0	10	0
(*Cran•Raspberry*) .	120	0	30.0	0	0	70	0
(*Langers*)	150	0	36.0	0	0	10	0
(*R.W. Knudsen*) . . .	130	0	32.0	0	0	20	0

Food and Measure	cal.	prot. (gms)	carbo. (gms)	fat (gms)	chol. (mgs)	sod. (mgs)	fiber (gms)
(*Snapple*)	120	0	29.0	0	0	10	0
frozen* (*Langers*) .	140	0	35.0	0	0	10	0
strawberry							
(*Cran•Strawberry*) .	120	0	30.0	0	0	80	0
tangerine							
(*Cran•Tangerine*) ..	130	0	35.0	0	0	35	0
Cranberry juice,							
8 fl. oz., except as noted:							
(*After the Fall* Cape							
Cod)	120	0	30.0	0	0	15	0
(*Apple & Eve* & More)	130	0	32.0	0	0	25	0
(*Apple & Eve* Naturally)	130	1.0	32.0	0	0	20	0
(*Langers/L&A* 100) ..	140	0	35.0	0	0	15	0
(*Mountain Sun* Pure) .	60	0	15.0	0	0	20	0
(*Northland*)	130	0	33.0	0	0	35	0
(*Ocean Spray* 100%) .	50	0	12.0	0	0	35	0
(*R.W. Knudsen* Nectar)	130	<1.0	31.0	0	0	40	0
(*R.W. Knudsen* Just							
Cranberry)	70	0	18.0	0	0	10	0
(*Walnut Acres* Organic)	110	0	26.0	0	0	15	0
frozen*:							
(*Cascadian Farm*							
Organic)	120	0	32.0	0	0	15	0
(*Langers*)	120	0	35.0	0	0	10	0
sparkling (*R.W.*							
Knudsen)	130	<1.0	31.0	0	0	45	0
Cranberry juice blend,							
8 fl. oz., except as							
noted:							
(*Ocean Spray* Premium/							
Organic)	140	0	35.0	0	0	35	0
(*Simply Nutritious Vita*							
Cranberry)	130	0	31.0	0	0	10	0
apple:							
(*Apple & Eve*)	130	1.0	33.0	0	0	20	0
(*Land O Lakes*) ...	120	0	30.0	0	0	15	0
(*Northland*)	130	0	33.0	0	0	35	0
berry, mixed:							
(*Langers* 100)	130	0	33.0	0	0	10	0
wild (*Apple & Eve*) .	130	0	33.0	0	0	25	0
blackberry (*Northland*)	140	0	35.0	0	0	35	0
blueberry:							
(*Apple & Eve*							
Organics)	130	0	31.0	0	0	25	0

Food and Measure	cal.	prot. (gms)	carbo. (gms)	fat (gms)	chol. (mgs)	sod. (mgs)	fiber (gms)
Cranberry juice blend, blueberry *(cont.)*							
(*Northland*)	140	0	34.0	0	0	35	0
(*Ocean Spray*)	140	0	36.0	0	0	35	0
(*R.W. Knudsen* Organic)	130	0	33.0	0	0	15	0
cherry (*Northland*) ...	140	0	35.0	0	0	35	0
grape:							
(*Apple & Eve*)	140	1.0	34.0	0	0	25	0
(*Langers* 100)	150	0	38.0	0	0	15	0
(*Northland*)	140	0	36.0	0	0	35	0
(*Ocean Spray*)	150	0	37.0	0	0	35	0
kiwi (*Ceres*)	110	0	28.0	0	0	14	0
peach mango (*Apple & Eve*)	120	0	31.0	0	0	20	0
pomegranate:							
(*Northland*)	140	0	34.0	0	0	25	0
(*Ocean Spray*)	140	0	34.0	0	0	35	0
(*R.W. Knudsen* Organic)	130	0	32.0	0	0	15	0
raspberry:							
(*After the Fall*)	130	1.0	32.0	0	0	10	0
(*Apple & Eve*)	120	1.0	26.0	0	0	20	0
(*Langers* 100)	145	0	36.0	0	0	15	0
(*Northland*)	140	0	34.0	0	0	35	0
(*Ocean Spray*)	140	0	34.0	0	0	35	0
(*Ocean Spray* Organic)	140	0	35.0	0	0	30	0
Cranberry juice cocktail, see "Cranberry drink"							
Cranberry juice concentrate:							
(*R.W. Knudsen*), 8 fl. oz.	45	0	18.0	0	0	25	0
(*Tree of Life*), 8 tsp. ..	110	0	28.0	0	0	0	0
Cranberry sauce, can/jar, ¼ cup, except as noted:							
(*R.W. Knudsen*), 1 tbsp.	25	0	6.0	0	0	0	0
all styles:							
(*S&W*)	100	0	26.0	0	0	35	1.0
(*Tree of Life* Organic)	100	0	26.0	0	0	35	1.0
jellied (*Ocean Spray*) .	110	0	25.0	0	0	10	1.0
whole (*Ocean Spray*) .	110	0	27.0	0	0	10	1.0
Cranberry sauce fruit blend, orange or raspberry (*Cran-Fruit*), ¼ cup	120	0	29.0	0	0	35	1.0

Food and Measure	cal.	prot. (gms)	carbo. (gms)	fat (gms)	chol. (mgs)	sod. (mgs)	fiber (gms)
Crayfish, mixed species:							
farmed, meat only:							
raw, 4 oz.	82	16.8	0	1.1	122	70	0
raw, 8 pcs., .95 oz.	19	4.0	0	.3	29	17	0
boiled or steamed,							
4 oz.	99	19.9	0	1.5	155	110	0
wild, meat only:							
raw, 4 oz.	87	18.1	0	1.1	129	66	0
raw, 8 pcs., .95 oz.	21	4.3	0	.3	31	16	0
boiled or steamed,							
4 oz.	93	19.0	0	1.4	151	107	0
Cream:							
half-and-half:							
(*Land O Lakes*							
Gourmet), 2 tbsp.	35	<1.0	1.0	3.5	10	15	0
(*Organic Valley*),							
2 tbsp.	40	<1.0	1.0	3.5	10	10	0
1 cup	315	7.2	10.4	27.8	89	98	0
1 tbsp.	20	.4	.6	1.7	6	6	0
nonfat (*Land O*							
Lakes), 2 tbsp. . . .	20	<1.0	3.0	0	0	30	0
nonfat (*Simply*							
Smart), 2 tbsp. .	15	<1.0	2.0	0	<5	30	0
light, coffee or table:							
1 cup	469	6.5	8.8	46.3	159	95	0
1 tbsp.	29	.4	.6	2.9	10	6	0
medium (25% fat):							
1 cup	583	5.9	8.3	59.8	209	88	0
1 tbsp.	37	.4	.5	3.8	13	6	0
sour, see "Cream, sour"							
whipped topping, see							
"Cream topping"							
whipping[1], light:							
1 cup	699	5.2	7.1	73.9	265	82	0
1 tbsp.	44	.3	.4	4.6	17	5	0
whipping[1], heavy:							
(*Land O Lakes*),							
1 tbsp.	50	0	0	5.0	20	5	0
(*Organic Valley*),							
1 tbsp.	50	0	0	6.0	20	5	0
1 cup	821	4.9	6.6	88.1	326	89	0
1 tbsp.	52	.3	.4	5.6	21	6	0

[1]Unwhipped; volume approximately doubled when whipped.

Food and Measure	cal.	prot. (gms)	carbo. (gms)	fat (gms)	chol. (mgs)	sod. (mgs)	fiber (gms)
Cream, clotted (*The Devon Cream Company*), 1 oz.	140	0	<1.0	15.0	45	5	0
Cream, sour, 2 tbsp., except as noted:							
(*Breakstone's* All Natural)	60	1.0	1.0	5.0	20	10	0
(*Friendship*)	60	1.0	1.0	5.0	20	15	0
(*Land O Lakes*)	60	1.0	2.0	6.0	20	40	0
(*Organic Valley*)	60	1.0	2.0	5.0	25	20	0
1 cup	493	7.3	9.8	48.2	102	123	0
light/low fat:							
(*Breakstone's*)	40	1.0	2.0	3.0	15	20	0
(*Friendship*)	40	1.0	3.0	2.5	10	25	0
(*Knudsen*)	30	2.0	2.0	2.0	10	20	0
(*Land O Lakes*) . . .	40	1.0	2.0	2.5	5	20	0
(*Organic Valley*) . . .	30	1.0	3.0	2.0	10	20	0
nonfat:							
(*Breakstone's*)	30	1.0	5.0	0	5	25	0
(*Friendship*)	25	2.0	4.0	0	0	20	0
(*Knudsen*)	30	2.0	5.0	0	5	25	0
(*Land O Lakes*) . . .	20	1.0	3.0	0	0	50	0
flavored (*Friendship*):							
onion, toasted	60	1.0	2.0	5.0	20	140	0
salsa	50	1.0	2.0	4.0	15	120	0
"Cream," sour, non-dairy (*Tofutti Sour Supreme*), 2 tbsp. . .	85	1.0	9.0	5.0	0	160	0
Cream gravy, see "Gravy, country"							
Cream of tartar, 1 tsp.	7	0	1.9	0	0	2	0
Cream topping, whipped, 2 tbsp.:							
(*Cool Whip*)	25	0	2.0	1.5	0	0	0
(*Cool Whip* Extra Creamy)	25	0	2.0	2.0	0	0	0
(*Cool Whip* Fat Free) .	15	0	3.0	0	0	5	0
(*Cool Whip* Lite/Sugar Free)	20	0	3.0	1.0	0	3	0
(*Land O Lakes* Light) .	20	0	1.0	1.5	5	0	0
(*Reddi Wip* Extra Creamy)	15	0	<1.0	1.5	5	0	0
(*Reddi Wip* Original) .	15	0	<1.0	1.0	<5	0	0
chocolate (*Cool Whip*)	25	0	2.0	1.5	0	0	0

Food and Measure	cal.	prot. (gms)	carbo. (gms)	fat (gms)	chol. (mgs)	sod. (mgs)	fiber (gms)
(*Reddi Wip*)	15	0	1.0	1.0	<5	0	0
strawberry or French vanilla (*Cool Whip*)	25	0	2.0	1.5	0	0	0
Creamer, nondairy:							
fluid, 1 tbsp.:							
(*Coffee-mate*)	20	0	2.0	1.0	0	0	0
(*Coffee-mate* Low Fat)	10	0	1.0	.5	0	5	0
(*Coffee-mate* Nonfat)	10	0	2.0	0	0	0	0
(*Silk*)	15	0	1.0	1.0	0	10	0
powder, 1 tsp.							
(*Coffee-mate*)	10	0	1.0	.5	0	0	0
(*Coffee-mate* Nonfat)	10	0	2.0	0	0	0	0
(*Cremora*)	10	0	1.0	.5	0	10	0
(*Cremora* Lite & Creamy)	10	0	1.0	0	0	5	0
Creamer, nondairy, flavored, fluid, 1 tbsp.:							
all varieties:							
(*Coffee-mate* Sugar Free)	15	0	1.0	1.0	0	30	0
(*International Delight* Fat Free) .	30	0	7.0	0	0	5	0
amaretto, cinnamon hazelnut, Irish crème, or vanilla toffee caramel (*International Delight*) ..	40	0	7.0	1.5	0	0	0
amaretto, cinnamon vanilla crème, crème brûlée, French vanilla, hazelnut, Irish crème, toffee nut, vanilla caramel, or vanilla nut (*Coffee-mate*) ..	35	0	5.0	1.5	0	10	0
butter pecan (*International Delight* Southern*)	40	0	7.0	1.5	0	10	0
chocolate caramel, white chocolate macadamia, French vanilla, or vanilla hazelnut (*International Delight*) ..	45	0	7.0	2.0	0	5	0

Food and Measure	cal.	prot. (gms)	carbo. (gms)	fat (gms)	chol. (mgs)	sod. (mgs)	fiber (gms)
Creamer, nondairy, flavored, fluid *(cont.)*							
chocolate raspberry (*Coffee-mate*)	35	0	5.0	1.5	0	15	0
coconut crème (*Coffee-mate*)	40	0	5.0	2.0	0	5	0
hazelnut:							
(*Coffee-mate* Nonfat)	25	0	5.0	0	0	0	0
(*International Delight*)	45	0	6.0	2.0	0	5	0
(*International Delight* Sugar Free)	20	0	1.0	2.0	0	0	0
hazelnut or French vanilla (*Silk*)	20	0	3.0	1.0	0	10	0
vanilla, French (*International Delight* Sugar Free)	20	0	1.0	0	0	5	0
Creamer, nondairy, flavored, powder (*Coffee-mate*), 4 tsp., except as noted:							
all flavors, sugar free, 1 tbsp.	30	0	2.0	2.5	0	15	0
chocolate, creamy ...	60	0	9.0	2.5	0	30	0
hazelnut	60	0	9.0	3.0	0	15	0
vanilla, French	60	0	9.0	2.5	0	15	0
vanilla, French, non-fat	50	0	11.0	0	0	15	0
vanilla caramel	60	0	9.0	3.0	0	15	0
Crème fraîche:							
(*Santè*), 2 tbsp.	100	<1.0	<1.0	11.0	40	10	0
(*Vermont Butter & Cheese*), 1 oz.	110	1.0	1.0	11.0	25	20	0
Creole sauce, see "Seafood sauce"							
Creole seasoning:							
(*Zatarain's*), ¼ tsp....	0	0	0	0	0	270	0
sauce base (*Zatarain's* Shrimp Creole), 2 tsp.	25	1.0	4.0	.5	0	480	0
Crepe, French style (*Frieda's*), .45-oz. pc.	46	1.0	8.0	1.0	6	71	0
Crepe, filled, dessert, frozen, 1 pc.:							
chocolate (*Chocolate Lover's Delight*), 1.75 oz.	170	3.0	18.0	9.0	>5	120	0

Food and Measure	cal.	prot. (gms)	carbo. (gms)	fat (gms)	chol. (mgs)	sod. (mgs)	fiber (gms)
mango (*Lupita's*), 1.3 oz.	100	2.0	14.0	4.0	10	200	1.0
strawberries and cream (*Lupita's*), 2.25 oz. .	140	2.0	19.0	7.0	0	60	1.0
Cress, garden, ½ cup:							
raw	8	.7	1.4	.2	0	4	.3
boiled, drained	16	1.3	2.6	.4	0	5	.5
Cress, water, see "Watercress"							
Croaker, meat only, raw, Atlantic, 4 oz. .	119	20.2	0	3.6	69	63	0
Croissant:							
butter, 1-oz. pc.	115	2.3	13.0	6.0	19	211	.7
apple, 2-oz. pc.	144	4.2	21.0	4.9	18	155	1.4
cheese, 1.5-oz. pc. ...	174	3.9	19.7	8.8	24	233	1.1
mini (*Toufayan*), 3 pcs., 1.65 oz. ...	190	5.0	22.0	9.0	0	240	1.0
Croissant, frozen, petite (*Sara Lee* French Style), 2 pcs., 2 oz.	200	4.0	23.0	10.0	15	290	<1.0
Crookneck squash:							
(*Frieda's* Baby), ⅔ cup, 3 oz.	15	1.0	3.0	0	0	0	1.0
sliced, ½ cup:							
raw, ends trimmed .	12	.6	2.6	.2	0	1	.7
boiled, drained	18	.8	3.9	.3	0	1	1.3
Crookneck squash, canned, cut, drained, no salt, ½ cup	14	.7	3.2	.1	0	5	1.1
Crookneck squash, frozen, boiled, sliced, ½ cup	24	1.2	5.3	.2	0	6	1.2
Croutons (see also "Salad toppers"), 2 tbsp. or ¼ oz., except as noted:							
Caesar:							
(*Cardini's*)	35	1.0	4.0	1.5	0	50	0
(*Chatham Village*) .	35	1.0	4.0	1.5	0	50	0
(*Marzetti's* Large Cut)	35	1.0	4.0	1.5	0	50	0
(*Mrs. Cubbison's*), 5 pcs.	35	<1.0	4.0	1.5	0	65	0
(*Pepperidge Farm* Classic), 6 pcs. .	30	<1.0	5.0	1.0	0	60	0

Food and Measure	cal.	prot. (gms)	carbo. (gms)	fat (gms)	chol. (mgs)	sod. (mgs)	fiber (gms)
Croutons (cont.)							
cheese and garlic:							
(*Chatham Village*)	40	1.0	3.0	2.5	0	60	0
(*Marzetti's* Large Cut)	40	1.0	3.0	2.5	0	60	0
(*Mrs. Cubbison's*),							
5 pcs.	30	1.0	5.0	1.0	0	90	0
4 cheese (*Pepper-*							
idge Farm), 6 pcs.	30	1.0	5.0	1.0	0	65	0
garlic (*Cardini's*)	35	1.0	4.0	1.5	0	55	0
garlic and butter:							
(*Chatham Village*)	35	1.0	4.0	1.5	0	55	0
(*Marzetti's*)	35	1.0	3.0	2.0	0	60	0
(*Marzetti's* Large Cut)	35	1.0	4.0	1.5	0	55	0
(*Mrs. Cubbison's*),							
5 pcs.	30	0	5.0	1.0	0	100	0
garlic and onion:							
(*Chatham Village*							
Fat Free)	30	1.0	5.0	0	0	85	0
(*Marzetti's* Large Cut)	30	1.0	5.0	0	0	85	0
herb, garden (*Chat-*							
ham Village)	35	1.0	4.0	1.5	0	55	0
Italian:							
(*Cardini's*)	30	1.0	4.0	1.5	0	80	0
(*Pepperidge Farm*							
Zesty), 6 pcs.	30	<1.0	5.0	1.0	0	55	0
onion and garlic:							
(*Mrs. Cubbison's*),							
5 pcs.	30	<1.0	5.0	1.0	0	100	0
(*Pepperidge Farm*),							
6 pcs.	30	<1.0	5.0	1.0	0	70	0
ranch:							
(*Chatham Village*							
Large Cut)	35	1.0	4.0	1.5	0	95	0
(*Marzetti's* Large Cut)	35	1.0	4.0	1.5	0	95	0
cool herb (*Mrs.*							
Cubbison's), 5 pcs.	30	<1.0	5.0	1.0	0	75	0
Romano cheese							
(*Cardini's*)	40	1.0	3.0	2.5	0	60	0
seasoned:							
(*Mrs. Cubbison's*),							
5 pcs.	30	<1.0	4.0	1.0	0	90	0
(*Mrs. Cubbison's*							
Fat Free), 5 pcs. . .	30	1.0	5.0	0	0	105	0

Food and Measure	cal.	prot. (gms)	carbo. (gms)	fat (gms)	chol. (mgs)	sod. (mgs)	fiber (gms)
(*Pepperidge Farm*), 6 pcs.	30	<1.0	5.0	1.0	0	75	0
whole grain (*Pepperidge Farm*), 6 pcs.	30	1.0	5.0	1.0	0	70	<1.0
Crowder peas, see "Peas, crowder"							
Crusting blend, see "Panko crumb coating mix"							
Cucumber, w/peel:							
(*Chiquita*), ⅓ medium, 3.5 oz.	15	1.0	3.0	0	0	0	1.0
(*Frieda's* Hothouse/ Japanese), ⅔ cup, 3 oz.	10	1.0	2.0	0	0	0	1.0
1 medium, 8¼" long .	38	2.1	8.3	.4	0	6	2.4
sliced, ½ cup	7	.4	1.4	.1	0	1	.4
Cucumber, pickled, see "Pickles"							
Cucumber dill dip seasoning (*Watkins*), 1 tsp.	10	0	2.0	0	0	230	0
Cucuzza squash (*Frieda's*), ¾ cup, 3 oz.	10	1.0	3.0	0	0	0	0
Cumin seed, ground, 1 tsp.	8	.4	.9	.5	0	4	.2
Cupcake, see "Cake, snack"							
Curacao, blue, non-alcoholic (*Angostura*), 1 fl. oz.	55	0	13.0	0	0	5	0
Currant juice, see "Black Currant juice"							
Currants:							
fresh, ½ cup:							
black, Europe	36	.8	8.6	.2	0	1	3.0
red or white	31	.8	7.7	.1	0	1	2.4
dried, Zante:							
(*Sun•Maid*), ¼ cup, 1.4 oz.	120	1.0	30.0	0	0	10	2.0
½ cup	204	2.9	53.3	.2	0	6	4.9

Food and Measure	cal.	prot. (gms)	carbo. (gms)	fat (gms)	chol. (mgs)	sod. (mgs)	fiber (gms)
Curry, vegetable, see "Vegetable dish, can or jar"							
Curry paste, 2 tbsp., except as noted:							
biryani (*Patak's*)	180	1.0	6.0	16.0	0	890	3.0
(*Roland* Laksa)	50	0	4.0	4.0	0	560	1.0
green:							
(*Roland*), 1 tbsp. . . .	25	0	3.0	1.5	0	390	1.0
(*A Taste of Thai*), 1 tsp.	15	0	1.5	1.0	0	200	0
garam Masala (*Patak's*), 2 tsp.	130	1.0	4.0	12.0	0	1080	0
hot, extra (*Patak's*) . . .	160	1.0	4.0	16.0	0	1130	0
Madras (*Patak's*)	160	1.0	4.0	16.0	0	1010	0
mild (*Patak's*)	170	1.0	5.0	16.0	0	900	0
Panang (*A Taste of Thai*), 1 tsp.	10	0	2.0	0	0	190	0
red:							
(*Mae Ploy*), 2 tsp. . .	13	1.0	2.0	0	0	600	0
(*Roland*), 1 tbsp. . .	25	0	3.0	1.5	0	360	1.0
(*A Taste of Thai*), 1 tsp.	10	0	1.0	1.0	0	340	0
tandoori:							
(*Neera's* Grilling), 2 tsp.	19	0	3.0	2.0	0	156	1.0
(*Patak's*)	30	1.0	5.0	1.0	0	800	1.0
tikka:							
(*Patak's*)	50	1.0	6.0	2.5	0	830	2.0
Masala (*Patak's*) . . .	120	1.0	8.0	10.0	0	970	2.0
vindaloo:							
(*Neera's*), 2 tsp. . . .	48	0	3.0	4.0	0	118	1.0
(*Patak's*)	160	1.0	4.0	16.0	0	1020	0
yellow:							
(*Roland*), 1 tbsp. . .	30	0	3.0	1.5	0	450	0
(*A Taste of Thai*), 1 tsp.	10	0	1.0	.5	0	135	0
Curry powder:							
1 tbsp.	20	.8	3.7	.9	0	3	1.0
1 tsp.	6	.3	1.2	.3	0	1	.3
Masala:							
(*Neera's*), 2 tsp. . . .	13	1.0	3.0	1.0	0	167	1.0
(*Neera's* Garam), ¼ tsp.	2	0	0	0	0	0	0

Food and Measure	cal.	prot. (gms)	carbo. (gms)	fat (gms)	chol. (mgs)	sod. (mgs)	fiber (gms)
Curry sauce (see also "Marinade" and "Thai sauce"), can/ jar (*Patak's*), ½ cup:							
hot chili and cumin ..	290	3.0	15.0	24.0	0	750	0
korma	220	4.0	12.0	17.0	0	670	1.0
Rogan Josh	190	3.0	12.0	14.0	0	750	1.0
tikka Masala	220	3.0	14.0	17.0	0	1000	1.0
vindaloo	320	3.0	14.0	27.0	0	790	1.0
Curry sauce, cooking ½ cup, except as noted:							
(*Ethnic Gourmet* Bombay Curry Simmer Sauce), 4 oz.	70	2.0	10.0	2.5	0	540	2.0
coconut (*Maya Kaimal*)	130	2.0	11.0	10.0	0	750	2.0
chicken:							
butter (*Devya Organic*)	100	4.0	19.0	3.5	0	190	5.0
butter (*Patak's*) . . .	150	1.0	13.0	11,0	5	480	1.0
mango (*Patak's*) . . .	120	1.0	14.0	6.0	5	480	1.0
tandoori (*Devya Organic*)	170	3.0	19.0	10.0	0	n.a.	3.0
Dopiaza (*Patak's*)	90	2.0	11.0	4.5	0	750	0
Jalfrezi:							
(*Patak's*)	140	2.0	15.0	8.0	0	620	1.0
(*Seeds of Change Organic*), ⅓ cup .	90	1.0	9.0	6.0	0	270	2.0
korma:							
(*Ethnic Gourmet* Delhi Simmer Sauce), 4 oz. . . .	100	2.0	9.0	7.0	10	500	2.0
(*Maya Kaimal* Classic)	150	2.0	11.0	9.0	10	650	3.0
(*Patak's*)	240	2.0	13.0	20.0	15	750	1.0
(*Seeds of Change Organic*), ⅓ cup .	140	1.0	9.0	11.0	10	290	1.0
Madras:							
(*Neera's*), 4 oz.	110	1.0	6.0	9.0	0	530	1.0
(*Seeds of Change Organic*), 3 oz. . .	60	1.0	8.0	4.0	0	240	1.0
Masala:							
(*Ethnic Gourmet* Calcutta), 4 oz. . .	90	2.0	10.0	4.5	5	500	1.0

Food and Measure	cal.	prot. (gms)	carbo. (gms)	fat (gms)	chol. (mgs)	sod. (mgs)	fiber (gms)
Curry sauce, cooking, masala *(cont.)*							
channa (*Devya* Organic)	190	3.0	17.0	14.0	0	450	4.0
mild (*Patak's*)	90	1.0	13.0	3.0	0	490	2.0
Rogan Josh (*Patak's*) .	90	2.0	12.0	4.0	0	750	2.0
spinach (*Ethnic Gourmet* Punjab Saag), 4 oz.	60	2.0	6.0	3.0	5	500	1.0
tamarind (*Maya Kaimal*)	130	1.0	7.0	12.0	0	380	2.0
tikka (*Neera's*), 4 oz. .	130	3.0	10.0	10.0	10	410	2.0
tikka Masala:							
(*Maya Kaimal*)	190	3.0	11.0	16.0	50	630	2.0
(*Patak's*)	120	1.0	12.0	8.0	0	900	0
(*Seeds of Change* Organic), 3 oz. . .	90	1.0	8.0	7.0	10	280	2.0
vegetable (*Devya* Organic)	150	2.0	14.0	14.0	0	490	3.0
vindaloo:							
(*Maya Kaimal*)	170	2.0	9.0	16.0	0	590	2.0
(*Neera's*), 4 oz.	140	2.0	14.0	9.0	0	590	2.0
Curry seasoning blend, dry (*Naturally India* Simmer Sauce), ⅙ pkg.:							
au chole	33	1.0	4.0	1.0	0	120	.3
biryani	36	1.0	5.0	1.0	0	120	.3
dum aloo	34	1.0	5.0	1.0	0	100	.3
korma	35	2.0	4.0	1.0	0	200	.4
makhanwala or tikka masala	41	1.0	4.0	1.0	0	130	.6
Cusk, meat only:							
raw, 4 oz.	99	21.6	0	.8	47	36	0
baked or broiled, 4 oz.	127	27.6	0	1.0	60	45	0
Custard apple, trimmed, 1 oz.	29	.5	7.1	.2	0	1	1.0
Custard marrow, see "Chayote"							
Cuttlefish, meat only:							
raw, 4 oz.	90	18.4	.9	.8	127	422	0
boiled or steamed, 4 oz.	179	36.8	1.9	1.6	254	844	0
Cuttlefish, canned, in ink sauce:							
(*Goya*), ¼ cup	120	8.0	2.0	9.0	15	350	0

Food and Measure	cal.	prot. (gms)	carbo. (gms)	fat (gms)	chol. (mgs)	sod. (mgs)	fiber (gms)
(*Roland*), ¼ cup	110	7.0	0	9.0	40	320	0
(*Vigo*), 2 oz.	130	9.0	2.0	10.0	44	250	0
Cuttlefish, dried, all varieties (*Roland*), 1 oz.	240	13.0	5.0	0	80	870	0

D

Food and Measure	cal.	prot. (gms)	carbo. (gms)	fat (gms)	chol. (mgs)	sod. (mgs)	fiber (gms)
Daikon, fresh, see "Radish, Oriental"							
Daikon, pickled (*Eden* Organic), 2 slices, .5 oz.	5	0	1.0	0	0	250	0
Daiquiri drink mixer:							
(*Angostura*), 2 fl. oz. . .	72	0	18.0	0	0	5	0
dry (*Bar-Tender's*), 2 pouches	130	0	16.0	0	0	30	0
frozen, 2 fl. oz.:							
banana (*Bacardi*) . .	140	0	36.0	0	0	5	0
peach (*Bacardi*) . . .	120	0	32.0	0	0	0	0
strawberry (*Angostura*), 8 fl. oz.	120	0	31.0	0	0	240	0
strawberry (*Bacardi*)	120	0	32.0	0	0	0	0
Dairy Queen/Brazier:							
burgers:							
bacon cheddar *Grillburger*	710	36.0	41.0	42.0	95	1450	2.0
DQ Original:							
burger	350	17.0	33.0	14.0	50	680	1.0
cheeseburger . . .	400	19.0	34.0	18.0	65	920	1.0
double	640	34.0	34.0	34.0	125	1230	1.0
double w/bacon	730	41.0	35.0	41.0	150	1550	1.0
DQ Ultimate	780	41.0	33.0	48.0	155	1390	1.0
mushroom Swiss *Grillburger*	680	29.0	39.0	42.0	75	950	2.0
¼ lb. *Chili Meltdown Grillburger*	600	29.0	41.0	34.0	70	1060	3.0
¼ lb. *Flame Thrower Grillburger*	840	34.0	41.0	59.0	105	1490	2.0
Chicken Strip Basket, 4 pc.:							
barbecue hot dip . .	1090	37.0	129.0	48.0	75	2680	9.0

Food and Measure	cal.	prot. (gms)	carbo. (gms)	fat (gms)	chol. (mgs)	sod. (mgs)	fiber (gms)
country gravy	1030	37.0	105.0	54.0	75	2400	8.0
wild Buffalo	1340	36.0	82.0	96.0	90	4820	9.0
hot dog	250	9.0	21.0	14.0	25	770	1.0
hot dog, chili cheese .	430	18.0	39.0	23.0	45	990	2.0
sandwich, chicken:							
crispy	530	22.0	47.0	29.0	55	1020	5.0
grilled	400	23.0	32.0	16.0	55	790	1.0
Grilled Flame							
Thrower	630	34.0	34.0	36.0	100	1580	2.0
sandwich, fish	420	17.0	54.0	20.0	30	1070	1.0
DQ fries:							
large	480	5.0	66.0	21.0	0	1000	7.0
medium	370	4.0	51.0	17.0	0	780	5.0
small	290	3.0	40.0	13.0	0	620	4.0
DQ onion rings	470	6.0	45.0	30.0	0	740	3.0
salad, no dressing:							
crispy chicken	420	28.0	30.0	22.0	70	960	6.0
grilled chicken	320	31.0	14.0	11.0	75	890	4.0
side salad	45	2.0	11.0	0	0	50	3.0
Arctic Rush slush,							
medium	310	0	63.0	0	0	0	0
Blizzard, medium:							
chocolate chip							
cookie	1030	17.0	151.0	40.0	70	530	1.0
Oreo cookie	690	13.0	103.0	26.0	45	560	1.0
Reese's cups	770	17.0	104.0	32.0	55	400	2.0
DQ soft serve:							
chocolate, ½ cup ..	150	4.0	22.0	5.0	15	75	0
vanilla, ½ cup	150	3.0	22.0	5.0	15	70	0
cone, medium:							
chocolate dip	490	8.0	61.0	23.0	30	170	0
vanilla	340	8.0	54.0	10.0	30	160	0
cone, waffle, soft serve:							
plain	430	9.0	68.0	13.0	35	160	0
chocolate coated ..	550	9.0	79.0	22.0	40	190	1.0
malt, chocolate,							
medium	900	19.0	157.0	21.0	65	460	0
MooLatte, 16 oz.:							
cappuccino	500	7.0	73.0	19.0	30	180	0
caramel	630	8.0	103.0	19.0	35	260	0
mocha	590	8.0	84.0	23.0	30	200	0
vanilla, French	570	7.0	90.0	18.0	30	170	0
novelties:							
Buster Bar	480	11.0	45.0	31.0	20	220	2.0

Food and Measure	cal.	prot. (gms)	carbo. (gms)	fat (gms)	chol. (mgs)	sod. (mgs)	fiber (gms)
Dairy Queen/Brazier, novelties *(cont.)*							
Chocolate Dilly bar .	240	4.0	24.0	15.0	15	70	1.0
DQ fudge bar	50	4.0	13.0	0	0	70	6.0
DQ sandwich	190	4.0	32.0	5.0	10	105	1.0
DQ vanilla orange bar	60	2.0	18.0	0	0	45	6.0
Starkiss	80	0	21.0	0	0	10	0
Royal Treats:							
banana split	530	8.0	98.0	14.0	30	180	3.0
Brownie Earthquake	740	10.0	149.0	28.0	60	370	1.0
Peanut Buster parfait	710	16.0	96.0	30.0	30	380	2.0
shake, vanilla, medium	780	17.0	136.0	20.0	60	300	0
sundae, medium:							
chocolate	410	7.0	72.0	10.0	30	190	0
strawberry	370	7.0	63.0	10.0	30	170	1.0
sundae, waffle bowl:							
chocolate covered							
strawberry	800	9.0	100.0	40.0	35	200	2.0
fab fudge	730	10.0	106.0	29.0	35	250	1.0
turtle	820	11.0	117.0	35.0	40	330	2.0
Dal, see "Lentil dish mix"							
Dandelion greens:							
raw (*Frieda's*), 3 oz. . .	40	2.0	8.0	0	0	65	3.0
raw, ½ cup chopped .	13	.8	2.6	.2	0	22	1.0
boiled, drained, chopped, ½ cup	17	1.0	3.3	.3	0	23	1.5
Danish, see "Cake"							
Dasheen, see "Taro"							
Date, dried:							
(*Dole*), 1.4 oz.	120	1.0	33.0	0	0	10	3.0
(*Earthbound Farm* Organic), 1.4 oz. . .	120	1.0	31.0	0	0	0	3.0
(*Frieda's* Medjool), 2–3 pcs., 1.4 oz. . .	120	1.0	31.0	0	0	0	3.0
(*Shiloh Farms* Organic Deglet/Deglet Noor), 5–6 pcs., 1.4 oz. . .	120	1.0	31.0	0	0	0	3.0
(*Sun•Maid*), ¼ cup, 1.4 oz.	110	1.0	30.0	0	0	0	4.0
(*Sunsweet*), 5–6 pcs., 1.4 oz.	120	1.0	30.0	0	0	0	3.0
10 pcs. , 2.9 oz.	228	1.6	61.0	.4	0	2	6.2
pitted, ½ cup	245	1.8	65.4	.5	0	3	6.7

Food and Measure	cal.	prot. (gms)	carbo. (gms)	fat (gms)	chol. (mgs)	sod. (mgs)	fiber (gms)
chopped, 1.4 oz.:							
(*Sun•Maid*), ¼ cup	120	1.0	33.0	0	0	5	3.0
(*Sunsweet*)	120	1.0	31.0	0	0	0	3.0
Date, Indian, see "Tamarindo"							
Delicata squash (*Frieda's*), ¾ cup, 3 oz.	30	1.0	7.0	0	0	0	1.0
Dessert bars, see "Cookie mix"							
Dill dip, 2 tbsp.:							
(*Litehouse* Dilly)	150	1.0	2.0	16.0	15	200	0
(*Marzetti's*)	120	1.0	2.0	13.0	20	200	0
(*Marzetti's* Light)	60	0	2.0	5.0	5	230	0
(*Marzetti's* Nonfat) . . .	30	1.0	6.0	0	0	300	0
creamy (*Marie's*)	100	1.0	2.0	10.0	15	140	0
Dill seed, 1 tsp.	6	.3	1.2	.3	0	<1	.4
Dill weed, fresh:							
5 sprigs	<1	<1.0	.1	<.1	0	1	<.1
1 cup	4	.3	.6	.1	0	5	.2
Dill weed, dried, 1 tsp.	3	.2	.6	<.1	0	2	.1
Dip, see specific listings							
Dipping sauce (see also specific listings), Indian (*Naturally India*), 1.1 oz.:							
chili, garlic, lemon . . .	75	2.0	11.0	3.0	0	235	2.0
mango, chili, cilantro .	97	.2	2.4	3.0	0	293	.2
mango, saffron, ginger	79	.1	20.0	.1	0	97	.1
tamarina, date, chili . .	67	.3	16.0	.1	0	237	.3
Dock:							
raw, chopped, 1 cup .	29	2.6	4.3	.9	9	5	3.9
boiled, drained, 4 oz. .	23	2.1	3.3	.7	0	3	<1.0
Dolphin fish, see "Mahi mahi"							
Domino's Pizza, ⅛ pie, except as noted:							
12" pie, 1 topping, w/sauce/cheese:							
deep dish	225	8.0	27.0	11.0	10	525	3.0
hand-tossed	170	7.0	24.0	5.5	10	350	1.0
thin crust	130	4.0	14.0	7.5	10	240	1.0
add 1 topping:							
bacon	40	4.0	0	2.5	10	115	0

Food and Measure	cal.	prot. (gms)	carbo. (gms)	fat (gms)	chol. (mgs)	sod. (mgs)	fiber (gms)
Domino's Pizza, 12" pie, 1 topping *(cont.)*							
banana pepper ..	0	0	0	0	0	130	0
beef	40	2.0	0	3.0	10	70	0
cheese, extra ...	25	2.0	1.0	2.0	5	85	0
chicken, grilled ..	15	2.0	0	0	5	90	0
garlic	10	0	1.0	0	0	0	0
green pepper or mushrooms ..	0	0	0	0	0	0	0
ham	10	2.0	0	0	5	100	0
jalapeño pepper .	0	0	0	0	0	100	0
olives, black	10	0	1.0	1.0	0	65	0
olives, green ...	15	0	0	1.5	0	95	0
onions	0	0	1.0	0	0	0	0
Philly meat	10	2.0	0	0	5	60	0
pineapple	10	0	2.0	0	0	0	0
pepperoni	40	2.0	0	3.5	5	140	0
sausage	45	2.0	1.0	3.5	5	130	0
12" pie, 2–3 toppings, w/sauce/cheese:							
deep dish	230	8.0	27.0	12.0	10	525	3.0
hand-tossed	215	9.0	30.0	8.0	10	335	1.0
thin crust	135	5.0	14.0	8.5	10	240	1.0
add 2–3 toppings:							
bacon	25	3.0	0	2.0	5	80	0
banana pepper ..	0	0	0	0	0	90	0
beef	25	1.0	0	2.5	5	50	0
cheese, extra ...	25	2.0	1.0	2.0	4	85	0
chicken, grilled ..	10	2.0	0	0	5	65	0
garlic	10	0	1.0	0	0	0	0
green pepper, onion or mushrooms ..	0	0	0	0	0	0	0
ham	10	1.0	0	0	4	75	0
jalapeño pepper .	0	0	0	0	0	65	0
olives, black	5	0	1.0	1.0	0	45	0
olives, green ...	10	0	0	1.0	0	65	0
pepperoni	40	2.0	0	3.5	10	140	0
Philly meat	10	2.0	0	0	4	60	0
pineapple	5	0	1.0	0	0	0	0
sausage	30	1.0	1.0	2.5	5	90	0
14" pie, 1 topping, w/sauce/cheese:							
deep dish	320	11.0	40.0	14.0	15	740	4.0

Food and Measure	cal.	prot. (gms)	carbo. (gms)	fat (gms)	chol. (mgs)	sod. (mgs)	fiber (gms)
hand-tossed	230	8.0	34.0	7.5	5	490	2.0
thin crust	180	7.0	20.0	9.5	5	340	2.0
add 1 topping:							
bacon	60	6.0	0	4.0	15	170	0
banana pepper . .	0	0	0	0	0	180	0
beef	50	3.0	0	4.5	10	100	0
cheese, extra . . .	30	2.0	1.0	2.5	5	120	0
chicken, grilled . .	20	3.0	0	.5	10	130	0
garlic	15	0	1.0	0	0	0	0
green pepper, onion or mushrooms . .	0	1.0	0	0	0	0	0
ham	15	2.0	0	.5	5	140	0
jalapeño pepper .	0	0	0	0	0	135	0
olives, black	10	0	1.0	.5	0	60	0
olives, green . . .	20	0	1.0	2.0	0	125	0
pepperoni	50	2.0	0	4.5	10	190	0
Philly meat	15	2.0	0	.5	5	85	0
pineapple	15	0	3.0	0	0	0	0
sausage	60	2.0	2.0	5.5	10	190	0
14" pie, 2–3 toppings, w/sauce/cheese:							
deep dish	320	10.0	40.0	19.0	15	740	5.0
hand-tossed	290	12.0	42.0	9.0	5	470	3.0
thin crust	180	7.0	20.0	9.5	5	340	2.0
add 2–3 toppings:							
bacon	40	4.0	0	3.0	10	125	0
banana pepper . .	0	0	0	0	0	120	0
beef	35	2.0	0	3.0	10	70	0
cheese, extra . . .	30	2.0	1.0	2.5	5	120	0
chicken, grilled . .	15	2.0	0	0	5	90	0
garlic	10	0	1.0	0	0	0	0
green pepper, onion or mushrooms . .	0	0	0	0	0	0	0
ham	10	2.0	0	.5	5	110	0
jalapeño pepper .	0	0	0	0	0.	90	0
olives, black	10	0	1.0	.5	0	60	0
olives, green . . .	10	0	0	1.0	0	85	0
pepperoni	50	2.0	0	4.5	10	190	0
Philly meat	15	2.0	0	.5	5	85	0
pineapple	10	0	2.0	0	0	0	0
sausage	45	2.0	1.0	3.5	5	130	0

Food and Measure	cal.	prot. (gms)	carbo. (gms)	fat (gms)	chol. (mgs)	sod. (mgs)	fiber (gms)
Domino's Pizza (cont.)							
12" *Feast* pie, w/sauce/cheese:							
deep dish	230	8.0	27.0	12.0	10	525	3.0
hand-tossed	215	9.0	31.0	8.0	10	335	1.0
thin crust	135	5.0	14.0	8.5	10	240	1.0
add *Feast* topping:							
America's Favorite	130	6.0	4.0	10.0	20	450	1.0
Bacon Cheese- burger	140	9.0	3.0	11.0	30	390	1.0
barbecue	130	7.0	8.0	8.0	20	360	0
Deluxe	100	5.0	4.0	8.0	15	380	1.0
ExtravaganZZa .	160	9.0	5.0	12.0	30	590	1.0
Hawaiian	90	6.0	5.0	6.0	15	390	1.0
MeatZZa	150	8.0	4.0	11.0	30	560	1.0
Pepperoni	130	7.0	4.0	11.0	25	530	1.0
Philly cheese steak	100	7.0	1.0	7.0	20	360	0
Vegi	80	5.0	4.0	6.0	15	340	1.0
14" *Feast* pie, w/sauce/cheese:							
deep dish	320	11.0	40.0	14.0	15	740	5.0
hand-tossed	290	12.0	42.0	9.0	5	470	3.0
thin crust	180	7.0	20.0	9.5	5	340	2.0
add *Feast* topping:							
America's Favorite	170	9.0	6.0	14.0	30	640	1.0
Bacon Cheese- burger	200	12.0	4.0	15.0	40	550	1.0
barbecue	170	9.0	11.0	11.0	30	500	0
Deluxe	130	7.0	5.0	10.0	20	500	1.0
ExtravaganZZa .	200	12.0	7.0	16.0	40	780	1.0
Hawaiian	130	8.0	7.0	8.0	25	550	1.0
MeatZZa	210	12.0	6.0	17.0	40	810	1.0
Pepperoni	180	10.0	5.0	15.0	35	730	1.0
Philly cheese steak	130	9.0	2.0	9.0	30	470	0
Vegi	120	7.0	6.0	8.0	20	480	1.0
10" *Oreo* dessert pie .	120	2.0	20.0	4.0	0	110	1.0
chicken, 1 serving:							
Buffalo Chicken Kickers	90	9.0	6.0	3.0	20	90	1.0
Buffalo wings:							
barbecue	230	17.0	6.0	14.0	50	410	0
hot	210	16.0	5.0	14.0	50	440	0
dipping cup:							
blue cheese	210	1.0	2.0	22.0	20	390	0

Food and Measure	cal.	prot. (gms)	carbo. (gms)	fat (gms)	chol. (mgs)	sod. (mgs)	fiber (gms)
hot	120	0	3.0	12.0	0	790	0
ranch	190	1.0	2.0	21.0	10	390	0
salad, ½ cont.:							
chicken Caesar	100	10.0	6.0	4.5	20	310	2.0
garden fresh	70	4.0	5.0	4.0	10	80	2.0
salad dressing, 1 pkt.:							
blue cheese	230	2.0	2.0	24.0	30	450	0
buttermilk ranch . . .	220	1.0	2.0	24.0	10	420	0
Caesar, creamy . . .	210	1.0	2.0	22.0	10	510	0
Italian, golden	220	0	2.0	23.0	0	370	0
Italian, light	20	0	2.0	1.0	0	780	0
sides, 1 pc. or pkt.:							
breadstick	110	2.0	11.0	6.0	0	100	0
cheesy bread	120	4.0	11.0	6.0	5	150	0
dipping sauce:							
garlic	440	0	0	49.0	0	390	0
marinara	25	1.0	5.0	0	0	260	1.0
Cinna Stix	120	2.0	14.0	6.0	0	85	1.0
icing, sweet, cup . .	250	0	57.0	3.0	0	0	0
Donuts, 1 pc., except as noted:							
plain (*Entenmann's Softee*), 1.5 oz. . . .	190	2.0	21.0	11.0	0	210	<1.0
chocolate frosted:							
(*Entenmann's*), 2.1 oz.	300	2.0	30.0	20.0	10	190	1.0
mini (*Entenmann's*), 1.1 oz.	160	1.0	15.0	11.0	5	90	<1.0
crullers (*Entenmann's Pop'ettes*), 2 pcs. . . .	210	1.0	25.0	12.0	10	140	0
crumb topped (*Entenmann's*), 2.1 oz. . . .	250	2.0	36.0	12.0	10	210	<1.0
devil's food crumb (*Entenmann's*), 2.1 oz.	250	2.0	35.0	12.0	10	200	1.0
donut holes (*Entenmann's Pop'ems*), 4 pcs.:							
chocolate frosted . .	320	2.0	28.0	23.0	10	180	1.0
glazed	220	2.0	30.0	10.0	0	170	0
powdered sugar . . .	250	3.0	31.0	13.0	0	230	<1.0
rainbow	210	2.0	25.0	9.0	10	130	<1.0
powdered sugar (*Entenmann's Softees*), 4 pcs. . . .	250	3.0	32.0	12.0	25	290	<1.0

Food and Measure	cal.	prot. (gms)	carbo. (gms)	fat (gms)	chol. (mgs)	sod. (mgs)	fiber (gms)
Dow gok, see "Yardlong bean"							
Dragon fruit (*Frieda's*), 3.5 oz.	60	2.0	0	1.5	0	60	0
Drum, freshwater, meat only:							
raw, 4 oz.	135	19.9	0	5.6	73	85	0
baked or broiled, 4 oz.	173	25.5	0	7.2	93	109	0
Duck, domesticated, roasted, 4 oz.:							
meat w/skin	382	21.5	0	32.1	95	67	0
meat only	228	26.6	0	12.7	101	74	0
young, Pekin:							
breast, meat w/skin	229	27.8	0	12.3	154	95	0
leg, meat w/skin	246	30.3	0	12.9	129	125	0
Duck, wild, raw:							
meat w/skin, 4 oz.	239	19.8	0	17.2	91	64	0
breast meat, 4 oz.	139	22.5	0	4.8	87	65	0
Duck breast fillet, raw, marinated (*Bell & Evans*), ½ pc., 3 oz.	160	19.0	0	8.0	105	510	0
Duck fat, 1 tbsp.	115	0	0	12.8	13	0	0
Duck sauce, see "Sweet and sour sauce"							
Dumpling, sweet, frozen (*Pepperidge Farm*):							
apple, 1 pc.	250	3.0	33.0	11.0	0	180	1.0
peach, 1 pc.	320	3.0	50.0	11.0	0	150	4.0
Dumpling squash, see "Sweet dumpling squash"							
Dunkin Donuts:							
breakfast sandwich:							
bacon/egg/cheese:							
bagel	540	18.0	69.0	18.0	200	1400	2.0
croissant	440	19.0	33.0	25.0	150	910	1.0
English muffin	360	17.0	36.0	16.0	200	1300	1.0
egg/cheese:							
bagel	470	20.0	65.0	15.0	190	1120	2.0
biscuit	540	16.0	53.0	29.0	125	1390	2.0
croissant	430	14.0	33.0	26.0	190	780	1.0
English muffin	280	15.0	34.0	9.0	140	1010	1.0
ham/egg/cheese:							
bagel	510	26.0	65.0	16.0	200	1390	2.0

Food and Measure	cal.	prot. (gms)	carbo. (gms)	fat (gms)	chol. (mgs)	sod. (mgs)	fiber (gms)
croissant	460	20.0	33.0	27.0	205	1040	1.0
English muffin ..	310	21.0	34.0	10.0	160	1270	1.0
omelet, supreme,							
croissant	530	21.0	35.0	33.0	255	1070	2.0
sausage/egg/cheese:							
bagel	660	28.0	63.0	35.0	225	1450	3.0
biscuit	800	24.0	54.0	52.0	235	1960	2.0
English muffin ..	530	23.0	37.0	32.0	235	1610	1.0
hash browns, 3 pc.	60	1.0	7.0	3.0	0	240	1.0
hash browns, 9 pc.	180	2.0	22.0	9.0	0	730	3.0
sandwich, flatbread:							
cheese, three	460	20.0	42.0	24.0	55	1000	2.0
ham/Swiss	350	20.0	41.0	12.0	35	1040	2.0
turkey/cheddar/							
bacon	360	20.0	41.0	13.0	35	1060	2.0
deli sandwiches:							
classics:							
ham/Swiss	360	23.0	44.0	11.0	45	1120	4.0
roast beef/Swiss	530	31.0	45.0	25.0	80	1290	4.0
tuna	550	29.0	49.0	26.0	35	830	4.0
turkey/cheese ...	510	35.0	45.0	22.0	65	1380	4.0
vegetarian	420	9.0	51.0	21.0	5	480	8.0
cravings:							
chicken, chipotle	620	49.0	49.0	26.0	110	1730	4.0
chicken bruschetta	580	42.0	48.0	25.0	85	1450	4.0
pastrami supreme	760	48.0	47.0	42.0	130	1990	5.0
turkey pesto	530	33.0	46.0	23.0	65	1630	4.0
favorites:							
avocado/turkey ..	500	38.0	49.0	22.0	40	1330	8.0
chicken Cordon							
Bleu	550	45.0	51.0	19.0	95	1370	4.0
Italian, toasted ..	630	35.0	49.0	34.0	90	2330	5.0
steak/cheese ...	510	30.0	45.0	23.0	75	1830	4.0
turkey bacon club	510	35.0	44.0	22.0	70	1770	4.0
deli salads:							
Caesar	390	10.0	14.0	33.0	35	980	3.0
chicken Caesar	520	34.0	16.0	36.0	85	1520	3.0
garden	240	12.0	24.0	12.0	30	430	5.0
Mediterranean	220	10.0	23.0	11.0	15	760	5.0
Oriental	580	30.0	39.0	35.0	45	1510	4.0
deli soups, 1 cup:							
broccoli cheese ...	180	7.0	10.0	13.0	40	1310	1.0
chicken noodle	140	8.0	20.0	3.5	45	840	1.0
chili w/beans	230	15.0	26.0	8.0	35	890	8.0

Food and Measure	cal.	prot. (gms)	carbo. (gms)	fat (gms)	chol. (mgs)	sod. (mgs)	fiber (gms)
Dunkin Donuts, deli soups (cont.)							
clam chowder	230	10.0	20.0	11.0	30	990	1.0
lasagna soup	250	11.0	21.0	13.0	35	810	2.0
pizza, personal:							
cheese	400	18.0	46.0	19.0	25	820	2.0
pepperoni	410	19.0	45.0	19.0	35	960	2.0
supreme	430	17.0	46.0	21.0	35	1010	2.0
bagel:							
plain	320	12.0	62.0	2.5	0	650	2.0
blueberry	330	10.0	66.0	2.5	0	600	2.0
cinnamon raisin ...	330	10.0	65.0	3.0	0	430	3.0
everything	370	14.0	67.0	6.0	0	650	3.0
multigrain........	410	16.0	67.0	8.0	0	580	9.0
onion	320	12.0	61.0	3.5	0	610	3.0
poppy seed	370	14.0	65.0	7.0	0	650	3.0
reduced carb							
w/cheese	380	25.0	45.0	12.0	20	780	14.0
salt	320	12.0	62.0	2.5	0	4520	2.0
sesame	380	14.0	64.0	8.0	0	650	3.0
wheat	330	12.0	62.0	4.0	0	610	4.0
biscuit	440	7.0	51.0	22.0	0	980	2.0
croissant, plain	270	6.0	30.0	14.0	0	300	1.0
cream cheese, 2 oz.:							
plain	190	4.0	4.0	17.0	55	190	0
plain, lite	120	4.0	5.0	9.0	30	280	0
blueberry,							
reduced fat	170	2.0	17.0	10.0	30	240	0
chive	170	4.0	4.0	17.0	45	230	2.0
salmon	170	4.0	2.0	17.0	45	180	0
strawberry	190	4.0	9.0	17.0	45	150	0
vegetable, garden ..	170	2.0	4.0	15.0	45	340	0
vegetable, lite	100	3.0	5.0	8.0	25	270	0
cookies, 4.5 oz.:							
chocolate chunk ...	540	7.0	80.0	23.0	50	550	3.0
oatmeal raisin	480	8.0	83.0	14.0	40	310	5.0
peanut butter cup ..	590	11.0	73.0	29.0	50	530	3.0
Danish:							
apple	330	4.0	32.0	20.0	30	260	1.0
cheese	340	4.0	30.0	22.0	35	270	1.0
strawberry cheese .	320	4.0	31.0	20.0	30	260	1.0
donut:							
apple crumb	320	4.0	46.0	13.0	0	360	2.0
apple 'n spice	260	4.0	35.0	11.0	0	350	2.0
Bavarian Kreme ...	250	4.0	35.0	11.0	0	350	1.0

Food and Measure	cal.	prot. (gms)	carbo. (gms)	fat (gms)	chol. (mgs)	sod. (mgs)	fiber (gms)
black raspberry ...	210	3.0	32.0	8.0	0	280	1.0
blueberry cake	290	3.0	35.0	16.0	10	400	1.0
blueberry crumb ..	330	4.0	48.0	13.0	0	360	2.0
Boston Kreme	270	4.0	38.0	12.0	0	370	1.0
chocolate, double ..	340	3.0	36.0	20.0	0	360	3.0
chocolate coconut .	370	3.0	42.0	21.0	0	380	3.0
chocolate frosted ..	230	4.0	29.0	11.0	0	320	2.0
chocolate frosted cake	330	4.0	36.0	19.0	15	260	2.0
chocolate glazed ..	340	3.0	39.0	19.0	0	360	2.0
chocolate Kreme filled	300	4.0	39.0	14.0	0	360	2.0
cinnamon cake	310	3.0	34.0	18.0	15	260	2.0
crueller, French ...	150	2.0	17.0	8.0	20	105	1.0
gingerbread	280	5.0	56.0	4.0	45	400	1.0
glazed	230	4.0	30.0	10.0	0	320	1.0
glazed cake	330	3.0	38.0	18.0	15	260	2.0
jelly filled	270	4.0	39.0	10.0	0	350	1.0
maple frosted	240	4.0	31.0	10.0	0	320	1.0
marble frosted	230	4.0	30.0	11.0	0	320	1.0
mini *M&M's*	270	4.0	39.0	12.0	0	360	1.0
old fashioned cake .	280	3.0	26.0	18.0	15	260	2.0
powdered cake	310	3.0	34.0	18.0	15	260	2.0
pumpkin glazed ...	280	4.0	52.0	6.0	20	460	1.0
strawberry frosted .	240	4.0	32.0	10.0	0	330	1.0
sugar raised	210	4.0	27.0	10.0	0	320	1.0
vanilla Kreme filled .	320	4.0	39.0	16.0	0	360	1.0
wheat glazed cake .	310	4.0	32.0	19.0	0	380	2.0
donut stick, cake:							
plain	310	4.0	29.0	20.0	15	280	2.0
chocolate, glazed ..	370	3.0	41.0	21.0	0	390	2.0
cinnamon	340	4.0	36.0	20.0	15	290	2.0
glazed	360	4.0	41.0	20.0	15	280	2.0
jelly	420	4.0	53.0	20.0	15	310	2.0
powdered	340	4.0	37.0	20.0	15	280	2.0
fancies:							
apple fritter	290	4.0	35.0	13.0	0	360	2.0
bow tie donut	300	4.0	34.0	17.0	0	340	1.0
chocolate iced Bismark	340	3.0	50.0	15.0	0	290	1.0
coffee roll, frosted .	340	4.0	33.0	20:0	0	340	1.0
éclair	300	3.0	39.0	15.0	0	290	1.0
glazed fritter	250	4.0	31.0	13.0	0	330	1.0

Food and Measure	cal.	prot. (gms)	carbo. (gms)	fat (gms)	chol. (mgs)	sod. (mgs)	fiber (gms)
Dunkin Donuts (cont.)							
Munchkins, 4 pcs.:							
cake, plain	230	3.0	21.0	15.0	10	210	2.0
cake, glazed	300	3.0	38.0	15.0	10	210	2.0
cake, powdered ...	260	3.0	29.0	15.0	10	210	2.0
chocolate cake,							
glazed	300	2.0	39.0	15.0	0	290	2.0
cinnamon cake	260	3.0	29.0	15.0	10	210	2.0
glazed	300	3.0	38.0	15.0	10	210	2.0
Munchkins, 5 pcs.:							
jelly filled	240	3.0	37.0	8.0	0	280	1.0
sugar raised	190	3.0	26.0	8.0	0	270	1.0
muffins:							
banana walnut	540	10.0	69.0	25.0	65	520	3.0
blueberry	470	8.0	73.0	17.0	60	500	2.0
blueberry,							
reduced fat	400	8.0	78.0	5.0	60	490	3.0
chocolate, triple ...	660	7.0	84.0	33.0	10	460	4.0
chocolate chip	630	10.0	89.0	26.0	70	560	2.0
coffee cake muffin .	580	9.0	78.0	19.0	65	520	1.0
corn	510	8.0	77.0	18.0	75	860	1.0
cranberry orange ..	440	8.0	66.0	17.0	65	480	3.0
English	160	6.0	31.0	1.5	0	340	2.0
honey bran raisin ..	480	8.0	79.0	15.0	60	480	5.0
pumpkin	560	6.0	82.0	24.0	15	480	3.0
Coolatta, 16 fl. oz.:							
cherry lime, SoBe .	250	0	62.0	0	0	65	0
coffee, w/cream ...	350	3.0	40.0	22.0	75	65	0
coffee, w/milk	210	4.0	42.0	4.0	15	80	0
coffee, w/2% milk .	190	4.0	41.0	2.0	10	80	0
coffee, w/skim milk	170	4.0	41.0	0	0	80	0
lemonade	240	0	59.0	0	0	35	0
orange, Tropicana .	370	1.0	92.0	0	0	50	3.0
strawberry fruit ...	290	0	72.0	0	0	30	1.0
vanilla bean	500	1.0	85.0	17.0	0	95	2.0
espresso drinks, hot:							
cappuccino	80	4.0	7.0	4.5	20	70	0
w/soy milk	70	4.0	6.0	2.5	0	80	1.0
w/soy milk, sugar	120	4.0	20.0	2.5	0	80	1.0
w/sugar	130	4.0	21.0	4.5	15	65	0
Turbo Hot	130	1.0	20.0	6.0	20	55	0
latte, hot, 10 fl. oz.:							
w/milk	120	6.0	10.0	6.0	25	95	0
w/milk, sugar	160	6.0	22.0	6.0	25	95	0

Food and Measure	cal.	prot. (gms)	carbo. (gms)	fat (gms)	chol. (mgs)	sod. (mgs)	fiber (gms)
w/soy milk	90	6.0	8.0	3.5	0	110	1.0
w/soy milk, sugar .	150	6.0	22.0	3.5	0	110	1.0
caramel crème	250	8.0	40.0	9.0	20	125	0
caramel swirl	230	8.0	36.0	6.0	25	140	0
caramel swirl, soy .	210	8.0	34.0	3.5	0	160	1.0
lite latte	70	6.0	10.0	0	5	80	0
mocha almond	290	8.0	46.0	10.0	20	115	1.0
mocha swirl, soy ..	210	7.0	35.0	4.5	0	130	2.0
pumpkin spice	220	8.0	34.0	6.0	20	125	0
vanilla	80	7.0	12.0	0	0	105	0
latte, iced, 16 fl. oz.:							
w/milk	120	6.0	11.0	7.0	25	105	0
w/milk, sugar	170	6.0	23.0	7.0	25	110	0
w/skim milk	70	7.0	11.0	0	0	110	0
w/skim milk, sugar	120	7.0	23.0	0	0	110	0
caramel crème	260	8.0	40.0	9.0	20	125	0
caramel swirl	240	8.0	37.0	7.0	25	150	0
w/skim milk	180	8.0	36.0	0	0	150	0
lite latte	80	7.0	13.0	0	0	110	0
mocha almond	290	8.0	46.0	10.0	20	115	1.0
mocha swirl	240	7.0	38.0	8.0	25	125	1.0
w/skim milk	180	7.0	37.0	1.0	0	115	1.0
Turbo Ice	120	1.0	14.0	7.0	20	25	0
smoothie, 16 fl. oz.:							
mango passion fruit	360	7.0	79.0	2.5	10	120	2.0
strawberry banana .	360	7.0	79.0	2.5	10	125	2.0
tropical fruit	360	7.0	77.0	2.5	10	110	1.0
wildberry	360	7.0	79.0	2.5	10	120	1.0
drinks, other:							
Dunkaccino	230	2.0	35.0	11.0	10	5	0
hot chocolate:							
10 fl. oz.	230	2.0	39.0	7.0	0	290	2.0
white, 10 fl. oz. .	230	2.0	37.0	9.0	0	290	0
vanilla chai	230	1.0	40.0	8.0	5	50	0
Durian, fresh:							
½ of 1.3-lb. fruit	442	4.4	81.5	16.0	0	3	11.4
chopped, ½ cup	179	1.8	32.9	6.5	0	2	4.6
Durian, frozen (Frieda's), 2.2-lb. fruit untrimmed ...	150	1.0	27.0	1.0	0	0	2.0
Dutch brand loaf, see "Lunch meat"							

E

Food and Measure	cal.	prot. (gms)	carbo. (gms)	fat (gms)	chol. (mgs)	sod. (mgs)	fiber (gms)
Éclair (*Entenmann's*), 2 pcs., 3.6 oz.	260	3.0	46.0	9.0	65	190	3.0
Éclair, frozen:							
(*Smart Ones*), 2-oz. pc.	140	3.0	24.0	4.0	30	180	1.0
mini (*Kozy Shack*), 5 pcs., 3.1 oz.	250	5.0	23.0	16.0	95	80	1.0
Edamame (see also "Soybean"), fresh (*Frieda's*), ½ cup in pod, 1 cup shelled .	100	8.0	10.0	3.0	0	10	3.0
Edamame, frozen:							
in pod:							
(*Cascadian Farm Organic*), ⅔ cup edible	120	10.0	9.0	5.0	0	10	3.0
(*C&W Soybeans*), 1 cup	110	9.0	12.0	3.5	0	0	9.0
(*Seapoint Farms/ Seapoint Farms Organic*), 2.6 oz. edible	100	8.0	9.0	3.0	0	30	4.0
shelled:							
(*Cascadian Farm Organic*), ⅔ cup	120	10.0	9.0	5.0	0	10	3.0
(*C&W Soybeans*), ½ cup	100	10.0	7.0	3.5	0	5	7.0
(*Seapont Farms Salted*), ½ cup ..	100	8.0	9.0	3.0	0	260	4.0
(*Seapoint Farms/ Seapoint Farms Organic*), ½ cup .	100	8.0	9.0	3.0	0	30	4.0
Edamame, roasted:							
(*Roland*), ¼ cup	130	13.0	9.0	4.0	0	230	7.0

Food and Measure	cal.	prot. (gms)	carbo. (gms)	fat (gms)	chol. (mgs)	sod. (mgs)	fiber (gms)
dry-roasted (*Seapoint Farms*):							
goji blend, 1 oz.	120	11.0	15.0	3.0	0	140	7.0
lightly salted, ¼ cup	130	14.0	10.0	4.0	0	150	8.0
wasabi, ¼ cup	130	14.0	9.0	4.5	0	130	7.0
Eel, meat only:							
raw, 4 oz.	209	20.9	0	3.2	143	58	0
baked or broiled, 4 oz.	268	26.8	0	17.0	183	74	0
Eel, smoked, canned in oil (*Roland*),							
3.66-oz. can	340	12.0	1.0	32.0	40	520	0
Egg, chicken:							
raw, 1 large:							
whole	75	6.3	.6	5.0	213	63	0
white only	17	3.5	.3	0	0	55	0
yolk only (w/small portion white) ..	59	2.8	.3	5.1	213	7	0
raw, brown (*Organic Valley*):							
extra large	80	7.0	<1.0	5.0	240	80	0
extra large, omega-3	80	7.0	<1.0	5.0	250	80	0
jumbo	90	8.0	<1.0	6.0	270	80	0
large	70	6.0	<1.0	5.0	215	65	0
large, omega-3	70	7.0	<1.0	5.0	225	85	0
medium	70	5.0	<1.0	4.5	185	55	0
raw, white only:							
(*Egg Beaters*), 3 tbsp.	25	5.0	1.0	0	0	75	0
(*Organic Valley*), ¼ cup	25	5.0	1.0	0	0	90	0
hard-boiled, chopped, 1 cup	210	17.1	1.5	14.4	578	169	0
Egg, chicken, dried:							
whole:							
1 oz.	168	13.0	1.4	11.9	544	148	0
stabilized, 1 oz. ...	174	13.7	.7	12.5	572	155	0
white, flakes, 1 oz. ...	100	21.8	1.2	<.1	0	328	0
yolk, 1 oz.	195	8.7	.1	17.4	830	26	0
Egg, duck, 1 egg	130	9.0	1.0	9.6	619	102	0
Egg, goose, 1 egg ...	267	20.0	1.9	19.1	1227	199	0
Egg, quail:							
fresh, 1 egg	14	1.2	<.1	1.0	76	13	0
canned (*Roland*), 6 eggs	80	6.0	1.0	6.0	110	90	0
Egg, substitute, ¼ cup:							
(*Better'n Eggs*)	30	6.0	1.0	0	0	115	0

Food and Measure	cal.	prot. (gms)	carbo. (gms)	fat (gms)	chol. (mgs)	sod. (mgs)	fiber (gms)
Egg substitute *(cont.)*							
(*Better'n Eggs* Plus) ..	35	6.0	1.0	0	0	115	0
(*Egg Beaters*)	30	6.0	1.0	0	0	115	0
(*Egg Beaters* Frozen) .	30	6.0	1.0	0	0	125	0
(*Morningstar Farms* Scramblers)	35	6.0	2.0	0	0	95	0
cheese, 3 (*Better'n Eggs*)	45	6.0	1.0	1.0	5	150	0
cheese and chive (*Egg Beaters*)	35	6.0	1.0	1.0	<5	210	0
garden vegetable (*Egg Beaters*)	30	6.0	1.0	0	0	160	0
ham and cheese (*Better'n Eggs*)	45	6.0	1.0	1.5	5	150	0
Southwestern (*Egg Beaters*)	30	6.0	1.0	0	0	180	0
Egg, turkey, 1 egg ...	135	10.8	.9	9.4	737	119	0
Egg breakfast, frozen (see also "Breakfast sandwich/pastry" and specific listings), 1 pkg.:							
omelet:							
asparagus/cheese (*Cedarlane Dr. Sears Zone*), 10 oz.	340	24.0	32.0	13.0	35	630	3.0
cheese (*Cedarland Dr. Sears Zone*), 9.5 oz.	350	25.0	31.0	14.0	40	720	2.0
ham/cheese (*Aunt Jemima*), 5.2 oz.	250	13.0	19.0	14.0	265	810	1.0
spinach/mushroom (*Cedarlane Dr. Sears Zone*), 10 oz.	320	23.0	29.0	13.0	30	510	2.0
scrambled, 6.8 oz.:							
ham (*Aunt Jemima*)	260	16.0	21.0	13.0	195	970	2.0
sausage (*Aunt Jemima*)	300	15.0	21.0	18.0	200	890	2.0
scrambled, hash browns:							
bacon (*Aunt Jemima*), 5.25 oz.	300	15.0	14.0	20.0	340	910	1.0

Food and Measure	cal.	prot. (gms)	carbo. (gms)	fat (gms)	chol. (mgs)	sod. (mgs)	fiber (gms)
sausage (*Aunt Jemima*), 6.25 oz.	360	16.0	15.0	26.0	385	940	1.0
Egg breakfast, vegetarian, scramble:							
(*Morningstar Farms* Classic), ¼ pkg.	60	6.0	8.0	.5	0	150	1.0
(*Morningstar Farms* Veggie Bites Country), 3 pcs., 3 oz.	180	11.0	17.0	8.0	10	550	2.0
Florentine (*Morningstar Farms* Veggie Bites), 3 pcs., 3 oz.	180	10.0	17.0	8.0	15	560	2.0
Egg roll (see also "Spring roll"):							
chicken, 6 pcs., 3 oz.:							
(*Michelina's*)	170	5.0	22.0	7.0	5	440	1.0
sweet and sour (*Michelina's*) ...	180	5.0	25.0	7.0	5	390	1.0
shrimp (*Michelina's*), 6 pcs., 3 oz.	170	4.0	23.0	7.0	5	360	1.0
spinach (*Health is Wealth*), 3-oz. pc. .	170	8.0	18.0	8.0	0	310	3.0
vegetable (*Empire*), 3-oz. pc.	110	3.0	15.0	4.5	0	470	2.0
Egg roll entree, frozen, vegetable (*Lean Cuisine One Dish Favorites*), 9-oz. pkg.	310	7.0	60.0	5.0	5	630	3.0
"Egg" salad, vegetarian, see "Tofu salad"							
Egg roll wrapper (see also "Wrappers"):							
(*Frieda's*), 2 pcs.	130	5.0	28.0	.5	0	250	1.0
(*Nasoya*), 3 pcs.	170	7.0	35.0	.5	10	410	1.0
Eggnog, dairy, ½ cup:							
(*Hood* Golden)	180	4.0	22.0	9.0	65	95	0
(*Hood* Light)	140	4.0	22.0	4.0	45	95	0
(*Organic Valley*)	180	5.0	18.0	10.0	90	85	0
cinnamon (*Hood*) ...	180	4.0	21.0	9.0	60	115	0
pumpkin (*Hood*)	180	4.0	22.0	9.0	60	115	0
vanilla (*Hood*)	180	4.0	22.0	9.0	65	95	0
Eggnog, canned (*Borden*), ½ cup ..	160	4.0	17.0	9.0	75	80	0

Food and Measure	cal.	prot. (gms)	carbo. (gms)	fat (gms)	chol. (mgs)	sod. (mgs)	fiber (gms)
Eggplant, fresh:							
raw:							
(*Frieda's* Chinese/							
Japanese), 3 oz. .	20	1.0	5.0	0	0	0	2.0
1" pcs., ½ cup	11	.4	2.5	.1	0	1	1.0
boiled, drained,							
1" cubes, ½ cup . . .	13	.4	3.2	.1	0	2	1.2
Eggplant appetizer:							
baba ghanoush:							
(*Peloponnese*),							
2 tbsp.	40	1.0	2.0	3.0	0	250	1.0
(*Sabra* Classic), 1 oz.	80	0	2.0	8.0	5	135	0
roasted (*Cedar's*							
Baba Ghannouj),							
2 tbsp.	45	1.0	5.0	3.0	0	70	1.0
caponata:							
(*Alessi*), ⅓ cup . . .	140	2.0	7.0	7.0	0	310	4.0
(*Campagna* Sicilian),							
1 tbsp.	10	0	1.0	0	0	20	0
(*Roland*), ⅓ cup . .	140	2.0	11.0	10.0	0	630	4.0
flame-roasted, w/red							
pepper (*Sabra*), 1 oz.	50	0	2.0	5.0	0	190	0
grilled, w/onion (*Sabra*),							
1 oz.	40	0	2.0	3.5	0	110	1.0
roasted, 2 tbsp.:							
(*Peloponnese* Meze)	20	1.0	3.0	1.0	0	200	0
(*Peloponnese*							
Spread)	30	0	3.0	2.5	0	240	0
sautéed, tomato sauce							
(*Sabra* Mediter-							
ranean), 1 oz.	80	1.0	5.0	7.0	0	410	1.0
stuffed (*Roland*), ¼ of							
14-oz. can	80	1.0	11.0	3.5	0	300	4.0
tapanade, 2 tbsp.:							
roasted (*Meditalia*) .	40	.4	.9	4.0	0	155	.1
tomato (*Meditalia*) .	25	.3	1.6	2.0	0	171	0
Eggplant entree,							
frozen, 1 pkg.,							
except as noted:							
(*Ethnic Gourmet*							
Bhartha), 11 oz. . . .	300	8.0	47.0	9.0	0	650	10.0
moussaka (*Cedarlane*),							
10 oz.	230	13.0	22.0	10.0	20	590	6.0

Food and Measure	cal.	prot. (gms)	carbo. (gms)	fat (gms)	chol. (mgs)	sod. (mgs)	fiber (gms)
Parmesan:							
(*Cedarlane*), ½ of 10-oz. pkg.	160	7.0	16.0	8.0	15	390	3.0
vegetable and cheese (*Cedarland Dr. Sears Zone*), 11.3 oz.	320	24.0	29.0	12.0	45	910	5.0
parmigiana:							
(*Celentano*), 10 oz. . .	480	13.0	37.0	31.0	40	710	8.0
(*Celentano*), ½ of 14-oz. pkg.	330	9.0	26.0	22.0	25	480	5.0
(*Celentano* Vegan), 10 oz.	410	12.0	41.0	22.0	0	460	8.0
and red pepper pie (*The Fillo Factory*), ½ of 10-oz pkg. . . .	230	4.0	35.0	9.0	0	310	3.0
rollettes, 10 oz.:							
(*Celentano*)	390	12.0	35.0	23.0	35	780	8.0
(*Celentano* Vegan) .	350	13.0	36.0	17.0	0	520	8.0
Eggplant entree, pkg. (*TastyBite* Punjab), ½ of 10-oz. pkg. . .	144	4.0	13.0	9.0	0	515	2.0
Eggplant pocket, frozen, and roasted red pepper (*Aunt Trudy's* Organic), 5-oz. pc.	210	4.0	34.0	7.0	0	310	3.0
Eggplant relish, Indian (*Patak's* Brinjal), 1 tbsp.	70	0	8.0	4.0	0	250	1.0
Eight ball squash (*Frieda's*), 1 cup, 4.4 oz.	18	2.0	4.0	0	0	4	1.0
Elderberries, ½ cup .	53	.5	13.3	.4	0	4	5.1
Elk, meat only, roasted, 4 oz.	166	34.2	0	2.2	83	69	0
Emu, ground, panbroiled, 4 oz. . .	185	32.2	0	5.3	99	74	0
Enchilada, frozen, w/sauce, 1 pc.:							
beef, shredded (*El Monterey*), 4 oz. . .	140	6.0	15.0	6.0	15	450	2.0

Food and Measure	cal.	prot. (gms)	carbo. (gms)	fat (gms)	chol. (mgs)	sod. (mgs)	fiber (gms)
Enchilada, frozen (cont.)							
cheese, w/tofu, (Helen's Kitchen), 5 oz.	150	5.1	20.2	9.1	10	300	5.2
chicken (El Monterey), 4 oz.	180	7.0	15.0	10.0	25	590	1.0
Enchilada dinner, frozen, 1 pkg.:							
baked (Michelina's Lean Gourmet), 8.5 oz.	300	11.0	47.0	8.0	15	750	6.0
black bean (Amy's Whole Meal), 10 oz.	330	9.0	53.0	8.0	0	740	9.0
cheese (Amy's Whole Meal), 9 oz.	350	15.0	38.0	15.0	30	680	6.0
Enchilada entree, frozen, 1 pkg., except as noted:							
(Amy's Bowls Santa Fe), 10 oz.	350	16.0	47.0	11.0	5	780	10.0
black bean and tofu (Cedarlane Meal Organic), 9 oz.	220	10.0	42.0	3.0	0	390	6.0
black bean/vegetable: (Amy's), ½ of 9.5-oz. pkg.	180	5.0	26.0	6.0	0	390	3.0
(Amy's Family Size), ⅐ of 35-oz. pkg.	170	5.0	26.0	5.0	0	390	3.0
(Amy's Light Sodium), ½ of 9.5-oz. pkg.	160	5.0	22.0	6.0	0	190	3.0
cheese: (Amy's), ½ of 9.5-oz. pkg.	240	10.0	18.0	14.0	35	440	2.0
(Amy's Family Size), ⅐ of 35-oz. pkg.	240	11.0	19.0	13.0	35	460	2.0
(Patio), 1 pkg.	390	12.0	58.0	13.0	10	1500	10.0
and vegetable (Cedarlane Dr. Sears Zone), 9.5 oz.	300	23.0	32.0	12.0	15	540	7.0
chicken: (Healthy Choice), 9 oz.	270	10.0	45.0	5.0	20	600	5.0

Food and Measure	cal.	prot. (gms)	carbo. (gms)	fat (gms)	chol. (mgs)	sod. (mgs)	fiber (gms)
(*Lean Cuisine One Dish Favorites*), 9 oz.	280	15.0	46.0	4.0	20	530	3.0
(*Old El Paso* Complete Skillet Meal), 1 cup*	210	10.0	35.0	4.0	15	750	4.0
(*Stouffer's* Party), ⅛ of 57-oz. pkg.	280	12.0	30.0	12.0	40	720	3.0
Monterey (*Smart Ones*), 9.5 oz. . .	310	12.0	41.0	10.0	25	730	5.0
Suiza (*Smart Ones*), 9 oz.	310	14.0	45.0	8.0	35	730	3.0
combo (*Patio*), 1 pkg.	380	11.0	57.0	12.0	5	1250	5.0
pie:							
black bean, cheese (*Cedarlane Dr. Sears Zone*), 11 oz.	300	24.0	34.0	12.0	20	750	8.0
3-layer (*Cedarlane Organic*), ½ of 11-oz. pkg.	215	13.0	27.0	7.0	15	595	3.0
vegetable (*Cedarlane Organic Low Fat*), ½ of 9-oz. pkg. . . .	140	9.0	20.0	3.0	10	310	3.0
Enchilada entree kit (*Old El Paso* Dinner), ¼ pkg.	160	3.0	28.0	4.0	0	1100	2.0
Enchilada sauce, ¼ cup:							
(*Ortega*)	10	<1.0	4.0	.5	0	340	<1.0
(*Pace*)	25	1.0	5.0	0	0	520	1.0
green:							
(*Las Palmas*)	25	0	3.0	1.5	0	340	0
mild (*La Victoria*) . .	15	0	3.0	0	0	310	1.0
mild (*Old El Paso*) .	20	0	3.0	1.0	0	340	0
hot (*Las Palmas*)	15	0	2.0	.5	0	330	0
hot, medium, or mild (*Old El Paso*)	20	1.0	3.0	1.0	0	270	0
mild (*Las Palmas*) . . .	20	0	2.0	.5	0	310	1.0
red:							
(*Las Palmas*)	20	0	2.0	.5	0	310	1.0
chili (*La Victoria*) . .	15	0	2.0	0	0	310	0
mild or hot (*La Victoria*)	25	0	2.0	1.5	0	330	0
tomato (*Las Palmas*) .	20	<1.0	5.0	0	0	290	<1.0

Food and Measure	cal.	prot. (gms)	carbo. (gms)	fat (gms)	chol. (mgs)	sod. (mgs)	fiber (gms)
Enchilada sauce mix:							
(*Lawry's*), 2 tsp.	20	<1.0	4.0	0	0	260	0
(*McCormick*), 2 tsp. . . .	15	0	3.0	0	0	280	0
Endive, chopped,							
½ cup	4	.3	.8	.1	0	6	.8
Endive, Belgian, see "Chicory, witloof"							
Epazote, raw, 2 sprigs	1	0	.3	0	0	172	.2
Eppaw, raw, ½ cup . .	75	2.3	15.8	.9	0	6	n.a.
Escargot, see "Snail, canned"							
Escarole, see "Endive"							
Etouffee sauce mix							
(*Zatarain's*), ½ cup*	35	1.0	7.0	0	0	440	1.0

F

Food and Measure	cal.	prot. (gms)	carbo. (gms)	fat (gms)	chol. (mgs)	sod. (mgs)	fiber (gms)
Fajita, refrigerated (*Tyson* Meal Kit):							
beef, 3.8 oz. pc.*	140	9.0	17.0	4.0	15	310	2.0
chicken, 3.8-oz. pc.*	130	8.0	17.0	3.5	15	350	2.0
Fajita entree, frozen, chicken:							
(*Birds Eye Voila!*), 1 cup*	150	10.0	13.0	6.0	25	730	3.0
(*Smart Ones* Supreme), 9.25-oz. pkg.	260	17.0	32.0	7.0	40	600	4.0
w/rice (*Michelina's Lean Gourmet*), 8-oz. pkg.	230	11.0	34.0	6.0	15	890	2.0
Fajita entree kit, ⅕ pkg. mix:							
(*Old El Paso* Dinner)	190	4.0	33.0	5.0	0	1040	1.0
(*Taco Bell* Dinner)	230	5.0	41.0	5.0	0	1000	2.0
Fajita sauce, see "Marinade"							
Fajita seasoning mix:							
(*Chi-Chi's*), ¼ pkg.	35	0	7.0	1.0	0	520	0
(*McCormick*), 2 tsp.	15	0	2.0	0	0	290	0
(*Old El Paso*), 2 tsp.	10	0	3.0	0	0	280	0
(*Ortega*), 1½ tsp.	20	0	3.0	0	0	430	0
Falafel mix:							
(*Casbah*), ⅓ cup	180	7.0	29.0	5.0	0	680	3.0
(*Fantastic*), ¼ cup	130	7.0	21.0	2.0	0	250	6.0
(*Near East*), ¼ cup	100	10.0	18.0	1.0	0	560	5.0
(*Near East*), about 2½ patties*	220	10.0	18.0	14.0	0	560	5.0
Farfalle pasta entree, frozen, 1 pkg.:							
basil pesto (*Helen's Kitchen*), 9 oz.	320	20.0	70	11.0	30	370	5.0

Food and Measure	cal.	prot. (gms)	carbo. (gms)	fat (gms)	chol. (mgs)	sod. (mgs)	fiber (gms)
Farfalle pasta entree *(cont.)*							
spinach pesto sauce (*Moosewood* Organic), 10 oz.	370	14.0	56.0	11.0	20	370	4.0
Farina, whole grain:							
dry, 1 oz.	105	3.0	22.1	.1	0	1	.8
cooked, 1 cup	116	3.4	24.6	.2	0	1	3.3
Farro (see also "Spelt") (*Roland*), ¼ cup	170	7.0	33.0	0	0	30	3.0
Fava bean, see "Broad bean"							
Feijoa, raw:							
(*Frieda's*), 5 oz.	70	2.0	15.0	1.0	0	0	0
w/skin, 2.3-oz. pc. . . .	25	.6	5.3	.4	0	2	0
pureed, ½ cup	60	1.5	12.9	1.0	0	4	0
Fennel, bulb, raw:							
(*Andy Boy*), 1 medium	73	5.8	17.0	.5	0	122	7.3
(*Frieda's*), ¾ cup, 3 oz.	25	1.0	6.0	0	0	45	0
8.3 oz.	72	2.9	17.1	.5	0	122	7.3
sliced, 1 cup	27	1.1	6.3	.2	0	45	2.7
Fennel seed, 1 tsp. . .	7	.3	1.1	.3	0	2	<1.0
Fenugreek seed, 1 tsp.	12	.9	2.2	.2	0	2	<1.0
Fettuccine:							
dry, see "Pasta"							
refrigerated, 1¼ cups:							
(*Buitoni*)	260	12.0	46.0	3.0	70	90	2.0
spinach (*Buitoni*) . .	260	12.0	46.0	3.0	70	90	2.0
Fettuccine dish mix, ⅔ cup mix, except as noted:							
Alfredo:							
(*Knorr Lipton Pasta Sides*)	240	8.0	39.0	6.0	10	920	1.0
(*Knorr Lipton Pasta Sides* Whole Grain)	300	10.0	39.0	4.0	10	790	4.0
(*Pasta Roni*), 1 cup*	450	11.0	47.0	25.0	5	1140	2.0
broccoli (*Knorr Lipton Pasta Sides*)	250	9.0	40.0	6.0	10	850	1.0
primavera (*Knorr Lipton Sides Plus*), ¾ cup	230	9.0	39.0	4.5	10	690	3.0

Food and Measure	cal.	prot. (gms)	carbo. (gms)	fat (gms)	chol. (mgs)	sod. (mgs)	fiber (gms)
butter:							
(*Knorr Lipton Pasta Sides*)	240	7.0	43.0	4.0	10	890	1.0
and herb (*Knorr Lipton Pasta Sides*) .	240	7.0	42.0	4.5	5	700	1.0
chicken:							
(*Knorr Lipton Pasta Sides*)	220	7.0	43.0	2.0	<5	790	1.0
(*Knorr Lipton Pasta Sides* Whole Grain)	270	9.0	44.0	2.5	5	650	4.0
broccoli (*Knorr Lipton Pasta Sides*) .	220	8.0	41.0	2.5	<5	740	2.0
creamy (*Knorr Lipton Pasta Sides*) .	230	7.0	40.0	4.0	5	710	1.0
curly, white cheddar broccoli sauce (*Annie's*), 2.5 oz. . .	250	10.0	48.0	3.0	5	450	1.0
Parmesan (*Knorr Lipton Pasta Sides*) . . .	230	9.0	43.0	4.5	10	760	1.0
Stroganoff (*Knorr Lipton Pasta Sides*) . . .	210	7.0	39.0	2.0	<5	840	1.0
Fettuccine entree, frozen (see also "Chicken entree, frozen"), Alfredo, 1 pkg.:							
(*Lean Cuisine One Dish Favorites*), 9.25 oz.	280	14.0	40.0	7.0	15	680	2.0
(*Michelina's Authentico Tuscan*), 8 oz.	300	12.0	36.0	12.0	35	700	2.0
(*Michelina's Budget Gourmet*), 8 oz. . . .	300	10.0	42.0	10.0	25	600	2.0
(*Seeds of Change* di Roma Organic), 10 oz.	320	19.0	45.0	7.0	20	640	4.0
(*Smart Ones*), 9.25 oz.	290	15.0	45.0	6.0	25	720	3.0
(*Stouffer's*), 11.5 oz. .	610	18.0	57.0	34.0	85	1030	5.0
Fettuccine entree, microwave, Alfredo (*Kraft It's Pasta Anytime*), 11.5 oz.	580	21.0	74.0	22.0	50	1800	4.0
Fiddlehead fern, fresh, raw, 4 oz.	39	5.2	6.3	.5	0	1	n.a.

Food and Measure	cal.	prot. (gms)	carbo. (gms)	fat (gms)	chol. (mgs)	sod. (mgs)	fiber (gms)
Fig, fresh:							
1 large, 2.3 oz.	47	.5	12.3	.2	0	1	2.1
1 medium, 1.8 oz. . . .	37	.4	9.6	.2	0	1	1.7
Fig, can/jar, in light syrup, ½ cup:							
(*Oregon* Kadota)	118	1.0	27.0	0	0	5	3.0
(*Roland* Kadota)	120	1.0	28.0	0	0	0	1.0
Fig, dried:							
(*Del Monte*), 2 pcs., 1.3 oz.	100	1.0	29.0	0	0	5	3.0
(*Shiloh Farms* Organic Black Mission), 5 pcs., 1.4 oz.	110	1.0	28.0	.5	0	5	4.0
(*Shiloh Farms* Organic Calimyrna), 2 pcs., 1.6 oz.	120	1.0	30.0	.5	0	5	4.0
(*Sun•Maid* Mission/ Calimyrna). ¼ cup, 1.4 oz.	120	1.0	28.0	0	0	0	5.0
10 figs, 6.6 oz.	477	5.7	122.2	2.2	0	20	17.4
Filberts, see "Hazelnuts"							
Fillo dough, frozen:							
sheets:							
(*Apollo*), 1.7 oz.	130	3.0	27.0	1.0	0	330	1.0
(*Athens* Twin Pack 9" x 14"), 2 oz. . .	180	4.0	37.0	1.5	0	230	1.0
(*Athens* 14" x 18"), 2 oz.	180	4.0	37.0	1.5	0	230	1.0
(*The Fillo Factory* Organic), 1.5 oz. . . .	130	4.0	28.0	1.0	0	160	1.0
extra thick (*Apollo* Country Style), 2-oz. sheet	200	4.0	34.0	4.5	0	470	1.0
shells:							
(*The Fillo Factory* Organic), .7-oz. pc.	80	2.0	13.0	2.0	0	55	0
mini (*Athens*), 2 pcs., .3 oz. . . .	35	0	4.0	2.0	0	25	0
mini (*The Fillo Factory* Organic), .4-oz. pc.	45	1.0	7.0	1.5	0	30	0
shredded:							
(*Athens/Apollo*), ⅛ of 12-oz. pkg.	120	3.0	22.0	1.5	0	115	<1.0

Food and Measure	cal.	prot. (gms)	carbo. (gms)	fat (gms)	chol. (mgs)	sod. (mgs)	fiber (gms)
(*The Fillo Factory Kataifi*), ⅛ of 1-lb. pkg.	180	5.0	35.0	2.0	0	140	4.0
Finishing sauce, 1 tbsp., except as noted:							
chipotle (*Roland*)	60	0	2.0	6.0	0	360	0
cranberry horseradish (*Roland*)	70	0	4.0	6.0	0	160	0
honey mustard (*McCormick*), ¼ cup ..	120	1.0	25.0	1.0	0	380	0
kalamata feta (*Roland*)	60	0	<1.0	6.0	0	200	0
mushroom, creamy (*McCormick*), ¼ cup	70	2.0	3.0	5.0	20	240	0
red Burgundy (*McCormick*), ¼ cup ..	30	1.0	3.0	1.0	0	380	0
wasabi (*Roland*)	60	0	1.0	6.0	0	350	0
yellow pepper (*Roland*)	50	0	2.0	5.0	0	200	0
Fireweed, leaves, fresh, 1 cup	24	1.1	4.4	.7	0	8	2.4
Fish, see specific listings							
Fish, canned (see also specific fish), steaks, in hot sauce (*Chicken of the Sea*), 3.75-oz. can	70	9.0	1.0	3.0	50	430	1.0
Fish cake, see "Fish entree" and specific fish listings							
Fish cake mix, crab, salmon, or tuna (*Zatarain's*), 4 tbsp.	110	4.0	23.0	1.0	0	440	2.0
Fish coating mix, see "Seafood coating mix"							
Fish dinner, frozen, lemon pepper (*Healthy Choice*), 10.7-oz. pkg.	310	13.0	53.0	4.5	20	440	5.0
Fish entree, frozen (see also specific fish listings):							
cakes, 2 pcs., 4 oz.:							
(*Kineret*)	160	4.0	23.0	6.0	5	310	1.0
(*Schooner*)	240	8.0	38.0	6.0	5	820	1.0

Food and Measure	cal.	prot. (gms)	carbo. (gms)	fat (gms)	chol. (mgs)	sod. (mgs)	fiber (gms)
Fish entree, frozen (cont.)							
fillet, beer batter:							
(Gorton's), 2 pcs.,							
3.6 oz.	250	8.0	17.0	17.0	20	600	1.0
(Gorton's Tenders),							
3 pcs., 3.4 oz. . .	230	8.0	18.0	14.0	20	650	3.0
(Mrs. Paul's/Van							
de Kamp's),							
2.1-oz. pc.	120	6.0	12.0	6.0	15	380	<1.0
(Mrs. Paul's Tenders),							
4 pcs., 4 oz.	230	11.0	22.0	11.0	25	710	1.0
fillet, battered:							
(Gorton's Crispy),							
2 pcs., 3.8 oz. . .	230	8.0	22.0	12.0	25	650	1.0
(Gorton's Tenders),							
3 pcs., 3.6 oz. . .	230	8.0	23.0	12.0	20	660	2.0
(Mrs. Paul's Crispy),							
2.5-oz. pc.	140	6.0	14.0	7.0	15	440	0
(Mrs. Paul's Crispy),							
3.5-oz. pc.	190	8.0	19.0	9.0	20	610	<1.0
(Mrs. Paul's/Van							
de Kamp's Tenders),							
4 pcs., 4 oz.	210	9.0	22.0	10.0	20	700	1.0
(Van de Kamp's							
Crispy 10 pc.),							
2.1-oz. pc.	120	5.0	12.0	16.0	10	370	<1.0
(Van de Kamp's							
Crispy 6 pc.),							
2 pcs., 3.5 oz. . .	190	8.0	20.0	9.0	20	620	<1.0
lemon pepper							
(Gorton's), 2 pcs.,							
3.7 oz.	270	8.0	20.0	18.0	20	580	1.0
fillet, breaded:							
(Gorton's Crunchy							
Golden), 2 pcs.,							
3.8 oz.	240	9.0	23.0	12.0	30	500	0
(Gorton's Tenders							
Extra Crunchy),							
3 pcs., 3.4 oz. . .	230	9.0	25.0	10.0	45	550	0
(Van de Kamp's							
12 Pc.), 2 pcs.,							
3.5 oz.	230	8.0	21.0	13.0	20	440	<1.0
(Van de Kamp's							
6 Pc.), 2 pcs., 4 oz.	270	10.0	25.0	15.0	25	520	1.0

Food and Measure	cal.	prot. (gms)	carbo. (gms)	fat (gms)	chol. (mgs)	sod. (mgs)	fiber (gms)
(*Van de Kamp's* Crisp & Healthy), 2 pcs., 3.7 oz. ..	150	8.0	25.0	1.5	20	470	1.0
garlic herb (*Gorton's*), 2 pcs., 3.7 oz. ..	230	9.0	22.0	12.0	30	770	0
lemon herb (*Gorton's*), 2 pcs., 3.7 oz. ..	240	9.0	21.0	13.0	25	720	0
potato crunch (*Gorton's*), 2 pcs., 3.7 oz.	240	9.0	20.0	14.0	25	790	2.0
ranch (*Gorton's*), 2 pcs., 3.7 oz. ..	240	9.0	22.0	13.0	30	650	0
fillet, crusted, 1 pkg.: Parmesan (*Lean Cuisine*), 9 oz. ..	290	15.0	40.0	8.0	30	650	4.0
tortilla (*Lean Cuisine*), 8 oz.	330	16.0	45.0	9.0	35	540	3.0
fillet, grilled (*Gorton's*), 3.8-oz. pc.: Cajun blackened ...	100	17.0	1.0	3.0	60	330	1.0
garlic butter or lemon pepper ...	100	17.0	1.0	3.0	70	290	1.0
lemon butter	100	17.0	1.0	3.0	75	320	1.0
fillet, w/mac and cheese (*Stouffer's*), 9-oz. pkg.	400	27.0	36.0	16.0	55	1050	4.0
lemon pepper (*Lean Cuisine*), 9-oz. pkg.	330	15.0	50.0	8.0	40	590	2.0
nuggets, fish shape: (*Mrs. Paul's*), 4 pcs., 4.25 oz.	270	12.0	27.0	13.0	30	430	1.0
(*Van de Kamp's*), 4 pcs., 4.25 oz. .	260	9.0	29.0	12.0	15	790	1.0
popcorn (*Mrs. Paul's/ Van de Kamp's*), 8 pcs., 4 oz.	220	11.0	18.0	12.0	30	480	2.0
portions, breaded (*Schooners's*), 3-oz. pc.	270	8.0	46.0	6.0	20	120	1.0
sticks, breaded: (*Gorton's* Crunchy Golden), 6 pcs., 3.6 oz.	250	11.0	20.0	14.0	20	380	2.0

Food and Measure	cal.	prot. (gms)	carbo. (gms)	fat (gms)	chol. (mgs)	sod. (mgs)	fiber (gms)
Fish entree, frozen, sticks, breaded *(cont.)*							
(*Mrs. Paul's* 30 pc.), 6 pcs., 3.8 oz. ..	250	10.0	25.0	12.0	25	390	1.0
(*Mrs. Paul's* 44/60 pc.), 6 pcs., 3.4 oz.	220	9.0	22.0	10.0	25	340	<1.0
(*Mrs. Paul's* Crunchy), 6 pcs., 3.4 oz.	220	9.0	22.0	10.0	25	340	<1.0
(*Mrs. Paul's* Healthy Selects), 6 pcs., 3.7 oz.	140	9.0	24.0	1.0	25	380	1.0
(*Mrs. Paul's/Van de Kamp's* X-Large), 4 pcs., 3.4 oz. ..	220	9.0	22.0	11.0	25	350	1.0
(*Schooner*), 4 pcs., 3.2 oz.	180	8.0	22.0	6.0	25	190	1.0
(*Van de Kamp's* 18/30 pc.), 6 pcs., 4 oz.	260	11.0	26.0	13.0	30	410	1.0
(*Van de Kamp's* 44/60 pc.), 6 pcs., 3.4 oz.	230	10.0	23.0	11.0	25	370	1.0
(*Van de Kamp's* Crisp & Healthy), 6 pcs., 3.7 oz. ..	140	9.0	24.0	1.0	25	380	1.0
mini (*Gorton's*), 13 pcs., 3.5 oz. .	230	9.0	21.0	12.0	20	330	0
tenders, 4 oz.:							
(*Gorton's* Extra Crunchy)	260	10.0	29.0	12.0	30	640	0
(*Gorton* Original Batter)	270	9.0	25.0	15.0	25	770	0
beer batter (*Gorton's*)	260	9.0	21.0	15.0	25	740	0
Fish seasoning mix, see "Seafood coating mix"							
Flageolets, canned fine green (*Roland*), ½ cup	130	7.0	23.0	1.0	0	390	6.0
Flageolets, dried, green (*Roland*), ¼ cup	120	8.0	21.0	0	0	10	9.0
Flan, see "Pudding"							

Food and Measure	cal.	prot. (gms)	carbo. (gms)	fat (gms)	chol. (mgs)	sod. (mgs)	fiber (gms)
Flatbread melts, frozen (*Lean Cuisine*), 6.5-oz. pkg.:							
chicken pesto	330	22.0	43.0	8.0	20	630	5.0
chicken Philly	330	21.0	41.0	8.0	25	650	5.0
chicken ranch club ...	330	21.0	41.0	9.0	20	640	4.0
steak, chophouse	330	21.0	40.0	9.0	30	570	4.0
Flatfish, meat only:							
raw, 4 oz.	104	21.4	0	1.4	54	92	0
baked or broiled, 4 oz.	133	27.4	0	1.7	77	119	0
Flax seed:							
(*Arrowhead Mills* Organic), 3 tbsp. ...	140	6.0	9.0	9.0	0	0	7.0
(*Hodgson Mill* Golden Organic), 2 tbsp. ...	65	3.0	4.0	4.0	0	0	4.0
(*Hodgson Mill* Milled), 2 tbsp.	60	3.0	4.0	5.0	0	0	4.0
(*Hodgson Mill* Travel Flax All Natural/ Organic), 1 pkt. ...	30	1.0	2.0	2.0	0	0	2.0
(*Spectrum* Organic Whole), 1½ tbsp. ...	80	3.0	5.0	5.0	0	0	4.0
brown (*Shiloh Farms* Organic), 3 tbsp. ...	140	5.0	11.0	10.0	0	0	6.0
golden:							
(*Arrowhead Mills* Organic), 3 tbsp. ...	160	8.0	10.0	10.0	0	10	9.0
(*Shiloh Farms* Organic), 1 tbsp. ...	61	2.0	3.0	4.0	0	0	3.0
roasted (*Shiloh Farms*), 2 tbsp. .	105	4.0	7.0	7.0	0	7	6.0
ground (*Spectrum* Organic), 2 tbsp. ...	80	3.0	5.0	5.0	0	0	4.0
Flax seed meal:							
(*Arrowhead Mills* Organic), 2 tbsp. ...	80	3.0	5.0	4.5	0	0	4.0
brown (*Nature's Path* FlaxPlus Organic), 2 tbsp.	70	3.0	5.0	5.0	0	5	4.0
w/herbs (*Spectrum* Flax Fiber), 1 tbsp. .	30	2.0	4.0	.5	0	0	4.0
Flounder, fresh, see "Flatfish"							

Food and Measure	cal.	prot. (gms)	carbo. (gms)	fat (gms)	chol. (mgs)	sod. (mgs)	fiber (gms)
Flounder entree, frozen, fillet:							
breaded, 1 pc.:							
(*Mrs. Paul's*), 2.7 oz.	150	8.0	12.0	7.0	25	290	1.0
(*Schooner*), 3.5 oz.	290	9.0	48.0	6.0	30	160	1.0
stuffed (*Oven Poppers*), 5-oz. pc.:							
broccoli, cheese ...	150	20.0	4.0	6.0	55	330	1.0
cheese, au gratin ..	220	24.0	5.0	11.0	75	450	1.0
crab	240	17.0	15.0	13.0	35	400	0
garlic, shrimp, and almonds	260	16.0	16.0	14.0	40	380	0
Flour, see "Wheat flour" and specific listings							
Focaccia, see "Bread"							
Focaccia, stuffed, frozen (*Cedarlane*), 4 oz.:							
Mediterranean	296	13.0	37.0	10.0	22	485	1.0
tomato and basil	275	14.0	33.0	9.0	14	528	2.0
veggie "pepperoni" ..	250	12.0	34.0	6.0	20	430	1.0
Foo qua, see "Balsam pear"							
Frankfurter, 1 link, 2 oz., except as noted:							
(*Ball Park* Bun Size/ Franks)	180	6.0	3.0	16.0	40	560	0
(*Ball Park* Fat Free), 1.8 oz.	40	5.0	4.0	0	10	420	0
(*Ball Park* Lite), 1.8 oz.	100	6.0	3.0	7.0	25	460	0
(*Ball Park Singles*), 1.6 oz.	150	5.0	2.0	13.0	30	450	0
(*Dietz & Watson*)	170	7.0	2.0	13.0	30	490	0
(*Dietz & Watson* Gourmet Lite)	60	7.0	5.0	1.5	15	390	0
(*Dietz & Watson* Wieners)	150	7.0	1.0	14.0	30	470	0
(*Farmland* Deli Style/ Premium)	180	6.0	2.0	17.0	50	620	0
(*Hatfield* Franks), 1.6 oz.	140	5.0	1.0	12.0	25	390	0
(*Hatfield* Jumbo)	170	7.0	2.0	16.0	35	490	0
(*Hatfield* Reduced Sodium)	150	7.0	2.0	13.0	30	350	0

Food and Measure	cal.	prot. (gms)	carbo. (gms)	fat (gms)	chol. (mgs)	sod. (mgs)	fiber (gms)
(*Healthy Choice*), 1.75 oz.	70	6.0	6.0	2.5	20	440	0
(*Oscar Mayer*), 1.6 oz.	130	5.0	1.0	12.0	35	540	0
(*Oscar Mayer* Bun Length/Jumbo) ...	170	6.0	0	16.0	45	680	0
(*Oscar Mayer* Wieners Light), 1.6 oz.	90	5.0	1.0	7.0	30	460	0
beef:							
(*Applegate Farms*), 1.5 oz.	70	6.0	0	4.5	20	430	0
(*Applegate Farms* Big Apple)	100	9.0	1.0	6.0	20	640	0
(*Applegate Farms* Organic), 1.5 oz.	100	8.0	1.0	7.0	30	390	0
(*Applegate Farms* Organic Great) ..	110	7.0	0	8.0	30	330	0
(*Ball Park* Bun Size)	180	6.0	3.0	16.0	35	550	0
(*Ball Park* Fat Free), 1.8 oz.	45	6.0	5.0	0	10	420	0
(*Ball Park* Franks) .	180	6.0	3.0	16.0	40	560	0
(*Ball Park* Lite), 1.8 oz.	100	6.0	3.0	7.0	25	450	0
(*Ball Park* Grill-master), 2.9 oz. .	250	9.0	3.0	23.0	50	780	0
(*Ball Park* Grillmaster Deli), 2.9 oz. ...	250	8.0	3.0	23.0	50	830	0
(*Ball Park* Grillmaster Hot 'N Spicy), 2.9 oz.	260	9.0	4.0	24.0	50	780	0
(*Ball Park* Singles), 1.6 oz.	150	5.0	3.0	13.0	30	440	0
(*Boar's Head* Lite), 1.6 oz.	90	7.0	0	6.0	25	270	0
(*Boar's Head* Natural Casing)	160	7.0	1.0	14.0	30	440	0
(*Boar's Head* Skinless), 1.6 oz.	120	6.0	0	11.0	20	350	0
(*Dietz & Watson*) ..	150	7.0	2.0	13.0	30	490	0
(*Dietz & Watson* Gourmet Lite) ...	60	7.0	5.0	1.5	15	390	0
(*Deitz & Watson* New York Style) .	160	7.0	2.0	14.0	30	490	0
(*Farmland* Premium)	180	7.0	3.0	16.0	35	610	0

Food and Measure	cal.	prot. (gms)	carbo. (gms)	fat (gms)	chol. (mgs)	sod. (mgs)	fiber (gms)
Frankfurter, beef *(cont.)*							
(*Farmland* Premium Black Angus) ...	180	6.0	3.0	15.0	30	530	0
(*Farmland* Twister) .	180	6.0	3.0	15.0	30	520	0
(*Hans' All Natural New York*), 1.5 oz.	90	6.0	0	8.0	25	280	0
(*Hebrew National*), 1.7 oz.	150	6.0	1.0	14.0	30	370	0
(*Hebrew National* Jumbo), 3 oz. ...	270	10.0	1.0	26.0	45	720	0
(*Hebrew National* 97% Fat Free), 1.7 oz.	45	6.0	3.0	1.5	15	400	0
(*Hebrew National* Quarter Pound Dinner), 4 oz. ...	350	13.0	1.0	32.0	70	990	0
(*Hebrew National* Reduced Fat), 1.7 oz.	120	6.0	0	10.0	25	360	0
(*Nathan's* Casing) ..	180	7.0	1.0	17.0	35	460	0
(*Oscar Mayer* Bun Length/Jumbo) .	180	6.0	2.0	170	35	580	0
(*Oscar Mayer* Light), 1.6 oz.	90	5.0	2.0	6.0	20	500	0
(*Oscar Mayer* XXL), 1.6 oz.	140	5.0	1.0	13.0	30	460	0
(*Oscar Mayer* XXL Deli Style/Premium), 2.7 oz. ...	230	9.0	1.0	22.0	50	740	0
(*Wranglers*)	170	7.0	1.0	15.0	35	560	0
cheese:							
(*Ball Park*)	180	6.0	3.0	16.0	40	560	0
(*Ball Park Singles*), 1.6 oz.	150	5.0	2.0	13.0	30	460	0
(*Farmland* Premium)	160	7.0	2.0	14.0	35	650	0
(*Hatfield*)	180	7.0	2.0	16.0	35	550	0
(*Oscar Mayer* Cheese Dogs), 1.6 oz. ..	140	5.0	1.0	13.0	35	540	0
(*Wranglers*)	170	7.0	1.0	15.0	35	610	0
chicken:							
(*Applegate Farms*), 1.5 oz.	70	7.0	0	4.5	30	430	0
(*Applegate Farms* Organic), 1.5 oz.	70	7.0	1.0	3.0	35	440	0

Food and Measure	cal.	prot. (gms)	carbo. (gms)	fat (gms)	chol. (mgs)	sod. (mgs)	fiber (gms)
(*Empire Kosher*) ..	100	6.0	0	7.0	50	550	0
(*Foster Farms*) ...	140	7.0	1.0	12.0	30	550	0
(*Hans' All Natural* California), 1.5 oz.	60	7.0	0	3.5	25	340	0
cocktail, beef, 5 pcs.:							
(*Boar's Head*)	170	8.0	0	15.0	30	430	0
(*Hebrew National*) .	180	7.0	1.0	16.0	40	450	0
hot and spicy (*Oscar Mayer XXL*), 2.7 oz.	210	10.0	1.0	19.0	45	750	0
pork (*Hans' All Natural* Chicago), 1.5 oz. ..	60	7.0	0	3.5	25	340	0
pork and beef:							
(*Boar's Head*)	150	7.0	0	14.0	25	460	0
(*Farmland* Premium Jumbo)	170	6.0	1.0	16.0	35	470	0
salmon (*A&B Famous*), 2 pcs., 2.6 oz.	170	9.0	4.0	14.0	30	510	0
smoked:							
(*Ball Park Grillmaster* Smokehouse), 2.9 oz.	260	9.0	3.0	24.0	50	790	0
(*Hormel* Smokies), 1 oz.	80	4.0	1.0	7.0	20	290	0
(*Johnsonville* Natural Casing), 1.7 oz.	150	6.0	1.0	14.0	40	410	0
(*Johnsonville* New Orleans), 2.7 oz.	230	9.0	2.0	20.0	40	630	0
(*Oscar Mayer XXL*), 2.7 oz.	240	9.0	1.0	23.0	45	680	0
(*Wranglers*)	170	7.0	1.0	15.0	35	560	0
beef (*Johnsonville* Stadium), 2.7 oz.	240	9.0	2.0	22.0	50	760	0
w/cheese (*Hormel* Smokies), 1 oz. ..	80	4.0	1.0	7.0	20	310	0
hickory (*Farmland* Hot Dogs), 1.2 oz.	110	3.0	1.0	10.0	30	370	0
hickory (*Farmland* Special Select) ..	170	6.0	2.0	17.0	50	620	0
hot (*Johnsonville* Hot Links), 2.7 oz.	230	9.0	2.0	20.0	40	630	0
hot, beef (*Johnson-ville* Hot Links), 2.7 oz.	230	9.0	2.0	20.0	40	620	0

Food and Measure	cal.	prot. (gms)	carbo. (gms)	fat (gms)	chol. (mgs)	sod. (mgs)	fiber (gms)
Frankfurter (cont.)							
turkey:							
(Applegate Farms), 1.5 oz.	60	6.0	0	4.0	25	300	0
(Applegate Farms Organic), 1.5 oz.	80	6.0	0	6.0	30	350	0
(Empire Kosher) ..	100	6.0	0	8.0	45	540	0
(Foster Farms)	140	7.0	1.0	12.0	25	560	0
(Louis Rich/Oscar Mayer), 1.6 oz. .	100	5.0	2.0	8.0	30	510	0
(Louis Rich/Oscar Mayer Bun Length)	120	6.0	3.0	10.0	35	640	0
cheese (Louis Rich/ Oscar Mayer), 1.6 oz.	100	6.0	2.0	8.0	30	490	0
smoked, white (Ball Park Bun Size), 1.8 oz.	45	6.0	5.0	0	10	420	0
uncured (Organic Prairie), 1.5 oz.:							
beef	120	5.0	0	11.0	25	360	0
chicken, fresh	100	7.0	1.0	6.0	35	480	0
chicken, frozen	70	7.0	1.0	4.5	30	500	0
pork and beef	130	5.0	0	12.0	25	390	0
turkey	80	8.0	1.0	6.0	25	480	0
"Frankfurter," vegeta-rian, 1 link or pc., except as noted:							
canned, 1.8 oz.:							
(Loma Linda Big Franks)	110	11.0	3.0	6.0	0	220	2.0
low fat (Loma Linda Big Franks)	80	12.0	3.0	2.5	0	240	2.0
frozen/refrigerated:							
(Morningstar Farms Veggie Dogs), 2 oz.	80	11.0	6.0	.5	0	580	1.0
(Tufurky Foot Long), 3.5 oz.	160	22.0	11.0	4.0	0	750	4.0
(Tofurky Franks), 1.6 oz.	80	11.0	5.0	2.0	0	390	3.0
(Worthington Leanies), 1.4 oz.	100	8.0	2.0	7.0	0	430	1.0
(Yves Hot Dogs), 1.6 oz.	50	10.0	2.0	.5	0	400	0

Food and Measure	cal.	prot. (gms)	carbo. (gms)	fat (gms)	chol. (mgs)	sod. (mgs)	fiber (gms)
(*Yves* Hot Dogs Jumbo), 2.7 oz.	110	16.0	5.0	3.0	0	460	0
(*Yves* The Good Dog), 1.6 oz.	70	8.0	1.0	3.5	0	430	0
(*Yves* Tofu Dogs), 1.3 oz.	45	8.0	2.0	1.0	0	300	0
chipotle (*Tofurky* Franks), 1.6 oz.	90	10.0	5.0	3.0	0	270	3.0
Frankfurter, wrapped:							
(*Hebrew National* Franks in a Blanket), 5 pcs., 2.9 oz.	290	9.0	8.0	24.0	40	690	1.0
in bagel (*Vienna Beef*), 5-oz. pc.	420	33.0	33.0	17.0	35	990	1.0
in bun, 3.4-oz. pc.:							
(*Oscar Mayer Fast Franks*)	290	10.0	21.0	19.0	45	790	1.0
beef (*Oscar Mayer Fast Franks*)	300	10.0	21.0	8.0	35	830	1.0
corn dogs, 1 pc.:							
(*Farmer John*)	220	7.0	19.0	12.0	25	530	1.0
(*Oscar Mayer*)	210	6.0	21.0	12.0	25	590	1.0
beef (*Farmer John*)	210	7.0	19.0	12.0	40	560	>1.0
cheese (*Foster Farms* Extreme)	180	7.0	15.0	8.0	35	490	1.0
chili cheese (*Foster Farms*)	200	6.0	24.0	9.0	20	470	0
honey crunchy (*Foster Farms*)	180	7.0	15.0	10.0	35	490	1.0
honey crunchy, jumbo (*Foster Farms*)	270	10.0	22.0	15.0	50	730	1.0
vegetarian, see "Corn dogs, vegetarian"							
French toast, frozen:							
(*Aunt Jemima* Home-style), 2 pcs.	220	8.0	37.0	4.5	77	350	1.0
cinnamon:							
(*Aunt Jemima*), 2 pcs.	220	7.0	37.0	4.5	75	360	1.0
sticks (*Aunt Jemima*), 5 pcs.	360	6.0	58.0	12.0	0	400	2.0
sticks, toaster, 2 pcs.:							
(*Eggo* Original)	220	5.0	36.0	6.0	20	530	1.0

Food and Measure	cal.	prot. (gms)	carbo. (gms)	fat (gms)	chol. (mgs)	sod. (mgs)	fiber (gms)
French toast, frozen, sticks *(cont.)*							
cinnamon (*Eggo*) ..	220	4.0	39.0	6.0	20	510	1.0
maple syrup (*Eggo*)	150	3.0	28.0	3.5	15	330	0
whole grain (*Aunt Jemima*), 2 pcs.	240	8.0	39.0	6.0	70	340	3.0
French toast breakfast, frozen, and sausage (*Aunt Jemima*), 5.5-oz. pkg.	350	13.0	40.0	16.0	105	610	2.0
Frog's legs, raw, 2 oz.	41	9.2	0	.2	28	32	0
Frosting, ready-to-spread, 2 tbsp.:							
(*Pillsbury Funfetti* Confetti)	150	0	25.0	6.0	0	70	0
all varieties, except milk chocolate (*Pillsbury Whipped Supreme*)	100	0	14.0	5.0	0	20	0
buttercream:							
(*Betty Crocker* Rich & Creamy)	140	0	23.0	5.0	0	70	0
(*Betty Crocker* Whipped)	110	0	14.0	6.0	0	25	0
cherry (*Betty Crocker* Rich & Creamy) ...	140	0	23.0	5.0	0	70	0
chocolate:							
(*Betty Crocker* Rich & Creamy)	140	1.0	18.0	8.0	0	105	<1.0
(*Betty Crocker* Whipped)	100	<1.0	14.0	5.0	0	55	1.0
(*Pillsbury Creamy Supreme*)	140	0	21.0	6.0	0	90	0
dark (*Betty Crocker* Rich & Creamy) .	140	1.0	18.0	8.0	0	105	<1.0
fudge (*Pillsbury Creamy Supreme*)	140	0	21.0	6.0	0	90	0
fudge (*Pillsbury Creamy Supreme Reduced Sugar*) .	120	0	16.0	8.0	0	75	1.0
milk (*Betty Crocker* Rich & Creamy) .	140	0	19.0	7.0	0	95	<1.0
milk (*Betty Crocker* Whipped)	100	0	14.0	4.5	0	50	0
milk (*Pillsbury Creamy Supreme*)	140	0	21.0	6.0	0	55	0

Food and Measure	cal.	prot. (gms)	carbo. (gms)	fat (gms)	chol. (mgs)	sod. (mgs)	fiber (gms)
milk (*Pillsbury* Whipped Supreme)	100	0	14.0	4.5	0	50	0
mousse (*Betty Crocker* Whipped)	90	0	14.0	4.5	0	55	1.0
chocolate chip, triple fudge (*Betty Crocker* Rich & Creamy) ...	140	1.0	22.0	5.0	0	90	<1.0
coconut pecan:							
(*Betty Crocker* Rich & Creamy)	140	0	18.0	7.0	0	55	<1.0
(*Pillsbury Creamy Supreme*)	160	1.0	17.0	10.0	0	60	<1.0
cream cheese:							
(*Betty Crocker* Rich & Creamy)	140	0	23.0	5.0	0	70	0
(*Betty Crocker* Whipped)	110	0	15.0	5.0	0	45	0
(*Pillsbury Creamy Supreme*)	150	0	24.0	6.0	0	70	0
chocolate (*Pillsbury Creamy Supreme*)	140	0	21.0	6.0	0	90	<1.0
lemon:							
(*Betty Crocker* Rich & Creamy)	140	0	23.0	5.0	0	70	0
(*Pillsbury Creamy Supreme*)	150	0	23.0	6.0	0	70	0
pink (*Pillsbury Funfetti*)	140	0	23.0	5.0	0	65	0
rainbow chip (*Betty Crocker* Rich & Creamy)	140	0	23.0	5.0	0	70	0
strawberry:							
(*Betty Crocker* Whipped)	110	0	15.0	5.0	0	25	0
(*Pillsbury Creamy Supreme*)	150	0	24.0	6.0	0	70	0
vanilla:							
(*Betty Crocker* Whipped)	110	0	15.0	5.0	0	25	0
(*Pillsbury Creamy Supreme*)	150	0	24.0	6.0	0	70	0
(*Pillsbury Creamy Supreme* Reduced Sugar)	120	0	18.0	7.0	0	60	0
(*Pillsbury Funfetti*) .	150	0	25.0	6.0	0	70	0

Food and Measure	cal.	prot. (gms)	carbo. (gms)	fat (gms)	chol. (mgs)	sod. (mgs)	fiber (gms)
Frosting, ready-to-spread, vanilla *(cont.)*							
French (*Pillsbury*							
Creamy Supreme)	160	0	25.0	6.0	0	75	0
or white (*Betty*							
Crocker Rich &							
Creamy)	140	0	23.0	5.0	0	70	0
or white (*Betty*							
Crocker Whipped)	110	0	15.0	5.0	0	25	0
whipped cream (*Betty*							
Crocker Whipped) .	100	0	15.0	5.0	0	25	0
Frosting mix:							
chocolate (*Dr. Oetker*							
Organic), 1/12 pkg...	110	0	26.0	0	0	65	0
fudge (*"Jiffy"*), 1/4 pkg.	150	<1.0	28.0	4.0	0	130	<1.0
vanilla (*Dr. Oetker*							
Organic), 1/12 pkg...	110	0	27.0	0	0	65	0
white:							
(*Betty Crocker* Home-							
style), 3 tbsp.	100	<1.0	24.0	0	0	55	0
(*"Jiffy"*), 1/4 pkg.	150	0	28.0	4.0	0	140	0
Fructose (*Tree of Life*),							
1 tsp.	15	0	4.0	0	0	0	0
Fruit, see specific							
listings							
Fruit, mixed, can/jar							
(see also "Fruit cock-							
tail"), 1/2 cup, except							
as noted:							
(*Dole* Fruit Bowl),							
4-oz. cont.	80	<1.0	19.0	0	0	10	1.0
in juice:							
(*Del Monte*), 4-oz. can	50	0	13.0	0	0	10	<1.0
(*Del Monte* Orchard							
Select)	80	<1.0	19.0	0	0	10	<1.0
chunky (*Del Monte*)	60	0	15.0	0	0	10	1.0
chunky (*S&W*							
Natural Style) ...	80	<1.0	19.0	0	0	20	3.0
tropical (*Del Monte*)	60	0	16.0	0	0	15	1.0
tropical (*Del Monte*),							
4-oz. cup	70	<1.0	18.0	0	0	5	<1.0
tropical (*Del Monte*							
Fruit Naturals							
Medley)	70	<1.0	18.0	0	0	5	<1.0

Food and Measure	cal.	prot. (gms)	carbo. (gms)	fat (gms)	chol. (mgs)	sod. (mgs)	fiber (gms)
in extra light syrup:							
(*Del Monte* Lite), 4-oz. can	50	0	13.0	0	0	10	<1.0
ambrosia salad (*SunFresh*)	70	0	16.0	0	0	5	2.0
chunky (*Del Monte* Lite)	60	0	15.0	0	0	10	1.0
citrus (*Del Monte/ SunFresh*)	80	0	20.0	0	0	20	0
in gelatin:							
cherry (*Del Monte*), 4.5-oz. cup	90	0	23.0	0	0	40	0
cherry or peach (*Dole*), 4.3-oz. cup	90	<1.0	23.0	0	0	25	<1.0
in light syrup:							
(*Del Monte*), 4-oz. cup	70	<1.0	18.0	0	0	10	<1.0
(*Del Monte*), 4-oz. can	80	0	20.0	0	0	10	<1.0
(*Dole* Jar)	80	0	21.0	0	0	5	1.0
cherry (*Del Monte*)	90	<1.0	22.0	0	0	10	<1.0
cherry (*Del Monte*), 4-oz. cup	70	<1.0	18.0	0	0	10	<1.0
cherry (*Del Monte* Very Cherry) ...	90	1.0	22.0	0	0	10	<1.0
citrus (*Del Monte*) .	80	0	20.0	0	0	20	0
in light syrup, tropical:							
(*Del Monte*)	80	0	21.0	0	0	10	1.0
(*Dole* Can)	90	0	21.0	0	0	10	0
(*Dole* Fruit Bowl), 4-oz. cont.	80	<1.0	19.0	0	0	10	2.0
(*Dole* Jar)	80	0	20.0	0	0	10	1.0
(*SunFresh* Salad) ..	80	1.0	20.0	0	0	10	0
w/fruit juice (*Sun-Fresh*)	80	0	21.0	0	0	10	1.0
w/passion fruit juice (*Roland*), 1 cup .	100	1.0	23.0	0	0	0	2.0
in heavy syrup, chunky (*Del Monte*)	100	0	24.0	0	0	10	1.0
Fruit, mixed, candied, 1 oz.	91	.1	23.4	0	0	28	.5
Fruit, mixed, dried, 1.4 oz., ¼ cup, except as noted:							
(*Mariani*)	100	2.0	24.0	0	0	25	3.0
(*Sun•Maid*)	100	1.0	26.0	0	0	35	3.0

Food and Measure	cal.	prot. (gms)	carbo. (gms)	fat (gms)	chol. (mgs)	sod. (mgs)	fiber (gms)
Fruit, mixed, dried (cont.)							
(*Sun•Maid* Bits)	120	1.0	29.0	0	0	20	2.0
(*Sunsweet* Orchard) ..	100	1.0	25.0	0	0	60	3.0
tropical mix:							
(*Sun•Maid* Trio) ...	140	0	34.0	0	0	75	1.0
(*SunRidge Farms*) .	130	2.0	32.0	.5	0	5	4.0
(*Sunsweet*), ⅓ cup	150	0	33.0	2.0	0	30	2.0
Fruit, mixed, frozen, ¾ cup:							
(*C&W* Ultimate)	50	1.0	13.0	0	0	5	2.0
(*Dole*)	60	0	16.0	0	0	0	2.0
(*Dole* Wildly Nutritious)	60	0	16.0	0	0	5	2.0
tropical:							
(*Dole* Island Blend)	70	0	18.0	0	0	15	2.0
(*Dole* Wildly Nutritious)	70	0	17.0	0	0	0	3.0
Fruit bar, frozen (see also "Ice bar," "Iced confection bar," and "Sorbet bar"), 1 bar:							
all varieties:							
(*Breyer's* Pure Fruit/ Pure Fruit Swirl) .	40	0	10.0	0	0	0	0
(*Breyer's* Pure Fruit No Sugar)	25	0	5.0	0	0	0	0
(*Dreyer's/Edy's* Value Pack No Sugar) .	30	0	8.0	0	0	0	1.0
banana:							
(*Blue Bunny*)	35	0	9.0	0	0	5	0
(*Blue Bunny* Goin' Bananas)	150	4.0	29.0	1.5	5	115	0
and cream (*Froz-Fruit*)	160	1.0	27.0	6.0	25	15	1.0
creamy (*Fruit-a-Freeze*) .	120	1.0	19.0	4.0	15	35	<1.0
creamy, chocolate dipped (*Fruit-a-Freeze*)	200	2.0	23.0	12.0	10	40	1.0
cherry (*Edy's* Value Pack)	70	0	17.0	0	0	0	0
coconut:							
(*Breyer's* Pure Fruit)	150	0	31.0	2.5	0	45	1.0
(*Dreyer's/Edy's*) ...	120	3.0	21.0	3.0	0	40	1.0
(*FrozFruit*)	150	1.0	14.0	10.0	25	20	<1.0

Food and Measure	cal.	prot. (gms)	carbo. (gms)	fat (gms)	chol. (mgs)	sod. (mgs)	fiber (gms)
(*Fruit-a-Freeze*) ...	160	2.0	20.0	9.0	15	45	<1.0
(*Palapa Azul*)	80	0	10.0	1.0	0	10	0
grape:							
(*Dreyer's/Edy's*) ...	80	0	20.0	0	0	0	0
(*Edy's* Value Pack) .	70	0	17.0	0	0	0	0
lemon lime swirl							
(*Breyer's* Pure Fruit)	45	0	11.0	0	0	0	0
lemonade (*Dreyer's/ Edy's*)	80	0	20.0	0	0	0	0
lime:							
(*Breyer's* Pure Fruit Single)	110	0	27.0	0	0	10	0
(*Dreyer's/Edy's*) ...	80	0	20.0	0	0	0	0
(*Dreyer's/Edy's* Value Pack)	60	0	13.0	0	0	0	0
(*Fruit-a-Freeze*) ...	70	0	17.0	0	0	0	0
double (*FrozFruit*) .	90	0	22.0	0	0	10	0
mango:							
(*Palapa Azul*)	70	0	18.0	0	0	0	0
(*FrozFruit* Chunky) .	80	0	21.0	0	0	10	<1.0
chili (*Palapa Azul*) .	70	0	17.0	0	0	290	0
pineapple (*Fruit-a- Freeze*)	70	0	16.0	0	0	0	0
orange (*Minute Maid*)	60	0	15.0	0	0	10	0
papaya (*Palapa Azul* Mexican*)	60	0	14.0	0	0	0	1.0
piña colada, creamy (*FrozFruit*)	180	1.0	21.0	10.0	30	20	<1.0
pineapple:							
(*Breyer's* Pure Fruit)	100	0	26.0	0	0	5	0
(*FrozFruit*)	80	0	21.0	0	0	10	<1.0
(*Palapa Azul*)	60	0	15.0	0	0	0	1.0
pomegranate cherry (*FrozFruit Superfruit*)	80	0	19.0	0	0	10	0
raspberry acai (*Froz- Fruit Superfruit*) ...	60	0	15.0	0	0	10	<1.0
strawberry:							
(*Breyer's* Pure Fruit)	45	0	11.0	0	0	0	0
(*Breyer's* Pure Fruit)	100	0	25.0	0	0	10	1.0
(*Dreyer's/Edy's*) ...	80	0	21.0	0	0	0	0
(*Dreyer's/Edy's* Value Pack)	60	0	13.0	0	0	0	0
(*FrozFruit* Chunky) .	70	0	18.0	0	0	10	<1.0
(*FrozFruit* No Sugar)	35	0	15.0	0	0	10	3.0

Food and Measure	cal.	prot. (gms)	carbo. (gms)	fat (gms)	chol. (mgs)	sod. (mgs)	fiber (gms)
Fruit bar, frozen, strawberry *(cont.)*							
(*FrozFruit* Strawberries & Cream)	160	<1.0	27.0	5.0	20	25	<1.0
(*Palapa Azul*)	50	0	13.0	0	0	0	1.0
creamy (*Fruit-a-Freeze*)	130	1.0	22.0	4.0	15	40	0
creamy, chocolate dipped (*Fruit-a-Freeze*)	210	2.0	26.0	12.0	10	40	<1.0
strawberry banana smoothie (*Dreyer's/Edy's*)	100	2.0	20.0	2.0	5	30	3.0
tangerine (*Dreyer's/Edy's*)	80	0	20.0	0	0	0	0
tropical:							
(*Edy's* Value Pack) .	70	0	17.0	0	0	0	0
(*FrozFruit*)	70	0	17.0	0	0	10	<1.0
smoothie (*Dreyer's/Edy's*)	110	2.0	21.0	2.0	5	25	3.0
watermelon (*Palapa Azul*)	50	0	14.0	0	0	0	0
Fruit cocktail, can or jar, ½ cup:							
(*Del Monte Carb Clever*)	40	0	11.0	0	0	10	<1.0
in juice:							
(*Del Monte* 100%) .	60	0	15.0	0	0	10	1.0
(*S&W* Natural Style)	80	0	20.0	0	0	20	2.0
w/liquid	55	.6	14.1	0	0	5	1.2
in extra light syrup (*Del Monte* Lite) . . .	60	0	15.0	0	0	10	1.0
in light syrup:							
(*S&W*)	70	0	18.0	0	0	15	1.0
w/liquid	72	.5	18.8	.1	0	7	1.4
in heavy syrup:							
(*Del Monte*)	100	0	24.0	0	0	10	1.0
w/liquid	91	.5	23.4	.1	0	7	1.2
Fruit crisps (*Flat Earth* Baked), 1 oz.:							
apple cinnamon	130	1.0	21.0	4.5	0	35	2.0
berry, wild	130	1.0	21.0	4.5	0	40	1.0
peach mango	130	1.0	21.0	4.5	0	35	1.0
Fruit dip, 2 tbsp.:							
caramel:							
(*Litehouse*)	110	1.0	25.0	1.5	0	125	0

Food and Measure	cal.	prot. (gms)	carbo. (gms)	fat (gms)	chol. (mgs)	sod. (mgs)	fiber (gms)
(*Litehouse* Lowfat) .	110	1.0	27.0	0	0	140	0
(*Marzetti's* Apple Dip Fat Free)	120	1.0	28.0	0	0	115	0
(*Marzetti's* Apple Dip Light)	100	1.0	26.0	1.5	5	75	0
(*Marzetti's* Apple Dip Old Fashioned) . .	140	0	22.0	6.0	5	75	0
chocolate (*Litehouse* Hershey's)	120	1.0	23.0	3.0	0	120	0
toffee (*Litehouse* Heath)	110	1.0	26.0	1.0	0	150	0
chocolate:							
(*Marzetti's*)	110	1.0	23.0	2.0	0	85	1.0
milk (*Baker's* Real) .	80	1.0	9.0	5.0	0	10	0
semisweet, dark (*Baker's* Real) . . .	70	1.0	9.0	4.5	0	5	1.0
yogurt (*Litehouse* Hershey's)	110	1.0	14.0	6.0	0	95	0
cream cheese:							
(*Marzetti's*)	70	0	10.0	3.0	15	85	0
strawberry (*Marzetti's*)	70	0	9.0	3.5	15	90	0
peanut butter caramel (*Marzetti's* Apple Dip)	120	2.0	17.0	5.0	0	150	1.0
strawberry, yogurt (*Litehouse*)	50	1.0	10.0	1.5	0	45	0
vanilla, yogurt:							
(*Litehouse*)	60	1.0	10.0	1.5	0	50	0
French (*Marzetti's* Light)	45	0	10.0	0	0	45	0
Fruit drink blend (see also specific listings), 8 fl. oz., except as noted:							
(*Odwalla AntioxDance*)	90	0	23.0	0	0	10	0
(*Odwalla Super Protein*)	190	10.0	35.0	1.0	0	180	1.0
(*Odwalla Superfood*) .	130	1.0	30.0	.5	0	10	0
(*Odwalla Superfood Amazing Purple*) . .	140	1.0	29.0	1.5	0	25	2.0
(*V8 Splash* Medley) . .	70	0	19.0	0	0	50	0
all flavors (*Special K₂O* Protein Water), 16 fl. oz.	50	5.0	13.0	0	0	40	5.0

Food and Measure	cal.	prot. (gms)	carbo. (gms)	fat (gms)	chol. (mgs)	sod. (mgs)	fiber (gms)
Fruit drink blend *(cont.)*							
lemon ginger echinacea							
(*Simply Nutritious*)	110	0	27.0	0	0	15	0
punch:							
(*AriZona*)	100	0	26.0	0	0	25	0
(*Capri Sun*)	110	0	30.0	0	0	20	0
(*Hi-C* Blast)	110	0	30.0	0	0	140	0
(*Langers* Cocktail) .	120	0	30.0	0	0	15	0
(*Minute Maid*)	120	0	31.0	0	0	35	0
(*Snapple*)	110	0	29.0	0	0	10	0
(*SoBe Power*)	110	0	27.0	0	0	15	0
(*SoBe Synergy*),							
11.5 fl. oz.	120	0	32.0	0	0	35	0
(*Tropicana*)	130	0	32.0	0	0	15	0
(*Tropicana* Light) . .	10	0	3.0	0	0	5	0
frozen* (*Minute Maid*)	110	0	30.0	0	0	0	0
tropical:							
(*Bolthouse Farms*							
C-Boost Smoothie)	152	1.0	36.0	0	0	15	<1.0
(*Minute Maid*							
Breakfast Blends)	120	0	30.0	0	0	15	0
(*Santa Cruz Organic*							
Box)	110	0	27.0	0	0	5	0
(*Tropical* Smoothie),							
11 fl. oz.	220	1.0	53.0	0	0	15	1.0
(*V8 Splash*)	70	0	18.0	0	0	50	0
colada (*V8 Splash*							
Smoothies)	100	3.0	21.0	0	0	50	1.0
tropical punch:							
(*Minute Maid*)	110	0	30.0	0	0	15	0
(*Tropicana*)	120	0	31.0	0	0	5	0
frozen* (*Minute*							
Maid)	100	0	28.0	0	0	0	0
Fruit glaze, see							
specific fruits							
Fruit juice blend (see							
also specific listings),							
8 fl. oz., except as noted:							
(*Bolthouse Farms* Green							
Goodess)	140	2.0	33.0	0	0	25	1.0
(*Ceres* Medley)	130	0	31.0	0	0	10	2.0
(*Langers* Autumn/							
Spring/Winter Blend)	120	0	30.0	0	0	10	0
(*Langers* Summer Blend)	125	0	31.0	0	0	10	0

Food and Measure	cal.	prot. (gms)	carbo. (gms)	fat (gms)	chol. (mgs)	sod. (mgs)	fiber (gms)
(*Minute Maid* Medley), 10 fl. oz.	140	0	36.0	0	0	26	0
(*Odwalla Mo' Beta*) ..	150	1.0	37.0	0	0	15	1.0
(*Odwalla Wellness*) ..	150	2.0	30.0	1.0	0	35	1.0
(*R.W. Knudsen* Razzleberry)	120	0	30.0	0	0	15	0
(*R.W. Knudsen* Razzleberry Box) ..	120	0	28.0	0	0	15	0
(*Simply Nutritious Mega Antioxidant*) .	120	0	29.0	0	0	20	0
(*Simply Nutritious Mega C*)	140	0	34.0	0	0	15	0
(*Simply Nutritious Mega Green*)	130	1.0	31.0	0	0	35	0
(*Simply Nutritious Morning Blend*) ...	130	1.0	30.0	0	0	25	0
(*Simply Nutritious Plum Boost*)	120	1.0	33.0	0	0	10	0
(*Simply Nutritious Vita Juice*)	120	1.0	31.0	0	0	40	<1.0
punch:							
(*Apple & Eve*)	120	0	29.0	0	0	20	0
(*Apple & Eve Organics*)	100	0	24.0	0	0	25	0
(*Minute Maid*), 6.75 fl. oz.	100	0	24.0	0	0	15	0
(*Mott's*), 6.75 fl.oz.	100	0	25.0	0	0	20	0
(*Snapple*), 11.5 fl. oz.	170	0	42.0	0	0	15	0
(*Tropicana*), 10 fl. oz.	170	<1.0	40.0	0	0	30	0
tropical:							
(*R.W. Knudsen* Juice Box)	120	0	29.0	0	0	15	0
(*Santa Cruz Organic*)	140	1.0	33.0	0	0	10	0
(*Veryfine* Fusion) ..	130	0	31.0	0	0	25	0
and carrot (*Dole Paradise Blend*) .	120	<1.0	29.0	0	0	4	0
Fruit pectin (*Slim Set/ Sure•Jell*), ⅛ tsp ..	0	0	0	0	0	0	0
Fruit protector (*Sure•Jell Ever Fresh*), ⅛ tsp.	5	0	<1.0	0	0	0	0
Fruit sauce, Asian, four (*Heaven and Earth*), 1 tbsp.	100	10.0	5.0	16.0	0	90	0

Food and Measure	cal.	prot. (gms)	carbo. (gms)	fat (gms)	chol. (mgs)	sod. (mgs)	fiber (gms)
Fruit snack (see also specific listings), 1 roll or pkg.:							
all fruits:							
(*Fruit by the Foot*), ¾ oz.	80	0	17.0	1.0	0	50	0
(*Fruit by the Foot Mini Feet*), .4 oz.	45	0	10.0	.5	0	30	0
(*Fruit Gushers*), .8-oz. pouch	90	0	20.0	1.0	0	55	0
(*Fruit Roll-Ups*), .5-oz. roll	50	0	12.0	1.0	0	55	0
(*Tropicana FruitWise*), .7-oz. strip	70	0	17.0	0	0	0	1.0
except apple, apricot, or mango (*Stretch Island* Fruit Leather), .5 oz.	45	0	12.0	0	0	0	1.0
apple (*Stretch Island* Fruit Leather), .5 oz.	45	0	12.0	0	0	5	1.0
apricot or mango (*Stretch Island* Fruit Leather), .5 oz.	45	0	11.0	0	0	0	1.0
cherry berry or orange citrus (*Tropicana FruitWise*), 1.4 oz. .	220	<1.0	36.0	0	0	10	2.0
strawberry (*Tropicana FruitWise*), 1.4 oz. .	140	0	36.0	0	0	10	2.0
Fruit spread (see also "Jam and preserves" and specific listings), all fruits, 1 tbsp.:							
(*Cascadian Farm Organic*)	40	0	10.0	0	0	0	0
(*Polaner* All Fruit) ..	40	0	10.0	0	0	0	0
(*Smucker's Simply Fruit*)	40	0	10.0	0	0	0	0
(*Sorrell Ridge*)	36	0	9.0	0	0	0	0
(*Tree of Life* Organic)	35	0	9.0	0	0	0	0
apricot (*Polaner* Fancy Fruit)	50	0	13.0	0	0	0	0
raspberry, seedless red (*Polaner* Fancy Fruit)	50	0	13.0	0	0	5	0

Food and Measure	cal.	prot. (gms)	carbo. (gms)	fat (gms)	chol. (mgs)	sod. (mgs)	fiber (gms)
strawberry:							
(*Smucker's*)	50	0	13.0	0	0	0	0
(*Smucker's* Reduced Sugar)	20	0	6.0	0	0	0	0
Fruit-nut mix, see "Trail mix"							
Fudge, see "Candy"							
Fudge topping, see "Chocolate topping"							
Fuki, see "Butterbur"							
Fuzzy navel, drink mixer, frozen (*Bacardi*), 2 fl. oz. . .	120	0	33.0	0	0	0	0

G

Food and Measure	cal.	prot. (gms)	carbo. (gms)	fat (gms)	chol. (mgs)	sod. (mgs)	fiber (gms)
Gai choy, see "Cabbage, mustard"							
Gai lan, see "Kale, Chinese"							
Galanga (*Frieda's*), ⅔ cup, 3 oz.	60	1.0	13.0	.5	0	10	2.0
Garbanzo bean:							
dry, ¼ cup:							
(*Arrowhead Mills* Organic)	160	9.0	27.0	2.5	0	10	8.0
(*Shiloh Farms* Organic)	170	10.0	29.0	2.0	0	10	6.0
boiled, ½ cup	134	7.3	22.5	2.1	0	6	2.9
pre-soaked (*Frieda's*), ⅓ cup, 3 oz.	150	7.0	23.0	3.0	0	230	22.0
Garbanzo bean, canned, ½ cup, except as noted:							
(*Allens/East Texas Fair* Chick Peas)	120	5.0	19.0	2.5	0	330	8.0
(*Bush's*)	105	6.0	20.0	2.0	0	470	5.0
(*Eden* Organic)	130	7.0	23.0	1.0	0	30	5.0
(*Progresso* Chick Peas)	100	5.0	17.0	1.5	0	280	4.0
(*Roland*)	110	7.0	20.0	1.0	0	350	7.0
(*S&W*)	80	7.0	19.0	1.0	0	460	5.0
(*S&W* Less Salt)	80	7.0	19.0	1.0	0	220	5.0
(*Westbrae Natural* Organic)	110	6.0	18.0	2.0	0	140	5.0
(*Zapata*), ⅔ cup	120	6.0	20.0	2.0	0	290	8.0
Garbanzo bean dish, pkg., w/potatoes (*Tamarind Tree* Au Chole), 9.25-oz. pkg.	350	12.0	63.0	6.0	0	620	9.0

Food and Measure	cal.	prot. (gms)	carbo. (gms)	fat (gms)	chol. (mgs)	sod. (mgs)	fiber (gms)
Garbanzos, roasted, seasoned (*Baja Express*), ⅓ cup, 1.1 oz.	110	5.0	17.0	3.0	0	210	5.0
Garlic, fresh: (*Frieda's* Elephant), chopped, 1 tbsp. ...	5	0	1.0	0	0	0	0
trimmed, 1 oz.	42	1.8	9.4	.1	0	5	.6
1 clove, .1 oz.	4	.2	1.0	<.1	0	1	.1
granulated/minced, 1 tsp.	13	.7	2.9	0	0	1	0
Garlic, in jars: chopped, in oil (*Delallo*), ¼ oz.	22	.3	1.5	1.8	0	<1	.2
cloves, w/herbs (*Roland*), 2 tbsp.	10	0	2.0	0	0	270	0
crushed (*McCormick* California), 1 tsp. ...	10	0	0	0	0	0	0
minced (*McCormick* California), 1 tsp. ...	15	0	0	.5	0	0	0
puree, regular or roasted, w/olive oil (*Alessi*), 1 tsp.	8	0	0	1.0	0	25	0
roasted: (*McCormick*), 1 tsp.	5	0	0	0	0	0	0
in oil (*Delallo*), ¼ oz.	36	.7	3.0	2.7	0	21	.1
Garlic bread, see "Bread, frozen/ refrigerated"							
Garlic bread sprinkle (*McCormick*), ¼ tsp.	5	0	0	0	0	30	0
Garlic dill dip seasoning (*Watkins*), 1 tsp.	10	0	2.0	0	0	95	0
Garlic herb seasoning: (*McCormick*), ¼ tsp. ..	0	0	0	0	0	50	0
Italian (*McCormick*), 1 tsp.	5	0	0	0	0	0	0
Garlic oil, olive oil (*McCormick*), 1 tsp.	10	0	0	.5	0	0	0
Garlic pâté (*Alessi*), 2 tbsp.	90	1.0	6.0	7.0	0	720	1.0

Food and Measure	cal.	prot. (gms)	carbo. (gms)	fat (gms)	chol. (mgs)	sod. (mgs)	fiber (gms)
Garlic pepper:							
(*McCormick* California), ¼ tsp.	0	0	0	0	0	105	0
(*McCormick* Grinder), ¼ tsp.	0	0	0	0	0	75	0
1 tsp.	8	.3	1.8	0	0	360	.3
w/red bell and black (*McCormick* California Style), ¼ tsp. ...	0	0	0	0	0	105	0
roasted, and bell pepper (*McCormick* Blends), 1 tsp.	10	0	2.0	0	0	370	0
Garlic powder, 1 tsp. ..	10	.5	2.3	0	0	1	0
Garlic relish, Indian, (*Patak's*), 1 tbsp. ...	45	0	4.0	3.0	0	300	0
Garlic salt, ¼ tsp.:							
(*McCormick*)	0	0	0	0	0	490	0
(*McCormick Season-All*)	0	0	0	0	0	260	0
w/parsley (*McCormick*)	0	0	0	0	0	220	0
sea salt (*McCormick* Grinder)	0	0	0	0	0	125	0
Garlic sauce, Asian (*Dai Day*), 2 tbsp. .	96	0	24.0	0	0	500	0
Garlic saffron spread (*Saratoga Garlic*), 1 tbsp.	80	0	<1.0	8.0	<5	60	0
Gefilte fish, in jars, w/out gel, 1 pc.:							
(*Manischewitz*), w/ ¼ carrot, 2.3 oz. ...	90	5.0	6.0	5.0	15	280	<1.0
(*Mother's*), 2 oz.	60	6.0	2.0	3.0	25	190	1.0
(*Yehuda* Sweet), 1.8 oz.	48	3.0	7.0	1.0	10	255	<1.0
whitefish and pike: (*Manischewitz*), 2.3 oz.	50	7.0	3.0	1.5	15	370	<1.0
(*Mother's*), 2 oz. ..	50	7.0	2.0	1.5	20	210	1.0
(*Rokeach*), 2 oz.	50	6.0	2.0	2.0	35	240	1.0
Gefilte fish, frozen, uncooked, except as noted:							
(*Ungar's*), 2 slices, 3/8", 1.8 oz.	65	6.0	3.5	3.0	25	230	0
pike/white, 2 oz.: (*A&B Famous*)	70	7.0	5.0	2.0	65	290	2.0

Food and Measure	cal.	prot. (gms)	carbo. (gms)	fat (gms)	chol. (mgs)	sod. (mgs)	fiber (gms)
(*A&B Famous* Homestyle)	80	6.0	7.0	3.5	50	220	<1.0
precooked (*A&B Famous*), 2 oz.	80	6.2	9.0	2.5	40	170	1.0
salmon:							
(*A&B Famous*), 2 oz.	140	12.0	4.0	8.0	20	260	1.0
(*Ungar's*), 2 slices, 3/8", 1.8 oz.	80	6.0	5.0	4.0	25	250	0
sweet, 2 oz.:							
(*A&B Famous*)	80	6.0	7.0	3.5	50	220	1.0
and savory (*A&B Famous* Hungarian)	80	6.0	9.0	2.5	40	170	1.0
Gelatin, unflavored (*Knox*), ¼ pkt.	5	2.0	0	0	0	0	0
Gelatin dessert, ready- to-eat, 3.5 oz.:							
all fruit flavors:							
(*Jell-O*)	70	1.0	17.0	0	0	40	0
(*Jell-O* Sugar Free) .	10	1.0	0	0	0	45	0
cherry and blue rasp- berry (*Jell-O X-Treme*)	70	0	17.0	0	0	40	0
cherry (*Hunt's Snack Pack* No Sugar) . . .	10	0	2.0	0	0	65	<1.0
fruit w/, see specific fruit listings							
strawberry/orange (*Hunt's Snack Pack*)	100	0	25.0	0	0	45	0
watermelon and green apple (*Jell-O X-Treme*)	100	0	24.0	0	0	45	0
Gelatin dessert mix, ½ cup*:							
all fruit flavors:							
(*Dr. Oetker Trio Treats*)	60	1.0	12.0	1.0	0	20	0
(*Jell-O*)	80	2.0	19.0	0	0	—¹	0
(*Jell-O* Sugar Free) .	10	1.0	0	0	0	—²	0
Gelatin substitute, unflavored (*Lieber's*), ¼ pkt, ½ cup*	80	0	21.0	0	0	45	0

¹*Sodium values vary between 75 and 120 mgs. according to flavor.*
²*Sodium values vary between 45 and 80 mgs. according to flavor.*

Food and Measure	cal.	prot. (gms)	carbo. (gms)	fat (gms)	chol. (mgs)	sod. (mgs)	fiber (gms)
Ginger, trimmed root:							
1 oz.	20	.5	4.3	.2	0	4	.6
chopped (*Frieda's*),							
1 tbsp.	0	0	1.0	0	0	0	0
sliced, ¼ cup	17	.4	3.6	.2	0	3	.5
Ginger, candied or							
crystallized:							
(*Frieda's*), 9 pcs., 1.1 oz.	100	0	26.0	0	0	10	0
(*SunRidge Farms*),							
¼ cup, 1.4 oz.	130	4.0	30.0	3.0	0	15	8.0
slices (*Roland*),							
5 pcs., 1 oz.	100	0	25.0	0	0	23	1.0
Ginger, ground, 1 tsp.	6	.2	1.3	.1	0	1	.2
Ginger, pickled:							
Japanese, 1 oz.	10	.1	2.1	<.1	0	105	0
sliced, w/shiso leaves							
(*Eden* Organic),							
1 tbsp., .5 oz.	20	0	4.0	0	0	100	<1.0
sushi (*Roland* Shoga),							
1 tbsp.	0	0	0	0	0	0	0
Ginger, in syrup, in							
jars (*Roland*), 4 pcs.	80	0	21.0	0	0	5	0
Ginger, Thai, see							
"Galanga"							
Ginger-mint sauce,							
Asian (*Heaven and*							
Earth), 1 tbsp.	35	0	9.0	0	0	10	1.0
Ginkgo nut, shelled:							
raw, 1 oz.	52	1.2	10.7	.5	0	2	<1.0
canned, drained, 1 oz.	32	.6	6.3	.5	0	87	2.6
dried, 1 oz.	99	2.9	20.6	.8	0	4	n.a.
Glacé, see "Fruit,							
mixed, candied"							
Glaze, see specific							
listings							
Glaze sauce, see							
"Grilling sauce" and							
"Marinade"							
Gluten, see "Wheat							
gluten"							
Gnocchi, potato, pkg.:							
(*Alessi*), 1 cup	240	5.0	55.0	.5	0	550	2.0
(*Bellino*), ¾ cup	170	4.0	35.0	1.0	0	660	3.0
(*Pastene*), ¾ cup	170	4.0	35.0	1.0	0	660	3.0

Food and Measure	cal.	prot. (gms)	carbo. (gms)	fat (gms)	chol. (mgs)	sod. (mgs)	fiber (gms)
(*Vigo*), 2 oz.	80	2.0	18.0	9.0	0	253	0
w/spinach (*Bellino*), ¾ cup	214	5.0	38.0	.6	0	680	3.0
Goat, meat only, roasted, 4 oz.	162	30.7	0	3.4	85	98	0
Gobo root, see "Burdock root"							
Goji berries, dried:							
(*Dole*), 1.1 oz.	110	4.0	22.0	0	0	105	2.0
(*Frieda's*), ⅓ pkg., 1 oz.	101	3.0	20.0	1.0	2	121	6.0
(*Shiloh Farms* Himalayan), ¼ cup	170	10.0	29.0	2.0	0	10	6.0
(*Tree of Life* Organic), 1 oz.	110	<4.0	25.0	0	0	130	<5.0
Goji punch (*Snapple*), 8 fl. oz.	80	0	18.0	0	0	25	0
Golden nugget squash (*Frieda's*), ¾ cup, 3 oz.	30	1.0	7.0	0	0	0	1.0
Goose, roasted:							
meat w/skin, 4 oz. ...	346	28.5	0	24.9	103	79	0
meat only, 4 oz.	270	32.9	0	14.4	109	86	0
Goose fat, 1 tbsp. ...	115	0	0	12.8	13	0	0
Goose liver, see "Liver" and "Pâté"							
Gooseberries, fresh, ½ cup	34	.7	7.6	.4	0	1	3.2
Gooseberries, canned, in light syrup (*Oregon*), ½ cup ..	90	<1.0	22.0	0	0	5	3.0
Gourd, boiled, ½ cup:							
dishcloth, 1" slices ...	50	.6	12.8	.3	0	18	<1.0
white-flower, 1" cubes	11	.4	2.7	<.1	0	1	<1.0
Gourd, dried, see "Kanpyo"							
Grains, mixed, whole, dry, ¼ cup:							
w/brown and wild rice (*RiceSelect Royal Blend*)	160	5.0	34.0	1.5	0	5	2.0
w/brown and red rice (*RiceSelect Royal Blend*)	160	4.0	33.0	1.5	0	5	2.0

Food and Measure	cal.	prot. (gms)	carbo. (gms)	fat (gms)	chol. (mgs)	sod. (mgs)	fiber (gms)
Grains, mixed, dish, mix (see also specific listings), 1 cup*:							
brown rice/wheat (*Near East*):							
barley, chicken herb	280	7.0	52.0	6.0	0	780	5.0
bulgur, roasted garlic	220	6.0	41.0	5.0	0	570	5.0
pecan and garlic ...	250	6.0	38.0	9.0	0	540	4.0
seven grain pilaf (*Seeds of Change* Organic)	280	8.0	59.0	2.0	0	770	7.0
wheat pilaf, w/orzo (*Near East*)	200	7.0	40.0	4.5	10	680	8.0
white rice/wheat, creamy Parmesan (*Near East*)	280	8.0	48.0	8.0	20	840	3.0
Grains, mixed, entree, frozen, seven grain Turkish pilaf (*Seeds of Change* Organic), 10-oz. pkg.	310	14.0	46.0	9.0	25	610	5.0
Granadilla, see "Passion fruit"							
Granola, see "Cereal"							
Granola/cereal bar, 1 bar, except as noted:							
(*Cinnamon Toast Crunch* Milk 'n Cereal)	180	3.0	33.0	4.0	0	140	1.0
(*Grape-Nuts* Trail Mix Crunch)	110	2.0	20.0	3.0	0	110	1.0
(*Odwalla Bar!* Super Protein)	230	16.0	31.0	4.5	0	160	4.0
(*Odwalla Bar!* Superfood)	230	4.0	43.0	4.0	0	110	3.0
all varieties (*Health Valley* Trail Mix Granola)	140	3.0	23.0	4.0	0	100	1.0
almond:							
(*Honey Bunches of Oats*)	140	2.0	25.0	4.0	0	100	1.0
(*Nature Valley* Sweet & Salty Granola)	160	3.0	22.0	7.0	0	170	3.0
roasted (*Nature Valley* Granola), 2 bars .	190	4.0	28.0	7.0	0	180	2.0

Food and Measure	cal.	prot. (gms)	carbo. (gms)	fat (gms)	chol. (mgs)	sod. (mgs)	fiber (gms)
sweet and salty (*Odwalla* Chewy Nut Bar)	220	7.0	22.0	11.0	0	65	6.0
toasted (*Barbara's* Crunchy Organic Granola), 2 bars .	200	4.0	27.0	8.0	0	60	3.o
apple:							
(*Back to Nature* Fruit & Grain)	110	2.0	20.0	2.0	0	85	<1.0
baked (*Quaker* Chewy Granola) .	90	1.0	19.0	1.5	0	85	1.0
baked, tarts (*Health Valley* Organic Cereal)	150	2.0	29.0	2.5	0	100	<1.0
cobbler (*Health Valley* Organic Cereal)	140	2.0	27.0	2.5	0	95	1.0
Dutch (*Health Valley* Moist & Chewy Granola)	100	1.0	20.0	1.5	0	10	<1.0
apple cinnamon:							
(*Barbara's* Fruit & Yogurt)	150	3.0	28.0	3.0	0	125	1.0
(*Barbara's Nature's Choice* Cereal) . .	140	2.0	28.0	2.0	0	80	1.0
(*Genisoy* Organic Soy)	160	8.0	26.0	3.0	0	85	2.0
(*Grape-Nuts* Trail Mix Crunch)	110	2.0	22.0	2.0	0	120	2.0
(*Nutri-Grain*)	140	1.0	26.0	3.0	0	105	2.0
(*Quaker* Oatmeal To Go)	220	4.0	43.0	4.0	15	210	5.0
apple crisp (*Nature Valley* Granola), 2 bars	180	4.0	29.0	6.0	0	160	2.0
apricot nut (*Nature's Path* Organic Granola)	160	3.0	26.0	5.0	0	85	2.0
banana bread (*Quaker* Oatmeal To Go) . . .	220	4.0	43.0	4.0	15	220	5.0
banana nut:							
(*Honey Bunches of Oats* Single), 1.23 oz.	140	2.0	24.0	4.0	0	115	1.0

Food and Measure	cal.	prot. (gms)	carbo. (gms)	fat (gms)	chol. (mgs)	sod. (mgs)	fiber (gms)
Granola/cereal bar, banana nut *(cont.)*							
(*Honey Bunches of Oats* 6 Pack), 1 oz.	110	2.0	20.0	3.5	0	80	1.0
(*Odwalla Bar!*)	240	4.0	41.0	6.0	0	115	5.0
walnut (*Back to Nature* Bakery Squares), 1.1 oz.	130	3.0	19.0	5.0	0	60	2.0
berry:							
(*Odwalla Bar! Berries GoMega*)	220	5.0	41.0	4.5	0	230	5.0
harvest (*Cascadian Farm* Granola Organic)	130	2.0	27.0	2.0	0	130	1.0
mixed (*Genisoy* Organic Soy) ...	160	8.0	26.0	3.0	0	85	2.0
mixed (*Nature Valley* Trail Mix)	140	2.0	26.0	3.5	0	80	1.0
mixed (*Nutri-Grain*)	140	1.0	26.0	3.0	0	105	<1.0
triple (*Barbara's Nature's Choice* Cereal)	150	2.0	29.0	2.0	0	85	2.0
wild (*Health Valley* Moist & Chewy Granola)	110	1.0	22.0	1.5	0	10	<1.0
berry and almond (*Nutri-Grain* Fruit & Nut)	120	3.0	22.0	3.5	0	100	3.0
blueberry:							
(*Barbara's Nature's Choice* Cereal) ..	150	2.0	29.0	2.0	0	85	2.0
(*Nutri-Grain*)	140	1.0	26.0	3.0	0	105	2.0
(*Special K*)	90	1.0	18.0	1.5	0	95	<1.0
apple (*Barbara's* Fruit & Yogurt)	150	3.0	29.0	3.0	0	125	1.0
cobbler (*Health Valley* Organic Cereal)	140	2.0	27.0	2.5	0	90	1.0
flax/soy (*Nature's Path Optimum Energy Organic*) .	200	7.0	37.0	3.0	0	115	5.0
tarts (*Health Valley* Organic Cereal) .	150	2.0	29.0	2.5	0	95	<1.0
brown sugar cinnamon:							
(*All-Bran*)	130	2.0	27.0	3.0	0	180	5.0

Food and Measure	cal.	prot. (gms)	carbo. (gms)	fat (gms)	chol. (mgs)	sod. (mgs)	fiber (gms)
(*Quaker* Oatmeal To Go)	220	4.0	43.0	4.0	15	230	5.0
(*Quaker Simple Harvest* Granola)	140	2.0	28.0	3.0	0	90	2.0
frosted (*Go-Tarts!*)	140	1.0	24.0	4.0	0	140	<1.0
caramel apple (*Save the Forest* Organic) ...	150	3.0	32.0	2.0	5	45	2.0
caramel chocolately chunk (*Rice Krispies Treats*)	180	1.0	31.0	5.0	<5	170	<1.0
caramel peanut (*Go-Lean* Roll!)	200	12.0	29.0	5.0	0	210	6.0
carob chip (*Barbara's Nature's Choice* Granola)	80	2.0	15.0	2.0	0	0	<1.0
carrot (*Odwalla Bar!*) .	220	4.0	43.0	4.0	0	115	4.0
cashew (*Nature Valley* Sweet & Salty Granola)	160	2.0	22.0	7.0	0	150	1.0
cherry:							
(*Barbara's Nature's Choice* Cereal) ..	150	2.0	28.0	2.0	0	80	1.0
(*Nutri-Grain*)	140	1.0	26.0	3.0	0	100	<1.0
red, tart (*Health Valley* Organic Cereal)	150	2.0	29.0	2.5	0	95	<1.0
cherry apple (*Barbara's* Fruit & Yogurt)	150	3.0	29.0	3.0	0	125	1.0
cherry pecan (*Back to Nature* Chewy Trail Mix), 1 oz.	120	2.0	19.0	5.0	0	70	2.0
chocolate:							
(*Genisoy* Protein Crunch)	150	15.0	16.0	7.0	0	280	1.0
(*Honey Bunches of Oats*)	140	2.0	26.0	3.0	0	150	1.0
(*Kudos M&M's* Granola)	100	1.0	17.0	3.0	0	80	1.0
(*Kudos Snickers* Granola)	100	1.0	16.0	3.0	0	70	1.0
(*South Beach Living* Cereal)	140	10.0	15.0	5.0	0	150	3.0
(*Special K* Chocolately Drizzle) ...	90	1.0	17.0	1.5	0	105	1.0

Food and Measure	cal.	prot. (gms)	carbo. (gms)	fat (gms)	chol. (mgs)	sod. (mgs)	fiber (gms)
Granola/cereal bar, chocolate *(cont.)*							
(*Special K* Snack Bar Delight)	110	4.0	16.0	3.0	0	80	<1.0
almond (*GoLean Crunchy!*)	170	8.0	27.0	5.0	0	210	5.0
almond or peanut (*Kellogg's Crunchy Sweet & Salty Granola*)	150	3.0	18.0	8.0	0	160	2.0
almond toffee (*Go-Lean* Chewy) . . .	290	13.0	45.0	6.0	0	250	6.0
caramel (*Genisoy Ultra*)	150	8.0	26.0	2.0	0	120	3.0
caramel (*GoLean Crunchy!*)	150	8.0	28.0	3.0	0	220	6.0
crème (*Hershey's SnackBarz*)	120	1.0	17.0	6.0	0	65	0
dark (*CocoaVia Granola*)	80	2.0	13.0	2.0	0	65	1.0
dark, almond (*CocoaVia* Granola)	80	1.0	13.0	2.0	0	60	1.0
dark, cherry (*Quaker* Chewy Granola) .	90	1.0	19.0	2.0	0	75	1.0
double (*Genisoy Natural Choice*) .	170	13.0	21.0	4.5	0	230	2.0
double (*Special K Protein Meal*) . . .	180	10.0	24.0	6.0	0	230	5.0
double (*Special K Protein Meal Variety Pack*) . . .	170	10.0	25.0	4.5	0	190	5.0
fudge, frosted (*Go-Tarts!*)	140	1.0	24.0	4.0	0	150	<1.0
fudge brownie (*Genisoy*)	240	14.0	35.0	5.0	0	210	2.0
mint, crispy (*Genisoy*)	240	14.0	37.0	4.5	0	150	2.0
peanut (*GoLean Crunchy!*)	180	9.0	30.0	5.0	0	250	6.0
peanut (*GoLean Roll!*)	190	12.0	28.0	5.0	0	230	6.0
peanut (*Snickers Marathon Energy Chewy*)	220	13.0	27.0	7.0	5	240	2.0

Food and Measure	cal.	prot. (gms)	carbo. (gms)	fat (gms)	chol. (mgs)	sod. (mgs)	fiber (gms)
peanut butter (*Genisoy* Natural Choice)	180	13.0	21.0	5.0	0	240	3.0
peanut butter (*Special K* Protein Meal) .	180	10.0	25.0	4.5	0	190	5.0
pretzel (*GoLean* Crunchy!)	160	11.0	28.0	3.0	0	250	5.0
w/pretzel (*Hershey's* Sweet & Salty Granola)	140	3.0	22.0	5.0	0	240	1.0
rich (*Genisoy* Organic Soy) . . .	160	9.0	25.0	3.0	0	85	3.0
raspberry (*Genisoy* Ultra)	160	11.0	28.0	2.0	0	115	3.0
tarts (*Health Valley* Organic Cereal) .	150	2.0	29.0	3.0	0	85	<1.0
turtle (*GoLean* Roll!)	190	12.0	28.0	5.0	0	200	6.0
chocolate chip/chunk:							
(*Cascadian Farm* Granola Organic)	140	2.0	25.0	3.0	0	125	1.0
(*Genisoy* Protein) . .	150	15.0	18.0	6.0	0	280	2.0
(*Health Valley* Low Fat Granola)	160	2.0	32.0	2.5	0	20	<1.0
(*Health Valley* Moist & Chewy Granola)	110	1.0	22.0	2.0	0	10	<1.0
(*Kudos* Granola) . . .	100	1.0	20.0	3.5	0	70	1.0
(*Odwalla Bar!* Chocowalla)	240	5.0	42.0	6.0	0	80	5.0
(*Quaker* Chewy Granola)	90	1.0	19.0	2.0	0	80	1.0
(*Quaker Chewy Dipps*)	140	2.0	22.0	5.0	0	80	1.0
(*Special K* Protein Meal)	180	10.0	25.0	4.0	0	190	5.0
(*Special K* Protein Meal Variety Pack)	170	10.0	24.0	6.0	0	230	5.0
dark (*Quaker Simple Harvest* Granola)	150	2.0	26.0	4.5	0	95	2.0
double (*Rice Krispies Treats*)	100	1.0	15.0	3.5	0	75	<1.0
frosted (*Go-Tarts!*)	140	1.0	24.0	4.5	0	140	<1.0
peanut (*Odwalla Bar!*)	250	8.0	38.0	7.0	0	180	4.0
cinnamon:							
(*Nature Valley* Granola), 2 bars .	180	4.0	29.0	6.0	0	160	2.0

Food and Measure	cal.	prot. (gms)	carbo. (gms)	fat (gms)	chol. (mgs)	sod. (mgs)	fiber (gms)
Granola/cereal bar, cinnamon *(cont.)*							
coffee cake (*GoLean Crunchy!*)	160	11.0	28.0	3.0	0	250	5.0
crisp (*Barbara's Crunchy Organic Granola*), 2 bars .	190	4.0	27.0	8.0	0	60	3.0
raisin (*South Beach Living* Cereal) . . .	140	10.0	15.0	5.0	5	150	3.0
cocoa (*Rice Krispies*) .	100	1.0	17.0	2.5	0	70	<1.0
cookies and cream:							
(*Genisoy* Natural Choice)	170	13.0	20.0	4.5	0	240	2.0
(*Genisoy* Soy Protein)	240	14.0	35.0	4.5	0	250	1.0
(*GoLean* Chewy) . .	290	13.0	50.0	6.0	0	200	6.0
cranberry:							
(*Nature's Path Optimum* Energy Zen Organic)	200	6.0	37.0	3.0	0	140	5.0
(*Odwalla Bar! Cranberry C Monster*)	220	4.0	44.0	3.0	0	85	3.0
cranberry almond:							
(*Back to Nature* Trail Mix)	120	2.0	19.0	4.5	0	70	2.0
(*Honey Bunches of Oats*)	110	2.0	20.0	3.0	0	80	1.0
(*South Beach Living* Granola)	140	10.0	15.0	5.0	0	135	3.0
cranberry and:							
ginger (*Nature's Path* Organic Granola)	160	3.0	27.0	4.0	0	75	3.0
raisins and peanut (*Nutri-Grain* Fruit & Nut)	120	3.0	22.0	3.5	0	115	3.0
date almond (*Health Valley* Low Fat Granola)	150	1.0	32.0	2.5	0	25	<1.0
fig cobbler (*Health Valley* Organic Cereal)	130	2.0	26.0	2.5	0	80	2.0
fruit and nut:							
(*Cascadian Farm* Granola Organic)	140	2.0	24.0	4.0	0	110	1.0
(*Nature Valley* Trail Mix)	140	3.0	25.0	4.0	0	80	1.0

Food and Measure	cal.	prot. (gms)	carbo. (gms)	fat (gms)	chol. (mgs)	sod. (mgs)	fiber (gms)
fudge sundae (*GoLean* Roll!)	190	12.0	27.0	5.0	0	260	6.0
honey almond flax (*TLC* Chewy Granola)	140	7.0	19.0	5.0	0	115	4.0
honey nut:							
(*Cheerios Crunch* Milk 'n Cereal)	160	3.0	28.0	4.0	0	120	1.0
(*Nature Valley* Healthy Heart Granola)	160	3.0	28.0	4.0	0	115	3.0
(*Quaker* Chewy Granola)	90	1.0	19.0	2.0	0	80	1.0
(*Special K*)	90	2.0	18.0	2.0	0	110	<1.0
roasted (*Quaker Simple Harvest*)	160	3.0	23.0	7.0	0	115	2.0
honey oat (*All-Bran*)	130	2.0	26.0	3.0	0	180	5.0
honey peanut yogurt (*Genisoy*)	250	14.0	36.0	6.0	0	160	1.0
lemon tart (*Genisoy* Natural Choice)	170	12.0	23.0	4.0	0	210	2.0
malted chocolate crisp (*GoLean* Chewy)	290	13.0	49.0	6.0	0	200	6.0
maple (*Country Choice* Organic Oatmeal Squares)	210	4.0	41.0	3.0	0	180	4.0
maple brown sugar (*Nature Valley* Granola), 2 bars	180	4.0	29.0	6.0	0	160	2.0
maple nut (*South Beach Living*)	140	10.0	15.0	5.0	5	160	3.0
mocha fudge, café (*Genisoy*)	230	14.0	34.0	4.0	0	150	1.0
multigrain:							
(*Cascadian Farm* Granola Organic)	130	2.0	27.0	2.0	0	150	1.0
(*Snickers* Marathon Energy Crunch)	220	10.0	32.0	7.0	5	210	2.0
nut, mixed, roasted (*Nature Valley* Sweet & Salty)	160	3.0	21.0	8.0	0	150	1.0
oatmeal (*Honey Maid*)	150	2.0	24.0	6.0	0	160	1.0
oatmeal raisin:							
(*All-Bran*)	120	2.0	27.0	2.5	0	170	5.0
(*Back to Nature* Bakery Squares)	120	3.0	20.0	4.0	0	60	1.0

Food and Measure	cal.	prot. (gms)	carbo. (gms)	fat (gms)	chol. (mgs)	sod. (mgs)	fiber (gms)
Granola/cereal bar, oatmeal raisin *(cont.)*							
(*Country Choice* Organic Oatmeal Squares)	180	4.0	41.0	3.0	0	180	4.0
(*Honey Maid*)	150	2.0	24.0	6.0	0	140	1.0
(*Nature Valley* Healthy Heart Granola)	150	3.0	30.0	2.0	0	95	3.0
(*Quaker* Chewy Granola)	90	1.0	19.0	1.5	0	80	1.0
(*Quaker* Oatmeal to Go)	220	4.0	43.0	4.0	15	240	5.0
(*Uncle Sam* Cereal)	180	9.0	28.0	3.0	0	135	3.0
cookie (*GoLean*) ...	280	13.0	49.0	5.0	0	140	6.0
oatmeal walnut (*GoLean* Roll!)	190	12.0	27.0	5.0	0	250	6.0
oats and:							
chocolate (*Fiber One* Chewy)	140	2.0	29.0	4.0	0	90	9.0
honey (*Barbara's* Crunchy Organic Granola), 2 bars .	190	4.0	27.0	8.0	0	60	3.0
honey (*Nature Valley* Granola), 2 bars .	180	4.0	29.0	6.0	0	160	2.0
nuts, honey (*Quaker* Sweet & Salty Crunch Granola), 2 bars	150	3.0	24.0	5.0	0	210	2.0
peanut butter (*Fiber One* Chewy)	140	3.0	28.0	4.5	0	105	9.0
orange chocolate (*Nature's Path Optimum* Energy Bar Organic)	220	5.0	37.0	6.0	0	120	4.0
peaches and berries (*Special K*)	90	1.0	18.0	2.0	0	85	<1.0
peanut:							
(*Nature Valley* Sweet & Salty Granola)	170	4.0	19.0	9.0	0	150	2.0
honey roasted (*Quaker* Sweet & Salty Crunch), 2 bars	150	3.0	23.0	6.0	0	170	2.0

Food and Measure	cal.	prot. (gms)	carbo. (gms)	fat (gms)	chol. (mgs)	sod. (mgs)	fiber (gms)
roasted or nut medley (*South Beach Living* Granola)	150	6.0	18.0	7.0	0	180	3.0
sweet and salty (*Odwalla* Chewy Nut Bar)	190	5.0	28.0	6.0	0	180	2.0
peanut butter:							
(*Barbara's* Crunchy Organic Granola), 2 bars	200	4.0	26.0	9.0	0	55	3.0
(*Genisoy* Protein)	150	15.0	18.0	4.5	0	260	2.0
(*Hershey's Snack-Barz*)	120	2.0	16.0	5.0	0	95	<1.0
(*Kellogg's Crunchy* Sweet & Salty Granola)	150	4.0	17.0	8.0	0	160	2.0
(*Kudos* Granola)	100	2.0	18.0	6.0	0	75	1.0
(*Nature Valley* Granola), 2 bars	180	5.0	30.0	7.0	0	190	2.0
(*Nature's Path* Organic Granola)	160	4.0	25.0	5.0	0	100	2.0
(*Nature's Path Optimum* Energy Bar Organic)	190	10.0	33.0	4.0	0	140	4.0
(*Quaker* Chewy Granola)	90	1.0	18.0	2.0	0	115	1.0
(*Quaker Chewy Dipps*)	150	2.0	19.0	7.0	0	100	1.0
(*Reese's* Sweet & Salty Granola)	240	7.0	26.0	13.0	0	260	2.0
(*South Beach Living* Cereal)	140	10.0	15.0	5.0	0	160	3.0
all varieties (*Health Valley*)	130	2.0	26.0	2.5	0	140	1.0
chip (*Cascadian Farm* Organic)	140	2.0	25.0	4.0	0	130	1.0
and chocolate (*GoLean* Chewy)	290	13.0	48.0	6.0	0	280	6.0
w/chocolate (*Reese's* Sweet & Salty Granola)	160	4.0	18.0	9.0	0	170	1.0
chocolately (*Rice Krispies Treats*)	100	1.0	15.0	3.5	0	90	<1.0
fudge (*Genisoy*)	240	14.0	34.0	7.0	0	130	2.0

Food and Measure	cal.	prot. (gms)	carbo. (gms)	fat (gms)	chol. (mgs)	sod. (mgs)	fiber (gms)
Granola/cereal bar, peanut butter *(cont.)*							
peanut (*TLC* Chewy Granola)	140	7.0	19.0	5.0	0	90	4.0
peanut crunch:							
(*Health Valley* Moist & Chewy Granola)	110	2.0	21.0	2.5	0	85	<1.0
(*Odwalla Bar!*)	240	8.0	37.0	7.0	0	210	3.0
pecan crunch (*Nature Valley* Granola), 2 bars	190	4.0	29.0	7.0	0	170	2.0
pomegranate cherry (*Nature's Path Optimum* Energy Organic)	230	4.0	39.0	5.0	0	140	4.0
pumpkin and flax:							
(*Nature's Path Flax Plus* Organic Granola)	150	3.0	27.0	3.5	0	90	2.0
spice (*TLC* Crunchy Granola), 2 bars .	180	6.0	26.0	6.0	0	150	4.0
w/raisins and hemp (*Nature's Path Hemp Plus* Organic Granola)	130	3.0	28.0	3.0	0	100	2.0
raspberry:							
(*Barbara's Nature's Choice* Cereal) ..	150	2.0	29.0	2.0	0	85	2.0
(*Genisoy* Protein) ..	150	15.0	19.0	4.5	0	220	2.0
(*Nutri-Grain*)	140	1.0	26.0	3.0	0	105	<1.0
streusel (*Quaker* Oatmeal to Go) ..	220	4.0	23.0	4.0	15	220	5.0
tarts (*Health Valley* Organic Cereal) .	150	2.0	30.0	3.0	0	95	<1.0
strawberry:							
(*Back to Nature* Fruit & Grain), 1.1 oz.	120	2.0	22.0	2.5	0	85	<1.0
(*Barbara's Nature's Choice* Cereal) ..	150	2.0	29.0	2.0	0	85	2.0
(*Genisoy* Ultra)	160	7.0	27.0	2.0	0	160	3.0
(*Honey Bunches of Oats* Single), 1.23 oz.	140	2.0	25.0	3.0	0	110	1.0
(*Honey Bunches of Oats* 6 Pack), 1 oz.	110	2.0	20.0	2.5	0	90	1.0
(*Nutri-Grain*)	140	1.0	26.0	3.0	0	120	2.0
(*Special K*)	90	1.0	18.0	1.5	0	95	<1.0

Food and Measure	cal.	prot. (gms)	carbo. (gms)	fat (gms)	chol. (mgs)	sod. (mgs)	fiber (gms)
(*Special K* Snack Bites), .8 oz. ...	90	1.0	18.0	2.0	0	130	<1.0
(*Special K* Protein Meal)	180	10.0	24.0	5.0	0	150	5.0
cobbler (*Health Valley* Organic Cereal)	130	2.0	26.0	2.5	0	85	1.0
frosted (*Go-Tarts!*)	140	1.0	25.0	3.5	0	140	<1.0
tarts (*Health Valley* Organic Cereal) .	140	2.0	28.0	2.5	0	95	<1.0
vanilla (*Quaker* Chewy Granola) .	90	1.0	19.0	1.5	0	75	1.0
strawberry apple (*Barbara's* Fruit & Yogurt)	150	3.0	28.0	3.0	0	125	1.0
strawberry pomegranate (*Odwalla Bar!*)	220	4.0	44.0	3.0	0	95	4.0
trail mix bar:							
(*Odwalla* Chewy Nut)	190	5.0	27.0	7.0	0	65	3.0
(*TLC* Chewy Granola)	140	6.0	20.0	5.0	0	105	4.0
tropical (*Genisoy* Ultra)	160	7.0	27.0	2.0	0	170	3.0
vanilla:							
chip (*Cascadian Farm* Organic) ..	140	2.0	26.0	3.0	0	95	1.0
crème sandwich (*Café Creations*) .	130	2.0	28.0	2.0	0	80	1.0
crisp (*Special K*) ..	90	2.0	17.0	1.5	0	100	<1.0
nut (*Nature Valley* Granola), 2 bars .	190	4.0	28.0	7.0	0	160	2.0
yogurt:							
blueberry, lemon, or strawberry (*Nature Valley* Granola)	140	2.0	26.0	3.5	0	110	1.0
strawberry or vanilla (*Nutri-Grain*) ...	140	1.0	26.0	3.0	0	105	1.0
strawberry vanilla (*GoLean* Cereal) .	290	13.0	50.0	5.0	0	200	6.0
vanilla (*Nature Valley* Granola)	140	2.0	26.0	3.5	0	130	1.0
Grape, fresh:							
(*Dole* Green), 1½ cups	90	1.0	24.0	1.0	0	0	1.0
(*Frieda's* Champagne), ½ cup, 3 oz.	50	1.0	15.0	0	0	0	1.0
American type (slipskin): 10 medium	15	.2	4.1	.1	0	tr.	.3

Food and Measure	cal.	prot. (gms)	carbo. (gms)	fat (gms)	chol. (mgs)	sod. (mgs)	fiber (gms)
Grape, fresh, American type (cont.)							
peeled and seeded, ½ cup	29	.3	7.9	.2	0	1	.6
European type (adherent skin):							
seeded, 1 lb.	287	2.7	72.0	2.3	0	7	2.7
seedless, 10 medium	36	.3	8.9	.3	0	1	.3
seedless or seeded, ½ cup	57	.5	14.2	.5	0	2	.5
Grape, canned, seedless, ½ cup:							
in light syrup (*Oregon Thompson*)	100	<1.0	23.0	0	0	0	1.0
in heavy syrup, w/liquid	94	.6	25.1	.1	0	6	.5
Grape drink, 8 fl. oz., except as noted:							
(*Apple & Eve* Concord)	130	0	35.0	0	0	10	0
(*Lincoln*)	130	0	32.0	0	0	45	0
(*Nantucket Nectars* Organic Concord) ..	130	0	31.0	0	0	35	0
(*Newman's Own* Gorilla Grape)	140	0	34.0	0	0	140	0
(*Santa Cruz Organic* Box)	100	0	23.0	0	0	10	0
(*SoBe Synergy*), 11.5 fl. oz.	120	0	32.0	0	0	10	0
(*Tropicana*)	150	<1.0	38.0	0	0	25	0
cocktail, frozen* (*Minute Maid*)	120	0	33.0	0	0	5	0
grapeade:							
(*AriZona*)	120	0	31.0	0	0	20	0
(*Nantucket Nectars*)	140	0	33.0	0	0	25	0
(*Snapple*)	120	0	29.0	0	0	10	0
punch:							
(*Minute Maid*)	120	0	32.0	0	0	15	0
(*Tropicana*)	120	0	29.0	0	0	25	0
white (*SoBe Elixir 3C* Concord)	120	0	31.0	0	0	25	0
Grape juice, 8 fl. oz., except as noted:							
(*Apple & Eve*), 6.75 fl. oz.	110	0	29.0	0	0	20	0
(*Apple & Eve Organics* Vintage Concord) ..	160	0	40.0	0	0	15	0

Food and Measure	cal.	prot. (gms)	carbo. (gms)	fat (gms)	chol. (mgs)	sod. (mgs)	fiber (gms)
(*Dole* Single Serve),							
15.2 fl. oz.	290	1.0	72.0	0	0	15	0
(*Fragile Planet* Organic)	160	0	40.0	0	0	15	0
(*Kedem*), 6.6 fl. oz. .	120	<1.0	29.0	0	0	15	0
(*L&A/Langers* Plus) ..	160	0	40.0	0	0	15	0
(*Minute Maid*), 10 fl. oz.	150	0	39.0	0	0	25	0
(*Mott's*), 6.75 fl. oz. ..	60	0	16.0	0	0	5	0
(*R.W. Knudsen*)	150	<1.0	37.0	0	0	15	0
(*R.W. Knudsen* Box) .	130	1.0	32.0	0	0	15	0
(*R.W. Knudsen*							
Concord Natural/							
Organic/Kosher/*Just*							
Concord Grape) ...	160	<1.0	40.0	0	0	15	0
(*Santa Cruz Organic*							
Concord)	160	<1.0	40.0	0	0	15	0
(*Snapple*), 11.5 fl. oz.	170	0	43.0	0	0	15	0
(*Welch's*)	170	0	42.0	0	0	20	0
frozen*:							
(*Cascadian Farm*							
Organic)	150	0	38.0	0	0	5	0
sweetened	128	.5	31.9	.2	0	5	.3
sparkling (*R.W. Knud-*							
sen Kosher)	120	<1.0	30.0	0	0	25	0
white grape:							
(*Langers* Plus)	160	0	40.0	0	0	15	0
(*Santa Cruz Organic*)	160	<1.0	39.0	0	0	10	0
(*Welch's*)	160	0	39.0	0	0	20	0
Grape juice blend, 8 fl. oz.,							
except as noted:							
acai (*Mountain Sun*) .	130	0	33.0	0	0	20	0
white grape:							
cherry (*Welch's*) ...	140	0	35.0	0	0	15	0
mango passion fruit	160	0	41.0	0	0	15	0
peach (*Welch's*) ...	160	0	39.0	0	0	15	0
pomegranate							
(*Welch's*)	140	0	36.0	0	0	15	0
raspberry (*Apple &*							
Eve), 6.75 fl. oz. .	100	0	21.0	0	0	15	0
Grape juice concen-							
trate, Concord (*Tree*							
of Life), 9 tsp.	160	<1.0	40.0	0	0	15	0
Grape leaves, fresh:							
1 cup	13	.8	2.4	.3	0	1	1.5
1 leaf	3	.2	.5	<.1	0	<1	.3

Food and Measure	cal.	prot. (gms)	carbo. (gms)	fat (gms)	chol. (mgs)	sod. (mgs)	fiber (gms)
Grape leaves, in jar							
(*Roland*), 3 leaves .	10	<1.0	2.0	0	0	480	0
Grape leaves, stuffed:							
(*Cedar's*), ½ cup, 5 oz.	260	3.0	26.0	16.0	0	940	7.0
(*Peloponnese* Dolmas),							
6 pcs.	180	3.0	20.0	8.0	0	650	3.0
(*Roland*), 5 pcs., 4.7 oz.	210	3.0	19.0	14.0	5	510	3.0
Grapefruit, fresh:							
(*Chiquita*), ½ medium	60	1.0	16.0	0	0	0	6.0
(*Del Monte*), ½ medium,							
5.4 oz.	60	1.0	16.0	0	0	0	6.0
all areas/varieties:							
½ large, 4.7 oz. . . .	53	1.1	13.4	.2	0	0	1.8
sections, 1 cup . . .	74	1.5	18.6	.2	0	0	2.5
all areas, pink/red:							
½ medium, 3¾" . . .	37	.7	9.5	.1	0	0	n.a.
sections, 1 cup . . .	69	1.3	17.7	.2	0	0	n.a.
all areas, white:							
½ medium, 3¾" . . .	39	.8	9.9	.1	0	0	1.3
sections, 1 cup . . .	76	1.3	17.7	.2	0	0	2.5
California/Arizona:							
pink/red, ½ medium,							
3¾"	46	.6	11.9	.1	0	1	1.4
pink/red, sections							
w/juice, 1 cup . .	85	1.2	22.3	.2	0	2	2.6
white, ½ medium,							
3¾"	43	1.0	10.7	.1	0	0	1.3
white, sections,							
w/juice, 1 cup . .	85	2.0	20.9	.2	0	0	2.6
Florida:							
pink/red, ½ medium,							
3¾"	37	.7	9.2	.1	0	0	1.4
pink/red, sections							
w/juice, 1 cup . .	69	1.3	17.3	.2	0	0	2.5
white, ½ medium,							
3¾"	38	.7	9.7	.1	0	0	.2
white, sections							
w/juice, 1 cup . .	74	1.5	18.8	.2	0	0	.4
Grapefruit, can/jar,							
all varieties, ½ cup,							
except as noted:							
in extra light syrup, red							
(*Del Monte Fruit*							
Naturals)	60	0	16.0	0	0	15	<1.0

Food and Measure	cal.	prot. (gms)	carbo. (gms)	fat (gms)	chol. (mgs)	sod. (mgs)	fiber (gms)
in light syrup:							
(*Roland*), ⅔ cup ..	100	0	24.0	0	0	25	0
red (*Del Monte*) ...	90	1.0	21.0	0	0	0	1.0
red (*SunFresh*)	80	1.0	19.0	0	0	10	2.0
w/liquid	76	.7	19.6	.1	0	3	.5
in water (*Roland*),							
⅔ cup	50	0	14.0	0	0	25	0
and orange sections,							
in syrup (*Roland*),							
⅔ cup	100	0	24.0	0	0	25	0
Grapefruit, Chinese,							
see "Pummelo"							
Grapefruit drink, ruby							
red, except as							
noted, 8 fl. oz.:							
(*Apple & Eve*)	130	0	32.0	0	0	10	0
(*Langers*)	130	0	33.0	0	0	10	0
(*Langers* Diet)	40	0	8.0	0	0	10	0
(*Langers* Low Carb) ..	40	0	10.0	0	0	10	0
(*Minute Maid*)	130	0	34.0	0	0	20	0
(*Ocean Spray* Cock-							
tail)	120	0	31.0	0	0	65	0
(*Ocean Spray* Light							
Ruby)	40	0	10.0	0	0	65	0
(*Tropicana*)	130	1.0	31.0	0	0	15	0
pink (*Tropicana Fruit							
Squeeze*), 15.2 fl. oz.	35	0	9.0	0	0	50	0
sweet (*Tropicana Pure							
Premium*)	130	1.0	31.0	0	0	20	0
Grapefruit juice, 8 fl. oz.,							
except as noted:							
(*Ocean Spray* White) .	90	0	21.0	0	0	35	0
(*Odwalla*)	90	2.0	20.0	0	0	5	0
(*R.W. Knudsen*)	100	1.0	24.0	0	0	10	0
(*R.W. Knudsen* Organic)	100	1.0	23.0	0	0	5	0
(*Simply Grapefruit*) ..	90	1.0	21.0	0	0	10	0
golden or ruby red							
(*Tropicana Pure							
Premium*)	90	1.0	22.0	0	0	0	0
pink:							
(*Ocean Spray* Blend)	110	0	28.0	0	0	35	0
(*Organic Valley*) ...	90	1.0	21.0	0	0	0	0
(*Tree Ripe*)	100	1.0	24.0	0	0	0	0

Food and Measure	cal.	prot. (gms)	carbo. (gms)	fat (gms)	chol. (mgs)	sod. (mgs)	fiber (gms)
Grapefruit juice *(cont.)*							
ruby red:							
(*Dole* Single Serve),							
15.2 fl. oz.	260	1.0	63.0	0	0	30	0
(*Florida's Natural*							
Calcium)	90	1.0	22.0	0	0	0	0
(*Ocean Spray* Blend)	130	0	32.0	0	0	35	0
(*R.W. Knudsen* Rio							
Red)	140	1.0	35.0	0	0	15	0
(*Tropicana*), 10 fl. oz.	170	0	42.0	0	0	20	0
canned, unsweetened	94	1.3	22.1	.3	0	3	.3
fresh, pink or white . .	96	1.2	22.7	.3	0	3	.3
frozen*:							
(*Minute Maid*)	100	0	25.0	0	0	0	0
unsweetened	101	1.4	24.0	.3	0	3	.3
Gravlax, see "Salmon,							
marinated"							
Gravy, see specific							
listings							
Gravy, country style							
canned (*Campbell's*):							
cream, ¼ cup	45	1.0	3.0	3.0	5	190	0
sausage, ¼ cup	70	2.0	4.0	5.0	5	270	0
Gravy mix (see also							
specific gravy							
listings), ¼ cup*:							
country style:							
(*McCormick* Original)	50	0	4.0	3.5	0	260	0
peppered (*McCor-*							
mick)	45	0	4.0	2.5	5	240	0
sausage flavor (*Mc-*							
Cormick)	45	0	4.0	3.0	0	300	0
homestyle (*McCormick*)	25	0	4.0	1.0	0	280	0
for steak:							
chipotle, savory							
(*McCormick*) . . .	40	0	4.0	1.5	0	430	0
cracked peppercorn							
(*McCormick*) . . .	35	0	5.0	.5	0	380	0
roasted garlic (*Mc-*							
Cormick)	35	0	5.0	.5	0	350	0
Great northern bean:							
dry (*Shiloh Farms*							
Organic), ¼ cup . . .	160	10.0	29.0	.5	0	5	18.0
boiled, ½ cup	104	7.3	18.6	.4	0	2	6.2

Food and Measure	cal.	prot. (gms)	carbo. (gms)	fat (gms)	chol. (mgs)	sod. (mgs)	fiber (gms)
Great northern bean, canned, ½ cup:							
(*Allens*)	100	6.0	19.0	.5	0	310	7.0
(*Bush's*)	80	6.0	17.0	0	0	460	6.0
(*Eden* Organic)	110	5.0	20.0	1.0	0	45	8.0
(*Furmano's*)	90	6.0	16.0	0	0	260	5.0
(*Luck's*)	130	7.0	20.0	2.0	0	370	6.0
(*Westbrae Natural* Organic)	100	7.0	19.0	0	0	140	6.0
w/sausage (*Trappey's*)	100	6.0	18.0	1.0	0	460	7.0
seasoned (*Glory*)	90	6.0	17.0	0	0	570	5.0
Green bean, fresh:							
raw:							
(*Del Monte*), ¾ cup	25	1.0	5.0	0	0	0	3.0
all varieties (*Frieda's* Snap Beans), 3 oz.	25	2.0	6.0	0	0	5	3.0
½ cup	17	1.0	3.9	.1	0	3	1.9
boiled, drained, ½ cup	22	1.2	4.9	.2	0	2	2.0
Green bean, can/jar, ½ cup:							
whole:							
(*Allens*)	30	1.0	6.0	0	0	460	3.0
(*Freshlike* Selects) .	35	2.0	7.0	0	0	380	3.0
whole, cut, or French:							
(*Del Monte*)	20	1.0	4.0	0	0	390	2.0
(*S&W*)	20	1.0	4.0	0	0	390	2.0
cut:							
(*Allens* No Salt) . . .	15	0	3.0	0	0	10	2.0
(*Allens/Sunshine*) . .	30	0	6.0	0	0	320	3.0
(*Freshlike*)	35	2.0	7.0	0	0	380	3.0
(*Freshlike* No Salt) .	25	2.0	4.0	0	0	0	2.0
(*Freshlike* Selects) .	30	2.0	5.0	0	0	370	2.0
(*Furmano's*)	20	1.0	4.0	0	0	336	2.0
(*Green Giant* 50% Less Sodium) . . .	20	1.0	4.0	0	0	200	1.0
(*Green Giant/Green Giant Kitchen Sliced*)	20	1.0	4.0	0	0	400	1.0
(*Westbrae Natural* Organic)	20	1.0	4.0	0	0	370	1.0
dilled (*S&W*), 1 oz.	20	0	5.0	0	0	125	1.0
w/liquid	18	1.0	4.2	.1	0	311	1.8
French style:							
(*Allens/Sunshine*) . .	25	1.0	4.0	0	0	300	2.0

Food and Measure	cal.	prot. (gms)	carbo. (gms)	fat (gms)	chol. (mgs)	sod. (mgs)	fiber (gms)
Green bean, can/jar, French style *(cont.)*							
(*Freshlike*)	20	1.0	3.0	0	0	380	3.0
(*Freshlike* No Salt) .	20	1.0	4.0	0	0	0	2.0
(*Green Giant*)	20	1.0	4.0	0	0	390	1.0
(*Westbrae Natural* Organic)	20	1.0	4.0	0	0	370	1.0
Italian cut:							
(*Allens* Shellouts) . .	50	3.0	9.0	0	0	320	3.0
(*Allens/Sunshine*) . .	35	1.0	7.0	0	0	320	3.0
(*Del Monte*)	30	1.0	6.0	0	0	390	3.0
(*Furmano's*)	20	1.0	3.0	0	0	330	1.0
seasoned (*Allens/ Sunshine*)	45	2.0	8.0	0	0	370	3.0
seasoned:							
(*Glory* Pole Beans) .	20	1.0	5.0	0	0	380	2.0
(*Glory* Sensibly) . . .	25	1.0	5.0	0	0	160	2.0
(*Glory* String Beans)	25	1.0	5.0	0	0	380	2.0
w/red pepper (*Del Monte*)	20	1.0	4.0	0	0	360	2.0
Green bean, frozen:							
whole, 1 cup:							
(*Birds Eye/Birds Eye Steamfresh*)	35	1.0	5.0	0	0	0	2.0
(*Cascadian Farm* Organic Petite) . .	25	1.0	5.0	0	0	95	2.0
(*C&W* Haricots Verts/ Petite)	35	1.0	5.0	0	0	0	2.0
(*Green Giant Select*)	30	1.0	5.0	0	0	0	2.0
cut:							
(*Birds Eye/Birds Eye Steamfresh*), ⅔ cup	30	1.0	5.0	0	0	0	2.0
(*Cascadian Farm* Organic), ¾ cup .	30	1.0	6.0	0	0	0	2.0
(*Green Giant*), ½ cup cooked	25	1.0	5.0	0	0	0	2.0
(*McKenzie's* Pole Beans), ½ cup . .	25	1.0	4.0	0	0	10	2.0
French cut (*C&W*), 1 cup	30	1.0	5.0	0	0	0	2.0
Italian cut (*Birds Eye/ C&W*), ¾ cup	35	1.0	5.0	0	0	0	2.0
boiled, drained, ½ cup .	19	1.0	4.4	.1	0	6	2.0

Food and Measure	cal.	prot. (gms)	carbo. (gms)	fat (gms)	chol. (mgs)	sod. (mgs)	fiber (gms)
Green bean combinations, canned, ½ cup:							
casserole (*Allens*) ...	40	2.0	6.0	1.0	0	270	1.0
and potatoes:							
(*Allens/Sunshine*) ..	50	2.0	10.0	0	0	160	2.0
(*Glory* Southern) ..	35	2.0	8.0	0	0	420	2.0
ham style flavor (*Del Monte*)	30	1.0	6.0	0	0	330	<1.0
and wax beans (*S&W*)	20	1.0	4.0	0	0	390	2.0
Green bean combinations, frozen:							
w/almonds:							
(*C&W*), 1 cup	80	3.0	12.0	2.0	0	270	4.0
(*Green Giant Simply Steam* No Sauce), ½ cup cooked ..	50	2.0	5.0	3.0	0	95	2.0
toasted (*Cascadian Farm Organic*), ¾ cup	70	3.0	10.0	3.0	0	115	4.0
toasted, lightly (*Birds Eye*), ¾ cup	80	3.0	8.0	4.0	0	410	3.0
baby, mixed, w/carrots (*Birds Eye*), 1 cup .	35	1.0	6.0	0	0	20	2.0
casserole (*Green Giant*), ⅔ cup	110	2.0	8.0	8.0	0	460	1.0
and spaetzle, in sauce (*Birds Eye* Bavarian), 1 cup	150	5.0	16.0	7.0	30	390	3.0
stir-fry (*Birds Eye* Crisp), 1 cup cooked	100	4.0	19.0	0	0	30	2.0
Green peas, see "Peas, green"							
Greens, see specific listings							
Greens, mixed, fresh (see also "Salad blend"), Southern blend (*Glory*), 2 cups	20	2.0	4.0	0	0	15	2.0
Greens, mixed, canned, ½ cup:							
(*Bush's*)	25	2.0	3.0	0	0	300	2.0
seasoned:							
(*Glory*)	35	1.0	4.0	0	0	490	2.0

Food and Measure	cal.	prot. (gms)	carbo. (gms)	fat (gms)	chol. (mgs)	sod. (mgs)	fiber (gms)
Greens, mixed, canned, seasoned *(cont.)*							
(*Glory* Sensibly) ...	20	1.0	4.0	0	0	240	2.0
(*Sunshine*)	45	4.0	6.0	.5	0	830	1.0
Grenadine, syrup:							
(*Angostura*), 1 tsp.	10	0	3.0	0	0	5	0
(*Roland*), 1 tbsp.	40	0	9.0	0	0	0	0
Grilling sauce (see also "Barbecue sauce," "Marinade," and specific listings), 1 tbsp.:							
apricot ginger (*Campagna* Grill & Glaze)	25	0	6.0	0	0	0	0
balsamic mustard seed (*Campagna* Grill & Glaze)	30	1.0	3.0	1.5	0	115	0
cranberry chipotle (*Campagna* Grill & Glaze)	5	0	1.0	0	0	0	0
hickory, smoked (*Campagna* Grill & Glaze)	10	0	2.0	0	0	20	0
Hunan, spicy (*House of Tsang* Smokehut)	40	0	8.0	.5	0	410	0
Kobe steak (*House of Tsang Hibachi Grill*)	50	0	3.0	4.0	0	600	0
peanut, Thai (*House of Tsang Hibachi Grill*)	50	1.0	4.0	3.0	0	280	0
pear Dijon (*Campagna* Grill & Glaze)	10	0	2.0	0	0	50	0
pepper Dijon (*Campagna* Grill & Glaze)	25	0	3.0	1.5	0	180	0
sesame, sweet ginger (*House of Tsang Hibachi Grill*)	40	0	8.0	1.0	0	410	0
teriyaki (*House of Tsang Hibachi Grill*)	40	0	10.0	0	0	520	0
Grits, see "Corn grits"							
Ground cherry, ½ cup	37	1.3	7.8	.5	0	n.a.	2.0
Grouper, meat only:							
raw, 4 oz.	104	22.0	0	1.2	42	60	0
baked or broiled, 4 oz.	134	28.2	0	1.5	53	60	0
Guacamole, frozen/ refrigerated, 2 tbsp.:							
(*Calavo* Authentic) ...	50	1.0	2.0	5.0	0	95	1.0

Food and Measure	cal.	prot. (gms)	carbo. (gms)	fat (gms)	chol. (mgs)	sod. (mgs)	fiber (gms)
(*Calavo* Authentic Frozen)	50	1.0	7.0	2.5	0	120	1.0
(*Calavo* Caliente)	40	<1.0	2.0	3.5	0	105	1.0
(*Calavo* Fiesta)	60	1.0	2.0	5.0	0	140	2.0
(*Calavo* Homestyle) . .	70	<1.0	3.0	6.0	0	70	1.0
(*Calavo* Original)	60	<1.0	6.0	4.0	0	120	1.0
(*Kraft*)	50	1.0	3.0	4.5	0	240	0
(*Marie's* Dip)	40	1.0	3.0	3.0	5	140	1.0
(*Marzetti's* Dip)	130	0	2.0	13.0	15	240	0
(*Santa Barbara*)	40	<1.0	3.0	4.0	0	100	0
hot/spicy (*Calavo*) . . .	80	<1.0	3.0	7.0	0	150	1.0
Mexican (*Calavo*)	70	<1.0	3.0	7.0	0	120	1.0
mild (*Calavo*)	70	<1.0	4.0	5.0	0	125	1.0
nondairy (*Tofutti* Sour Supreme)	85	1.0	9.0	5.0	0	160	0
pico de gallo (*Calavo*)	40	<1.0	2.0	3.5	0	100	1.0
spicy (*Calavo*)	45	<1.0	4.0	3.0	0	110	1.0
Western (*Calavo*)	50	0	6.0	3.0	0	110	1.0
Guacamole seasoning:							
(*Lawry's*), ½ tsp. . . .	0	0	1.0	0	0	130	0
(*McCormick*), ½ tsp. .	10	0	1.0	0	0	80	0
Guava (see also "Feijoas"), fresh:							
(*Frieda's*), 3-oz. pc. . .	45	1.0	10.0	.5	0	0	5.0
1 medium, 4 oz.	45	.7	10.7	.5	0	2	4.9
½ cup	42	.7	9.8	.5	0	2	4.5
strawberry, ½ cup . . .	85	.7	21.2	.7	0	45	7.8
Guava, can/jar, in syrup:							
whole (*Herdez*), 4 pcs., 4.5 oz.	190	0	32.0	0	0	10	5.0
sliced (*Vigo* Shells), ⅕ of 18-oz. can . . .	200	0	51.0	0	0	10	3.0
Guava drink blend (*Nantucket Nectars*), 8 fl. oz.	130	0	33.0	0	0	25	0
Guava juice (*Ceres*), 8 fl. oz.	120	0	30.0	0	0	10	0
Guava nectar (*Apple & Eve*), 8 fl. oz. . . .	130	0	32.0	0	0	35	0
Guava sauce, ½ cup .	43	.4	11.3	.2	0	4	4.3
Guava strawberry juice (*R.W. Knudsen*), 8 fl. oz.	120	1.0	28.0	0	0	25	<1.0

Food and Measure	cal.	prot. (gms)	carbo. (gms)	fat (gms)	chol. (mgs)	sod. (mgs)	fiber (gms)
Guavadilla, see "Passionfruit"							
Guinea hen, raw:							
meat w/skin, 4 oz.	179	26.5	0	7.3	84	86	0
meat only, 4 oz.	125	23.4	0	2.8	71	78	0
Gumbo base mix (*Zatarain's*), 1 cup*	45	1.0	9.0	0	0	800	1.0
Gyoza wrappers (*Frieda's*), ⅔ cup, 3 oz.	10	1.0	2.0	0	0	0	1.0
Gyros mix, dry (*Casbah*), .65 oz. ..	70	2.0	14.0	.5	0	560	2.0

H

Food and Measure	cal.	prot. (gms)	carbo. (gms)	fat (gms)	chol. (mgs)	sod. (mgs)	fiber (gms)
Habas, see "Broad bean, mature"							
Haddock, meat only:							
raw, 4 oz.	99	21.5	0	.8	65	78	0
baked or broiled, 4 oz.	127	27.5	0	1.1	84	99	0
smoked, 4 oz.	132	28.6	0	1.1	87	865	0
Haddock, frozen, raw fillet (*Matlaw's*), 3 oz.	81	14.0	0	2.0	49	37	0
Haddock entree, frozen, fillets:							
battered (*Van de Kamp's*), 2 pcs., 3.7 oz.	210	9.0	21.0	11.0	20	580	2.0
breaded, 1 pc.:							
(*Mrs. Paul's*), 4 oz.	220	12.0	17.0	11.0	10	430	1.0
(*Schooner*), 3.5 oz.	160	7.0	20.0	6.0	20	230	1.0
Hake, see "Whiting"							
Halibut, meat only:							
Atlantic/Pacific, 4 oz.:							
raw	124	23.6	0	2.6	37	61	0
baked or broiled . .	159	30.3	0	3.3	46	78	0
Greenland, 4 oz.							
raw	211	16.3	0	15.7	52	91	0
baked or broiled . . .	271	20.9	0	20.1	67	117	0
Halvah, 1 oz.:							
chocolate (*Cedar's*) . .	148	4.0	16.0	8.0	0	31	0
pistachio (*Cedar's*) . . .	133	3.0	14.0	7.0	0	28	0
vanilla (*Cedar's*)	129	3.0	15.0	7.0	0	30	0
Ham, fresh, meat only, 4 oz., except as noted:							
whole leg, roasted:							
lean w/fat	310	30.4	0	20.0	107	68	0
lean w/fat, diced, 1 cup	369	36.2	0	23.8	127	81	0
lean only	239	33.4	0	10.7	107	73	0

Food and Measure	cal.	prot. (gms)	carbo. (gms)	fat (gms)	chol. (mgs)	sod. (mgs)	fiber (gms)
Ham, fresh *(cont.)*							
lean only, diced,							
1 cup	285	39.7	0	12.7	127	86	0
rump half, roasted:							
lean w/fat	286	32.7	0	16.2	109	70	0
lean only	235	35.1	0	9.2	109	74	0
shank half, roasted:							
lean w/fat	328	28.7	0	22.7	104	67	0
lean only	244	32.0	0	11.9	104	73	0
Ham, cured:							
whole leg, lean w/fat:							
unheated, 4 oz. ...	279	21.0	.1	21.0	64	1456	0
unheated, chopped							
or diced, 1 cup ..	344	25.9	.1	25.9	78	1798	0
roasted, 4 oz.	276	24.5	0	19.0	70	1346	0
roasted, chopped							
or diced, 1 cup ..	341	30.2	0	23.5	86	1661	0
whole leg, lean only:							
unheated, 4 oz. ...	167	25.3	.1	6.5	59	1719	0
unheated, chopped							
or diced, 1 cup ..	206	31.3	0	8.0	73	2122	0
roasted, 4 oz.	178	28.4	0	6.2	62	1505	0
roasted, chopped or							
diced, 1 cup	219	35.1	0	7.7	77	1858	0
boneless (11% fat):							
unheated, 4 oz. ...	206	19.9	3.5	12.0	65	1493	0
roasted, 4 oz.	202	25.7	0	10.2	67	1701	0
roasted, chopped or							
diced, 1 cup	249	31.7	0	12.6	83	2100	0
boneless, extra lean							
(5% fat):							
unheated, 4 oz. ...	149	21.9	1.1	5.6	53	1620	0
roasted, 4 oz.	164	23.7	1.7	6.3	60	1364	0
roasted, chopped or							
diced, 1 cup	203	29.3	2.1	7.7	74	1684	0
Ham, refrigerated/							
canned, 3 oz.,							
except as noted:							
(*Black Bear* European							
Classic)	110	14.0	1.0	5.0	40	720	0
(*Bilinski* Champagne) .	150	11.0	1.0	12.0	45	390	0
(*Cure 81*)	100	15.0	0	4.5	45	890	0
(*Curemaster*)	80	14.0	0	2.5	40	950	0

Food and Measure	cal.	prot. (gms)	carbo. (gms)	fat (gms)	chol. (mgs)	sod. (mgs)	fiber (gms)
(*Black Label* Can)	100	14.0	1.0	4.0	40	1050	0
(*Farmer John* Bone-In), 2 oz.	110	9.0	3.0	7.0	30	910	0
(*Hatfield* Breakfast Slices), 4-oz. slice .	130	17.0	4.0	4.0	45	1110	0
(*Hatfield* Country Made Half/Quarter)	100	14.0	3.0	3.0	40	900	0
(*Hatfield* Country Made Whole)	100	14.0	3.0	3.0	40	870	0
(*Hatfield* Traditional Dinner Ham)	100	14.0	3.0	3.0	40	870	0
(*Hormel* Dinner), 2 oz.	70	10.0	2.0	2.0	30	550	0
(*Spiral Cure 81*)	130	16.0	1.0	7.0	50	1060	0
brown sugar (*Cure 81*)	100	14.0	2.0	3.5	40	890	0
cubed/julienne strips (*Farmland*), 2 oz. . .	60	9.0	3.0	2.0	30	750	0
diced, 2 oz.:							
(*Farmland*)	70	9.0	3.0	2.0	30	720	0
(*Hormel Pillow Pack*)	60	10.0	1.0	2.0	30	580	0
honey/honey cured:							
(*Black Bear*)	110	15.0	3.0	3.0	45	680	0
(*Dietz & Watson* Dinner), 3.5 oz. .	80	10.0	2.0	3.0	45	750	0
(*Hatfield* Boneless Dinner)	110	13.0	7.0	3.0	20	660	0
maple brown sugar glazed (*Tyson*), 5 oz.	180	17.0	18.0	4.5	60	780	0
patties, 2-oz. pc.:							
(*Hormel*)	180	7.0	1.0	16.0	40	620	0
and cheese (*Hormel*)	180	7.0	0	17.0	40	520	0
roast (*Farmland* Steamship)	140	16.0	2.0	7.0	60	850	0
semiboneless:							
(*Black Bear*)	130	14.0	1.0	8.0	45	720	0
(*Dietz & Watson*) . .	130	16.0	3.0	6.0	45	760	0
(*Hatfield*)	120	12.0	2.0	7.0	25	400	0
smoked:							
(*Bilinski* Champagne)	150	11.0	1.0	12.0	45	390	0
(*Farmland* Bone-in Picnic), 4.5 oz. . .	250	17.2	.9	20.2	74	1700	0
(*Farmland* Boneless)	90	13.0	1.0	4.0	40	1080	0
(*Farmland* Classic Cure)	100	15.0	2.0	3.0	50	1030	0

Food and Measure	cal.	prot. (gms)	carbo. (gms)	fat (gms)	chol. (mgs)	sod. (mgs)	fiber (gms)
Ham, refrigerated/canned, smoked *(cont.)*							
(*Farmland* Maple River)	120	13.0	1.0	8.0	45	1110	0
(*Farmland* Picnic), 4.5 oz.	250	15.0	2.0	20.0	70	1590	0
(*Farmland* Pit Style)	110	13.0	2.0	5.1	45	1040	0
(*Farmland* Tradition)	110	13.0	2.0	6.0	40	1110	0
(*Farmland* w/Water)	90	11.0	2.0	4.0	35	950	0
Black Forest (*Hatfield* Dinner)	100	14.0	3.0	4.0	40	840	0
hardwood (*Organic Prairie*)	110	19.0	<1.0	3.0	40	940	0
honey cure (*Carando*)	100	15.0	4.0	2.0	50	850	0
smoked, hickory:							
(*Farmland*)	140	14.0	3.0	8.0	50	1150	0
(*Farmland* Original Sliced)	130	14.0	2.0	7.0	50	830	0
(*Smithfield* Sliced) .	100	14.0	5.0	2.0	25	970	0
peppered (*Farmland* Original)	130	15.0	2.0	6.0	50	1020	0
spiral sliced:							
(*Dietz & Watson*), 2 oz.	140	16.0	3.0	7.0	50	690	0
(*Farmer John* Bone-in), 2 oz. . .	90	12.0	3.0	4.0	35	480	0
(*Farmland* Grillable)	140	16.0	2.0	7.0	60	850	0
brown sugar glaze (*Farmland*)	140	17.0	5.0	6.0	55	880	0
hardwood smoked (*Organic Prairie*)	110	19.0	<1.0	3.0	40	940	0
hickory smoked (*Farmland* Bone-in Quarter)	140	17.0	2.0	7.0	60	1040	0
honey cure (*Farmland* Bone-in Quarter)	160	16.0	2.0	10.0	60	880	0
w/honey glaze pkt. (*Hatfield*)	150	15.0	3.0	9.0	30	840	0
smoked (*Black Bear*)	130	14.0	1.0	8.0	45	720	0
steak:							
(*Black Bear* Boneless)	90	14.0	2.0	3.0	40	690	0
(*Dietz & Watson*), 2 oz.	110	19.0	2.0	3.0	55	690	0

Food and Measure	cal.	prot. (gms)	carbo. (gms)	fat (gms)	chol. (mgs)	sod. (mgs)	fiber (gms)
(*Farmer John* Boneless), 2 oz. .	50	9.0	2.0	1.0	25	540	0
(*Hatfield* Hardwood Griller)	90	14.0	2.0	1.5	20	690	0
(*Hatfield* Traditional)	90	14.0	2.0	1.5	20	700	0
(*Hatfield Special Selects*)	90	14.0	0	1.5	20	600	0
brown sugar mustard (*Hatfield*)	110	14.0	7.0	1.5	20	710	0
hickory smoked (*Hatfield*)	110	14.0	5.0	1.5	20	860	0
honey (*Hatfield*) . . .	110	14.0	7.0	1.5	20	670	0
maple (*Hatfield*) . . .	110	14.0	6.0	1.5	20	730	0
mesquite (*Hatfield* Griller)	110	14.0	4.0	3.0	20	820	0
sliced (*Farmer John* Bone-In)	160	13.0	4.0	11.0	45	1370	0
Ham and cheese loaf: (*Farmland* w/Cheese), 1 oz.	110	5.0	2.0	9.0	30	470	0
(*Farmland* Loaf), 1.3-oz. slice	100	5.0	2.0	9.0	30	470	0
(*Hansel 'n Gretel*), 2 oz.	130	7.0	3.0	14.0	30	840	0
Ham and cheese sandwich, frozen, 1 pc.: cheddar (*OscarMayer Deli Creations*), 6.8 oz.	430	28.0	48.0	15.0	55	1550	5.0
honey ham/Swiss (*Oscar Mayer Deli Creations*), 6.8 oz. .	440	28.0	51.0	14.0	55	1490	4.0
Swiss (*South Beach Living* Hot Melts), 5.65 oz.	320	24.0	37.0	11.0	40	950	8.0
Ham croquettes, frozen (*Goya*), 3 pcs.	280	13.0	30.0	12.0	30	730	3.0
Ham entree, frozen, sausage Jambalaya: (*Glory* Savory Singles), 11-oz. pkg.	400	17.0	42.0	18.0	50	1320	2.0
(*Glory* Savory Family Size), 1 cup	370	16.0	38.0	16.0	45	1210	2.0
Ham glaze: (*Ah-So*), 2 tbsp.	50	0	13.0	0	0	15	0

Food and Measure	cal.	prot. (gms)	carbo. (gms)	fat (gms)	chol. (mgs)	sod. (mgs)	fiber (gms)
Ham glaze *(cont.)*							
(*Crosse & Blackwell*), 1 tbsp.	30	0	7.0	0	0	25	0
(*Polynesian*), 2 tbsp. . .	60	0	16.0	0	0	200	0
(*Reese's*), 1 tbsp.	20	0	5.0	0	0	55	0
(*Saucy Susan*), 2 tbsp.	80	0	19.0	0	0	260	1.0
brown sugar/spice (*Boar's Head*), 2 tbsp.	120	0	30.0	0	0	95	0
Ham lunch meat (see also "Proscuitto"), 2 oz., except as noted:							
(*Boar's Head* Deluxe) .	60	9.0	2.0	1.0	25	590	0
(*Boar's Head* Deluxe Lower Sodium) . . .	60	10.0	2.0	1.0	25	460	0
(*Di Lusso* Deluxe) . . .	50	9.0	2.0	1.0	25	670	0
(*Dietz & Watson* Chef Carved)	70	10.0	2.0	2.0	30	500	0
(*Dietz & Watson* Classic Trim & Tied)	70	12.0	1.0	2.5	35	400	0
(*Dietz & Watson* Tiffany)	50	11.0	0	1.0	30	520	0
(*Farmer John*)	50	10.0	1.0	1.5	20	700	0
(*Farmer John* Roll) . . .	60	10.0	1.0	1.5	25	450	0
(*Farmland*), 4 slices, 1.8 oz.	60	9.0	2.0	1.0	30	550	0
(*Farmland* Special Select)	60	9.2	.7	1.9	27	690	0
(*Hansel 'n Gretel* Deluxe)	65	9.0	1.0	2.0	25	560	0
(*Hatfield Deli Choice* Ham Off the Bone) .	70	10.0	2.0	2.0	25	470	0
(*Healthy Deli* All Natural)	70	10.0	2.0	1.5	29	470	0
(*Healthy Deli* Zero Carb Deluxe)	60	9.0	0	1.5	20	480	0
baked:							
(*Healthy Choice* Tub), 2 slices, 2 oz. . . .	60	10.0	1.0	1.5	25	460	0
(*Healthy Choice Deli Thin*), 6 slices, 1.9 oz.	60	9.0	1.0	1.5	25	470	0
Black Forest:							
(*Applegate Farms*) .	50	10.0	0	1.5	35	480	0
(*Applegate Farms* Deli Counter) . . .	50	10.0	0	1.5	35	530	0
(*Boar's Head*)	60	10.0	2.0	1.0	30	580	0

Food and Measure	cal.	prot. (gms)	carbo. (gms)	fat (gms)	chol. (mgs)	sod. (mgs)	fiber (gms)
(*Di Lusso*)	60	10.0	1.0	2.0	30	580	0
(*Dietz & Watson*) ..	80	11.0	1.0	3.0	35	530	0
(*Healthy Deli*)	60	10.0	1.0	1.5	20	480	0
(*Hormel*)	60	10.0	0	2.0	30	560	0
(*Hormel Natural Choice*)	60	11.0	0	2.0	35	530	0
boiled (*Oscar Mayer*), 2.2 oz.	60	10.0	1.0	2.0	30	820	0
brown sugar:							
(*Di Lusso*)	80	10.0	5.0	2.0	25	560	0
(*Hormel Natural Choice*)	70	11.0	2.0	2.0	35	520	0
(*Oscar Mayer* Deli Fresh Thin Sliced)	70	10.0	4.0	1.5	25	830	0
honey (*Farmer John*), 1.3-oz. slice	45	7.0	2.0	1.0	15	410	0
Cajun style (*Dietz & Watson*)	60	10.0	1.0	1.5	30	570	0
capicola/cappy:							
(*Applegate Farms* Dry Cure Coppa), 5 slices, 1 oz.	60	8.0	0	3.0	25	400	0
(*Black Bear*)	50	10.0	1.0	1.0	30	590	0
(*Boar's Head*)	60	10.0	3.0	1.5	15	590	0
(*Carando* Hot), 1 oz.	70	9.0	1.0	3.0	30	730	0
(*Hansel 'n Gretel*) .	60	9.0	2.0	1.5	20	280	0
(*Healthy Deli*)	60	9.0	2.0	1.5	20	480	0
hot (*Di Lusso*)	60	9.0	0	2.5	30	670	0
hot (*Dietz & Watson* Capocolla), 1 oz.	60	8.0	1.0	5.0	25	540	0
hot or sweet (*Boar's Head* Capocollo), 1 oz.	80	7.0	0	7.0	15	590	0
sweet (*Dietz & Watson* Capocolla), 1 oz.	60	8.0	1.0	3.0	22	750	0
and cheese, see "Ham and cheese loaf"							
chopped:							
(*Black Bear*)	100	9.0	1.0	6.0	35	530	0
(*Farmer John*), 1.3-oz. slice	40	6.0	1.0	1.5	15	350	0
(*Farmland* Deli Favorites), 1 oz. .	70	4.0	2.0	6.0	15	400	0

Food and Measure	cal.	prot. (gms)	carbo. (gms)	fat (gms)	chol. (mgs)	sod. (mgs)	fiber (gms)
Ham lunch meat, chopped *(cont.)*							
(*Farmland* Deli Style), 1 oz.	80	4.0	2.0	6.0	20	400	0
(*Hormel*)	140	7.0	3.0	11.0	30	690	0
(*Oscar Mayer/Oscar Mayer* Smoke Flavor), 1 oz. . . .	50	4.0	1.0	3.0	15	340	0
cinnamon apple (*Healthy Deli*)	70	9.0	4.0	1.5	20	480	0
cooked:							
(*Alpine Lace*)	60	9.0	2.0	1.5	25	600	0
(*Black Bear*)	60	9.0	2.0	1.0	30	600	0
(*Dietz & Watson* Imported)	70	10.0	1.0	1.0	25	420	0
(*Dietz & Watson* Gourmet Lite) . . .	50	12.0	0	.5	30	430	0
(*Farmland* Deli Favorites), 1 oz. .	25	4.0	1.0	1.0	15	370	0
(*Farmland* Deli Style), 1 oz.	30	4.0	1.0	1.0	15	370	0
(*Hatfield Deli Choice* Imported)	60	9.0	2.0	1.5	10	410	0
(*Hatfield Deli Choice* Premium)	70	10.0	2.0	1.5	25	730	0
(*Healthy Choice* Hearty Slices), 1 oz.	30	5.0	1.0	1.0	15	240	0
(*Healthy Choice Deli Thin*), 4 slices, 1.9 oz.	60	9.0	2.0	1.5	25	450	0
(*Hormel*)	60	10.0	1.0	2.0	30	630	0
(*Hormel Natural Choice*)	60	10.0	1.0	1.5	30	520	0
(*Oscar Mayer* Deli Fresh), 1 oz.	30	5.0	0	1.0	15	340	0
(*Tyson*), 2 slices, 1.6 oz.	45	9.0	0	1.5	20	740	0
shaved (*Tyson*) . . .	60	10.0	0	1.5	25	760	0
fresh ham, see "Pork lunch meat"							
glazed:							
(*Hansel 'n Gretel*) .	60	10.0	2.0	1.5	20	620	0
(*Healthy Deli* Deluxe)	60	10.0	2.0	1.5	20	480	0
honey/honey cured:							
(*Alpine Lace*)	60	9.0	2.0	1.5	25	600	0

Food and Measure	cal.	prot. (gms)	carbo. (gms)	fat (gms)	chol. (mgs)	sod. (mgs)	fiber (gms)
(Applegate Farms) .	70	10.0	3.0	1.5	30	450	0
(Black Bear)	70	10.0	4.0	1.5	30	540	0
(Di Lusso)	60	10.0	1.0	2.0	30	580	0
(Dietz & Watson) ..	70	10.0	3.0	2.0	25	600	0
(Healthy Deli)	60	9.0	2.0	1.5	20	480	0
(Hormel)	70	10.0	3.0	2.0	30	560	0
(Hormel Natural Choice Sliced) ..	70	10.0	3.0	1.5	25	520	0
(Oscar Mayer Deli Fresh), ¼ of 10-oz. pkg.	60	11.0	2.0	1.5	35	800	0
(Oscar Mayer 96% Fat Free), 2.2 oz.	70	11.0	2.0	2.0	30	770	0
(Tyson), 2 slices, 1.6 oz.	50	9.0	1.0	1.5	25	740	0
chopped (Oscar Mayer), 1 oz. ...	60	4.0	4.0	3.5	15	320	0
shaved (Tyson) ...	60	9.0	1.0	1.5	30	760	0
honey maple:							
(Di Lusso)	60	10.0	2.0	2.0	30	570	0
(Healthy Choice Hearty Slices), 1-oz. slice	30	5.0	1.0	1.0	15	170	0
(Healthy Choice Deli Thin), 4 slices, 1.9 oz.	60	9.0	2.0	1.5	25	450	0
honey mustard (Healthy Choice Deli Thin), 4 slices, 1.9 oz.	60	9.0	3.0	1.5	25	450	0
honey peppered (Farmland Special Select)	60	9.0	1.0	1.5	30	650	0
jalapeño (Healthy Deli)	60	8.0	3.0	1.5	15	480	0
maple:							
(Applegate Farms Deli Counter) ...	50	10.0	2.0	1.5	35	520	0
(Healthy Deli Vermont)	60	9.0	3.0	1.5	20	460	0
glazed (Boar's Head Honey Coat)	60	10.0	3.0	1.0	20	570	0
pepper/peppered:							
(Boar's Head)	60	10.0	2.0	1.0	20	560	0
(Dietz & Watson) ..	70	10.0	3.0	1.5	35	590	0

Food and Measure	cal.	prot. (gms)	carbo. (gms)	fat (gms)	chol. (mgs)	sod. (mgs)	fiber (gms)
Ham lunch meat, pepper/peppered (cont.)							
(Hatfield Deli Choice)	70	10.0	3.0	1.5	15	470	0
(Healthy Deli)	60	9.0	2.0	1.5	20	470	0
pesto Parmesan (Boar's Head)	70	12.0	1.0	2.5	30	550	0
prosciuttini:							
(Dietz & Watson) . . .	60	10.0	1.0	1.5	30	570	0
peppered (Black Bear)	50	9.0	1.0	1.5	25	590	0
rosemary:							
(Black Bear)	70	11.0	1.0	2.5	30	520	0
(Dietz & Watson) . .	70	11.0	0	3.0	35	500	0
sun-dried tomato (Boar's Head) . . .	70	10.0	2.0	2.5	10	590	0
smoked:							
(Boar's Head Sweet Slice)	100	15.0	1.0	3.5	30	780	0
(Hormel Natural Choice Sliced) . .	60	10.0	1.0	1.5	25	520	0
(Oscar Mayer Deli Fresh), ¼ of 10-oz. pkg.	60	11.0	0	1.5	30	790	0
(Oscar Mayer 96% Fat Free), 2.2 oz.	50	10.0	0	1.0	15	730	0
(Oscar Mayer 97% Fat Free Thin Sliced)	50	10.0	0	1.5	25	720	0
double (Di Lusso) .	70	11.0	1.0	2.0	30	550	0
double (Healthy Deli)	60	10.0	1.0	1.5	20	470	0
double (Hormel) . .	60	10.0	0	2.0	30	560	0
hardwood (Organic Prairie)	70	10.0	1.0	2.5	35	250	0
shaved (Oscar Mayer Deli Fresh), ⅕ of 9-oz. pkg.	45	9.0	0	1.0	25	640	0
spiced, see "Lunch meat"							
tavern:							
(Black Bear)	60	10.0	1.0	1.5	30	590	0
(Boar's Head) . . . : .	60	10.0	2.0	1.0	30	580	0
(Dietz & Watson) . .	60	10.0	1.0	1.5	30	570	0
(Dietz & Watson Gourmet Lite) . . .	60	10.0	1.0	1.5	30	450	0
(Hatfield Deli Choice)	70	9.0	3.0	2.0	25	590	0
(Healthy Deli)	60	10.0	1.0	1.5	20	470	0

Food and Measure	cal.	prot. (gms)	carbo. (gms)	fat (gms)	chol. (mgs)	sod. (mgs)	fiber (gms)
honey cured (*Black Bear*)	60	10.0	1.0	1.5	30	620	0
honey cured (*Dietz & Watson*)	60	10.0	1.0	1.5	30	570	0
tomato and basil:							
(*Black Bear*)	70	11.0	1.0	2.5	30	520	0
(*Dietz & Watson*) ..	70	11.0	1.0	2.0	30	520	0
uncured:							
(*Applegate Farms*) .	60	11.0	0	1.5	35	480	0
(*Applegate Farms* Organic)	50	10.0	0	1.5	35	530	0
Virginia:							
(*Applegate Farms*) .	50	9.0	1.0	1.5	30	480	0
(*Black Bear*)	60	9.0	3.0	1.0	25	560	0
(*Black Bear* Lite) ..	60	9.0	3.0	1.0	25	460	0
(*Boar's Head*)	60	9.0	2.0	1.0	25	590	0
(*Dietz & Watson*) ..	60	9.0	2.0	.2	30	560	0
(*Dietz & Watson* Lite)	60	9.0	2.0	1.5	25	450	0
(*Hansel 'n Gretel*)	65	10.0	2.0	2.0	25	600	0
(*Hatfield Deli Choice*)	80	9.0	4.0	2.0	25	610	0
(*Hormel Natural Choice*)	60	11.0	0	2.0	35	530	0
smoked (*Healthy Choice Deli Thin*), 4 slices, 1.9 oz. ..	60	9.0	2.0	1.5	25	470	0
Ham patties, see "Ham, refrigerated/canned"							
Ham spread, deviled (*Hormel Cure 81*), 4 tbsp., 2 oz.	150	9.0	2.0	12.0	40	430	0
Hamburger, see "Beef sandwich"							
"Hamburger," vegetarian, see "Burger, vegetarian"							
Hamburger entree mix, 1 cup*, except as noted:							
(*Annie's* Organic Skillet Meal):							
cheeseburger, macaroni	350	28.0	27.0	13.0	50	670	1.0
lasagna cheesy	280	23.0	26.0	9.0	35	670	1.0
Stroganoff	320	25.0	24.0	13.0	45	620	1.0

Food and Measure	cal.	prot. (gms)	carbo. (gms)	fat (gms)	chol. (mgs)	sod. (mgs)	fiber (gms)
Hamburger entree mix *(cont.)*							
(Hamburger Helper):							
cheddar melt	310	20.0	29.0	13.0	55	820	1.0
cheese, three	350	23.0	35.0	13.0	60	780	1.0
cheeseburger:							
bacon	380	24.0	38.0	15.0	60	840	1.0
macaroni	300	20.0	27.0	13.0	50	870	1.0
macaroni, double	330	22.0	30.0	13.0	60	750	1.0
chili cheese	340	22.0	33.0	13.0	60	730	1.0
chili macaroni	290	20.0	29.0	11.0	55	750	1.0
enchilada, cheesy . .	350	20.0	40.0	13.0	55	680	<1.0
hash browns,							
cheesy	400	21.0	39.0	19.0	55	610	2.0
jambalaya, cheesy .	330	22.0	30.0	14.0	60	850	1.0
lasagna	270	19.0	26.0	11.0	50	900	0
lasagna, 4 cheese .	330	22.0	31.0	13.0	60	850	1.0
pasta, beef	270	20.0	24.0	11.0	55	810	1.0
penne, tomato basil	300	20.0	31.0	11.0	55	720	1.0
Philly cheesesteak .	320	21.0	25.0	14.0	55	770	1.0
potato, baked,							
cheesy	310	20.0	29.0	13.0	55	820	2.0
potato, Stroganoff .	290	20.0	25.0	12.0	60	810	1.0
quesadilla, double							
cheese	350	21.0	40.0	12.0	55	880	<1.0
Salisbury	280	20.0	26.0	11.0	55	830	1.0
sausage, Italian,							
flavor	290	20.0	29.0	11.0	55	840	1.0
shells, cheesy Italian	350	22.0	37.0	13.0	60	1000	1.0
spaghetti	280	20.0	26.0	11.0	55	870	1.0
Stroganoff	330	23.0	31.0	13.0	60	880	1.0
taco, beef	280	18.0	29.0	11.0	50	890	1.0
taco, crunchy	300	19.0	27.0	14.0	55	800	<1.0
Stroganoff, creamy,							
w/pasta *(Campbell's*							
Supper Bakes),							
1/6 pkg.	190	6.0	33.0	4.0	10	740	1.0
Hamburger seasoning							
(Mrs. Dash Grilling							
Blend), 1/4 tsp.	0	0	1.0	0	0	0	0
Hard sauce *(Crosse &*							
Blackwell), 2 tbsp. .	180	0	25.0	8.0	20	70	0
Hazelnut, shelled:							
(Diamond), 1/4 cup . . .	190	4.0	5.0	18.0	0	0	3.0

Food and Measure	cal.	prot. (gms)	carbo. (gms)	fat (gms)	chol. (mgs)	sod. (mgs)	fiber (gms)
raw, ¼ cup:							
(*Shiloh Farms* Organic)	190	5.0	5.0	16.0	0	0	4.0
(*Tree of Life*)	210	4.0	5.0	21.0	0	0	3.0
dried:							
1 oz.	179	3.7	4.4	17.8	0	1	1.7
chopped, 1 cup ...	727	15.0	17.6	72.0	0	3	7.0
dry-roasted, salted, 1 oz.	188	2.8	5.1	18.8	0	221	<2.0
oil-roasted, salted, 1 oz.	187	4.1	5.4	18.1	0	223	1.8
chopped (*Planters*), 2-oz. pkg.	350	7.0	9.0	35.0	0	0	5.0
Hazelnut beverage (*Pacific*), 8 fl. oz. ...	110	2.0	18.0	3.5	0	120	1.0
Hazelnut butter:							
(*Nutella*), 2 tbsp.	190	3.0	22.0	11.0	0	15	1.0
creamy (*Kettle Roaster Fresh*), 1 oz.	180	4.0	5.0	17.0	0	0	3.0
Head cheese:							
(*Boar's Head*), 2 oz. .	90	10.0	<1.0	5.0	65	420	0
(*Farmer John*), 1.4-oz. slice	100	8.0	0	7.0	30	400	0
(*Hansel 'n Gretel*), 2 oz.	90	9.0	2.0	5.0	35	960	0
pork, 2 oz.	88	7.7	0	6.1	39	465	0
Heart, braised or simmered, 4 oz.:							
beef	199	32.6	.5	6.4	219	71	0
chicken, broiler-fryer .	210	30.0	.1	9.0	274	54	0
lamb	210	28.3	2.2	9.0	282	71	0
pork	168	26.8	.5	5.7	251	40	0
turkey	201	30.3	2.3	6.9	256	62	0
veal	211	33.0	.1	7.7	200	66	0
Herbs, see specific listings							
Herbs, mixed, seasoning, ¼ tsp.:							
(*McCormick* Seasoning Blend), 1 tsp.	5	0	1.0	0	0	220	0
Italian (*McCormick* Grinder), ¼ tsp.	0	0	0	0	0	15	0
Herring, fresh, 4 oz.:							
Atlantic, meat only:							
raw	180	20.4	0	10.3	68	102	0
baked or broiled ...	230	26.1	0	13.1	87	130	0

Food and Measure	cal.	prot. (gms)	carbo. (gms)	fat (gms)	chol. (mgs)	sod. (mgs)	fiber (gms)
Herring, fresh *(cont.)*							
kippered	246	27.9	0	14.0	93	1041	0
pickled	297	16.1	10.9	20.4	15	987	0
lake, see "Cisco"							
Pacific, meat only:							
raw	224	18.6	0	15.8	87	84	0
baked or broiled ...	284	23.8	0	20.2	112	108	0
Herring, canned (see							
also "Herring, pickled"							
and "Sardine"):							
in horseradish sauce							
(*Roland*), ¼ cup ..	120	7.0	2.0	9.0	45	200	0
in hot sauce, 1 can:							
(*Beach Cliff* Fish							
Steaks Louisiana),							
3.75 oz.	150	17.0	2.0	8.0	75	470	0
(*Brunswick* Fish							
Steaks Louisiana),							
3.75 oz.	160	19.0	2.0	7.0	75	480	0
(*Brunswick* Seafood							
Snacks Louisiana),							
3.5 oz.	140	16.0	2.0	8.0	70	450	0
kippered:							
(*Beach Cliff/ Bruns-*							
wick Seafood							
Snacks), 3 oz. ..	130	16.0	0	8.0	65	460	0
(*Roland* Snacks),							
3.25-oz. can	190	19.0	0	13.0	60	390	0
smoked (*Bar Harbor*),							
¼ cup	110	11.0	0	8.0	35	230	0
lemon, cracked pepper							
(*Brunswick* Seafood							
Snacks), 3-oz. can .	130	15.0	0	8.0	60	250	0
lobster sauce (*Roland*),							
¼ cup	100	8.0	2.0	6.0	45	190	0
mushroom sauce							
(*Roland*), ¼ cup ..	80	8.0	2.0	4.5	45	240	0
mustard sauce, 1 can:							
(*Beach Cliff* Fish							
Steaks), 3.75 oz. .	160	17.0	2.0	9.0	80	450	0
(*Brunswick* Fish							
Steaks), 3.75 oz. .	160	21.0	2.0	9.0	80	420	0
smoked:							
(*Roland*), ¼ cup ..	110	11.0	0	8.0	35	230	0

Food and Measure	cal.	prot. (gms)	carbo. (gms)	fat (gms)	chol. (mgs)	sod. (mgs)	fiber (gms)
golden (*Brunswick* Seafood Snacks), 2.8-oz. can	130	16.0	0	8.0	60	240	0
in soybean oil, drained:							
(*Beach Cliff* Fish Steaks 3.75 oz.), 3.3 oz.	190	19.0	0	13.0	90	300	0
(*Brunswick* Fish Steaks 3.75 oz.), 3.4 oz.	200	20.0	0	13.0	80	310	0
w/hot green chilies or jalapeños (*Beach Cliff* Fish Steaks 3.75 oz.), 3.3 oz.	190	19.0	0	12.0	85	310	0
w/hot tabasco pepper (*Brunswick* Fish Steaks 3.75 oz.), 3.4 oz.	200	20.0	1.0	13.0	80	240	0
teriyaki sauce (*Brunswick* Seafood Snacks), 3.5-oz. can	160	16.0	5.0	8.0	70	800	0
tomato basil sauce (*Brunswick* Seafood Snacks), 3.5-oz. can	140	16.0	2.0	8.0	70	420	0
tomato sauce (*Roland*), ¼ cup	100	7.0	2.0	7.0	15	250	0
in water, drained (*Brunswick* Fish Steaks 3.75 oz.), 3.3 oz.	150	19.0	0	8.0	115	240	0
in wine sauce (*Roland*), ¼ cup	100	8.0	2.0	7.0	45	230	0
Herring, kippered, see "Herring" and "Herring, canned"							
Herring, pickled, in jars:							
in cream sauce:							
(*Acme/Blue Hill Bay*), 5 pcs., 2 oz.	90	5.0	7.0	5.0	13	450	1.0
(*Nathan's* Snacks), ¼ cup, 2 oz.	120	6.0	11.0	6.0	40	680	0
in wine sauce:							
(*Acme/Blue Hill Bay*), 5 pcs., 2 oz.	85	8.0	7.0	3.0	18	550	1.0

Food and Measure	cal.	prot. (gms)	carbo. (gms)	fat (gms)	chol. (mgs)	sod. (mgs)	fiber (gms)
Herring, pickled, in wine sauce *(cont.)*							
(*Nathan's*), ¼ cup	90	5.0	7.0	4.0	25	420	0
(*Skansen* Tidbits), 5 pcs., 2 oz.	85	8.0	7.0	3.0	18	550	<1.0
Herring oil, see "Oil"							
Hibiscus drink, cooler, 8 fl. oz.:							
(*R.W. Knudsen*)	100	0	25.0	0	0	10	0
(*Santa Cruz Organic*)	100	<1.0	24.0	0	0	40	0
Hickory nut, dried, shelled, 1 oz.	187	3.6	5.2	18.3	0	tr.	1.8
Hiziki, see "Seaweed"							
Hoisin sauce:							
(*House of Tsang*), 1 tsp.	15	0	4.0	0	0	120	0
(*Ka•Me*), 2 tbsp.	70	1.0	15.0	0	0	370	0
(*Mee Tu*), 2 tbsp.	80	0	19.0	0	0	260	1.0
(*Polynesian* Chinese BBQ), 2 tbsp.	40	0	10.0	0	0	160	0
(*Roland*), 1 tbsp.	50	0	10.0	0	0	410	0
1 tbsp.	35	.5	7.1	.5	0	258	.4
raspberry (*Heaven and Earth*), 1 tbsp.	20	0	4.0	0	0	140	0
Hollandaise sauce, in jars, 2 tbsp.:							
(*Melba*)	90	1.0	1.0	9.0	80	410	0
(*Reese*)	110	0	1.0	11.0	30	60	0
Hollandaise sauce mix (*McCormick*), 1 tsp.	15	0	1.0	0	15	110	0
Hominy, dry, white (*Goya*), ¼ cup	180	4.0	39.0	0	0	0	0
Hominy, canned:							
golden, ½ cup:							
(*Allens/Allens* Pepi-Hominy)	120	2.0	27.0	.5	0	340	4.0
(*Bush's*)	60	1.0	13.0	0	0	550	3.0
white, ½ cup:							
(*Allens*)	100	2.0	22.0	.5	0	340	4.0
(*Busch's*)	70	1.0	14.0	1.0	0	530	4.0
Hominy grits, see "Corn grits"							
Hommus, see "Hummus"							
Honey, 1 tbsp.:							
(*Aunt Sue's/Grandma's/ Sue Bee*)	60	0	17.0	0	0	0	0

Food and Measure	cal.	prot. (gms)	carbo. (gms)	fat (gms)	chol. (mgs)	sod. (mgs)	fiber (gms)
raw, all varieties (*Tree of Life*)	60	0	17.0	0	0	0	0
Honey bun, see "Bun, sweet"							
Honey butter, see "Butter, flavored"							
Honey mustard, see "Mustard blend" and "Pretzel dip"							
Honey roll sausage, beef, 1 oz.	52	5.3	.6	3.0	14	375	0
Honey vanilla cream dip (*Marie's*), 2 tbsp.	60	1.0	5.0	4.5	15	20	0
Honeycomb (*Frieda's*), ½ cup, 3 oz.	260	0	70.0	0	0	0	0
Honeydew melon:							
(*Chiquita*), ¹⁄₁₀ melon .	50	1.0	13.0	0	0	35	1.0
(*Del Monte*), ¹⁄₁₀ melon, 4.7 oz.	50	1.0	13.0	0	0	35	1.0
(*Dole*), ¹⁄₁₀ melon	50	1.0	13.0	0	0	35	1.0
¹⁄₁₀ melon, 7" x 2"	46	.6	11.8	.1	0	13	.8
cubed, 1 cup	60	.8	15.6	.2	0	17	1.0
Horned melon (*Frieda's Kiwano*), 3.5-oz. melon	25	1.0	3.0	0	0	0	1.0
Horseradish, fresh:							
leafy tips, ½ cup:							
raw, chopped	6	.9	.8	.1	0	1	.2
boiled, drained, chopped	13	1.1	2.3	.2	0	2	.4
pods, ½ cup:							
raw, sliced	19	1.1	4.3	.1	0	21	1.6
boiled, drained, sliced	21	1.2	4.8	.1	0	25	2.5
Horseradish, prepared, 1 tsp., except as noted:							
(*Boar's Head*)	0	0	0	0	0	30	0
(*Zatarain's*), 1 tbsp. . . .	15	0	2.0	0	0	90	0
hot:							
chunky (*Dietz & Watson*)	10	0	0	1.0	0	0	0
creamy (*Dietz & Watson*)	0	0	0	0	0	30	0
extra (*Silver Spring*)	0	0	0	0	0	10	0

Food and Measure	cal.	prot. (gms)	carbo. (gms)	fat (gms)	chol. (mgs)	sod. (mgs)	fiber (gms)
Horseradish dip (*Marzetti's* Veggie Dip), 2 tbsp.	110	1.0	3.0	11.0	15	190	0
Horseradish mustard, see "Mustard blend"							
Horseradish sauce, 1 tsp., except as noted:							
(*Boar's Head* Pub Style)	15	0	1.0	1.5	5	15	0
(*Kraft*)	15	0	1.0	1.5	0	40	0
(*Marzetti*), 1 tbsp. ...	50	0	3.0	4.5	5	110	0
cranberry (*Dietz & Watson*)	10	0	0	1.0	0	0	0
smoky (*Dietz & Watson*)	5	0	<1.0	0	0	120	0
Hot dog, see "Frankfurter"							
Hot dog sauce, see "Chili sauce"							
Hot fudge sauce, see "Chocolate topping"							
Hot sauce (see also specific listings), 1 tsp., except as noted:							
(*Búfalo* Picante Clasica)	0	0	0	0	0	210	0
(*Búfalo* Picante Especial)	0	0	0	0	0	140	0
(*Da'Bomb* Beyond Insanity), 2 tsp.	0	0	0	0	0	0	0
(*Da'Bomb* Ground Zero/ The Final Answer), 2 tsp.	10	0	2.0	0	0	0	0
(*Frank's RedHot*)	0	0	0	0	0	200	0
(*Glory*)	0	0	0	0	0	120	0
(*La Victoria* Salsa Brava), 1 tbsp.	0	0	0	0	0	25	0
(*Tabasco*)	0	0	0	0	0	30	0
(*Taco Bell*)	0	0	0	0	0	50	0
(*TryMe* Tennessee Sunshine)	0	0	0	0	0	160	0
(*TryMe* Yucatan Sunshine)	0	0	0	0	0	125	0
(*TryMe* Tiger Sauce Original)	10	0	2.0	0	0	140	0
(*Watkins* Calypso) ...	10	0	3.0	0	0	25	0

Food and Measure	cal.	prot. (gms)	carbo. (gms)	fat (gms)	chol. (mgs)	sod. (mgs)	fiber (gms)
(*Watkins* Inferno), 2 tbsp.	35	0	8.0	0	0	800	0
(*Zapata*)	0	0	0	0	0	240	0
balsamic (*Roland*), 1 tbsp.	10	0	3.0	0	0	0	0
cayenne:							
(*Cajun Bayou*)	0	0	1.0	0	0	199	0
honey (*Pain is Good*)	15	0	3.0	0	0	55	0
chili (*Roland*)	5	0	1.0	0	0	190	0
chipotle (*Búfalo*)	0	0	0	0	0	150	0
garlic:							
(*Pain is Good*)	0	0	1.0	0	0	70	0
(*Tabasco*)	0	0	0	0	0	140	0
lemon (*Roland* Piri-Piri)	0	0	0	0	<1	0	0
green pepper (*Emeril's* Kicked Up)	0	0	0	0	0	140	0
habanero, peach (*Prairie Thyme* Ambrosia), 1 tbsp. .	35	0	9.0	0	0	5	0
Louisiana style (*Pain is Good*)	5	0	1.0	0	0	75	0
jalapeño:							
(*Búfalo*)	0	0	0	0	0	115	0
(*Cajun Bayou*)	0	0	1.0	0	0	100	0
(*La Victoria*), 1 tbsp.	5	0	1.0	0	0	140	0
(*Pain is Good* Harissa)	5	0	1.0	0	0	35	0
(*Watkins*)	0	0	0	0	0	140	0
raspberry (*Prairie Thyme* Ambrosia Original/Fiery), 1 tbsp.	35	0	9.0	0	0	5	0
wasabi (*Pain is Good*)	5	0	3.0	0	0	50	0
Jamaican style (*Pain is Good*)	0	0	0	0	0	70	0
mild (*Taco Bell*)	0	0	0	0	0	40	0
red or wing sauce (*Emeril's/Emeril's* Kicked Up)	0	0	0	0	0	140	0
Hubbard squash:							
raw:							
(*Frieda's* Blue/Orange), ¾ cup, 3 oz.	35	2.0	7.0	0	0	5	2.0
1 cup	46	2.3	10.1	.6	0	8	2.7

Food and Measure	cal.	prot. (gms)	carbo. (gms)	fat (gms)	chol. (mgs)	sod. (mgs)	fiber (gms)
Hubbard squash *(cont.)*							
baked, cubed, ½ cup	51	2.5	11.0	.6	0	8	2.9
boiled, drained, mashed, ½ cup	35	1.8	7.6	.4	0	6	3.4
Hummus, 2 tbsp., except as noted:							
(*Athenos* Greek)	50	1.0	5.0	3.0	0	160	1.0
(*Athenos* Original)	50	1.0	5.0	3.0	0	160	<1.0
(*Athenos* NeoClassic Original)	80	2.0	5.0	5.0	0	180	1.0
(*Cedar's* Organic)	60	2.0	5.0	3.0	0	95	1.0
(*Cedar's* Original)	60	2.0	5.0	4.0	0	95	1.0
(*Cedar's* Smooth n' Creamy)	70	2.0	4.0	5.0	0	80	1.0
(*Emerald Valley* Organic Traditional)	50	2.0	7.0	2.0	0	200	2.0
(*Guiltless Gourmet* Original)	50	2.0	8.0	1.5	0	110	2.0
(*Marzetti's* Oriental)	45	2.0	4.0	3.0	0	100	1.0
(*Tribe* All Natural Classic)	50	2.0	4.0	3.5	0	130	1.0
(*Tribe* Organic Classic)	50	2.0	4.0	3.5	0	100	1.0
artichoke garlic (*Athenos*)	50	1.0	4.0	3.0	0	180	<1.0
artichoke olive:							
(*Cedar's* Kalamata)	60	2.0	5.0	3.0	0	105	1.0
(*Cedar's* Smooth n' Creamy Kalamata)	70	1.0	5.0	5.0	0	90	1.0
artichoke spinach:							
(*Cedar's*)	70	2.0	5.0	4.0	0	105	1.0
(*Cedar's* Smooth n' Creamy)	50	1.0	3.0	3.5	0	70	1.0
chili:							
(*Tribe* Organic)	50	2.0	4.0	3.5	0	115	1.0
cracked (*Tribe* All Natural)	50	1.0	3.0	3.5	0	135	1.0
chili pepper, roasted (*Cedar's*)	35	2.0	6.0	.5	0	115	1.0
chipotle, spicy (*Tribe* All Natural)	45	1.0	3.0	3.0	0	130	1.0
cucumber dill (*Athenos*)	45	1.0	5.0	3.0	0	160	<1.0
dill (*Tribe* All Natural Savory)	50	2.0	4.0	3.5	0	125	1.0

Food and Measure	cal.	prot. (gms)	carbo. (gms)	fat (gms)	chol. (mgs)	sod. (mgs)	fiber (gms)
eggplant, roasted:							
(*Athenos*)	45	<1.0	4.0	3.0	0	210	<1.0
(*Tribe* All Natural) ..	35	1.0	3.0	2.5	0	150	1.0
w/40 spices (*Tribe* All Natural)	50	1.0	3.0	3.5	0	140	1.0
w/garbanzos (*Sabra* Merakesh), 1 oz. ...	90	2.0	4.0	8.0	0	150	1.0
garlic:							
(*Cedar's* Garlic Lovers)	40	2.0	5.0	1.5	0	100	1.0
(*Cedar's* Garlic Lovers Organic) .	45	2.0	5.0	2.0	0	115	1.0
(*Sabra*), 1 oz.	80	2.0	4.0	6.0	0	135	1.0
and parsley (*Athenos NeoClassic*)	80	2.0	5.0	5.0	0	200	1.0
garlic, roasted:							
(*Athenos*)	50	1.0	5.0	3.0	0	230	<.10
(*Cedar's* Smooth n' Creamy)	60	1.0	4.0	4.5	0	80	1.0
(*Guiltless Gourmet*)	50	2.0	8.0	1.5	0	110	2.0
(*Tribe* All Natural) ..	50	2.0	4.0	3.5	0	130	1.0
(*Tribe* Organic)	50	2.0	4.0	3.5	0	100	1.0
chive (*Cedar's*)	40	2.0	5.0	1.5	0	100	1.0
Greek olive (*Emerald Valley* Organic) ..	60	2.0	6.0	3.0	0	190	2.0
horseradish:							
(*Cedar's*)	60	2.0	6.0	3.5	0	85	1.0
(*Tribe* All Natural) ..	50	2.0	4.0	3.5	0	120	1.0
jalapeño:							
(*Tribe* All Natural) ..	50	1.0	4.0	3.5	0	120	2.0
smoked, and garlic (*Emerald Valley* Organic)	50	2.0	8.0	2.0	0	145	1.5
and water chestnuts (*Cedar's*)	60	1.0	4.0	4.5	0	180	2.0
lemon:							
(*Cedar's* Zesty)	60	2.0	5.0	3.5	0	85	1.0
(*Sabra*), 1 oz.	80	2.0	4.0	6.0	0	150	1.0
(*Tribe* All Natural Zesty)	50	1.0	4.0	3.0	0	130	1.0
olive:							
black (*Athenos*) ...	50	1.0	4.0	3.0	0	170	<1.0
Calamata (*Tribe* All Natural)	50	1.0	4.0	3.5	0	140	1.0

Food and Measure	cal.	prot. (gms)	carbo. (gms)	fat (gms)	chol. (mgs)	sod. (mgs)	fiber (gms)
Hummus *(cont.)*							
onion, French (*Tribe* All Natural)	50	1.0	4.0	3.5	0	120	1.0
pepper, red, roasted:							
(*Athenos*)	50	1.0	5.0	3.0	0	150	<1.0
(*Cedar's*)	50	2.0	5.0	3.0	0	80	3.0
(*Cedar's* Organic) ..	45	2.0	5.0	2.0	0	120	1.0
(*Cedar's* Smooth n' Creamy)	60	1.0	5.0	4.5	0	75	1.0
(*Emerald Valley* Organic)	50	2.0	6.0	2.5	0	160	2.0
(*Marzetti's*)	45	2.0	4.0	2.5	0	135	1.0
(*Tribe* All Natural) ..	40	1.0	3.0	2.5	0	125	1.0
(*Tribe* Organic)	40	1.0	3.0	2.5	0	95	1.0
w/red pepper, parsley (*Athenos Neo-Classic*)	80	2.0	5.0	6.0	0	130	1.0
pepper, three, spicy (*Athenos*)	50	1.0	5.0	3.0	0	230	<1.0
pesto:							
(*Athenos*)	50	1.0	5.0	3.0	0	160	<1.0
(*Cedar's*)	70	2.0	6.0	4.5	0	180	1.0
pine nuts, roasted (*Cedar's* Smooth n' Creamy)	70	2.0	4.0	5.0	0	80	1.0
sesame seeds, parsley (*Athenos NeoClassic*)	80	2.0	5.0	6.0	0	160	1.0
scallion:							
(*Athenos*)	50	1.0	5.0	3.0	0	190	<1.0
(*Tribe* All Natural) ..	50	1.0	4.0	3.5	0	125	1.0
spinach and feta (*Emerald Valley* Organic)	50	2.0	6.0	2.0	0	190	1.0
tomato basil:							
(*Tribe* All Natural) ..	50	1.0	3.0	4.0	0	115	1.0
sun-dried (*Cedar's*)	35	2.0	6.0	.5	0	115	1.0
sun-dried (*Cedar's* Organic)	60	2.0	11.0	1.0	0	150	2.0
vegetable:							
(*Cedar's* Organic) ..	45	2.0	5.0	2.0	0	120	1.0
garden (*Cedar's*) ..	60	2.0	5.0	3.5	0	90	1.0
garden (*Tribe* All Natural)	50	1.0	3.0	3.5	0	120	1.0

Food and Measure	cal.	prot. (gms)	carbo. (gms)	fat (gms)	chol. (mgs)	sod. (mgs)	fiber (gms)
Hummus mix, dry:							
(*Casbah*), 2 tbsp.* ...	50	2.0	5.0	2.0	0	160	1.0
(*Fantastic*), .5 oz.	60	3.0	7.0	2.0	0	200	2.0
Hunter sauce mix							
(*McCormick*), 1 tsp.	25	0	4.0	0	0	270	0
Hush puppies, frozen:							
(*Delta Pride*), 3 pcs. ...	140	2.0	21.0	5.0	0	470	n.a.
(*McKenzie's Gold King*), 2 oz.	190	2.0	23.0	10.0	0	470	2.0
jalapeño (*Delta Pride*), 3 pcs.	130	2.0	20.0	5.0	0	470	n.a.
Hush puppy mix:							
(*Golden Dipt* Fry Easy Corn Meal Mix), ¼ cup	120	2.0	26.0	.5	0	540	0
(*Martha White*), ¼ cup	110	3.0	25.0	0	20	610	1.0
(*Zatarain's*), 3 tbsp. ...	100	2.0	23.0	.5	0	320	1.0
Hyacinth bean, immature, boiled, drained, ½ cup	22	1.3	4.1	.1	0	1	n.a.
Hyacinth bean, dried, boiled, ½ cup	114	7.9	20.1	.6	0	7	n.a.

I

Food and Measure	cal.	prot. (gms)	carbo. (gms)	fat (gms)	chol. (mgs)	sod. (mgs)	fiber (gms)
Ice, Italian, 6 fl. oz., except as noted:							
all flavors, except lemon and orange (*Lindy's Homemade*)	80	0	20.0	0	0	0	0
cherry:							
(*Luigi's*)	130	0	32.0	0	0	15	<1.0
(*Luigi's* No Sugar), 4 fl. oz.	70	0	20.0	0	0	10	0
lemon:							
(*Luigi's*)	120	0	30.0	0	0	10	<1.0
(*Luigi's* No Sugar), 4 fl. oz.	60	0	20.0	0	0	10	0
and cherry (*Turkey Hill Venice*), 4 fl. oz.	100	0	24.0	0	0	0	0
lemon or orange (*Lindy's Homemade*)	80	0	21.0	0	0	0	0
lemon strawberry (*Luigi's*)	120	0	31.0	0	0	10	<1.0
mango:							
(*Luigi's*)	130	0	33.0	0	0	35	0
(*Turkey Hill Venice*), 4 fl. oz.	100	0	23.0	0	0	30	0
piña colada (*Luigi's*) . .	130	0	33.0	0	0	40	0
pomegranate blueberry w/acai (*Turkey Hill Venice*), 4 fl. oz. . . .	110	0	28.0	0	0	5	0
raspberry (*Turkey Hill Venice*), 4 fl. oz. . . .	100	0	24.0	0	0	0	0
Ice bar (see also "Fruit bar" and "Iced confection bar"), 1 bar:							
(*Blue Bunny* Twin Pops)	70	0	18.0	0	0	10	0

Food and Measure	cal.	prot. (gms)	carbo. (gms)	fat (gms)	chol. (mgs)	sod. (mgs)	fiber (gms)
(*Blue Bunny Bomb Pop Original*)	50	0	11.0	0	0	5	0
(*Blue Bunny Jarritos Bomb Pop*)	45	0	11.0	0	0	10	0
all flavors:							
(*Popsicle*)	45	0	11.0	0	0	0	0
(*Popsicle* ACE Juice Pops)	50	0	12.0	0	0	5	0
(*Popsicle* Rainbow)	40	0	10.0	0	0	5	0
(*Popsicle* Super Twin)	60	0	14.0	0	0	5	0
spicy:							
(*Lucas Chamoy*) . .	60	0	16.0	0	0	480	0
(*Lucas Pelucas*) . . .	70	0	17.0	0	0	580	0
Ice cream, ½ cup:							
(*Ben & Jerry's Americone Dream*)	280	4.0	32.0	15.0	60	100	0
(*Ben & Jerry's Chubby Hubby*)	330	7.0	31.0	20.0	55	150	1.0
(*Ben & Jerry's Dave Matthews Band Magic Brownie*) . . .	240	4.0	29.0	12.0	60	80	0
(*Ben & Jerry's Dublin Mudslide*)	260	4.0	29.0	15.0	60	80	1.0
(*Ben & Jerry's everything but the . . .*) . .	300	5.0	31.0	19.0	50	80	1.0
(*Ben & Jerry's Fossil Fuel*)	300	4.0	32.0	18.0	55	85	1.0
(*Ben & Jerry's Half Baked*)	270	4.0	33.0	13.0	45	85	1.0
(*Ben & Jerry's Karamel Sutra*)	270	4.0	32.0	14.0	50	75	1.0
(*Ben & Jerry's Phish Food*)	270	4.0	37.0	12.0	30	80	1.0
(*Ben & Jerry's Phish Food* Light)	210	4.0	37.0	6.0	25	90	1.0
(*Ben & Jerry's Turtle Soup*)	280	4.0	30.0	15.0	60	100	1.0
(*Ben & Jerry's Vermonty Python*)	310	4.0	30.0	19.0	60	90	1.0
(*Blue Bunny Bunny Tracks*)	170	3.0	20.0	10.0	20	70	<1.0
(*Blue Bunny Bunny Tracks* Light)	130	3.0	21.0	5.0	10	70	3.0

Food and Measure	cal.	prot. (gms)	carbo. (gms)	fat (gms)	chol. (mgs)	sod. (mgs)	fiber (gms)
Ice cream (cont.)							
(*Dreyer's/Edy's Butterfinger* Loaded)	130	3.0	19.0	5.0	5	65	1.0
(*Dreyer's/Edy's Nestlé Turtles* Grand)	160	3.0	18.0	9.0	25	50	0
(*Dreyer's/Edy's Slow Churned French Silk*)	130	3.0	20.0	4.5	20	70	1.0
almond, toasted, fudge (*Blue Bunny*)	160	3.0	18.0	9.0	25	55	<1.0
almond praline:							
(*Dreyer's/Edy's* Grand)	150	2.0	20.0	7.0	25	85	0
(*Dreyer's/Edy's Slow Churned*)	120	3.0	19.0	4.0	20	80	0
Baily's Irish Cream (*Häagen-Dazs*)	260	5.0	21.0	17.0	100	50	0
Banana Foster (*Häagen-Dazs*)	260	4.0	28.0	15.0	100	90	0
banana fudge walnut (*Ben & Jerry's Chunky Monkey*) . .	290	4.0	30.0	17.0	55	45	1.0
banana split:							
(*Ben & Jerry's*) . . .	270	4.0	30.0	15.0	60	55	1.0
(*Blue Bunny*)	140	2.0	19.0	7.0	20	50	0
(*Häagen-Dazs*)	280	4.0	31.0	16.0	90	70	0
(*Turkey Hill*)	150	2.0	19.0	7.0	25	40	1.0
(*Turkey Hill* Light) .	110	3.0	19.0	2.5	5	50	1.0
black raspberry:							
(*Turkey Hill*)	140	2.0	18.0	7.0	25	45	0
chip (*Häagen-Dazs*)	280	5.0	24.0	18.0	100	55	0
chocolate (*Breyer's* All Natural)	150	3.0	20.0	7.0	15	35	0
black walnut:							
(*Blue Bunny* Ozark)	150	2.0	18.0	7.0	25	60	0
(*Häagen-Dazs*)	300	5.0	21.0	22.0	105	85	0
brownie, chocolate caramel (*Breyer's* All Natural)	150	4.0	23.0	4.5	25	85	1.0
brownie, chocolate fudge:							
(*Ben & Jerry's Chocolate Fudge Brownie*)	250	4.0	31.0	12.0	35	75	2.0
(*Ben & Jerry's Chocolate Fudge Brownie* Organic)	240	3.0	29.0	13.0	50	50	<1.0

Food and Measure	cal.	prot. (gms)	carbo. (gms)	fat (gms)	chol. (mgs)	sod. (mgs)	fiber (gms)
(*Blue Bunny Super Fudge Brownie Light*)	120	3.0	22.0	3.0	10	50	3.0
(*Breyer's Cyclone*)	150	2.0	22.0	6.0	15	55	1.0
(*Breyer's Double Churn* No Sugar)	90	3.0	20.0	1.5	5	85	4.0
(*Dreyer's/Edy's* Loaded)	120	3.0	19.0	4.0	10	55	1.0
double (*Dreyer's/ Edy's*)	170	3.0	20.0	9.0	25	45	1.0
brownie, vanilla fudge (*Breyer's All Natural*)	150	3.0	20.0	7.0	15	45	1.0
brownie batter (*Ben & Jerry's*)	300	5.0	33.0	17.0	65	115	1.0
butter almond (*Breyer's All Natural*)	150	3.0	15.0	9.0	20	100	0
butter pecan:							
(*Ben & Jerry's*)	280	4.0	21.0	20.0	65	105	0
(*Blue Bunny*)	150	2.0	16.0	8.0	25	85	0
(*Breyer's All Natural*)	160	3.0	14.0	10.0	20	110	0
(*Breyer's Carb Smart*)	140	2.0	10.0	11.0	20	100	3.0
(*Breyer's Double Churn* Light)	120	2.0	16.0	5.0	10	105	0
(*Breyer's Double Churn* No Sugar)	110	2.0	14.0	6.0	10	105	4.0
(*Dreyer's/Edy's* Grand)	170	3.0	16.0	10.0	25	95	0
(*Dreyer's/Edy's Slow Churned*)	120	3.0	16.0	5.0	20	80	0
(*Häagen-Dazs*)	310	5.0	21.0	23.0	110	110	<1.0
(*Turkey Hill*)	160	2.0	15.0	10.0	25	95	0
w/chocolate (*Dove Pleasure*)	290	4.0	25.0	20.0	45	80	1.0
caramel:							
(*Breyer's Cyclone Caramel Tracks*)	140	2.0	19.0	7.0	15	85	0
(*Breyer's Double Churn* Light Caramel Tracks)	140	2.0	22.0	4.5	10	100	0
(*Dreyer's/Edy's Slow Churned* Delight)	120	3.0	19.0	3.5	20	50	0
(*Dreyer's/Edy's Ultimate Caramel Cup* Grand)	170	2.0	22.0	8.0	20	55	0

Food and Measure	cal.	prot. (gms)	carbo. (gms)	fat (gms)	chol. (mgs)	sod. (mgs)	fiber (gms)
Ice cream, caramel *(cont.)*							
(*Häagen-Dazs Reserve* De Sel) ...	280	4.0	28.0	17.0	85	160	0
(*Papaya Azul*)	250	4.0	37.0	10.0	35	105	0
caramel cone:							
(*Häagen-Dazs*)	320	4.0	32.0	19.0	100	190	0
(*Häagen-Dazs* Light)	250	6.0	39.0	8.0	50	130	0
caramel pecan:							
w/chocolate (*Dove* Perfection)	300	4.0	30.0	18.0	50	95	1.0
praline crunch (*Breyer's* All Natural)	160	3.0	22.0	7.0	20	110	0
cherry, black (*Turkey Hill*)	130	2.0	18.0	6.0	25	40	0
cherry chocolate chip:							
(*Ben & Jerry's Cherry Garcia*)	240	4.0	27.0	14.0	60	50	1.0
(*Breyer's* Very Chocolate Cherry)	140	3.0	22.0	4.5	10	60	1.0
(*Dove* Chocolate Cherry Courtship)	270	4.0	27.0	15.0	45	55	1.0
(*Dreyer's/Edy's* Grand)	160	2.0	19.0	8.0	20	40	0
(*Dreyer's/Edy's* Slow Churned)	120	3.0	18.0	4.0	20	50	0
cherry fudge ripple (*Turkey Hill* No Sugar/Fat)	80	3.0	22.0	0	0	70	4.0
cherry vanilla:							
(*Breyer's* All Natural)	140	3.0	17.0	6.0	20	40	0
(*Dreyer's/Edy's* Grand)	140	2.0	17.0	7.0	25	35	0
(*Häagen-Dazs*)	240	4.0	23.0	15.0	100	60	0
chocolate:							
(*Ben & Jerry's*) ...	250	4.0	25.0	15.0	40	50	2.0
(*Blue Bunny*)	130	2.0	17.0	7.0	25	55	.0
(*Blue Bunny* Gelato)	180	3.0	24.0	8.0	10	50	<1.0
(*Breyer's* All Natural)	140	3.0	16.0	7.0	20	40	1.0
(*Breyer's* All Natural Extra Creamy) ..	120	4.0	18.0	4.0	30	55	1.0
(*Breyer's* Organic) .	140	3.0	17.0	7.0	20	30	1.0
(*Breyer's Carb Smart*)	120	2.0	10.0	8.0	20	55	3.0
(*Breyer's* Double Churn Light)	100	2.0	17.0	3.5	10	55	1.0
(*Breyer's Goya*) ...	130	3.0	21.0	4.0	10	55	1.0

Food and Measure	cal.	prot. (gms)	carbo. (gms)	fat (gms)	chol. (mgs)	sod. (mgs)	fiber (gms)
(*Ciao Bella* Gelato) .	240	5.0	25.0	15.0	45	60	<1.0
(*Dove* Unconditional)	290	4.0	31.0	17.0	40	65	2.0
(*Dreyer's/Edy's* Grand)	150	3.0	17.0	8.0	25	35	1.0
(*Dreyer's/Edy's Slow Churned*)	110	3.0	16.0	3.5	20	45	1.0
(*Dreyer's/Edy's Slow Churned* No Sugar)	95	3.0	14.0	3.0	10	60	2.0
(*Good Humor*)	120	2.0	16.0	6.0	15	40	1.0
(*Häagen-Dazs*)	270	5.0	22.0	18.0	115	60	1.0
(*Häagen-Dazs* Dutch Light)	190	4.0	33.0	5.0	55	95	<1.0
(*Häagen-Dazs* Mayan)	310	5.0	29.0	19.0	90	55	1.0
(*Häagen-Dazs Reserve* Amazon Valley)	290	5.0	25.0	19.0	105	45	0
(*Palapa Azul*)	280	4.0	42.0	13.0	30	45	2.0
(*Sheer Bliss*)	320	6.0	32.0	19.0	65	65	0
(*Stonyfield* Organic)	250	3.0	21.0	17.0	60	35	0
(*Turkey Hill* All Natural)	150	3.0	18.0	8.0	30	45	0
chocolate, triple:							
(*Breyer's* All Natural)	150	3.0	17.0	8.0	20	60	1.0
(*Breyer's* Double Churn No Sugar)	110	2.0	17.0	5.0	10	45	4.0
(*Dreyer's/Edy's Slow Churned* No Sugar)	110	3.0	17.0	3.5	10	65	2.0
(*Häagen-Dazs*)	330	5.0	31.0	21.0	95	105	<1.0
chocolate almond fudge (*Blue Bunny* No Sugar)	120	3.0	13.0	8.0	25	35	3.0
chocolate caramel:							
(*Blue Bunny*)	150	2.0	20.0	7.0	25	80	0
w/chips (*Turkey Hill Dulce de Chocolate* Light)	130	2.0	25.0	3.0	5	160	1.0
chocolate chip:							
(*Blue Bunny*)	140	2.0	15.0	7.0	25	55	0
(*Blue Bunny* Gelato)	200	4.0	26.0	9.0	15	80	0
(*Breyer's* All Natural)	160	3.0	17.0	8.0	20	40	1.0
(*Dreyer's/Edy's* Grand)	170	3.0	18.0	9.0	25	45	0
(*Dreyer's/Edy's Slow Churned*)	120	3.0	17.0	4.5	20	50	0
(*Turkey Hill* Light) .	120	3.0	17.0	4.5	10	65	1.0

Food and Measure	cal.	prot. (gms)	carbo. (gms)	fat (gms)	chol. (mgs)	sod. (mgs)	fiber (gms)
Ice cream, chocolate chip *(cont.)*							
chocolate (*Häagen-Dazs*)	300	5.0	26.0	20.0	105	55	2.0
chunky (*Blue Bunny*)	160	3.0	19.0	9.0	25	55	0
malt (*Turkey Hill Light*)	120	3.0	20.0	3.5	10	85	1.0
chocolate chip cookie dough:							
(*Ben & Jerry's*) . . .	270	4.0	32.0	14.0	65	80	0
(*Ben & Jerry's Light*)	200	4.0	35.0	6.0	35	80	2.0
(*Blue Bunny*)	160	2.0	21.0	7.0	20	75	0
(*Blue Bunny Premium*)	190	3.0	23.0	10.0	35	80	0
(*Breyer's All Natural*)	160	3.0	20.0	8.0	20	50	0
(*Breyer's Cyclone*) .	160	2.0	21.0	8.0	15	65	1.0
(*Dreyer's/Edy's Grand*)	180	3.0	21.0	9.0	25	55	0
(*Dreyer's/Edy's Nestlé Toll House Loaded*)	130	2.0	21.0	4.5	10	45	1.0
(*Dreyer's/Edy's Slow Churned*)	130	3.0	20.0	4.5	20	60	0
(*Häagen-Dazs*)	310	4.0	29.0	20.0	95	125	0
(*Turkey Hill*)	160	2.0	20.0	8.0	25	80	0
(*Turkey Hill Light*) .	120	3.0	20.0	3.5	10	85	1.0
chocolate fudge:							
(*Dreyer's/Edy's Slow Churned Sugar Free*)	100	3.0	16.0	3.0	10	65	2.0
chunk (*Dreyer's/Edy's Slow Churned*) . .	120	3.0	18.0	4.5	20	50	0
chunks w/nuts (*Ben & Jerry's New York Super Fudge Chunk*)	300	5.0	29.0	19.0	35	55	2.0
sundae (*Edy's Grand*)	170	3.0	20.0	9.0	20	50	0
chocolate hazelnut (*Ciao Bella* Gelato) .	260	5.0	25.0	18.0	45	60	2.0
chocolate marshmallow (*Turkey Hill*)	160	2.0	24.0	6.0	20	100	1.0
chocolate mocha silk (*Breyer's Double Churn* Light)	130	3.0	19.0	4.5	20	50	1.0
chocolate peanut butter:							
(*Häagen-Dazs*)	360	8.0	27.0	24.0	100	100	2.0
(*Turkey Hill* Cup) . .	180	3.0	18.0	11.0	25	90	1.0

Food and Measure	cal.	prot. (gms)	carbo. (gms)	fat (gms)	chol. (mgs)	sod. (mgs)	fiber (gms)
chocolate raspberry:							
cheesecake (*Blue Bunny* Light) ...	100	2.0	18.0	2.5	10	50	3.0
swirl (*Stonyfield* Organic)	230	3.0	25.0	13.0	50	30	1.0
truffle, white (*Häagen-Dazs*) ..	310	5.0	32.0	18.0	105	65	1.0
cinnamon:							
(*Ben & Jerry's* Bun)	290	4.0	36.0	15.0	60	120	0
dulce de leche (*Häagen-Dazs*) ..	290	5.0	29.0	16.0	90	85	0
coconut, toasted, sesame brittle (*Häagen-Dazs Reserve*)	300	4.0	31.0	18.0	85	65	<1.0
coffee:							
(*Ben & Jerry's*) ...	230	4.0	21.0	14.0	70	60	0
(*Blue Bunny* Premium Coffee Break)	130	2.0	16.0	7.0	25	45	0
(*Breyer's* All Natural)	130	3.0	15.0	7.0	20	40	0
(*Breyer's* Organic) .	140	4.0	15.0	7.0	25	40	0
(*Dreyer's/Edy's* Grand)	140	2.0	15.0	8.0	25	40	0
(*Dreyer's/Edy/s Slow Churned*)	105	3.0	15.0	3.5	20	45	0
(*Häagen-Dazs*)	270	5.0	21.0	18.0	120	70	0
(*Häagen-Dazs* Light)	210	5.0	32.0	7.0	65	85	0
(*Sheer Bliss* Mediterranean)	260	3.0	25.0	18.0	65	65	0
(*Starbucks* Classic)	230	5.0	26.0	12.0	65	50	0
(*Stonyfield* Organic Gotta Have Java)	250	3.0	22.0	16.0	60	45	0
(*Turkey Hill* Colombian)	140	2.0	16.0	7.0	25	45	0
(*Turkey Hill All Natural Recipe*)	140	3.0	16.0	8.0	30	50	0
almond fudge (*Starbucks*)	250	5.0	29.0	13.0	60	65	1.0
cappuccino (*Breyer's* Double Churn Fat Free)	110	3.0	26.0	0	0	100	3.0
caramel cappuccino swirl (*Starbucks*)	240	4.0	30.0	12.0	65	100	0
chocolate chip (*Starbucks* Java Chip)	250	4.0	29.0	13.0	60	55	0

Food and Measure	cal.	prot. (gms)	carbo. (gms)	fat (gms)	chol. (mgs)	sod. (mgs)	fiber (gms)
Ice cream, coffee *(cont.)*							
espresso (*Blue Bunny* Gelato) ..	170	3.0	26.0	7.0	10	55	0
espresso (*Ciao Bella* Gelato)	210	3.0	23.0	13.0	45	70	0
espresso chip (*Edy's* Grand)	150	2.0	17.0	8.0	25	50	0
fudge brownie (*Starbucks*)	190	4.0	25.0	11.0	65	55	6.0
latte (*Starbucks* Low Fat)	170	5.0	30.0	3.0	10	60	0
toffee crunch (*Ben & Jerry's* Heath) ..	280	4.0	29.0	16.0	60	115	0
cookie dough, see "chocolate chip cookie dough," above							
cookie jar (*Breyer's*) ..	140	3.0	23.0	4.0	10	80	1.0
w/cookies (*Breyer's Oreo*)	160	2.0	20.0	8.0	20	75	0
cookies and cream:							
(*Ben & Jerry's* Sweet Cream Organic) .	250	4.0	24.0	15.0	60	95	0
(*Blue Bell*)	180	4.0	21.0	9.0	30	100	0
(*Blue Bunny*)	150	2.0	20.0	7.0	25	85	0
(*Breyer's* All Natural)	160	3.0	19.0	8.0	20	85	0
(*Breyer's* All Natural Creamery)	140	3.0	21.0	5.0	30	95	0
(*Breyer's Cyclone*) .	150	2.0	19.0	8.0	15	60	1.0
(*Breyer's* Double Churn Light)	120	2.0	20.0	4.0	10	80	0
(*Dreyer's/Edy's* Grand)	160	3.0	19.0	8.0	25	50	0
(*Dreyer's/Edy's* Loaded)	110	2.0	18.0	3.5	5	50	1.0
(*Dreyer's/Edy's* Slow Churned)	120	3.0	18.0	4.0	20	60	0
(*Good Humor*)	120	2.0	16.0	6.0	15	50	0
(*Häagen-Dazs*)	270	5.0	23.0	17.0	105	95	0
(*Stonyfield* Organic)	270	3.0	27.0	16.0	55	105	0
(*Turkey Hill*)	150	2.0	19.0	8.0	25	60	0
corn, sweet (*Palapa Azul*)	160	3.0	19.0	9.0	25	45	0
crème brûlée:							
(*Ben & Jerry's*) ...	310	4.0	36.0	17.0	90	90	0
(*Häagen-Dazs*)	280	4.0	23.0	19.0	120	75	0

Food and Measure	cal.	prot. (gms)	carbo. (gms)	fat (gms)	chol. (mgs)	sod. (mgs)	fiber (gms)
crème caramel (*Stony-field* Organic)	250	3.0	29.0	14.0	55	80	0
dulce de leche:							
(*Breyer's* All Natural)	150	3.0	20.0	6.0	20	105	0
(*Breyer's Goya*) . . .	130	2.0	23.0	3.0	10	110	0
(*Ciao Bella* Gelato) .	243	3.0	27.0	14.0	39	72	0
(*Dreyer's/Edy's* Grand)	150	2.0	20.0	7.0	25	50	0
(*Häagen-Dazs*)	290	5.0	28.0	17.0	100	95	0
(*Häagen-Dazs* Light)	220	5.0	33.0	7.0	60	110	0
eggnog (*Dreyer's/Edy's* Slow Churned)	110	2.0	18.0	3.0	20	40	0
espresso, see "coffee," above							
flan (*Palapa Azul*) . . .	200	4.0	24.0	11.0	90	45	0
fried (*Breyer's*)	140	3.0	22.0	4.0	10	170	0
fudge:							
hot, sundae (*Blue Bunny*)	150	3.0	19.0	7.0	20	65	0
ripple (*Turkey Hill*) .	140	2.0	20.0	6.0	25	55	0
swirl (*Dreyer's/Edy's* Grand)	150	2.0	19.0	7.0	25	50	0
tracks (*Dreyer's/Edy's* Grand)	180	3.0	18.0	11.0	25	60	0
tracks (*Dreyer's/Edy's* Slow Churned) . .	120	3.0	18.0	4.5	20	50	0
green tea:							
(*Häagen-Dazs*)	250	5.0	20.0	17.0	105	50	0
white chocolate chunk (*Ciao Bella* Gelato)	219	3.0	24.0	14.0	44	72	0
hazelnut gelato:							
(*Blue Bunny*)	170	4.0	23.0	7.0	15	65	0
(*Ciao Bella*)	240	3.0	24.0	15.0	45	70	<1.0
honey, Hawaiian lehua, and sweet cream (*Häagen-Dazs* Reserve)	270	4.0	26.0	17.0	100	60	0
ice cream sandwich (*Dreyer's/Edy's* Nestlé Grand)	150	3.0	19.0	7.0	25	75	0
lemon pie (*Turkey Hill* Southern)	160	2.0	22.0	7.0	25	105	0
macadamia brittle (*Häagen-Dazs*)	300	4.0	25.0	20.0	110	110	0

Food and Measure	cal.	prot. (gms)	carbo. (gms)	fat (gms)	chol. (mgs)	sod. (mgs)	fiber (gms)
Ice cream (cont.)							
mango:							
(Häagen-Dazs)	250	4.0	28.0	14.0	85	50	<1.0
and cream (Breyer's Goya)	120	2.0	20.0	3.0	10	50	0
mint chocolate chip:							
(Blue Bell)	170	4.0	18.0	9.0	35	60	0
(Blue Bunny Mint Bon Bon)	130	2.0	16.0	7.0	25	60	0
(Blue Bunny Mint Chip)	140	2.0	17.0	7.0	25	55	0
(Breyer's All Natural)	160	3.0	17.0	8.0	20	40	1.0
(Breyer's Double Churn Light) ...	130	2.0	19.0	4.5	10	50	1.0
(Ciao Bella Gelato) .	230	4.0	25.0	14.0	40	65	1.0
(Dreyer's/Edy's Grand)	170	3.0	18.0	9.0	25	45	0
(Dreyer's/Edy's Slow Churned)	120	3.0	17.0	4.5	20	50	0
(Good Humor)	120	2.0	16.0	6.0	15	45	0
(Häagen-Dazs)	300	5.0	26.0	19.0	105	85	<1.0
(Häagen-Dazs Light)	230	6.0	34.0	8.0	55	65	0
(Turkey Hill)	160	2.0	17.0	9.0	25	45	1.0
(Turkey Hill All Natural Recipe) .	160	3.0	18.0	9.0	25	45	0
cookie (Ben & Jerry's)	250	4.0	26.0	14.0	60	100	0
chunk (Ben & Jerry's)	270	4.0	26.0	17.0	65	55	1.0
chunk (Dove)	300	4.0	30.0	18.0	45	75	1.0
mocha almond fudge:							
(Dreyer's Grand) ..	160	3.0	17.0	9.0	25	45	0
(Dreyer's/Edy's Slow Churned)	120	3.0	16.0	4.5	20	45	0
mocha chip (Häagen-Dazs)	290	5.0	25.0	19.0	100	55	0
mud pie (Starbucks) .	240	4.0	32.0	11.0	55	85	1.0
Neapolitan:							
(Ben & Jerry's Neapolitan Dynamite)	250	4.0	29.0	13.0	45	70	1.0
(Blue Bunny)	130	2.0	16.0	6.0	25	50	0
(Dreyer's/Edy's Grand)	140	2.0	16.0	7.0	25	35	0
(Dreyer's/Edy's Slow Churned)	100	3.0	15.0	3.0	20	40	0
(Good Humor)	110	2.0	14.0	5.0	15	40	0
(Turkey Hill)	140	3.0	17.0	7.0	25	45	0

Food and Measure	cal.	prot. (gms)	carbo. (gms)	fat (gms)	chol. (mgs)	sod. (mgs)	fiber (gms)
(*Turkey Hill All Natural Recipe*) .	140	3.0	17.0	8.0	30	45	0
oatmeal cookie chunk (*Ben & Jerry's*) ...	260	4.0	30.0	14.0	55	115	1.0
peach:							
(*Breyer's* All Natural)	120	2.0	17.0	5.0	15	30	0
cobbler (*Ben & Jerry's*)	220	3.0	28.0	11.0	50	55	0
and cream (*Häagen-Dazs*)	240	3.0	29.0	12.0	75	55	0
peanut brittle (*Turkey Hill* No Sugar)	120	5.0	19.0	6.0	0	105	5.0
peanut butter:							
(*Turkey Hill* Light Mania)	130	3.0	19.0	5.0	10	95	1.0
brownie (*Blue Bunny* Sensation)	170	3.0	18.0	10	25	90	<1.0
fudge (*Blue Bunny* Light)	130	3.0	18.0	5.0	10	75	3.0
fudge (*Blue Bunny* No Sugar)	150	3.0	15.0	10	25	70	4.0
fudge (*Breyer's* Double Churn Light)	140	4.0	19.0	5.0	10	100	1.0
ripple (*Turkey Hill*) .	170	3.0	16.0	11.0	25	90	1.0
swirl (*Breyer's* Tracks)	170	4.0	19.0	9.0	10	90	1.0
peanut butter cup:							
(*Ben & Jerry's*) ...	340	6.0	28.0	24.0	55	125	1.0
(*Breyer's Reese's*) .	160	3.0	24.0	6.0	10	105	1.0
(*Dreyer's/Edy's* Grand)	180	3.0	19.0	10.0	20	75	0
(*Dreyer's/Edy's* Slow Churned)	130	3.0	17.0	6.0	20	65	0
chocolate (*Dreyer's/ Edy's* Loaded) ..	140	3.0	18.0	6.0	10	70	2.0
pear, caramelized, and toasted pecan (*Häagen-Dazs*)	270	4.0	30.0	15.0	75	50	1.0
pecan pralines and cream (*Blue Bell*) ..	200	3.0	25.0	9.0	30	80	0
peppermint (*Dreyer's/ Edy's* Slow Churned)	110	3.0	17.0	3.5	20	40	0
pineapple coconut:							
(*Häagen-Dazs*)	230	4.0	25.0	13.0	90	55	0
(*Häagen-Dazs* Light)	210	5.0	37.0	4.5	45	40	0

Food and Measure	cal.	prot. (gms)	carbo. (gms)	fat (gms)	chol. (mgs)	sod. (mgs)	fiber (gms)
Ice cream *(cont.)*							
pistachio:							
(*Ben & Jerry's Pistachio Pistachio*) ..	250	5.0	22.0	16.0	65	55	1.0
(*Blue Bunny* Gelato)	180	4.0	24.0	8.0	10	70	0
(*Ciao Bella* Gelato) .	250	4.0	24.0	15.0	40	85	<1.0
(*Häagen-Dazs*)	290	5.0	22.0	20.0	110	80	<1.0
almond (*Blue Bunny* Premium)	150	3.0	15.0	8.0	25	50	<1.0
pomegranate:							
(*Sheer Bliss*)	300	4.0	33.0	19.0	65	70	0
chip (*Häagen-Dazs Reserve*)	280	4.0	31.0	16.0	80	65	<1.0
w/dark chocolate chip (*Sheer Bliss*) ...	320	4.0	35.0	20.0	55	70	0
raspberry chocolate chip/chunk:							
(*Ben & Jerry's* Light)	180	3.0	32.0	5.0	25	60	2.0
(*Dove* Irresistibly) .	240	3.0	29.0	13.0	30	40	1.0
(*Dreyer's/Edy's Slow Churned* Royale)	120	3.0	18.0	4.0	20	45	0
(*Turkey Hill* Light) .	120	3.0	19.0	4.0	5	50	1.0
rocky road:							
(*Blue Bunny*)	150	3.0	21.0	7.0	20	90	0
(*Blue Bunny* No Sugar)	130	4.0	21.0	6.0	15	65	2.0
(*Breyer's* All Natural)	160	3.0	20.0	8.0	15	40	1.0
(*Breyer's Carb Smart*)	130	3.0	12.0	10.0	20	70	3.0
(*Breyer's Double Churn* Light)	130	3.0	22.0	4.5	10	45	1.0
(*Dreyer's/Edy's* Grand)	170	3.0	19.0	10.0	30	35	1.0
(*Dreyer's/Edy's Slow Churned*)	120	3.0	17.0	4.0	20	40	0
(*Häagen-Dazs*)	300	5.0	29.0	18.0	90	75	1.0
(*Turkey Hill*)	170	3.0	23.0	8.0	20	125	1.0
root beer (*Breyer's A&W* Float)	130	2.0	20.0	4.5	15	35	0
rum raisin:							
(*Häagen-Dazs*)	270	4.0	22.0	17.0	110	60	0
(*Turkey Hill*)	140	2.0	19.0	6.0	25	55	0
s'mores (*Ben & Jerry's*)	290	4.0	33.0	16.0	30	65	1.0
spumoni (*Dreyer's/ Edy's* Grand)	150	3.0	16.0	8.0	25	40	0

Food and Measure	cal.	prot. (gms)	carbo. (gms)	fat (gms)	chol. (mgs)	sod. (mgs)	fiber (gms)
strawberry:							
(*Ben & Jerry's*) ...	230	4.0	26.0	13.0	65	50	0
(*Ben & Jerry's* Organic)	200	3.0	20.0	12.0	55	40	0
(*Breyer's* All Natural)	120	2.0	15.0	5.0	15	30	0
(*Blue Bunny*)	120	2.0	17.0	6.0	25	50	0
(*Ciao Bella* Gelato) .	180	3.0	21.0	10.0	40	55	1.0
(*Dreyer's/Edy's* Grand Real)	130	2.0	16.0	6.0	20	30	0
(*Dreyer's/Edy's* Slow Churned)	110	2.0	18.0	3.0	15	40	0
(*Häagen-Dazs*)	250	4.0	23.0	16.0	95	65	<1.0
and cream (*Ben & Jerry's* Light) ...	150	3.0	29.0	3.5	25	50	2.0
and cream (*Turkey Hill*)	120	2.0	16.0	6.0	20	35	1.0
double (*Blue Bunny* No Sugar)	110	3.0	18.0	4.0	15	60	2.0
double (*Blue Bunny* Premium Pint) ..	160	3.0	21.0	7.0	35	40	0
marble (*Blue Bunny*)	130	2.0	17.0	6.0	25	55	0
and vanilla ice cream (*Blue Bell*)	160	3.0	23.0	7.0	30	50	0
strawberry banana (*Breyer's Dora the Explorer*)	120	2.0	24.0	2.0	5	35	0
strawberry cheesecake:							
(*Ben & Jerry's*) ...	240	3.0	27.0	13.0	45	40	0
(*Blue Bunny*)	130	2.0	20.0	5.0	20	50	0
(*Breyer's Sara Lee*)	150	2.0	22.0	5.0	10	70	0.
(*Turkey Hill* Light) .	120	2.0	20.0	3.5	10	105	0
strawberry shortcake (*Good Humor*)	130	1.0	23.0	4.5	5	55	0
sundae cone (*Dreyer's/ Edy's Nestlé Drumstick* Grand) .	180	3.0	19.0	10.0	25	45	0
tin roof sundae:							
(*Blue Bunny*)	150	2.0	19.0	8.0	25	80	0
(*Turkey Hill*)	150	2.0	19.0	8.0	25	65	0
toffee:							
(*Breyer's Heath*) ...	180	2.0	22.0	9.0	20	125	0
(*Häagen-Dazs* English)	350	4.0	33.0	22.0	110	150	0

Food and Measure	cal.	prot. (gms)	carbo. (gms)	fat (gms)	chol. (mgs)	sod. (mgs)	fiber (gms)
Ice cream, toffee *(cont.)*							
bar crunch (*Dreyer's/ Edy's* Grand) ...	160	2.0	21.0	8.0	25	55	0
toffee pudding, sticky (*Häagen-Dazs*)	300	4.0	30.0	18.0	95	75	0
turtle sundae:							
(*Blue Bunny* Home-made)	180	4.0	21.0	9.0	35	70	0
(*Blue Bunny* Home-made Pint)	240	4.0	28.0	13.0	40	105	0
(*Blue Bunny* No Sugar)	140	3.0	20.0	7.0	20	80	2.0
vanilla:							
(*Ben & Jerry's*) ...	230	4.0	22.0	14.0	70	60	0
(*Ben & Jerry's* Organic)	220	3.0	18.0	14.0	65	50	0
(*Blue Bunny*)	130	2.0	16.0	7.0	25	60	0
(*Blue Bunny* New York)	130	2.0	16.0	7.0	25	60	0
(*Blue Bunny* No Sugar/Fat)	80	4.0	20.0	0	<5	70	5.0
(*Blue Bunny* Prem-ium)	140	3.0	16.0	8.0	30	50	0
(*Blue Bunny* Prem-ium All Natural) .	160	3.0	16.0	9.0	55	50	0
(*Blue Bunny* Prem-ium Pint)	150	3.0	16.0	8.0	40	50	0
(*Breyer's* All Natural)	140	3.0	15.0	7.0	20	40	0
(*Breyer's* All Natural Creamery Extra Creamy)	120	3.0	17.0	4.0	30	50	0
(*Breyer's* All Natural Homemade)	140	3.0	16.0	7.0	35	55	0
(*Breyer's* Lactose Free)	130	2.0	14.0	7.0	20	35	0
(*Breyer's Carb Smart*)	110	2.0	10.0	8.0	20	30	3.0
(*Breyer's* Double Churn Fat Free) .	90	3.0	21.0	0	0	50	3.0
(*Breyer's* Double Churn Light) ...	100	2.0	17.0	3.0	10	55	0
(*Breyer's* Double Churn No Sugar)	80	2.0	14.0	4.0	10	40	4.0
(*Breyer's Goya*) ...	120	2.0	19.0	3.5	10	60	0
(*Ciao Bella* Gelato) .	210	3.0	22.0	12.0	45	70	0

Food and Measure	cal.	prot. (gms)	carbo. (gms)	fat (gms)	chol. (mgs)	sod. (mgs)	fiber (gms)
(*Dreyer's* Grand) ..	150	2.0	14.0	10.0	35	35	0
(*Dreyer's/Edy's* Slow Churned)	100	3.0	15.0	3.5	20	45	0
(*Edy's* Grand)	140	2.0	15.0	8.0	25	35	0
(*Good Humor* Classic)	110	2.0	14.0	5	15	40	0
(*Häagen-Dazs*)	270	5.0	21.0	18.0	120	70	0
(*Stonyfield* Organic)	240	3.0	21.0	16.0	60	45	0
(*Turkey Hill* Original)	140	2.0	16.0	7.0	30	45	0
double (*Dreyer's/ Edy's* Grand) ...	140	3.0	16.0	7.0	35	40	0
vanilla, French:							
(*Blue Bell*)	160	4.0	19.0	8.0	75	60	0
(*Blue Bunny*)	140	2.0	16.0	8.0	55	55	0
(*Blue Bunny* Family)	140	2.0	15.0	7.0	55	50	0
(*Blue Bunny* Premium)	150	3.0	17.0	8.0	55	50	0
(*Breyer's* All Natural)	140	3.0	15.0	8.0	45	40	0
(*Breyer's* Double Churn No Sugar)	90	2.0	14.0	4.5	30	45	4.0
(*Dreyer's/Edy's* Grand)	150	2.0	16.0	9.0	50	35	0
(*Dreyer's/Edy's* Slow Churned)	100	3.0	15.0	3.5	30	45	0
(*Turkey Hill*)	140	2.0	16.0	7.0	50	45	0
vanilla, w/chocolate:							
chip (*Häagen-Dazs*)	290	5.0	26.0	18.0	105	75	0
chunks, and brownie (*Dove* Chocolate & Brownie Affair) ..	300	4.0	30.0	19.0	50	65	1.0
swirl (*Dreyer's/Edy's Slow Churned* No Sugar)	100	3.0	14.0	3.0	10	65	2.0
swirl/chunks (*Dove* Chocolate Soul) .	290	4.0	29.0	18.0	45	75	1.0
vanilla bean:							
(*Blue Bell* Natural) .	180	4.0	21.0	8.0	35	65	0
(*Breyer's* Organic) .	140	3.0	15.0	7.0	20	40	0
(*Breyers* Double Churn Light)	100	2.0	17.0	3.0	10	50	0
(*Dove* Beyond)	240	4.0	23.0	15.0	50	60	0
(*Dreyer's/Edy's* Grand)	140	2.0	15.0	8.0	25	35	0
(*Dreyer's/Edy's* Slow Churned)	100	3.0	15.0	3.5	20	45	0
(*Häagen-Dazs*)	290	5.0	26.0	18.0	105	75	0
(*Häagen-Dazs* Light)	200	5.0	29.0	7.0	65	55	0

Food and Measure	cal.	prot. (gms)	carbo. (gms)	fat (gms)	chol. (mgs)	sod. (mgs)	fiber (gms)
Ice cream, vanilla bean *(cont.)*							
(*Turkey Hill*)	140	2.0	16.0	7.0	30	45	0
(*Turkey Hill* Light) .	100	3.0	16.0	2.5	10	65	1.0
(*Turkey Hill* No Sugar/Fat)	70	3.0	19.0	0	0	75	5.0
(*Turkey Hill* All Natural Recipe) .	140	2.0	16.0	8.0	30	50	0
vanilla caramel fudge (*Ben & Jerry's*) . . .	270	4.0	31.0	14.0	65	100	0
vanilla chai (*Stoneyfield Organic*)	240	3.0	21.0	16.0	60	45	0
vanilla and chocolate:							
(*Blue Bunny*)	130	2.0	16.0	6.0	25	60	0
(*Breyer's* All Natural)	140	3.0	16.0	7.0	20	40	0
(*Dreyer's/Edy's Slow Churned*)	100	3.0	13.0	3.5	20	45	0
(*Edy's* Grand)	150	3.0	16.0	8.0	25	30	0
(*Turkey Hill*)	140	2.0	17.0	7.0	25	45	0
vanilla and chocolate and strawberry:							
(*Breyer's* All Natural)	130	3.0	16.0	7.0	20	40	0
(*Breyer's* Double Churn Light)	100	2.0	17.0	3.0	10	50	0
(*Breyer's* Double Churn* No Sugar)	80	2.0	14.0	4.0	10	40	4.0
vanilla fudge:							
(*Häagen-Dazs*)	290	5.0	26.0	18.0	100	95	0
brownie (*Häagen-Dazs*) . .	300	5.0	28.0	19.0	105	100	0
vanilla fudge twirl:							
(*Blue Bunny*)	140	2.0	18.0	6.0	25	60	0
(*Breyer's* All Natural)	130	3.0	17.0	6.0	15	50	0
(*Breyer's* Organic) .	140	3.0	19.0	6.0	15	35	1.0
(*Good Humor*)	120	2.0	19.0	5.0	15	50	1.0
vanilla and orange sherbet, see "Sherbet"							
vanilla pomegranate:							
(*Sheer Bliss*)	320	3.0	33.0	17.0	60	65	0
and blueberry (*Sheer Bliss*) . . .	290	3.0	32.0	16.0	55	60	0
vanilla Swiss almond (*Häagen-Dazs*)	300	5.0	24.0	20.0	105	75	<1.0
vanilla toffee (*Ben & Jerry's Heath*)	290	4.0	29.0	17.0	65	110	0

Food and Measure	cal.	prot. (gms)	carbo. (gms)	fat (gms)	chol. (mgs)	sod. (mgs)	fiber (gms)
"Ice cream," nondairy, ½ cup:							
almond pecan (*It's So Delicious*)	140	2.0	24.0	4.5	0	175	3.0
banana, w/chocolate (*Purely Decadent*) .	230	2.0	31.0	13.0	0	15	5.0
"butter" pecan:							
(*Organic So Delicious*)	160	2.0	22.0	7.0	0	90	3.0
(*Soy Dream*)	150	1.0	19.0	9.0	0	140	<1.0
(*Tofutti Better Pecan*)	210	1.0	21.0	13.0	0	220	0
carob:							
almond (*Rice Dream*)	190	0	27.0	9.0	0	75	1.0
peppermint (*It's Soy Delicious*)	115	2.0	24.0	1.5	0	130	2.0
chai (*It's Soy Delicious*)	110	2.0	25.0	1.5	0	160	2.0
cherry (*Purely Decadent* Nirvana)	190	1.0	32.0	9.0	0	15	5.0
chocolate:							
(*It's Soy Delicious Awesome*)	115	2.0	24.0	1.5	0	130	2.0
(*Organic So Delicious* Velvet) . . .	130	2.0	23.0	3.5	0	50	1.0
(*Purely Decadent Obsession*)	210	2.0	36.0	9.0	0	15	5.0
(*Soy Dream*)	120	1.0	17.0	6.0	0	110	1.0
(*Temptation Fair Trade Certified*) .	210	1.0	27.0	14.0	0	40	1.0
chocolate almond (*It's Soy Delicious*)	140	3.0	23.0	4.5	0	165	3.0
chocolate brownie almond (*Purely Decadent*)	210	3.0	34.0	10.0	0	75	6.0
chocolate caramel chai (*Rice Dream* Supreme)	150	1.0	24.0	7.0	0	75	2.0
chocolate chip cookie dough (*Temptation*)	230	1.0	27.0	13.0	0	57	1.0
chocolate coffee (*It's Soy Delicious*)	110	1.0	25.0	1.5	0	105	2.0
chocolate fudge (*Soy Dream*)	130	1.0	18.0	7.0	0	115	1.0
chocolate peanut butter:							
(*It's Soy Delicious*) .	135	3.0	24.0	3.5	0	155	3.0
(*Organic So Delicious*)	140	2.0	23.0	4.5	0	60	2.0

Food and Measure	cal.	prot. (gms)	carbo. (gms)	fat (gms)	chol. (mgs)	sod. (mgs)	fiber (gms)
"Ice cream," nondairy *(cont.)*							
cocoa marble fudge							
(*Rice Dream* Organic)	180	<1.0	31.0	6.0	0	90	1.0
coconut (*Purely Deca-*							
dent Craze)	240	3.0	31.0	12.0	0	60	6.0
coffee (*Temptation Fair*							
Trade Certified) . . .	200	1.0	25.0	14.0	0	40	0
cookie:							
(*Purely Decadent*							
Avalanche)	200	2.0	34.0	9.0	0	70	5.0
(*Rice Dream* Cookies							
'n Dream)	170	1.0	24.0	8.0	0	85	0
dough (*Purely Deca-*							
dent Gluten Free)	230	1.0	36.0	8.0	0	75	5.0
cookies and "cream"							
(*Organic So Deli-*							
cious)	150	2.0	26.0	4.0	0	80	3.0
dulce de leche (*Organic*							
So Delicious)	140	1.0	26.0	3.0	0	130	2.0
espresso (*It's Soy*							
Delicious)	115	2.0	23.0	1.5	0	130	2.0
green tea:							
(*It's Soy Delicious*) .	110	2.0	24.0	1.5	0	130	2.0
(*Soy Dream*)	140	<1.0	18.0	8.0	0	125	<1.0
(*Temptation Fair*							
Trade Certified) .	200	1.0	24.0	13.0	0	35	0
mango raspberry (*It's*							
Soy Delicious)	110	1.0	25.0	1.5	0	105	2.0
mint, chunky, w/choco-							
late (*Purely Decadent*							
Madness)	200	2.0	35.0	8.0	0	30	6.0
mint carob chip (*Rice*							
Dream)	170	1.0	25.0	8.0	0	85	0
mint chocolate chip:							
(*Purely Decadent*) .	190	1.0	27.0	8.0	0	45	5.0
(*Temptation*)	220	1.0	40.0	14.0	0	40	0
mint fudge, marble							
(*Organic So Deli-*							
cious)	140	1.0	27.0	3.0	0	55	2.0
mocha fudge:							
(*Organic So*							
Delicious)	130	2.0	26.0	3.0	0	85	3.0
(*Soy Dream*)	140	<1.0	21.0	7.0	0	120	<1.0

Food and Measure	cal.	prot. (gms)	carbo. (gms)	fat (gms)	chol. (mgs)	sod. (mgs)	fiber (gms)
almond (*Purely Decadent*)	200	3.0	32.0	9.0	0	45	6.0
Neapolitan:							
(*Organic So Delicious*)	120	2.0	23.0	3.5	0	55	2.0
(*Rice Dream*)	150	1.0	23.0	6.0	0	100	1.0
orange vanilla swirl (*Rice Dream*)	160	1.0	22.0	7.0	0	90	0
peach cobbler (*Temptation*)	230	1.0	31.0	14.0	0	80	1.0
peach pie (*Rice Dream*)	150	0	23.0	6.0	0	55	1.0
peanut butter (*Purely Decadent* Zig Zag) .	230	3.0	32.0	13.0	0	50	5.0
pistachio almond (*It's Soy Delicious*)	130	3.0	23.0	4.5	0	200	3.0
pomegranate chip (*Purely Decadent*) .	200	1.0	33.0	8.0	0	40	5.0
praline pecan (*Purely Decadent*)	210	2.0	33.0	10.0	0	50	5.0
raspberry:							
(*It's Soy Delicious*) .	115	1.0	25.0	1.5	0	120	2.0
à la mode (*Purely Decadent*)	200	2.0	34.0	7.0	0	70	5.0
rocky road (*Purely Decadent*)	190	2.0	31.0	8.0	0	85	5.0
strawberry:							
(*Organic So Delicious*)	120	1.0	23.0	3.0	0	55	3.0
(*Purely Decadent*) .	170	1.0	33.0	4.5	0	30	4.0
(*Rice Dream* Organic)	150	0	25.0	5.0	0	75	0
(*Temptation*)	200	1.0	24.0	13.0	0	35	0
swirl (*Soy Dream*) .	140	<1.0	20.0	7.0	0	125	<1.0
turtle (*Purely Decadent* Trails)	200	1.0	31.0	8.0	0	85	5.0
vanilla:							
(*It's Soy Delicious*) .	110	2.0	24.0	1.5	0	130	2.0
(*Purely Decadent* Purely)	170	1.0	29.0	8.0	0	20	6.0
(*Rice Dream* Organic)	140	0	22.0	6.0	0	75	0
(*Soy Dream*)	140	<1.0	17.0	8.0	0	125	<1.0
creamy (*Organic So Delicious*)	130	1.0	24.0	3.0	0	55	3.0
French (*Soy Dream*)	140	<1.0	17.0	8.0	0	125	<1.0
French (*Temptation*)	200	1.0	24.0	18.0	0	35	1.0

Food and Measure	cal.	prot. (gms)	carbo. (gms)	fat (gms)	chol. (mgs)	sod. (mgs)	fiber (gms)
"Ice cream," nondairy (cont.)							
vanilla almond, Swiss:							
(*Purely Decadent*) .	200	2.0	31.0	9.0	0	90	6.0
(*Rice Dream*)	150	<1.0	25.0	8.0	0	80	<1.0
vanilla fudge:							
(*It's Soy Delicious*) .	120	2.0	25.0	1.5	0	130	2.0
swirl (*Soy Dream*) .	140	<1.0	20.0	7.0	0	120	<1.0
vanilla gingersnap							
(*Rice Dream*)	150	0	22.0	6.0	0	65	1.0
vanilla hazelnut fudge							
(*Rice Dream*)	150	0	22.0	7.0	0	60	1.0
Ice cream bar (see also "Iced confection bar"), 1 bar:							
(*Ben & Jerry's Half Baked*)	360	5.0	46.0	18.0	50	150	2.0
(*Blue Bunny Supremes Bunny Tracks*)	220	3.0	22.0	14.0	15	75	<1.0
(*Blue Bunny Sweet Freedom Supremes* Turtle Sundae)	160	2.0	17.0	12.0	10	60	1.0
(*Twix* Single)	170	2.0	19.0	10.0	10	50	0
almond, toasted:							
(*Good Humor*)	180	2.0	22.0	10.0	10	30	1.0
(*Good Humor* Single)	240	2.0	30.0	12.0	10	40	1.0
brownie, fudge (*Blue Bunny Super Fudge Brownie*)	200	2.0	23.0	12.0	15	55	0
caramel, w/chocolate:							
(*Klondike Nascar*) .	260	3.0	31.0	14.0	15	150	1.0
(*Klondike Nascar* Single)	310	4.0	37.0	17.0	15	170	1.0
crisps (*Blue Bunny* Crunch)	150	2.0	14.0	10.0	15	50	0
cherry, w/chocolate:							
(*Ben & Jerry's Cherry Garcia*) . .	270	4.0	28.0	19.0	35	35	1.0
(*Klondike*)	250	2.0	24.0	17.0	20	55	0
chocolate, w/chocolate:							
(*Klondike*)	250	3.0	21.0	17.0	20	45	1.0
dark (*Häagen-Dazs*)	300	4.0	24.0	21.0	70	40	<1.0
triple (*Dove*)	340	4.0	35.0	22.0	30	50	3.0
triple (*Klondike*) . . .	240	3.0	27.0	14.0	10	75	1.0

Food and Measure	cal.	prot. (gms)	carbo. (gms)	fat (gms)	chol. (mgs)	sod. (mgs)	fiber (gms)
chocolate éclair:							
(*Blue Bunny*)	240	3.0	30.0	12.0	15	125	0
(*Good Humor*)	160	2.0	21.0	8.0	5	55	1.0
(*Good Humor* Single)	220	2.0	30.0	11.0	10	75	1.0
chocolate sundae							
(*Blue Bunny Choco-*							
late Sundae Crunch)	170	2.0	21.0	9.0	15	85	0
coffee, almond crunch							
(*Häagen-Dazs*)	310	4.0	23.0	22.0	75	65	<1.0
cookies and cream:							
(*Dreyer's/Edy's Slow*							
Churned)	150	2.0	20.0	8.0	3	45	1.0
(*Good Humor* Single)	90	2.0	18.0	1.5	5	55	2.0
cookie coated (*Good*							
Humor)	190	2.0	21.0	11.0	10	80	1.0
cookie coated (*Good*							
Humor Oreo) ...	250	3.0	28.0	15.0	15	150	1.0
dulce de leche, choco-							
late (*Häagen-Dazs*) .	300	4.0	28.0	19.0	60	70	0
mango and cream:							
(*Breyer's Goya*) ...	100	2.0	18.0	2.0	5	30	1.0
(*Breyer's Goya* Single)	120	3.0	22.0	3.0	10	45	1.0
mint, w/chocolate:							
(*Klondike York* Pep-							
permint Pattie) ..	220	3.0	22.0	14.0	10	55	1.0
dark (*Häagen-Dazs*)	290	4.0	23.0	20.0	65	30	1.0
Neapolitan, w/chocolate							
(*Klondike*)	250	3.0	22.0	17.0	20	55	1.0
peanut butter:							
(*Blue Bunny Peanut*							
Butter Panic) ...	230	4.0	19.0	16.0	15	95	<1.0
(*Blue Bunny Sweet*							
Freedom)	160	3.0	17.0	11.0	10	60	2.0
(*Good Humor*							
Reese's)	310	4.0	27.0	21.0	15	85	1.0
(*Klondike Reese's*) .	260	4.0	26.0	16.0	10	95	1.0
pomegranate,							
w/chocolate:							
(*Sheer Bliss*)	250	2.0	25.0	17.0	35	40	<1.0
dark (*Häagen-Dazs*							
Reserve)	280	3.0	27.0	18.0	55	35	1.0
raspberry, black (*Blue*							
Bunny Sweet Free-							
dom)	90	1.0	9.0	7.0	10	25	2.0

Food and Measure	cal.	prot. (gms)	carbo. (gms)	fat (gms)	chol. (mgs)	sod. (mgs)	fiber (gms)
Ice cream bar *(cont.)*							
raspberry cheesecake (*Blue Bunny Sweet Freedom Supremes*)	150	2.0	15.0	10.0	10	55	2.0
rocky road (*Breyer's Double Churn* Light)	180	4.0	23.0	9.0	5	80	3.0
strawberries and cream:							
(*Breyer's Goya*) ...	80	2.0	14.0	2.0	5	30	0
(*Breyer's Goya* Single)	100	2.0	17.0	3.0	10	40	0
strawberry:							
(*Blue Bunny Strawberry Sundae Crunch*)	170	2.0	20.0	9.0	15	55	0
(*Blue Bunny Sweet Freedom Lites*) ..	90	2.0	10.0	6.0	<5	30	2.0
strawberry cheesecake (*Klondike Sara Lee*)	290	2.0	29.0	18.0	15	85	0
strawberry shortcake:							
(*Blue Bunny*)	230	2.0	29.0	12.0	15	75	0
(*Good Humor*)	170	1.0	21.0	9.0	5	50	0
(*Good Humor* Single)	230	2.0	30.0	12.0	10	85	1.0
(*Popsicle*)	170	1.0	21.0	9.0	5	50	0
toffee w/chocolate:							
(*Blue Bunny* English Toffee Bar)	130	1.0	12.0	9.0	15	40	0
(*Blue Bunny* Royal Toffee Crunch) ..	190	2.0	17.0	13.0	20	60	0
(*Blue Bunny* Heath 2 oz.)	190	2.0	16.0	13.0	20	40	0
(*Blue Bunny* Heath 3.2 oz.)	300	3.0	26.0	21.0	35	65	0
vanilla w/chocolate:							
(*Breyer's Carb Smart*)	170	2.0	9.0	15.0	15	45	2.0
(*Breyer's Double Churn* Light)	160	3.0	21.0	8.0	5	45	3.0
(*Breyer's Double Churn* No Sugar)	150	4.0	18.0	9.0	5	35	3.0
(*Breyer's Carb Smart*)	170	2.0	9.0	15.0	15	45	2.0
(*Dreyer's/Edy's Slow Churned Nestlé Crunch* Coated) .	150	2.0	19.0	8.0	3	30	1.0
(*Good Humor* Single)	260	3.0	24.0	17.0	20	50	0

Food and Measure	cal.	prot. (gms)	carbo. (gms)	fat (gms)	chol. (mgs)	sod. (mgs)	fiber (gms)
(*Klondike* Original) .	250	3.0	22.0	17.0	20	55	0
(*Klondike Slim-a-Bear*)	100	1.0	11.0	6.0	5	20	2.0
(*Klondike Slim-a-Bear* Low Fat) ...	100	2.0	21.0	1.5	0	65	2.0
(*Klondike Slim-a-Bear* No Sugar) .	170	4.0	21.0	9.0	5	65	4.0
(*Popsicle*)	180	2.0	15.0	12.0	10	35	1.0
candy center crunch (*Good Humor*) ..	310	3.0	24.0	23.0	15	80	1.0
cookies (*Klondike Oreo*)	260	3.0	26.0	17.0	15	120	1.0
creamy (*Dreyer's/Edy's Slow Churned*)	160	2.0	19.0	8.0	3	25	1.0
crisps (*Blue Bunny Crunch*)	260	3.0	24.0	18.0	25	75	0
crisps (*Blue Bunny Sweet Freedom Lites*)	90	2.0	10.0	6.0	5	35	2.0
crisps (*Breyer's Double Churn Krunch* No Sugar)	150	4.0	18.0	9.0	5	60	3.0
crisps (*Crunch*) ...	220	2.0	18.0	15.0	15	55	0
crisps (*Klondike Krunch*)	250	3.0	22.0	17.0	20	55	0
crisps (*Klondike Krunch* Single) ..	260	3.0	24.0	17.0	15	65	0
crisps (*Klondike Slim-a-Bear Krunch* No Sugar)	170	4.0	22.0	10.0	5	85	4.0
dark (*Breyer's All Natural Single*) ..	260	4.0	25.0	17.0	30	45	1.0
dark (*Dove*)	320	4.0	32.0	21.0	35	40	2.0
dark (*Good Humor*)	180	2.0	15.0	13.0	15	30	0
dark (*Häagen-Dazs*)	300	4.0	23.0	21.0	70	45	<1.0
dark (*Klondike*) ...	250	3.0	22.0	17.0	20	50	1.0
milk (*Ben & Jerry's*)	310	4.0	26.0	21.0	45	60	1.0
milk (*Blue Bunny Homemade*)	150	2.0	13.0	11.0	20	35	0
milk (*Blue Bunny Homemade Single*)	190	3.0	16.0	13.0	30	50	0
milk (*Blue Bunny Big Star Bars*) ..	110	1.0	11.0	7.0	5	30	0

Food and Measure	cal.	prot. (gms)	carbo. (gms)	fat (gms)	chol. (mgs)	sod. (mgs)	fiber (gms)
Ice cream bar, vanila w/chocolate *(cont.)*							
milk (*Blue Bunny Big Star Bars Single*)	130	2.0	13.0	8.0	5	40	0
milk (*Dove*)	330	4.0	31.0	21.0	40	60	1.0
milk (*Good Humor*)	180	2.0	15.0	13.0	15	45	0
milk (*Häagen-Dazs*)	290	4.0	22.0	21.0	75	55	0
milk, w/almonds (*Dove*)	340	6.0	28.0	23.0	35	135	1.0
vanilla w/almonds:							
(*Ben & Jerry's*) ...	330	5.0	28.0	22.0	60	120	2.0
(*Blue Bunny Sweet Freedom*)	160	2.0	11.0	14.0	15	20	3.0
(*Breyer's All Natural Single*)	290	5.0	24.0	20.0	25	65	2.0
(*Breyer's Carb Smart*)	180	3.0	9.0	15.0	15	40	2.0
(*Breyer's Double Churn Light*)	170	4.0	21.0	9.0	5	55	3.0
(*Häagen-Dazs*)	320	5.0	22.0	12.0	75	55	<1.0
(*Klondike Hershey*)	240	4.0	23.0	15.0	10	75	1.0
vanilla w/root beer (*Blue Bunny Root Beer Float*)	80	<1.0	14.0	2.0	10	25	0
Ice cream bar, miniature, coated (*Dove*), 5 pcs., 3.1 oz.:							
dark chocolate	300	4.0	32.0	20.0	45	40	2.0
milk chocolate	300	4.0	30.0	20.0	30	55	1.0
"Ice cream" bar, nondairy, 1 bar:							
chocolate caramel chai (*Rice Dream*) .	240	<1.0	28.0	15.0	0	65	2.0
fudge:							
(*So Delicious Sugar Free*)	80	2.0	12.0	5.0	0	50	6.0
(*Sweet Nothings*) ..	100	1.0	23.0	0	0	5	0
creamy (*Organic So Delicious*)	140	3.0	25.0	4.0	0	25	2.0
creamy (*So Delicious*)	90	2.0	17.0	2.0	0	45	2.0
mango raspberry (*Sweet Nothings*) ..	100	1.0	23.0	0	0	10	0
orange or raspberry (*So Delicious*)	80	1.0	18.0	1.5	0	30	2.0

Food and Measure	cal.	prot. (gms)	carbo. (gms)	fat (gms)	chol. (mgs)	sod. (mgs)	fiber (gms)
vanilla:							
almond (*Purely Decadent Soy Delicious*)	210	2.0	26.0	10.0	0	10	4.0
and almonds (*Organic So Delicious*)	300	4.0	32.0	17.0	0	30	2.0
w/chocolate (*Purely Decadent Soy Delicious* Purely)	200	2.0	26.0	9.0	0	10	3.0
w/chocolate (*Rice Dream*)	230	1.0	24.0	15.0	0	70	<1.0
w/chocolate (*So Delicious* Sugar Free)	150	2.0	15.0	14.0	0	50	6.0
creamy, w/chocolate (*Organic So Delicious*)	260	3.0	31.0	13.0	0	25	1.0
w/nuts (*Rice Dream Nutty Bar*)	320	5.0	27.0	24.0	0	65	2.0
vanilla hazelnut fudge (*Rice Dream*)	240	<1.0	28.0	15.0	0	55	2.0
Ice cream bites, chocolate coated:							
caramel (*Dreyer's/ Edy's Dibs*), 26 pcs.	440	3.0	35.0	32.0	20	80	1.0
chocolate, 26 pcs.:							
(*Breyer's Hershey's Kisses* Poppers) .	470	5.0	34.0	35.0	25	80	2.0
(*Dreyer's/Edy's Dibs*)	420	4.0	28.0	32.0	30	75	1.0
coffee (*Dreyer's/Edy's Dibs*), 26 pcs.	400	4.0	31.0	29.0	25	65	1.0
cookie crumb (*Breyer's Oreo* Poppers), 27 pcs.	410	4.0	38.0	27.0	15	190	1.0
cookes and cream:							
(*Dreyer's/Edy's Dibs*), 26 pcs.	410	4.0	33.0	29.0	20	95	1.0
(*Good Humor* Poppers), 3.2-fl.oz. cont. . .	340	3.0	30.0	23.0	15	130	1.0
mint (*Dreyer's/Edy's Dibs*), 26 pcs.	420	3.0	29.0	32.0	25	65	0
peanut butter:							
(*Breyer's Reese's Peanut Butter Cup* Poppers), 27 pcs.	470	5.0	35.0	34.0	20	110	1.0

Food and Measure	cal.	prot. (gms)	carbo. (gms)	fat (gms)	chol. (mgs)	sod. (mgs)	fiber (gms)
Ice cream bites, peanut butter *(cont.)*							
(*Dreyer's/Edy's Dibs*), 26 pcs.	510	7.0	32.0	39.0	20	170	2.0
rocky road (*Dreyer's/ Edy's Dibs*), 26 pcs.	400	5.0	29.0	29.0	25	75	2.0
strawberry (*Dreyer's/ Edy's Dibs*), 26 pcs.	390	4.0	31.0	28.0	30	60	1.0
toffee (*Breyer's Heath Poppers*), 27 pcs. .	410	3.0	32.0	30.0	20	120	1.0
vanilla:							
(*Breyer's Hershey's Poppers*), 27 pcs.	430	5.0	31.0	31.0	25	65	1.0
(*Breyer's Hershey's Kisses Poppers*), 26 pcs.	460	5.0	33.0	34.0	25	70	1.0
(*Dreyer's/Edy's Dibs*), 26 pcs.	420	3.0	29.0	32.0	25	65	0
(*Dreyer's/Edy's Dibs Nestlé Crunch Coated*), 26 pcs. .	380	3.0	29.0	28.0	25	90	0
(*Dreyer's/Edy's Dibs Nestlé Drumstick Coated*), 26 pcs. .	390	3.0	29.0	29.0	25	90	0
(*Klondike Movie Bites*), 4.5-oz. pkg.	290	3.0	24.0	21.0	20	55	0
Ice cream cone, filled, 1 pc.:							
(*Blue Bunny Bunny Tracks King Size*) . .	410	7.0	51.0	21.0	35	180	2.0
(*Drumstick Baby Ruth*)	450	5.0	47.0	27.0	35	170	1.0
(*Good Humor* Giant King Single)	390	7.0	44.0	21.0	30	135	2.0
(*Good Humor* King Single)	250	4.0	30.0	13.0	15	100	1.0
caramel (*Blue Bunny The Champ!*)	350	7.0	40.0	19.0	35	140	1.0
cherry, fudge chunks (*Ben & Jerry's Cherry Garcia*)	310	5.0	41.0	16.0	45	110	1.0
chocolate, chocolate cookie (*Blue Bunny The Champ!* Chocolate Lovers)	300	5.0	38.0	15.0	40	130	1.0
chocolate, triple:							
(*Drumstick* King Size)	430	5.0	44.0	25.0	35	130	2.0

Food and Measure	cal.	prot. (gms)	carbo. (gms)	fat (gms)	chol. (mgs)	sod. (mgs)	fiber (gms)
brownie (*Good Humor* Giant King)	410	6.0	56.0	20.0	25	135	2.0
chocolate chip cookie dough (*Ben & Jerry's*)	380	5.0	47.0	20.0	45	170	1.0
cookies and cream:							
(*Drumstick Simply Dipped*)	330	4.0	40.0	17.0	20	110	1.0
(*Good Humor Oreo*)	220	3.0	32.0	10.0	15	120	1.0
fried (*Klondike Choco Taco*)	290	3.0	39.0	14.0	10	190	1.0
mint cookie crunch (*Drumstick Simply Dipped*)	330	4.0	39.0	17.0	20	120	1.0
strawberry (*Blue Bunny The Champ!*)	270	3.0	36.0	13.0	25	90	0
sundae:							
(*Blue Bunny* Classic)	270	4.0	32.0	14.0	25	105	1.0
(*Good Humor* Single)	260	4.0	29.0	15.0	15	80	1.0
(*Good Humor* Variety Pack)	240	4.0	30.0	15.0	5	85	1.0
chocolate (*Drumstick*)	360	5.0	33.0	23.0	25	100	1.0
chocolate (*Drumstick* Variety Pack)	360	5.0	36.0	22.0	25	100	1.0
peanut butter fudge (*Drumstick*)	360	6.0	36.0	21.0	20	120	2.0
vanilla (*Drumstick*) .	340	4.0	33.0	21.0	20	90	1.0
vanilla caramel (*Drumstick*)	360	5.0	36.0	22.0	25	100	1.0
vanilla fudge (*Drumstick*)	340	6.0	36.0	19.0	20	100	2.0
vanilla fudge (*Turkey Hill*)	320	6.0	33.0	18.0	20	120	2.0
vanilla nutty (*Blue Bunny*)	250	5.0	34.0	11.0	10	120	1.0
vanilla, w/chocolate:							
(*Drumstick Simply Dipped*)	320	4.0	38.0	17.0	20	110	1.0
swirls (*Drumstick* King Size)	330	6.0	39.0	17.0	20	120	1.0
vanilla, chocolate, nuts:							
(*Blue Bunny The Champ!*)	280	6.0	23.0	19.0	35	60	1.0
(*Klondike*)	280	5.0	30.0	16.0	15	85	1.0

Food and Measure	cal.	prot. (gms)	carbo. (gms)	fat (gms)	chol. (mgs)	sod. (mgs)	fiber (gms)
Ice cream cone, vanilla, chocolate, nuts *(cont.)*							
caramel (*Klondike*) .	300	5.0	34.0	17.0	15	105	1.0
fudge (*Klondike*) ..	300	5.0	34.0	16.0	15	110	1.0
vanilla brownie (*Blue Bunny*)	440	5.0	56.0	22.0	50	150	1.0
Ice cream cone/cup, unfilled, 1 pc.:							
bowl or cup, waffle (*Keebler*)	50	<1.0	10.0	1.0	0	25	0
cone:							
chocolate (*Oreo*) ..	60	1.0	12.0	.5	0	75	0
sugar (*Comet*)	50	1.0	11.0	0	0	20	0
sugar (*Keebler*) . . .	50	1.0	10.0	.5	0	55	0
cup:							
(*Comet*)	20	0	4.0	0	0	10	0
(*Keebler*)	15	0	4.0	0	0	20	0
fudge dipped (*Keebler Fudge Shoppe*)	35	0	6.0	1.5	0	20	0
rainbow (*Comet*) ..	20	0	4.0	0	1	10	0
Ice cream cup, filled, 10 fl. oz., except as noted:							
chocolate brownie fudge (*Good Humor Cyclone*)	390	6.0	60.0	16.0	30	125	2.0
cookies and cream:							
(*Breyer's Double Churn 100 Calorie*), 4 fl. oz.	100	3.0	20.0	1.5	5	60	3.0
(*Good Humor Cyclone*)	380	5.0	48.0	20.0	30	150	1.0
(*Popsicle Zone*) . . .	290	5.0	43.0	12.0	30	160	1.0
vanilla, w/chocolate strawberry swirl (*Good Humor Swirlwind*), 6 fl. oz.	160	4.0	31.0	2.5	10	110	0
vanilla, w/root beer (*Barq's Floatz*), 4 fl. oz.	120	<1.0	22.0	3.0	10	25	0
vanilla fudge (*Breyer's Double Churn* 100 Calorie), 4 fl. oz. ..	100	3.0	20.0	1.5	5	55	3.0

Food and Measure	cal.	prot. (gms)	carbo. (gms)	fat (gms)	chol. (mgs)	sod. (mgs)	fiber (gms)
Ice cream dessert (*Smart Ones*), 1 serving:							
brownie à la mode . . .	200	5.0	36.0	4.0	25	160	3.0
sundaes:							
chocolate chip cookie dough . . .	170	3.0	32.0	3.0	5	100	1.0
mint chocolate chip	150	4.0	28.0	3.0	5	130	1.0
mocha fudge	160	3.0	27.0	4.0	5	85	1.0
Ice cream pie, see "Ice cream sandwich"							
Ice cream sandwich, w/chocolate wafers, except as noted, 1 pc:							
caramel swirl, vanilla wafers (*Healthy Choice*)	150	3.0	30.0	2.0	10	115	1.0
chocolate (*Klondike*) .	100	2.0	21.0	1.5	0	65	3.0
chocolate w/almond:							
(*Blue Bunny* Mississippi Mud)	190	3.0	27.0	8.0	15	180	<1.0
(*Blue Bunny Big Mississippi Mud*)	280	5.0	39.0	12.0	30	230	<1.0
chocolate chip:							
malt (*Turkey Hill*) . .	210	3.0	32.0	8.0	20	190	1.0
mint (*Turkey Hill* No Sugar)	160	4.0	31.0	4.5	5	140	5.0
cookies and cream:							
(*Blue Bunny*)	250	4.0	36.0	10.0	20	310	2.0
(*Breyer's Double Churn* Light)	140	3.0	30.0	1.5	0	100	3.0
fudge (*Healthy Choice*)	140	4.0	24.0	3.0	10	110	3.0
Neapolitan:							
(*Blue Bunny*)	180	3.0	26.0	7.0	20	160	0
(*Good Humor* Giant)	250	4.0	38.0	9.0	20	130	1.0
peanut butter ripple (*Turkey Hill*)	220	4.0	28.0	10.0	20	200	1.0
strawberry, vanilla wafer:							
(*Blue Bunny Big Double Strawberry*)	270	4.0	41.0	10.0	30	160	0
cheesecake (*Turkey Hill*)	190	3.0	30.0	7.0	20	130	1.0
shortcake (*Blue Bunny*)	180	2.0	28.0	7.0	15	135	0

Food and Measure	cal.	prot. (gms)	carbo. (gms)	fat (gms)	chol. (mgs)	sod. (mgs)	fiber (gms)
Ice cream sandwich (cont.)							
vanilla:							
(*Blue Bunny*)	170	3.0	24.0	7.0	20	150	0
(*Blue Bunny Big Vanilla*)	260	4.0	39.0	10.0	35	160	0
(*Breyer's Double Churn* Light)	130	3.0	28.0	1.5	0	85	3.0
(*Healthy Choice*) . .	130	3.0	25.0	2.0	5	115	2.0
(*Good Humor*)	160	2.0	26.0	5.0	10	90	0
(*Good Humor* Giant)	250	4.0	38.0	9.0	20	125	1.0
(*Klondike*)	180	3.0	29.0	6.0	15	100	0
(*Klondike* Original Single)	290	5.0	44.0	11.0	25	150	1.0
(*Klondike Slim-a-Bear*)	100	2.0	21.0	1.5	0	65	2.0
(*Klondike Slim-a-Bear* No Sugar) .	100	3.0	20.0	2.0	5	90	2.0
bean (*Turkey Hill*) .	190	3.0	29.0	7.0	20	95	1.0
bean (*Turkey Hill* Light)	160	3.0	32.0	3.0	10	95	3.0
chocolate chip (*Blue Bunny Chips Galore!*)	310	3.0	40.0	16.0	35	170	1.0
vanilla, w/cookies:							
(*Turkey Hill Moose Tracks*)	320	4.0	41.0	17.0	30	150	2.0
chocolate (*Klondike Oreo*)	230	3.0	35.0	9.0	10	310	2.0
chocolate chip (*Blue Bunny Big Bopper*)	460	6.0	60.0	23.0	55	290	1.0
chocolate chip (*Breyer's Mrs. Fields*)	460	5.0	68.0	19.0	20	300	1.0
chocolate chip (*Good Humor*) . .	280	3.0	41.0	13.0	10	190	1.0
chocolate chunk (*Turkey Hill*)	320	3.0	44.0	15.0	30	290	1.0
vanilla wafer (*Blue Bunny*)	180	4.0	25.0	8.0	30	130	0
vanilla and chocolate (*Turkey Hill* Double Decker)	190	3.0	30.0	7.0	20	105	1.0

Food and Measure	cal.	prot. (gms)	carbo. (gms)	fat (gms)	chol. (mgs)	sod. (mgs)	fiber (gms)
vanilla fudge chip, w/fudge swirl cookie (*Ben & Jerry's* 'Wich)	340	4.0	45.0	17.0	55	220	1.0
"Ice cream" sandwich, nondairy, w/chocolate wafers, except as noted, 1 pc.:							
chocolate:							
(*Organic So Delicious* Low Fat) ..	160	3.0	27.0	3.0	0	105	2.0
(*Rice Dream* Pie) ..	330	3.0	40.0	19.0	0	50	2.0
(*So Delicious* Low Fat)	150	3.0	27.0	3.0	0	105	2.0
(*So Delicious* Low Fat Mini)	90	2.0	17.0	2.0	0	70	1.0
(*Soy Dream* Li'l Dreamers)	100	1.0	15.0	4.5	0	60	<1.0
mint:							
(*Organic So Delicious* Low Fat) ..	150	3.0	28.0	3.0	0	125	2.0
(*Rice Dream* Pie) ..	330	3.0	40.0	19.0	0	50	2.0
chocolate chip (*Organic So Delicious*)	260	3.0	41.0	10.0	0	70	2.0
mint or mocha, coated (*Organic So Delicious* Mania)	265	3.0	32.0	14.0	0	130	2.0
mocha (*Rice Dream* Pie)	330	3.0	40.0	18.0	0	50	2.0
mocha or vanilla, coated (*Purely Decadent* Mania)	240	3.0	31.0	12.0	0	100	3.0
Neapolitan:							
(*Organic So Delicious* Low Fat) ..	150	3.0	28.0	3.0	0	110	2.0
(*So Delicious* Low Fat Mini)	90	2.0	18.0	2.0	0	70	1.0
peanut butter (*Organic So Delicious*)	160	3.0	27.0	4.5	0	115	2.0
vanilla:							
(*Organic So Delicious* Big Buddy)	240	4.0	42.0	8.0	0	190	2.0
(*Organic So Delicious/So Delicious* Low Fat)	150	3.0	28.0	3.0	0	105	2.0
(*Rice Dream* Pie) ..	320	3.0	40.0	17.0	0	80	1.0

Food and Measure	cal.	prot. (gms)	carbo. (gms)	fat (gms)	chol. (mgs)	sod. (mgs)	fiber (gms)
"Ice cream" sandwich, nondairy, vanilla *(cont.)*							
(*So Delicious* Low Fat Mini)	90	2.0	17.0	2.0	0	70	1.0
(*Soy Dream* Li'l Dreamers)	100	1.0	15.0	4.0	0	60	0
oatmeal cookie (*Organic So Delicious*)	265	3.0	32.0	14.0	0	130	2.0
vanilla chocolate chip (*Organic So Delicious*)	260	3.0	41.0	10.0	0	60	2.0
Ice cream and sherbet or sorbet, see "Sherbet" and "Sorbet bar"							
Ice cream topping, see "Topping, dessert" and specific flavors							
Iced confection bar, dairy (see also "'Ice cream' bar, nondairy" and "Fruit bar"), 1 bar:							
cappuccino, creamy (*Fruit-a-Freeze*) . . .	140	2.0	21.0	6.0	20	50	0
coffee:							
fudge (*Frappuccino Java Fudge*)	130	4.0	25.0	2.0	5	50	4.0
vanilla (*Starbucks Frappuccino* Caffe Vanilla No Sugar Low Fat)	110	4.0	20.0	1.5	5	45	9.0
cucumber chili (*Palapa Azul*)	40	0	10.0	0	0	180	0
fudge:							
(*Blue Bunny* Big) . .	110	3.0	21.0	1.5	5	75	0
(*Breyer's Carb Smart*)	100	2.0	9.0	7.0	20	50	1.0
(*Fudgsicle*), 1.65 fl. oz.	60	1.0	12.0	1.5	0	50	0
(*Fudgsicle*), 2.5 fl. oz.	100	2.0	17.0	2.0	0	75	1.0
(*Fudgsicle* Fat Free)	80	2.0	13.0	0	0	60	1.0
(*Fudgsicle* Low Fat)	60	1.0	12.0	1.5	0	50	0
(*Fudgsicle* No Sugar)	80	3.0	19.0	1.5	0	95	4.0
(*Healthy Choice*) . .	80	3.0	13.0	1.0	5	60	0
(*Klondike Slim-a-Bear*)	100	3.0	19.0	2.5	5	65	4.0

Food and Measure	cal.	prot. (gms)	carbo. (gms)	fat (gms)	chol. (mgs)	sod. (mgs)	fiber (gms)
mocha:							
(*Starbucks Frappuccino* Low Fat) . . .	120	4.0	22.0	2.0	10	50	3.0
swirl (*Healthy Choice*)	90	2.0	17.0	1.5	5	50	1.0
orange sherbet:							
(*Cool Tubes*)	110	0	24.0	1.0	5	30	0
(*Popsicle Pop-Ups*)	90	1.0	18.0	1.0	5	20	0
orange sherbet/vanilla ice cream:							
(*Blue Bunny Orange Dream Bars*)	80	1.0	16.0	1.5	5	35	0
(*Creamsicle*), 2.7 fl. oz.	110	1.0	21.0	2.0	5	40	0
(*Creamsicle* Low Fat)	70	1.0	30.0	1.0	5	25	0
(*Creamsicle* No Sugar)	45	1.0	10.0	.5	<5	25	2.0
or raspberry sherbet (*Creamsicle*), 1.65 fl. oz.	70	1.0	13.0	1.0	5	25	0
or raspberry sherbet (*Creamsicle*), 2.5 fl. oz.	100	1.0	20.0	1.5	5	35	0
raspberry orange crème:							
(*Blue Bunny*)	100	3.0	19.0	1.0	5	65	0
(*Blue Bunny Health Smart*)	70	1.0	17.0	0	0	35	4.0
strawberry crème (*Blue Bunny Health Smart*)	60	1.0	16.0	0	0	35	4.0
vanilla, w/fruit ice (*Breyer's* Pure Fruit & Cream)	60	1.0	12.0	.5	0	30	0
Icing, see "Frosting"							
Indian entree, frozen (see also "Vegetable entree" and specific listings), 1 pkg.:							
matter paneer (*Amy's* Meal), 10 oz.	320	11.0	54.0	8.0	5	780	6.0
matter tofu (*Amy's* Meal), 9.5 oz.	260	12.0	37.0	8.0	0	680	5.0
paneer tikka (*Amy's* Meal), 9.5 oz.	320	8.0	36.0	18.0	20	550	5.0

J

Food and Measure	cal.	prot. (gms)	carbo. (gms)	fat (gms)	chol. (mgs)	sod. (mgs)	fiber (gms)
Jack in the Box:							
breakfast:							
biscuit:							
bacon/egg/cheese	430	17.0	34.0	25.0	220	1100	1.0
chicken	450	15.0	42.0	24.0	30	980	2.0
chicken, spicy . .	460	21.0	44.0	22.0	40	1020	2.0
sausage	440	12.0	32.0	29.0	35	870	2.0
sausage/egg/							
cheese	740	27.0	35.0	55.0	280	1430	2.0
Breakfast Jack	290	17.0	29.0	12.0	220	760	1.0
bacon	300	16.0	29.0	14.0	215	730	1.0
sausage	450	20.0	29.0	28.0	245	840	1.0
burrito:							
meaty	620	33.0	40.0	36.0	450	1480	5.0
meaty w/salsa . .	610	32.0	39.0	36.0	450	1360	5.0
sirloin/egg	790	37.0	52.0	48.0	450	1320	6.0
sirloin/egg w/salsa	790	37.0	54.0	48.0	450	1440	6.0
croissant, sausage .	580	21.0	37.0	39.0	255	770	2.0
croissant, supreme	450	18.0	36.0	25.0	235	860	1.0
French toast sticks:							
blueberry, 4	450	8.0	59.0	20.0	0	550	3.0
original, 4	470	7.0	58.0	23.0	25	450	4.0
hash brown, 1	150	1.0	13.0	10.0	0	230	2.0
sandwich:							
ciabatta	710	36.0	63.0	36.0	440	1730	3.0
Extreme Sausage	670	29.0	31.0	48.0	290	1300	2.0
ultimate	570	34.0	49.0	27.0	445	1700	2.0
burgers:							
cheeseburger:							
bacon, junior . . .	400	19.0	31.0	23.0	55	860	1.0
sirloin bacon . . .	1120	54.0	63.0	73.0	190	2620	4.0
sirloin/Swiss . . .	1070	53.0	61.0	71.0	180	1850	4.0
ultimate	1010	40.0	53.0	71.0	125	1580	2.0

Food and Measure	cal.	prot. (gms)	carbo. (gms)	fat (gms)	chol. (mgs)	sod. (mgs)	fiber (gms)
ultimate, bacon .	1090	46.0	53.0	77.0	140	2040	2.0
ultimate, sour-dough	950	38.0	36.0	73.0	125	1360	2.0
ciabatta:							
bacon/cheese single	870	31.0	66.0	54.0	90	1550	4.0
bacon/cheese double	1120	45.0	66.0	76.0	135	1670	4.0
sirloin/cheddar . .	770	43.0	65.0	38.0	110	1310	4.0
hamburger	280	14.0	30.0	12.0	30	580	1.0
w/cheese	330	16.0	31.0	15.0	45	770	1.0
deluxe	350	15.0	32.0	18.0	40	600	2.0
deluxe w/cheese .	440	19.0	34.0	25.0	65	970	2.0
Jumbo Jack	600	21.0	51.0	35.0	45	940	3.0
w/cheese	690	25.0	54.0	42.0	70	1310	3.0
sirloin steak melt . .	640	36.0	34.0	40.0	100	1490	2.0
Sourdough Jack . . .	710	27.0	36.0	51.0	75	1230	3.0
chicken/fish:							
chicken club, sour-dough, grilled . . .	530	36.0	34.0	28.0	85	1430	3.0
chicken fajita pita, w/out salsa	280	21.0	30.0	9.0	60	1110	2.0
chicken sandwich . .	400	15.0	38.0	21.0	35	730	2.0
w/bacon	440	19.0	39.0	24.0	40	970	2.0
w/cheese	430	17.0	40.0	24.0	45	880	1.0
chicken strips:							
crispy, 4	500	35.0	36.0	25.0	80	1260	3.0
grilled, 4	180	37.0	3.0	2.0	125	700	0
Chipotle Chicken Ciabatta:							
crispy, spicy	750	37.0	75.0	34.0	80	1650	5.0
grilled	690	44.0	65.0	28.0	105	1850	4.0
fish & chips:							
large	830	21.0	92.0	42.0	35	1530	6.0
medium	660	18.0	70.0	34.0	35	1250	5.0
small	570	17.0	58.0	30.0	35	1100	4.0
Jack's Spicy Chicken	620	25.0	61.0	31.0	50	1100	4.0
w/cheese	700	29.0	62.0	37.0	70	1410	4.0
extras/snacks:							
bacon cheddar potato wedges . .	720	21.0	52.0	48.0	45	1360	4.0
Beef Monster Taco .	240	8.0	20.0	14.0	20	390	3.0
beef taco, regular . .	160	5.0	15.0	8.0	15	270	2.0

Food and Measure	cal.	prot. (gms)	carbo. (gms)	fat (gms)	chol. (mgs)	sod. (mgs)	fiber (gms)
Jack in the Box, extras/snacks _(cont.)_							
chicken bites, spicy:							
7 pcs.	290	18.0	21.0	14.0	45	660	3.0
16 pcs.	650	41.0	49.0	33.0	100	1500	6.0
egg roll, 1 pc.	130	5.0	15.0	6.0	5	310	2.0
egg roll, 3 pcs.	400	14.0	44.0	19.0	15	920	6.0
fries, natural cut:							
large	640	9.0	77.0	33.0	0	1180	9.0
medium	450	6.0	54.0	23.0	0	830	6.0
small	340	5.0	41.0	17.0	0	620	5.0
fries, seasoned curly:							
large	550	8.0	60.0	31.0	0	1200	6.0
medium	400	6.0	45.0	23.0	0	890	5.0
small	270	4.0	30.0	15.0	0	590	3.0
fruit cup	90	1.0	22.0	0	0	20	2.0
jalapeños, stuffed:							
3 pcs.	230	7.0	22.0	13.0	20	690	2.0
7 pcs.	530	15.0	51.0	30.0	45	1600	4.0
mozzarella sticks:							
3 pcs.	240	11.0	21.0	12.0	25	420	1.0
6 pcs.	483	20.0	39.0	27.0	46	1018	2.0
onion rings, 8	500	6.0	51.0	30.0	0	420	3.0
sampler trio	750	35.0	65.0	39.0	85	1760	5.0
salad, w/out dressing, condiments:							
chicken, Asian:							
crispy	330	21.0	34.0	13.0	40	650	7.0
grilled	160	22.0	18.0	1.5	65	870	5.0
chicken, Southwest:							
crispy	480	30.0	44.0	23.0	70	1040	9.0
grilled	320	31.0	27.0	12.0	90	760	7.0
chicken club:							
crispy	480	33.0	28.0	27.0	80	1060	6.0
grilled	320	34.0	11.0	16.0	105	780	4.0
side salad	50	3.0	5.0	3.0	10	60	2.0
sauces/dressing:							
dipping sauce:							
barbecue	45	0	11.0	0	0	330	0
Buffalo, _Franks Red Hot_	10	0	2.0	0	0	840	0
buttermilk house	130	0	3.0	13.0	10	210	0
marinara, zesty .	15	0	4.0	0	0	200	0
sweet and sour .	45	0	11.0	0	0	160	0
teriyaki	60	2.0	13.0	0	0	460	0

Food and Measure	cal.	prot. (gms)	carbo. (gms)	fat (gms)	chol. (mgs)	sod. (mgs)	fiber (gms)
dressing:							
Asian sesame . . .	230	1.0	20.0	17.0	0	780	0
bacon ranch	320	2.0	4.0	33.0	35	810	0
balsamic, low fat	40	0	6.0	2.0	0	600	0
ranch	390	1.0	4.0	41.0	30	590	0
ranch, lite	190	1.0	3.0	18.0	25	700	0
Southwest, creamy	270	1.0	4.0	27.0	30	1060	0
mayo-onion sauce .	90	0	1.0	10.0	5	85	0
salsa	5	0	1.0	0	0	105	0
soy sauce	5	1.0	1.0	0	0	480	0
syrup, *Log Cabin* . .	190	0	49.0	0	0	35	0
taco sauce	0	0	0	0	0	80	0
tartar sauce	210	0	2.0	22.0	20	370	0
condiments:							
almonds:							
sliced, ranch . . .	100	4.0	3.0	9.0	0	130	2.0
slivered	110	4.0	4.0	9.0	0	5	2.0
cheese:							
American, slice .	45	2.0	1.0	3.5	10	180	0
cheddar, .75 oz. .	90	5.0	1.0	7.0	20	135	0
Swiss, .75 oz. . .	80	6.0	0	7.0	25	n.a.	0
Swiss style, slice	40	2.0	1.0	3.0	10	150	0
corn sticks, spicy . .	130	2.0	20.0	5.0	0	150	<1.0
croutons, seasoned	100	2.0	11.0	5.0	0	230	0
grape jelly	35	0	9.0	0	0	10	0
sour cream	60	1.0	2.0	5.0	15	25	<1.0
spread, *Country*							
Crock	25	0	0	2.5	0	45	0
whipped topping . .	110	0	5.0	10.0	0	15	0
wonton strips	110	2.0	13.0	6.0	0	45	0
shakes, ice cream:							
chocolate, 16 oz. . .	720	12.0	89.0	35.0	130	270	1.0
egg nog, 16 oz. . . .	730	11.0	90.0	35.0	115	240	0
Oreo, 16 oz.	770	12.0	88.0	40.0	115	370	1.0
strawberry, 16 oz. .	730	11.0	91.0	35.0	115	240	0
vanilla, 16 oz.	650	11.0	70.0	35.0	115	230	0
desserts:							
cheesecake	310	7.0	34.0	16.0	55	220	0
chocolate overload							
cake	300	4.0	57.0	7.0	40	360	2.0
Jackfruit, fresh,							
trimmed, 1 oz. . . .	27	.4	6.8	.1	0	1	.5
Jackfruit, canned, in							
syrup, ½ cup	82	.3	21.3	.1	0	10	.8

Food and Measure	cal.	prot. (gms)	carbo. (gms)	fat (gms)	chol. (mgs)	sod. (mgs)	fiber (gms)
Jalapeño, see "Pepper, jalapeño"							
Jalapeño sauce, see "Hot sauce" and specific listings							
Jalapeño raspberry sauce (*Fiesta*), 2 tbsp.	20	4.0	3.0	1.0	0	220	6.0
Jam and preserves (see also "Fruit spreads"), 1 tbsp.:							
all fruits:							
(*Knott's Berry Farm*)	50	0	13.0	0	0	0	0
(*Smucker's*)	50	0	13.0	0	0	0	0
(*Smucker's* Low Sugar)	25	0	6.0	0	0	0	0
(*Smucker's* Sugar Free)	10	0	5.0	0	0	0	0
except blackberry (*Polaner* Fancy Fruit)	50	0	13.0	0	0	0	0
except blackberry guava (*Campagna*)	40	0	10.0	0	0	0	0
blackberry (*Polaner* Fancy Fruit)	50	0	13.0	0	0	5	0
blackberry guava (*Campagna*)	45	0	11.0	0	0	0	0
orange marmalade:							
(*Cascadian Farm* Organic)	45	0	11.0	0	0	0	0
(*Crosse & Blackwell*)	50	0	13.0	0	0	0	0
raspberry or strawberry (*Cascadian Farms* Organic)	40	0	10.0	0	0	5	0
Jambalaya entree, frozen:							
(*Contessa*):							
w/sauce, 8 oz.	240	15.0	29.0	7.0	50	1120	2.0
w/out sauce, 6 oz. . .	180	14.0	25.0	3.0	50	400	2.0
(*Zatarain's* New Orleans), 12-oz. pkg.	400	18.0	69.0	5.0	30	1440	2.0
Java plum:							
3 medium, .4 oz.	5	.1	1.4	<.1	0	1	<1.0
seeded, ½ cup	41	.5	10.5	.2	0	9	<1.0

Food and Measure	cal.	prot. (gms)	carbo. (gms)	fat (gms)	chol. (mgs)	sod. (mgs)	fiber (gms)
Jelly, fruit, 1 tbsp.:							
all fruits, except grape and currant							
(*Smucker's*)	50	0	13.0	0	0	0	0
apple mint:							
(*Great Expectations*)	50	0	13.0	0	0	5	0
or guava (*Crosse & Blackwell*)	50	0	13.0	0	0	0	0
grape:							
(*Campagna*)	45	0	12.0	0	0	0	0
(*Smucker's Squeeze*)	50	0	13.0	0	0	5	0
grape and currant							
(*Smucker's*)	50	0	13.0	0	0	5	0
guava (*Goya*)	58	0	14.0	0	0	0	0
Jelly, hot pepper:							
(*Campagna*), 1 tbsp. .	50	0	13.0	0	0	0	0
(*Reese*), 1 tbsp.	50	0	13.0	0	0	35	0
Jerk sauce, see "Barbecue sauce" and "Marinade"							
Jerk seasoning (see also "Rubs"):							
(*McCormick* Caribbean), ¼ tsp.	0	0	0	0	0	70	0
spice paste (*Neera's* Jamaican), 2 tsp. ...	15	1.0	4.0	0	0	290	1.0
Jerusalem artichoke:							
(*Frieda's Sunchoke*), ½ cup, 3 oz.	70	2.0	14.0	0	0	0	1.0
sliced, ½ cup	57	1.5	13.1	<.1	0	3	1.2
Jew's ear, see "Pepeao"							
Jicama, see "Yam bean"							
Jujube:							
raw, seeded, 1 oz. ...	22	.3	5.7	.1	0	1	n.a.
dried, 1 oz.	81	1.0	20.1	.3	0	3	n.a.
Jute, potherb, ½ cup:							
raw	5	.7	.8	<.1	0	1	n.a.
boiled, drained	16	1.6	3.1	.1	0	5	.9

K

Food and Measure	cal.	prot. (gms)	carbo. (gms)	fat (gms)	chol. (mgs)	sod. (mgs)	fiber (gms)
Kabocha squash							
(*Frieda's*), 3 oz. . . .	30	1.0	7.0	0	0	0	1.0
Kahn choy, see "Celery, Chinese"							
Kale, fresh:							
(*Glory*), 2.8 oz.	40	3.0	8.0	.5	0	35	2.0
raw, chopped, ½ cup .	17	1.1	3.4	.2	0	15	.7
boiled, drained,							
chopped, ½ cup . . .	18	1.2	3.7	.3	0	5	3.6
Kale, canned, ½ cup:							
chopped (*Bush's*)	30	2.0	4.0	0	0	330	2.0
seasoned (*Glory*)	35	2.0	5.0	.5	0	490	1.0
seasoned (*Sunshine*) .	35	3.0	5.0	.5	0	830	1.0
Kale, frozen, boiled, drained, chopped,							
½ cup	20	1.9	3.4	.3	0	10	1.3
Kale, Chinese, fresh:							
(*Frieda's* Chinese Broccoli), 1 cup, 3 oz.	15	2.0	3.0	0	0	15	0
cooked, 1 cup	19	1.0	3.3	.6	0	6	2.2
Kale, Scotch, ½ cup:							
raw, chopped	14	1.0	2.8	.2	0	24	.6
boiled, drained,							
chopped	18	1.2	3.7	.3	0	29	.8
Kamranga, see "Carambola"							
Kamut, grain (*Shiloh Farms* Organic),							
¼ cup	170	6.0	35.0	1.0	0	0	9.0
Kamut flakes (see also "Cereal"), (*Shiloh Farms* Organic),							
½ cup	140	6.0	28.0	.5	0	0	4.0

Food and Measure	cal.	prot. (gms)	carbo. (gms)	fat (gms)	chol. (mgs)	sod. (mgs)	fiber (gms)
Kamut flour							
(*Arrowhead Mills Organic*), ⅓ cup ...	130	5.0	25.0	1.0	0	0	4.0
Kanpo, dried:							
.2-oz. strip	16	.5	4.1	<.1	0	1	n.a.
½ cup	70	2.3	15.6	.1	0	4	n.a.
Kasha, see "Buck wheat groats"							
Kefir (*Lifeway*), 8 fl. oz., plain:							
whole milk, organic ..	160	10.0	12.0	8.0	30	125	3.0
low fat, organic	110	14.0	12.0	2.5	10	125	3.0
Helios, organic	120	8.0	12.0	4.0	15	85	2.0
Ketchup, 1 tbsp.:							
(*Annie's Naturals Organic*)	15	0	3.0	0	0	150	0
(*Del Monte*)	15	0	4.0	0	0	190	0
(*Heinz*)	15	0	4.0	0	0	190	0
(*Hunt's*)	15	0	4.0	0	0	180	0
(*Muir Glen Organic*) ..	20	0	4.0	0	0	230	0
jalapeño (*Fiesta*)	15	0	3.0	0	0	210	0
KFC, 1 serving:							
Extra Crispy:							
breast	440	34.0	15.0	27.0	105	970	0
drumstick	160	12.0	6.0	10.0	55	370	0
thigh	370	18.0	12.0	28.0	85	850	0
whole wing	170	12.0	6.0	11.0	55	350	1.0
Original Recipe:							
breast	360	37.0	7.0	21.0	115	1020	0
breast, no skin/ breading	140	29.0	1.0	2.0	65	520	0
drumstick	130	12.0	2.0	8.0	65	350	0
thigh	330	20.0	8.0	24.0	110	870	0
whole wing	170	12.0	6.0	11.0	55	350	1.0
bowls/pies:							
chicken and biscuit bowl	870	29.0	88.0	44.0	60	2420	7.0
pot pie	770	33.0	70.0	40.0	115	1680	5.0
KFC Famous Bowls:							
potato/gravy	740	27.0	80.0	35.0	60	2350	7.0
rice/gravy	620	26.0	67.0	28.0	60	2150	6.0
popcorn:							
individual	400	21.0	22.0	26.0	60	1160	3.0

Food and Measure	cal.	prot. (gms)	carbo. (gms)	fat (gms)	chol. (mgs)	sod. (mgs)	fiber (gms)
KFC, popcorn (cont.)							
kids	290	16.0	16.0	19.0	40	850	2.0
large	550	29.0	30.0	35.0	80	1600	3.0
strips, 2 pcs.	240	20.0	11.0	13.0	50	800	0
strips, 3 pcs.	350	29.0	16.0	19.0	70	1190	0
wings, 5 pcs.:							
Buffalo, fiery	380	21.0	19.0	24.0	105	1480	2.0
honey barbecue	390	21.0	23.0	24.0	105	830	3.0
Hot Wings	350	20.0	14.0	24.0	105	740	2.0
sweet/spicy	400	21.0	24.0	24.0	105	760	2.0
teriyaki	480	22.0	40.0	25.0	105	830	2.0
boneless:							
Buffalo, fiery	420	28.0	33.0	20.0	65	2260	3.0
honey barbecue	450	28.0	41.0	20.0	65	1880	4.0
sweet/spicy	440	27.0	38.0	19.0	65	1700	3.0
teriyaki	500	28.0	50.0	21.0	65	1730	3.0
sides, individual:							
baked beans	220	8.0	45.0	1.0	0	730	7.0
biscuit, 2 oz.	220	4.0	24.0	11.0	0	640	1.0
coleslaw	180	1.0	22.0	10.0	5	270	3.0
corn on cob, 3"	70	2.0	13.0	1.5	0	5	3.0
corn on cob, 5.5"	150	5.0	26.0	3.0	0	10	7.0
green beans	50	2.0	7.0	1.5	5	570	2.0
macaroni and cheese	180	8.0	18.0	8.0	15	800	0
potato salad	180	2.0	22.0	9.0	5	470	2.0
potato wedges	260	4.0	33.0	13.0	0	740	3.0
potatoes, mashed	110	2.0	17.0	4.0	0	320	1.0
w/gravy	140	2.0	20.0	5.0	0	560	1.0
rice, seasoned	150	4.0	32.0	1.0	0	630	2.0
sandwiches:							
double crunch	470	27.0	38.0	23.0	55	1190	2.0
honey barbecue	280	22.0	40.0	3.5	60	780	3.0
KFC Snacker	290	15.0	29.0	13.0	30	680	2.0
Buffalo	260	15.0	31.0	8.0	25	860	1.0
cheese, ultimate	280	15.0	30.0	11.0	25	780	1.0
fish	330	17.0	31.0	15.0	60	710	1.0
w/out sauce	290	17.0	29.0	12.0	60	610	1.0
honey barbecue	210	14.0	32.0	3.0	40	530	2.0
Tender Roast	380	37.0	29.0	13.0	80	1180	2.0
w/out sauce	300	37.0	28.0	4.5	70	1060	2.0
Twister:							
crispy	550	26.0	49.0	28.0	55	1500	3.0
oven-roasted	420	28.0	40.0	17.0	60	1250	3.0
w/out sauce	330	28.0	39.0	7.0	50	1120	3.0

Food and Measure	cal.	prot. (gms)	carbo. (gms)	fat (gms)	chol. (mgs)	sod. (mgs)	fiber (gms)
salad, no dressing or croutons:							
BLT, crispy	330	28.0	18.0	17.0	65	1130	4.0
BLT, roasted	200	29.0	8.0	6.0	65	880	4.0
Caesar, crispy	350	29.0	16.0	19.0	70	1080	3.0
Caesar, roasted ...	220	30.0	6.0	8.0	70	830	3.0
side salad	15	1.0	2.0	0	0	10	1.0
KFC Parmesan garlic croutons, 1 pkt.	60	2.0	8.0	3.0	0	135	0
salad dressing, 1 pkt.:							
Hidden Valley:							
Italian, light	45	0	6.0	2.5	0	660	0
ranch, fat free ..	35	1.0	8.0	0	0	410	0
ranch, original ..	200	1.0	3.0	20.0	25	470	0
KFC creamy Parmesan Caesar	260	2.0	4.0	26.0	15	540	0
dessert:							
apple pie, mini, 3 ..	370	2.0	44.0	20.0	0	260	2.0
double chocolate chip cake	330	4.0	41.0	16.0	50	260	1.0
Lil' Bucket:							
chocolate cream .	280	3.0	38.0	13.0	0	230	3.0
lemon crème ...	410	7.0	61.0	15.0	0	270	2.0
strawberry cake .	210	2.0	33.0	7.0	10	125	1.0
Sweet Life cookie:							
chocolate chip ..	160	2.0	23.0	7.0	10	95	1.0
oatmeal raisin ..	150	2.0	24.0	5.0	5	135	1.0
sugar	160	2.0	23.0	6.0	5	120	0
Teddy Grahams ...	90	1.0	15.0	3.0	0	95	1.0
Kidney beans:							
dry (*Shiloh Farms* Organic), ¼ cup ...	70	9.0	22.0	0	0	0	14.0
boiled, ½ cup	112	7.6	20.1	.4	0	2	6.5
Kidney beans, canned, ½ cup:							
green, see "Flageolets"							
red:							
(*Eden* Organic)	100	8.0	18.0	0	0	15	10.0
(*Furmano's*)	100	7.0	18.0	0	0	380	5.0
(*Luck's*)	110	6.0	22.0	0	0	370	6.0
(*Progresso*)	110	8.0	20.0	0	0	340	60
(*Roland*)	110	9.0	18.0	0	0	430	7.0
(*S&W*)	100	7.0	23.0	.5	0	460	6.0

Food and Measure	cal.	prot. (gms)	carbo. (gms)	fat (gms)	chol. (mgs)	sod. (mgs)	fiber (gms)
Kidney beans, canned, red *(cont.)*							
(*Van Camp's* New Orleans Style) . .	90	6.0	19.0	0	0	450	6.0
red, dark:							
(*Allens*)	130	8.0	22.0	.5	0	310	8.0
(*Bush's*)	105	7.0	22.0	0	0	260	8.0
(*Progresso*)	110	8.0	20.0	0	0	340	6.0
(*Trappey's*)	120	1.0	28.0	0	0	470	5.0
(*Van Camp's*)	90	7.0	19.0	0	0	730	6.0
red, light:							
(*Allens/Trappey's*) .	120	6.0	22.0	.5	0	340	8.0
(*Bush's*)	100	7.0	22.0	0	0	260	7.0
(*Furmano's*)	100	6.0	17.0	0	0	380	5.0
bacon (*Trappey's*) .	130	7.0	23.0	1.0	0	350	7.0
chili (*Trappey's*) . . .	110	6.0	20.0	1.0	0	510	7.0
jalapeño (*Trappey's*)	110	6.0	19.0	1.0	0	420	6.0
white, cannellini:							
(*Bush's*)	110	7.0	18.0	.5	0	300	6.0
(*Eden* Organic)	100	6.0	17.0	1.0	0	40	5.0
(*Furmano's*)	90	6.0	16.0	0	0	430	5.0
(*Progresso*)	110	8.0	20.0	0	0	340	6.0
Kidney beans, sprouted, raw, ½ cup	27	3.9	3.8	.5	0	6	<1.0
Kidneys, braised:							
beef, 4 oz.	163	28.9	1.1	3.9	439	152	0
lamb, 4 oz.	155	26.8	1.1	4.1	641	171	0
pork, 4 oz.	171	28.8	0	5.3	544	91	0
pork, chopped, 1 cup .	211	35.6	0	6.6	673	111	0
veal, 4 oz.	185	29.8	0	6.4	897	125	0
Kielbasa, 2 oz., except as noted:							
(*Applegate Farms* Organic), 3-oz. link .	190	12.0	2.0	14.0	50	600	0
(*Black Bear* Polska Rope/Link)	150	8.0	2.0	12.0	30	420	0
(*Boar's Head*)	120	9.0	0	10.0	50	440	0
(*Carando* Polska)	170	7.0	2.0	15.0	n.a.	580	0
(*Hatfield* Loop)	150	7.0	2.0	12.0	30	420	0
(*Healthy Choice* Polska)	80	7.0	6.0	2.5	25	480	0
smoked (*Farmland* Polska Rope)	180	6.0	3.0	16.0	35	580	0
turkey (*Jennie-O*)	70	9.0	1.0	3.0	35	550	0
"Kielbasa," vegetarian (*Tofurky*), 3.5 oz. . .	240	26.0	12.0	12.0	0	650	8.0

Food and Measure	cal.	prot. (gms)	carbo. (gms)	fat (gms)	chol. (mgs)	sod. (mgs)	fiber (gms)
Kim chee, 2 oz.:							
(*Frieda's*), ¼ cup	15	1.0	2.0	0	0	340	1.0
mild (*King's*)	15	1.0	2.0	0	0	240	1.0
Kippers, see "Herring"							
Kiwi, fresh:							
(*Del Monte*), 2 med-ium, 5.2 oz.	100	2.0	24.0	1.0	0	0	4.0
(*Frieda's/Frieda's Baby/ Gold*), 5 oz.	90	1.0	21.0	.5	0	5	5.0
1 large, 3.7 oz.	55	.9	13.5	.4	0	4	3.1
1 medium, 3.1 oz. ...	46	.8	11.3	.3	0	4	2.6
Kiwi, canned, in syrup (*Roland*), ½ cup ..	150	0	38.0	0	0	35	4.0
Kiwi drink blend, 8 fl. oz.:							
berry (*Nantucket Nectars*)	120	0	29.0	0	0	25	0
pear (*Snapple*)	10	0	2.0	0	0	35	0
raspberry or strawberry (*Langers* Cocktail) .	120	0	29.0	0	0	0	0
strawberry:							
(*AriZona*)	120	0	29.0	0	0	20	0
(*R.W. Knudsen*) ...	120	0	29.0	0	0	15	0
(*Snapple*)	110	0	28.0	0	0	10	0
(*SoBe Synergy*), 11.5-fl.-oz. can ..	120	0	32.0	0	0	15	0
frozen* (*Langers*) .	120	0	30.0	0	0	15	0
tangerine (*Apple & Eve*)	120	0	29.0	0	0	25	0
Knockwurst, 1 link:							
(*Black Bear*), 3.2 oz. .	240	11.0	0	21.0	40	650	0
(*Dietz & Watson*), 2 oz.	240	12.0	0	21.0	50	770	0
beef:							
(*Boar's Head*), 4 oz.	310	15.0	1.0	27.0	70	950	0
(*Hebrew National*), 3 oz.	260	10.0	1.0	24.0	55	810	0
beef and pork (*Boar's Head*), 3.2 oz.	240	11.0	0	21.0	40	650	0
Kohlrabi:							
raw (*Frieda's*), ⅔ cup, 3 oz.	25	1.0	5.0	0	0	15	3.0
raw, sliced, ½ cup ...	19	1.2	4.3	.1	0	14	2.5
boiled, drained, sliced, ½ cup	24	1.5	5.5	.1	0	17	.9

Food and Measure	cal.	prot. (gms)	carbo. (gms)	fat (gms)	chol. (mgs)	sod. (mgs)	fiber (gms)
Krispy Kreme:							
donut, 1 pc.:							
apple fritter	380	4.0	47.0	20.0	5	220	2.0
cake, powdered . . .	290	3.0	37.0	14.0	20	320	<1.0
cake, traditional . . .	230	3.0	25.0	13.0	20	320	<1.0
Caramel Kreme							
Crunch	380	4.0	49.0	19.0	10	170	<1.0
cheesecake,							
New York	340	4.0	34.0	20.0	15	200	<1.0
chocolate, glazed:							
cake	300	3.0	42.0	15.0	20	250	2.0
cruller	290	2.0	37.0	15.0	15	240	<1.0
chocolate, iced:							
cake	280	3.0	36.0	14.0	20	320	<1.0
custard filled . . .	300	3.0	35.0	17.0	5	150	<1.0
glazed	250	3.0	33.0	12.0	5	100	<1.0
kreme filled	350	3.0	39.0	20.0	5	140	<1.0
w/sprinkles	270	3.0	38.0	12.0	5	100	<1.0
cinnamon, glazed . .	210	2.0	24.0	12.0	5	100	<1.0
cinnamon apple filled	290	3.0	32.0	16.0	5	150	<1.0
cinnamon bun	260	3.0	28.0	16.0	5	125	<1.0
cinnamon twist . . .	240	3.0	23.0	15.0	5	130	<1.0
cruller, glazed	240	2.0	26.0	14.0	15	240	<1.0
dulce de leche	300	3.0	31.0	18.0	5	160	<1.0
glazed, original	200	2.0	22.0	12.0	5	95	<1.0
kreme filled, glazed	340	3.0	39.0	20.0	5	140	<1.0
lemon filled, glazed	290	3.0	35.0	16.0	5	135	<1.0
maple iced glazed .	240	2.0	32.0	12.0	5	100	<1.0
pumpkin spice cake	300	2.0	42.0	14.0	20	250	<1.0
raspberry filled,							
glazed	300	3.0	36.0	16.0	5	125	<1.0
sour cream, glazed	300	2.0	43.0	13.0	20	250	<1.0
strawberry filled,							
powdered	290	3.0	33.0	16.0	5	135	<1.0
sugar	200	2.0	21.0	12.0	5	95	0
donut holes, glazed, 4 pcs.:							
blueberry	220	3.0	27.0	12.0	20	280	<1.0
cake, plain or							
chocolate	210	2.0	29.0	10.0	15	240	<1.0
original	200	2.0	25.0	11.0	5	90	<1.0
pumpkin spice	210	2.0	29.0	10.0	15	240	<1.0
chillers, fruity, no							
whipped cream:							
berry, 12 oz.	170	0	43.0	0	0	10	0

Food and Measure	cal.	prot. (gms)	carbo. (gms)	fat (gms)	chol. (mgs)	sod. (mgs)	fiber (gms)
orange, 12 oz.	180	0	43.0	0	0	10	0
orange, 20 oz.	300	0	71.0	0	0	10	0
chillers, Kremey, w/whipped cream, 12 oz.:							
Berries & Kreme ..	620	3.0	92.0	28.0	30	220	<1.0
chocolate, chocolate	670	4.0	104.0	29.0	30	320	2.0
lemon sherbet	630	3.0	95.0	28.0	30	220	<1.0
mocha dream	670	3.0	105.0	28.0	30	320	1.0
Oranges & Kreme .	630	3.0	92.0	28.0	30	220	<1.0
Kumquat, fresh:							
(*Frieda's*), 5 oz.	90	1.0	23.0	0	0	10	9.0
1 medium, .7 oz.	12	.2	3.1	<.1	0	1	1.3
seeded, 1 oz.	18	.3	4.7	<.1	0	2	1.9
Kumquat, canned, in extra heavy syrup (*Roland*), 2 pcs. ...	80	0	20.0	0	0	20	0
Kuri squash, see "Red kuri squash"							
Kuzu root starch (*Eden* Organic), 1 tbsp. ...	30	0	8.0	0	0	0	0

L

Food and Measure	cal.	prot. (gms)	carbo. (gms)	fat (gms)	chol. (mgs)	sod. (mgs)	fiber (gms)
Lamb, choice grade, trimmed to ¼" fat, meat only, 4 oz., except as noted:							
cubed, leg/shoulder:							
braised or stewed .	253	38.2	0	10.0	122	79	0
broiled	211	31.8	0	8.3	102	86	0
foreshank, braised:							
lean w/fat	276	32.2	0	15.3	120	82	0
lean only	212	35.2	0	6.8	118	84	0
ground:							
raw	320	18.8	0	26.5	83	67	0
broiled	321	28.1	0	22.3	110	92	0
broiled, 1 cup	328	28.7	0	23.1	113	94	0
leg, whole, roasted:							
lean w/fat	293	29.0	0	18.7	105	75	0
lean w/fat, 1 slice, 3" diam. x ¼" . . .	73	7.2	0	4.7	26	19	0
lean only	217	32.1	0	8.8	101	77	0
lean only, 3" slice . .	54	8.0	0	2.2	25	19	0
leg, shank, roasted:							
lean w/fat	255	29.9	0	14.1	102	74	0
lean w/fat, 1 slice, 3" diam. x ¼" . . .	64	7.5	0	3.5	26	18	0
lean only	204	31.9	0	7.6	99	75	0
lean only, 3" slice . .	51	8.0	0	1.9	25	19	0
leg, sirloin, roasted:							
lean w/fat	331	27.9	0	23.4	110	77	0
lean w/fat, 1 slice, 3" diam. x ¼" . . .	83	7.0	0	5.9	27	19	0
lean only	231	32.1	0	10.4	104	81	0
lean only, 3" slice . .	58	8.0	0	2.6	26	20	0
loin chop, broiled:							
lean w/fat, 2¼ oz. (4.2 oz. raw w/bone)	201	16.1	0	14.7	64	49	0

Food and Measure	cal.	prot. (gms)	carbo. (gms)	fat (gms)	chol. (mgs)	sod. (mgs)	fiber (gms)
lean w/fat	358	28.5	0	26.2	113	87	0
lean only, 1.6 oz. (4.2 oz. raw w/bone and fat) .	100	13.9	0	4.5	44	39	0
lean only	245	34.0	0	11.0	108	95	0
loin, roasted:							
lean w/fat	350	25.6	0	26.8	108	73	0
lean only	229	30.2	0	11.1	99	75	0
rib:							
broiled, lean w/fat . .	409	25.1	0	33.6	112	86	0
broiled, lean only . .	266	31.5	0	14.7	103	96	0
roasted, lean w/fat . .	407	24.0	0	33.8	110	83	0
roasted, lean only .	263	29.7	0	15.1	100	92	0
shoulder, whole:							
braised, lean w/fat . .	390	32.5	0	27.8	132	85	0
braised, lean only . .	321	37.2	0	10.0	133	90	0
roasted, lean w/fat .	313	25.5	0	22.6	104	75	0
roasted, lean only .	231	28.3	0	12.2	99	77	0
Lamb's quarters, boiled, drained, chopped, ½ cup . . .	29	2.9	4.5	.6	0	26	1.9
Landjaeger (*Dietz & Watson*), 1 oz.	130	8.0	0	11.0	25	430	0
Lard (*Farmer John*), 1 tbsp.	120	0	0	13.0	10	0	0
Lasagna entree, frozen, 1 pkg., except as noted:							
Alfredo:							
(*Michelina's Authentico*), 9 oz.	340	12.0	38.0	15.0	40	700	2.0
w/broccoli (*Michelina's Budget Gourmet*), 8 oz. .	300	10.0	36.0	12.0	30	560	2.0
bake (*Healthy Choice*), 9 oz.	240	11.0	38.0	4.5	10	600	5.0
Bolognese (*Smart Ones*), 9 oz.	270	14.0	43.0	4.0	15	540	3.0
cheese:							
(*Amy's*), 10.3 oz. . .	380	20.0	44.0	14.0	45	680	4.0
(*Celentano*), ½ of 14-oz. pkg.	300	14.0	38.0	10.0	30	710	5.0
(*Celentano* Light), 10 oz.	340	18.0	52.0	7.0	30	800	7.0

Food and Measure	cal.	prot. (gms)	carbo. (gms)	fat (gms)	chol. (mgs)	sod. (mgs)	fiber (gms)
Lasagna entree, frozen, cheese (cont.)							
Florentine bake (Lean Cuisine One Dish Favorites), 10 oz.	260	14.0	35.0	7.0	20	680	4.0
cheese, five:							
(Lean Cuisine One Dish Favorites Classic), 11.5 oz.	320	19.0	44.0	8.0	25	690	4.0
(Michelina's Lean Gourmet), 8 oz. .	290	13.0	50.0	5.0	10	560	8.0
(Stouffer's), 10.75 oz.	370	21.0	39.0	14.0	35	960	4.0
(Stouffer's Homestyle), ½ of 18.25-oz. pkg.	330	18.0	33.0	14.0	35	870	3.0
cheese, four:							
(Michelina's Authentico), 8 oz.	280	12.0	43.0	7.0	25	490	3.0
layered (Michelina's Authentico), 8 oz.	280	12.0	46.0	7.0	10	650	8.0
cheese, three (Michelina's Authentico), 8.5 oz.	330	14.0	48.0	10.0	15	580	8.0
cheese and chicken (Cedarlane Dr. Sears Zone), 11 oz.	340	24.0	35.0	12.0	115	790	3.0
chicken:							
(Stouffer's), ⅕ of 39-oz. pkg.	330	15.0	33.0	15.0	30	830	3.0
Florentine (Lean Cuisine One Dish Favorites), 10 oz.	290	21.0	37.0	6.0	25	650	3.0
w/chicken scaloppini (Lean Cuisine), 10 oz.	290	19.0	35.0	8.0	30	580	5.0
eggplant Portobello mushroom (Seeds of Change Calabrese Organic), 10 oz. . . .	270	13.0	42.0	6.0	15	770	4.0
Florentine (Smart Ones), 10.5 oz. . . .	290	15.0	35.0	9.0	30	580	4.0
meat sauce:							
(Lean Cuisine One Dish Favorites), 10.5 oz.	320	19.0	44.0	7.0	30	690	4.0
(Michelina's Budget Gourmet), 8 oz. .	260	10.0	35.0	8.0	15	660	3.0

Food and Measure	cal.	prot. (gms)	carbo. (gms)	fat (gms)	chol. (mgs)	sod. (mgs)	fiber (gms)
(*Smart Ones* Traditional), 10.5 oz. . .	300	17.0	43.0	6.0	25	780	5.0
(*Stouffer's*), 10.5 oz.	350	24.0	38.0	11.0	40	930	3.0
(*Stouffer's* Bake), 11.5 oz.	380	18.0	47.0	13.0	40	1080	5.0
(*Stouffer's* Italiano), ½ of 19-oz. pkg. .	290	16.0	30.0	12.0	35	690	3.0
(*Stouffer's* Italiano Family), ⅕ of 38-oz. pkg.	280	15.0	30.0	11.0	35	680	3.0
(*Stouffer's* Family), ⅕ of 38-oz. pkg.	290	18.0	27.0	12.0	35	730	2.0
(*Stouffer's* Party), 1/12 of 96-oz. pkg.	330	23.0	27.0	14.0	45	820	2.0
cheese, four (*Michelina's Authentico*), 9 oz. . . .	320	14.0	40.0	10.0	35	740	3.0
cheese, three (*Michelina's Authentico*), 8.5 oz. . . .	340	17.0	52.0	9.0	25	940	8.0
layered (*Michelina's Authentico*), 8 oz.	310	16.0	46.0	8.0	25	940	7.0
layered (*Michelina's Lean Gourmet*), 8 oz.	310	15.0	49.0	6.0	20	890	8.0
mozzarella (*Michelina's Budget Gourmet Classics/Zap'ems*), 8 oz.	260	9.0	39.0	7.0	20	540	3.0
spinach (*Seeds of Change* di Parma Organic), 10 oz. . . .	340	20.0	40.0	10.0	35	750	4.0
tomato sauce, sausage (*Stouffer's*), 10.9 oz.	410	18.0	41.0	19.0	50	930	4.0
vegetable: (*Amy's*), 9.5 oz. . . .	310	16.0	35.0	12.0	20	680	5.0
(*Amy's* Light Sodium), 9.5 oz.	290	15.0	41.0	8.0	15	340	4.0
(*Cedarlane Dr. Sears Zone*), 11 oz. . . .	310	24.0	33.0	12.0	15	910	5.0
(*Stouffer's*), 10.5 oz.	390	17.0	40.0	18.0	25	730	4.0
(*Stouffer's* Family), 1/12 of 96-oz. pkg.	320	16.0	35.0	13.0	25	1010	3.0

Food and Measure	cal.	prot. (gms)	carbo. (gms)	fat (gms)	chol. (mgs)	sod. (mgs)	fiber (gms)
Lasagna entree, frozen, vegetable *(cont.)*							
garden (*Amy's*), 10.3 oz.	290	13.0	41.0	9.0	20	720	5.0
garden (*Cedarlane* Organic Lowfat), ½ of 10-oz. pkg. .	180	10.0	26.0	3.0	10	390	2.0
primavera (*Michelina's Zap'ems*), 8 oz. .	270	9.0	38.0	9.0	20	550	2.0
tofu (*Amy's*), 9.5 oz.	310	13.0	41.0	11.0	0	680	6.0
vegetarian:							
(*Boca*), 10.5 oz. . . .	290	21.0	42.0	5.0	15	880	5.0
(*Yves* Bowl), 10.5 oz.	300	17.0	51.0	3.0	0	650	4.0
w/meatless ground round (*Cedarlane*), 10 oz.	380	25.0	45.0	12.0	35	570	3.0
primavera (*Celentano* Organic), 10 oz. .	270	15.0	40.0	5.0	0	590	7.0
Lasagne entree, microwave, 1 cont.:							
cheese (*Hamburger Helper* Single)	210	8.0	33.0	4.5	5	580	1.0
w/meat sauce:							
(*Hormel* Microcup), 7.5 oz.	210	14.0	31.0	5.0	10	840	3.0
(*Hormel Compleats*), 10 oz.	280	13.0	42.0	7.0	50	1100	3.0
Lasagne entree, pkg.:							
(*Chef Boyardee* Kit), ⅙ pkg.	210	9.0	35.0	4.0	10	620	3.0
pasta bake (*Betty Crocker Complete Meals*), ⅕ pkg.	250	9.0	46.0	3.0	10	1030	2.0
Lecithin granules:							
(*Shiloh Farms*), 2 tbsp.	70	0	1.0	5.0	0	0	0
(*Tree of Life*), 1 tbsp. .	55	0	1.0	4.0	0	2	0
Leek, w/lower leaf portion, fresh:							
raw:							
(*Frieda's*), 3 oz. . . .	50	1.0	12.0	0	0	15	2.0
9.9-oz. leek	76	1.9	17.6	.4	0	25	2.2
chopped, ½ cup . . .	32	.8	7.4	.2	0	10	.9
boiled, drained:							
4.4-oz. leek	38	.2	9.5	.3	0	12	1.2
chopped, ½ cup . . .	16	.4	4.0	.1	0	5	.5

Food and Measure	cal.	prot. (gms)	carbo. (gms)	fat (gms)	chol. (mgs)	sod. (mgs)	fiber (gms)
Leek, freeze-dried, 1 tbsp.	1	<.1	.2	tr.	0	<1	<1.0
Lemon, fresh:							
(*Del Monte*), 2 oz. . . .	15	0	5.0	0	0	5	1.0
2⅛" lemon, 3.8 oz. . . .	22	1.3	11.6	.3	0	3	n.a.
1 wedge, ¼ medium .	5	.3	2.9	.1	0	1	n.a.
peeled, 2⅛" lemon . . .	17	.6	5.4	.2	0	1	1.6
Lemon, preserved, in brine (*Roland*), 1 pc.	5	0	1.0	0	0	200	<1.0
Lemon curd (*Crosse & Blackwell*), 1 tbsp.	50	0	13.0	0	0	0	0
Lemon drink (see also "Lemonade"):							
(*Santa Cruz Organic Box*), 8 fl. oz.	120	0	29.0	0	0	10	0
(*Tropicana Fruit Squeeze Summer*), 15.2-fl.-oz. bottle . .	35	0	8.0	0	0	50	0
Lemon drink blend ginger echinacea (*Santa Cruz Organic*), 8 fl. oz.	100	<1.0	25.0	0	0	10	0
Lemongrass, fresh, sliced, 1 cup	66	.5	16.9	.3	0	4	n.a.
Lemongrass, in jars sliced (*Roland*), 1 tbsp.	5	0	2.0	0	0	10	0
Lemongrass sauce, see "Marinade"							
Lemon herb seasoning (*McCormick*), ¼ tsp.	0	0	0	0	0	190	0
Lemon juice, fresh:							
½ cup	31	.5	10.5	0	0	1	.5
1 tbsp.	4	.1	1.3	0	0	<1	.1
Lemon pepper:							
(*Lawry's*), ¼ tsp.	0	0	0	0	0	80	0
1 tsp.	7	.2	1.5	0	0	425	.3
w/garlic and onion (*McCormick* California Style), ¼ tsp.	0	0	0	0	0	30	0
Lemonade, 8 fl. oz., except as noted:							
(*Apple & Eve*)	130	0	32.0	0	0	5	0
(*AriZona*)	110	0	27.0	0	0	25	0
(*Earthbound Farm Organic*)	126	1.0	31.0	0	0	10	0

Food and Measure	cal.	prot. (gms)	carbo. (gms)	fat (gms)	chol. (mgs)	sod. (mgs)	fiber (gms)
Lemonade *(cont.)*							
(*Minute Maid*), 12 fl. oz.	150	0	42.0	0	0	15	0
(*Minute Maid 12%*) ..	110	0	31.0	0	0	15	0
(*Minute Maid 3%*) ...	100	0	28.0	0	0	15	0
(*Nantucket Nectars* Squeezed)	110	0	28.0	0	0	20	0
(*Newman's Own* Lightly Sweetened)	80	0	20.0	0	0	40	0
(*Newman's Own* Virgin Old Fashioned Roadside/Organic) .	110	0	27.0	0	0	40	0
(*Odwalla*)	110	0	28.0	0	0	10	0
(*R.W. Knudsen* Box) .	130	1.0	32.0	0	0	15	0
(*Santa Cruz Organic*) .	100	0	24.0	0	0	0	0
(*Simply Lemonade*) ..	120	0	30.0	0	0	15	0
(*Snapple*)	110	0	28.0	0	0	50	0
(*SoBe Synergy*), 11.5 fl. oz.	120	0	32.0	0	0	15	0
(*Tropicana* Homestyle), 12 fl. oz.	180	<1.0	43.0	0	0	30	0
(*Tropicana* Juice Drink)	120	0	29.0	0	0	20	0
(*Tropicana* Orchard) ..	120	0	31.0	0	0	20	0
(*Turkey Hill*)	120	0	29.0	0	0	10	0
pink:							
(*Minute Maid 13%*)	110	0	29.0	0	0	15	0
(*Minute Maid* Cooler)	90	0	25.0	0	0	15	0
(*Newman's Own* Virgin)	110	0	27.0	0	0	40	0
(*Snapple*)	110	0	27.0	0	0	50	0
or strawberry kiwi (*Turkey Hill*)	110	0	29.0	0	0	10	0
frozen*:							
(*Cascadian Farm* Organic)	110	0	28.0	0	0	15	0
pink or white (*Minute Maid*) ..	110	0	29.0	0	0	0	0
sparkling (*Santa Cruz* Organic)	100	0	26.0	0	0	0	0
tea, see "Tea, iced"							
Lemonade fruit blend, 8 fl. oz.:							
cranberry:							
(*Bolthouse Farms*) .	130	1.0	34.0	0	0	5	<1.0

Food and Measure	cal.	prot. (gms)	carbo. (gms)	fat (gms)	chol. (mgs)	sod. (mgs)	fiber (gms)
(*Honest Ade* Organic)	48	0	12.0	0	0	5	0
white (*Langers*) ...	120	0	30.0	0	0	15	0
limeade:							
(*Minute Maid* Limonada)	120	0	33.0	0	0	15	0
(*Turkey Hill* Limonada)	120	0	29.0	0	0	10	0
frozen* (*Minute Maid* Limonada)	90	0	25.0	0	0	0	0
mango (*Bolthouse Farms*)	120	<1.0	30.0	0	0	0	<1.0
prickly pear (*Bolthouse Farms*)	130	1.0	34.0	0	0	5	<1.0
raspberry:							
(*Langers*)	120	0	29.0	0	0	0	0
(*Minute Maid*)	120	0	32.0	0	0	15	0
(*Santa Cruz Organic*)	100	0	24.0	0	0	0	0
frozen* (*Minute Maid*)	110	0	29.0	0	0	15	0
strawberry (*Santa Cruz Organic*)	100	0	24.0	0	0	0	0
Lemonade mix* (*Country Time*), 8 fl. oz.:							
pink or white	60	0	16.0	0	0	25	0
raspberry	80	0	19.0	0	0	0	0
strawberry	80	0	20.0	0	0	0	0
Lentil, ¼ cup, except as noted:							
dry (*Shiloh Farms* Organic):							
black Beluga	200	12.0	34.0	3.0	0	9	9.0
brown	230	18.0	40.0	1.0	0	4	16.0
French	160	10.0	30.0	0	0	0	3.0
green	150	11.0	27.0	0	0	15	7.0
red, split	150	11.0	27.0	0	0	15	7.0
dry, green:							
(*Arrowhead Mills* Organic)	150	10.0	27.0	1.0	0	5	7.0
(*Roland*)	120	10.0	20.0	0	0	5	5.0
dry, red (*Arrowhead Mills* Organic)	170	13.0	28.0	1.0	0	5	7.0
cooked, ½ cup	115	8.9	19.9	.4	0	2	7.8

Food and Measure	cal.	prot. (gms)	carbo. (gms)	fat (gms)	chol. (mgs)	sod. (mgs)	fiber (gms)
Lentil, canned, ½ cup:							
(*Westbrae Natural*							
Organic)	100	8.0	17.0	0	0	150	9.0
w/onion, bay leaf							
(*Eden* Organic)	90	8.0	13.0	0	0	210	4.0
rice and (*Eden* Organic)	120	4.0	23.0	1.0	0	120	2.0
Lentil, sprouted, raw,							
½ cup	40	3.4	8.4	.2	0	4	n.a.
Lentil dish, mix:							
(*Neera's* Dal and							
Seasoning), 1 cup*	140	11.0	23.0	1.0	0	4	12.0
(*Neera's* Urad and							
Channa Dal), 1 cup*	104	8.0	18.0	1.0	0	4	9.0
rice and, see "Rice							
dish mix"							
pilaf (*Casbah*), ¼ cup	150	9.0	32.0	.5	0	440	6.0
pilaf, w/rice:							
(*Near East*), 2 oz. . .	180	11.0	36.0	.5	0	630	8.0
(*Near East*), 1·cup*	200	11.0	36.0	3.5	10	660	8.0
Lentil entree, frozen,							
w/linguine (*Seeds*							
of Change Moroccan							
Tagine Organic),							
10-oz. pkg.	320	10.0	52.0	8.0	0	780	8.0
Lentil entree, pkg.,							
½ of 10-oz. pkg.,							
except as noted:							
(*Tasty Bite* Bengal) . . .	158	6.0	16.0	8.0	0	439	8.0
(*Tasty Bite* Jodhpur) .	106	6.0	12.0	4.0	0	664	7.0
w/red beans (*Tasty*							
Bite Madras)	127	6.0	14.0	5.0	3	455	5.0
spicy, w/beans							
(*Tamarind Tree* Dal							
Makhani), 9.25 oz. . .	330	14.0	55.0	6.0	5	670	14.0
vegetables (*Tamarind*							
Tree Channa Dal							
Masala), 9.25-oz. . .	340	13.0	62.0	5.0	0	700	10.0
Lettuce (see also							
"Salad blend"):							
bibb or Boston:							
1 head, 5" diam. . . .	21	2.1	3.8	.4	0	8	1.6
2 inner leaves	2	.2	.4	<.1	0	1	.5
butter (Dole), ½ head,							
3 oz.	10	1.0	3.0	0	0	0	1.0

Food and Measure	cal.	prot. (gms)	carbo. (gms)	fat (gms)	chol. (mgs)	sod. (mgs)	fiber (gms)
butterhead (*Frieda's Limestone*), 3 oz. . .	10	1.0	2.0	0	0	10	1.0
iceberg:							
(*Dole*), ⅙ medium .	15	1.0	3.0	0	0	10	1.0
1 head, 6" diam.	70	5.4	11.3	1.0	0	48	7.5
1 leaf, .7 oz.	3	.2	.4	<.1	0	2	.3
shredded (*Fresh Express Shreds!*), 1½ cups, 3.1 oz.)	15	1.0	3.0	0	0	10	1.0
shredded, 1 cup . . .	7	.6	1.2	.1	0	3	.8
leaf/loose-leaf, shredded:							
(*Del Monte*), 1½ cups, 3 oz. . .	15	1.0	4.0	0	0	30	2.0
½ cup	5	.4	1.0	.1	0	3	.5
green (*Dole*), ¼ head, 3.2 oz.	15	1.0	3.0	0	0	25	1.0
mâche (*Earthbound Farm* Organic), 3 oz.	30	2.0	5.0	0	0	20	2.0
romaine or cos:							
(*Dole*), 6 leaves, 3 oz.	20	1.0	3.0	0	0	0	1.0
1 inner leaf	1	.2	.2	0	0	1	.2
shredded, ½ cup . .	4	.5	.7	.1	0	2	.5
romaine, chopped (*Dole* Fresh Discoveries), 3 oz. .	15	1.0	3.0	0	0	5	1.0
romaine hearts, 3 oz.:							
(*Andy Boy*), 6 leaves	20	1.0	3.0	0	0	0	1.0
(*Dole*)	15	1.0	3.0	0	0	10	1.0
(*Dole* Organic)	15	1.0	3.0	0	0	5	1.0
(*Earthbound Farm* Organic)	10	1.0	2.0	0	0	1	1.0
(*Fresh Express* Organic)	15	1.0	2.0	0	0	5	1.0
baby (*Fresh Express*)	15	1.0	3.0	0	0	5	1.0
chopped (*Fresh Express*)	15	1.0	3.0	0	0	5	2.0
Lima beans:							
immature, ½ cup:							
raw, trimmed	88	5.3	15.7	.7	0	6	3.8
boiled, drained	104	5.8	20.1	.3	0	14	4.5
mature, dry:							
baby (*Shiloh Farms* Organic), ¼ cup .	70	8.0	23.0	0	0	15	15.0
baby, boiled, ½ cup	115	7.3	21.2	.3	0	2	7.0

Food and Measure	cal.	prot. (gms)	carbo. (gms)	fat (gms)	chol. (mgs)	sod. (mgs)	fiber (gms)
Lima beans (cont.)							
large (*Shiloh Farms*							
Organic), ¼ cup .	70	7.0	22.0	0	0	20	12.0
large, boiled, ½ cup	108	7.3	19.6	.4	0	2	6.6
Lima beans, canned							
(see also "Butter							
beans"), ½ cup:							
(*Luck's* Fat Free)	120	7.0	22.0	0	0	400	5.0
(*Luck's* Giant)	130	7.0	22.0	1.5	0	370	5.0
(*S&W*)	80	4.0	15.0	0	0	390	4.0
baby, seasoned (*Glory*)	100	6.0	18.0	0	0	570	6.0
green:							
(*Allens/East Texas*							
Fair)	120	7.0	23.0	0	0	370	8.0
(*Del Monte*)	80	4.0	15.0	0	0	390	4.0
w/bacon (*Trappey's*)	120	6.0	22.0	1.0	0	330	6.0
green, baby:							
(*Freshlike/Freshlike*							
Selects)	140	9.0	26.0	.5	0	270	7.0
(*Veg-All*)	90	4.0	15.0	1.0	0	330	3.0
green and white (*Allens*)	110	6.0	20.0	1.0	0	280	9.0
white, w/bacon (*Trappey's*)	130	8.0	21.0	1.5	0	350	6.0
Lima beans, frozen,							
½ cup, except as noted:							
baby:							
(*Birds Eye/C&W/*							
C&W Petite)	110	6.0	20.0	0	0	240	5.0
(*Green Giant Simply*							
Steam No Sauce),							
½ cup cooked . .	80	4.0	15.0	0	0	170	3.0
(*McKenzie's*)	110	6.0	22.0	.5	0	140	5.0
baby, in butter sauce							
(*Green Giant*), ⅔ cup	100	5.0	18.0	1.5	<5	420	5.0
Fordhook (*Birds Eye*) .	100	6.0	18.0	0	0	5	4.0
Lime, fresh:							
(*Del Monte*), 2.4 oz. . .	20	0	7.0	0	0	0	2.0
(*Frieda's* Key Lime),							
3-oz. lime	25	1.0	9.0	0	0	0	2.0
2"-diam. lime	20	.5	7.1	.1	0	1	1.9
peeled, seeded, 1 oz. .	9	.2	3.0	.1	0	1	.8
Lime drink, 8 fl. oz.,							
except as noted:							
w/yerba mate (*Honest Tea*							
Organic Sublime Lime)	40	0	10.0	0	0	5	0

Food and Measure	cal.	prot. (gms)	carbo. (gms)	fat (gms)	chol. (mgs)	sod. (mgs)	fiber (gms)
limeade:							
(*Honest Ade* Organic)	48	0	12.0	0	0	5	0
(*Newman's Own* Virgin)	140	0	34.0	0	0	35	0
(*Odwalla Summertime Lime*)	120	0	29.0	0	0	10	0
(*Santa Cruz Organic*)	100	0	26.0	0	0	0	0
(*Simply Limeade*) ..	120	0	31.0	0	0	15	0
cherry (*Minute Maid*)	120	0	34.0	0	0	15	0
sparkling (*Santa Cruz Organic*) ...	100	0	26.0	0	0	0	0
raspberry (*Tropicana Fruit Squeeze*), 15.2 fl. oz.	35	0	9.0	0	0	50	0
Lime juice, fresh:							
½ cup	33	.5	11.1	.1	0	1	.5
1 tbsp.	4	.1	1.4	<.1	0	tr.	.1
Lime juice, bottled:							
sweetened, 1 tsp.:							
(*Angostura*)	5	0	1.0	0	0	0	0
(*Roland*)	10	0	2.0	0	0	0	0
unsweetened, 2 tbsp. ..	6	<.1	2.0	<.1	0	5	.1
Lime relish, Indian:							
hot (*Patak's*), 1 tbsp. .	35	0	2.0	3.0	0	560	1.0
mild (*Patak's*), 1 tbsp. .	30	0	0	3.0	0	530	0
Limeade, see "Lime drink							
Ling, meat only:							
raw, 4 oz.	99	21.5	0	.7	45	153	0
baked or broiled, 4 oz.	126	27.6	0	.9	58	196	0
Ling cod, meat only:							
raw, 4 oz.	96	20.0	0	1.2	59	67	0
baked or broiled, 4 oz.	124	25.7	0	1.5	76	86	0
Lingonberries, in jars, in syrup w/pectin (*Roland*), 2 tbsp. ...	70	0	16.0	0	0	5	1.0
Linguine:							
dry, see "Pasta"							
refrigerated (*Buitoni*), 1¼ cups	240	10.0	45.0	2.5	50	20	2.0
Linguine entree, frozen, w/clams, shrimp (*Michelina's Authentico*), 8-oz. pkg.	320	13.0	49.0	7.0	40	250	3.0

Food and Measure	cal.	prot. (gms)	carbo. (gms)	fat (gms)	chol. (mgs)	sod. (mgs)	fiber (gms)
Liquor[1], 1 fl. oz.:							
80 proof	64	0	0	0	0	tr.	0
90 proof	73	0	0	0	0	tr.	0
100 proof	82	0	0	0	0	tr.	0
Litchi, see "Lychee"							
Liver:							
beef, panfried, 4 oz. . .	246	30.3	8.9	9.1	547	120	0
calves (veal), 4 oz.:							
braised	218	32.2	4.3	7.1	579	88	0
panfried	219	31.0	5.1	7.4	550	96	0
chicken, simmered:							
4 oz.	189	27.7	1.0	7.4	638	86	0
chopped, 1 cup . . .	219	34.1	1.2	7.6	883	71	0
chicken, panfried, 4 oz.	195	29.2	1.3	7.3	640	104	0
duck, raw, 1 oz.	39	5.3	1.0	1.3	146	n.a.	0
goose, raw, 1 oz.	38	4.6	1.8	1.2	146	40	0
lamb, braised, 4 oz. . .	249	34.7	2.9	10.0	568	64	0
lamb, panfried, 4 oz. .	270	29.0	4.3	14.3	559	141	0
pork, braised, 4 oz. . .	187	29.5	4.3	5.0	403	56	0
turkey, simmered:							
4 oz.	192	27.2	3.9	6.7	710	73	0
chopped, 1 cup . . .	237	33.6	4.8	8.3	876	89	0
"Liver," vegetarian,							
chopped (*Sabra*), 1 oz.	70	1.0	2.0	6.0	30	70	0
Liverwurst (see also "Braunschweiger"), 2 oz.:							
(*Boar's Head* Strassburger)	170	8.0	1.0	15.0	85	560	0
(*Farmer John*)	160	8.0	3.0	12.0	55	460	0
(*Hansel 'n Gretel*) . . .	170	9.0	4.0	13.0	95	730	0
w/bacon (*Farmer John*)	160	8.0	3.0	12.0	55	460	0
smoked (*Boar's Head*)	170	8.0	1.0	15.0	45	620	0
Lo bok, see "Radish, Oriental"							
Lobster, northern, meat only:							
raw, 4 oz.	102	21.3	.6	1.0	108	n.a.	0
boiled or steamed:							
4 oz.	111	23.2	1.5	.7	82	431	0
1 cup, 5.1 oz.	142	29.7	1.9	.9	104	551	0

[1] Includes all pure distilled liquors: bourbon, brandy, gin, rum, scotch, tequila, vodka, etc.

Food and Measure	cal.	prot. (gms)	carbo. (gms)	fat (gms)	chol. (mgs)	sod. (mgs)	fiber (gms)
"Lobster," imitation, chunk or salad style (*Louis Kemp Lobster Delights*), ½ cup, 3 oz.	70	7.0	10.0	0	5	460	1.0
Lobster, spiny, see "Spiny lobster"							
Lobster cake, frozen (*Matlaw's*), 2 oz.	130	8.0	15.0	4.5	35	270	<1.0
Lobster sauce, canned (*Progresso*), ½ cup	100	3.0	6.0	7.0	5	430	2.0
Loganberries, fresh, 1 cup	89	1.4	21.5	.9	0	1	n.a.
Long bean, see "Yardlong bean"							
Long John Silver's:							
fish/seafood:							
cod, baked, 1 pc.	120	22.0	1.0	4.5	90	240	0
clams, breaded, 3-oz. box	320	9.0	26.0	19.0	35	1190	2.0
fish, battered, 1 pc.	260	12.0	17.0	16.0	35	790	<1.0
flounder, 1 pc.	250	12.0	26.0	11.0	35	910	2.0
lobster bites, buttered, 3.5-oz. box	250	14.0	27.0	9.0	65	560	2.0
shrimp:							
battered, 1 pc.	45	2.0	3.0	3.0	15	160	0
popcorn, 3-oz. box	270	9.0	23.0	16.0	75	570	1.0
Chicken Plank, 1 pc.	140	8.0	9.0	8.0	20	480	<1.0
dipping sauce, 1 oz.:							
cocktail	25	0	6.0	0	0	250	0
tartar	100	0	4.0	9.0	15	250	0
sandwiches:							
chicken	360	14.0	40.0	15.0	25	900	3.0
fish	470	18.0	48.0	23.0	45	1210	3.0
Ultimate Fish Sandwich	530	21.0	49.0	28.0	60	1400	3.0
salad, no dressing:							
chicken club	510	28.0	35.0	30.0	65	1550	5.0
shrimp and seafood	260	18.0	22.0	12.0	85	820	4.0
salad dressing, 1 pkt.:							
Italian, lite	20	0	3.0	1.0	0	780	0
ranch, garden	230	1.0	2.0	24.0	10	400	0
Thousand Island	220	0	7.0	21.0	25	350	0
sides/starters:							
clam chowder, bowl	170	4.0	19.0	8.0	15	1220	<1.0

Food and Measure	cal.	prot. (gms)	carbo. (gms)	fat (gms)	chol. (mgs)	sod. (mgs)	fiber (gms)
Long John Silver's, sides/starters *(cont.)*							
coleslaw, 4 oz.	200	1.0	15.0	15.0	20	340	3.0
cheesesticks, 3 pcs.	140	4.0	12.0	8.0	10	320	1.0
corn cobbette, 1 pc.	90	3.0	14.0	3.0	0	0	3.0
Crumblies, 1 oz.	170	1.0	14.0	12.0	0	420	1.0
fries, large	390	4.0	56.0	17.0	0	580	5.0
fries, regular	230	3.0	34.0	10.0	0	350	3.0
hush puppies, 1 pc.	60	1.0	9.0	2.5	0	200	1.0
lobster stuffed crab cake, 1 pc.	170	6.0	16.0	9.0	30	390	1.0
rice, 4 oz.	180	3.0	34.0	3.5	0	540	3.0
dessert pie, 1 pc.:							
chocolate cream	310	5.0	24.0	22.0	15	170	1.0
pecan	370	4.0	55.0	15.0	40	190	2.0
pineapple cream	290	4.0	39.0	13.0	15	210	1.0
Longan, fresh:							
(*Frieda's*), 20 pcs.	38	0	10.0	.1	0	0	0
seeded, 1 oz.	17	.4	4.3	<.1	0	<1	.3
Longan, canned, in heavy syrup							
(*Roland*), 2 tbsp.	25	0	6.0	0	0	0	0
Longan, dried, 1 oz.	81	1.4	21.0	.1	0	14	<1.0
Loquat:							
(*Frieda's*), 5 oz.	70	1.0	17.0	0	0	0	2.0
1 large, .7 oz.	9	<.1	2.4	0	0	tr.	.3
cubed, 1 cup	70	.6	18.1	.3	0	1	2.5
peeled, seeded, 1 oz.	13	.1	3.4	.1	0	<1	.5
Loquat, canned, in syrup (*Roland*), 2 tbsp.	20	0	5.0	0	0	0	0
Lotus root:							
raw:							
(*Frieda's*), 1 cup, 3 oz.	50	2.0	15.0	0	0	35	4.0
10 slices	60	2.1	14.0	.1	0	32	4.0
trimmed, 1 oz.	16	.7	4.9	<.1	0	11	1.4
boiled, drained, ½ cup	40	1.0	9.6	<.1	0	27	1.9
Lotus root, dried (*Eden* Organic), about 5 slices, .4 oz.	35	1.0	8.0	0	0	25	2.0
Lotus seeds:							
raw, 1 oz.	25	1.2	4.9	.2	0	<1	n.a.
dried, 1 oz.	94	4.4	18.3	.6	0	1	n.a.
fried, 1 cup	106	4.9	20.6	.6	0	1	n.a.
Lox, see "Salmon, smoked"							

Food and Measure	cal.	prot. (gms)	carbo. (gms)	fat (gms)	chol. (mgs)	sod. (mgs)	fiber (gms)
Lunch meat (see also specific listings), loaf, 2 oz.:							
(*Dietz & Watson* Roll)	70	10.0	1.0	2.5	35	550	0
deluxe loaf:							
(*Black Bear*)	140	7.0	3.0	11.0	30	510	0
(*Dietz & Watson*) . .	130	7.0	3.0	10.0	35	480	0
Dutch:							
(*Boar's Head*)	150	7.0	2.0	12.0	25	610	0
pepper (*Hatfield Deli Choice*)	120	8.0	3.0	8.0	25	510	0
honey roll (*Dietz & Watson*)	70	9.0	4.0	2.0	30	620	0
jalapeño (*Hansel 'n Gretel*)	150	5.0	6.0	12.0	30	910	0
macaroni and cheese (*Hansel 'n Gretel*) .	160	7.0	8.0	12.0	30	890	0
mission (*Farmer John*)	60	10.0	1.0	1.5	25	450	0
olive loaf:							
(*Black Bear*)	140	7.0	3.0	11.0	30	580	0
(*Boar's Head*)	130	6.0	<1.0	12.0	20	630	0
(*Dietz & Watson*) . .	120	6.0	7.0	8.0	20	580	0
(*Hansel 'n Gretel*) .	180	6.0	7.0	14.0	35	850	0
pepper loaf:							
(*Black Bear*)	140	7.0	3.0	11.0	30	520	0
(*Dietz & Watson*) . .	140	7.0	4.0	11.0	30	520	0
pickle/red pepper:							
(*Black Bear*)	140	7.0	3.0	11.0	30	580	0
(*Boar's Head*)	150	6.0	2.0	13.0	30	500	0
(*Dietz & Watson*) . .	120	6.0	7.0	8.0	10	580	0
spiced:							
(*Farmland* Sandwich)	130	5.0	3.3	10.6	20	690	0
(*Hansel 'n Gretel*) .	180	7.0	6.0	15.0	40	840	0
ham (*Boar's Head*) .	120	7.0	1.0	10.0	30	570	0
ham (*Di Lusso*) . . .	140	8.0	1.0	11.0	35	680	0
ham (*Hormel*)	140	8.0	1.0	11.0	35	690	0
Lunch meat, canned (*Spam*), 2 oz.:							
classic	180	8.0	2.0	16.0	40	800	0
classic less salt	180	7.0	1.0	16.0	40	580	0
lite	110	9.0	1.0	8.0	40	580	0
w/bacon	180	7.0	1.0	16.0	40	590	0
w/cheese	170	8.0	1.0	15.0	40	720	0
garlic	160	8.0	1.0	14.0	40	600	0

Food and Measure	cal.	prot. (gms)	carbo. (gms)	fat (gms)	chol. (mgs)	sod. (mgs)	fiber (gms)
Lunch meat, canned (cont.)							
honey, golden grill ...	190	7.0	5.0	15.0	35	470	0
hot and spicy	180	7.0	2.0	16.0	40	600	0
smoked	170	8.0	2.0	15.0	40	610	0
turkey	80	8.0	2.0	4.0	30	450	0
Lunch "meat," vegetarian, frozen (*Worthington Wham*),							
3 slices, 2 oz.	110	10.0	3.0	7.0	0	400	0
Lupin, boiled, ½ cup .	98	12.9	8.2	2.4	0	3	2.3
Lychee, fresh:							
(*Frieda's*), 6–8 pcs.,							
3.5 oz.	60	1.0	14.0	0	0	0	1.0
1 fruit, .3 oz.	6	.1	1.6	0	0	0	.1
shelled:							
1 cup	125	1.6	31.4	.8	0	2	2.5
1 oz.	19	.2	4.7	.1	0	<1	.4
Lychee, canned, in heavy syrup							
(*Roland*), 2 tbsp. ...	30	0	7.0	0	0	5	0
Lychee, dried, 10 fruits,							
.7 oz.	69	1.0	17.7	.3	0	0	1.2
Lychee juice (*Ceres*							
Litchi), 8 fl. oz.	120	0	30.0	0	0	10	0

M

Food and Measure	cal.	prot. (gms)	carbo. (gms)	fat (gms)	chol. (mgs)	sod. (mgs)	fiber (gms)
Macadamia nut butter,							
roasted (*MaraNatha*),							
2 tbsp.	230	2.0	4.0	24.0	0	0	3.0
Macadamias:							
(*Planters*), 1 oz.	200	2.0	4.0	21.0	0	55	3.0
raw, whole/halves:							
(*Shiloh Farms*							
Organic), 1 oz. . .	201	2.0	4.0	21.0	0	1	2.0
(*Tree of Life*), ¼ cup,							
1.2 oz.	230	3.0	5.0	24.0	0	0	2.0
1 oz.	204	2.2	3.9	21.5	0	1	2.4
¼ cup	241	2.7	4.6	25.4	0	2	2.9
chopped:							
(*Diamond*), ¼ cup .	220	2.0	4.0	23.0	0	0	3.0
(*Planters*), 2 oz. . . .	400	5.0	8.0	42.0	0	0	5.0
dried, shelled:							
1 oz.	199	2.4	3.9	20.9	0	1	2.6
¼ cup	235	2.8	4.6	24.7	0	2	3.1
dry-roasted (*Mauna Loa*),							
1 oz.	230	2.0	4.0	24.0	0	105	2.0
whole/halves, ¼ cup	241	2.6	4.5	25.5	0	1	2.7
oil-roasted, 1 oz.	204	2.1	3.7	21.7	0	2	n.a.
Macadamias, flavored							
(see also "Candy"):							
coffee glazed (*Mauna*							
Loa Kona), 1 oz. . . .	180	1.0	12.0	15.0	<5	75	1.0
honey-roasted (*Mauna*							
Loa), 1 oz.	180	2.0	9.0	16.0	0	85	2.0
onion garlic (*Mauna Loa*							
Maui), .5 oz.	100	1.0	2.0	11.0	0	85	1.0
Macaroni (see also							
"Pasta"):							
uncooked:							
2 oz.	210	7.3	42.4	.9	0	4	1.4

Food and Measure	cal.	prot. (gms)	carbo. (gms)	fat (gms)	chol. (mgs)	sod. (mgs)	fiber (gms)
Macaroni, uncooked *(cont.)*							
elbow, 1 cup	389	13.4	78.4	1.7	0	8	2.5
enriched, 2 oz.	213	11.3	38.3	1.3	0	5	1.4
whole wheat, 2 oz. . .	198	.3	42.8	.8	0	5	4.7
cooked, 1 cup:							
enriched, elbows . .	197	6.7	39.7	.9	0	1	1.8
enriched, spirals . .	189	6.4	38.0	.9	0	1	1.7
small shells	162	5.5	32.6	.8	0	1	1.8
vegetable, enriched,							
spirals	172	6.1	35.7	.2	0	8	5.8
whole wheat, elbows	174	7.5	37.2	.8	0	4	3.9
Macaroni entree, can,							
microwave, or pkg.,							
1 cont., except							
as noted:							
and beef, 1 cup:							
(*Chef Boyardee* Mini							
Beef Micro)	240	8.0	33.0	8.0	15	950	3.0
(*Chef Boyardee*							
Beefaroni)	240	9.0	30.0	9.0	20	960	3.0
(*Chef Boyardee*							
Beefaroni Micro)	250	10.0	31.0	9.0	25	920	3.0
(*Chef Boyardee* Big							
Beefaroni)	260	12.0	32.0	9.0	20	860	4.0
and cheddar (*Kraft Bistro*							
Deluxe), ⅓ of							
10-oz. pkg.	310	12.0	40.0	11.0	35	860	3.0
and cheese:							
(*Hormel*), 7.5 oz. . .	270	12.0	32.0	11.0	35	710	1.0
(*Kraft Easy Mac*							
Micro), 2.05 oz. .	230	7.0	42.0	4.0	5	550	1.0
(*Kraft Easy Mac*							
Extreme Cheese							
Micro), 2.05 oz. .	230	7.0	42.0	4.0	5	520	1.0
w/bacon (*Kraft Easy*							
Mac Micro),							
2.05 oz.	220	7.0	38.0	4.5	5	580	1.0
portobello mushroom							
(*Kraft Bistro Deluxe*),							
⅓ of 10-oz. pkg.	310	12.0	40.0	11.0	35	800	3.0
three, Italian (*Kraft*							
Bistro Deluxe), ⅓							
of 10-oz. pkg. . .	310	12.0	40.0	11.0	30	920	3.0

Food and Measure	cal.	prot. (gms)	carbo. (gms)	fat (gms)	chol. (mgs)	sod. (mgs)	fiber (gms)
tomato, sun-dried, and Parmesan (*Kraft Bistro Deluxe*), ⅓ of 10-oz. pkg.	300	12.0	40.0	11.0	30	870	3.0
cheesy burger (*Chef Boyardee*), 1 cup ..	200	9.0	30.0	5.0	15	820	3.0
chili (*Chef Boyardee* Chili Mac), 1 cup ..	260	9.0	26.0	13.0	20	970	3.0
Macaroni entree, frozen, 1 pkg., except as noted: and beef:							
(*Blake's* Organic), 8 oz.	220	15.0	22.0	8.0	30	620	2.0
(*Lean Cuisine One Dish Favorites*), 9.5 oz.	310	20.0	38.0	9.0	30	630	3.0
(*Michelina's Budget Gourmet/Zap'ems*), 8 oz.	280	12.0	33.0	10.0	25	690	2.0
cheesy (*Birds Eye Voila!* Family Skillets), 1 cup* .	370	14.0	44.0	15.0	25	970	1.0
and cheese:							
(*Amy's*), 9 oz.	410	16.0	47.0	16.0	40	590	3.0
(*Amy's* 20 oz.), 1 cup	360	14.0	41.0	14.0	45	590	3.0
(*Amy's* Light Sodium), 9 oz.	400	16.0	47.0	16.0	40	290	3.0
(*Cedarlane* Organic Lowfat), 9 oz. ...	270	17.0	42.0	3.0	10	680	2.0
(*Glory* Savory), 11 oz.	480	21.0	47.0	23.0	90	1300	1.0
(*Glory* Savory Family Size), 1 cup	390	17.0	38.0	18.0	70	1050	<1.0
(*Healthy Choice*), 9.1 oz.	210	9.0	32.0	4.0	5	600	4.0
(*Lean Cuisine One Dish Favorites*), 10 oz.	290	15.0	41.0	7.0	20	620	2.0
(*Michelina's Authentico*), 8 oz.	230	9.0	40.0	3.5	10	540	2.0
(*Michelina's Budget Gourmet/Zap'ems*), 8 oz.	310	12.0	42.0	10.0	20	730	2.0
(*Michelina's Lean Gourmet*), 10 oz.	270	10.0	47.0	3.5	10	520	2.0

Food and Measure	cal.	prot. (gms)	carbo. (gms)	fat (gms)	chol. (mgs)	sod. (mgs)	fiber (gms)
Macaroni entree, frozen, and cheese *(cont.)*							
(*Shedd's Spread Country Crock*), 1 cup	370	14.0	40.0	17.0	40	940	1.0
(*Smart Ones*), 10 oz.	270	11.0	52.0	2.0	<5	790	2.0
(*Stouffer's*), 6 oz. or ½ of 10-oz. pkg. . .	350	15.0	34.0	17.0	25	920	2.0
(*Stouffer's Family*), ¼ of 40-oz. pkg. . .	350	15.0	34.0	17.0	30	920	2.0
3 cheese (*Moosewood Organic*), 10 oz. . .	400	17.0	35.0	17.0	35	670	2.0
3 cheese (*Smart Ones*), 9 oz.	300	14.0	48.0	6.0	10	570	3.0
asiago/cheddar (*Helen's Kitchen*), 9 oz.	325	15.0	43.0	8.0	25	620	3.0
w/beef (*Michelina's Authentico* Cheeseburger Mac*), 8 oz.	350	17.0	38.0	12.0	40	720	2.0
w/broccoli (*Stouffer's*), 12 oz.	480	22.0	52.0	20.0	35	1000	5.0
cheddar, sharp (*Michelina's Authentico*), 10 oz. . .	420	17.0	50.0	16.0	40	950	2.0
cheddar/Romano (*Michelina's Budget Gourmet*), 8 oz. . .	260	10.0	40.0	7.0	15	550	2.0
w/ham (*Michelina's Authentico*), 8 oz.	330	17.0	33.0	13.0	45	960	2.0
rice pasta (*Amy's* Rice Mac & Cheese), 9 oz.	400	16.0	47.0	16.0	50	590	1.0
and chili, see "Chili entree"							
meat sauce (*Organic Classics*), 10 oz. . . .	340	16.0	49.0	9.0	20	580	3.0
vegetarian, soy cheese:							
(*Amy's*), 9 oz.	370	16.0	42.0	15.0	0	500	4.0
(*Yves Bowl*), 10.5 oz.	340	13.0	52.0	9.0	0	880	3.0
Macaroni entree mix							
(see also "Pasta dish mix" and specific pasta listings), dry mix, except as noted:							
Alfredo:							
(*Kraft Easy Mac Micro*), 2.05 oz. .	220	7.0	39.0	4.5	5	590	1.0

Food and Measure	cal.	prot. (gms)	carbo. (gms)	fat (gms)	chol. (mgs)	sod. (mgs)	fiber (gms)
cheesy (Kraft Dinner), ⅓ of 7.25-oz. pkg.	260	9.0	49.0	2.5	5	650	2.0
and cheddar:							
(*Annie's* Wisconsin Micro), ¾ cup*	230	9.0	40.0	4.5	10	570	<1.0
(*Annie's Simply Organic*), 2.5 oz.	240	10.0	48.0	2.0	5	740	2.0
(*Kraft* Deluxe), ¼ of 14-oz. pkg.	320	12.0	45.0	10.0	15	930	1.0
(*Kraft* Deluxe Half the Fat), ¼ of 14-oz. pkg.	290	13.0	50.0	4.5	15	850	2.0
sharp (*Kraft* Deluxe), ¼ of 14-oz. pkg.	320	12.0	47.0	9.0	15	840	2.0
wheat (*Kraft* Harvest), ½ of 6-oz. pkg.	290	12.0	58.0	2.5	5	750	2.0
white (*Annie's* Micro), ½ cup	230	9.0	40.0	4.5	10	560	<1.0
white (*Kraft*), ⅓ of 7.3-oz. pkg.	260	10.0	48.0	2.5	10	580	2.0
and cheese:							
(*Annie's* Classic), 2.5 oz	270	10.0	47.0	4.0	10	530	2.0
(*Annie's* Classic Organic), 2.5 oz.	270	10.0	46.0	4.5	10	520	2.0
(*Annie's* Single Serve Micro), ¾ cup*	230	9.0	40.0	4.5	10	560	<1.0
(*Kraft* Dinner), ⅓ of 7.25-oz. pkg.	260	9.0	48.0	3.5	15	580	1.0
(*Kraft* Thick 'n Creamy), ⅓ of 7.25-oz. pkg.	250	9.0	50.0	2.0	5	580	2.0
4 (*Annie's* Creamy Deluxe), 1 cup*	320	14.0	45.0	11.0	30	750	2.0
4 (*Kraft* Deluxe), ¼ of 14-oz. pkg.	320	12.0	46.0	10.0	15	890	2.0
3 (*Kraft*), ⅓ of 7.25-oz. pkg.	260	9.0	49.0	2.5	5	610	2.0
whole wheat pasta (*Hodgson Mill*), 2 oz.	255	11.0	45.0	.5	<5	570	6.0

Macaroni and cheese, see "Macaroni dish" and "Macaroni entree"

Food and Measure	cal.	prot. (gms)	carbo. (gms)	fat (gms)	chol. (mgs)	sod. (mgs)	fiber (gms)
Mace, ground, 1 tsp. .	8	.1	.9	.6	0	1	.1
Mackerel, meat only:							
Atlantic, 4 oz.:							
raw	230	21.1	0	15.8	80	102	0
baked or broiled . . .	297	27.0	0	20.2	85	94	0
king, 4 oz.:							
raw	119	23.0	0	2.3	61	179	0
baked or broiled . . .	152	29.5	0	2.9	77	230	0
Pacific/Jack, 4 oz.:							
raw	179	22.8	0	9.0	53	98	0
baked or broiled . . .	228	29.2	0	11.5	68	125	0
Spanish, 4 oz.:							
raw	158	21.9	0	7.2	86	67	0
baked or broiled . . .	179	26.8	0	7.2	83	75	0
Mackerel, canned,							
Jack, drained:							
(*Orleans*), 2 oz.	90	13.0	0	4.0	55	280	0
in oil, boneless, skin-							
less (*Roland*), 2 oz. .	80	14.0	0	3.0	35	330	0
in tomato sauce							
(*Chicken of the Sea*),							
¼ cup	70	10.0	2.0	3.0	45	250	0
in water, ⅓ cup:							
(*Chicken of the Sea*)	90	13.0	0	4.0	55	280	0
(*Roland*)	90	13.0	0	4.0	45	240	0
Mackerel, salted, 2 oz.	171	10.4	0	14.1	53	2492	0
Mahi mahi, fresh,							
meat only:							
raw, 4 oz.	97	21.0	0	.8	83	99	0
raw, vacuum pack							
(*Peter Pan*), 4 oz. . .	101	21.3	0	1.0	97	145	0
baked or broiled, 4 oz.	124	26.0	0	1.0	107	128	0
Malanga, fresh:							
(*Frieda's*), 3 oz.	90	1.0	23.0	0	0	10	2.0
sliced, ½ cup	66	1.0	16.0	.3	0	14	1.0
Malt syrup, see							
"Barley malt syrup"							
Mammy apple:							
½ of 25-oz. fruit	216	2.1	52.9	2.1	0	63	12.7
peeled, seeded, 1 oz. .	14	.1	3.5	.1	0	4	.9
Mandarin orange,							
see "Tangerine"							
Mango, fresh:							
(*Dole*), ½ medium . . .	70	0	17.0	0	0	0	1.0

Food and Measure	cal.	prot. (gms)	carbo. (gms)	fat (gms)	chol. (mgs)	sod. (mgs)	fiber (gms)
10.6-oz. fruit, 7.3 oz.							
trimmed	135	1.1	35.2	.6	0	4	3.7
sliced, 1 cup	107	8.4	28.1	.5	0	2	3.0
Mango, can/jar:							
in light syrup, ½ cup:							
(*SunFresh*)	70	0	19.0	0	0	15	<1.0
sliced (*Roland*)	90	0	22.0	0	0	15	1.0
in syrup, sliced							
(*Herdez*), 2 pcs.	170	0	30.0	0	0	10	1.0
Mango, dried, 1.4 oz.,							
except as noted:							
(*Sunsweet* Philippine)	130	1.0	30.0	.5	0	220	2.0
(*Sunsweet* Thailand)	140	0	34.0	0	0	20	1.0
spears (*SunRidge Farms*),							
4 pcs., 1.4 oz.	140	1.0	36.0	.5	0	0	4.0
unsweetened:							
slices (*SunRidge*							
Farms Organic)	25	0	7.0	0	0	0	<1.0
slices (*Tree of Life*)	30	0	7.0	0	0	0	<1.0
Mango, frozen, chunks,							
¾ cup:							
(*C&W* Ultimate)	90	1.0	24.0	0	0	0	3.0
(*Dole*)	90	0	24.0	0	0	0	3.0
Mango drink, 8 fl. oz.:							
(*Apple & Eve* Nectar)	140	0	33.0	0	0	25	0
(*Langers* Mongo)	120	0	30.0	0	0	0	0
(*Snapple* Madness)	110	0	29.0	0	0	10	0
Mango drink blend,							
8 fl. oz.:							
(*AriZona* Mucho)	100	0	27.0	0	0	20	0
mangosteen (*Apple &*							
Eve)	120	0	30.0	0	0	15	0
melon (*SoBe Nirvana*)	120	0	29.0	0	0	15	0
orange (*Langers*)	130	0	33.0	0	0	0	0
passion fruit (*SoBe Fuerte*)	130	0	35.0	0	0	10	0
peach (*V8 Splash*)	80	0	20.0	0	0	40	0
Mango juice (*R.W.*							
Knudsen Organic							
Nectar), 8 fl. oz.	120	0	29.0	0	0	15	0
Mango juice blend,							
8 fl. oz.:							
(*After the Fall*)	150	1.0	37.0	0	0	15	0
(*Apple & Eve* Tropicals							
Passion)	130	0	33.0	0	0	25	0

Food and Measure	cal.	prot. (gms)	carbo. (gms)	fat (gms)	chol. (mgs)	sod. (mgs)	fiber (gms)
Mango juice blend *(cont.)*							
(*Ceres*)	120	0	30.0	0	0	10	1.0
(*Odwalla Mango Tango* Smoothie)	150	1.0	34.0	1.0	0	10	0
lime (*Dole* Fiesta)	120	<1.0	30.0	0	0	15	0
peach (*R.W. Knudsen*)	130	<1.0	31.0	0	0	50	0
Mango relish, Indian (see also "Chutney") (*Patak's*), 1 tbsp.:							
hot, extra	45	0	3.0	4.0	0	760	1.0
mild	40	0	1.0	4.0	0	660	0
w/lime, chili	40	0	0	4.0	0	410	0
Mangosteen, canned in syrup, ½ cup	70	.4	6.7	5.7	0	7	1.8
Manicotti dinner, frozen, 4 cheese (*Healthy Choice*), 11.75-oz. pkg.	380	16.0	63.0	6.0	25	600	8.0
Manicotti entree, frozen, 1 pkg., except as noted: cheese, w/sauce:							
(*Celentano*), 10 oz. .	420	18.0	51.0	15.0	40	1030	7.0
(*Celentano*), ½ of 14-oz. pkg.	310	14.0	39.0	10.0	35	710	4.0
(*Celentano* Light), 10 oz.	330	17.0	51.0	6.0	25.0	800	7.0
(*Michelina's Authentico*), 8.5 oz.	300	14.0	31.0	13.0	40	860	2.0
4 cheese (*Healthy Choice*), 10 oz. . .	270	12.0	44.0	4.5	15	450	5.0
3 cheese (*Stouffer's*), 9 oz.	360	18.0	41.0	14.0	70	920	2.0
Florentine (*Celentano* Light), 10 oz. . . .	330	16.0	52.0	6.0	25	660	8.0
cheese, w/out sauce (*Celentano*), ½ of 14-oz. pkg.	360	20.0	43.0	11.0	60	800	2.0
spinach and broccoli (*Celentano* Organic Vegan), 10 oz.	300	18.0	42.0	6.0	0	670	8.0
Manioc, see "Yuca"							
Maple syrup, pure:							
(*Roland*), ¼ cup	200	0	53.0	0	0	5	0
(*Tree of Life*), ¼ cup .	200	0	53.0	0	0	10	0

Food and Measure	cal.	prot. (gms)	carbo. (gms)	fat (gms)	chol. (mgs)	sod. (mgs)	fiber (gms)
Margarine (see also "Butter blend"), 1 tbsp.:							
soft tub/spread:							
(*Blue Bonnet*)	60	0	0	7.0	0	125	0
(*Blue Bonnet* Light)	40	0	0	4.5	0	90	0
(*Country Morning Blend*)	100	0	0	11.0	0	80	0
(*Fleischmann's*) ...	70	0	0	8.0	0	75	0
(*Fleischmann's* Light)	40	0	0	4.5	0	90	0
(*I Can't Believe It's Not Butter!*)	80	0	0	8.0	0	90	0
(*I Can't Believe It's Not Butter!* Light)	50	0	0	5.0	0	85	0
(*Land O Lakes*) ...	100	0	0	11.0	0	125	0
(*Land O Lakes Fresh Buttery Taste*) ...	70	0	0	8.0	0	80	0
(*Parkay* Light)	45	0	0	5.0	0	75	0
(*Parkay* Original) ..	80	0	0	9.0	0	110	0
(*Parkay* Soft Spread)	60	0	0	7.0	0	90	0
(*Shedd's Spread Country Crock*) .	60	0	0	7.0	0	110	0
(*Shedd's Spread Country Crock Churn*)	80	0	0	8.0	0	95	0
(*Shedd's Spread Country Crock Light/Plus Calcium/ Vitamins*)	50	0	0	5.0	0	85	0
(*Shedd's Spread Country Crock Omega Plus*) ...	70	0	0	8.0	0	100	0
squeeze:							
(*I Can't Believe It's Not Butter!*)	60	0	0	7.0	0	80	0
whipped (*Shedd's Spread Country Crock*)	60	0	0	7.0	0	85	0
stick:							
(*Blue Bonnet*)	80	0	0	9.0	0	110	0
(*Blue Bonnet* Light)	50	0	0	5.0	0	80	0
(*Country Morning Spread*)	100	0	0	11.0	0	90	0

Food and Measure	cal.	prot. (gms)	carbo. (gms)	fat (gms)	chol. (mgs)	sod. (mgs)	fiber (gms)
Margarine, stick *(cont.)*							
(*I Can't Believe It's Not Butter!*)	90	0	0	10.0	0	95	0
(*I Can't Believe It's Not Butter!* Light) . . .	50	0	0	6.0	0	85	0
(*Land O Lakes*) . . .	100	0	0	11.0	0	105	0
(*Land O Lakes Fresh Buttery Taste*) . . .	90	0	0	10.0	0	95	0
Margarine, flavored (*Shedd's Spread Country Crock*), 1 tbsp.:							
apple cinnamon	60	0	2.0	6.0	0	45	0
blueberry	50	0	2.0	5.0	0	35	0
cinnamon or maple . .	60	0	3.0	6.0	0	45	0
Margarita drink mixer:							
(*Angostura*), 4 fl. oz. . .	80	0	30.0	0	0	5	0
(*Jose Cuervo*), 4 fl. oz.	100	0	24.0	0	0	80	0
dry (*Bar-Tender's*), 2 pouches	90	0	21.0	0	0	70	0
frozen, 2 fl. oz.:							
(*Bacardi*)	90	0	25.0	0	0	0	0
(*No Worries*)	95	0	24.0	0	0	60	0
Marinade (see also "Barbecue sauce," "Grilling sauce" and specific listings), 1 tbsp., except as noted:							
(*A.1.* Chicago)	20	0	3.0	1.0	0	270	0
(*A.1.* New York)	20	0	5.0	0	0	230	0
(*House of Tsang* Mandarin)	25	0	6.0	0	0	680	0
(*Neera's* Kashmiri), 1 tsp.	18	0	5.0	1.0	0	69	0
(*Patak's* Sweet & Smoky)	25	0	6.0	0	0	190	0
(*Spiedie* State Fair) . .	15	0	1.0	1.5	0	160	0
(*World Harbors Amalfi Coast* Otalian Grill), 2 tbsp.	25	0	4.0	1.0	0	300	0
abobo (*Acadia Naturals* Honey Ancho), 2 tbsp.	40	0	9.0	0	0	320	0
Cajun:							
(*A.1.* New Orleans) .	25	0	5.0	0	0	180	0
(*Litehouse*), 2 tbsp.	35	0	7.0	.5	0	410	0

Food and Measure	cal.	prot. (gms)	carbo. (gms)	fat (gms)	chol. (mgs)	sod. (mgs)	fiber (gms)
cherry soy (*World Harbors* Cheriyaki Glaze), 2 tbsp.	50	0	14.0	0	0	390	0
chili and lime (*Lawry's* Mexican)	15	0	3.0	0	0	240	0
chimichurri (*World Harbors* Argentine), 2 tbsp.	40	0	9.0	0	0	180	0
Chinese (*Mee Tu* All Purpose)	25	0	7.0	0	0	120	0
chipotle:							
(*Lawry's* Baja)	15	0	4.0	0	0	390	0
hickory maple (*Emeril's*)	35	0	2.0	3.0	0	75	0
Southwest (*Mrs. Dash* 10 Minute)	35	0	2.0	3.0	0	75	0
cilantro lime wasabi (*Acadia Naturals*), 2 tbsp.	35	0	4.0	0	0	150	0
curry, Madras (*Acadia Naturals* Garam Masala), 2 tbsp.	60	0	12.0	0	0	210	0
fajita:							
(*World Harbors* Mexican), 2 tbsp.	45	0	10.0	0	0	290	0
medium (*Zapata*) . .	5	0	<1.0	0	0	125	0
garlic, roasted:							
(*Acadia Naturals* Tuscan Grill)	10	0	2.0	0	0	105	0
balsamic (*Consorzio*)	30	0	6.0	.5	0	260	0
garlic herb (*Mrs. Dash* 10 Minute Zest) . . .	25	0	3.0	3.0	0	0	0
garlic lime:							
(*Lawry's* Havana) . .	10	0	2.0	0	0	330	0
(*Mrs. Dash* 10 Minute)	30	0	4.0	1.0	0	0	0
ginger:							
sesame (*Simply Tsang*)	50	0	9.0	2.0	0	630	0
spicy (*Annie's Naturals* Organic), 2 tbsp.	35	1.0	3.0	2.0	0	450	0
Hawaiian (*Lawry's*) . .	25	0	5.0	0	0	250	0

Food and Measure	cal.	prot. (gms)	carbo. (gms)	fat (gms)	chol. (mgs)	sod. (mgs)	fiber (gms)
Marinade *(cont.)*							
herb and garlic:							
(*Ken's*)	20	0	3.0	1.0	0	370	0
(*Lawry's*)	10	0	2.0	0	0	420	0
roasted (*Newman's Own*)	20	0	3.0	1.0	0	370	0
honey Dijon:							
(*Lawry's*)	20	0	4.0	0	0	440	0
(*World Harbors* Mont St. Michel), 2 tbsp.	30	0	7.0	0	0	230	0
honey ginger (*Patak's*)	20	0	5.0	0	0	180	0
Italian garlic steak (*Lawry's*)	10	0	2.0	0	0	400	0
jerk:							
(*A.1. Jamaican*) . . .	25	0	5.0	.5	0	190	0
(*Lawry's* Caribbean)	25	0	5.0	0	0	430	0
(*Simply Tsang* Jamaican)	60	0	8.0	3.5	0	400	0
(*World Harbors* Jamaican), 2 tbsp.	70	0	18.0	0	0	200	0
raspberry (*Acadia Naturals*)	20	0	4.0	0	0	85	0
lemon garlic (*Spiedie Garlicious*)	47	3.0	3.0	4.0	0	225	0
lemon herb peppercorn (*Mrs. Dash* 10 Minute)	25	0	2.0	2.0	0	0	0
lemon pepper:							
(*Ken's*)	10	0	2.0	0	0	350	0
(*Lawry's*)	10	0	2.0	0	0	390	0
(*Newman's Own*) . .	15	0	3.0	0	0	300	0
and garlic (*World Harbors* Maine's Own), 2 tbsp. . . .	35	0	8.0	0	0	140	0
herbed (*Emeril's*) . .	70	0	1.0	8.0	0	55	0
lemon rosemary garlic (*Emeril's* Gaaahlic) .	70	0	1.0	8.0	0	120	0
lime, Baja (*Consorzio Organic*)	25	0	1.0	2.5	0	180	<1.0
mango:							
(*World Harbors* Island), 2 tbsp. . . .	60	0	14.0	0	0	190	0
cilantro (*Consorzio Organic*)	20	0	3.0	.5	0	130	0
golden (*Patak's*) . . .	20	0	5.0	0	0	160	0

Food and Measure	cal.	prot. (gms)	carbo. (gms)	fat (gms)	chol. (mgs)	sod. (mgs)	fiber (gms)
maple wasabi (*World Harbors* Pacific Fusion), 2 tbsp. ...	45	0	8.0	0	0	370	0
mesquite:							
(*Ken's*)	20	0	4.0	1.0	0	330	0
(*Lawry's*)	5	0	1.0	0	0	350	0
grille (*Mrs. Dash* 10 Minute)	25	0	2.0	1.5	0	0	0
w/lime (*Newman's Own*)	20	0	3.0	1.0	0	190	0
mojo (*World Harbors* Cuban), 2 tbsp. ...	25	0	5.0	1.0	0	300	0
orange herb poppyseed (*Emeril's*)	150	0	4.0	15.0	0	170	0
pepper, red (*Lawry's* Louisiana)	10	0	2.0	0	0	390	0
sesame (*Emeril's* Asian)	140	<1.0	4.0	14.0	0	340	0
sesame ginger:							
(*Ken's*)	25	0	6.0	0	0	390	0
(*Lawry's*)	30	0	7.0	0	0	580	0
sesame orange (*Consorzio*)	25	0	5.0	.5	0	150	0
steak:							
(*Annie's Naturals* Organic), 2 tbsp. .	50	<1.0	5.0	3.5	0	470	0
(*Simply Tsang* Japanese Steakhouse)	40	0	6.0	1.5	0	770	0
and chop (*Lawry's*) .	5	0	1.0	0	0	400	0
sweet and sour (*Simply Tsang*)	50	0	13.0	0	0	420	0
tequila lime (*Lawry's*)	15	0	4.0	0	0	490	0
teriyaki:							
(*A.1.*)	25	0	5.0	0	0	490	0
(*Ah-So*)	30	0	6.0	0	0	280	0
(*Annie's Naturals* Organic)	30	0	6.0	.5	0	340	0
(*Ken's*)	20	0	4.0	0	0	260	0
(*Consorzio* California)	35	1.0	8.0	0	0	310	0
(*Lawry's*)	20	0	5.0	0	0	560	0
(*Newman's Own*) ..	25	0	6.0	0	0	330	0
(*Simply Tsang*)	45	0	11.0	0	0	690	0

Food and Measure	cal.	prot. (gms)	carbo. (gms)	fat (gms)	chol. (mgs)	sod. (mgs)	fiber (gms)
Marinade, teriyaki *(cont.)*							
(*World Harbors* Maui Mountain), 2 tbsp.	70	0	17.0	0	0	270	0
blueberry (*Acadia Naturals*)	30	0	6.0	0	0	125	0
ginger (*Emeril's*) ..	25	<1.0	4.0	.5	0	240	0
honey (*Ken's*)	25	0	6.0	0	0	250	0
hot (*World Harbors* Maui Mountain), 2 tbsp.	70	0	17.0	0	0	300	0
spicy (*Mrs. Dash* 10 Minute)	25	0	5.0	1.0	0	0	0
tomato, smoky (*Annie's Naturals* Organic), 2 tbsp.	60	0	1.0	6.0	0	160	0
vegetable, roasted (*Emeril's*)	150	0	2.0	16.0	0	200	0
Marinade seasoning mix, 1 tsp., except as noted:							
beef, tenderizing (*Lawry's*), ¾ tsp. ...	0	0	<1.0	0	0	550	0
chipotle pepper (*Grill Mates*)	10	0	2.0	0	0	520	0
citrus (*Grill Mates* Baja)	10	0	1.0	0	0	310	0
garlic, herbs, wine (*Grill Mates*)	5	0	1.0	0	0	430	0
herb, zesty (*Grill Mates*)	10	0	1.0	0	0	260	0
hickory barbecue (*Grill Mates*)	15	0	0	0	0	340	0
meat:							
(*Adolph's/Lawry's* Marinade in Minutes), ¾ tsp..	5	0	1.0	0	0	380	0
(*McCormick*)	15	0	2.0	0	0	240	0
mesquite (*Grill Mates*), 2 tsp.	15	0	2.0	0	0	610	0
peppercorn and garlic (*Grill Mates*)	5	0	1.0	0	0	340	0
Southwest (*Grill Mates*), 2 tsp.	15	0	2.0	0	0	440	0
steak, ½ tsp.:							
(*Grill Mates* Montreal)	0	0	0	0	0	350	0
(*Grill Mates* Montreal 25% Less Sodium)	0	0	0	0	0	260	0

Food and Measure	cal.	prot. (gms)	carbo. (gms)	fat (gms)	chol. (mgs)	sod. (mgs)	fiber (gms)
teriyaki (*Grill Mates*) .	15	0	2.0	0	0	290	0
tomato, garlic, basil (*Grill Mates*)	5	0	1.0	0	0	330	0
Marionberry, see "Blackberry, dried"							
Marjoram, dried, 1 tsp.	2	.1	.4	<.1	0	<1	.1
Marmalade, see "Jam and preserves"							
Marrow squash, raw, trimmed, 1 oz.	4	.2	1.0	<.1	0	n.a.	<1.0
Marshmallow topping:							
(*Jet-Puffed* Crème), 1 tbsp.	40	0	11.0	0	0	10	0
(*Marshmallow Fluff*), 2 tbsp.	60	0	15.0	0	0	10	0
(*Smucker's*), 2 tbsp. . .	110	0	28.0	0	0	5	0
Martini drink mixer, bottled (*Master of Mixers Martini Gold*), 2 fl. oz.:							
chocolate	80	0	20.0	0	0	45	0
lemon drop	74	0	22.0	0	0	40	0
Masa, see "Cornmeal"							
Matai, see "Water chestnut"							
Matzo, see "Cracker"							
Matzo ball mix:							
(*Manischewitz*), 2 tbsp.	50	1.0	11.0	0	0	700	1.0
and soup mix, 1 tbsp.:							
(*Manischewitz*)	40	1.0	9.0	.5	0	1290	1.0
(*Streit's*)	50	<1.0	12.0	0	0	880	0
Matzo meal, see "Cracker crumbs/meal"							
Mayonnaise, in jars, 1 tbsp.:							
(*Blue Plate*)	100	0	0	11.0	10	80	0
(*Cains* All Natural) . . .	100	0	0	11.0	5	75	0
(*Cains* Light)	50	0	2.0	4.5	5	130	0
(*Cains* Reduced Fat) . .	30	0	3.0	2.0	0	130	0
(*Hellmann's/Best Foods* Real)	90	0	0	10.0	5	90	0
(*Hellmann's/Best Foods* Canola Cholestrol Free)	45	0	<1.0	4.5	0	90	0
(*Hellmann's/Best Foods* Light)	45	0	<1.0	4.5	<5	120	0

Food and Measure	cal.	prot. (gms)	carbo. (gms)	fat (gms)	chol. (mgs)	sod. (mgs)	fiber (gms)
Mayonnaise *(cont.)*							
(*Hellmann's/Best Foods* Mayonesa con Jugo de Limón)	90	0	0	10.0	15	85	0
(*Hellmann's/Best Foods* Reduced Fat)	20	0	2.0	2.0	0	125	0
(*Kraft* Light 32 oz.) ..	40	0	1.0	5.0	5	95	0
(*Kraft* Light 16 oz.) ..	40	0	1.0	3.5	5	90	0
(*Kraft* Light Squeeze 24 oz.)	45	0	2.0	4.0	5	95	0
(*Kraft* Light Squeeze 18 oz.)	50	0	1.0	4.0	5	95	0
(*Kraft* Real 32 oz.) ...	100	0	0	11.0	10	85	0
(*Kraft* Real 16/48/32 oz. Big Mouth Jar/ Squeeze)	90	0	0	10.0	5	70	0
(*Nasoya Nayonaise*) ..	35	<1.0	1.0	3.5	0	115	0
chipotle, smoked (*French's GourMayo*)	50	0	1.0	5.0	10	115	0
Dijon:							
(*Nasoya Nayonaise*)	30	<1.0	1.0	3.0	0	140	0
(*Spectrum* Organic)	90	0	1.0	10.0	10	90	0
dressing:							
(*Kraft* Fat Free)	10	0	2.0	0	0	120	0
(*Miracle Whip*)	40	0	2.0	3.0	5	125	0
(*Miracle Whip* Fat Free)	15	0	3.0	0	0	125	0
(*Miracle Whip* Light)	20	0	2.0	1.5	5	135	0
(*Miracle Whip* Light 16 oz.)	25	0	3.0	1.5	5	140	0
spicy, smoked jalapeño (*Fiesta*) .	60	3.0	12.0	.5	0	390	0
garlic, roasted (*Spectrum* Organic)	100	0	0	11.0	10	30	0
hot and spicy (*Kraft* Real)	100	0	0	11.0	5	85	0
olive oil (*Spectrum* Organic)	100	0	0	11.0	5	75	0
wasabi:							
garlic (*Spectrum* Organic)	100	0	0	11.0	10	65	0
horseradish (*French's* GourMayo)	50	0	2.0	5.0	10	115	0

Food and Measure	cal.	prot. (gms)	carbo. (gms)	fat (gms)	chol. (mgs)	sod. (mgs)	fiber (gms)
Mayonnaise, refrigerated, 1 tbsp.:							
(*Delouis fils*)	110	0	0	12.0	30	70	0
garlic (*Delouis Fils* Aioli)	102	0	0	11.2	27	97	0
McDonald's:							
breakfast:							
Big Breakfast	730	28.0	50.0	47.0	555	1550	3.0
w/large biscuit . .	790	28.0	55.0	51.0	555	1660	4.0
biscuit, regular	260	5.0	33.0	12.0	0	740	2.0
bacon/egg/cheese	430	16.0	37.0	24.0	240	1230	2.0
chicken	420	18.0	41.0	20.0	35	1200	2.0
sausage	430	11.0	34.0	27.0	30	1080	2.0
sausage/egg	510	18.0	36.0	33.0	250	1170	2.0
biscuit, large	320	5.0	39.0	16.0	0	850	3.0
bacon/egg/cheese	520	19.0	43.0	30.0	245	1520	3.0
chicken	480	18.0	47.0	24.0	35	1310	3.0
sausage	480	11.0	39.0	31.0	30	1190	3.0
sausage/egg	570	18.0	42.0	37.0	250	1280	3.0
burrito, sausage . . .	300	12.0	26.0	16.0	130	830	1.0
burrito, *McSkillet:*							
w/sausage	610	27.0	44.0	36.0	410	1390	3.0
w/steak	570	32.0	44.0	30.0	430	1470	3.0
deluxe breakfast, no syrup/							
margarine	1080	36.0	110.0	55.0	575	2130	6.0
w/large biscuit . .	1140	36.0	115.0	59.0	575	2250	7.0
eggs, scrambled, 2	170	15.0	1.0	11.0	520	180	0
hash browns	140	1.0	15.0	8.0	0	290	2.0
hotcakes, no syrup/							
margarine	350	8.0	60.0	9.0	20	590	3.0
w/sausage	520	15.0	61.0	24.0	50	930	3.0
hotcake syrup pkt. . .	180	0	45.0	0	0	20	0
margarine, 2 pats . .	40	0	0	4.5	0	55	0
McGriddles:							
bacon/egg/cheese	420	16.0	48.0	19.0	240	1190	2.0
sausage	420	11.0	44.0	22.0	35	1030	2.0
sausage/egg/ cheese	560	20.0	48.0	32.0	265	1360	2.0
McMuffin:							
egg	300	18.0	30.0	12.0	260	820	2.0
sausage	370	14.0	29.0	22.0	45	850	2.0
sausage/egg	450	21.0	30.0	27.0	285	920	2.0
muffin, English	160	5.0	27.0	3.0	0	280	2.0
preserves/jam	35	0	9.0	0	0	0	0

Food and Measure	cal.	prot. (gms)	carbo. (gms)	fat (gms)	chol. (mgs)	sod. (mgs)	fiber (gms)
McDonald's *(cont.)*							
burgers/sandwiches:							
Big Mac	540	25.0	45.0	29.0	75	1040	3.0
Big N' Tasty	460	24.0	37.0	24.0	70	720	3.0
w/cheese	510	27.0	38.0	28.0	85	960	3.0
cheeseburger	300	15.0	33.0	12.0	40	750	2.0
double	440	25.0	34.0	23.0	80	1150	2.0
chicken, crispy:							
classic	550	27.0	61.0	22.0	50	1200	3.0
club	660	35.0	62.0	30.0	75	1480	4.0
ranch BLT	600	31.0	63.0	24.0	65	1510	3.0
Southern style ..	420	24.0	40.0	19.0	50	1090	1.0
chicken, grilled:							
classic	420	32.0	51.0	10.0	70	1190	3.0
club	530	40.0	52.0	17.0	90	1470	4.0
ranch BLT	470	36.0	53.0	12.0	80	1500	3.0
Filet-O-Fish	380	15.0	38.0	18.0	35	660	2.0
hamburger	250	12.0	31.0	9.0	25	520	2.0
McChicken	360	14.0	40.0	16.0	40	790	1.0
McRib	500	22.0	44.0	26.0	70	980	3.0
Quarter Pounder ..	410	24.0	37.0	19.0	65	730	2.0
w/cheese	510	29.0	40.0	26.0	90	1190	3.0
w/cheese, double	740	48.0	40.0	42.0	155	1380	3.0
Snack Wrap, crispy:							
chipotle barbecue ..	330	14.0	27.0	15.0	25	800	1.0
honey mustard	330	14.0	35.0	16.0	30	780	1.0
ranch	340	14.0	33.0	17.0	30	810	1.0
Snack Wrap, grilled:							
chipotle barbecue ..	260	18.0	28.0	9.0	45	830	1.0
honey mustard	260	18.0	27.0	9.0	45	800	1.0
ranch	270	18.0	26.0	10.0	45	830	1.0
Chicken McNuggets:							
4 pcs.	170	10.0	10.0	10.0	25	450	0
6 pcs.	250	15.0	15.0	15.0	35	670	0
10 pcs.	420	25.0	26.0	24.0	60	1120	0
McNuggets sauce:							
barbecue	50	0	12.0	0	0	260	0
honey	50	0	12.0	0	0	0	0
hot mustard	60	1.0	9.0	2.5	5	250	2.0
sweet 'n sour ...	50	0	12.0	0	0	150	0
Chicken Selects:							
3 pcs.	400	22.0	25.0	23.0	50	1000	0
5 pcs.	670	37.0	42.0	39.0	85	1660	0

Food and Measure	cal.	prot. (gms)	carbo. (gms)	fat (gms)	chol. (mgs)	sod. (mgs)	fiber (gms)
Selects sauce:							
Buffalo, spicy ...	70	0	1.0	7.0	0	960	2.0
chipotle barbecue	70	0	18.0	0	0	260	1.0
honey mustard ..	70	1.0	13.0	2.5	5	170	0
ranch, creamy ..	200	0	2.0	22.0	10	320	0
fries:							
large	570	6.0	70.0	30.0	0	330	7.0
medium	380	4.0	47.0	20.0	0	220	5.0
small	250	2.0	30.0	13.0	0	140	3.0
ketchup pkt.	10	0	3.0	0	0	100	0
salt pkt.	0	0	0	0	0	270	0
salad, no dressing:							
Asian	150	8.0	15.0	7.0	0	35	5.0
w/crispy chicken	430	27.0	33.0	22.0	50	900	5.0
w/grilled chicken	300	32.0	23.0	10.0	65	890	5.0
bacon ranch	140	9.0	10.0	7.0	25	300	3.0
w/crispy chicken	390	29.0	22.0	22.0	75	1020	3.0
w/grilled chicken	260	33.0	12.0	9.0	90	1010	3.0
Caesar	90	7.0	9.0	4.0	10	180	3.0
w/crispy chicken	350	26.0	21.0	18.0	60	890	3.0
w/grilled chicken	220	30.0	12.0	6.0	75	890	3.0
fruit/walnut, pkg. ...	210	4.0	31.0	8.0	5	60	2.0
Southwest	140	6.0	20.0	4.5	10	150	6.0
w/crispy chicken	450	26.0	40.0	21.0	55	970	6.0
w/grilled chicken	320	30.0	30.0	9.0	70	960	6.0
side salad	20	1.0	4.0	0	0	10	1.0
croutons, butter garlic	60	2.0	10.0	1.5	0	140	1.0
dressing (*Newman's Own*), 1.5 fl. oz.:							
balsamic vinaigrette	40	0	4.0	3.0	0	730	0
Caesar, creamy ...	190	2.0	4.0	18.0	20	500	0
ranch	170	1.0	9.0	15.0	20	530	0
sesame ginger	90	1.0	15.0	2.5	0	740	0
Southwest, creamy	100	1.0	11.0	6.0	20	340	0
shakes:							
McFlurry, 12 fl. oz.:							
M&M's	620	14.0	96.0	20.0	55	190	1.0
Oreo	550	13.0	88.0	17.0	50	250	1.0
Triple Thick, 16 oz.:							
chocolate	580	13.0	102.0	14.0	50	250	1.0
strawberry	560	13.0	97.0	13.0	50	170	0
vanilla	550	13.0	96.0	13.0	50	190	0
desserts/sundaes:							
apple dippers	35	0	8.0	0	0	0	0

Food and Measure	cal.	prot. (gms)	carbo. (gms)	fat (gms)	chol. (mgs)	sod. (mgs)	fiber (gms)
McDonald's, desserts/sundaes *(cont.)*							
apple pie	270	3.0	36.0	12.0	0	190	4.0
caramel dip	70	0	15.0	.5	5	35	0
cinnamon melts ...	460	6.0	66.0	19.0	15	370	3.0
cone, vanilla	150	4.0	24.0	3.5	15	60	0
cookies:							
chocolate chip ..	160	2.0	22.0	7.0	10	90	1.0
McDonaldland ..	250	4.0	42.0	8.0	0	270	1.0
McDonaldland							
chocolate chip	270	3.0	39.0	11.0	35	170	1.0
oatmeal raisin ..	150	2.0	22.0	6.0	10	135	1.0
sugar	150	2.0	21.0	6.0	5	110	0
fruit/yogurt parfait .	160	4.0	31.0	2.0	5	85	1.0
w/out granola ...	130	4.0	25.0	2.0	5	55	0
sundaes:							
hot caramel	340	7.0	60.0	8.0	30	160	0
hot fudge	330	8.0	54.0	10.0	25	180	2.0
strawberry	280	6.0	49.0	6.0	25	95	1.0
sundae peanuts ...	45	2.0	2.0	3.5	0	0	1.0
iced coffee, medium:							
regular	200	1.0	30.0	8.0	30	60	0
caramel	190	1.0	27.0	8.0	30	115	0
hazelnut	190	1.0	29.0	8.0	30	60	0
vanilla	190	1.0	29.0	8.0	30	60	0
Meat, potted, see "Meat spread"							
Meat loaf, refrigerated, 5 oz.:							
beef, seasoned (*Tyson*)	320	14.0	16.0	23.0	60	600	0
and gravy (*Hormel*) ..	190	16.0	11.0	9.0	40	920	0
w/tomato sauce (*Hormel*)	260	22.0	13.0	13.0	60	870	1.0
Meat loaf dinner, frozen, 1 pkg.:							
(*Healthy Choice* Complete), 12 oz...	300	15.0	40.0	8.0	50	590	9.0
(*Stouffer's* Homestyle), 16 oz.	610	34.0	46.0	32.0	65	1230	5.0
Meat loaf entree, frozen, 1 pkg., except as noted:							
w/gravy:							
(*South Beach Living*), 9 oz.	210	16.0	17.0	9.0	50	910	4.0
(*Stouffer's*), ⅙ of 33-oz. pkg.	200	18.0	8.0	11.0	30	650	1.0

Food and Measure	cal.	prot. (gms)	carbo. (gms)	fat (gms)	chol. (mgs)	sod. (mgs)	fiber (gms)
and vegetable medley (*Organic Classics*), 9.5 oz.	310	17.0	17.0 ·	20.0	60	650	5.0
w/potato, gravy:							
(*Michelina's Authentico*), 8 oz.	370	13.0	25.0	21.0	60	1020	2.0
(*Michelina's Lean Gourmet*), 8 oz. .	180	11.0	21.0	6.0	35	860	2.0
(*Smart Ones*), 9.5 oz.	250	22.0	23.0	8.0	45	880	3.0
(*Stouffer's*), 9.9 oz. .	340	22.0	19.0	20.0	80	780	2.0
w/potato and green beans (*Swanson Angus*), 11 oz.	380	15.0	30.0	22.0	45	1210	4.0
and whipped potato (*Lean Cuisine* Comfort Classics), 9.375 oz.	250	21.0	26.0	7.0	35	570	4.0
Meat loaf entree, microwave, w/potato, gravy (*Hormel Compleats*), 10 oz. .	310	18.0	34.0	11.0	45	1380	4.0
"Meat" loaf entree, vegetarian, frozen, 1 pkg.:							
(*Amy's* Veggie Loaf Whole Meal), 10 oz.	290	9.0	47.0	8.0	0	690	7.0
(*Amy's* Veggie Loaf Whole Meal Light Sodium), 10 oz.	280	9.0	47.0	7.0	0	340	7.0
(*Hain Vegetarian Classics*), 10 oz.	300	32.0	39.0	6.0	0	400	16.0
Meat loaf seasoning:							
(*Adolph's/Lawry's* Meal Makers), 1 tbsp....	25	<1.0	5.0	0	0	380	0
(*Lawry's*). 1 tbsp.	30	<1.0	7.0	0	0	470	<1.0
(*McCormick*), 1 tsp. ...	15	0	2.0	0	0	350	0
(*McCormick Bag 'n Season*), 2 tsp.	15	1.0	2.0	0	0	390	0
(*Mrs. Cubbison's*), 1 tbsp.	30	0	4.0	.5	0	430	0
Meat spread (see also specific listings):							
(*Spam* Spread), 4 tbsp., 2 oz.	140	8.0	1.0	12.0	40	570	0

Food and Measure	cal.	prot. (gms)	carbo. (gms)	fat (gms)	chol. (mgs)	sod. (mgs)	fiber (gms)
Meat spread (cont.)							
potted (Goya), ¼ cup .	80	8.0	0	5.0	55	550	0
potted (Libby's), ¼ cup	120	8.0	0	9.0	40	410	0
Meat tenderizer:							
(Adolph's Original),							
¼ tsp.	0	0	0	0	0	380	0
(McCormick), ¼ tsp. .	0	0	0	0	0	400	0
(Watkins Meat Magic),							
1 tsp.	5	0	1.0	0	0	180	0
seasoned, ¼ tsp.:							
(Adolph's)	0	0	0	0	0	450	0
(McCormick)	0	0	0	0	0	300	0
Meatball, frozen/							
refrigerated, 3 oz.,							
except as noted:							
(Mama Lucia), 4 pcs.,							
3.2 oz.	280	11.0	8.0	23.0	50	640	0
(Organic Classics),							
3 pcs.	180	17.0	5.0	11.0	50	430	1.0
(Rosina), 3 pcs.	240	14.0	5.0	19.0	40	640	1.0
(Rosina Organic), 6 pcs.	200	15.0	5.0	13.0	25	540	3.0
beef, Italian style							
(Shady Brook Farms),							
3 pcs.	260	15.0	5.0	20	55	510	1.0
chicken:							
Italian style (Tyson),							
6 pcs.	180	13.0	6.0	11.0	45	610	2.0
teriyaki pineapple							
(Aidells), 4 pcs. .	190	15.0	10.0	10.0	80	750	2.0
sausage (Rosina),							
6 pcs.	270	13.0	4.0	22.0	45	620	2.0
turkey:							
(Foster Farms Home-							
style), 3 pcs. . . .	160	18.0	3.0	9.0	30	280	0
(Perdue), 4 pcs. . . .	180	15.0	.5	10	45	520	0
(Rosina), 3 pcs. . . .	170	12.0	5.0	11.0	70	650	1.0
Italian style (Foster							
Farms), 3 pcs. . .	160	16.0	5.0	8.0	40	380	0
Italian style (Shady							
Brook Farms),							
3 pcs.	190	17.0	6.0	10.0	65	600	<1.0
turkey/chicken:							
chipotle (Aidells),							
4 pcs.	140	13.0	2.0	9.0	85	740	2.0

Food and Measure	cal.	prot. (gms)	carbo. (gms)	fat (gms)	chol. (mgs)	sod. (mgs)	fiber (gms)
sun-dried tomato (*Aidells*), 4 pcs. .	160	14.0	4.0	10.0	80	550	1.0
"Meatball," vegetarian, canned (*Loma Linda Tender Rounds*), 6 pcs., 2.8 oz.	120	13.0	6.0	4.5	0	340	1.0
"Meatball," vegetarian, frozen:							
(*Gardenburger* Mama Mia), 6 pcs., 3 oz. .	110	12.0	7.0	4.5	0	400	4.0
(*Nate's* Meatless Classic), 3 pcs., 1.5 oz.	90	8.0	5.0	4.5	0	270	2.0
(*Veggie Patch*), 3 pcs., 3 oz.	120	16.0	7.0	4.5	0	480	4.0
garlic portobello (*Veggie Patch*), 4 pc., 3 oz. .	130	16.0	6.0	4.5	0	460	3.0
Italian (*Nate's* Zesty), 3 pcs., 1.5 oz.	90	9.0	4.0	4.5	0	340	2.0
mushroom (*Nate's* Savory), 3 pcs., 1.5 oz.	100	8.0	6.0	4.5	0	230	2.0
Meatball entree, canned, stew (*Dinty Moore*), 1 cup	250	13.0	19.0	15.0	40	1050	1.0
Meatball entree, frozen (see also specific pasta entrees), Swedish, 1 pkg.:							
(*Michelina's Authentico*), 10 oz. .	500	20.0	48.0	23.0	75	990	3.0
(*Michelina's Lean Gourmet*), 8.5 oz. .	310	14.0	42.0	9.0	25	620	2.0
(*Smart Ones*), 9.1 oz.	270	20.0	35.0	5.0	30	730	3.0
(*Stouffer's*), 11.5 oz. . .	560	32.0	47.0	27.0	100	1250	3.0
w/pasta (*Lean Cuisine One Dish Favorites*), 9⅛ oz.	280	23.0	30.0	7.0	50	630	2.0
Meatball entree, microwave, Swedish, w/pasta, cream sauce (*Hormel Compleats*), 10-oz. cont.	350	15.0	32.0	18.0	60	980	0
Meatball seasoning/sauce mix, Swedish (*McCormick*), 2 tsp. seasoning and 1 tsp. sauce mix	45	0	4.0	1.0	0	790	0

Food and Measure	cal.	prot. (gms)	carbo. (gms)	fat (gms)	chol. (mgs)	sod. (mgs)	fiber (gms)
Meatball wontons, w/cheese (*Original Rangoon Rangoons*), 3 pcs.	220	11.0	32.0	6.0	15	390	1.0
Melba sauce (*Roland*), 2 tbsp.	100	0	24.0	0	0	0	0
Melogold (*Frieda's*), ½ fruit, 5.9 oz.	50	0	13.0	0	0	0	2.0
Melon, see specific melon listings							
Melon balls, frozen, cantaloupe/honeydew, ½ cup	28	.7	6.9	.2	0	27	.6
Melon berry juice (*Snapple*), 11.5 fl. oz.	180	0	44.0	0	0	15	0
Mexican beans, see "Pinto beans" and specific listings							
Mexican dip, frozen, 5 layer (*Cedarlane Organic*), 2 tbsp. . .	60	3.0	4.0	3.0	10	100	1.0
Mexican entree (see also specific listings), frozen, 9.5-oz. pkg.:							
(*Amy's* Casserole) . . .	470	11.0	70.0	16.0	20	780	7.0
(*Amy's* Casserole Light Sodium)	370	12.0	48.0	16.0	20	390	7.0
Mexican sauce (see also "Mole sauce," "Salsa," and specific listings) (*Mrs. Renfro's*), 2 tbsp.:							
habanero	15	0	3.0	0	0	310	0
habanero mango	15	0	4.0	0	0	170	0
hot	10	0	2.0	0	0	210	0
mild	10	0	3.0	0	0	240	0
Mexican seasoning (*Chi-Chi's* Fiesta Restaurante), 1 tsp. .	10	0	2.0	0	0	290	0
Mexican squash (*Frieda's*), ½ cup, 3 oz.	35	1.0	9.0	0	0	0	2.0
Milk, 8 fl. oz.: buttermilk:							
(*Friendship*)	120	9.0	12.0	4.0	15	125	0

Food and Measure	cal.	prot. (gms)	carbo. (gms)	fat (gms)	chol. (mgs)	sod. (mgs)	fiber (gms)
(*Hood* Nonfat)	90	9.0	13.0	0	<5	220	0
(*Organic Valley*) ...	100	8.0	12.0	2.5	15	250	0
cultured	99	8.1	11.7	2.2	9	257	0
whole:							
(*Cool Moos*)	150	8.0	12.0	8.0	35	120	0
(*Land O Lakes*) ...	150	8.0	12.0	8.0	35	125	0
(*Land O Lakes Dairy Ease*)	160	8.0	11.0	9.0	20	125	0
(*Organic Valley*) ...	150	8.0	12.0	8.0	30	120	0
(*Organic Valley* Non-homogenized) ..	150	8.0	12.0	8.0	35	125	0
3.3% fat	150	8.0	11.4	8.2	33	120	0
reduced fat, 2%:							
(*Cool Moos*)	120	8.0	12.0	5.0	20	125	0
(*Land O Lakes*) ...	120	8.0	12.0	5.0	20	125	0
(*Land O Lakes Dairy Ease*)	130	9.0	12.0	5.0	15	130	0
(*Organic Valley*) ...	130	8.0	13.0	5.0	20	125	0
(*Organic Valley Lactose Free*) ...	130	8.0	13.0	5.0	20	120	0
(*Organic Valley* Ultra Pasturized)	130	8.0	12.0	5.0	20	120	0
2% fat	121	8.1	11.7	4.7	18	122	0
2%, protein fortified	137	9.7	13.5	4.9	19	145	0
low fat, 1%:							
(*Land O Lakes*) ...	100	8.0	13.0	2.5	15	125	0
(*Organic Valley*) ...	110	8.0	13.0	2.5	15	125	0
(*Organic Valley Lactose Free*) ...	110	8.0	14.0	2.5	10	125	0
1% fat	102	8.0	11.7	2.6	10	123	0
1%, protein fortified	119	9.7	13.6	2.9	10	143	0
skim/fat free:							
(*Land O Lakes*) ...	90	8.0	13.0	0	<5	125	0
(*Land O Lakes Dairy Ease*)	90	8.0	12.0	0	5	125	0
(*Organic Valley*) ...	90	8.0	13.0	0	5	125	0
(*Organic Valley Lactose Free*) ...	90	8.0	14.0	0	5	130	0
8 fl. oz.	86	8.4	11.9	.4	4	126	0
Milk, canned, 2 tbs.:							
condensed, sweetened:							
(*Carnation*)	130	3.0	22.0	3.0	10	45	0
(*Eagle Brand/ Magnolia*)	130	3.0	23.0	3.0	10	40	0

Food and Measure	cal.	prot. (gms)	carbo. (gms)	fat (gms)	chol. (mgs)	sod. (mgs)	fiber (gms)
Milk, canned *(cont.)*							
(*Eagle Brand* Low Fat)	120	3.0	23.0	1.5	5	40	0
(*Eagle Brand* Nonfat)	110	3.0	24.0	0	<5	40	0
evaporated:							
(*Carnation*)	40	2.0	3.0	2.0	10	30	0
(*Carnation* Lowfat) .	25	2.0	3.0	.5	5	35	0
(*Carnation* Skim) . .	25	2.0	4.0	0	0	40	0
(*Pet*)	40	2.0	3.0	2.0	10	30	0
(*Pet* Skim)	25	2.0	4.0	0	0	40	0
Milk, chocolate, see "Milk, flavored"							
Milk, dry:							
buttermilk, sweet cream, 1 tbsp.	25	2.2	3.2	.4	4	34	0
buttermilk blend (*Organic Valley*), 3 tbsp.	110	10.0	16.0	1.0	25	45	0
whole, 1 oz.	141	7.5	10.9	7.6	27	105	0
whole, 1 cup	635	33.7	49.2	34.2	124	475	0
nonfat:							
(*Carnation*), ⅓ cup	80	8.0	12.0	0	<5	125	0
(*Organic Valley*), 3 tbsp.	90	9.0	13.0	0	<5	130	0
regular, 1 cup	435	43.4	62.4	.9	24	642	0
instant, 3.2-oz. pkt. .	244	23.9	35.5	.5	12	373	0
Milk, flavored, 8 fl. oz., except as noted:							
banana, reduced fat (*Nesquik*)	200	7.0	30.0	5.0	20	120	0
cherry, w/chocolate (*Ben & Jerry's Cherry Garcia*)	320	6.0	47.0	12.0	40	130	0
chocolate:							
(*Ben & Jerry's Chocolate Fudge Brownie*)	340	6.0	51.0	12.0	40	105	0
(*Hershey's* Creamy MilkShake)	270	10.0	43.0	8.0	20	140	1.0
reduced fat (*Hershey's*)	200	8.0	31.0	5.0	20	135	1.0
reduced fat (*Land O Lakes* Swiss 2%)	190	8.0	26.0	5.0	20	220	<1.0
reduced fat (*Nesquik*)	200	8.0	32.0	5.0	15	150	<1.0

Food and Measure	cal.	prot. (gms)	carbo. (gms)	fat (gms)	chol. (mgs)	sod. (mgs)	fiber (gms)
reduced fat (*Nesquik* Milkshake)	170	8.0	26.0	5.0	15	180	<1.0
reduced fat (*Organic Valley*)	170	8.0	24.0	5.0	20	250	<1.0
low fat (*Cool Moos*)	180	8.0	32.0	2.5	10	210	0
low fat (*Hershey's* No Sugar)	120	11.0	15.0	2.5	5	170	1.0
low fat (*Organic Valley*)	160	9.0	27.0	2.5	15	290	1.0
low fat (*Smart Balance* 1%)	150	9.0	26.0	1.0	5	150	0
skim (*Nesquik*)	160	8.0	32.0	0	0	150	<1.0
skim (*Land O Lakes*)	160	8.0	31.0	0	<5	220	<1.0
skim, rich (*CocoaVia*), 5.65 fl. oz.	150	6.0	28.0	3.0	5	135	3.0
chocolate, double, reduced fat (*Nesquik*)	200	8.0	30.0	5.0	15	170	<1.0
cookies and cream: (*Hershey's* Shake) .	280	10.0	45.0	7.0	20	180	0
cookies and milk shake, reduced fat (*Nesquik*)	180	8.0	26.0	5.0	20	170	1.0
strawberries and cream (*Frappuccino*), 9.5 fl. oz.	230	7.0	38.0	6.0	25	180	<1.0
strawberry: (*Hershey's* Shake) .	280	9.0	44.0	7.0	20	220	0
(*Land O Lakes*) ...	190	7.0	22.0	8.0	30	125	0
reduced fat (*Hershey's*)	200	8.0	30.0	5.0	15	130	0
reduced fat (*Nesquik*)	200	8.0	33.0	5.0	15	120	0
reduced fat (*Nesquik* Milkshake) .	170	8.0	25.0	5.0	20	140	<1.0
low fat (*Cool Moos*)	160	8.0	27.0	2.5	10	140	0
low fat (*Organic Valley*)	150	8.0	27.0	2.5	15	120	2.0
vanilla: (*Frappuccino*), 9.5 fl. oz.	200	6.0	37.0	3.0	15	100	0
(*Hershey's* Shake) .	320	9.0	55.0	7.0	20	240	0
reduced fat (*Nesquik* Very)	200	8.0	30.0	5.0	15	120	0
Milk, goat, fresh, 8 fl. oz.	168	8.7	10.9	10.1	28	122	0

Food and Measure	cal.	prot. (gms)	carbo. (gms)	fat (gms)	chol. (mgs)	sod. (mgs)	fiber (gms)
"Milk," nondairy, see "Soy beverage" and specific listings							
Milk, human, 8 fl. oz.	172	2.9	16.9	10.8	34	42	0
Milk, sheep, 8 fl. oz. . .	265	14.7	13.1	17.2	66	108	0
Milkfish, meat only:							
raw, 4 oz.	168	23.3	0	7.6	59	82	0
baked or broiled, 4 oz.	215	29.8	0	9.8	76	104	0
Millet, grain:							
dry, ¼ cup:							
(Shiloh Farms Organic)	150	5.0	34.0	1.5	0	0	3.0
hulled (Arrowhead Mills Organic) . .	150	4.0	33.0	1.5	0	0	1.0
cooked, 4 oz.	135	4.0	26.8	1.1	0	2	1.5
Millet flour (Arrowhead Mills Organic), ⅓ cup	130	4.0	26.0	1.5	0	0	3.0
Mincemeat, see "Pie filling"							
Mint, fresh:							
peppermint, 2 tbsp. . . .	2	.1	.5	0	0	.1	<.1
spearmint, 2 tbsp. . . .	5	.4	.9	.1	0	3	.7
Mint, dried, spearmint, 1 tbsp.	5	.3	.8	.1	0	6	.5
Mint drink mixer (Angostura), 2 fl. oz.	80	0	18.0	0	0	5	0
Mint sauce (Crosse & Blackwell), 1 tsp. . . .	5	0	2.0	0	0	0	0
Mirin, see "Wine, cooking"							
Miso, 1 tbsp., except as noted:							
(Eden Organic Hacho)	40	3.0	4.0	1.5	0	680	<1.0
(Eden Organic Shiro) .	30	1.0	6.0	.5	0	330	<1.0
½ cup	284	16.3	38.6	8.4	0	5032	7.6
barley (Westbrae Natural Bag), 1 tsp.	10	0	2.0	0	0	310	0
brown rice:							
(Eden Organic Genmai)	25	2.0	3.0	.5	0	780	2.0
(Westbrae Natural Bag), 1 tsp.	10	<1.0	<1.0	0	0	250	0
(Westbrae Natural Organic Tub), 1 tsp.	10	<1.0	2.0	0	0	220	<1.0

Food and Measure	cal.	prot. (gms)	carbo. (gms)	fat (gms)	chol. (mgs)	sod. (mgs)	fiber (gms)
red (*Westbrae Natural* Organic Mellow), 1 tsp.	10	0	2.0	0	0	210	<1.0
soy and barley (*Eden* Organic Mugi)	25	2.0	4.0	.5	0	640	<1.0
soybean (*Westbrae Natural*), 1 tsp.	10	<1.0	0	.5	0	280	0
white (*Westbrae Natural* Organic Mellow), 1 tsp.	10	<1.0	2.0	0	0	180	<1.0
Miso condiment, see "Tekka"							
Mochi (*Grainaissance Mochi* Bake & Serve), 1.5 oz., ⅛ pkg.:							
cashew-date	110	2.0	24.0	2.0	0	35	0
chocolate brownie	130	3.0	24.0	2.0	0	35	0
original or wheatgrass/ mugwort	110	2.0	24.0	1.0	0	0	0
pizza	110	2.0	24.0	1.0	0	65	0
raisin-cinnamon	120	2.0	25.0	1.0	0	35	0
sesame-garlic	110	2.0	23.0	1.5	0	20	0
super seed	120	3.0	23.0	2.0	0	35	0
Mojito drink mixer:							
(*Angostura*), 3 fl. oz.	80	0	20.0	0	0	15	0
(*Stirrings*), 2 fl. oz.	80	0	20.0	0	0	0	0
frozen (*Bacardi*), 2 fl. oz.	110	0	30.0	0	0	0	0
traditional, passion fruit or mango (*Rose's*), 3 fl. oz.	80	0	20.0	0	0	40	0
Molasses, 1 tbsp.:							
(*Brer Rabbit* Full Flavored)	60	0	15.0	0	0	10	0
(*Grandma's*)	50	0	12.0	0	0	0	0
(*Plantation* Barbados)	60	0	15.0	0	0	0	0
blackstrap:							
(*Brer Rabbit*)	60	1.0	13.0	0	0	65	0
(*Plantation*)	42	0	11.0	0	0	10	0
(*Plantation* Organic)	60	0	13.0	0	0	0	0
(*Tree of Life*)	45	0	11.0	0	0	15	0
Molasses blend (*Mrs. Renfro's* Country Syrup), ¼ cup	240	0	61.0	0	0	15	0

Food and Measure	cal.	prot. (gms)	carbo. (gms)	fat (gms)	chol. (mgs)	sod. (mgs)	fiber (gms)
Mole sauce (*Doña Maria*), 2 tbsp.:							
original	230	3.0	12.0	15.0	0	460	2.0
condiment	200	3.0	10.0	13.0	0	400	2.0
green (verde)	240	5.0	10.0	18.0	0	660	2.0
Monkfish, meat only:							
raw, 4 oz.	86	16.4	0	1.7	29	21	0
baked or broiled, 4 oz.	110	21.0	0	2.2	36	26	0
Monosodium glutamate (MSG) (*McCormick Flavor Enhancer*), ¼ tsp.	0	0	0	0	0	125	0
Moose, meat only, roasted, 4 oz.	152	33.2	0	1.1	88	78	0
Mortadella, 2 oz.:							
(*Black Bear*)	150	10.0	2.0	14.0	30	490	0
(*Boar's Head*)	160	9.0	0	14.0	30	560	0
(*Dietz & Watson*)	150	9.0	0	14.0	30	560	0
beef and pork	174	9.2	1.7	14.2	31	698	0
w/pistachios:							
(*Boar's Head*)	170	10.0	2.0	14.0	30	560	0
(*Dietz & Watson*) . .	150	9.0	0	14.0	30	500	0
Mothbean, boiled, 4 oz.	133	8.9	23.8	.6	0	11	n.a.
Moussaka, see "Eggplant entree"							
Mousse, chocolate, frozen (*Smart Ones*), 2.7 oz.	180	7.0	28.0	4.0	<5	100	3.0
Mousse mix:							
chocolate:							
dark, truffle (*Dr. Oetker*), 3 tbsp. . .	100	2.0	15.0	3.5	0	90	1.0
double (*Dr. Oetker Supreme*), 3 tbsp.	130	3.0	21.0	4.0	0	45	1.0
milk (*Dr. Oetker*), 3 tbsp.	100	2.0	15.0	3.5	0	50	0
chocolate raspberry (*Dr. Oetker*), 3 tbsp.	130	2.0	21.0	4.0	0	30	1.0
mocha (*Dr. Oetker*), 2 tbsp.	70	1.0	13.0	2.5	0	80	0
pistachio (*Dr. Oetker Supreme*), 2 tbsp. .	100	1.0	19.0	2.0	0	25	0
strawberry:							
(*Dr. Oetker*), 2 tbsp.	80	.4	13.0	3.0	0	140	0

Food and Measure	cal.	prot. (gms)	carbo. (gms)	fat (gms)	chol. (mgs)	sod. (mgs)	fiber (gms)
(*Dr. Oetker* Light), 1 tbsp.	35	1.0	4.0	2.0	0	120	0
vanilla, French:							
(*Dr. Oetker*), 2 tbsp.	90	.4	15.0	3.0	0	130	0
(*Dr. Oetker* Light), 1 tbsp.	30	0	3.0	2.0	0	80	0
MSG, see "Monosodium glutamate"							
Muffin, 1 pc.:							
corn, 2 oz.	174	3.6	29.0	4.8	15	297	1.9
English:							
(*Bays* Original)	140	5.0	27.0	1.5	0	530	1.0
(*Cobblestone Mill*)	140	5.0	27.0	1.0	0	270	1.0
(*Crystal Farms*)	130	4.0	27.0	1.0	0	240	1.0
(*Pepperidge Farm*)	130	5.0	25.0	1.5	0	170	1.0
(*Thomas'* Double Fiber)	110	4.0	26.0	.5	0	220	5.0
(*Thomas'* Original)	120	4.0	25.0	1.0	0	200	1.0
(*Thomas'* Super Size)	190	7.0	38.0	2.0	0	280	2.0
cinnamon raisin (*Thomas'*)	140	4.0	29.0	1.0	0	170	1.0
honey wheat (*Bays*)	130	5.0	25.0	1.5	0	500	2.0
multigrain (*Thomas'*)	150	5.0	27.0	2.5	0	160	2.0
oatmeal and honey (*Thomas'*)	130	5.0	25.0	1.0	0	180	2.0
raisin (*Sun•Maid*)	170	5.0	36.0	.5	0	180	2.0
sourdough (*Bays*)	130	5.0	26.0	1.5	0	500	2.0
whole grain (*Thomas'*)	130	5.0	26.0	1.0	0	220	2.0
whole wheat (*Pepperidge Farm*)	140	6.0	26.0	1.5	0	210	3.0
whole wheat (*Roman Meal*)	140	6.0	29.0	1.0	0	320	3.0
whole wheat (*Thomas'*)	120	5.0	23.0	1.0	0	220	3.0
oat bran, 2 oz.	154	4.0	27.5	4.2	0	224	2.6
Muffin, frozen, chocolate chip (*Smart Ones*), 2.5-oz. pc.	190	4.0	39.0	2.0	0	320	2.0
Muffin, toaster, see "Toaster pastry and muffins"							

Food and Measure	cal.	prot. (gms)	carbo. (gms)	fat (gms)	chol. (mgs)	sod. (mgs)	fiber (gms)
Muffin mix (see also "Bread mix, sweet"), 1 pc.* except as noted:							
almond poppy seed (*Krusteaz*)	170	3.0	30.0	4.5	20	240	<1.0
apple cinnamon:							
(*Dr. Oetker* Organic), ¹⁄₁₂ pkg.	120	2.0	28.0	0	0	190	0
(*"Jiffy"*), ¼ cup . . .	160	2.0	26.0	5.0	<5	320	0
(*Krusteaz*)	170	2.0	31.0	4.0	<5	280	1.0
(*Krusteaz* Fat Free) .	140	2.0	32.0	0	0	280	2.0
(*Martha White*), ¼ cup	140	1.0	24.0	4.0	20	150	0
(*Martha White* Low Fat), ¼ cup	130	1.0	27.0	2.0	20	135	<1.0
(*Martha White* Whole Grain), ¼ cup . . .	140	2.0	24.0	4.0	20	150	1.0
(*Pillsbury* Pouch), ¼ cup	160	2.0	28.0	4.5	5	170	0
w/flax seed (*Hodgson Mill*), ¼ cup	120	5.0	25.0	1.5	0	80	3.0
apple streusel (*Betty Crocker*)	200	3.0	34.0	6.0	20	250	1.0
banana (*Krusteaz* Fat Free)	140	2.0	33.0	0	0	290	2.0
banana nut:							
(*Betty Crocker* Box) .	180	4.0	27.0	6.0	20	240	<1.0
(*Betty Crocker* Pouch)	150	2.0	26.0	4.0	0	280	<1.0
(*"Jiffy"*), ¼ cup . . .	150	2.0	24.0	6.0	<5	310	<1.0
(*Krusteaz*)	220	3.0	34.0	9.0	35	260	1.0
(*Martha White*), ¼ cup	150	2.0	25.0	5.0	20	220	<1.0
(*Martha White* Whole Grain), ¼ cup . . .	150	2.0	25.0	5.0	20	220	2.0
(*Pillsbury* Pouch), ¼ cup	150	2.0	25.0	5.0	5	220	<1.0
berry:							
(*Martha White* Wildberry), ¼ cup	140	1.0	24.0	4.0	20	150	0
triple (*Betty Crocker* Pouch)	150	2.0	27.0	3.5	0	270	0
wild (*Pillsbury* Pouch), ¼ cup	160	2.0	29.0	4.5	5	170	1.0

494

Food and Measure	cal.	prot. (gms)	carbo. (gms)	fat (gms)	chol. (mgs)	sod. (mgs)	fiber (gms)
blackberry or blueberry (*Martha White*), ¼ cup	140	1.0	24.0	4.0	20	150	n.a.
blueberry:							
(*Betty Crocker* Pouch)	150	2.0	27.0	3.5	0	270	0
(*Betty Crocker* Twice the Blueberries) .	180	3.0	30.0	5.0	35	240	1.0
(*"Jiffy"*), ¼ cup . . .	160	2.0	26.0	5.0	<5	320	0
(*Krusteaz* Fat Free) .	130	2.0	31.0	0	0	280	2.0
(*Martha White* Low Fat), ¼ cup	130	1.0	27.0	2.0	20	135	<1.0
(*Pillsbury* Pouch), ¼ cup	160	2.0	28.0	4.5	5	170	0
(*Pillsbury* Ultimate), 1/12 pkg.	190	1.0	34.0	5.0	0	210	0
wild (*Betty Crocker*)	190	3.0	27.0	7.0	35	220	1.0
wild (*Krusteaz*)	220	2.0	31.0	10.0	20	260	1.0
wild, whole wheat (*Hodgson Mill*), ¼ cup	145	5.0	32.0	1.0	0	206	4.0
blueberry cheesecake (*Martha White*), ¼ cup	150	2.0	22.0	6.0	20	180	n.a.
bran, ¼ cup:							
(*Hodgson Mill*) . . .	130	4.0	28.0	1.0	0	200	3.0
date (*"Jiffy"*)	140	2.0	24.0	4.5	<5	270	2.0
honey (*Martha White*), ¼ cup	150	2.0	26.0	4.0	20	210	3.0
caramel apple streusel (*Pillsbury* Ultimate), 1/12 pkg.	200	1.0	37.0	4.5	0	210	<1.0
carrot (*Pillsbury* Pouch), ¼ cup	150	2.0	29.0	3.5	5	200	1.0
chocolate, double (*Betty Crocker*) . . .	200	3.0	31.0	7.0	20	220	0
chocolate chip:							
(*Betty Crocker*) . . .	160	2.0	26.0	5.0	0	300	1.0
(*Krusteaz*)	230	3.0	34.0	9.0	35	260	1.0
(*Martha White*), ¼ cup	150	2.0	25.0	5.0	20	160	<1.0
(*Pillsbury* Pouch), ¼ cup	170	2.0	28.0	5.0	5	180	<1.0

Food and Measure	cal.	prot. (gms)	carbo. (gms)	fat (gms)	chol. (mgs)	sod. (mgs)	fiber (gms)
Muffin mix, chocolate chip *(cont.)*							
chocolate *(Martha White)*, ¼ cup	150	2.0	25.0	5.0	20	160	1.0
chocolate fudge *(Pillsbury Ultimate)*, ¹⁄₁₂ pkg.	190	2.0	33.0	6.0	0	200	1.0
cinnamon streusel *(Betty Crocker)*	210	3.0	29.0	9.0	35	240	0
corn, ¼ cup:							
(Glory)	170	2.0	25.0	4.0	0	340	<1.0
(Hodgson Mill)	130	4.0	27.0	.5	0	240	3.0
("Jiffy")	150	2.0	27.0	4.5	<5	340	<1.0
honey *(Krusteaz)*	110	2.0	20.0	2.5	0	200	<1.0
honey *(Krusteaz Fat Free)*	120	2.0	27.0	0	0	410	1.0
yellow *(Martha White)*	140	2.0	26.0	3.0	20	230	1.0
cranberry orange:							
(Krusteaz Fat Free)	140	2.0	32.0	0	0	280	2.0
(Martha White), ¼ cup	140	1.0	25.0	4.0	20	150	0
lemon blueberry *(Krusteaz)*	190	2.0	29.0	7.0	20	250	<1.0
lemon poppy seed:							
(Betty Crocker Pouch)	130	2.0	22.0	3.5	0	190	0
(Betty Crocker Sunkist Box)	200	3.0	30.0	8.0	20	210	0
(Krusteaz)	170	3.0	30.0	4.5	20	280	<1.0
(Martha White), ¼ cup	150	2.0	27.0	4.0	20	160	<1.0
(Pillsbury Pouch), ¼ cup	150	2.0	27.0	4.0	5	160	<1.0
oat bran *(Krusteaz)*	180	3.0	31.0	4.5	0	300	1.0
oatmeal *(Dr. Oetker Organic)*, ¹⁄₁₂ pkg.	150	3.0	32.0	1.0	0	190	1.0
raspberry *("Jiffy")*, ¼ cup	160	2.0	26.0	6.0	<5	320	0
strawberry, ¼ cup:							
(Martha White)	140	1.0	24.0	4.0	20	150	1.0
(Martha White Low Fat)	130	1.0	27.0	2.0	20	140	1.0
(Pillsbury Pouch)	160	2.0	28.0	4.5	5	170	0
strawberry cheesecake *(Martha White)*, ¼ cup	150	2.0	22.0	6.0	20	180	<1.0

Food and Measure	cal.	prot. (gms)	carbo. (gms)	fat (gms)	chol. (mgs)	sod. (mgs)	fiber (gms)
whole wheat (*Hodgson Mill*), ¼ cup	130	4.0	27.0	.5	0	206	3.0
Muffin sandwich, see "Breakfast sandwich/ pastry"							
Mulberries, fresh:							
10 berries, ½ oz.	7	.2	1.5	.1	0	2	.3
½ cup	31	1.0	6.9	.3	0	7	1.2
Mulberries, dried, white hunza (*Shiloh Farms*), ⅓ cup	130	1.0	32.0	.5	0	0	7.0
Mullet, striped, meat only:							
raw , 4 oz.	133	22.0	0	4.3	56	74	0
baked or broiled, 4 oz.	170	28.1	0	5.5	71	81	0
Multigrain pilaf, pkg. (*Tasty Bite*), ½ of 10-oz. pkg.	200	9.0	33.0	5.0	0	440	4.0
Mung bean:							
dry (*Shiloh Farms Organic*), ¼ cup ...	160	11.0	28.0	.5	0	0	9.0
boiled, ½ cup	106	7.1	19.3	.4	0	2	7.7
Mung bean sprouts:							
raw, 1 cup	31	3.2	6.2	.2	0	6	1.9
boiled, drained, ½ cup	13	1.3	2.6	.1	0	6	.5
Mung bean sprouts, canned, drained, 1 cup	15	1.8	2.7	<.1	0	175	1.0
Mungo bean, boiled, ½ cup	95	6.8	16.5	.5	0	7	5.8
Mushroom (see also specific listings), common:							
raw:							
(*Del Monte*), 5 medium, 3 oz. ..	20	3.0	3.0	0	0	0	1.0
(*Dole*), ½ cup, 1.2 oz.	9	1.0	1.0	0	0	0	0
pcs. or slices, ½ cup	9	1.0	1.5	.2	0	1	.4
boiled, drained, pcs., ½ cup	21	1.7	4.0	.4	0	2	1.7
can or jar, all styles, ½ cup:							
(*Green Giant*)	25	2.0	4.0	0	0	440	1.0

Food and Measure	cal.	prot. (gms)	carbo. (gms)	fat (gms)	chol. (mgs)	sod. (mgs)	fiber (gms)
Mushroom, can or jar, all styles *(cont.)*							
(*Roland*)	30	2.0	4.0	0	0	550	3.0
drained	19	1.5	3.9	.5	0	332	1.9
w/liquid	20	2.0	3.0	0	0	400	<1.0
Mushroom, abalone,							
canned (*Roland*),							
½ cup	30	2.0	6.0	0	0	390	2.0
Mushroom, breaded,							
frozen:							
w/mozzarella:							
(*Morningstar Farms*							
Veggie Bites),							
3 pcs., 3 oz.	190	9.0	16.0	10.0	10	550	1.0
portobello (*Veggie*							
Patch Bites),							
3 pcs., 2.6 oz. . .	160	7.0	17.0	8.0	10	330	4.0
w/roasted garlic (*Alexia*							
Mushroom Bites),							
2 oz.	110	3.0	16.0	4.0	0	280	1.0
Mushroom, cepes							
(see also "Mushroom,							
porcini), canned							
(*Roland*), ½ cup . .	25	1.0	4.0	.5	0	240	2.0
Mushroom, chanterelle:							
canned (*Roland*),							
½ cup	25	1.0	4.0	.5	0	240	2.0
dried (*Frieda's*), 2 pcs.,							
.14 oz.	15	1.0	2.0	0	0	0	1.0
Mushroom, cloud ear,							
dried:							
.2-oz. pc.	13	.4	3.3	<.1	0	2	3.2
½ cup	39	1.3	10.2	.1	0	5	9.8
Mushroom, crimini,							
brown, or Italian,							
raw, .5-oz. pc.	3	.4	.6	0	0	1	<.1
Mushroom, enoki,							
fresh:							
(*Frieda's*), .9 oz.	10	1.0	2.0	0	0	0	1.0
trimmed, 1 oz.	10	.2	2.0	.1	0	1	.7
1 large, 4 ⅛" long . . .	2	.1	.4	<.1	0	<1	<1.0
Mushroom, golden,							
canned (*Roland*),							
½ cup	30	2.0	6.0	0	0	390	2.0

Food and Measure	cal.	prot. (gms)	carbo. (gms)	fat (gms)	chol. (mgs)	sod. (mgs)	fiber (gms)
Mushroom, maltake, dried (*Eden* Organic), .4 oz., about 10 pcs.	35	2.0	7.0	0	0	0	4.0
Mushroom, marinated, can or jar:							
(*Vigo*), 3 pcs.	15	1.0	1.0	.5	0	135	0
pickled, cocktail (*Fanci Food*), 1 oz.	10	1.0	0	0	0	360	0
pickled (escababeche):							
(*Herdez*), 2 tbsp. . . .	10	0	1.0	0	0	310	0
(*Sabores Aztecas*), 2.1 oz.	45	0	1.0	5.0	0	312	1.0
Mushroom, morel, dried (*Frieda's*), 3 pcs. .14 oz.	15	1.0	2.0	0	0	0	0
Mushroom, oyster: fresh:							
1 large, 5.2 oz.	55	6.1	9.2	.8	0	46	3.6
1 small, .5 oz.	6	.6	.9	.1	0	5	.4
canned (*Roland*), ½ cup	20	1.0	4.0	0	0	330	2.0
dried (*Frieda's*), 3 pcs., .14 oz.	15	1.0	2.0	0	0	0	0
Mushroom, pickled, see "Mushroom, marinated"							
Mushroom, porcini, dried:							
(*Frieda's*), 5 pcs., .14 oz.	15	1.0	2.0	0	0	0	1.0
(*Roland*), ¼ cup	30	3.0	4.0	0	0	0	2.0
(*Roland* Porcini Cepes), ½ cup	50	5.0	6.0	1.0	0	70	3.0
Mushroom, portobello:							
fresh, 1 oz.	7	.7	1.4	<.1	0	2	.4
dried (*Frieda's*), 7 pcs., .14 oz.	0	1.0	1.0	0	0	0	0
grilled, 1 oz.	10	1.1	1.4	.2	0	3	.7
Mushroom, shiitake: fresh, raw (*Frieda's*), 3.5 oz.	290	9.0	75.0	1.0	0	15	11.0
fresh, cooked, 4 medium or ½ cup pcs. . .	40	1.1	10.4	.2	0	3	1.5

Food and Measure	cal.	prot. (gms)	carbo. (gms)	fat (gms)	chol. (mgs)	sod. (mgs)	fiber (gms)
Mushroom, shiitaki *(cont.)*							
dried:							
(*Frieda's*), ¼ cup,							
.14 oz.	10	0	3.0	0	0	0	0
(*Roland*), ¼ cup . .	30	2.0	5.0	0	0	0	2.0
4 medium, .5 oz. . .	44	1.4	11.3	.2	0	2	1.7
whole or sliced (*Eden* Organic), 6 pcs.,							
.4 oz.	35	2.0	7.0	0	0	0	5.0
Mushroom, straw:							
canned:							
drained, ½ cup . . .	29	3.5	4.2	.6	0	350	2.3
whole or broken							
(*Roland*), ½ cup	20	2.0	3.0	0	0	380	2.0
dried (*Frieda's* Padi Straw), 6 pcs., .14 oz.	15	1.0	2.0	0	0	0	0
Mushroom, wild mix:							
can or jar (*Roland* Wild Forest), ½ cup	25	1.0	3.0	.5	0	240	1.0
dried:							
(*Alessi*), ¼ of .5-oz. pkg.	6	0	2.0	0	0	0	0
(*Roland*), ¼ cup . .	30	2.0	5.0	0	0	0	2.0
Mushroom, wood ear, dried (*Frieda's*), 3 pcs., .14 oz.	15	0	2.0	0	0	0	0
Mushroom antipasto, balsamic fennel (*Campagna*), 1 tbsp.	10	0	1.0	.5	0	0	0
Mushroom batter mix (*Don's Chuck Wagon*), ¼ cup	95	3.0	21.0	0	0	706	1.0
Mushroom gravy, can or jar, ¼ cup:							
(*Campbell's*)	20	0	3.0	1.0	<5	280	0
(*Pacific* Natural)	25	0	4.0	.5	0	270	0
rich (*Heinz* Home Style)	20	<1.0	3.0	.5	0	320	0
Mushroom gravy mix, ¼ cup*:							
(*McCormick*)	20	0	2.0	.5	0	260	0
and herb (*McCormick* for Steak)	40	1.0	5.0	1.0	5	220	0

Food and Measure	cal.	prot. (gms)	carbo. (gms)	fat (gms)	chol. (mgs)	sod. (mgs)	fiber (gms)
Mushroom sauce, shiitake (*Annie Chun's*), 1 tbsp. . . .	15	1.0	3.0	0	0	190	0
Mushroom-leek pocket, frozen (*Aunt Trudy's* Organic), 5-oz. pc. .	190	5.0	32.0	6.0	0	380	3.0
Muskrat, meat only, roasted, 4 oz.	265	34.1	0	13.3	88	78	0
Mussels, blue, meat only:							
raw, 4 oz.	98	13.5	4.2	2.5	32	324	0
raw, 1 cup	129	17.9	3.4	5.5	42	429	0
boiled or steamed, 4 oz.	195	27.0	8.4	5.1	64	418	0
Mussels, can/jar: à la nicoise (*Roland*), ⅓ cup	60	10.0	3.0	2.0	35	220	0
marinated, in oil: (*Roland*), ⅓ cup . .	75	11.0	0	4.0	25	290	0
spiced (*Vigo* Escabeche), 2 oz. .	75	11.0	0	4.0	25	250	0
smoked, cherrywood, in oil (*Roland*), ¼ cup	110	13.0	0	7.0	40	270	0
in tomato sauce, spices (*Roland*), ⅓ cup . .	60	6.0	4.0	2.0	30	540	0
in water (*Roland*), ¼ cup	50	10.0	1.0	1.5	20	220	0
Mustard, prepared, 1 tsp., except as noted: (*Jack Daniel's* Old No. 7)	5	0	0	0	0	70	0
Asian style (*Westbrae Natural*)	5	0	0	0	0	110	0
brown:							
(*Eden* Organic)	0	0	<1.0	0	0	80	0
spicy (*Grey Poupon*)	0	0	0	0	0	50	0
spicy (*Grey Poupon* Hearty)	0	0	0	0	0	55	0
spicy (*Gulden's*) . . .	5	0	0	0	0	50	0
Chinese, hot:							
(*Mee Tu*)	2	0	1.0	0	0	40	0
(*Polyunesian*)	2	0	1.0	0	0	40	0
(*Roland*)	0	0	1.0	0	0	40	0
coarse ground (*Grey Poupon*)	10	0	0	0	0	120	0
Creole (*Zatarain's*) . . .	10	0	<1.0	.5	0	150	0

Food and Measure	cal.	prot. (gms)	carbo. (gms)	fat (gms)	chol. (mgs)	sod. (mgs)	fiber (gms)
Mustard prepared *(cont.)*							
deli style:							
(*Boar's Head*)	0	0	0	0	0	40	0
(*Emeril's* New York)	5	0	0	0	0	50	0
(*Grey Poupon*)	5	0	0	0	0	50	0
(*Hebrew National*) .	4	0	0	0	0	65	0
Dijon:							
(*Annie's Naturals*							
Organic)	0	0	0	0	0	120	0
(*Bornier*)	5	0	0	.5	0	130	0
(*Dietz & Watson*							
Whole Grain) ...	5	0	1.0	0	0	110	0
(*Emeril's*)	5	0	1.0	0	0	120	0
(*Grey Poupon/Grey*							
Poupon Country)	5	0	0	0	0	120	0
(*Jack Daniel's* Stone							
Ground)	5	0	0	0	0	150	0
(*Maille* Original) ...	5	0	0	.5	0	105	0
(*Roland* Traditional							
European)	5	0	0	.5	0	100	0
(*Tree of Life* Organic)	0	0	0	0	0	65	0
(*Westbrae Natural*)	0	0	0	0	0	65	0
extra hot (*Maille*) ..	10	0	1.0	.5	0	115	0
grained, w/wine							
(*Roland*)	10	0	0	.5	0	105	0
green peppercorn or							
w/herbs (*Roland*)	10	0	0	.5	0	130	0
hickory (*Jack Daniel's*)	5	0	0	0	0	125	0
kobe style (*Roland*) ..	0	0	1.0	0	0	40	0
spicy (*Jack Daniel's*							
Southwest)	0	0	0	0	0	80	0
stone ground:							
(*Dietz & Watson*) ..	0	0	2.0	0	0	80	0
(*Westbrae Natural*)	0	0	0	0	0	65	0
or yellow (*Tree of*							
Life Organic) ...	0	0	0	0	0	55	0
sweet and hot (*Dietz*							
& Watson)	10	0	1.0	0	0	80	0
yellow:							
(*Annie's Naturals*							
Organic)	0	0	0	0	0	55	0
(*Eden* Organic)	0	0	0	0	0	80	0
(*French's*)	0	0	0	0	0	55	0

Food and Measure	cal.	prot. (gms)	carbo. (gms)	fat (gms)	chol. (mgs)	sod. (mgs)	fiber (gms)
Mustard blends, 1 tsp.:							
Champagne dill (*Dietz & Watson*)	5	0	<1.0	0	0	120	0
cranberry honey (*Dietz & Watson*)	5	0	3.0	0	0	30	0
honey:							
(*Annie's Naturals Organic*)	10	0	2.0	0	0	40	0
(*Boar's Head*)	10	0	2.0	0	0	25	0
(*Dietz & Watson*) . .	20	0	4.0	0	0	30	0
(*Emeril's*)	10	0	1.0	0	0	25	0
(*Grey Poupon*)	10	0	1.0	0	0	5	0
(*Gulden's* Zesty) . . .	10	0	2.0	0	0	35	0
(*Hellmann's/Best Foods*)	10	0	2.0	0	0	25	0
Dijon (*Jack Daniel's*) .	10	0	2.0	0	0	70	0
Dijon (*Roland*)	10	0	1.0	0	0	65	0
horseradish:							
(*Annie's Naturals Organic*)	5	0	1.0	0	0	90	0
(*Emeril's*)	5	0	0	0	0	60	0
(*Jack Daniel's*)	5	0	0	0	0	75	0
jalapeño (*Dietz & Watson*)	0	0	1.0	0	0	80	0
mayonnaise (*Dijonnaise*)	5	0	1.0	0	0	70	0
wasabi (*Dietz & Watson*)	5	0	0	0	0	105	0
Mustard cabbage, see "Cabbage, mustard"							
Mustard greens, fresh:							
raw (*Glory*), 2 cups . .	20	2.0	4.0	0	0	20	3.0
raw, chopped:							
(*Del Monte*), 1½ cups, 3 oz. . . .	25	2.0	3.0	0	0	40	1.0
1 oz. or ½ cup	7	.8	1.4	.1	0	7	.6
boiled, drained, ½ cup	11	1.6	1.5	.2	0	11	1.4
Mustard greens, canned, ½ cup:							
chopped (*Bush's*)	25	2.0	3.0	0	0	400	2.0
seasoned:							
(*Glory*)	35	2.0	3.0	0	0	490	1.0
(*Sunshine*)	45	4.0	6.0	.5	0	830	1.0
Mustard greens, frozen, chopped boiled, drained, 1 cup	30	3.4	4.7	.4	0	38	4.2

Food and Measure	cal.	prot. (gms)	carbo. (gms)	fat (gms)	chol. (mgs)	sod. (mgs)	fiber (gms)
Mustard powder, 1 tsp.	9	.5	.3	.6	0	<1	<1.0
Mustard seeds, 1 tsp.	15	.8	1.2	1.0	0	<1	<1.0
Mustard spinach:							
raw, chopped, 1 cup .	33	3.3	5.9	.5	0	32	4.2
boiled, drained,							
chopped, 1 cup ...	29	3.1	5.0	.4	0	25	3.6
Mustard tallow, 1 tbsp.	115	0	0	12.8	13	0	0

N

Food and Measure	cal.	prot. (gms)	carbo. (gms)	fat (gms)	chol. (mgs)	sod. (mgs)	fiber (gms)
Nacho snack, frozen (*Amy's*), ½ of 6-oz. pkg., 5–6 pcs.	210	9.0	26.0	8.0	20	460	<1.0
Nacho snack kit (*Taco Bell Ultimate Nachos*), ¼ of 18.5-oz. pkg. . .	280	7.0	31.0	14.0	10	1010	3.0
Name yam (*Frieda's*), ¾ cup, 3 oz.	100	1.0	24.0	0	0	10	3.0
Nan, see "Bread"							
Natto, ½ cup	187	15.6	12.6	9.7	0	6	4.8
Navy beans:							
dry (*Shiloh Farms Organic*), ¼ cup . . .	170	12.0	32.0	.5	0	5	13.0
boiled, ½ cup	129	7.9	24.0	.5	0	1	3.3
Navy beans, canned, ½ cup:							
(*Allens*)	110	6.0	19.0	1.0	0	380	6.0
(*Bush's*)	80	6.0	17.0	0	0	470	7.0
(*Eden* Organic)	110	7.0	20.0	0	0	15	7.0
w/bacon:							
(*Trappey's*)	110	5.0	18.0	1.5	0	420	6.0
jalapeño (*Trappey's*)	110	5.0	17.0	1.5	0	420	6.0
Navy beans, sprouted, ½ cup	35	3.2	6.8	.4	0	14	n.a.
Nectarine:							
(*Del Monte*), 1 medium, 4.9 oz.	70	1.0	16.0	0	0	0	2.0
1 medium, 2½" diam.	67	1.3	16.0	.6	0	<1	2.2
sliced, ½ cup	34	.7	8.1	.3	0	<1	1.1
Noni berry drink (*Snapple*), 8 fl. oz. . .	10	0	1.0	0	0	35	0
Noni juice (*Tree of Life*), 2 tbsp.	15	0	4.0	0	0	10	0

Food and Measure	cal.	prot. (gms)	carbo. (gms)	fat (gms)	chol. (mgs)	sod. (mgs)	fiber (gms)
Noodle, Asian, 2 oz, dry, except as noted:							
bean thread:							
(*Roland*), 2-oz. pkg.	200	0	49.0	0	0	0	0
(*Roland*), 1.8-oz. nest	180	0	43.0	0	0	0	0
cellophane or long rice	200	.1	48.8	<.1	0	6	<1.0
Chinese or Japanese style (*Nasoya*), 1 cup	210	8.0	43.0	.5	0	410	2.0
chow mein:							
(*Annie Chun's*)	200	8.0	39.0	1.0	0	350	3.0
fresh (*Frieda's*), 4 oz.	332	9.0	70.0	1.0	0	468	1.0
chow mein, dried, ½ cup	119	1.9	13.0	6.9	0	99	.9
crispy (*Frieda's*), ½ cup, 1 oz.	160	1.0	17.0	6.0	0	160	1.0
lo mein (*Roland* Organic)	190	5.0	40.0	1.0	0	170	1.0
rice:							
(*Annie Chun's* Original/Pad Thai)	210	2.0	50.0	0	0	75	0
(*A Taste of Thai* Thin/Wide)	200	3.0	46.0	0	0	0	2.0
(*Roland* Hsinchu), 1 cup	230	0	57.0	0	0	120	0
canned (*La Choy*), ½ cup	130	2.0	21.0	4.0	0	350	<1.0
sticks (*Roland* Pad Thai)	200	3.0	46.0	0	0	20	2.0
soba:							
(*Annie Chun's*)	200	8.0	39.0	1.0	0	390	3.0
(*Eden* Organic)	200	8.0	38.0	1.5	0	70	2.0
buckwheat (*Roland*)	200	7.0	40.0	1.0	0	170	1.0
buckwheat (*Eden* 100%)	200	6.0	43.0	1.0	0	5	3.0
buckwheat (*Eden* 40%)	190	8.0	37.0	1.0	0	490	3.0
kamut (*Eden* Organic)	200	7.0	38.0	1.0	0	60	3.0
lotus root (*Eden*) ..	190	9.0	37.0	1.0	0	470	4.0
mugwort (*Eden*) ...	190	8.0	37.0	.5	0	550	2.0
spelt (*Eden* Organic)	200	9.0	37.0	1.5	0	50	2.0
wild yam (*Eden* Jinenjo)	190	9.0	37.0	.5	0	510	2.0

Food and Measure	cal.	prot. (gms)	carbo. (gms)	fat (gms)	chol. (mgs)	sod. (mgs)	fiber (gms)
soba, cooked, 1 cup ..	113	5.8	24.4	.1	0	40	n.a.
somen:							
uncooked	203	6.5	42.2	.5	0	1049	2.4
cooked, 1 cup	230	7.0	48.5	.3	0	284	n.a.
sweet and sour, canned							
(La Choy), 1 cup ..	150	6.0	29.0	2.0	20	790	5.0
thin cut, fresh							
(Azumaya), 1 cup ..	210	8.0	43.0	.5	0	400	2.0
udon:							
(Eden Japanese) ..	190	8.0	37.0	1.5	0	660	3.0
(Eden Organic)	180	8.0	38.0	1.5	0	120	5.0
(Roland Organic) ..	190	5.0	40.0	1.0	0	170	1.0
brown rice (Eden) .	190	8.0	38.0	1.0	0	510	2.0
kamut (Eden Organic)	200	10.0	37.0	1.5	0	55	3.0
spelt (Eden Organic)	200	8.0	39.0	1.0	0	75	2.0
wheat and rice							
(Eden Organic) ..	200	8.0	38.0	2.0	0	80	3.0
udon, cooked, 4 oz. ...	115	2.8	23.0	.6	0	51	n.a.
wide cut (Azumaya),							
1 cup	210	8.0	43.0	.5	0	410	2.0
Noodle, Chinese,							
Japanese, or Thai,							
see "Noodle, Asian"							
Noodle, egg:							
dry, 2 oz.:							
all varieties (Amish							
Kitchen)	220	8.0	38.0	4.0	115	10	1.0
all varieties, except							
yolk free and							
whole wheat							
(Inn Maid)	220	8.0	38.0	4.0	115	10	1.0
enriched	216	7.9	40.3	2.4	54	12	1.5
spelt, whole grain							
(VitaSpelt Organic)	200	9.0	38.0	3.0	45	15	5.0
whole wheat							
(Hodgson Mill) .	190	10.0	34.0	2.0	30	20	4.0
whole wheat (Inn							
Maid)	210	8.0	38.0	3.0	70	0	2.0
yolk free (Inn Maid)	210	8.0	40.0	.5	0	20	2.0
cooked:							
1 cup	212	7.6	39.7	2.4	53	11	1.8
spinach, 1 cup	211	8.1	38.8	2.5	52	20	3.7

Food and Measure	cal.	prot. (gms)	carbo. (gms)	fat (gms)	chol. (mgs)	sod. (mgs)	fiber (gms)
Noodle, egg, frozen, ½ cup, except as noted:							
(*Reames* Home Style)	170	5.0	32.0	2.0	70	10	1.0
(*Reames* Home Style 12-oz. pkg.)	170	5.0	32.0	2.0	65	10	1.0
(*Reames* Golden Ribbon), 1⅓ cups	210	8.0	39.0	2.5	90	15	1.0
chicken noodle soup kit (*Reames* Hearty Home Style), 3 oz.	130	7.0	22.0	1.5	40	1020	1.0
dumplings, flat (*Reames* Home Style)	180	6.0	34.0	2.5	75	10	1.0
precooked (*Reames*), 1 cup	240	10.0	45.0	2.5	75	25	2.0
yolk free (*Reames* Home Style)	180	5.0	31.0	.5	0	10	1.0
Noodle, spelt, all varieties (*VitaSpelt* Organic), 2 oz.	190	9.0	39.0	1.0	0	15	2.0
Noodle entree, frozen, 1 pkg.:							
Asian, stir-fry (*Amy's*), 10 oz.	290	9.0	50.0	7.0	0	630	4.0
and chicken, see "Chicken entree, frozen"							
w/chicken, peas, carrots (*Michelina's Authentico*), 8 oz.	260	13.0	34.0	10.0	70	760	2.0
ginger stir-fry (*Seeds of Change* Organic), 10 oz.	260	9.0	47.0	3.0	35	680	4.0
pad Thai, 10 oz.:							
w/chicken (*Ethnic Gourmet*)	410	20.0	66.0	7.0	25	830	3.0
w/shrimp (*Ethnic Gourmet*)	410	17.0	70.0	7.0	55	850	3.0
w/tofu (*Ethnic Gourmet*)	420	13.0	73.0	8.0	0	720	3.0
Thai peanut, spicy (*Seeds of Change* Organic), 10 oz.	350	17.0	51.0	9.0	50	620	5.0

Food and Measure	cal.	prot. (gms)	carbo. (gms)	fat (gms)	chol. (mgs)	sod. (mgs)	fiber (gms)
Noodle entree,							
microwave or pkg.:							
(*Annie Chun's* Kung							
Pao Micro Bowl),							
½ of 9-oz. bowl ...	240	7.0	40.0	5.0	0	630	1.0
and chicken, see							
"Chicken entree,							
microwave"							
pad Thai (*Annie Chun's*							
Micro Bowl), ½ of							
9-oz. bowl	230	7.0	45.0	4.5	0	710	1.0
peanut sauce (*Annie*							
Chun's Micro Bowl),							
½ of 9-oz. bowl) ..	280	8.0	40.0	11.0	0	340	1.0
ramen noodles (*Annie*							
Chun's Noodle							
Express), ½ of							
7-oz. tray:							
chow mein	160	5.0	27.0	4.0	0	510	1.0
curry, Singapore ..	160	4.0	28.0	3.0	0	550	2.0
spicy Szechuan ...	170	4.0	29.0	3.0	0	470	1.0
teriyaki	160	5.0	31.0	2.0	0	510	1.0
Thai peanut	200	6.0	29.0	7.0	0	300	1.0
teriyaki (*Annie Chun's*							
Micro Bowl), ½ of							
8.2-oz. bowl	200	6.0	38.0	2.5	0	440	1.0
Noodle entree mix:							
beef lo mein (*Knorr*							
Lipton Asian Sides),							
¾ cup	230	9.0	42.0	2.5	50	900	2.0
coconut ginger (*A*							
Taste of Thai), 1 cup*	280	5.0	53.0	7.0	0	680	1.0
chow mein, ⅓ pkg.:							
(*Annie Chun's* Classic							
Organic)	240	8.0	42.0	4.0	0	560	1.0
garlic black bean							
(*Annie Chun's*) ..	250	8.0	43.0	4.5	0	690	1.0
peanut sesame							
(*Annie Chun's*							
Organic)	280	9.0	42.0	8.0	0	390	1.0
teriyaki (*Annie*							
Chun's Organic) .	250	8.0	43.0	4.5	0	600	1.0
curry, red (*A Taste of*							
Thai), 1 cup*	280	4.0	51.0	8.0	5	820	2.0

Food and Measure	cal.	prot. (gms)	carbo. (gms)	fat (gms)	chol. (mgs)	sod. (mgs)	fiber (gms)
Noodle entree mix *(cont.)*							
pad Thai:							
(*Annie Chun's*),							
⅓ pkg.	230	3.0	53.0	1.0	0	780	0
(*A Taste of Thai*),							
1 cup*	240	5.0	48.0	2.0	0	740	2.0
(*A Taste of Thai* for							
Two), ½ pkg. . . .	345	5.0	89.0	.5	0	395	3.5
peanut, Thai (*A Taste*							
of Thai), 1 cup* . . .	330	7.0	53.0	10.0	0	490	1.0
sesame, Thai:							
(*Knorr Lipton Asian*							
Sides), ½ pkg. . .	230	8.0	42.0	3.5	50	820	2.0
toasted, stir-fry (*Thai*							
Kitchen Noodles &							
Sauce), 1 cup* . .	280	5.0	54.0	5.0	0	1016	.5
soba, w/soy ginger							
sauce (*Annie Chun's*							
Organic), ⅓ pkg. . .	240	8.0	41.0	4.0	0	600	1.0
Szechuan (*A Taste of*							
China), 1 cup*	250	5.0	44.0	5.0	0	750	2.0
teriyaki (*Knorr Lipton*							
Asian Sides), ½ pkg.	250	8.0	46.0	3.0	50	900	2.0
Nopales/Nopalitos,							
see "Cactus pads"							
Nori, see "Seaweed"							
Nut butter, see							
specific nut listings							
Nut butter, mixed							
(*Peanut Better*							
Organic), 2 tbsp. . .	190	8.0	5.0	17.0	0	135	3.0
Nutmeg, ground, 1 tsp.	12	.1	1.1	.8	0	tr.	.1
Nuts, see specific							
listings							
Nuts, mixed, 1 oz.,							
except as noted:							
(*Fisher* Less Than 50%							
Peanuts)	180	6.0	5.0	16.0	0	110	2.0
(*Frito-Lay* Deluxe) . . .	170	4.0	6.0	16.0	0	115	2.0
(*Kettle* Deluxe)	170	5.0	7.0	14.0	0	70	2.0
(*Planters*)	170	6.0	5.0	15.0	0	110	2.0
(*Planters* Deluxe)	170	5.0	6.0	15.0	0	105	2.0
(*Planters* Deluxe Lightly							
Salted)	170	5.0	6.0	15.0	0	50	2.0

Food and Measure	cal.	prot. (gms)	carbo. (gms)	fat (gms)	chol. (mgs)	sod. (mgs)	fiber (gms)
(*Planters* Lightly Salted)	170	6.0	5.0	15.0	0	55	2.0
(*Planters* Nut-rition), 1.1 oz.	150	4.0	17.0	8.0	0	45	3.0
(*Planters* Nut-rition Energy Mix)	180	5.0	10.0	14.0	0	95	3.0
(*Planters* Nut-rition Lightly Salted)	170	6.0	5.0	16.0	0	40	3.0
(*Tree of Life* Deluxe), ¼ cup, 1.1 oz.	130	4.0	14.0	8.0	0	0	2.0
(*SunRidge Farms* Fancy), 1.1 oz.	190	5.0	6.0	17.0	0	85	3.0
cashew mix:							
almonds, macadamias (*Planters* Nut-rition Lightly Salted), ¾ oz.	170	5.0	6.0	15.0	0	50	2.0
almonds, pecans (*Planters* Select)	170	5.0	6.0	16.0	0	95	2.0
sesame, w/peanuts (*Planters*)	160	5.0	9.0	13.0	0	240	2.0
glazed (*Beer Nuts*) . . .	180	7.0	4.0	15.0	0	60	2.0
honey (*SunRidge Farms*), 1.1 oz.	170	6.0	6.0	14.0	0	0	2.0
honey-roasted:							
(*Kettle*)	150	5.0	9.0	12.0	0	35	2.0
(*Planters*)	160	5.0	9.0	12.0	0	120	2.0
macadamia mix:							
(*Mauna Loa* Mixed Nuts)	180	5.0	6.0	16.0	0	85	2.0
almond (*Mauna Loa*)	180	6.0	4.0	17.0	0	85	3.0
cashew (*Mauna Loa*)	180	4.0	6.0	17.0	0	85	2.0
cashew, almonds (*Planters* Select)	180	4.0	6.0	17.0	0	95	2.0
pecans, cashews, pistachios (*Planters* Pecan Lovers)	180	4.0	6.0	17.0	0	70	2.0
tamari, roasted (*SunRidge Farms*), 1.1 oz.	160	7.0	6.0	14.0	0	85	2.0

O

Food and Measure	cal.	prot. (gms)	carbo. (gms)	fat (gms)	chol. (mgs)	sod. (mgs)	fiber (gms)
Oat (see also "Cereal"):							
(*Shiloh Farms* Organic							
Steel Cut), ¼ cup ..	170	6.0	29.0	3.0	0	5	5.0
whole grain, 1 oz. ...	110	4.8	18.8	2.0	0	1	3.0
rolled or oatmeal:							
dry (*Shiloh Farms*							
Organic Rolled),							
½ cup	160	6.0	26.0	3.0	0	5	4.0
dry, 1 oz.	109	4.5	19.0	1.8	0	1	2.9
cooked, 1 cup	145	6.1	25.3	2.3	0	2	4.0
Oat beverage, 8 fl. oz.:							
(*Pacific* Organic)	130	4.0	24.0	2.5	0	105	2.0
vanilla (*Pacific* Organic)	130	4.0	25.0	2.5	0	110	2.0
Oat bran, dry:							
(*Shiloh Farms* Organic),							
⅓ cup	150	8.0	23.0	2.5	0	0	7.0
1 oz.	70	4.9	18.8	2.0	0	1	4.5
Oat flour:							
(*Arrowhead Mills*							
Organic), ⅓ cup ...	120	4.0	21.0	3.0	0	0	3.0
(*Shiloh Farms*), ⅓ cup	120	5.0	20.0	2.0	0	0	4.0
bran, ¼ cup:							
(*Hodgson Mill*) ...	110	3.0	23.0	2.0	0	0	3.0
(*Hodgson Mill* Blend)	110	3.0	24.0	1.0	0	0	3.0
(*Hodgson Mill*							
Organic)	110	4.0	22.0	2.0	0	0	3.0
Oat groats, ¼ cup:							
(*Arrowhead Mills*							
Organic)	160	7.0	28.0	3.0	0	0	4.0
(*Shiloh Farms*							
Organic)	160	6.0	29.0	3.0	0	0	4.0
Oco (*Frieda's*), ½ cup,							
3 oz.	70	2.0	15.0	0	0	5	1.0

Food and Measure	cal.	prot. (gms)	carbo. (gms)	fat (gms)	chol. (mgs)	sod. (mgs)	fiber (gms)
Ocean perch, Atlantic, meat only:							
raw, 4 oz.	107	21.1	0	1.9	48	85	0
baked or broiled, 4 oz.	137	27.1	0	2.4	61	109	0
Octopus, meat only:							
raw, 4 oz.	93	16.9	2.5	1.2	54	261	0
boiled or steamed, 4 oz.	186	33.8	5.0	2.4	109	522	0
Octopus, canned:							
in soy/olive oil (*Vigo*), 4 oz.	100	14.0	3.0	4.0	40	250	0
smoked (*Roland* Sliced), 3.66-oz. can	240	11.0	2.0	20.0	35	960	0
w/tomato sauce, vegetables (*Roland*), ½ of 4-oz. can	120	8.0	4.0	8.0	40	280	0
Oheloberry, ½ cup ..	20	.3	4.8	.2	0	1	n.a.
Oil, 1 tbsp., except as noted:							
(*House of Tsang Mongolian Fire*), 1 tsp. .	45	0	0	5.0	0	0	0
all varieties:							
(*Eden*)	120	0	0	14.0	0	0	0
(*Hain*)	120	0	0	14.0	0	0	0
almond, canola, cocoa butter, corn, cottonseed, hazelnut, oat, palm, or poppy seed	120	0	0	13.6	0	0	0
avocado or mustard ..	124	0	0	14.0	0	0	0
avocado, grape seed, nut, pumpkinseed, or rice (*Roland*) ...	130	0	0	14.0	0	0	0
butter oil	112	<.1	0	12.7	33	0	0
chili, chive, garlic, ginger, olive, truffle, or sesame (*Roland*) ..	120	0	0	14.0	0	0	0
chili, hot, or sesame (*House of Tsang*), 1 tsp.	45	0	0	5.0	0	0	0
coconut	117	0	0	13.6	0	0	0
cod liver	123	0	0	13.6	78	0	0
flax seed (*Arrowhead Mills*)	130	0	0	14.0	0	0	0
herring	123	0	0	13.6	104	0	0
menhaden	123	0	0	16.3	85	0	0

Food and Measure	cal.	prot. (gms)	carbo. (gms)	fat (gms)	chol. (mgs)	sod. (mgs)	fiber (gms)
Oil (cont.)							
olive, peanut, safflower, sesame, soybean, sunflower, vegetable, or walnut	120	0	0	14.0	0	0	0
salmon	123	0	0	13.6	66	0	0
sardine	123	0	0	13.6	97	0	0
wok (House of Tsang)	130	0	0	14.0	0	0	0
Okra, fresh:							
raw:							
(Frieda's Red), 3.5 oz.	33	2.0	8.0	.2	0	8	3.0
sliced, ½ cup	19	1.0	3.8	.1	0	4	1.3
boiled, drained, 8 pods, 3" x ⅝"	27	1.6	6.1	.1	0	5	2.1
boiled drained, sliced, ½ cup	25	1.5	5.8	.1	0	4	2.0
Okra, canned, ½ cup:							
cut (Allens/Trappey's) .	30	1.0	6.0	0	0	400	3.0
gumbo (Trappey's Creole)	35	2.0	6.0	0	0	290	3.0
w/tomatoes:							
(Allens/Trappey's) .	30	1.0	5.0	0	0	380	3.0
(Glory Sensibly Seasoned)	30	1.0	6.0	0	0	170	2.0
and corn (Allens) ..	30	1.0	6.0	0	0	280	4.0
and corn (Glory Sensibly Seasoned)	35	1.0	8.0	0	0	150	2.0
and corn (Trappey's)	30	<1.0	6.0	0	0	280	4.0
Okra, frozen, ½ cup:							
whole or cut (McKenzie's)	25	1.0	5.0	0	0	35	3.0
boiled, drained, sliced .	34	1.9	7.5	.3	0	3	2.6
breaded (McKenzie's Gold King)	90	3.0	n.a.	.5	0	350	n.a.
w/tomatoes, onions (McKenzie's)	20	1.0	4.0	0	0	30	2.0
Olive, pickled:							
(Vigo Party Mix), 2 pcs.	40	0	1.0	4.0	0	260	0
black, oil cured:							
(Roland), 4 pcs. ..	50	0	5.0	5.0	0	330	2.0
(Vigo), 4 pcs.	80	0	7.0	6.0	0	420	1.0
black, ripe, pitted:							
whole, large (Lindsay), .5 oz.	25	0	1.0	2.5	0	115	0

Food and Measure	cal.	prot. (gms)	carbo. (gms)	fat (gms)	chol. (mgs)	sod. (mgs)	fiber (gms)
whole, large (*Roland*), 4 pcs.	20	0	1.0	1.5	0	110	1.0
whole, medium (*Roland*), 5 pcs.	30	0	1.0	1.5	0	110	1.0
sliced (*Lindsay*), 2 tbsp.	25	0	1.0	2.5	0	125	0
sliced (*Roland*), 1 tbsp.	20	0	1.0	1.5	0	110	1.0
Greek, whole:							
(*Peloponnese* Atalanti), 3 pcs.	40	0	1.0	4.0	0	220	0
black (*Lindsay* Kalamata), 3 pcs., .5 oz.	25	0	<1.0	2.5	0	240	0
black (*Pelopennese* Amfissa), 3 pcs.	45	0	1.0	4.5	0	200	0
black (*Peloponnese* Kalamata), 5 pcs.	45	0	1.0	4.5	0	210	0
black (*Roland* Kalamata), 3 pcs.	40	0	2.0	3.5	0	160	0
black (*Roland* Mt. Pelion), 2 pcs.	30	0	2.0	2.5	0	160	0
black (*Vigo*), 4 pcs.	40	0	1.0	4.0	0	260	0
black (*Vigo* Calamata), 4 pcs.	35	5	2.0	3.0	0	270	0
black, 10 medium	65	.4	1.7	6.9	0	631	0
black, 10 extra large	89	.6	2.3	9.5	0	868	0
black, pitted, 1 oz.	96	.6	2.5	10.2	0	932	0
blonde (*Roland*), 2 pcs.	30	0	2.0	2.5	0	260	0
green (*Peloponnese* Ionian), 3 pcs.	25	0	1.0	2.5	0	250	0
green (*Roland* Mt. Pelion), 3 pcs.	15	0	2.0	1.0	0	190	0
mixed (*Roland* Greek Country), 3 pcs.	20	0	0	2.0	0	240	0
green, w/pits:							
(*Vigo* Sicilian), 2 pcs.	15	0	1.0	1.0	0	330	0
(*Vigo* Spanish Queen/ Colossal), 2 pcs.	20	0	1.0	1.5	0	290	0
10 small	33	.4	.4	3.6	0	686	.7
10 large	45	.5	.5	4.9	0	926	1.0
10 giant	76	.9	.9	8.3	0	1572	1.7

Food and Measure	cal.	prot. (gms)	carbo. (gms)	fat (gms)	chol. (mgs)	sod. (mgs)	fiber (gms)
Olive (cont.)							
green, chopped (*Vigo* Salad Manzanilla), .5 oz.	25	0	1.0	2.5	0	230	0
green, cracked:							
(*Peloponnese*), 4 pcs.	30	0	1.0	2.5	0	250	0
spiced (*Roland*), 3 pcs.	30	0	1.0	3.0	0	210	0
green, pitted:							
(*Lindsay* Ripe Select), 5 medium, .5 oz. .	25	0	1.0	2.5	0	115	0
queen (*Roland*), 3 pcs.	15	0	1.0	1.5	0	170	0
w/lemon slices (*Roland*), 3 pcs.	25	0	2.0	2.0	0	200	1.0
w/pimiento, sliced (*Lindsay*), 2 tbsp.	25	0	<1.0	2.5	0	330	0
seasoned (*Vigo*), 2 pcs.	20	0	1.0	1.5	0	290	0
mixed (*Peloponnese* Country), 4 pcs. . . .	30	0	1.0	3.0	0	250	0
niçoise (*Roland*), 5 pcs.	45	0	3.0	4.0	0	125	1.0
Picholine (*Roland*), 5 pcs.	25	0	2.0	2.0	0	200	1.0
Provencal, w/herbs or hot pepper (*Roland*), 3 pcs.	25	0	2.0	1.5	0	160	1.0
salad, w/pimento (*Pompeian*), 1 tbsp., .5 oz.	25	0	1.0	2.5	0	240	0
stuffed, green:							
almonds (*Roland*), 4 pcs.	35	0	1.0	3.5	0	310	0
anchovies (*Roland*), 5 pcs.	25	0	1.0	2.0	0	170	0
capers, queen (*Roland*), 2 pcs.	20	0	1.0	1.5	0	330	0
cheese, in oil (*Roland* Greek), ½ cup	520	3.0	7.0	54.0	0	640	3.0
garlic, queen (*Roland*), 2 pcs.	20	0	1.0	1.5	0	300	0

Food and Measure	cal.	prot. (gms)	carbo. (gms)	fat (gms)	chol. (mgs)	sod. (mgs)	fiber (gms)
jalapeño (*Roland*), 2 pcs.	25	0	1.0	2.5	0	330	0
jalapeño (*Vigo*), 2 pcs.	25	0	0	2.0	0	95	0
piri piri (*Roland*), 2 pcs.	20	0	1.0	1.5	0	310	0
onion or triple stuffed (*Roland*), 5 pcs.	25	0	1.0	2.0	0	330	0
stuffed, pimento: (*Roland* Jar), 5 pcs.	25	0	1.0	2.5	0	330	0
Manzanilla (*Lindsay*), 5 pcs., .5 oz.	25	0	<1.0	2.5	0	330	0
Manzanilla (*Roland*), 5 pcs.	25	0	0	2.5	0	230	0
queen (*Lindsay*), 2 pcs., .5 oz.	15	0	<1.0	1.5	0	310	0
queen (*Roland*), 2 pcs.	25	0	1.0	2.5	0	330	0
Olive antipasto, and vegetables (*Peloponnese*), ⅓ cup	35	1.0	2.0	3.0	0	740	0
Olive loaf, see "Lunch meat"							
Olive oil, see "Oil"							
Olive paste or pâté see "Olive spread"							
Olive sauce, green (*Italia In Tavola*), 2 tbsp.	90	0	0	10.0	0	970	0
Olive spread:							
(*Divina* Kalamata), 1 tsp.	15	0	0	2.0	0	150	0
(*Peloponnese* Kalamata), 1 tsp.	15	0	0	1.5	0	160	0
(*Roland* Greek Kalamata), 1 tbsp.	60	0	3.0	6.0	0	450	1.0
paste, 1 tbsp.:							
black (*Roland*)	40	0	0	4.0	0	180	0
green (*Roland*)	30	0	0	3.0	0	180	0
pâté, 2 tbsp.:							
black (*Alessi*)	187	1.0	2.0	19.0	0	817	1.0
green (*Alessi*)	160	1.0	2.0	17.0	0	460	1.0
Olive tapanade:							
black:							
(*Meditalia*), 2 tbsp.	42	.3	1.0	4.1	0	328	0
(*Roland*), 1 tbsp.	45	0	0	4.0	2	270	1.0

Food and Measure	cal.	prot. (gms)	carbo. (gms)	fat (gms)	chol. (mgs)	sod. (mgs)	fiber (gms)
Olive tapanade (cont.)							
and black fig (*Campagna*),							
1 tbsp.	35	0	3.0	2.5	0	105	0
green:							
(*Meditalia*), 2 tbsp. .	54	.5	1.3	5.2	0	306	.4
(*Roland*), 1 tbsp. . . .	40	0	1.0	4.0	2	250	1.0
Onion, fresh/stored:							
raw:							
(*Del Monte*),							
1 medium, 5.2 oz. .	60	2.0	14.0	0	0	5	3.0
(*Frieda's* Boiler/							
Cipolline), 3 pcs.,							
3 oz.	30	1.0	7.0	0	0	0	2.0
(*Frieda's* Hawaiian							
Maui), ⅓ cup,							
1.1 oz.	10	0	3.0	0	0	5	1.0
(*Frieda's* Pearl),							
⅔ cup, 3 oz. . . .	30	1.0	7.0	0	0	0	2.0
1 oz.	11	.3	2.4	<.1	0	1	.5
chopped, ½ cup . . .	30	.9	6.9	0.1	0	2	1.4
chopped, 1 tbsp. . .	4	.1	.9	<.1	0	tr.	.2
boiled, drained:							
chopped, ½ cup . . .	46	1.4	10.7	.2	0	3	1.5
chopped, 1 tbsp. . .	7	.2	1.5	<.1	0	<1	.2
Onion, can/jar:							
whole:							
(*Aunt Nellie's* Holland							
Style), ½ cup . . .	40	<1.0	8.0	0	0	410	1.0
baby (*Roland*),							
⅔ cup	24	1.0	5.0	0	0	300	2.0
w/balsamic vinegar							
(*Roland*), 2 tbsp. . .	20	0	5.0	0	0	55	0
cocktail:							
(*Crosse & Blackwell*),							
1 tbsp.	5	0	1.0	0	0	250	0
(*Roland*), 2 tbsp. . .	0	0	1.0	0	0	55	0
(*Vigo*), 1 pc.	0	0	0	0	0	30	0
Onion, dried:							
flakes, 1 tbsp.	16	.5	4.2	<.1	0	1	.5
minced, 1 tsp.	7	.2	1.9	0	0	<1	.2
Onion, french fried,							
canned, 2 tbsp.:							
(*French's* Original) . . .	45	0	3.0	3.5	0	60	0
cheddar (*French's*) . . .	45	0	3.0	3.5	0	65	0

Food and Measure	cal.	prot. (gms)	carbo. (gms)	fat (gms)	chol. (mgs)	sod. (mgs)	fiber (gms)
Onion, frozen (see also "Onion rings"):							
whole:							
(*C&W* Petite), ⅔ cup	30	0	6.0	0	0	10	<1.0
boiled, drained, ½ cup	30	.7	7.0	0	0	8	1.5
pearl, white (*Birds Eye*), ⅔ cup	30	0	6.0	0	0	10	1.0
chopped:							
boiled, drained, 1 tbsp.	4	.1	1.0	<.1	0	2	.2
w/peppers (*Mc-Kenzie's* Seasoning Mix), 1 oz.	10	1.0	2.0	0	0	10	0
Onion, green, raw, trimmed:							
bulb, w/top, 2 oz.	18	1.0	4.0	0	0	9	1.5
chopped:							
(*Del Monte*), ¼ cup	10	0	2.0	0	0	5	1.0
½ cup	16	.9	3.7	.1	0	8	1.3
1 tbsp.	2	.1	.4	<.1	0	1	.2
Onion dip, 2 tbsp., except as noted:							
French:							
(*Bravo*)	60	1.0	3.0	5.0	0	220	0
(*Frito-Lay*)	60	1.0	4.0	5.0	15	230	0
(*Gibble's*)	60	1.0	3.0	5.0	0	220	0
(*Kraft*)	60	1.0	3.0	4.5	0	220	0
(*Marzetti's*)	120	1.0	2.0	12.0	20	220	0
(*Marzetti's* Light) ..	60	0	3.0	6.0	5	230	0
roasted (*Marie's*) ..	100	1.0	2.0	10.0	15	220	0
green (*Kraft*)	60	1.0	3.0	4.5	0	170	0
sour cream (*Gibble's*)	60	1.0	2.0	5.0	20	250	0
Onion dip mix:							
French:							
(*Lay's*), 2 tbsp.* ...	60	1.0	3.0	6.0	15	230	0
(*McCormick*), ¾ tsp.	5	0	0	0	0	140	0
green:							
(*Bravo*), ¾ tsp.	5	0	1.0	0	0	180	0
(*Lay's*), 2 tbsp.* ...	60	1.0	3.0	6.0	15	170	0
Onion gravy mix (Mc-Cormick), ¼ cup* .	20	0	3.0	.5	0	340	0
Onion nuggets, frozen, w/cheese, breaded (*Kineret*), 3½ pcs., 2.8 oz.	150	5.0	20.0	5.0	10	490	6.0

Food and Measure	cal.	prot. (gms)	carbo. (gms)	fat (gms)	chol. (mgs)	sod. (mgs)	fiber (gms)
Onion powder, 1 tsp. . .	7	.2	1.7	0	0	1	.1
Onion relish, sweet (*Vidalia Valley*), 1 tbsp.	11	0	3.0	0	0	0	0
Onion ring batter mix, ¼ cup dry:							
(*Don's Chuck Wagon*)	100	3.0	21.0	0	0	690	1.0
(*Golden Dipt* Fry Easy Batter)	100	1.0	20.0	0	0	660	0
(*Zatarain's*)	100	2.0	22.0	.5	0	700	1.0
Onion rings, frozen, breaded:							
(*Alexia Onion Rings*), 6 pcs., 3 oz.	230	4.0	28.0	12.0	0	230	4.0
(*Kineret*), 6 pcs., 3.2 oz.	180	3.0	26.0	8.0	0	250	2.0
(*McKenzie's*), 3.25 oz.	220	3.0	28.0	10.0	0	210	6.0
heated, 10 rings	289	3.8	27.1	19.0	0	17	2.9
Onion salt (*McCormick*), ¼ tsp.	0	0	0	0	0	450	0
Onion sauce, 1 tbsp.:							
(*Boar's Head* Sweet Vidalia)	10	0	2.0	0	0	15	0
(*Sabrett* Pushcart) . . .	10	0	3.0	0	0	105	0
Onion snack chips, see "Snack chips"							
Onion, Welsh, 1 oz. . .	10	.5	1.8	.1	0	5	<1.0
Opo squash (*Frieda's*), ⅔ cup, 3 oz.	10	1.0	3.0	0	0	0	0
Opossum, meat only, roasted, 4 oz.	251	34.3	0	11.6	146	66	0
Orange, fresh:							
(*Dole*), 5.4-oz. fruit . .	70	1.0	21.0	0	0	0	7.0
(*Frieda's* Blood Moro/ Cara Cara), 5 oz. . .	70	1.0	16.0	0	0	0	3.0
(*Frieda's* Seville), 3 oz.	40	1.0	10.0	0	0	0	2.0
all varieties:							
3¹⁄₁₆" fruit, 6.5 oz. . . .	87	1.7	21.6	.2	0	0	4.4
sections, 1 cup . . .	85	1.7	21.2	.2	0	0	4.3
California navel:							
2⅞" fruit, 5 oz.	65	1.4	16.3	.1	0	1	3.4
sections, 1 cup . . .	76	1.7	19.2	.2	0	2	4.0
California Valencia:							
2⅝" fruit, 4.25 oz. . .	59	1.3	14.4	.4	0	0	3.0
sections, 1 cup . . .	88	1.9	21.4	.5	0	0	4.5

Food and Measure	cal.	prot. (gms)	carbo. (gms)	fat (gms)	chol. (mgs)	sod. (mgs)	fiber (gms)
Florida:							
2¹¹⁄₁₆" fruit, 5 oz.	65	1.0	16.3	.3	0	1	3.4
sections, 1 cup . . .	85	1.3	21.4	.4	0	1	4.4
Orange, blood, drink mixer (*Angostura*), 2 fl. oz.	70	0	18.0	0	0	5	0
Orange, canned:							
in syrup (*Vigo* Shells), ⅕ of 18-oz. can . . .	200	0	51.0	0	0	10	3.0
mandarin, see "Tangerine"							
Orange drink, 8 fl. oz., except as noted:							
(*Hi-C Blast*)	120	0	32.0	0	0	140	0
(*Minute Maid Light*) . .	50	0	13.0	0	0	15	0
(*Santa Cruz Organic*) .	100	0	25.0	0	0	10	0
(*Tropicana* Light 'n Healthy)	50	<1.0	13.0	0	0	10	0
orange flavor:							
(*Bright & Early*) . . .	110	0	30.0	0	0	20	0
frozen* (*Bright & Early*)	110	0	29.0	0	0	10	0
orangeade:							
(*AriZona*)	100	0	27.0	0	0	20	0
(*Minute Maid*), 12 fl. oz.	160	0	43.0	0	0	35	0
(*Minute Maid 10%*)	110	0	30.0	0	0	15	0
(*Minute Maid 3%*) .	110	0	29.0	0	0	25	0
(*Snapple*)	120	0	29.0	0	0	10	0
(*Tropicana*)	130	0	33.0	0	0	0	0
(*Turkey Hill*)	120	0	30.0	0	0	10	0
Orange drink blend, 8 fl. oz., except as noted:							
carrot:							
(*Apple & Eve*)	130	0	32.0	0	0	20	0
(*SoBe Elixir 3C*) . .	90	0	24.0	0	0	10	0
cream, w/herbs (*SoBe Tsunami*)	100	0	25.0	0	0	25	0
mango:							
(*Apple & Eve*)	120	0	30.0	0	0	30	0
(*Nantucket Nectars*)	120	0	30.0	0	0	25	0
(*Newman's Own* Tango)	150	0	37.0	0	0	5	0

Food and Measure	cal.	prot. (gms)	carbo. (gms)	fat (gms)	chol. (mgs)	sod. (mgs)	fiber (gms)
Orange drink blend, mango *(cont.)*							
(*SoBe Lizard* Lightning)	130	0	33.0	0	0	20	0
w/mangosteen (*Honest Ade* Organic)	48	0	12.0	0	0	5	0
pineapple (*Lincoln*) ..	130	0	32.0	0	0	70	0
pineapple mango (*Nantucket Nectars*)	120	1.0	30.0	0	0	30	0
Orange juice, 8 fl. oz., except as noted:							
(*Apple & Eve*)	110	1.0	27.0	0	0	10	0
(*Bolthouse Farms*) ...	110	3.0	24.0	0	0	25	>1.0
(*Dole*)	120	<1.0	27.0	0	0	10	0
(*Land O Lakes*)	110	1.0	25.0	0	0	45	0
(*Land O Lakes* Calcium)	120	1.0	29.0	0	0	0	0
(*Minute Maid* Extra Vitamins C&E)	120	2.0	27.0	0	0	15	0
(*Minute Maid* Low Acid/ Country/Home Squeezed Style/ Original/Original Calcium/Pulp Free) .	110	2.0	27.0	0	0	15	0
(*Minute Maid* Multi-Vitamin)	120	2.0	27.0	0	0	20	0
(*Minute Maid* Original), 10 fl. oz.	140	2.0	20.0	0	0	20	0
(*Minute Maid* Active) .	120	2.0	28.0	0	0	15	0
(*Minute Maid* Heart Wise)	110	2.0	27.0	0	0	20	0
(*Nantucket Nectars* Premium)	110	2.0	26.0	0	0	0	0
(*Odwalla*)	110	1.0	25.0	0	0	15	0
(*Organic Valley*)	120	2.0	26.0	0	0	0	0
(*Organic Valley* Calcium)	110	2.0	26.0	0	0	0	0
(*R.W. Knudsen*)	110	2.0	26.0	0	0	10	0
(*Simply Orange*)	110	2.0	26.0	0	0	0	0
(*Tropicana* Organics) .	120	1.0	28.0	0	0	25	0
(*Tropicana Pure Premium* Fiber) ...	120	2.0	29.0	0	0	0	3.0
(*Tropicana Pure Premium* Omega-3)	120	2.0	26.0	.5	0	0	0
(*Veryfine*)	120	0	28.0	0	0	20	0

Food and Measure	cal.	prot. (gms)	carbo. (gms)	fat (gms)	chol. (mgs)	sod. (mgs)	fiber (gms)
all varieties, except Fiber and Omega-3 (*Tropicana Pure Premium*)	110	2.0	26.0	0	0	0	0
canned	105	1.5	24.5	.4	0	5	.5
chilled	110	2.0	25.1	.7	0	3	.5
fresh	112	1.7	25.8	.5	0	2	.5
frozen*:							
(*Cascadian Farm Organic*)	110	1.0	27.0	0	0	0	0
(*Langer's*)	120	0	29.0	0	0	15	0
(*Minute Maid* Low Acid)	110	2.0	27.0	0	0	15	0
all varieties, except low acid (*Minute Maid*)	110	0	27.0	0	0	0	0
Orange juice blend, 8 fl. oz., except as noted:							
carrot:							
(*R.W. Knudsen Organic*)	120	1.0	29.0	0	0	35	0
(*Walnut Acres Organic*)	110	0	27.0	0	0	30	0
mango:							
(*R.W. Knudsen*) ...	120	1.0	30.0	0	0	5	0
(*Santa Cruz Organic*)	130	1.0	32.0	0	0	15	0
(*Snapple*), 11.5 fl. oz.	160	0	44.0	0	0	15	0
peach mango or strawberry banana: (*Dole*)	120	<1.0	28.0	0	0	10	0
pineapple:							
(*Santa Cruz Organic*)	130	0	31.0	0	0	20	0
(*Tropicana Pure Premium*)	130	2.0	31.0	0	0	0	0
strawberry banana (*Tropicana Pure Premium*)	130	2.0	30.0	0	0	0	0
tangerine:							
(*Apple & Eve*), 6.75 fl. oz.	100	0	25.0	0	0	20	0
(*Apple & Eve* Tropicals)	120	0	30.0	0	0	30	0
(*Tropicana Pure Premium*)	110	2.0	25.0	0	0	0	0
(*Veryfine*)	120	0	30.0	0	0	20	0

Food and Measure	cal.	prot. (gms)	carbo. (gms)	fat (gms)	chol. (mgs)	sod. (mgs)	fiber (gms)
Orange juice blend *(cont.)*							
tropical *(Minute Maid)*, 11.5-fl.-oz. can	180	0	46.0	0	0	30	0
frozen*:							
passion fruit *(Minute Maid Passion)*	130	0	31.0	0	0	5	0
tangerine *(Minute Maid)*	110	0	27.0	0	0	0	0
Orange roughy, see "Roughy, orange"							
Oregano, dried, 1 tsp.	3	.1	.5	0	0	0	.1
Oriental 5-spice *(Tone's)*, 1 tsp.	9	.3	1.9	.3	0	2	.5
Orzo entree, frozen *(Seeds of Change Athenian Organic)*, 10-oz. pkg.	300	15.0	42.0	9.0	25	520	5.0
Ostrich, ground, pan-broiled, 4 oz. ...	187	22.9	0	10.0	81	82	0
Oyster, meat only, 4 oz., except as noted:							
Eastern, farmed:							
raw	67	5.9	6.3	1.8	29	202	0
baked or broiled ...	90	7.9	8.3	2.4	43	185	0
Eastern, wild:							
raw, 1 lb.	310	32.0	17.7	11.1	238	957	0
raw, 6 medium, 3 oz.	57	5.9	3.3	2.1	44	177	0
baked or broiled ...	82	9.4	5.4	2.2	56	277	0
steamed or poached	155	16.0	8.9	5.6	119	478	0
Pacific:							
raw	92	10.7	5.6	2.6	57	120	0
raw, steamed, or poached, 1 medium.	41	4.7	2.5	1.2	25	53	0
boiled or steamed .	185	21.4	11.2	5.2	113	240	0
Oyster, canned:							
whole:							
(Bumble Bee), 2 oz.	70	7.0	3.0	3.0	45	140	0
(Chicken of the Sea), 2 oz.	80	7.0	6.0	3.0	35	220	0
(Yankee Clipper), ¼ cup	60	8.0	3.0	2.0	10	220	1.0

Food and Measure	cal.	prot. (gms)	carbo. (gms)	fat (gms)	chol. (mgs)	sod. (mgs)	fiber (gms)
Eastern, wild:							
w/liquid, 4 oz.	78	8.0	4.4	2.8	62	127	0
w/liquid, 1 cup	170	17.5	9.7	6.1	136	277	0
Oyster, smoked,							
canned:							
in oil, drained:							
(*Brunswick* 3 oz.),							
2.3 oz.	150	12.0	7.0	8.0	40	240	0
(*Bumble Bee*), 2 oz.	120	10.0	6.0	7.0	35	210	0
(*Chicken of the Sea*),							
3.75-oz. can	170	10.0	8.0	8.0	45	280	0
(*Yankee Clipper*							
Cocktail/Tiny/Extra							
Tiny), 3-oz. can	140	8.0	5.0	10.0	35	260	<1.0
in water (*Chicken of*							
the Sea), 4.75-oz.							
can	120	12.0	10.0	3.0	55	400	0
teriyaki (*Chicken of the*							
Sea), 3.75-oz. can .	120	12.0	12.0	3.0	55	470	1.0
Oyster plant,							
see "Salsify"							
Oyster sauce, Asian,							
1 tbsp.:							
(*House of Tsang*)	30	0	7.0	0	0	600	0
(*Polynesian*)	5	.3	1.0	0	0	390	0
(*Roland*)	15	0	4.0	0	0	730	0
Oyster and shrimp							
sauce (*TryMe*							
Caribbean Clipper),							
1 tsp.	10	0	2.0	0	0	140	0
Oyster stew, see							
"Soup, condensed"							

P

Food and Measure	cal.	prot. (gms)	carbo. (gms)	fat (gms)	chol. (mgs)	sod. (mgs)	fiber (gms)
Pad Thai entree, see "Noodle entree"							
Pad Thai sauce, see "Thai sauce"							
Paella entree, frozen (*Contessa*), w/seasoning, 1½ cups*	220	19.0	29.0	3.0	55	890	3.0
Palm, hearts of, can or jar:							
(*Roland* Organic Can), ½ cup	20	3.0	2.0	0	0	330	2.0
(*Roland* Organic Jar), ½ cup	40	3.0	6.0	0	0	590	4.0
(*Vigo/Vigo* Salad), ⅓ of 14-oz. can	15	2.0	1.0	0	0	420	2.0
marinated, ½ cup:							
(*Fanci Food*)	60	4.0	8.0	1.0	0	770	4.0
(*Roland*)	100	1.0	6.0	8.0	0	410	1.0
Pancake, frozen, 3 pcs., except as noted:							
(*Aunt Jemima*)	240	5.0	41.0	6.0	35	500	1.0
(*Aunt Jemima* Mini), 5 pcs.	240	7.0	44.0	4.5	25	500	2.0
(*Pillsbury* Original)	250	6.0	49.0	4.0	10	450	2.0
blueberry:							
(*Eggo*)	270	5.0	46.0	8.0	15	770	1.0
(*Pillsbury*)	230	5.0	46.0	3.5	10	430	2.0
buttermilk:							
(*Aunt Jemima*)	240	6.0	41.0	6.0	30	490	1.0
(*Aunt Jemima* Low Fat)	200	5.0	39.0	3.0	25	460	1.0
(*Eggo*)	280	6.0	46.0	9.0	15	580	1.0

Food and Measure	cal.	prot. (gms)	carbo. (gms)	fat (gms)	chol. (mgs)	sod. (mgs)	fiber (gms)
(*Pillsbury*)	240	6.0	47.0	4.0	10	470	2.0
mini (*Pillsbury*), 11 pcs.	250	4.0	42.0	7.0	10	560	<1.0
chocolate (*Pillsbury Chocolate Burst*) ..	280	5.0	51.0	7.0	10	400	2.0*
maple (*Pillsbury Maple Burst*)	290	5.0	53.0	7.0	10	410	2.0
mini (*Eggo*), 11 pcs. .	260	5.0	42.0	8.0	10	550	1.0
whole grain (*Aunt Jemima*)	240	5.0	42.0	6.0	20	460	3.0
whole wheat (*Nutri-Grain*)	240	6.0	40.0	7.0	0	370	3.0
Pancake, mix, 3 cakes*, except as noted:							
(*Aunt Jemima* Original), ⅓ cup	150	4.0	33.0	.5	0	470	1.0
(*Aunt Jemima* Original Complete), ⅓ cup .	160	5.0	32.0	1.5	5	470	1.0
(*Betty Crocker* Original Complete)	200	5.0	40.0	2.5	10	520	1.0
(*Bisquick* Original), ⅓ cup	160	3.0	26.0	5.0	0	490	<1.0
(*Bisquick Shake 'n Pour*)	220	6.0	42.0	3.0	0	800	1.0
(*Hungry Jack* Extra Light/Fluffy), ⅓ cup	150	4.0	30.0	2.0	n.a.	600	<1.0
(*Hungry Jack* Original), ⅓ cup	150	4.0	31.0	1.5	n.a.	550	<1.0
(*Krusteaz* No Sugar) .	210	6.0	42.0	2.0	5	590	1.0
(*Krusteaz* Original) ...	250	7.0	34.0	10.0	80	580	1.0
(*Shake 'n Pour*)	220	6.0	42.0	3.0	0	800	1.0
apple spice (*Krusteaz*), 2 cakes*, 4"	210	6.0	40.0	3.0	0	620	3.0
blueberry (*Hungry Jack Easy Packs*), ½ cup	200	5.0	40.0	2.5	n.a.	640	1.0
buckwheat:							
(*Arrowhead Mills* Organic), ⅓ cup .	170	7.0	29.0	2.0	0	290	7.0
(*Aunt Jemima*), ¼ cup	100	4.0	23.0	1.0	0	580	3.0
(*Hodgson Mill*), ⅓ cup	140	5.0	28.0	1.0	0	290	3.0

Food and Measure	cal.	prot. (gms)	carbo. (gms)	fat (gms)	chol. (mgs)	sod. (mgs)	fiber (gms)
Pancake, mix *(cont.)*							
buttermilk:							
(*Arrowhead Mills*							
Organic)	140	6.0	27.0	1.0	5	340	2.0
(*Aunt Jemima*),							
⅓ cup	110	4.0	23.0	.5	0	480	1.0
(*Aunt Jemima*							
Complete),⅓ cup	160	5.0	31.0	2.0	10	460	1.0
(*Betty Crocker*							
Complete)	200	5.0	40.0	2.5	10	530	1.0
(*Hungry Jack*), ⅓ cup	150	4.0	31.0	1.5	n.a.	630	<1.0
(*Hungry Jack*							
Complete)	150	4.0	31.0	1.5	n.a.	550	<1.0
(*Hungry Jack Easy*							
Packs), ½ cup . .	200	5.0	40.0	2.0	n.a.	710	1.0
(*"Jiffy"* Complete),							
⅓ cup	170	3.0	30.0	4.5	<5	380	<1.0
(*Krusteaz*)	210	6.0	42.0	2.0	5	560	1.0
(*Martha White Flap-*							
Stax), ½ cup . . .	240	5.0	44.0	5.0	20	590	<1.0
apple cinnamon							
(*Arrowhead Mills*							
Organic), ¼ cup .	130	5.0	27.0	.5	5	340	2.0
whole wheat							
(*Hodgson Mill*),							
⅓ cup	120	4.0	28.0	1.0	0	321	4.0
chocolate chip							
(*Krusteaz*)	210	5.0	41.0	3.0	<5	480	2.0
gluten-free (*Arrowhead*							
Mills Organic),							
¼ cup	150	2.0	36.0	0	0	290	0
kamut (*Arrowhead*							
Mills Organic), ¼ cup	140	6.0	24.0	2.0	0	200	4.0
multigrain, ¼ cup:							
(*Arrowhead Mills*							
Organic)	130	5.0	27.0	1.0	5	260	3.0
chocolate chip							
(*Arrowhead Mills*							
Organic)	140	4.0	26.0	2.5	5	240	3.0
oat bran:							
(*Arrowhead Mills*							
Organic), ¼ cup .	120	7.0	21.0	2.0	0	75	6.0
(*Krusteaz* Low Fat),							
2 cakes*, 4"	230	6.0	45.0	3.0	0	390	4.0

Food and Measure	cal.	prot. (gms)	carbo. (gms)	fat (gms)	chol. (mgs)	sod. (mgs)	fiber (gms)
wheat and honey (*Krusteaz*)	220	8.0	42.0	1.5	5	550	4.0
whole wheat blend (*Aunt Jemima*), ¼ cup	120	4.0	26.0	.5	0	620	3.0
wild rice (*Arrowhead Mills* Organic), ¼ cup	130	6.0	28.0	1.0	0	70	2.0
Pancake breakfast, frozen, 1 pkg., except as noted:							
and bacon (*Aunt Jemima*), 6.8 oz. ...	450	14.0	61.0	17.0	65	1100	3.0
and sausage:							
(*Aunt Jemima*), 6.8 oz.	480	14.0	58.0	22.0	90	1040	2.0
(*Jimmy Dean* Breakfast Bowls), 8.6 oz.	710	13.0	93.0	31.0	45	890	3.0
minis (*Jimmy Dean*), 3 pcs., 2.5 oz. ...	260	5.0	19.0	18.0	30	510	0
Pancake syrup, 4 tbsp. or ¼ cup:							
(*Aunt Jemima*)	210	0	52.0	0	0	120	0
(*Aunt Jemima* Lite) ..	100	0	26.0	0	0	190	1.0
(*Eggo*)	240	0	60.0	0	0	35	0
(*Eggo* Lite)	110	0	27.0	0	0	180	0
(*Hungry Jack*)	210	0	52.0	0	0	140	0
(*Hungry Jack* Lite) ...	100	0	24.0	0	0	180	0
butter flavor:							
(*Aunt Jemima* Lite)	100	0	26.0	0	0	210	1.0
(*Aunt Jemima* Rich)	210	0	53.0	0	0	210	0
(*Eggo* Buttery)	160	0	41.0	0	0	90	0
(*Hungry Jack*)	210	0	52.0	0	0	200	0
(*Hungry Jack* Lite) .	100	0	24.0	0	0	180	0
butter pecan (*Eggo*) ..	220	0	55.0	0	0	120	0
cinnamon French toast (*Eggo*)	160	0	41.0	0	0	90	0
Pancetta, see "Bacon, Italian"							
Pancreas, braised:							
beef, 4 oz.	307	30.7	0	19.5	297	68	0
lamb, 4 oz.	265	25.9	0	17.1	454	59	0
pork, 4 oz.	248	32.3	0	12.2	357	48	0
veal (calves), 4 oz. ...	290	33.0	0	16.6	n.a.	77	0

Food and Measure	cal.	prot. (gms)	carbo. (gms)	fat (gms)	chol. (mgs)	sod. (mgs)	fiber (gms)
Panera Bread:							
breakfast egg soufflé:							
four cheese	470	16.0	35.0	30.0	150	700	2.0
spinach/artichoke ..	560	21.0	37.0	36.0	140	990	2.0
spinach/bacon	530	19.0	36.0	34.0	135	910	2.0
turkey sausage/							
potato	450	14.0	36.0	28.0	115	600	2.0
breakfast sandwich:							
bacon/egg/cheese .	510	28.0	44.0	24.0	215	1060	2.0
egg/cheese	380	18.0	43.0	14.0	190	620	2.0
sausage/egg/cheese	540	26.0	44.0	27.0	220	980	2.0
bread, artisan, 2 oz.:							
cheese, 3, miche ..	140	5.0	25.0	2.0	5	290	1.0
ciabatta	460	16.0	84.0	5.0	0	760	3.0
country miche	130	5.0	26.0	.5	0	300	1.0
focaccia, asiago ...	160	5.0	23.0	5.0	5	230	1.0
French miche	130	5.0	26.0	.5	0	330	1.0
rye, stone-milled							
miche	120	4.0	25.0	.5	0	340	2.0
sesame semolina							
miche	130	4.0	27.0	.5	0	330	1.0
three seed demi ...	150	5.0	26.0	2.5	0	290	2.0
whole-grain miche .	150	6.0	29.0	1.5	0	300	3.0
bread, specialty, 2 oz.:							
asiago cheese loaf .	160	7.0	22.0	4.0	10	320	1.0
challah	180	6.0	34.0	2.5	10	290	1.0
cinnamon raisin ...	170	4.0	33.0	3.0	0	230	1.0
French, XL loaf	150	6.0	28.0	2.0	5	310	1.0
honey wheat	170	5.0	31.0	2.5	0	270	2.0
sourdough, XL loaf	140	5.0	28.0	.5	0	290	1.0
sunflower	180	6.0	27.0	6.0	0	280	2.0
tomato basil	140	5.0	27.0	.5	0	330	1.0
bagel, 1 pc.:							
plain	310	10.0	61.0	1.5	0	480	2.0
apple, Dutch, raisin .	340	7.0	73.0	2.5	0	590	2.0
asiago cheese	370	15.0	61.0	6.0	10	630	2.0
blueberry	350	11.0	71.0	2.0	0	520	3.0
chocolate chip	390	11.0	73.0	6.0	0	500	3.0
cinnamon crunch ..	420	10.0	76.0	8.0	0	490	2.0
everything	310	11.0	61.0	2.0	0	610	2.0
French toast	390	11.0	74.0	5.0	0	680	2.0
sesame	330	11.0	60.0	4.5	0	450	3.0
whole grain	350	12.0	67.0	3.0	5	410	5.0

Food and Measure	cal.	prot. (gms)	carbo. (gms)	fat (gms)	chol. (mgs)	sod. (mgs)	fiber (gms)
cream cheese, veggie, reduced fat, 2 oz. . . .	120	5.0	3.0	10.0	30	210	1.0
soup, 8 oz.:							
black bean, low fat .	150	8.0	28.0	1.0	0	920	6.0
broccoli cheddar . .	230	8.0	14.0	16.0	45	970	1.0
chicken, cream of, and wild rice . . .	200	5.0	19.0	12.0	35	970	<1.0
chicken noodle	100	5.0	15.0	2.0	15	1080	1.0
clam chowder	320	6.0	11.0	28.0	100	740	1.0
onion, French, no cheese/croutons .	90	2.0	13.0	3.0	10	1560	2.0
potato, baked	230	5.0	21.0	14.0	45	720	2.0
tomato, creamy . . .	290	5.0	29.0	18.0	40	920	3.0
turkey chickpea chili	180	10.0	22.0	5.0	25	800	7.0
vegetable, garden . .	90	4.0	17.0	.5	0	860	2.0
sandwiches, ½ portion, except as noted:							
asiago roast beef . .	360	24.0	29.0	16.0	60	640	1.0
Bacon Turkey Bravo	410	25.0	43.0	15.0	55	1460	2.0
chicken Caesar on three cheese	380	22.0	39.0	16.0	70	800	2.0
chicken tomesto on three cheese	310	21.0	40.0	8.0	40	760	3.0
chicken bacon Dijon panini on French	340	27.0	32.0	18.0	75	770	1.0
chicken salad on whole grain	290	15.0	35.0	13.0	10	790	8.0
chipotle chicken on French	400	22.0	25.0	24.0	70	900	2.0
Frontago Chicken panini, whole portion, 12.75 oz.	800	45.0	80.0	32.0	100	2150	5.0
ham and Swiss on stone-milled rye .	390	22.0	38.0	16.0	55	1200	3.0
Italian combo	530	29.0	53.0	24.0	85	1410	3.0
Mediterranean veggie	310	11.0	50.0	7.0	5	730	5.0
portobello mozzarella panini	330	13.0	41.0	12.0	20	640	2.0
Smokehouse Turkey panini on focaccia	400	26.0	40	15.0	50	1310	2.0
tuna salad on whole grain	430	14.0	45.0	22.0	20	770	6.0

Food and Measure	cal.	prot. (gms)	carbo. (gms)	fat (gms)	chol. (mgs)	sod. (mgs)	fiber (gms)
Panera Bread, sandwiches *(cont.)*							
turkey, Sierra, on							
cheese focaccia .	480	19.0	40.0	27.0	45	990	2.0
turkey artichoke							
panini	350	20.0	44.0	11.0	45	1170	3.0
turkey breast,							
smoked, on							
sourdough	240	15.0	25.0	9.0	30	840	1.0
salad, ½ portion:							
apple chicken, Fuji .	260	16.0	17.0	13.0	45	450	3.0
Caesar	200	6.0	13.0	14.0	25	310	2.0
grilled chicken . .	250	18.0	13.0	14.0	60	520	2.0
classic café	90	1.0	9.0	5.0	0	135	2.0
chicken, Asian							
sesame	210	16.0	16.0	10.0	35	450	2.0
Fandango salad . . .	200	7.0	14.0	14.0	15	280	2.0
Greek	220	5.0	7.0	20.0	10	690	3.0
salmon, grilled	160	11.0	15.0	6.0	25	360	3.0
fruit cup, small	70	1.0	19.0	0	0	15	1.0
Crispani, ⅓ pizza:							
cheese, three	350	15.0	37.0	16.0	35	590	2.0
chicken, barbecue .	380	20.0	42.0	15.0	50	970	2.0
Italian meat classic	390	17.0	38.0	18.0	40	990	2.0
mushroom, wild . . .	350	13.0	38.0	16.0	30	600	2.0
pepperoni	390	17.0	38.0	18.0	30	870	2.0
sausage/roasted							
pepper	380	15.0	38.0	18.0	40	730	2.0
tomato basil	330	13.0	38.0	13.0	20	590	2.0
pastries/sweets:							
bear claw	460	10.0	49.0	27.0	85	310	2.0
brownie:							
caramel pecan . .	470	5.0	59.0	24.0	80	170	2.0
very chocolate . .	460	5.0	61.0	22.0	80	180	2.0
cinnamon roll	610	9.0	90.0	27.0	80	340	5.0
cobblestone	590	6.0	107.0	12.0	0	510	3.0
cookies:							
chocolate chipper	410	5.0	55.0	20.0	55	290	2.0
nutty	430	5.0	51.0	24.0	50	270	3.0
chocolate duet,							
w/walnuts	400	6.0	52.0	22.0	50	290	3.0
nutty oatmeal							
raisin	340	5.0	50.0	14.0	45	270	3.0
shortbread	350	3.0	36.0	21.0	55	160	1.0
croissant, French . .	240	5.0	25.0	14.0	35	170	1.0

Food and Measure	cal.	prot. (gms)	carbo. (gms)	fat (gms)	chol. (mgs)	sod. (mgs)	fiber (gms)
lemon poppy mini Bundt cake	460	6.0	63.0	20.0	95	440	0
muffin:							
blueberry, wild- ...	400	6.0	59.0	16.0	60	240	1.0
reduced fat ...	360	6.0	61.0	10.0	55	220	1.0
carrot walnut ...	430	8.0	61.0	19.0	55	380	2.0
chocolate chip ..	270	4.0	40.0	12.0	35	140	1.0
pumpkin	530	6.0	82.0	20.0	30	430	2.0
pastry:							
caramel apple ...	400	7.0	51.0	19.0	60	300	2.0
cheese, artisan ..	380	7.0	38.0	22.0	25	330	1.0
cherry, artisan ..	420	8.0	51.0	21.0	10	330	1.0
cherry cheese ring	210	3.0	26.0	11.0	40	120	1.0
chocolate, artisan	340	6.0	37.0	20.0	10	230	2.0
chocolate crumb	470	9.0	64.0	21.0	45	260	3.0
pecan braid	410	6.0	48.0	22.0	5	230	2.0
strawberry citrus	310	6.0	37.0	16.0	10	270	1.0
pecan roll	620	9.0	74.0	35.0	45	270	2.0
pineapple upside-down mini Bundt	520	6.0	74.0	25.0	80	570	2.0
scone:							
blueberry, wild ..	410	6.0	63.0	15.0	60	360	2.0
cherry, tart	380	9.0	58.0	16.0	65	370	2.0
cinnamon chip ..	530	8.0	67.0	27.0	110	310	2.0
orange	460	8.0	65.0	24.0	110	290	1.0
drinks, frozen/iced, large size:							
I.C. caramel	720	6.0	102.0	30.0	90	200	0
I.C. mocha	700	8.0	111.0	29.0	80	150	3.0
iced chai latte	150	6.0	25.0	3.5	15	75	0
iced green tea	130	0	30.0	0	0	10	0
lemonade	130	1.0	31.0	0	0	10	0
mango passion fruit smoothie	360	1.0	92	.5	0	25	2.0
strawberry smoothie	290	1.0	62.0	1.5	5	230	5.0
drinks, hot/espresso:							
caffee latte	110	7.0	11.0	4.5	20	95	0
caffee mocha	410	10.0	61.0	17.0	45	140	2.0
cappuccino	110	7.0	11.0	4.5	20	95	0
caramel latte	430	9.0	53.0	18.0	55	180	0
chai tea latte .....,	190	7.0	31.0	4.0	15	85	0
hot chocolate	410	11.0	61.0	17.0	50	150	2.0

Food and Measure	cal.	prot. (gms)	carbo. (gms)	fat (gms)	chol. (mgs)	sod. (mgs)	fiber (gms)
Panini, frozen, 6 oz.:							
chicken:							
asiago (*Stouffer's Corner Bistro*) ..	460	21.0	45.0	22.0	45	930	7.0
basil (*Healthy Choice*)	310	25.0	41.0	5.0	15	600	5.0
club (*Lean Cuisine*)	320	24.0	34.0	9.0	35	880	3.0
grilled, Italian (*Stouffer's Corner Bistro*)	350	20.0	31.0	17.0	35	610	3.0
smoked (*Healthy Choice*)	310	25.0	42.0	4.5	10	580	5.0
Southwest (*Lean Cuisine*)	280	20.0	32.0	7.0	30	730	3.0
Southwest (*Stouffer's Corner Bistro*) ..	360	20.0	31.0	16.0	45	920	3.0
Tuscan (*Lean Cuisine*)	320	22.0	41.0	7.0	25	590	3.0
spinach, mushroom (*Lean Cuisine*) ..	280	21.0	32.0	8.0	25	690	5.0
Italian deli (*Stouffer's Corner Bistro*)	520	19.0	51.0	27.0	50	1100	4.0
Philly cheesesteak:							
(*Healthy Choice*) ..	310	24.0	43.0	4.5	10	600	6.0
(*Lean Cuisine*)	330	21.0	42.0	9.0	25	690	4.0
(*Stouffer's Corner Bistro*)	340	20.0	33.0	16.0	40	680	3.0
steak/cheddar/mushroom (*Lean Cuisine*)	330	21.0	33.0	9.0	35	730	3.0
tomato/basil/mozzarella (*Healthy Choice*) ..	310	23.0	42.0	4.5	10	600	6.0
turkey, smoked, club (*Stouffer's Corner Bistro*)	360	24.0	31.0	16.0	55	920	3.0
Panko crumbs:							
(*Ian's*), ¼ cup	70	2.0	15.0	0	0	32	.5
(*Roland*), ⅓ cup	80	2.0	15.0	0	0	75	0
Italian seasoned (*Ian's*), ¼ cup	70	2.0	15.0	0	0	137	2.0
Panko crumb coating mix (*McCormick Crusting Blends*), 1⅓ tbsp.:							
French onion/pepper/ herb	45	4.0	7.0	0	0	390	0
garlic/lemon/rosemary	45	3.0	7.0	0	0	400	0
Italian herb/cheese ...	40	3.0	5.0	1.0	5	390	0
Season-All	30	1.0	6.0	0	0	290	0

Food and Measure	cal.	prot. (gms)	carbo. (gms)	fat (gms)	chol. (mgs)	sod. (mgs)	fiber (gms)
Papa John's, ⅛ pie:							
original crust, 12":							
cheese	210	9.0	27.0	8.0	15	510	1.0
cheese, six	300	14.0	36.0	12.0	25	730	2.0
chicken, Hawaiian							
barbecue	240	11.0	33.0	8.0	20	690	1.0
chicken Alfredo ...	220	11.0	26.0	9.0	20	520	1.0
chicken and bacon,							
barbecue	240	11.0	32.0	8.0	20	690	1.0
garden fresh	200	8.0	28.0	7.0	10	490	2.0
Italian, spicy	260	11.0	27.0	8.0	20	680	2.0
Italian meats trio ..	250	12.0	27.0	8.0	25	740	2.0
the meats	240	11.0	27.0	11.0	20	640	1.0
meats, Tuscan	240	11.0	27.0	8.0	20	650	2.0
pepperoni	220	9.0	27.0	9.0	15	570	1.0
sausage	240	9.0	26.0	11.0	15	580	2.0
spinach Alfredo ...	200	8.0	26.0	8.0	15	450	1.0
spinach Alfredo							
chicken tomato .	210	10.0	27.0	8.0	20	490	2.0
the works	230	10.0	28.0	8.0	15	610	2.0
original crust, 14":							
cheese	300	13.0	39.0	11.0	20	750	2.0
cheese, six	320	15.0	38.0	13.0	25	780	2.0
chicken, Hawaiian							
barbecue	340	16.0	46.0	11.0	30	960	2.0
chicken Alfredo ...	310	15.0	36.0	12.0	30	720	2.0
chicken and bacon,							
barbecue	340	15.0	44.0	11.0	30	960	2.0
garden fresh	280	11.0	40.0	9.0	15	680	2.0
Italian, spicy	370	15.0	39.0	11.0	30	960	4.0
Italian meats trio ..	340	16.0	38.0	11.0	30	1030	2.0
the meats	350	15.0	38.0	16.0	30	920	2.0
meats, Tuscan	340	15.0	39.0	11.0	25	900	3.0
pepperoni	310	13.0	38.0	13.0	20	800	2.0
sausage	330	13.0	37.0	15.0	20	810	3.0
spinach Alfredo ...	280	11.0	36.0	11.0	20	630	2.0
spinach Alfredo							
chicken tomato .	290	13.0	37.0	11.0	25	670	2.0
the works	330	14.0	39.0	11.0	25	890	3.0
pan crust, 12":							
cheese	380	14.0	39.0	15.0	20	980	<1.0
cheese, six	400	16.0	40.0	21.0	25	1020	1.0
chicken, Hawaiian							
barbecue	420	16.0	46.0	16.0	30	1190	1.0

Food and Measure	cal.	prot. (gms)	carbo. (gms)	fat (gms)	chol. (mgs)	sod. (mgs)	fiber (gms)
Papa John's, pan crust *(cont.)*							
chicken Alfredo ...	380	15.0	36.0	16.0	30	950	2.0
chicken and bacon, barbecue	410	16.0	44.0	16.0	30	1190	1.0
garden fresh	360	12.0	40.0	13.0	15	910	2.0
Italian, spicy	450	16.0	39.0	15.0	30	1190	3.0
Italian meats trio ..	440	17.0	40.0	20.0	30	1300	2.0
the meats	420	16.0	38.0	19.0	30	1140	1.0
meats, Tuscan	430	16.0	40.0	11.0	25	1150	2.0
pepperoni	400	14.0	38.0	17.0	20	1050	1.0
sausage	410	13.0	38.0	19.0	20	1040	2.0
spinach Alfredo ...	360	12.0	36.0	15.0	20	860	1.0
spinach Alfredo chicken tomato .	380	14.0	37.0	16.0	25	910	2.0
the works	400	15.0	39.0	15.0	25	1100	2.0
thin crust, 14":							
cheese	240	10.0	22.0	13.0	20	500	1.0
cheese, six	250	12.0	21.0	14.0	25	570	1.0
chicken, Hawaiian barbecue	290	13.0	31.0	14.0	30	740	1.0
chicken Alfredo ...	240	12.0	20.0	13.0	30	470	1.0
chicken and bacon, barbecue	290	13.0	29.0	14.0	30	740	<1.0
garden fresh	210	8.0	23.0	11.0	15	430	2.0
Italian, spicy	320	12.0	24.0	14.0	30	740	3.0
Italian meats trio ..	280	13.0	22.0	12.0	30	820	2.0
the meats	300	13.0	23.0	18.0	30	700	2.0
meats, Tuscan	280	12.0	22.0	12.0	25	690	2.0
pepperoni	260	10.0	23.0	15.0	20	580	1.0
sausage	280	10.0	22.0	17.0	20	590	2.0
spinach Alfredo ...	220	8.0	19.0	13.0	20	370	1.0
spinach Alfredo chicken tomato .	230	10.0	21.0	13.0	25	430	1.0
the works	280	12.0	24.0	14.0	25	670	2.0
sides:							
breadstick, 1	140	4.0	26.0	2.0	0	260	1.0
breadstick, garlic Parmesan, 1	170	5.0	26.0	6.0	0	370	1.0
cheese sticks, 2 ...	370	15.0	42.0	16.0	25	830	2.0
chicken strips, 2 ..	160	10.0	10.0	8.0	25	350	0
wings, 2	160	14.0	1.0	11.0	90	680	<1.0
dipping sauce, 1 oz.:							
barbecue	40	0	11.0	0	0	240	0

Food and Measure	cal.	prot. (gms)	carbo. (gms)	fat (gms)	chol. (mgs)	sod. (mgs)	fiber (gms)
blue cheese	170	1.0	1.0	18.0	20	240	0
Buffalo	15	0	2.0	.5	0	890	0
cheese	70	1.0	1.0	6.0	0	150	0
garlic	150	0	0	17.0	0	310	0
honey mustard . .	150	0	5.0	15.0	10	120	0
pizza	20	0	3.0	0	0	140	0
ranch	110	1.0	1.0	11.0	10	250	0
desserts:							
sweetreat, ½ pie:							
apple twist	350	6.0	54.0	9.0	0	550	1.0
cinna swirl	390	6.0	53.0	14.0	0	580	1.0
sweetsticks, 4 pcs.:							
caramel	520	12.0	91.0	12.0	5	730	3.0
cinnamon	570	12.0	98.0	15.0	0	750	3.0
Papadum chips (*Baji Natural*), 1 oz.:							
cilantro, tangy	120	4.0	17.0	4.5	0	410	1.0
mango chutney	120	4.0	18.0	4.5	0	380	1.0
tandoori	120	4.0	17.0	4.5	0	450	1.0
yogurt dill, creamy . . .	120	4.0	17.0	4.5	0	460	1.0
Papaya, fresh:							
(*Frieda's* Golden Sunrise/Mexican), 1 cup, 5 oz.	50	1.0	14.0	0	0	0	3.0
1 lb., 3½" x 5⅛"	117	1.9	29.8	.4	0	8	5.5
cubed, 1 cup	55	.9	13.7	.2	0	4	2.5
mashed, 1 cup	90	1.4	22.6	.3	0	7	4.1
Papaya, can/jar:							
in extra light syrup (*SunFresh*), ½ cup .	70	1.0	17.0	0	0	5	1.0
in light syrup, chunks (*Roland*), ½ cup . .	70	0	18.0	0	0	10	0
in heavy syrup, chunks (*Vigo*), ⅕ of 18-oz. can	220	0	57.0	0	0	10	1.0
Papaya, dried, spears (*Tree of Life*), 1.2 oz.	38	1.0	10.0	0	0	3	2.0
Papaya drink (*Lincoln* Punch), 8 fl. oz. . .	130	0	32.0	0	0	75	0
Papaya juice, 8 fl. oz.:							
(*Ceres*)	120	0	31.0	0	0	15	0
(*L&A* Delight)	130	1.0	32.0	0	0	10	1.0
(*R.W. Knudsen* Nectar)	130	<1.0	31.0	0	0	35	0
creamed (*R.W. Knudsen*)	40	<1.0	10.0	0	0	10	2.0

Food and Measure	cal.	prot. (gms)	carbo. (gms)	fat (gms)	chol. (mgs)	sod. (mgs)	fiber (gms)
Papaya nectar:							
(*Goya*), 12 fl. oz.	220	0	56.0	0	0	25	1.0
canned, 8 fl. oz.	143	.4	36.3	.4	0	12	1.5
Paprika, 1 tsp.	6	.3	1.2	.3	0	1	.6
Parmesan-herb seasoning (*McCormick* Blends), ½ tsp.	5	0	0	0	0	55	0
Parsley, fresh:							
10 sprigs	4	.3	.6	.1	0	6	.3
chopped, ½ cup	11	.9	1.9	.2	0	17	1.0
Parsley, dried:							
1 tsp.	1	.1	.2	.1	0	1	.2
freeze-dried, 1 tbsp. ...	1	.1	.2	<.1	0	2	.2
Parsley root:							
(*Frieda's*), ⅔ cup, 3 oz.	10	2.0	2.0	.5	0	70	1.0
1 oz.	3	.8	.7	.2	0	28	.4
Parsnip:							
raw, sliced:							
(*Frieda's*), 1 cup ...	100	2.0	24.0	0	0	10	7.0
½ cup	50	.8	12.1	.2	0	7	3.3
boiled, drained:							
1 medium, 9"	130	2.1	31.3	.5	0	17	6.4
sliced, ½ cup	63	1.0	15.2	.2	0	8	3.1
Parsnip chips, 1 oz.:							
(*Terra*)	150	2.0	13.0	10.0	0	50	5.0
(*Trader Joe's* Lightly Salted)	150	2.0	13.0	10.0	0	50	5.0
Passion fruit, fresh:							
(*Frieda's*), 5 oz.	140	3.0	33.0	1.0	0	40	15.0
purple, 1 medium ...	18	.4	4.2	.1	0	5	1.9
purple, trimmed, ½ cup	115	.3	27.5	.8	0	33	12.2
Passion fruit juice, 8 fl. oz.:							
(*Ceres*)	130	0	32.0	0	0	15	0
fresh, purple	126	1.0	33.6	.1	0	15	.5
fresh, yellow	148	1.7	35.7	.4	0	15	.5
Passion fruit juice blend, apple and carrot (*Bolthouse Farms*), 8 fl. oz. ...	120	2.0	29.0	0	0	95	2.0
Passion fruit nectar (*Goya*), 12 fl. oz. ..	230	0	57.0	0	0	5	0

Food and Measure	cal.	prot. (gms)	carbo. (gms)	fat (gms)	chol. (mgs)	sod. (mgs)	fiber (gms)
Pasta (see also "Macaroni" and "Noodles"), dry, 2 oz., except as noted:							
plain	211	7.3	42.6	.9	0	4	1.4
all styles:							
(*Alessi*)	210	6.0	44.0	1.0	0	0	2.0
(*Delverde*)	200	7.0	41.0	.5	0	0	1.0
alphabets, vegetable							
(*Eden* Organic)	210	9.0	40.0	2.0	0	20	4.0
angel hair:							
(*DeBoles* Natural) ..	210	7.0	41.0	1.0	0	0	1.0
(*DeBoles* Organic) .	210	7.0	43.0	1.0	0	5	1.0
garlic parsley							
(*DeBoles* Natural)	210	7.0	41.0	1.0	0	5	2.0
garlic parsley							
(*DeBoles* Organic)	210	7.0	42.0	1.0	0	15	2.0
tomato basil							
(*DeBoles* Natural)	210	7.0	41.0	1.0	0	0	1.0
tomato basil							
(*DeBoles* Organic)	210	7.0	43.0	1.0	0	5	2.0
tomato pesto							
(*DeBoles* Organic)	210	7.0	42.0	1.0	0	10	1.0
whole wheat							
(*Hodgson Mill*) .	210	9.0	41.0	1.0	0	10	6.0
whole wheat, w/flax							
(*DeBoles*)	190	6.0	38.0	1.5	0	0	6.0
bows or wheels, whole wheat (*Hodgson Mill* Veggie*)	190	8.0	40.0	1.0	0	15	6.0
corn:							
angel hair (*Westbrae Natural*)	210	4.0	46.0	1.5	0	15	0
elbow or spaghetti (*DeBoles*)	200	4.0	43.0	2.0	0	15	5.0
ditalini, kamut (*Eden* Organic)	210	10.0	38.0	1.5	0	0	6.0
elbows:							
(*DeBoles* Organic) .	210	7.0	43.0	1.0	0	5	1.0
kamut whole grain (*Eden* Organic), ½ cup	210	10.0	38.0	1.5	0	0	6.0
whole wheat (*Hodgson Mill*) .	210	9.0	41.0	1.0	0	10	6.0

Food and Measure	cal.	prot. (gms)	carbo. (gms)	fat (gms)	chol. (mgs)	sod. (mgs)	fiber (gms)
Pasta *(cont.)*							
fettuccine:							
(*DeBoles* Natural) ..	210	7.0	41.0	1.0	0	0	1.0
(*DeBoles* Organic) .	210	7.0	43.0	1.0	0	5	1.0
basil (*al dente* Carba-Nada)	140	12.0	24.0	1.0	10	20	6.0
basil, fiesta, garlic parsley, lemon chive, or peppercorn (*al dente*) ..	210	8.0	42.0	1.0	15	15	2.0
egg (*al dente*)	210	8.0	41.0	1.5	30	10	2.0
egg, lemon pepper or garlic (*al dente* Carba-Nada)	140	12.0	24.0	1.0	15	20	6.0
spinach (*al dente*) .	210	8.0	41.0	1.0	10	20	2.0
spinach (*DeBoles* Organic)	210	7.0	43.0	1.0	0	20	3.0
whole wheat (*Hodgson Mill*) .	210	9.0	41.0	1.0	0	10	6.0
whole wheat blend plus flax (*al dente*)	190	7.0	34.0	2.5	10	5	6.0
gemelli:							
(*Eden* Organic Twisted Pair) ...	210	8.0	40.0	2.0	0	0	5.0
spelt and buckwheat (*Eden* Organic) ..	210	6.0	41.0	2.0	0	15	4.0
kuzu (*Eden* Organic) .	200	0	48.0	0	0	0	2.0
lasagna:							
(*DeBoles* Organic), 2.5 oz., ¼ pkg...	260	9.0	54.0	1.0	0	5	1.0
(*Vigo*)	200	6.0	42.0	1.0	0	0	2.0
precooked (*Vigo*), 3 pcs.	200	8.0	40.0	.5	0	0	2.0
whole wheat (*Hodgson Mill*) .	210	9.0	41.0	1.0	0	10	6.0
lentil bean (*Papadini's* Hi-Protein)	190	13.0	33.0	1.0	0	34	5.0
linguine:							
(*DeBoles* Natural) ..	210	7.0	41.0	1.0	0	0	1.0
(*DeBoles* Organic) .	210	7.0	43.0	1.0	0	5	1.0
roasted garlic or spicy sesame (*al dente*)	210	8.0	42.0	1.0	15	15	2.0

Food and Measure	cal.	prot. (gms)	carbo. (gms)	fat (gms)	chol. (mgs)	sod. (mgs)	fiber (gms)
mung bean (*Eden* Harusame)	190	0	47.0	0	0	5	0
orzo, ⅓ cup:							
(*RiceSelect* Original)	210	7.0	42.0	1.0	0	0	2.0
tri-color (*RiceSelect*)	210	7.0	42.0	1.0	0	20	2.0
whole wheat (*RiceSelect*)	195	7.0	39.0	1.0	0	0	9.0
penne:							
ancient grain (*DeBoles* Organic)	200	7.0	41.0	1.0	0	0	5.0
whole wheat (*Hodgson Mill*) .	210	9.0	40.0	1.0	0	10	6.0
radiatore, whole wheat:							
(*Hodgson Mill*) ...	210	9.0	34.0	1.0	0	10	6.0
or rotini (*Hodgson Mill* Veggie)	210	9.0	41.0	1.0	0	15	6.0
ribbons:							
artichoke (*Eden* Organic)	210	9.0	40.0	1.5	0	10	2.0
eggless (*DeBoles* Organic)	210	7.0	43.0	1.0	0	5	1.0
parsley garlic or saffron (*Eden* Organic)	210	9.0	40.0	1.5	0	0	3.0
spinach (*Eden* Organic)	210	8.0	41.0	1.0	0	30	5.0
vegetable (*Eden* Organic)	210	9.0	40.0	1.5	0	35	3.0
yolkless, whole wheat (*Hodgson Mill*) .	210	10.0	34.0	1.0	0	15	5.0
rice:							
(*Eden* Bifun)	200	5.0	44.0	.5	0	5	0
all styles (*Lundberg* Organic)	210	4.0	44.0	2.0	0	5	3.0
all styles, except lasagna (*DeBoles*)	210	4.0	46.0	.5	0	15	<1.0
lasagna (*DeBoles* Oven Ready), 2.5 oz.	260	5.0	56.0	.5	0	15	1.0
rigatoni, kamut and buckwheat (*Eden* Organic)	200	9.0	39.0	1.5	0	10	5.0
shells:							
(*DeBoles* Organic) .	210	7.0	43.0	1.0	0	5	1.0

Food and Measure	cal.	prot. (gms)	carbo. (gms)	fat (gms)	chol. (mgs)	sod. (mgs)	fiber (gms)
Pasta, shells *(cont.)*							
mini rainbow *(Rice-Select)*, ¼ cup ..	195	7.0	39.0	0	0	8	2.0
vegetable, small *(Eden* Organic) ..	210	9.0	40.0	2.0	0	20	4.0
whole wheat *(Hodgson Mill)* .	210	9.0	40.0	1.0	0	10	6.0
spaghetti:							
(DeBoles Natural) ..	210	7.0	41.0	1.0	0	0	1.0
(DeBoles Organic) .	210	7.0	43.0	1.0	0	5	1.0
kamut *(Eden* Organic)	210	10.0	38.0	1.5	0	0	6.0
parsley garlic *(Eden* Organic)	210	8.0	41.0	1.0	0	0	5.0
spinach *(DeBoles* Organic)	210	7.0	43.0	1.0	0	20	3.0
spaghetti, whole wheat:							
(Eden Organic 100% Whole Grain) ...	210	10.0	40.0	1.5	0	0	6.0
(Hodgson Mill) ...	210	9.0	41.0	1.0	0	10	6.0
spinach *(Hodgson Mill)*	210	9.0	41.0	1.0	0	25	5.0
thin *(Hodgson Mill)*	210	9.0	40.0	1.0	0	10	6.0
spelt:							
ribbons, spaghetti, or ziti rigati *(Eden* Organic) ..	210	7.0	41.0	2.0	0	10	5.0
white, all styles, except spaghetti *(VitaSpelt* Organic)	210	9.0	42.0	.5	0	0	2.0
white, spaghetti *(VitaSpelt* Organic)	190	8.0	42.0	1.0	0	0	5.0
whole grain, all styles *(VitaSpelt* Organic)	190	8.0	40.0	1.5	0	0	5.0
spirals:							
flax rice *(Eden* Organic)	200	9.0	40.0	2.0	0	10	4.0
kamut *(Eden* Organic)	210	10.0	38.0	1.5	0	0	6.0
kamut vegetable *(Eden* Organic) ..	210	8.0	40.0	2.0	0	45	6.0
rye *(Eden* Organic) .	200	6.0	44.0	0	0	10	8.0
spinach *(Eden* Organic)	210	8.0	41.0	1.0	0	30	5.0

Food and Measure	cal.	prot. (gms)	carbo. (gms)	fat (gms)	chol. (mgs)	sod. (mgs)	fiber (gms)
vegetable (*Eden* Organic)	200	8.0	40.0	1.0	0	15	2.0
whole wheat:							
all styles, except angel hair (*DeBoles* Organic)	210	7.0	42.0	1.5	0	10	5.0
w/flax seed, all styles (*Hodgson Mills* Organic)	200	9.0	40.0	2.0	0	10	6.0
Pasta, cooked (see also "Macaroni"):							
corn, 1 cup	176	3.7	39.1	1.0	0	1	3.4
spaghetti, 1 cup:							
plain	197	6.7	39.7	.9	0	1	2.4
protein fortified ...	230	11.3	44.3	.3	0	7	2.4
spinach	182	6.4	36.6	.9	0	20	n.a.
whole wheat	174	7.5	37.2	.6	0	4	6.3
Pasta, refrigerated (see also specific pastas) plain:							
uncooked:							
w/egg, 2 oz.	163	6.4	31.0	1.3	41	15	2.0
spinach, w/egg, 2 oz.	164	6.4	31.6	1.2	41	15	n.a.
cooked, 4 oz.:							
w/egg	149	5.8	28.3	1.2	37	7	n.a.
spinach, w/egg	147	5.7	28.4	1.1	37	7	n.a.
Pasta dish, frozen (see also "Pasta entree, frozen" and specific pastas), 1 cup cooked, except as noted:							
broccoli, Alfredo sauce (*Green Giant*)	210	9.0	34.0	4.0	<5	780	3.0
broccoli, carrots:							
cheese sauce (*Green Giant*)	200	8.0	35.0	4.0	5	950	3.0
sugar snap peas, garlic sauce (*Green Giant*) ...	200	6.0	36.0	4.0	5	760	3.0
vegetables, cheese sauce (*Birds Eye*), 1 cup	170	7.0	27.0	4.0	0	380	1.0

Food and Measure	cal.	prot. (gms)	carbo. (gms)	fat (gms)	chol. (mgs)	sod. (mgs)	fiber (gms)
Pasta dish mix (see also "Pasta salad mix" and specific pastas), 1 cup*, except as noted:							
Alfredo:							
(*Zatarain's* Dinner Mix)	140	5.0	22.0	3.5	5	680	0
whole wheat (*Annie's D.W.*), 2.5 oz. . . .	260	10.0	48.0	3.5	10	550	5.0
butter and:							
herb (*Annie's* Organic)	290	11.0	43.0	9.0	25	770	2.0
herb (*Pasta Roni* Italiano)	300	9.0	40.0	12.0	5	860	2.0
garlic (*Pasta Roni*) .	250	8.0	39.0	8.0	5	760	2.0
cheddar broccoli:							
(*Knorr Lipton Pasta Sides*), ½ of 4.8-oz. pkg.	250	9.0	48.0	2.0	5	810	2.0
white (*Pasta Roni*) .	300	9.0	38.0	13.0	5	770	2.0
and cheese:							
(*Annie's Bunny Pasta with Yummy Cheese*), 2.5 oz. .	270	10.0	48.0	4.5	10	550	1.0
nacho (*Knorr Lipton Fiesta Sides*), ¾ cup	230	8.0	44.0	2.5	<5	690	1.0
Parmesan (*Annie's Organic Peace Pasta*), 2.5 oz. . .	260	11.0	47.0	3.5	10	600	1.0
chicken:							
(*Pasta Roni*)	300	9.0	39.0	12.0	5	1060	2.0
Asian garlic (*Pasta Roni*)	280	7.0	39.0	11.0	0	1100	2.0
quesadilla (*Pasta Roni*)	310	10.0	40.0	13.0	5	860	2.0
garlic:							
Alfredo (*Pasta Roni*)	350	11.0	48.0	13.0	10	1100	2.0
creamy (*Pasta Roni*)	330	9.0	39.0	16.0	5	880	2.0
gumbo (*Zatarain's* Dinner Mix)	120	4.0	23.0	.5	0	690	2.0
jalapeño Jack (*Knorr Lipton Fiesta Sides*), ¾ cup	230	8.0	44.0	2.5	<5	510	2.0

Food and Measure	cal.	prot. (gms)	carbo. (gms)	fat (gms)	chol. (mgs)	sod. (mgs)	fiber (gms)
mushrooms in sauce							
(*Pasta Roni Nature's Way*)	280	9.0	39.0	10.0	5	710	2.0
olive oil and Italian herbs (*Pasta Roni Nature's Way*)	250	8.0	38.0	8.0	5	800	2.0
Parmesan, creamy (*Pasta Roni Nature's Way* Parmesano) ..	280	9.0	41.0	9.0	5	580	2.0
scampi (*Zatarain's* Dinner Mix)	110	4.0	21.0	.5	0	470	1.0
sour cream and chive (*Pasta Roni*)	310	8.0	38.0	15.0	5	880	2.0
Stroganoff (*Pasta Roni*)	350	9.0	47.0	15.0	0	1020	2.0
tomato Parmesan:							
(*Knorr Lipton Italian Sides*), ¾ cup ..	240	9.0	41.0	4.5	5	750	2.0
(*Pasta Roni*)	270	9.0	40.0	9.0	5	930	2.0
Pasta entree, can or pkg. (see also "Pasta entree, microwave" and specific pastas), 1 cup, except as noted:							
(*SpaghettiOs*)	180	6.0	37.0	1.0	5	630	3.0
(*SpaghettiOs* A to Z's)	180	6.0	36.0	1.0	<5	880	3.0
(*SpaghettiOs* Plus Calcium)	170	6.0	35.0	1.0	5	620	3.0
cheese, nacho (*Chef Boyardee Twistaroni*)	220	8.0	32.0	7.0	15	950	2.0
chili cheese (*Chef Boyardee Twistaroni*)	220	9.0	32.0	6.0	15	950	2.0
w/franks:							
(*SpaghettiOs*)	230	9.0	27.0	10.0	20	930	5.0
(*SpaghettiOs* A to Z's)	220	9.0	32.0	6.0	20	990	2.0
meat sauce (*SpaghettiOs*)	180	8.0	32.0	2.0	10	890	3.0
w/meatballs:							
(*Chef Boyardee* Mini Bites Rings)	240	9.0	30.0	9.0	20	940	2.0
(*SpaghettiOs*)	240	11.0	32.0	8.0	15	660	4.0
(*SpaghettiOs* A to Z's)	260	11.0	33.0	9.0	20	990	3.0
(*SpaghettiOs Cars*) .	240	11.0	32.0	8.0	15	890	3.0

Food and Measure	cal.	prot. (gms)	carbo. (gms)	fat (gms)	chol. (mgs)	sod. (mgs)	fiber (gms)
Pasta entree, can or pkg. *(cont.)*							
tomato and beef							
(*Chef Boyardee*							
Twistaroni)	230	8.0	38.0	5.0	10	850	2.0
tomato cheese sauce:							
(*Annie's All Stars/							
BernieO's* Organic)	150	4.0	31.0	1.0	0	680	<1.0
(*Annie's Arthur							
Loops* Organic) .	150	5.0	32.0	1.0	0	670	1.0
w/soy "meatballs"							
(*Annie's P'Sghetti							
Loops* Organic) .	190	9.0	29.0	4.0	0	650	2.0
Stroganoff, creamy,							
w/beef, ⅕ pkg.:							
(*Banquet Homestyle							
Bakes*)	310	12.0	28.0	17.0	25	980	2.0
(*Betty Crocker							
Complete Meals*)	200	10.0	30.0	4.5	15	760	1.0
Pasta entree, frozen/ refrigerated (see also "Pasta dish, frozen" and specific pastas), 1 pkg., except as noted:							
and beans (*Moosewood* Organic Pasta e Fagioli), 10 oz.	230	9.0	39.0	3.0	0	180	6.0
broccoli, Parmesan (*Moosewood* Organic), 10 oz.	380	14.0	52.0	13.0	30	380	4.0
cheese, four (*Shedd's Country Crock*), 1 cup	380	15.0	41.0	17.0	40	1060	2.0
w/chicken, see "chicken entree, frozen"							
w/pesto (*Ethnic Gourmet Trofie*), 10 oz.	550	15.0	49.0	33.0	5	800	5.0
primavera:							
(*Smart Ones*), 9 oz.	280	12.0	44.0	6.0	10	700	6.0
Parmesan (*Michelina's Budget Gourmet*), 8 oz.	280	10.0	47.0	4.5	10	480	3.0
tomato sauce, chunky (*Shedd's Spread Country Crock*), 1 cup	320	9.0	40.0	13.0	5	710	4.0

Food and Measure	cal.	prot. (gms)	carbo. (gms)	fat (gms)	chol. (mgs)	sod. (mgs)	fiber (gms)
wheels/cheese (Michelina's Budget Gourmet/ Zap'ems), 8 oz. ...	350	13.0	48.0	11.0	20	780	2.0
Pasta entree, microwave, 1 cont.:							
Alfredo (Bowl Appetit!)	360	13.0	53.0	11.0	15	850	1.0
cheddar broccoli (Bowl Appetit!)	330	11.0	49.0	11.0	10	1000	2.0
chicken flavor (Bowl Appetit!)	260	9.0	42.0	6.0	10	790	2.0
garden salsa (Hormel Pasta Cup)	120	5.0	23.0	.5	0	650	2.0
garlic Parmesan (Bowl Appetit!)	320	11.0	50.0	9.0	10	1010	1.0
Italian style (Hormel Pasta Cup)	210	7.0	25.0	10.0	10	1500	1.0
lemon pepper (Hormel Pasta Cup)	240	9.0	25.0	10.0	35	1220	2.0
Pasta flour, see "Semolina flour"							
Pasta salad mix:							
(Suddenly Salad Classic), 1 cup* ...	240	6.0	37.0	8.0	0	830	2.0
Caesar:							
(Kraft Pasta Salad), ¼ pkg.	190	7.0	36.0	2.0	5	520	2.0
(Suddenly Salad), 1 cup*	250	6.0	34.0	10.0	0	620	1.0
chipotle ranch (Suddenly Salad), ⅔ cup*	260	6.0	29.0	14.0	0	470	1.0
garlic Parmesan (Kraft Pasta Salad), ¼ pkg.	180	7.0	34.0	1.5	5	450	2.0
Italian:							
(Kraft Pasta Salad), ¼ pkg.	160	7.0	31.0	1.5	0	330	2.0
creamy (Suddenly Salad), ¾ cup* .	320	7.0	33.0	19.0	15	530	2.0
Parmesan, creamy (Suddenly Salad), 1 cup*	370	6.0	32.0	25.0	20	460	2.0
ranch:							
(Kraft Pasta Salad Gourmet Favorites Santa Fe), ⅕ pkg.	130	5.0	25.0	1.0	0	290	2.0

Food and Measure	cal.	prot. (gms)	carbo. (gms)	fat (gms)	chol. (mgs)	sod. (mgs)	fiber (gms)
Pasta salad mix, ranch *(cont.)*							
bacon (*Kraft Pasta Salad* Classic), ¼ pkg.	170	7.0	34.0	1.0	0	310	2.0
bacon (*Suddenly Salad*), ¾ cup* .	330	7.0	31.0	20.0	15	490	1.0
tuna (*Kraft Pasta Salad*), ⅛ pkg. . .	300	9.0	27.0	18.0	15	410	1.0
Pasta sauce (see also specific sauces), tomato, ½ cup, except as noted:							
(*Eden* Organic)	80	3.0	12.0	2.5	0	320	3.0
(*Eden* Organic Pizza/ Pasta)	65	2.0	9.0	2.5	0	300	5.0
(*Emeril's* Kicked Up) .	70	1.0	9.0	3.0	0	400	2.0
(*Emeril's* Sicilian Gravy)	90	1.0	10.0	5.0	0	520	1.0
(*Furmano's* Spaghetti)	50	2.0	9.0	1.0	0	440	2.0
(*Hunt's* Italian)	50	2.0	11.0	1.0	0	560	3.0
(*Hunt's* No Sugar) . . .	35	1.0	6.0	0	0	580	2.0
(*Hunt's* Traditional) . .	50	2.0	10.0	0	0	560	3.0
(*Newman's Own* Socka- rooni)	70	2.0	12.0	2.0	0	520	<1.0
(*Prego* Chunky Garden Combo)	70	2.0	13.0	1.5	0	470	3.0
(*Prego* Traditional) . . .	80	2.0	13.0	3.0	0	580	3.0
(*Prego* Traditional Heart Smart)	100	2.0	15.0	3.0	0	430	3.0
arrabiata:							
(*Cucina Antica*) . . .	45	1.0	6.0	2.0	0	239	1.0
(*Delallo*)	120	1.0	6.0	11.0	0	510	2.0
(*Mama Capri*)	80	3.0	6.0	5.0	0	650	2.0
(*Seeds of Change* di Roma)	80	1.0	6.0	6.0	0	370	2.0
artichoke hearts and asiago (*Mom's*) . . .	90	3.0	7.0	6.0	5	410	3.0
arugula, baby (*Cucina Antica*)	38	1.0	4.0	2.0	0	230	1.0
balsamic and onion (*Seeds of Change* Modena Organic) . .	80	1.0	7.0	5.0	0	330	2.0
basil, sweet (*Classico* Traditional)	80	2.0	15.0	1.5	0	500	3.0

Food and Measure	cal.	prot. (gms)	carbo. (gms)	fat (gms)	chol. (mgs)	sod. (mgs)	fiber (gms)
basil, tomato and:							
(*Amy's* Organic) ...	110	2.0	11.0	6.0	0	580	3.0
(*Bertolli*)	80	2.0	13.0	2.0	0	520	3.0
(*Classico*)	60	2.0	11.0	1.0	0	310	2.0
(*Cucina Antica*) ...	35	1.0	4.0	2.0	0	246	1.0
(*Del Monte*)	70	2.0	16.0	1.0	0	600	3.0
(*Delallo*)	120	1.0	5.0	11.0	0	510	2.0
(*Muir Glen* Organic)	60	2.0	12.0	1.0	0	370	2.0
(*Newman's Own* Bombolina)	90	2.0	13.0	4.5	0	620	<1.0
(*Newman's Own* Organic)	90	2.0	12.0	4.5	0	650	<1.0
(*Prego* Organic) ...	80	2.0	13.0	2.5	0	470	4.0
(*Seeds of Change* Organic Genovese)	60	2.0	9.0	3.5	0	360	2.0
spicy (*Classico*) ...	90	2.0	12.0	3.5	0	490	3.0
basil and garlic:							
(*Mama Capri*)	90	1.0	5.0	7.0	0	450	2.0
(*Prego*)	80	2.0	12.0	2.5	0	420	3.0
w/cheese:							
5 (*Newman's Own*)	80	3.0	10.0	3.0	5	610	<1.0
5 (*Classico*)	90	3.0	11.0	3.5	0	490	3.0
4 (*Del Monte*)	70	2.0	15.0	1.5	0	680	3.0
4 (*Hunt's*)	50	3.0	10.0	1.0	0	580	3.0
4 (*Muir Glen* Organic)	80	4.0	1.0	3.0	5	380	2.0
3 (*Prego*)	80	3.0	14.0	1.5	<5	430	3.0
3 (*Seeds of Change* Organic Romagna)	90	4.0	9.0	5.0	5	460	2.0
w/cheese and garlic (*Hunt's*)	50	3.0	9.0	1.0	0	600	2.0
eggplant, spicy (*Seeds of Change* Sicilian Organic)	90	2.0	10.0	6.0	0	540	3.0
garlic, roasted:							
(*Amy's* Organic) ...	130	2.0	13.0	8.0	0	470	3.0
(*Barilla*)	70	2.0	12.0	1.0	0	510	2.0
(*Classico*)	60	2.0	11.0	1.0	0	220	2.0
(*Delallo*)	90	1.0	7.0	7.0	0	300	2.0
(*Emeril's* Gaaahlic) .	70	2.0	9.0	3.0	0	480	2.0
(*Monique's*)	80	2.0	10.0	3.5	0	340	2.0
(*Muir Glen* Organic Garlic)	60	2.0	12.0	1.0	0	380	2.0
(*Newman's Own*) ..	70	2.0	11.0	2.5	0	580	<1.0
and herb (*Prego*) ..	90	2.0	13.0	3.5	0	560	3.0

Food and Measure	cal.	prot. (gms)	carbo. (gms)	fat (gms)	chol. (mgs)	sod. (mgs)	fiber (gms)
Pasta sauce, garlic, roasted *(cont.)*							
Parmesan (*Prego*)	70	3.0	13.0	1.0	5	480	3.0
and peppers (*Newman's Own*)	70	2.0	11.0	2.5	0	460	4.0
tomato and (*Newman's Own*)	70	2.0	11.0	2.5	0	580	<1.0
garlic, tomato and *Seeds of Change* Tuscan Organic)	60	2.0	77.0	2.5	0	650	2.0
garlic and:							
basil (*Mom's*)	70	2.0	7.0	3.0	0	380	2.0
basil (*Rising Moon Organics*)	60	2.0	9.0	2.5	0	400	2.0
chanterelles (*Rising Moon Organics*)	45	2.0	10.0	0	0	440	2.0
herb (*Del Monte*)	60	2.0	11.0	1.5	0	490	<1.0
herb (*Hunt's*)	40	2.0	8.0	1.0	0	610	3.0
Merlot (*Rising Moon Organics*)	45	2.0	9.0	0	0	400	2.0
mushroom (*Amy's* Organic)	120	3.0	10.0	7.0	5	680	3.0
onion (*Del Monte*)	80	2.0	16.0	1.0	0	490	2.0
onion (*Hunt's*)	50	2.0	10.0	0	0	470	3.0
green pepper/mushroom (*Del Monte*)	80	2.0	16.0	1.0	0	490	3.0
herb:							
(*Newman's Own* Organic)	90	2.0	13.0	4.0	0	660	<1.0
Italian (*Del Monte* Chunky)	60	2.0	12.0	1.0	0	520	<1.0
Italian (*Muir Glen* Organic)	60	2.0	11.0	1.0	0	350	2.0
7 (*Ragú Robusto*)	80	2.0	12.0	3.5	0	550	2.0
tomato and (*Muir Glen* Organic Chunky)	60	2.0	11.0	1.0	0	350	2.0
hot and spicy (*Newman's Own* Fra Diavolo)	70	0	10.0	3.0	0	510	3.0
leek and tomato (*Monique's*)	90	3.0	10.0	4.0	0	360	2.0
marinara:							
(*Alessi* Smooth/ Chunky)	100	2.0	6.0	9.0	0	420	2.0

Food and Measure	cal.	prot. (gms)	carbo. (gms)	fat (gms)	chol. (mgs)	sod. (mgs)	fiber (gms)
(*Amy's* Organic Family)	80	1.0	10.0	3.0	0	590	3.0
(*Amy's* Organic Light Sodium)	40	1.0	7.0	1.0	0	100	1.0
(*Barilla*)	70	2.0	12.0	1.5	0	460	2.0
(*Delallo*)	120	1.0	5.0	11.0	0	510	2.0
(*Emeril's*)	90	2.0	11.0	4.0	0	700	3.0
(*Mama Capri*)	120	2.0	5.0	10.0	0	440	2.0
(*Monique's*)	80	2.0	10.0	3.5	0	340	2.0
(*Newman's Own*) . .	70	2.0	12.0	2.0	0	510	<1.0
(*Newman's Own* Organic)	70	2.0	12.0	2.0	0	550	<1.0
(*Prego*)	100	2.0	11.0	5.0	0	550	4.0
(*Seeds of Change* di Venezia Organic)	60	1.0	6.0	3.5	0	380	2.0
Cabernet (*Muir Glen* Organic)	60	2.0	11.0	1.0	0	360	2.0
Cabernet (*Newman's Own*)	70	2.0	10.0	3.0	0	590	<1.0
eggplant (*Cucina Antica*)	35	1.0	4.0	2.0	0	246	1.0
garlic (*Cucina Antica*)	36	1.0	4.0	2.0	0	246	1.0
garlic basil (*Frutti Di Bosco*)	60	2.0	10.0	2.5	0	310	2.0
mushroom (*Newman's Own*)	70	2.0	12.0	2.0	0	520	<1.0
roasted red pepper (*Cucina Antica*) .	40	1.0	6.0	2.0	0	248	1.0
meat:							
(*Chef Boyardee*) . . .	80	3.0	10.0	3.5	5	750	2.0
(*Del Monte*)	60	3.0	14.0	1.0	2	720	3.0
(*Hunt's*)	60	3.0	11.0	1.0	0	610	3.0
(*Prego*)	130	2.0	19.0	5.0	5	570	3.0
meatball, mini (*Prego*)	110	4.0	13.0	5.0	5	650	3.0
Merlot (*Vino de Milo* Tuscan), 4 oz.	35	1.0	7.0	.5	0	270	2.0
mushroom:							
(*Del Monte*)	60	2.0	14.0	.5	0	630	2.0
(*Hunt's*)	45	2.0	10.0	.5	0	590	3.0
(*Prego* Chunky Garden Supreme)	90	2.0	13.0	3.0	0	510	3.0
(*Prego* Fresh)	90	2.0	14.0	3.0	0	550	3.0
(*Prego* Heart Smart)	100	2.0	15.0	3.0	0	410	3.0
(*Prego* Organic) . . .	70	2.0	13.0	2.5	0	470	4.0

Food and Measure	cal.	prot. (gms)	carbo. (gms)	fat (gms)	chol. (mgs)	sod. (mgs)	fiber (gms)
Pasta sauce, mushroom *(cont.)*							
porcini (*Delallo*) . . .	140	1.0	10.0	11.0	0	530	2.0
porcini (*Seeds of Change* di Apennine Organic) . . .	60	1.0	6.0	4.5	0	370	2.0
portobello (*Muir Glen* Organic) . . .	50	2.0	10.0	0	0	350	2.0
portobello shiraz (*Vino de Milo*), 4 oz.	40	2.0	8.0	.5	0	320	2.0
triple (*Classico*) . . .	80	3.0	12.0	2.0	0	390	3.0
mushroom and:							
garlic (*Prego*)	80	2.0	13.0	2.5	0	470	3.0
green pepper (*Prego* Chunky Garden) .	90	2.0	13.0	3.0	0	470	3.0
onion (*Emeril's*) . . .	100	1.0	11.0	6.0	0	640	1.0
ripe olives (*Classico*)	60	2.0	1..0	1.0	0	390	2.0
olive and caper (*Monique's*)	80	2.0	9.0	4.0	0	410	2.0
olive oil and garlic (*Bertolli*)	90	3.0	14.0	3.0	0	500	3.0
onion and garlic:							
(*Newman's Own*) . .	60	2.0	12.0	1.5	0	530	<1.0
(*Prego*)	100	2.0	12.0	4.5	0	480	3.0
(*Prego* Chunky Garden)	90	2.0	13.0	3.0	0	470	3.0
caramelized, roasted garlic (*Classico*) .	90	2.0	13.0	3.5	0	480	3.0
and garlic (*Tree of Life* Fat Free) . . .	40	2.0	8.0	0	0	260	<1.0
pepper, red:							
roasted (*Emeril's*) . .	60	1.0	7.0	3.0	0	390	2.0
roasted, and garlic (*Prego*)	90	2.0	13.0	3.5	0	530	3.0
spicy (*Classico*) . . .	60	2.0	7.0	1.5	0	300	2.0
w/pesto (*Delallo* Pomadoro)	150	4.0	6.0	12.0	10	310	1.0
pesto, tomato and:							
(*Newman's Own*) . .	80	2.0	10.0	4.0	0	640	<1.0
spicy (*Classico*) . . .	90	3.0	11.0	4.0	0	470	2.0
pinot grigio (*Vino de Milo*), 4 oz.	50	1.0	8.0	2.0	0	420	2.0
primavera (*Delallo* Low Fat)	70	1.0	9.0	3.5	0	490	2.0
puttanesca:							
(*Alessi*)	100	2.0	6.0	9.0	0	470	2.0

Food and Measure	cal.	prot. (gms)	carbo. (gms)	fat (gms)	chol. (mgs)	sod. (mgs)	fiber (gms)
(Amy's)	45	2.0	6.0	2.0	0	680	1.0
(Cucina Antica) ...	54	1.0	6.0	3.0	0	248	1.0
(Delallo)	130	1.0	5.0	12.0	0	270	2.0
(Emeril's)	80	2.0	9.0	5.0	0	760	2.0
(Fruitti Di Bosco) ..	60	2.0	8.0	3.5	0	470	2.0
(Seeds of Change Organic)	80	2.0	8.0	6.0	0	690	2.0
ricotta Parmesan (Prego)	90	3.0	13.0	3.0	5	470	3.0
sausage, Italian:							
(Hunt's)	60	2.0	10.0	1.5	0	610	3.0
and garlic (Prego) .	100	3.0	13.0	3.5	5	500	3.0
w/pepper and onion (Classico)	90	5.0	13.0	2.0	5	470	2.0
and peppers (Newman's Own)	90	4.0	11.0	4.0	10	630	<1.0
spinach and:							
cheese (Classico Florentine)	80	3.0	7.0	5.0	5	560	2.0
garlic (Classico Organic)	60	2.0	10.0	1.0	0	340	2.0
tomato:							
fire-roasted (Muir Glen Organic) ...	70	2.0	12.0	2.0	0	390	2.0
fire-roasted, and garlic (Classico) .	50	2.0	10.0	.5	0	320	2.0
herbs and spices (Classico Organic)	70	2.0	12.0	1.0	0	350	2.0
sun-dried (Classico)	80	2.0	11.0	3.0	0	390	2.0
vegetable, garden:							
(Muir Glen Organic)	60	2.0	10.0	1.0	0	350	2.0
(Seeds of Change Piemonte Organic)	60	1.0	7.0	3.5	0	300	2.0
vodka:							
(Bertolli)	150	3.0	12.0	9.0	25	730	2.0
(Classico)	150	3.0	12.0	10.0	10	500	3.0
(Cucina Antica) ...	66	1.0	4.0	5.0	18	232	1.0
(Delallo)	80	2.0	6.0	5.0	10	530	1.0
(Emeril's)	130	2.0	13.0	8.0	10	490	2.0
(Mama Capri)	140	3.0	5.0	12.0	15	550	1.0
(Newman's Own) ..	110	5.0	11.0	5.0	5	440	0
w/olives and vermouth (Mom's)	110	3.0	6.0	8.0	20	290	<1.0

Food and Measure	cal.	prot. (gms)	carbo. (gms)	fat (gms)	chol. (mgs)	sod. (mgs)	fiber (gms)
Pasta sauce, refrigerated (see also specific sauces), tomato (*Buitoni*), ½ cup:							
arrabbiata	90	1.0	8.0	6.0	0	610	2.0
marinara	70	1.0	10.0	3.0	0	560	2.0
marinara, roasted garlic	60	2.0	10.0	1.5	0	530	2.0
tomato herb Parmesan	130	4.0	10.0	8.0	10	740	2.0
vodka	100	2.0	7.0	7.0	20	610	1.0
Pasta sauce mix, spaghetti, 1 tbsp. dry, except as noted:							
(*Lawry's* Extra Rich & Thick)	30	<1.0	7.0	0	0	620	<1.0
(*Lawry's* Original), 1½ tbsp.	25	0	6.0	0	0	600	0
(*McCormick* Italian Style), 1⅓ tbsp.	35	0	7.0	0	0	740	0
(*McCormick* Thick & Zesty)	25	0	6.0	0	0	620	0
Pastrami, beef, 2 oz., except as noted:							
(*Black Bear*)	90	11.0	2.0	4.0	30	630	0
(*Black Bear* Brisket) ..	80	10.0	2.0	4.0	30	610	0
(*Boar's Head* Brisket) .	90	12.0	2.0	4.0	30	670	0
(*Boar's Head* Red) ...	80	12.0	1.0	3.0	35	610	0
(*Boar's Head* Round) .	70	12.0	1.0	2.5	30	580	0
(*Di Lusso*)	100	10.0	1.0	6.0	35	680	0
(*Dietz & Watson* Brisket)	70	12.0	1.0	2.5	30	590	0
(*Dietz & Watson* Spiced)	70	11.0	1.0	5.0	30	500	0
(*Healthy Deli*)	80	11.0	3.0	3.0	30	480	0
(*Hebrew National* First Cut)	80	11.0	1.0	3.0	30	520	0
Pastry, puff (see also "Fillo dough"), frozen:							
sheet:							
(*Kineret*), 2-oz. sq.	250	3.0	20.0	18.0	0	140	<1.0
(*Pepperidge Farm*), ⅙ sheet	170	3.0	14.0	11.0	0	200	<1.0
shell:							
(*Pepperidge Farm*), 1 pc.	190	4.0	16.0	13.0	0	230	<1.0
mini (*Pepperidge Farm*), 4 pcs.	180	3.0	15.0	9.0	0	290	1.0

Food and Measure	cal.	prot. (gms)	carbo. (gms)	fat (gms)	chol. (mgs)	sod. (mgs)	fiber (gms)
Pâté, see specific listings							
Pâté, liver, can/jar:							
2 oz.	179	8.0	.6	15.7	143	390	0
1 tbsp.	41	1.9	.2	3.6	33	91	0
chicken liver:							
2 oz.	113	7.5	3.7	7.3	219	216	0
1 tbsp.	26	1.8	.9	1.7	51	51	0
fois gras w/truffles:							
(*Maison Roland* Bloc 14.8 oz.), 2 oz.	220	5.0	0	22.0	630	240	0
(*Maison Roland* Bloc 11 oz.), 2 oz.	220	4.0	0	24.0	540	300	0
goose liver, smoked:							
2 oz.	259	6.4	2.6	24.6	84	390	0
1 tbsp.	60	1.5	.6	5.7	20	91	0
truffle flavor, 2 oz. ...	183	6.3	3.5	16.0	59	452	0
Pâté, liver, refrigerated, pork, 2 oz.:							
w/black peppercorns (*Tour Eiffel*)	140	7.0	3.0	11.0	55	400	1.0
w/champagne (*Marcel & Henri* Pâté de Campagne)	210	7.0	1.0	19.0	80	370	<1.0
Peach, fresh:							
(*Dole*), 1 medium, 3.5 oz.	40	1.0	10.0	0	0	0	2.0
(*Frieda's Donut/Frieda's* Late Season), 5 oz.	60	1.0	16.0	0	0	0	3.0
2½" peach, 4 per lb. .	37	.6	9.7	.1	0	0	1.7
sliced, 1 cup.	73	1.2	18.9	.2	0	0	3.4
Peach, can/jar, halves or slices, ½ cup, except as noted:							
(*Del Monte Carb Clever*)	30	1.0	7.0	0	0	10	1.0
in juice:							
(*Del Monte* 100%) .	60	0	15.0	0	0	10	1.0
(*S&W* Natural Style)	80	1.0	19.0	0	0	20	1.0
chunks (*Del Monte Fruit Naturals*) ..	70	<1.0	17.0	0	0	10	<1.0
diced (*Del Monte* 100%), 4-oz. can	60	0	13.0	0	0	10	<1.0

Food and Measure	cal.	prot. (gms)	carbo. (gms)	fat (gms)	chol. (mgs)	sod. (mgs)	fiber (gms)
Peach, can/jar *(cont.)*							
in extra light syrup:							
(*Del Monte* Lite Cling)	60	0	15.0	0	0	10	1.0
(*Del Monte* Lite Freestone)	60	0	14.0	0	0	10	1.0
diced (*Del Monte* Lite), 4-oz. can . .	50	0	13.0	0	0	10	<1.0
in light syrup:							
(*Del Monte Orchard Select*)	80	<1.0	20.0	0	0	10	<1.0
(*Dole* Sliced)	80	1.0	17.0	0	0	10	1.0
(*S&W*)	70	0	17.0	0	0	10	1.0
diced (*Del Monte*), 4-oz. cup	70	<1.0	17.0	0	0	10	<1.0
diced (*Dole* Fruit Bowl), 4-oz. cup .	70	<1.0	18.0	0	0	15	1.0
raspberry flavor (*Del Monte*)	80	<1.0	20.0	0	0	10	<1.0
spiced (*Del Monte* Harvest Spice) . .	80	<1.0	21.0	0	0	10	<1.0
strawberry-banana flavor (*Del Monte*), 4-oz. cup	70	<1.0	17.0	0	0	10	<1.0
white (*Roland*)	70	0	16.0	0	0	5	1.0
in light syrup, chunks:							
(*S&W* Sun)	80	<1.0	20.0	0	0	20	1.0
(*S&W* Tropical) . . .	80	<1.0	19.0	0	0	15	0
cinnamon brown sugar (*S&W* Sweet Memory) .	80	<1.0	19.0	0	0	15	<1.0
hybrid (*S&W* Snow)	80	<1.0	20.0	0	0	15	1.0
in heavy syrup:							
(*Del Monte*)	100	0	24.0	0	0	10	1.0
diced (*Del Monte*), 4-oz. can	80	0	20.0	0	0	10	<1.0
spiced, whole (*Del Monte*)	100	0	24.0	0	0	10	<1.0
in gelatin, 4.5 oz. cont., except as noted:							
peach (*Del Monte*)	90	0	22.0	0	0	40	0
raspberry (*Del Monte*),	90	0	23.0	0	0	40	0
strawberry (*Dole*), 4.3 oz.	90	<1.0	23.0	0	0	25	<1.0

Food and Measure	cal.	prot. (gms)	carbo. (gms)	fat (gms)	chol. (mgs)	sod. (mgs)	fiber (gms)
strawberry banana (*Del Monte* Lite),	60	0	14.0	0	0	40	0
and crème (Dole Parfait), 4.3-oz. cup	110	0	23.0	2.0	0	10	1.0
Peach, dried:							
(*Sun•Maid*), ¼ cup ...	100	2.0	25.0	0	0	0	3.0
(*Sunsweet*), 3 pcs., 1.4 oz.	110	2.0	25.0	0	0	0	3.0
sulfured:							
halves, ½ cup	191	2.9	49.1	.6	0	6	6.6
10 halves, 4.6 oz. ...	311	4.7	79.7	1.0	0	9	10.7
Peach, frozen, sliced:							
(*Cascadian Farm* Organic), 1 cup ...	50	<1.0	14.0	0	0	0	2.0
(*C&W* Ultimate), ¾ cup	50	1.0	13.0	0	0	0	2.0
(*Dole*), ¾ cup	50	1.0	13.0	0	0	0	2.0
(*Tree of Life* Organic), ¾ cup	40	1.0	11.0	.5	0	0	<2.0
sweetened, ½ cup ...	118	.8	30.0	.2	0	8	1.8
canned, 8 fl. oz.	135	.7	34.7	<.1	0	17	1.5
Peach drink blend, 8 fl. oz.:							
mangosteen (*Snapple*)	80	0	18.0	0	0	25	0
punch (*Tropicana* Orchard)	130	0	33.0	0	0	5	0
Peach glaze, 3 tbsp.:							
(*Litehouse*)	70	0	17.0	0	0	45	0
(*Marzetti's*)	60	0	15.0	0	0	65	0
Peach juice, 8 fl. oz.:							
(*After the Fall* Georgia)	130	1.0	31.0	0	0	15	0
(*Ceres*)	120	0	30.0	0	0	5	0
(*R.W. Knudsen* Nectar)	130	1.0	31.0	0	0	15	0
(*Santa Cruz Organic* Nectar)	120	0	29.0	0	0	10	0
Peach juice blend, 8 fl. oz.:							
mango (*Apple & Eve Organics*)	130	0	31.0	0	0	25	0
orange (*Nantucket Nectars*)	130	0	31.0	0	0	25	0
Peach nectar:							
(*Goya*), 12 fl. oz.	220	1.0	54.0	0	0	25	2.0
canned, 8 fl. oz.	135	.7	34.7	<.1	0	17	1.5

Food and Measure	cal.	prot. (gms)	carbo. (gms)	fat (gms)	chol. (mgs)	sod. (mgs)	fiber (gms)
Peach-apricot sauce							
(*Saucy Susan*), 2 tbsp.	80	0	19.0	0	0	260	1.0
Peanut, shelled, 1 oz., except as noted:							
(*Beer Nuts* Kettle Cooked)	185	8.0	6.0	15.0	0	60	2.0
(*Beer Nuts* Original) . .	170	7.0	7.0	14.0	0	80	2.0
(*Frito-Lay* Salted), 1.75-oz. pkg.	280	14.0	9.0	24.0	0	200	4.0
(*Frito-Lay* Salted in Shell)	160	7.0	6.0	14.0	0	170	2.0
(*Kettle* Salted)	170	8.0	4.0	15.0	0	120	3.0
(*Planters* Cocktail) . . .	170	7.0	6.0	14.0	0	115	2.0
(*Planters* Cocktail Lightly Salted)	170	7.0	5.0	15.0	0	55	2.0
(*Planters* Roasted in Shell Salted)	160	7.0	5.0	14.0	0	135	2.0
(*Planters* Salted)	170	7.0	5.0	14.0	0	115	2.0
(*Reese's Really Nuts!* Roasted), .5-oz. pkg.	80	4.0	3.0	7.0	0	85	1.0
(*Shiloh Farms* Organic Raw Redskin), ¼ cup, 1.2 oz.	190	9.0	7.0	16.0	0	0	3.0
barbecue (*Beer Nuts* Crunch Nuts)	130	4.0	18.0	4.5	0	110	2.0
boiled, salted	90	3.8	6.0	6.2	0	213	2.5
Cajun (*Beer Nuts* Devil Crunch Nuts)	140	4.0	15.0	6.0	0	140	1.0
dry-roasted:							
(*Fisher*)	170	7.0	8.0	14.0	0	190	2.0
(*Frito-Lay*), 1.75-oz. pkg. . . .	280	12.0	17.0	18.0	0	300	5.0
(*Planters*)	160	7.0	6.0	13.0	0	190	2.0
(*Planters* 14/16 oz.)	170	8.0	5.0	14.0	0	190	2.0
(*Planters* Lightly Salted)	170	8.0	5.0	14.0	0.	95	2.0
(*Planters* Lightly Salted 14/16 oz.)	160	7.0	5.0	14.0	0	95	2.0
½ cup	428	17.3	15.7	36.3	0	4	5.8
honey (*Planters*) . .	150	7.0	8.0	12.0	0	95	2.0
glazed (*Beer Nuts* Old Fashioned)	140	8.0	6.0	14.0	0	60	2.0
honey mustard (*Beer Nuts* Crunch Nuts) .	140	4.0	19.0	5.0	0	55	1.0

Food and Measure	cal.	prot. (gms)	carbo. (gms)	fat (gms)	chol. (mgs)	sod. (mgs)	fiber (gms)
honey-roasted:							
(*Fisher*)	170	7.0	7.0	13.0	0	70	2.0
(*Frito-Lay*), 1.75-oz. pkg.	250	11.0	11.0	20.0	0	130	3.0
(*Kettle*)	150	6.0	6.0	12.0	0	35	2.0
(*Planters*)	160	6.0	8.0	13.0	0	95	2.0
(*Planters* 12 oz.)	160	6.0	8.0	13.0	0	115	2.0
(*Planters* Party Size 34.5 oz.)	160	7.0	6.0	13.0	0	190	2.0
honey dry-roasted:							
(*Planters* 12 oz.)	150	6.0	7.0	12.0	0	110	2.0
(*Planters* 24 oz.)	160	6.0	7.0	13.0	0	110	2.0
hot and spicy:							
(*Beer Nuts*)	160	7.0	6.0	13.0	0	160	2.0
(*Frito-Lay*), 1.1 oz.	190	7.0	6.0	16.0	0	250	2.0
oil-roasted:							
(*Fisher*)	170	7.0	5.0	15.0	0	130	2.0
½ cup	419	19.0	13.6	35.5	0	4	6.6
sesame (*Beer Nuts* Crunch Nuts)	130	4.0	15.0	6.0	0	90	2.0
Spanish:							
(*Kettle*)	160	8.0	5.0	14.0	0	120	2.0
raw (*Diamond*), ¼ cup	220	10.0	5.0	19.0	0	10	4.0
raw (*Kettle*)	160	7.0	4.0	14.0	0	5	3.0
raw (*Planters*)	150	7.0	6.0	13.0	0	5	3.0
sweet and crunchy (*Planters*)	140	4.0	16.0	7.0	0	20	2.0
Peanut butter (see also "Peanut Spread"), 2 tbsp., except as noted:							
(*Jif* To Go), 2¼-oz. cont.	390	15.0	15.0	32.0	0	270	4.0
(*Skippy* Squeez' It)	190	7.0	7.0	17.0	0	160	2.0
chunky or creamy:							
(*Arrowhead Mills* Natural/Organic)	190	8.0	6.0	17.0	0	0	2.0
(*Kettle* Organic), 1 oz.	170	7.0	5.0	14.0	0	0	2.0
(*MaraNatha* Natural)	190	7.0	8.0	15.0	0	135	2.0
(*MaraNatha* Organic)	200	7.0	7.0	16.0	0	75	2.0
(*Santa Cruz Organic* Dark/Light Roast)	210	8.0	6.0	16.0	0	50	2.0
(*Smucker's*)	210	8.0	6.0	16.0	0	120	2.0
blended (*Tree of Life* Organic)	190	7.0	7.0	15.0	0	55	2.0

Food and Measure	cal.	prot. (gms)	carbo. (gms)	fat (gms)	chol. (mgs)	sod. (mgs)	fiber (gms)
Peanut butter, chunky or creamy (cont.)							
honey sweetened (*Arrowhead Mills*)	190	7.0	7.0	16.0	0	100	2.0
chunky/crunchy:							
(*Jif* Extra)	190	8.0	7.0	16.0	0	130	2.0
(*Jif* Reduced Fat) ..	190	8.0	15.0	12.0	0	220	2.0
(*Skippy Super Chunk*)	190	7.0	7.0	16.0	0	120	2.0
(*Skippy Super Chunk Natural*)	180	7.0	6.0	17.0	0	125	2.0
(*Skippy Super Chunk Reduced Fat*) ...	180	7.0	15.0	12.0	0	160	2.0
(*Tree of Life* Organic)	180	7.0	6.0	15.0	0	45	3.0
coarse ground (*Peanut Better* Organic):							
chocolate, deep ...	170	6.0	11.0	13.0	0	5	2.0
cinnamon currant ..	180	7.0	9.0	14.0	0	0	3.0
hickory smoked ...	190	9.0	5.0	16.0	0	135	3.0
molasses	180	8.0	8.0	14.0	0	0	2.0
onion parsley	180	8.0	6.0	15.0	0	115	3.0
praline	180	8.0	8.0	15.0	0	0	3.0
rosemary garlic ...	180	8.0	7.0	15.0	0	85	3.0
spicy Southwest ...	190	8.0	7.0	17.0	0	100	5.0
Thai ginger red pepper	180	8.0	7.0	15.0	0	110	3.0
vanilla cranberry ..	170	7.0	9.0	13.0	0	0	2.0
creamy:							
(*Jif*)	190	8.0	7.0	16.0	0	150	2.0
(*Jif* Reduced Fat) ..	190	8.0	15.0	12.0	0	250	2.0
(*Simply Jif*)	190	8.0	6.0	16.0	0	65	2.0
(*Reese's*)	200	8.0	7.0	16.0	0	140	3.0
(*Skippy*)	190	7.0	7.0	16.0	0	150	2.0
(*Skippy* Natural) ...	180	7.0	6.0	16.0	0	150	2.0
(*Skippy* Reduced Fat)	180	7.0	15.0	12.0	0	170	2.0
(*Smucker's* Reduced Fat)	200	9.0	12.0	12.0	0	120	2.0
(*Tree of Life* Organic)	190	8.0	7.0	16.0	0	45	1.0
w/honey:							
(*Jif*)	190	6.0	11.0	15.0	0	120	2.0
(*Smucker's*)	200	7.0	9.0	16.0	0	30	2.0
chunky (*Skippy*) ..	190	7.0	6.0	16.0	0	105	2.0
creamy (*Skippy*) ..	190	7.0	7.0	17.0	0	125	2.0
Peanut butter baking chips, .5 oz.:							
(*Hershey's Reese's* Chips)	80	3.0	7.0	4.5	0	35	<1.0

Food and Measure	cal.	prot. (gms)	carbo. (gms)	fat (gms)	chol. (mgs)	sod. (mgs)	fiber (gms)
(*SunSpire*)	80	1.0	9.0	4.0	0	35	0
w/milk chocolate:							
(*Hershey's Reese's* Pieces)	80	1.0	9.0	4.5	0	15	0
(*Nestlé Toll House*)	70	<1.0	9.0	4.5	0	25	0
swirled (*Nestlé Toll House*)	75	<1.0	8.0	4.5	0	20	0
Peanut butter sandwich, frozen, 1 pc.:							
(*Smucker's Uncrustables*)	200	7.0	18.0	11.0	0	250	2.0
and honey on wheat (*Smucker's Uncrustables*)	210	6.0	26.0	9.0	0	230	2.0
grape jelly or strawberry jam (*Smucker's Uncrustables*)	210	7.0	25.0	9.0	0	260	2.0
Peanut butter topping (*Reese's* Shell), 2 tbsp.	210	<1.0	17.0	17.0	0	70	1.0
Peanut butter–jelly:							
grape or strawberry (*Smucker's Goober*), 3 tbsp.	240	7.0	24.0	13.0	0	140	2.0
Peanut flour, 1 cup:							
defatted	196	31.3	20.8	.3	0	9	9.5
low fat	257	20.3	18.8	13.1	0	0	9.5
Peanut sauce (see also "Grilling sauce"), 2 tbsp., except as noted:							
(*Annie Chun's*)	120	4.0	10.0	7.0	0	230	1.0
(*Heaven and Earth*), 1 tbsp.	100	<10.0	5.0	16.0	0	90	0
(*San-J* Thai)	70	3.0	8.0	2.5	0	740	2.0
satay:							
(*Roland*)	80	2.0	12.0	3.0	0	680	2.0
(*A Taste of Thai*) ..	80	1.0	9.0	4.5	0	180	1.0
Peanut sauce mix (*A Taste of Thai*), ¼ pkt.	45	1.0	7.0	1.5	0	190	1.0
Peanut spread (see also "Peanut butter"), 2 tbsp.:							
(*Peanut Wonder*)	100	4.0	13.0	2.5	0	190	0

Food and Measure	cal.	prot. (gms)	carbo. (gms)	fat (gms)	chol. (mgs)	sod. (mgs)	fiber (gms)
Peanut spread *(cont.)*							
(Peanut Wonder Low Sodium)	100	4.0	13.0	2.5	0	95	0
honey *(MaraNatha* Natural)	180	7.0	10.0	14.0	0	70	2.0
Pear, fresh, w/peel:							
(Dole), 1 medium, 5.9 oz.	100	1.0	25.0	1.0	0	0	4.0
1 large, 2 per lb.	123	.8	31.6	.8	0	0	5.0
Bartlett, 1 medium, 2½ per lb.	98	.7	25.1	.7	0	1	4.0
sliced, ½ cup	49	.3	12.5	.3	0	1	2.0
Pear, Asian:							
(Frieda's), 5 oz.	60	1.0	15.0	0	0	0	5.0
1 medium, 2¼" x 2½" diam.	51	.6	13.0	.3	0	0	4.4
Pear, can/jar, ½ cup halves or slices, except as noted:							
(Del Monte Carb Clever)	40	0	10.0	0	0	10	1.0
baby, whole, in syrup *(Roland)*	80	0	21.0	0	0	10	1.0
in juice:							
(Del Monte 100%) .	60	0	15.0	0	0	10	1.0
(S&W Natural Style)	80	0	21.0	0	0	10	2.0
w/liquid	62	.4	16.0	.1	0	5	2.0
in extra light syrup:							
(Del Monte Lite) . . .	60	0	15.0	0	0	10	1.0
diced *(Del Monte* Lite), 4-oz. can . .	50	0	13.0	0	0	10	<1.0
in kiwi-berry gelatin *(Dole* Reduced Sugar), 4.3-oz. cup	60	<1.0	16.0	0	0	70	1.0
in light syrup:							
(S&W)	80	0	19.0	0	0	10	2.0
Bartlett *(Del Monte* Orchard Select) .	80	<1.0	20.0	0	0	10	2.0
w/liquid	72	.2	19.0	<.1	0	6	2.0
chunks *(S&W* Sun)	80	<1.0	20.0	0	0	10	<1.0
cinnamon *(Del Monte)*	80	0	21.0	0	0	10	1.0
diced *(Dole* Fruit Bowl), 4-oz. cup .	70	<1.0	18.0	0	0	10	1.0
in heavy syrup:							
(Del Monte)	100	0	24.0	0	0	10	1.0

Food and Measure	cal.	prot. (gms)	carbo. (gms)	fat (gms)	chol. (mgs)	sod. (mgs)	fiber (gms)
w/liquid	98	.3	25.5	.2	0	7	2.1
diced (*Del Monte*),							
4-oz. can	80	0	20.0	0	0	10	<1.0
Pear, dried:							
(*Shiloh Farms* Organic),							
3 pcs., 1.1 oz.	150	1.0	26.0	0	0	5	5.0
2 oz.	149	1.1	39.5	.4	0	4	4.3
sulfured:							
halves, ½ cup	236	1.7	62.7	.6	0	5	6.8
stewed, ½ cup	162	1.2	43.1	.4	0	4	8.2
Pear juice, 8 fl. oz.:							
(*Ceres*)	120	0	31.0	0	0	10	2.0
(*R.W. Knudsen* Organic)	150	<1.0	38.0	0	0	10	<1.0
(*R.W. Knudsen* Organic							
Box)	120	0	30.0	0	0	15	<1.0
(*Santa Cruz Organic*							
Nectar 100%)	120	0	31.0	0	0	30	0
sparkling (*R.W.*							
Knudsen Organic) .	120	0	29.0	0	0	15	0
Pear nectar:							
(*Goya*), 12 fl. oz.	240	1.0	59.0	0	0	20	2.0
canned, 8 fl. oz.	150	.3	39.4	<.1	0	10	1.5
Peas, see specific							
listings							
Peas, black-eyed, see							
"Black-eyed peas"							
Peas, cream, canned,							
(*East Texas Fair*),							
½ cup	100	6.0	17.0	1.0	0	460	5.0
Peas, crowder, canned,							
½ cup:							
(*Allens/East Texas Fair*)	110	6.0	19.0	1.0	0	460	8.0
(*Bush's*)	110	7.0	18.0	1.0	0	500	5.0
Peas, edible-podded,							
fresh:							
raw:							
(*Frieda's* Snow),							
1 cup, 3 oz.	35	2.0	6.0	0	0	0	2.0
in pods (*Frieda's*							
Sugar Snap),							
⅔ cup, 3 oz. ...	35	2.0	6.0	0	0	0	2.0
raw, w/sauce, ½ cup:							
(*Frieda's* Snow) ...	40	2.0	8.0	0	0	180	2.0
(*Frieda's* Sugar Snap)	35	2.0	8.0	0	0	180	2.0

Food and Measure	cal.	prot. (gms)	carbo. (gms)	fat (gms)	chol. (mgs)	sod. (mgs)	fiber (gms)
Peas, edible podded *(cont.)*							
boiled, drained,							
½ cup	34	2.6	5.6	.2	0	3	2.2
Peas, edible podded, frozen:							
sugar snap:							
(*Birds Eye/C&W*),							
⅔ cup	40	2.0	7.0	0	0	0	2.0
(*Cascadian Farm Organic*), ¾ cup .	35	2.0	6.0	0	0	140	2.0
(*Green Giant Select*), ¾ cup	40	2.0	9.0	0	0	0	2.0
(*Green Giant Simply Steam* No Sauce), ⅔ cup	40	2.0	10.0	0	0	95	2.0
boiled, drained, ½ cup	42	2.8	7.2	.3	0	4	2.5
Peas, edible podded, combinations, frozen, sugar snap, 1 cup:							
baby carrots, cauliflower, broccoli (*C&W Vegetable Stand Combinations*)	30	1.0	5.0	0	0	25	2.0
stir-fry, w/carrots, onion, mushrooms (*Birds Eye*)	40	1.0	7.0	0	0	30	2.0
Peas, field, canned, (see also "Peas, crowder" and "Peas, purple hull"), ½ cup:							
w/bacon (*Trappey's*) ..	90	6.0	15.0	1.0	0	380	5.0
w/jalapeño (*East Texas Fair* Pepper Peas) ..	120	6.0	22.0	1.0	0	580	6.0
w/pork (*East Texas Fair* Peas & Pork)	110	6.0	19.0	1.5	0	540	5.0
seasoned (*Glory*)	90	6.0	17.0	.5	0	570	3.0
w/snaps:							
(*Allens East Texas Fair/Sunshine*) ..	120	6.0	21.0	1.0	0	300	6.0
(*Bush's*)	80	5.0	16.0	0	0	430	2.0
and bacon (*Trappey's*)	110	6.0	19.0	1.0	0	380	4.0
seasoned (*Glory*) ..	90	6.0	17.0	.5	0	570	3.0
Peas, field, frozen (*McKenzie's*), ½ cup	110	7.0	21.0	.5	0	10	4.0

Food and Measure	cal.	prot. (gms)	carbo. (gms)	fat (gms)	chol. (mgs)	sod. (mgs)	fiber (gms)
Peas, green, fresh:							
raw, in pod, 1 lb.	140	9.3	24.9	.7	0	8	8.8
raw, shelled, ½ cup ..	59	3.9	10.4	.3	0	3	3.7
boiled, drained, ½ cup	67	4.3	12.5	.2	0	2	4.4
Peas, green, can or jar, ½ cup:							
(*Del Monte*)	60	3.0	13.0	0	0	390	4.0
(*Del Monte* Very Young Small)	60	3.0	10.0	0	0	360	4.0
(*Freshlike* Selects Petite)	90	5.0	16.0	.5	0	410	5.0
(*Freshlike* Tender Garden)	110	6.0	19.0	.5	0	370	6.0
(*Freshlike* Tender Garden No Salt) ...	110	6.0	19.0	.5	0	10	6.0
(*Green Giant* Sweet) ..	60	4.0	12.0	0	0	400	3.0
(*Green Giant* Sweet 50% Less Sodium)	60	4.0	11.0	0	0	200	3.0
(*LeSueur* Early)	60	4.0	12.0	0	0	380	3.0
(*Roland* Extra Fine) ..	120	7.0	21.0	.5	0	450	6.0
(*Roland* Petits Pois) ..	80	6.0	19.0	.5	0	420	7.0
(*S&W* Petit Pois)	60	3.0	10.0	0	0	360	4.0
(*S&W* Young)	60	3.0	13.0	0	0	390	4.0
drained	59	3.8	10.7	.3	0	214	3.5
seasoned, w/liquid ...	57	3.5	10.5	.3	0	288	2.8
Peas, green, combinations, can/jar:							
and carrots, ½ cup:							
(*Del Monte*)	60	2.0	11.0	0	0	360	2.0
(*Freshlike*)	60	4.0	11.0	0	0	350	3.0
(*Roland*)	80	4.0	19.0	.5	0	480	4.0
(*S&W*)	60	2.0	11.0	0	0	360	2.0
w/liquid	48	2.8	10.8	.3	0	332	2.6
and onions, ½ cup:							
(*Freshlike* Selects) .	60	3.0	11.0	0	0	440	3.0
(*S&W*)	40	3.0	11.0	0	0	530	3.0
w/liquid	31	2.0	5.1	.2	0	265	1.4
Peas, green, combinations, frozen, ⅔ cup, except as noted:							
and carrots:							
(*Cascadian Farm* Organic)	50	2.0	10.0	0	0	75	3.0
(*C&W* Early Harvest Petite/Baby)	60	3.0	10.0	0	0	150	3.0

Food and Measure	cal.	prot. (gms)	carbo. (gms)	fat (gms)	chol. (mgs)	sod. (mgs)	fiber (gms)
Peas, green, combinations, frozen, and carrots (cont.)							
boiled, drained, ½ cup	38	2.7	8.1	.3	0	54	2.5
and corn, carrots, sugar snap peas (C&W Vegetable Stand Combinations)	50	2.0	10.0	0	0	70	2.0
and mushrooms, garlic seasoned (Birds Eye Steamfresh), ¾ cup	80	4.0	12.0	2.0	0	340	3.0
and pearl onions:							
(Cascadian Farm Organic), ¾ cup .	60	4.0	11.0	0	0	160	3.0
(C&W Petite)	60	4.0	11.0	0	0	160	3.0
(Green Giant Simply Steam No Sauce), ½ cup	60	3.0	10.0	0	0	80	2.0
baby (Birds Eye) ..	60	4.0	12.0	0	0	0	3.0
baby, and vegetables (Birds Eye), ¾ cup	40	2.0	7.0	0	0	20	2.0
in sauce (Birds Eye)	90	5.0	17.0	0	0	510	4.0
boiled, drained, ½ cup	41	2.3	7.8	.2	0	33	2.0
Peas, green, dish, Indian, pkg., 5 oz.:							
w/cheese (Tasty Bite Peas Paneer)	155	3.0	7.2	9.9	13	351	6.3
in sauce (Tasty Bite Agra Peas & Greens)	138	4.0	9.0	10.0	3.0	417	4.0
Peas, green, dried, rehydrated (Frieda's), ⅓ cup, 3 oz.	130	9.0	22.0	0	0	290	9.0
Peas, green, frozen, ⅔ cup, except as noted:							
(Birds Eye Baby)	70	4.0	12.0	0	0	0	4.0
(Birds Eye Garden/ Birds Eye Steamfresh Sweet)	70	5.0	12.0	0	0	0	4.0
(Birds Eye Steamfresh Singles), 3.25 oz. ..	70	5.0	13.0	0	0	0	4.0
(Cascadian Farm Organic Garden/Sweet)	70	4.0	12.0	0	0	95	4.0
(Cascadian Farm Purely Steam Organic Petite)	50	4.0	10.0	1.0	0	90	4.0

Food and Measure	cal.	prot. (gms)	carbo. (gms)	fat (gms)	chol. (mgs)	sod. (mgs)	fiber (gms)
(*C&W* Petite)	70	4.0	12.0	0	0	200	4.0
(*C&W Early Harvest/* Organic/No Salt Petite)	70	4.0	12.0	0	0	0	4.0
(*Green Giant* Sweet) ..	70	5.0	12.0	0	0	135	4.0
(*Green Giant Select* Baby Sweet/Early) .	50	5.0	11.0	.5	0	95	4.0
(*Green Giant Simply Steam* No Sauce Baby Sweet)	60	4.0	13.0	.5	0	190	4.0
(*Tree of Life* Organic) .	70	5.0	12.0	0	0	100	4.0
Alfredo (*C&W*), ½ cup	110	6.0	11.0	5.0	15	380	4.0
in butter sauce (*Green Giant* Baby Sweet), ¾ cup	80	5.0	14.0	1.5	<5	440	4.0
Peas, green, snack:							
(*Calbee Salad Snack* Snapea Crisps), 1 oz., about 22 pcs.	150	5.0	14.0	8.0	0	125	2.0
wasabi:							
(*Roland*), ⅓ cup ..	120	5.0	19.0	5.0	0	270	2.0
(*SunRidge Farms*), ¼ cup.........	120	7.0	20.0	1.0	0	75	2.0
(*Tree of Life*), ¼ cup	120	5.0	17.0	4.0	0	130	2.0
Peas, pigeon, see "Pigeon peas"							
Peas, purple hull, canned, ½ cup:							
(*Allens/East Texas Fair*)	120	7.0	21.0	1.0	0	350	6.0
(*Bush's*)	90	6.0	19.0	0	0	460	5.0
Peas, purple hull, frozen (*McKenzie's*), ½ cup	110	7.0	21.0	.5	0	10	4.0
Peas, split, see "Split peas"							
Peas, sprouted:							
raw, ½ cup	77	5.3	17.0	.4	0	12	n.a.
boiled, drained, 4 oz. .	134	8.0	24.8	.6	0	3	3.7
Peas, sugar snap or snow, see "Peas, edible-podded"							
Peas, sweet, see "Peas, green"							

Food and Measure	cal.	prot. (gms)	carbo. (gms)	fat (gms)	chol. (mgs)	sod. (mgs)	fiber (gms)
Peas, wasabi, see "Peas, green, snack"							
Peas, white acre, canned (*East Texas Fair*), ½ cup	100	6.0	17.0	1.0	0	460	5.0
Peas and carrots or onions, see "Peas, green, combinations"							
Pecan, shelled:							
(*Diamond*), ¼ cup	210	3.0	4.0	22.0	0	0	3.0
(*Fisher*), 1 oz.	200	3.0	4.0	20.0	0	0	2.0
(*Shiloh Farms* Organic), ¼ cup, 1.1 oz.	200	3.0	4.0	20.0	0	0	3.0
1 oz.	190	2.2	5.2	19.2	0	<1	2.2
halves:							
(*Shiloh Farms*), ⅓ cup, 1.2 oz.	220	3.0	6.0	22.0	0	0	3.0
(*Tree of Life*), .9 oz.	200	2.0	4.0	20.0	0	0	2.0
1 cup	721	8.4	19.7	73.1	0	1	8.2
halves or pieces:							
(*Planters*), 1 oz.	190	3.0	4.0	20.0	0	0	3.0
or chips (*Planters*), 2-oz. pkg.	390	5.0	9.0	40.0	0	5	7.0
chopped, 1 cup	794	9.2	21.7	80.5	0	1	9.0
dry-roasted:							
unsalted, 1 oz.	201	2.7	3.8	21.1	0	<1	2.7
unsalted, 1 cup	781	10.5	14.9	81.7	0	11	10.5
oil-roasted:							
unsalted, 1 oz.	203	2.7	3.7	21.3	0	<1	2.7
unsalted, 1 cup	787	10.5	14.3	82.8	0	11	10.5
Pecan flour, 1 oz.	93	9.1	14.4	.4	0	tr.	n.a.
Pecan topping, in syrup (*Smucker's*), 1 tbsp.	160	1.0	19.0	9.0	0	0	0
Pectin, see "Fruit pectin"							
Penne entree, frozen, 1 pkg., except as noted:							
(*Jeff Nathan Creations* Siciliano), 12 oz.	340	16.0	41.0	12.0	30	840	5.0
Alfredo, tomato sauce (*Michelina's Budget Gourmet/Zap'ems* Penne Rosa), 8 oz.	340	12.0	46.0	11.0	30	530	2.0

Food and Measure	cal.	prot. (gms)	carbo. (gms)	fat (gms)	chol. (mgs)	sod. (mgs)	fiber (gms)
w/chicken or shrimp, see "Chicken entree" and "Shrimp entree"							
Italian sausage (*Michelina's Budget Gourmet/Zap'ems*), 8 oz.	280	10.0	41.0	7.0	10	410	3.0
marinara (*Seeds of Change* Venetian Organic), 10 oz. . . .	300	12.0	40.0	8.0	10	730	4.0
primavera (*Michelina's Lean Gourmet*), 8 oz.	280	11.0	43.0	6.0	15	480	3.0
puttanesca (*Moosewood* Organic), 10 oz.	300	8.0	45.0	10.0	0	300	2.0
w/sauce, meatballs (*Organic Classics*), 10 oz.	360	19.0	45.0	12.0	35	690	4.0
w/tomato basil sauce (*Lean Cuisine One Dish Favorites*), 10 oz.	260	9.0	51.0	2.5	0	210	4.0
vegetarian: (*Yves* Bowl), 10.5 oz.	210	12.0	36.0	1.5	0	730	4.0
w/roasted vegetables (*Celentano* 70% Organic), 10 oz. .	300	11.0	54.0	5.0	0	290	8.0
vodka (*Contessa*), w/sauce, 7 oz.	330	16.0	34.0	13.0	20	660	3.0
w/out sauce, 4 oz. . .	170	13.0	26.0	1.5	20	125	2.0
Penne entree mix Alfredo cheese sauce (*Annie's*), 2.5 oz. . .	270	11.0	47.0	4.0	10	500	1.0
Pepeao, raw, sliced, 1 cup	25	.5	6.7	0	0	9	n.a.
Pepeao, dried, 1 cup	72	1.2	19.5	.1	0	17	n.a.
Pepper, seasoning: black, 1 tsp.:							
ground	6	.3	1.7	.1	0	1	.7
whole	8	.3	1.9	0	0	1	.8
chili, 1 tsp.	9	.3	1.2	.3	0	<1	.7
red or cayenne, 1 tsp.	6	.2	1.0	.3	0	1	.7
white, 1 tsp.	7	.3	1.7	.1	0	0	.2
Pepper, ancho, dried, .6-oz. pepper	48	2.0	8.7	1.4	0	7	3.7
Pepper, banana, fresh, 1.2-oz. pc.	9	.6	1.8	.2	0	4	1.1

Food and Measure	cal.	prot. (gms)	carbo. (gms)	fat (gms)	chol. (mgs)	sod. (mgs)	fiber (gms)
Pepper, banana, in jars, sliced (*Roland*), ¼ cup	0	0	0	0	0	980	0
Pepper, bell, see "Pepper, sweet"							
Pepper, cherry, in jars: hot or sweet (*B&G*), 1-oz. pc.	10	0	2.0	0	0	310	0
sliced, in oil (*B&G*), 1 oz., about 7 pcs. .	28	0	0	2.8	0	310	0
sweet (*Vigo*), 4 pcs. . . .	10	0	2.0	0	0	480	0
Pepper, cherry, stuffed, w/proscuitto and provolone, marinated (*Boar's Head*), 2 oz. .	60	2.0	1.0	5.0	10	490	0
Pepper, chili, fresh, green and red:							
1 medium, 1.6 oz. . . .	18	.9	4.3	.1	0	3	.7
chopped, ½ cup	30	1.5	7.1	.2	0	5	1.1
Pepper, chili, can/jar (see also specific listings):							
whole, green, 1 pc.:							
(*Chi-Chi's*), 1.2 oz. . .	10	0	2.0	0	0	100	0
(*Las Palmas*), 1.2 oz.	10	0	2.0	0	0	230	1.0
(*Old El Paso*), 1.2 oz.	10	0	2.0	0	0	230	0
(*Ortega*), 1.2 oz. pc. .	10	<1.0	2.0	0	0	140	<1.0
fire-roasted (*La Victoria*), 1.2 oz.	5	0	1.0	0	0	190	<1.0
mild (*Zapata*)	5	0	1.0	0	0	85	0
large, 2.6 oz.	15	.7	3.7	<.1	0	856	1.0
whole, green, ½ cup .	15	.5	3.2	.1	0	276	1.2
chopped:							
(*Old El Paso*), 2 tbsp.	5	0	1.0	0	0	110	<1.0
w/liquid, ½ cup . . .	17	.6	4.2	.1	0	n.a.	1.3
diced, green, 2 tbsp.:							
(*Chi-Chi's*)	10	0	2.0	0	0	85	0
(*Las Palmas*)	5	0	1.0	0	0	110	1.0
(*Ortega*)	5	<1.0	1.0	0	0	70	0
(*Pace*)	10	0	2.0	0	0	100	<1.0
fire-roasted (*La Victoria* 4 oz.) . .	7	0	1.0	0	0	75	0
fire-roasted (*La Victoria* 7 oz.) . .	10	1.0	2.0	0	0	120	<1.0

Food and Measure	cal.	prot. (gms)	carbo. (gms)	fat (gms)	chol. (mgs)	sod. (mgs)	fiber (gms)
mild (*Zapata*)	5	0	1.0	0	0	75	0
strips, green (*Las Palmas*), 1.3-oz. pc.	10	0	2.0	0	0	240	1.0
Pepper, chili, dried:							
(*Frieda's* Ancho/del Arbol/Guajillo), .5 oz.	50	2.0	8.0	0	0	5	2.0
(*Frieda's* California Anaheim Chiles), .5 oz.	50	4.0	7.0	0	0	7	2.0
(*Frieda's* California Anaheim Chiles), 2 tbsp.	15	0	2.0	0	0	15	0
(*Frieda's* Japones Chiles), .5 oz.	50	4.0	7.0	0	0	5	2.0
sun-dried, hot, 2 pcs.	3	.1	.8	.1	0	1	.3
Pepper, chipotle, canned, in Adobo sauce (*Roland*), 2 tbsp.	20	0	1.0	1.0	0	130	1.0
Pepper, Greek (*Vigo*), 1 pc.	10	0	2.0	0	0	330	1.0
Pepper, green or red, sweet, see "Pepper, sweet"							
Pepper, hot, in jars:							
(*B&G* Sandwich Toppers/ Ring), 7 pcs., 1 oz.	0	0	1.0	0	0	310	0
chopped (*B&G*), 1 tsp., .5 oz.	5	0	1.0	0	0	120	0
Pepper, Hungarian, fresh, .94-oz. pc. . .	8	.2	1.8	.1	0	<1.	n.a.
Pepper, jalapeño, fresh, .5-oz. pc.	4	.2	.8	.1	0	<1	.4
Pepper, jalapeño, can/ jar:							
whole:							
(*Chi-Chi's*), 2 pcs., 1.1 oz.	10	0	2.0	0	0	190	0
(*Herdez*), 3 pcs., 1.25 oz.	15	0	1.0	0	0	620	1.0
(*Las Palmas*), 2 pcs., 1.3 oz.	15	<1.0	2.0	0	0	190	0
(*Mrs. Renfro's*), 1.1-oz. pc.	5	0	0	0	0	410	0
(*Old El Paso*), 2 pcs., .9 oz.	5	0	1.0	0	0	380	0

Food and Measure	cal.	prot. (gms)	carbo. (gms)	fat (gms)	chol. (mgs)	sod. (mgs)	fiber (gms)
Pepper, jalapeño, can/jar, whole *(cont.)*							
(*Ortega*), 2 pcs., .9 oz.	10	<1.0	2.0	0	0	20	0
(*Vigo*), 2 pcs.	5	0	2.0	0	0	330	1.0
chopped:							
(*B&G*), 2 tbsp.	5	0	1.0	0	0	120	0
w/liquid, ¼ cup . . .	7	.2	1.2	.2	0	434	.8
diced:							
(*Ortega*), 2 tbsp. . .	10	<1.0	2.0	0	0	25	0
(*Zapata*), 4 tbsp. . .	5	0	1.0	0	0	250	0
fire-roasted (*La Victoria*), 2 tbsp.	0	0	<1.0	0	0	150	0
sliced:							
(*B&G*), 7 pcs., 1 oz.	0	0	<1.0	0	0	190	0
(*Herdez*), ¼ cup . . .	10	0	1.0	0	0	630	0
(*La Victoria* Nacho), 14 pcs., 1.1 oz. .	5	0	<1.0	0	0	350	0
(*Las Palmas*), 3 tbsp.	10	<1.0	2.0	0	0	210	0
(*Mrs. Renfro's* Nacho), 12 pcs., 1 oz.	5	0	0	0	0	410	0
(*Old El Paso* Pickled), 2 tbsp.	5	0	1.0	0	0	190	<1.0
(*Ortega*), 1 oz.	5	<1.0	<1.0	0	0	300	<1.0
(*Pace* Nacho), 1 oz.	5	0	1.0	0	0	300	<1.0
(*Roland*), ¼ cup . .	5	0	1.0	0	0	640	1.0
(*Vigo*), 14 pcs.	5	0	2.0	0	0	330	1.0
(*Zapata* Nacho), 4 tbsp.	5	0	<1.0	0	0	530	0
w/liquid, ¼ cup . . .	9	.3	1.6	.3	0	568	.9
green or red (*Chi-Chi's* Wheels), ¼ cup . .	10	0	2.0	0	0	190	0
Pepper, pasilla, dried, 2 pcs., .5 oz.	48	1.7	7.2	2.2	0	12	3.8
Pepper, piquillo, in jars: (*Vigo*), 3 pcs.	20	0	4.0	0	0	135	1.0
whole or sliced (*Roland* Organic), ½ cup . . .	45	1.0	10.0	0	0	150	3.0
Pepper, poblano, see "Pepper, chili, can/jar"							
Pepper, roasted, see "Pepper, sweet, can/jar"							
Pepper, serrano, fresh:							
whole, .2-oz. pc.	2	.1	.4	<.1	0	2	.2
chopped, ½ cup	17	.9	3.5	.5	0	5	1.9

Food and Measure	cal.	prot. (gms)	carbo. (gms)	fat (gms)	chol. (mgs)	sod. (mgs)	fiber (gms)
Pepper, serrano, in jars, whole (*Herdez*), 4 pcs, 1.25 oz.	15	0	1.0	0	0	570	1.0
Pepper, stuffed (*Roland*), pkg:							
green, w/cheese, ½ cup	440	4.0	13.0	42.0	<5	1320	6.0
green, w/rice, spices 1 pc.	90	2.0	13.0	3.0	0	190	2.0
red, w/cheese, ½ cup	470	3.0	9.0	47.0	10	710	3.0
Pepper, stuffed, frozen, w/meat, sauce:							
(*Stouffer's*), ½ of 15.5-oz. pkg.	150	8.0	17.0	6.0	15	750	2.0
(*Stouffer's* Family), ¼ of 32-oz. pkg. . .	210	11.0	20.0	9.0	20	1180	3.0
casserole (*Michelina's Authentico*), 8 oz. . .	280	11.0	32.0	10.0	30	940	2.0
Pepper, sweet, fresh:							
green and/or red:							
raw (*Chiquita*), 5.2-oz. pc.	30	1.0	7.0	0	0	0	2.0
raw, 1 medium, 3¾" x 3" or ½ cup chopped	20	.7	4.8	.1	0	1	1.3
raw, sliced, 1 cup . .	25	.8	5.9	.2	0	2	1.7
boiled, drained, 1 medium	20	.7	4.9	.1	0	1	.9
boiled, drained, chopped, 1 tbsp.	3	.1	.8	<.1	0	<1	.1
boiled, drained, strips, ½ cup	19	.6	4.6	.1	0	1	.8
yellow, raw:							
1 large, 5" x 3"	50	1.9	11.8	.4	0	4	1.7
10 strips, 1.8 oz. . .	14	.5	3.3	.1	0	1	.5
Pepper, sweet, can/jar (see also "Pimiento"):							
fried (*B&G*), 1 oz.	25	0	2.0	1.5	0	169	1.0
green, spicy salad (*Peloponnese* Toursi), 1 oz.	10	0	2.0	0	0	690	1.0
red:							
in water, drained, ½ cup	13	.6	2.7	.2	0	958	.8
roasted (*Frieda's*), 1-oz. pc.	35	1.0	5.0	0	0	280	0

Food and Measure	cal.	prot. (gms)	carbo. (gms)	fat (gms)	chol. (mgs)	sod. (mgs)	fiber (gms)
Pepper, sweet, can/jar, red *(cont.)*							
roasted (*Peloponnese* Sweet Florina), 1 oz.	10	0	2.0	0	0	150	0
roasted (*Roland*), ½ cup	30	1.0	5.0	0	0	310	1.0
roasted (*Vigo*), 1 oz.	10	0	1.0	0	0	50	0
roasted, w/garlic, dill, oil (*Roland*), 1 oz.	40	2.0	2.0	0	0	115	0
roasted, strips (*Peloponnese* Florina), 1 oz.	10	0	2.0	0	0	260	0
strips (*B&G*), 1 oz. . .	20	0	5.0	0	0	75	0
red and yellow, fire-roasted (*Alessi*), 1 oz.	10	0	1.0	0	0	50	0
roasted (*B&G*), 1 oz.:							
w/balsamic vinegar	10	0	2.0	0	0	70	0
w/oregano/garlic ..	15	0	1.0	1.5	0	75	0
salad, w/oregano/garlic (*B&G*), 1 oz.	20	0	5.0	0	0	75	0
Pepper, sweet, freeze-dried, red or green, ¼ cup	5	.3	1.1	<.1	0	3	.3
Pepper, sweet, frozen:							
sliced, stir-fry, w/onion (*Birds Eye*), 1 cup .	25	1.0	5.0	0	0	10	1.0
strips (*C&W*), ¾ cup .	25	1.0	4.0	0	0	10	1.0
chopped, 1 oz.	6	.3	1.2	.1	0	1	.5
Pepper, sweet, seasoning, ¼ tsp.:							
Italian, and onion (*McCormick*)	0	0	0	0	0	50	0
smoky (*McCormick*) .	0	0	0	0	0	55	0
Pepper dip, red, roasted (*Marzetti's* Veggie Dip), 2 tbsp.	120	1.0	2.0	12.0	20	260	0
Pepper relish, sweet (*Grandmother's*), 1 tbsp.	20	0	5.0	0	0	105	0
Pepper sauce, see "Hot sauce," and specific listings							
Pepper spread, red:							
(*Peloponnese*), 1 tbsp.	15	0	0	1.5	0	90	0
(*Roland*), 2 tbsp.	30	0	5.0	1.0	0	0	0

Food and Measure	cal.	prot. (gms)	carbo. (gms)	fat (gms)	chol. (mgs)	sod. (mgs)	fiber (gms)
Pepper steak, see "Beef entree, frozen"							
Peppercorns, green, in vinegar or brine (*Roland*), 1 tbsp:	10	0	2.0	0	0	55	1.0
Pepperoncini, in jars:							
(*B&G*), 1 oz., about 3 pcs.	10	0	2.0	0	0	330	0
(*Roland*), 1 pc.	10	0	2.0	0	0	330	1.0
(*Roland* Golden), 3 pcs.	0	0	1.0	0	0	460	<1.0
Pepperoni, 1 oz., except as noted:							
(*Applegate Farms*)	120	7.0	0	10.0	30	490	0
(*Applegate Farms* Deli Counter), 2 oz.	230	13.0	1.0	19.0	60	980	0
(*Carando* Cubes/Link/ Grande)	130	5.0	1.0	11.0	30	540	0
(*Carando* Lower Fat)	80	8.0	1.0	5.0	20	600	0
(*Carando* Sliced)	140	6.0	0	12.0	30	530	0
(*Carnado* Snack Stick), 1.5-oz. pc.	200	8.0	1.0	18.0	45	830	0
(*Di Lusso*), 2 oz.	280	10.0	0	26.0	70	940	0
(*Farmland*)	130	5.0	1.0	11.0	30	540	0
(*Hansel 'n Gretel*), 2 oz.	240	12.0	2.0	20.0	50	860	0
(*Hormel* Chunk/Sliced/ Mild/Hot & Spicy)	140	5.0	0	13.0	35	490	0
(*Hormel* Twin)	140	5.0	0	13.0	30	500	0
(*Rosa Grande*)	140	5.0	0	13.0	30	500	0
all varieties, except thick sliced (*Hormel* Pillow Pack)	140	5.0	0	13.0	35	490	0
sandwich style (*Boar's Head*)	130	6.0	1.0	11.0	25	480	0
thick sliced (*Hormel* Pillow Pack)	140	5.0	0	13.0	35	470	0
turkey, see "Turkey pepperoni"							
uncured (*Hormel* Natural Choice*), 1.1 oz.	150	5.0	0	14.0	35	510	0
"Pepperoni," vege- tarian (*Yves*), 6 slices, 1.7 oz.	80	14.0	4.0	0	0	390	0
Perch, meat only:							
raw, 4 oz.	103	22.0	0	1.1	102	70	0

Food and Measure	cal.	prot. (gms)	carbo. (gms)	fat (gms)	chol. (mgs)	sod. (mgs)	fiber (gms)
Perch *(cont.)*							
baked or broiled, 4 oz.	133	28.2	0	1.3	130	90	0
ocean, see "Ocean perch"							
Perch, frozen, raw *(Matlaw's)*, 2 fillets, 4 oz.	100	21.0	0	1.0	100	65	0
Persimmon, fresh:							
(Frieda's Fuyu/Hachiya/ Sharon), 5 oz.	100	1.0	26.0	0	0	0	5.0
Japanese, 1 medium .	118	1.0	31.2	.3	0	3	6.0
native, 1 medium, 1.1 oz.	32	.2	8.4	.1	0	<1	n.a.
Persimmon, dried:							
(Frieda's Fuyu), ⅓ cup, 1.4 oz.	140	1.0	35.0	0	0	10	3.0
Japanese, 1 oz.	78	.4	20.8	.2	0	1	4.1
Pesto paste *(Amore)*, 2 tbsp.	110	<1.0	3.0	10.0	0	630	0
Pesto sauce, in jars:							
artichoke, w/roasted garlic *(Campagna)*, 1 tbsp.	40	1.0	1.0	3.5	0	40	<1.0
basil:							
(Alessi), 2 tbsp. . . .	175	2.0	4.0	18.0	0	490	0
(Campagna), 1 tbsp.	70	2.0	1.0	6.0	5	120	0
(Classico), ½ cup .	230	3.0	6.0	21.0	0	720	1.0
(Roland), 1 tbsp. . .	90	1.0	2.0	9.0	1	45	0
olive and sun-dried tomato *(Campagna)*, 1 tbsp.	45	0	2.0	4.0	0	65	0
tomato, sun-dried:							
(Classico), ¼ cup . .	90	3.0	8.0	5.0	0	630	1.0
(Roland), 1 tbsp. . .	80	0	2.0	8.0	0	40	0
Pesto sauce, refrigerated *(Buitoni)*, ¼ cup:							
basil	300	7.0	6.0	28.0	20	540	2.0
basil, reduced fat	240	7.0	9.0	19.0	15	540	2.0
tomato, sun-dried . . .	210	4.0	9.0	18.0	5	360	2.0
Pesto sauce mix *(McCormick)*, 2 tsp. . . .	10	1.0	1.0	0	0	480	0
Pheasant:							
raw, 4 oz.:							
meat w/skin	205	25.7	0	10.5	81	45	0
meat only	151	26.7	0	4.1	75	42	0

Food and Measure	cal.	prot. (gms)	carbo. (gms)	fat (gms)	chol. (mgs)	sod. (mgs)	fiber (gms)
raw, breast, 6.4 oz. ..	243	44.4	0	5.9	106	60	0
1 leg, 3.8 oz.	143	23.8	0	4.6	112	48	0
cooked, meat w/skin, 4 oz.	280	36.7	0	13.7	101	49	0
Phyllo, see "Fillo dough"							
Picante sauce (see also "Salsa"), 2 tbsp.:							
(*Pace*)	10	0	2.0	0	0	210	<1.0
(*Pace* Organic)	10	0	2.0	0	0	220	<1.0
hot (*Ortega*)	10	0	2.0	0	0	210	0
medium (*Ortega*)	10	0	2.0	0	0	130	0
mild (*Ortega*)	10	0	2.0	0	0	220	0
mild or medium (*Chi-Chi's*)	10	0	2.0	0	0	150	0
Pickle, cucumber, 1 oz., except as noted:							
bread and butter:							
(*B&G*)	25	0	6.0	0	0	190	0
(*B&G* Toppers)	30	0	7.0	0	0	120	0
(*Cascadian Farm* Organic)	30	0	8.0	0	0	110	0
(*Claussen* Chips) ..	20	0	4.0	0	0	180	0
cornichon (*Roland* Gherkins), 6 pcs. ..	5	0	1.0	0	0	360	1.0
deli style:							
(*B&G* New York) ..	0	0	1.0	0	0	190	0
spears (*B&G* Zesty)	0	0	1.0	0	0	170	0
dill:							
all varieties (*Roland*)	5	0	1.0	0	0	280	0
baby (*Cascadian Farm* Organic) ..	5	0	1.0	0	0	300	0
chips, hamburger (*Del Monte*)	0	0	0	0	0	370	0
hamburger (*B&G* Toppers)	0	0	<1.0	0	0	200	0
whole or halves (*Del Monte*)	5	0	1.0	0	0	370	1.0
whole or hamburger chips (*B&G*)	0	0	0	0	0	320	0
dill, kosher:							
(*B&G* No Salt)	10	0	2.0	0	0	0	0
(*Cascadian Farm* Organic)	5	1.0	0	0	0	300	0
(*Claussen* Halves) .	5	0	0	0	0	330	0

Food and Measure	cal.	prot. (gms)	carbo. (gms)	fat (gms)	chol. (mgs)	sod. (mgs)	fiber (gms)
Pickle, dill, kosher *(cont.)*							
all varieties (*Claussen*)	5	0	1.0	0	0	330	0
all varieties, except							
no salt (*B&G*) ...	0	0	0	0	0	200	0
burger slices							
(*Claussen*), .8 oz.	5	0	1.0	0	0	300	0
mini (*Claussen*),							
.8 oz.	5	0	1.0	0	0	290	0
sandwich slices							
(*Claussen*), 1.2 oz.	5	0	1.0	0	0	420	0
spears (*Claussen*),							
1.2 oz.	5	0	1.0	0	0	330	0
tiny (*Del Monte*) ...	5	0	1.0	0	0	240	<1.0
dill, Polish (*B&G*							
Toppers)	0	0	<1.0	0	0	160	0
garlic, hearty:							
whole (*Claussen*							
Deli Style)	5	0	1.0	0	0	270	0
slices (*Claussen*							
Deli Style), 1.2 oz.	5	0	1.0	0	0	320	0
sour, garlic (*Dietz &*							
Watson)	3	0	1.0	0	0	250	0
sour, half:							
(*B&G*)	0	0	0	0	0	270	0
(*Claussen* New York							
Deli)	5	0	1.0	0	0	260	0
new (*Dietz & Watson*)	4	0	1.0	0	0	210	0
sweet:							
(*B&G* Tiny Treats) .	40	0	10.0	0	0	160	0
all styles (*Del Monte*)	40	0	10.0	0	0	210	<1.0
gherkins (*Claussen*),							
.9 oz.	30	0	7.0	0	0	210	0
gherkins, whole, or							
mixed (*B&G*) ...	35	0	9.0	0	0	115	0
Pickle relish (see also							
specific listings),							
cucumber, 1 tbsp.:							
(*B&G* Emerald)	15	0	4.0	0	0	120	0
(*Crosse & Blackwell*							
Branston)	25	0	7.0	0	0	160	0
dill (*B&G*)	0	0	0	0	0	270	0
hamburger:							
(*B&G*)	15	0	4.0	0	0	150	0
(*Del Monte*)	20	0	5.0	0	0	125	<1.0

Food and Measure	cal.	prot. (gms)	carbo. (gms)	fat (gms)	chol. (mgs)	sod. (mgs)	fiber (gms)
hot dog:							
(B&G)	20	0	5.0	0	0	75	0
(Del Monte)	15	0	4.0	0	0	140	<1.0
India (B&G)	15	0	4.0	0	0	140	0
sweet:							
(B&G)	15	0	4.0	0	0	120	0
(Claussen)	15	0	3.0	0	0	85	0
(Del Monte)	20	0	5.0	0	0	125	0
(Tree of Life Organic)	15	0	4.0	0	0	120	0
(Wickles)	20	0	5.0	0	0	140	0
Pickling spice (Tone's), 1 tsp.	10	.3	1.2	.6	0	1	.3
Pie, apple (Entenmann's Homestyle), ⅛ pie .	380	3.0	57.0	16.0	0	400	2.0
Pie, frozen, ⅛ pie, except as noted:							
apple:							
(Amy's), ½ of 8-oz. pie	230	2.0	37.0	8.0	25	135	2.0
(Mrs. Smith's Slices), ½ pkg., 1 pc. . . .	270	2.0	36.0	13.0	0	290	1.0
(Sara Lee Oven Ready)	340	3.0	47.0	16.0	0	330	2.0
crumb (Mrs. Smith's Dutch)	370	3.0	51.0	17.0	0	200	2.0
banana crème (Edwards), ⅛ pie . .	480	4.0	51.0	29.0	15	340	<1.0
blueberry:							
(Mrs. Smith's)	330	3.0	43.0	16.0	0	360	2.0
(Sara Lee), ⅛ pie . .	350	3.0	50.0	16.0	0	350	2.0
coconut crème (Edwards)	460	4.0	51.0	27.0	15	330	2.0
coconut custard (Mrs. Smith's)	300	6.0	32.0	16.0	65	280	1.0
lemon meringue (Mrs. Smith's)	290	2.0	47.0	11.0	40	190	<1.0
lime, key:							
(Edward's)	450	6.0	58.0	22.0	50	310	0
(Edward's Slices), ½ pkg., 1 pc. . . .	330	4.0	42.0	16.0	35	250	0
mince (Mrs. Smith's) .	370	3.0	52.0	17.0	0	380	2.0
Oreo cream (Edward's Slices), ½ pkg., 1 pc.	290	3.0	32.0	17.0	10	220	<1.0

Food and Measure	cal.	prot. (gms)	carbo. (gms)	fat (gms)	chol. (mgs)	sod. (mgs)	fiber (gms)
Pie, frozen *(cont.)*							
pumpkin:							
(*Mrs. Smith's*)	290	5.0	38.0	14.0	45	310	1.0
(*Mrs. Smith's* Hearty)	280	5.0	38.0	13.0	45	280	2.0
strawberries and cream							
(*Sara Lee*)	350	3.0	42.0	20.0	0	160	1.0
sweet potato (*Mrs.*							
Smith's)	350	4.0	44.0	18.0	40	210	1.0
turtle (*Edward's*)	390	4.0	46.0	22.0	10	270	1.0
Pie, mix *(Jell-O* No Bake), ⅙ pkg., except as noted:							
chocolate silk, double	190	2.0	34.0	6.0	0	390	2.0
w/cookies	280	2.0	48.0	8.0	0	440	2.0
peanut butter cup,							
⅛ pkg.	290	4.0	39.0	15.0	0	310	2.0
pumpkin pie style,							
⅛ pkg.	130	1.0	30.0	1.5	0	340	1.0
Pie crust (see also "Pastry shell"), ⅛ of 9" crust, except as noted:							
(*Pet•Ritz*)	80	1.0	9.0	4.0	0	70	0
(*Pillsbury*)	110	<1.0	12.0	7.0	<5	140	0
chocolate:							
(*Arrowhead Mills* Organic)	110	1.0	14.0	6.0	0	95	<1.0
(*Ready Crust*)	100	1.0	14.0	4.5	0	110	<1.0
cookie, ⅙ crust:							
(*Nilla*)	140	1.0	18.0	8.0	5	85	0
(*Oreo*)	130	1.0	19.0	7.0	0	170	1.0
deep dish (*Pet•Ritz*) ..	90	1.0	11.0	5.0	<5	85	0
graham cracker:							
(*Arrowhead Mills* Organic)	110	1.0	14.0	5.0	0	65	<1.0
(*Honey Maid*), ⅙ crust	150	1.0	18.0	8.0	0	115	0
(*Ready Crust* 9") ..	110	1.0	14.0	5.0	0	115	<1.0
(*Ready Crust* 10"), ⅒ crust	130	1.0	18.0	6.0	0	140	<1.0
(*Ready Crust* Reduced Fat) ...	100	1.0	15.0	3.5	0	100	0
mini (*Ready Crust*), .8-oz. crust	110	1.0	15.0	5.0	0	125	<1.0

Food and Measure	cal.	prot. (gms)	carbo. (gms)	fat (gms)	chol. (mgs)	sod. (mgs)	fiber (gms)
shortbread (*Ready Crust*)	110	1.0	14.0	5.0	0	110	0
Pie crust mix:							
(*Betty Crocker*), ¼ crust*	160	4.0	33.0	2.0	0	340	1.0
("*Jiffy*"), ¹⁄₁₆ pkg.	80	<1.0	8.0	5.0	<5	120	0
Pie filling, ⅓ cup, except as noted:							
apple:							
(*Lucky Leaf* Lite) ..	30	0	7.0	0	0	10	0
(*Lucky Leaf/ Musselman's*) ...	90	0	22.0	0	0	40	2.0
apricot (*Lucky Leaf*) .	90	0	22.0	0	0	55	0
banana crème (*Musselman's*)	110	0	28.0	0	0	75	0
blackberry (*Lucky Leaf* Premium)	90	0	23.0	0	0	65	3.0
blueberry:							
(*Lucky Leaf* Premium)	100	0	24.0	0	0	45	1.0
(*Lucky Leaf/ Musselman's*) ...	90	0	22.0	0	0	50	1.0
cherry:							
(*Lucky Leaf* Lite) ..	35	0	8.0	0	0	15	0
(*Lucky Leaf/ Musselman's*) ...	100	0	24.0	0	0	40	0
dark sweet (*Lucky Leaf*)	140	0	35.0	0	0	15	0
chocolate crème (*Musselman's*)	100	0	25.0	0	0	95	0
coconut crème:							
(*Lucky Leaf*)	110	1.0	25.0	2.0	0	140	3.0
(*Musselman's*)	110	0	25.0	1.0	0	90	0
lemon:							
(*Lucky Leaf*)	120	0	29.0	1.0	15	220	0
(*Musselman's*)	120	0	30.0	0	0	220	0
lemon crème:							
(*Lucky Leaf*)	130	0	31.0	1.0	10	220	0
(*Musselman's*)	100	0	25.0	0	0	160	0
lime, key (*Lucky Leaf/ Musselman's*)	130	0	31.0	0	0	210	0
mince/mincemeat:							
(*Crosse & Blackwell*), ¼ cup	180	<1.0	43.0	0	0	220	0
(*None Such*)	190	0	45.0	.5	0	230	0

Food and Measure	cal.	prot. (gms)	carbo. (gms)	fat (gms)	chol. (mgs)	sod. (mgs)	fiber (gms)
Pie filling, mince/mincemeat *(cont.)*							
w/brandy and rum (*Crosse & Blackwell*), ¼ cup	180	<1.0	43.0	0	0	230	0
w/brandy and rum (*None Such*)	200	0	47.0	1.0	0	250	0
condensed (*None Such*), 4 tsp. . . .	150	0	36.0	.5	0	230	1.0
peach (*Lucky Leaf*) . .	80	0	21.0	0	0	30	0
pineapple (*Lucky Leaf*)	100	0	23.0	0	0	35	1.0
pumpkin:							
(*Libby's* Pie Mix) . .	90	1.0	20.0	.5	0	120	3.0
(*Tree of Life* Pie Mix Organic), ½ cup .	100	0	25.0	0	0	5	2.0
raisin (*Lucky Leaf*) . .	90	0	22.0	0	0	75	1.0
raspberry, red (*Lucky Leaf* Premium)	80	0	19.0	0	0	35	2.0
strawberry (*Lucky Leaf/ Musselman's*)	80	0	20.0	0	0	50	1.0
vanilla crème (*Musselman's*)	100	0	23.0	1.0	0	80	0
Pie filling mix, see "Pudding and pie filling mix"							
Pierogi, frozen, 3 pcs., 4.25 oz., except as noted:							
potato/cheddar:							
(*Mrs. T.'s*)	180	6.0	34.0	2.5	5	530	1.0
bacon, mini (*Mrs. T.'s*), 7 pcs., 3 oz.	140	5.0	25.0	3.0	5	450	1.0
broccoli (*Mrs. T.'s*) .	200	6.0	33.0	4.5	5	560	2.0
jalapeño (*Mrs. T.'s*)	180	6.0	34.0	2.5	10	540	1.0
mini (*Mrs. T.'s*), 7 pcs., 3 oz.	130	4.0	25.0	1.5	5	360	1.0
potato/cheese:							
(*Golden*), 3 pcs., 4 oz.	240	9.0	39.0	5.0	0	250	<1.0
American (*Mrs. T.'s*)	210	8.0	32.0	6.0	15	570	1.0
four (*Mrs. T.'s*)	230	6.0	36.0	7.0	10	570	1.0
four, mini (*Mrs. T.'s*), 7 pcs., 3 oz.	150	4.0	27.0	4.5	5	390	1.0
potato/onion:							
(*Mrs. T.'s*)	170	5.0	34.0	2.0	5	420	1.0

Food and Measure	cal.	prot. (gms)	carbo. (gms)	fat (gms)	chol. (mgs)	sod. (mgs)	fiber (gms)
(*Golden*), 3 pcs., 4 oz.	180	4.0	35.0	3.0	0	200	<1.0
potato/sour cream/ chive (*Mrs. T.'s*)	210	6.0	34.0	5.0	15	510	1.0
sauerkraut (*Mrs. T.'s*)	150	4.0	30.0	1.5	5	770	1.0
Pig's feet (see also "Pork, pickled"):							
simmered, 4 oz.	220	21.8	0	14.1	113	34	0
pickled, 2 oz.:							
(*Hormel*)	80	7.0	0	6.0	45	590	0
jalapeño (*Hormel*)	80	7.0	0	6.0	45	580	0
Pigeon peas, fresh:							
raw, ½ cup	105	5.5	18.4	1.3	0	4	3.2
boiled, drained, ½ cup	86	4.6	15.0	1.1	0	3	2.5
Pigeon peas, canned, green (*Roland*), ½ cup	80	4.0	15.0	0	0	610	4.0
Pigeon peas, dried, boiled, ½ cup	102	5.7	19.5	.3	0	5	3.9
Pignolia nuts, see "Pine nuts"							
Pike, meat only:							
northern, 4 oz.:							
raw	100	21.8	0	.8	44	44	0
baked or broiled	128	28.0	0	1.0	57	56	0
walleye, 4 oz.:							
raw	105	21.7	0	1.4	98	58	0
baked or broiled	135	27.8	0	1.8	125	74	0
Pili nuts, shelled, dried, 1 oz.	204	3.1	1.1	22.6	0	4	<1.0
Pimiento, can or jar:							
whole:							
(*Roland*), 6.5-oz. can	20	1.0	3.0	0	0	120	1.0
(*Roland* Del Piquillo), ½ cup	50	2.0	11.0	.5	0	180	1.0
whole or diced (*Roland*), ½ cup	30	1.0	5.0	0	0	310	1.0
Piña colada drink, see "Pineapple drink blend"							
Piña colada drink mixer:							
(*Angostura*), 8 fl. oz.	120	0	31.0	0	0	240	0

Food and Measure	cal.	prot. (gms)	carbo. (gms)	fat (gms)	chol. (mgs)	sod. (mgs)	fiber (gms)
Piña colada drink mixer *(cont.)*							
(*Daily's*), 3 fl. oz.	155	0	35.0	2.0	<5	55	0
(*Malibu*), 2.33 fl. oz. .	110	0	28.0	1.0	0	10	1.0
(*Master of Mixers*),							
4 fl. oz.	140	0	34.0	0	0	25	0
(*Roland/Costamar*),							
3 fl. oz.	120	1.0	17.0	6.0	0	30	0
(*Vigo*), 3 fl. oz.	120	1.0	17.0	6.0	0	30	0
frozen (*Bacardi*), 2 fl. oz.	170	0	36.0	4.0	0	20	0
Pine nuts, dried, shelled:							
(*Alessi*), 1 oz.	210	5.0	0	20.0	0	0	1.0
(*Diamond*), ¼ cup . . .	200	4.0	4.0	20.0	0	0	1.0
(*Frieda's*), ¼ cup, 1.1 oz.	150	7.0	4.0	15.0	0	0	1.0
(*Planters*), 2-oz. pkg. .	320	13.0	8.0	28.0	0	0	3.0
(*SunRidge Farms*),							
¼ cup, 1.1 oz.	160	7.0	5.0	14.0	0	5	1.0
pignolia:							
(*Alessi*), 4 tbsp. . . .	210	5.0	0	20.0	0	0	1.0
(*Shiloh Farms*),							
¼ cup, 1.3 oz. . .	190	4.0	9.0	15.0	0	0	4.0
1 oz.	160	6.8	4.0	14.2	0	1	1.3
1 tbsp.	49	2.1	1.2	4.4	0	<1	.4
pinyon:							
1 oz.	178	3.3	5.5	17.3	0	20	3.0
10 kernels	6	.1	.2	.6	0	1	.1
Pineapple, fresh:							
(*Dole*), 2 slices,							
3" diam. x ¾"	60	1.0	16.0	0	0	10	1.0
(*Frieda's* Zulu Queen							
Baby), 1 cup, 5 oz. .	70	1.0	17.0	.5	0	0	2.0
whole, 1 lb.	231	1.8	58.5	2.0	0	5	5.7
diced, ½ cup	38	.3	9.6	.3	0	<1	.9
Pineapple, can/jar,							
½ cup, except as							
noted:							
(*Dole*), 4-oz. bowl . . .	60	<1.0	16.0	0	0	10	1.0
in juice:							
chunks (*Del Monte*)	70	0	17.0	0	0	10	1.0
chunks (*Del Monte*							
Fruit Naturals) . .	70	<1.0	18.0	0	0	5	<1.0
chunks (*SunFresh*) .	70	0	18.0	0	0	10	<1.0
chunks or tidbits							
(*Dole*)	60	0	15.0	0	0	10	1.0
crushed (*Dole*)	70	0	17.0	0	0	10	1.0

Food and Measure	cal.	prot. (gms)	carbo. (gms)	fat (gms)	chol. (mgs)	sod. (mgs)	fiber (gms)
crushed (*Roland*) .	70	0	17.0	0	0	10	1.0
sliced (*Del Monte*), 2 pcs.	60	0	16.0	0	0	10	1.0
sliced (*Dole*), 2 pcs.	60	0	15.0	0	0	10	1.0
sliced or tidbits (*Roland*)	70	1.0	17.0	0	0	10	1.0
tidbits (*Del Monte* Bowl), 4 oz.	70	<1.0	18.0	0	0	5	<1.0
tidbits (*Del Monte* Pull-Top), 4 oz. .	50	<1.0	15.0	0	0	10	<1.0
wedges (*Del Monte*)	70	0	17.0	0	0	10	1.0
in light syrup:							
chunks (*Dole*)	80	0	21.0	0	0	0	1.0
sliced (*Roland*) . . .	108	1.0	26.0	0	0	16	1.0
in heavy syrup:							
chunks (*Dole*)	90	<1.0	24.0	0	0	10	1.0
chunks or crushed (*Del Monte*)	90	0	24.0	0	0	10	1.0
sliced (*Del Monte*), 2 pcs.	90	0	23.0	0	0	10	1.0
sliced (*Dole*), 2 pcs.	90	<1.0	24.0	0	0	10	1.0
and crème (*Dole* Parfait), 2.3-oz. cup . .	110	0	24.0	2.0	0	5	0
in lime gelatin (*Dole* Fruit Bowls), 4.3-oz. cup	90	<1.0	23.0	0	0	95	0
Pineapple, dried:							
(*Amport Foods*), 7 pcs., 1.5 oz.	140	1.0	36.0	0	0	0	1.0
(*Sunsweet*), ⅓ cup, 1.4 oz.	130	0	34.0	0	0	25	1.0
Pineapple, frozen, chunks, ¾ cup:							
(*Dole*)	100	0	25.0	0	0	0	2.0
(*Dole* Organic)	70	0	18.0	0	0	0	2.0
Pineapple drink blend, 8 fl. oz.:							
coconut (*R.W. Knudsen*) . . .	170	1.0	39.0	1.0	0	50	<1.0
(*Santa Cruz Organic*)	130	1.0	30.0	.5	0	20	0
(*SoBe Liz Bizz Piña Colada*)	130	0	32.0	0	0	50	0
orange (*Tropicana*) . . .	130	<1.0	32.0	0	0	25	0

Food and Measure	cal.	prot. (gms)	carbo. (gms)	fat (gms)	chol. (mgs)	sod. (mgs)	fiber (gms)
Pineapple drink blend *(cont.)*							
orange guava:							
(*Langers*) . . . . :	130	0	30.0	0	0	0	0
(*Nantucket Nectars*)	120	0	29.0	0	0	25	0
Pineapple guava, see "Feijoas"							
Pineapple juice, 8 fl. oz.:							
(*Ceres*)	120	0	29.0	0	0	5	2.0
(*Dole* Can), 6 fl.oz. . . .	110	1.0	26.0	0	0	0	0
(*Dole* Chilled)	130	<1.0	30.0	0	0	10	0
(*Langers*)	120	0	33.0	0	0	15	0
(*R.W. Knudsen* Nectar)	140	1.0	35.0	0	0	20	0
(*R.W. Knudsen* Organic)	120	0	28.0	0	0	15	0
frozen:							
(*Dole*), ¼ cup	130	<1.0	30.0	0	0	10	0
diluted	130	1.0	31.9	<.1	0	3	.5
Pineapple juice blend, 8 fl. oz., except as noted:							
coconut (*L&A/Langers*)	140	0	28.0	3.0	0	55	1.0
orange:							
(*Dole* Can), 6 fl. oz.	100	0	24.0	0	0	0	0
(*Dole* Chilled)	120	<1.0	29.0	0	0	10	0
orange banana:							
(*Apple & Eve* Tropicals)	120	1.0	30.0	0	0	30	0
(*Dole* Can), 6 fl. oz.	100	0	25.0	0	0	15	0
(*Dole* Chilled)	130	<1.0	30.0	0	0	10	0
(*Nantucket Nectars*)	140	<1.0	34.0	0	0	30	0
(*Tropicana*)	130	<1.0	32.0	0	0	25	0
frozen (*Dole*), ¼ cup	130	<1.0	30.0	0	0	10	0
orange strawberry:							
(*Dole*)	120	<1.0	29.0	0	0	10	0
frozen (*Dole*), ¼ cup	120	<1.0	29.0	0	0	10	0
Pineapple topping (*Smucker's*), 2 tbsp.	110	0	27.0	0	0	0	0
Pink bean, dried, boiled, ½ cup	125	7.6	23.5	.4	0	2	4.5
Pink bean, canned w/chili, onion, cumin (*S&W* Pinquitos), ½ cup .	80	6.0	20.0	.5	0	480	6.0
Pinto bean:							
dry (*Arrowhead Mills* Organic), ¼ cup . . .	150	9.0	27.0	0	0	0	10.0
boiled, ½ cup	117	7.0	21.8	.4	0	1	7.3

Food and Measure	cal.	prot. (gms)	carbo. (gms)	fat (gms)	chol. (mgs)	sod. (mgs)	fiber (gms)
Pinto bean, canned (see also "Chili Beans" and "Refried beans"), ½ cup:							
(*Allens*)	110	5.0	20.0	1.0	0	290	7.0
(*Bush's*)	110	6.0	19.0	0	0	390	6.0
(*Bush's* Frijoles Pintos)	80	6.0	18.0	0	0	450	7.0
(*Eden* Organic)	100	6.0	18.0	1.0	0	15	6.0
(*Luck's*)	130	7.0	21.0	2.0	0	380	6.0
(*Luck's* Fat Free)	110	7.0	21.0	0	0	400	6.0
(*S&W*)	100	6.0	22.0	0	0	220	7.0
(*Westbrae Natural* Organic)	100	6.0	19.0	0	0	140	7.0
w/bacon: (*Trappey's*)	120	6.0	20.0	1.0	0	270	7.0
and jalapeño (*Trappey's* Jalapinto)	120	6.0	22.0	1.0	0	540	8.0
seasoned (*Bush's*) .	120	6.0	17.0	2.5	5	530	6.0
w/onion (*Luck's*)	140	7.0	23.0	2.0	0	370	6.0
w/pork: (*Bush's*)	120	6.0	17.0	2.5	5	530	6.0
(*Luck's*)	130	7.0	21.0	2.0	0	380	6.0
seasoned: (*Glory*)	100	6.0	18.0	0	0	570	6.0
(*Glory* Sensibly) . . .	100	6.0	18.0	0	0	250	6.0
spicy (*Eden* Organic) .	120	6.0	24.0	1.0	0	200	7.0
w/tomato, corn, chili (*Del Monte Savory Sides* Rio Grande) .	70	2.0	14.0	0	0	470	2.0
Pinto bean, frozen, boiled, drained, ⅓ of 10-oz. pkg. . .	152	8.8	29.0	.5	0	78	8.1
Pinto bean seasoning mix (*Zatarain's*), ½ cup*	20	1.0	4.0	0	0	460	0
Pipian sauce (*Doña Maria*), 2 tbsp.	250	4.0	5.0	20.0	0	580	3.0
Pistachio nut, shelled, except as noted: (*Frito-Lay* Salted in Shell), 1 pkg.	150	4.0	7.0	13.0	0	180	3.0
(*Shiloh Farms* Organic Split), 1 oz.	156	6.0	8.0	12.0	0	0	3.0

Food and Measure	cal.	prot. (gms)	carbo. (gms)	fat (gms)	chol. (mgs)	sod. (mgs)	fiber (gms)
Pistachio nut *(cont.)*							
(*Sunkist*), ½ cup, 1.1 oz.	170	6.0	8.0	14.0	0	160	3.0
dried, 1 oz.	164	5.8	7.1	13.7	0	2	3.1
dry-roasted:							
(*Planters*), 1 oz. . . .	170	5.0	6.0	14.0	0	190	3.0
unsalted, 1 oz.	162	6.1	7.8	13.0	0	2	2.9
unsalted, ¼ cup . . .	183	6.8	8.9	14.7	0	3	3.3
roasted:							
(*Shiloh Farms* Or-							
ganic Salted),							
¼ cup	190	6.0	9.0	14.0	0	220	3.0
(*SunRidge Farms*),							
1.1 oz.	170	6.0	8.0	14.0	0	120	3.0
(*Tree of Life*), ¼ cup,							
1.1 oz.	180	4.0	8.0	16.0	0	230	3.0
(*Tree of Life* Organic),							
1 oz.	180	<6.0	8.0	14.0	0	115	3.0
Pita, see "Bread"							
Pita chips, 1 oz.:							
(*Athenos* Original) . . .	120	3.0	19.0	4.0	0	270	0
(*Garden of Eatin'*							
Greek Isle)	130	3.0	19.0	4.5	0	280	1.0
(*Stacy's* Multigrain) . .	140	3.0	19.0	6.0	0	240	2.0
(*Stacy's Simply Naked*)	130	3.0	19.0	5.0	0	270	2.0
Asian spice (*Garden							
of Eatin'*)	130	3.0	18.0	5.0	0	350	1.0
cinnamon sugar							
(*Stacy's*)	140	3.0	20.0	5.0	0	115	2.0
garlic (*New York Style*)	130	3.0	17.0	5.0	0	440	1.0
garlic, roasted, and							
herb (*Athenos*)	120	3.0	19.0	4.0	0	290	0
hot (*Stacy's* Texarkana)	130	3.0	19.0	5.0	0	260	2.0
maple sugar cinnamon							
(*New York Style*) . .	130	3.0	18.0	5.0	0	90	1.0
Parmesan garlic herb:							
(*Snyder's* MultiGrain)	140	4.0	19.0	5.0	0	280	3.0
(*Stacy's*)	140	4.0	19.0	5.0	0	200	2.0
pesto and sun-dried							
tomato (*Stacy's*) . . .	130	3.0	19.0	5.0	0	250	2.0
sea salt:							
(*Garden of Eatin'*) .	130	3.0	18.0	5.0	0	340	1.0
(*New York Style*) . .	130	3.0	17.0	5.0	0	340	1.0
(*Snyder's* MultiGrain)	140	4.0	18.0	5.0	0	160	3.0

Food and Measure	cal.	prot. (gms)	carbo. (gms)	fat (gms)	chol. (mgs)	sod. (mgs)	fiber (gms)
spicy (*New York Style* Mediterranean)	130	3.0	18.0	5.0	0	200	1.0
sun-dried tomato and herb (*Snyder's* Multi-Grain)	140	4.0	17.0	5.0	0	350	3.0
whole wheat:							
(*Athenos*)	120	4.0	18.0	4.0	0	270	2.0
(*New York Style* Natural)	120	3.0	17.0	5.0	0	350	3.0
Pitanga:							
1 medium, .3 oz.	2	.1	.5	<.1	0	<1	<1.0
½ cup	29	.7	6.5	.3	0	3	<1.0
Pitaya, see "Dragon fruit"							
Pizza, frozen, 1 pie or pkg., except as noted:							
(*Ristorante* Generosa), ¼ pkg.	230	8.0	21.0	13.0	20	680	1.0
(*Ristorante* Pomodori), ¼ pkg.	190	7.0	20.0	8.0	10	470	1.0
(*Ristorante* Speciale), ¼ pkg.	200	9.0	19.0	10.0	15	510	1.0
bacon cheeseburger:							
(*Jack's*), ¼ pie	290	15.0	29.0	13.0	30	750	2.0
(*Jack's* Naturally Rising), ⅙ pie ..	320	16.0	41.0	11.0	25	710	3.0
Cajun (*California Pizza Kitchen* Self-Rising), ⅓ pie	260	14.0	29.0	9.0	25	630	2.0
Canadian bacon:							
(*Jack's*), ⅓ pie	330	18.0	38.0	13.0	40	760	3.0
(*Jack's* Naturally Rising), ⅙ pie ..	290	14.0	41.0	8.0	25	600	3.0
(*Tombstone*), ¼ pie	320	17.0	37.0	12.0	35	720	4.0
(*Totino's Crisp Crust Party Pizza*), ½ pie	320	13.0	34.0	15.0	10	910	1.0
cheese:							
(*Amy's*), ⅓ pie	310	12.0	38.0	12.0	15	590	2.0
(*Amy's* Single)	410	18.0	49.0	17.0	20	720	3.0
(*Cedarlane Dr. Sears Zone*)	380	27.0	39.0	14.0	30	700	6.0
(*DiGiorno* Thin Crust), ¼ pie	340	14.0	38.0	15.0	25	720	4.0
(*Ellio's*), 2 pcs.	290	13.0	42.0	6.0	15	530	3.0

Food and Measure	cal.	prot. (gms)	carbo. (gms)	fat (gms)	chol. (mgs)	sod. (mgs)	fiber (gms)
Pizza, frozen, cheese *(cont.)*							
(*Ellio's* Micro)	380	17.0	56.0	10.0	15	620	4.0
(*Ellio's* Round), ⅓ pie	320	15.0	47.0	7.0	15	580	3.0
(*Empire Kosher* Mini 4.2 oz.)	250	11.0	38.0	5.0	10	560	0
(*Jack's*), ⅓ pie	320	15.0	38.0	13.0	30	610	3.0
(*Jack's* Naturally Rising), ⅕ pie . .	340	14.0	49.0	9.0	20	580	3.0
(*Jack's* Super), ¼ pie	320	16.0	30.0	15.0	35	700	3.0
(*Jeno's Crisp 'n Tasty*)	440	16.0	47.0	21.0	15	1060	2.0
(*Michelina's Zap 'ems*)	390	14.0	41.0	19.0	25	720	2.0
(*Ristorante* Mozzarella), ¼ pkg. .	220	9.0	19.0	11.0	20	440	1.0
(*Tombstone* Brick Oven 18.2 oz.), ¼ pie	320	15.0	29.0	17.0	40	710	3.0
(*Tombstone* Brick Oven 16 oz.), ⅓ pie	350	17.0	38.0	15.0	35	680	3.0
(*Tombstone* Garlic Bread), ⅙ pie . . .	350	15.0	40.0	14.0	25	540	3.0
(*Tombstone* Harvest Wheat Thin), ⅓ pie	300	17.0	37.0	10.0	25	620	3.0
(*Totino's Crisp Crust Party Pizza*), ½ pie	320	12.0	34.0	15.0	10	760	1.0
extra (*Tombstone* 11.25 oz.), ½ pie	360	17.0	42.0	14.0	30	680	4.0
extra (*Tombstone* 20.5 oz.), ¼ pie .	350	18.0	37.0	15.0	40	660	4.0
rice crust (*Amy's*), ⅓ pie	300	11.0	31.0	14.0	15	590	2.0
cheese, five:							
(*Michelina's Lean Gourmet*)	290	15.0	42.0	7.0	10	840	2.0
tomato (*California Pizza Kitchen* 27.2 oz.), ⅙ pie .	350	18.0	35.0	15.0	35	770	2.0
tomato (*California Pizza Kitchen* 12.58 oz.), ⅓ pie	320	18.0	29.0	15.0	35	720	1.0
tomato (*Kashi*), ⅓ pie	290	14.0	37.0	9.0	20	570	4.0

Food and Measure	cal.	prot. (gms)	carbo. (gms)	fat (gms)	chol. (mgs)	sod. (mgs)	fiber (gms)
cheese, four:							
(*California Pizza Kitchen* Crispy Thin), ⅓ pie	330	17.0	31.0	16.0	35	690	2.0
(*Casa di Mama*), ¼ pie	210	9.0	25.0	8.0	20	670	2.0
(*DiGiorno*), ⅙ pie ..	310	15.0	40.0	11.0	20	830	3.0
(*DiGiorno* Thin Crust), ⅕ pie	300	15.0	34.0	11.0	25	660	3.0
(*DiGiorno Harvest Wheat Rising Crust*), ⅙ pie ...	270	15.0	35.0	9.0	15	620	4.0
(*DiGiorno Rising Crust*), ⅓ pie ...	270	13.0	34.0	9.0	20	710	2.0
(*DiGiorno Rising Crust* Micro), ½ pie	370	15.0	44.0	15.0	15	720	3.0
(*Empire Kosher*), ⅓ pie	210	11.0	32.0	6.0	20	440	1.0
(*Healthy Choice* Café Selections), 6 oz.	370	25.0	58.0	3.0	5	470	4.0
(*Lean Cuisine*)	360	17.0	55.0	8.0	10	690	2.0
(*Ristorante* Quattro Formaggi), ¼ pkg.	230	9.0	21.0	130	25	480	1.0
(*Smart Ones*)	390	19.0	56.0	10.0	20	830	4.0
(*South Beach Living* Wheat Crust) ...	340	31.0	36.0	11.0	20	650	10.0
cheese, three:							
(*Heaven's Bistro*), ⅓ pie	240	13.0	42.0	2.0	5	630	4.0
(*Tombstone* Thin Crust), ¼ pie ...	310	16.0	28.0	15.0	40	660	3.0
(*Totino's Crisp Crust Party Pizza*), ½ pie	330	13.0	33.0	16.0	25	720	1.0
cornmeal crust (*Amy's*), ⅓ pie ..	370	10.0	41.0	19.0	10	580	2.0
"cheese," vegetarian:							
(*Amy's* Soy Cheeze), ⅓ pie	290	12.0	37.0	11.0	0	590	2.0
(*Tofutti Pizza Pizzaz*), ⅓ pie	175	7.0	24.0	5.0	0	320	0
cheese/pesto, whole-wheat crust (*Amy's*), ⅓ pie	360	13.0	37.0	18.0	15	680	2.0

Food and Measure	cal.	prot. (gms)	carbo. (gms)	fat (gms)	chol. (mgs)	sod. (mgs)	fiber (gms)
Pizza, frozen *(cont.)*							
chicken:							
Greek recipe (*Michelina's Authentico*)	360	12.0	40.0	17.0	20	780	3.0
fajita (*California Pizza Kitchen Thin*), ⅓ pie	280	16.0	30.0	11.0	35	570	2.0
garlic (*California Pizza Kitchen*), ⅓ pie	280	16.0	30.0	11.0	35	570	2.0
garlic (*California Pizza Kitchen Thin*), ⅓ pie	290	17.0	31.0	11.0	35	540	2.0
garlic, roasted (*Kashi*), ⅓ pie ..	300	16.0	39.0	9.0	30	650	4.0
garlic, roasted (*Lean Cuisine*) ..	340	20.0	49.0	7.0	20	670	2.0
garlic, roasted (*Michelina's Authentico*)	360	13.0	41.0	160	25	690	2.0
Jamaican jerk (*California Pizza Kitchen*), ⅓ pie .	270	15.0	33.0	9.0	30	720	2.0
spicy, supreme (*DiGiorno Rising Crust*), ⅙ pie ...	320	17.0	40.0	10.0	30	910	3.0
Thai (*California Pizza Kitchen 27.9 oz.*), ⅙ pie	310	16.0	38.0	11.0	20	790	3.0
Thai (*California Pizza Kitchen 12.9 oz.*), ⅓ pie	280	15.0	34.0	10.0	20	780	2.0
tomato and spinach, grilled (*DiGiorno Thin Crispy*), ⅕ pie	260	16.0	33.0	8.0	25	550	2.0
and vegetable (*South Beach Living Wheat Crust*) ...	330	30.0	37.0	10.0	25	600	10.0
chicken, barbecue:							
(*California Pizza Kitchen 28 oz.*), ⅙ pie	310	17.0	38.0	9.0	30	780	2.0

Food and Measure	cal.	prot. (gms)	carbo. (gms)	fat (gms)	chol. (mgs)	sod. (mgs)	fiber (gms)
(*California Pizza Kitchen* 12.96 oz.), ⅓ pie	270	16.0	33.0	9.0	30	650	2.0
(*California Pizza Kitchen* Thin), ⅓ pie	290	17.0	35.0	9.0	30	560	2.0
(*Heaven's Bistro*), ⅓ pie	270	16.0	48.0	2.0	15	790	4.0
(*Lean Cuisine*)	350	19.0	50.0	8.0	20	620	2.0
combination:							
(*Jeno's Crisp 'n Tasty*)	490	17.0	50.0	25.0	20	1160	2.0
(*Totino's Crisp Crust Party Pizza*), ½ pie	380	14.0	34.0	21.0	15	940	1.0
deluxe:							
(*Casa di Mama*), ¼ pie	220	11.0	21.0	10.0	20	690	1.0
(*Lean Cuisine*)	350	19.0	50.0	8.0	20	530	3.0
(*South Beach Living* Wheat Crust)	340	30.0	37.0	11.0	25	650	10.0
(*Tombstone* Brick Oven), ¼ pie	280	14.0	30.0	12.0	30	560	2.0
(*Tombstone* 13.15 oz.), ⅓ pie	270	13.0	29.0	12.0	25	530	3.0
(*Tombstone* 23.6 oz.), ⅕ pie	290	14.0	31.0	12.0	30	580	3.0
hamburger:							
(*Jack's* Original), ¼ pie	280	14.0	29.0	12.0	30	580	2.0
(*Tombstone*), ⅓ pie	350	18.0	37.0	15.0	35	720	4.0
(*Totino's Crisp Crust Party Pizza*), ½ pie	360	15.0	35.0	19.0	20	800	1.0
Hawaiian (*California Pizza Kitchen*), ⅓ pie	260	14.0	31.0	9.0	20	750	2.0
Margherita:							
(*Amy's*), ⅓ pie	240	10.0	27.0	10.0	10	480	2.0
(*California Pizza Kitchen* Thin), ⅓ pie	290	13.0	31.0	13.0	20	520	2.0
(*Lean Cuisine*)	340	14.0	50.0	9.0	5	540	3.0
(*Michelina's Authentico*)	360	13.0	41.0	17.0	20	660	2.0
meat, four, ⅕ pie:							
(*DiGiorno* Thin Crispy)	320	13.0	37.0	13.0	35	830	2.0
(*Tombstone*)	310	15.0	30.0	14.0	35	690	3.0

Food and Measure	cal.	prot. (gms)	carbo. (gms)	fat (gms)	chol. (mgs)	sod. (mgs)	fiber (gms)
Pizza, frozen *(cont.)*							
meat, three:							
(*Casa di Mama*),							
¼ pie	220	10.0	23.0	9.0	20	750	2.0
(*DiGiorno* Cheese							
Stuffed Crust),							
⅙ pie	340	14.0	34.0	16.0	35	940	2.0
(*DiGiorno* Deep							
Dish), ⅙ pie	310	13.0	32.0	15.0	25	790	2.0
(*DiGiorno* Rising							
Crust), ⅙ pie . . .	360	17.0	40.0	15.0	30	1000	3.0
(*DiGiorno* Rising							
Crust Micro),							
½ pie	420	17.0	44.0	19.0	25	910	4.0
(*Jack's* Naturally							
Rising), ⅙ pie . .	330	14.0	41.0	12.0	25	640	3.0
(*Lean Cuisine*)	370	20.0	51.0	9.0	25	630	2.0
(*Tombstone* Cheese							
Stuffed), ⅙ pie . .	320	15.0	34.0	14.0	30	750	4.0
(*Totino's Crisp Crust*							
Party Pizza), ½ pie	350	13.0	34.0	18.0	15	870	1.0
meatball:							
marinara (*DiGiorno*							
Rising Crust							
2 Pack), ⅙ of							
1 pie	330	16.0	42.0	12.0	30	870	3.0
mini (*Totino's Crisp*							
Crust Party Pizza),							
½ pie	350	13.0	34.0	18.0	10	790	1.0
Mediterranean:							
(*California Pizza*							
Kitchen Thin),							
⅓ pie	280	12.0	36.0	11.0	15	580	4.0
(*Kashi*), ⅓ pie	290	15.0	37.0	9.0	20	640	5.0
cornmeal crust							
(*Amy's*), ⅓ pie . .	360	12.0	45.0	15.0	15	680	3.0
Mexican style:							
(*Jack's* Original),							
¼ pie	290	13.0	29.0	14.0	30	720	3.0
(*Totino's Crisp Crust*							
Party Pizza), ½ pie	370	16.0	34.0	19.0	20	790	2.0
mini (*Cedarlane* Bistro),							
3 pcs., 4 oz.	280	10.0	27.0	15.0	25	660	2.0

Food and Measure	cal.	prot. (gms)	carbo. (gms)	fat (gms)	chol. (mgs)	sod. (mgs)	fiber (gms)
mushroom:							
(*Empire Kosher*), ⅓ pie	210	6.0	32.0	4.0	10	380	1.0
(*Lean Cuisine* Gourmet)	320	15.0	49.0	7.0	5	660	2.0
(*Ristorante* Funghi), ¼ pkg.	220	7.0	20.0	12.0	10	510	1.0
mushroom/olive:							
(*Amy's*), ⅓ pie	250	10.0	33.0	9.0	10	560	2.0
(*Amy's* Single)	450	18.0	56.0	19.0	20	780	3.0
pepperoni:							
(*DiGiorno*), ⅙ pie	360	17.0	40.0	16.0	35	1010	2.0
(*DiGiorno* Cheese Stuffed Crust), ⅕ pie	370	19.0	40.0	16.0	40	1030	3.0
(*DiGiorno* Deep Dish), ⅙ pie	340	14.0	32.0	18.0	35	920	2.0
(*DiGiorno* Thin Crust), ⅕ pie	310	15.0	34.0	12.0	35	790	2.0
(*DiGiorno* Harvest Wheat Thin Crust), ⅕ pie	270	15.0	32.0	9.0	25	620	4.0
(*DiGiorno* Harvest Wheat Rising Crust), ⅙ pie	260	15.0	36.0	8.0	15	620	4.0
(*DiGiorno* Rising Crust 12.7 oz.), ⅓ pie	290	14.0	35.0	11.0	25	810	2.0
(*DiGiorno* Rising Crust 29.6 oz.), ⅙ pie	360	16.0	39.0	16.0	35	1050	3.0
(*DiGiorno* Rising Crust Micro), ½ pie	400	16.0	44.0	18.0	20	840	3.0
Ellio's), 2 pcs.	310	13.0	40.0	10.0	20	620	2.0
(*Healthy Choice* Café Selections), 6 oz.	370	24.0	58.0	4.5	10	540	5.0
(*Heaven's Bistro*), ⅓ pie	250	15.0	42.0	2.0	10	730	4.0
(*Jack's*), ⅓ pie	390	18.0	38.0	19.0	45	890	3.0
(*Jack's* Naturally Rising), ⅙ pie	330	14.0	41.0	13.0	30	680	3.0
(*Jack's* Original), ½ pie	370	16.0	36.0	18.0	45	830	3.0
(*Jeno's Crisp 'n Tasty*)	490	16.0	50.0	26.0	20	1170	2.0

Food and Measure	cal.	prot. (gms)	carbo. (gms)	fat (gms)	chol. (mgs)	sod. (mgs)	fiber (gms)
Pizza, frozen, pepperoni *(cont.)*							
(*Lean Cuisine*)	370	20.0	53.0	9.0	30	690	4.0
(*Michelina's Lean Gourmet*)	300	14.0	41.0	9.0	20	970	2.0
(*Michelina's Zap 'ems*)	410	13.0	41.0	22.0	25	880	2.0
(*Smart Ones*)	390	24.0	50.0	11.0	40	840	4.0
(*South Beach Living* Wheat Crust) ...	350	31.0	36.0	12.0	25	700	9.0
(*Tombstone* Brick Oven), ¼ pie ...	310	14.0	29.0	16.0	40	720	2.0
(*Tombstone* Garlic Bread), ⅙ pie ...	370	15.0	40.0	17.0	30	670	3.0
(*Tombstone* 12 oz.), ⅓ pie	280	13.0	28.0	14.0	30	620	3.0
(*Tombstone* 21.6 oz.), ¼ pie	290	14.0	30.0	13.0	30	590	3.0
(*Tombstone* Thin Crust), ¼ pie ...	320	15.0	28.0	18.0	40	780	3.0
(*Tombstone* Harvest Wheat Thin), ¼ pie	260	15.0	29.0	10.0	25	610	3.0
(*Totino's Crisp Crust Party Pizza*), ½ pie	360	12.0	33.0	10.0	10	870	2.0
(*Totino's Crisp Crust Party Pizza* Classic), ½ pie	370	13.0	33.0	20.0	15	950	1.0
(*Totino's Crisp Crust Party Pizza* Trio), ½ pie	370	13.0	33.0	21.0	15	980	1.0
cheese supreme (*Tombstone* Deep Dish), ½ of 1 pie	500	16.0	51.0	25.0	35	1030	3.0
spicy (*Casa di Mama*), ¼ pie	190	8.0	22.0	8.0	15	750	2.0
pepperoni/mushroom (*Jack's* Original), ¼ pie	300	14.0	29.0	15.0	35	680	2.0
pepperoni/sausage:							
(*Jack's*), ½ pie	370	16.0	36.0	18.0	45	810	3.0
(*Tombstone* 12.5 oz.), ⅓ pie	290	14.0	29.0	14.0	30	650	3.0
(*Tombstone* 21.4 oz.), ¼ pie	370	18.0	37.0	17.0	40	800	4.0
pesto:							
(*Amy's*), ⅓ pie	310	12.0	39.0	12.0	10	480	2.0
(*Amy's* Single)	440	12.0	39.0	19.0	15	780	2.0

Food and Measure	cal.	prot. (gms)	carbo. (gms)	fat (gms)	chol. (mgs)	sod. (mgs)	fiber (gms)
sausage:							
(*Heaven's Bistro*), ⅓ pie	250	14.0	42.0	3.0	10	630	4.0
(*Jack's*), ¼ pie	290	13.0	29.0	13.0	30	560	3.0
(*Jack's* Naturally Rising), ⅙ pie	330	13.0	41.0	12.0	25	580	3.0
(*Jeno's Crisp 'n Tasty*)	480	16.0	50.0	24.0	20	1130	2.0
(*Tombstone* Brick Oven Classic), ¼ pie	290	14.0	29.0	13.0	30	590	2.0
(*Tombstone* Double Top), ⅙ pie	310	17.0	27.0	16.0	40	700	3.0
(*Tombstone* Original Classic 22.1 oz.), ⅕ pie	290	14.0	30.0	13.0	30	590	3.0
(*Tombstone* Original Classic 12.05 oz.), ⅓ pie	270	13.0	29.0	12.0	25	540	3.0
(*Tombstone* Thin Crust), ¼ pie	330	17.0	29.0	17.0	40	760	3.0
(*Totino's* Crisp Crust Party Pizza), ½ pie	360	14.0	34.0	19.0	15	810	1.0
Italian (*DiGiorno* Rising Crust), ⅙ pie	350	16.0	39.0	15.0	30	950	3.0
Italian, sweet/tangy (*California Pizza Kitchen* Thin), ⅓ pie	290	14.0	31.0	12.0	25	570	2.0
spicy Italian (*Jack's*), ⅓ pie	380	18.0	38.0	17.0	40	720	3.0
sausage/mushroom:							
(*Jack's*), ¼ pie	290	13.0	29.0	14.0	30	570	3.0
(*Tombstone*), ⅕ pie	290	15.0	30.0	13.0	30	590	3.0
sausage/pepperoni:							
(*DiGiorno Rising Crust*), ⅙ pie	360	17.0	40.0	15.0	30	980	3.0
(*Ellio's*), 2 pcs.	310	14.0	41.0	10.0	15	610	4.0
(*Jack's*), ¼ pie	300	14.0	29.0	15.0	35	660	2.0
(*Jack's* Naturally Rising Combination), ⅙ pie	330	14.0	41.0	13.0	30	640	3.0
(*Tombstone* Brick Oven), ¼ pie	320	15.0	29.0	17.0	40	710	3.0

Food and Measure	cal.	prot. (gms)	carbo. (gms)	fat (gms)	chol. (mgs)	sod. (mgs)	fiber (gms)
Pizza, frozen, sausage/pepperoni *(cont.)*							
(*Tombstone* Double Top), ⅙ pie	330	17.0	26.0	18.0	45	780	3.0
and mushroom (*California Pizza Kitchen Self-Rising*), ⅓ pie	290	14.0	30.0	13.0	25	730	2.0
and mushroom (*Jack's* Naturally Rising), ⅙ pie ..	340	14.0	41.0	13.0	30	640	3.0
Sicilian:							
(*California Pizza Kitchen* Thin), ⅓ pie	310	17.0	30.0	14.0	30	920	2.0
(*Michelina's Authentico*)	400	15.0	40.0	20.0	30	860	2.0
spinach:							
(*Amy's*), ⅓ pie	310	12.0	38.0	12.0	15	590	2.0
(*Amy's* Single)	440	19.0	54.0	18.0	20	780	3.0
(*Ristorante*), ¼ pkg.	220	7.0	21.0	12.0	10	570	2.0
cheese (*Cedarlane Dr. Sears Zone*) .	370	26.0	40.0	14.0	30	710	7.0
garlic (*DiGiorno* Thin Crust), ¼ pie ...	330	13.0	39.0	14.0	20	650	5.0
mushroom garlic (*DiGiorno* Rising Crust), ⅙ pie ...	300	14.0	40.0	9.0	20	780	3.0
rice crust (*Amy's*), ⅓ pie	350	7.0	37.0	21.0	0	580	4.0
supreme:							
(*DiGiorno* Cheese Stuffed Crust), ⅙ pie	350	18.0	35.0	16.0	35	950	3.0
(*DiGiorno* Deep Dish), ⅙ pie	320	14.0	33.0	15.0	30	810	2.0
(*DiGiorno* Thin Crust), ⅕ pie	300	14.0	36.0	12.0	30	740	3.0
(*DiGiorno* Harvest Wheat), ⅕ pie ..	250	13.0	32.0	8.0	20	520	4.0
(*DiGiorno* Rising Crust 14.3 oz.), ⅓ of 1 pie	320	15.0	35.0	14.0	30	900	3.0
(*DiGiorno* Rising Crust 32.7 oz.), ⅙ of 1 pie	370	17.0	40.0	16.0	30	1000	3.0

Food and Measure	cal.	prot. (gms)	carbo. (gms)	fat (gms)	chol. (mgs)	sod. (mgs)	fiber (gms)
(*DiGiorno Rising Crust* Micro), ½ pie	410	16.0	45.0	18.0	25	860	4.0
(*Ellio's*), 2 pcs.	310	15.0	41.0	10.0	20	630	5.0
(*Jack's*), ¼ pie	300	14.0	29.0	15.0	35	650	3.0
(*Jeno's Crisp 'n Tasty*)	490	17.0	49.0	25.0	20	1150	2.0
(*Healthy Choice* Café Selections)	360	22.0	56.0	4.0	5	460	5.0
(*Tombstone*), ⅕ pie	300	14.0	31.0	14.0	30	640	3.0
(*Tombstone* Brick Oven), ¼ pie . . .	320	15.0	29.0	16.0	40	700	3.0
(*Tombstone* Garlic Bread), ⅙ pie . . .	360	14.0	41.0	15.0	25	610	3.0
(*Tombstone* Harvest Wheat* Thin), ¼ pie	260	15.0	29.0	10.0	25	600	3.0
(*Totino's Crisp Crust Party Pizza*), ½ pie	360	14.0	34.0	19.0	15	840	1.0
taco (*Tombstone*), ¼ pie	330	14.0	38.0	14.0	35	960	3.0
supreme/pepperoni (*Tombstone* Half & Half), ⅕ pie	330	15.0	31.0	16.0	35	730	3.0
vegetable/veggie:							
(*Amy's* Combo), ⅓ pie	300	10.0	36.0	13.0	10	680	1.0
(*Empire Kosher* Supreme), ⅓ pie	250	12.0	38.0	5.0	15	460	2.0
(*Ristorante*), ¼ pie .	190	7.0	21.0	9.0	15	570	2.0
(*Tombstone* Light), ⅕ pie	230	13.0	31.0	6.0	10	510	4.0
grilled (*Heaven's Bistro*), ⅓ pie . . .	230	13.0	42.0	1.0	0	530	4.0
vegetable, roasted:							
(*Amy's*), ⅓ pie	270	6.0	42.0	9.0	0	490	2.0
(*Amy's* Single)	410	11.0	62.0	14.0	0	780	5.0
(*Bravissimo!* All Natural), ⅓ pie . .	210	6.0	41.0	3.5	0	470	3.0
(*Cedarlane Dr. Sears* Zone)	380	27.0	39.0	14.0	30	710	7.0
(*DiGiorno Harvest Wheat*), ⅙ pie . .	240	12.0	35.0	6.0	10	490	4.0
(*Lean Cuisine*)	310	14.0	52.0	5.0	5	530	3.0
white (*California Pizza Kitchen* Crispy Thin), ⅓ pie	290	15.0	31.0	12.0	25	600	2.0

Food and Measure	cal.	prot. (gms)	carbo. (gms)	fat (gms)	chol. (mgs)	sod. (mgs)	fiber (gms)
Pizza, frozen (cont.)							
the works (*Jack's Naturally Rising*), ⅙ pie	330	14.0	42.0	12.0	25	590	3.0
Pizza, bagel, frozen, 4 pcs., 3.1 oz., except as noted:							
cheese:							
(*Empire Kosher*), 2.25-oz. pc.	130	7.0	19.0	3.0	10	330	<1.0
three (*Bagel Bites*)	210	9.0	30.0	6.0	15	580	2.0
cheese and pepperoni (*Bagel Bites*)	220	9.0	30.0	7.0	15	480	2.0
cheese, sausage, and pepperoni (*Bagel Bites*)	200	8.0	29.0	6.0	10	580	2.0
Pizza, flatbread, 1 pc.:							
chicken/bacon/spinach (*Stouffer's Corner Bistro*)	470	21.0	57.0	17.0	35	540	2.0
Margherita (*Stouffer's Corner Bistro*)	470	18.0	59.0	18.0	30	500	3.0
steak fajita (*Stouffer's Corner Bistro*)	470	20.0	58.0	17.0	40	480	3.0
Pizza, French bread, frozen, 1 pc.:							
cheese:							
(*Healthy Choice*)	350	20.0	55.0	5.0	5	600	5.0
(*Lean Cuisine*)	310	18.0	46.0	7.0	15	670	4.0
(*Stouffer's*)	360	14.0	43.0	15.0	20	530	4.0
extra (*Stouffer's*)	400	16.0	44.0	18.0	25	630	4.0
five (*Stouffer's*)	420	17.0	44.0	20.0	35	600	3.0
deluxe:							
(*Lean Cuisine*)	310	16.0	44.0	9.0	20	700	3.0
(*Stouffer's*)	430	15.0	44.0	21.0	25	820	4.0
meat, three (*Stouffer's*)	470	19.0	43.0	25.0	40	990	4.0
pepperoni:							
(*Healthy Choice*)	350	22.0	54.0	4.5	10	600	5.0
(*Lean Cuisine*)	290	15.0	43.0	8.0	20	650	3.0
(*Stouffer's*)	410	15.0	43.0	20.0	25	810	4.0
pepperoni/mushroom (*Stouffer's*)	430	16.0	44.0	21.0	25	920	4.0
sausage (*Stouffer's*)	420	15.0	43.0	21.0	25	730	4.0

Food and Measure	cal.	prot. (gms)	carbo. (gms)	fat (gms)	chol. (mgs)	sod. (mgs)	fiber (gms)
sausage/pepperoni (*Stouffer's*)	460	17.0	43.0	24.0	30	880	4.0
supreme (*Healthy Choice*)	340	20.0	53.0	4.0	10	600	4.0
vegetable, grilled (*Stouffer's*)	340	13.0	44.0	12.0	15	570	4.0
white (*Stouffer's*)	470	22.0	44.0	23.0	40	900	4.0
Pizza, stuffed/pocket (see also "Pizza snack"), frozen, 1 pc., 4.5 oz., except as noted:							
cheese:							
(*Amy's* Pocket)	300	14.0	42.0	9.0	15	450	4.0
(*Amy's* Toaster Pops), 1.9 oz.	150	5.0	23.0	5.0	5	220	1.0
(*Jack's Pizza Bursts* Super), 3 oz. . . .	250	9.0	25.0	13.0	20	440	1.0
and tomato (*Aunt Trudy's*), 5 oz. . .	320	11.0	36.0	15.0	20	490	2.0
"cheese," soy (*Amy's* Cheeze Pocket) . . .	260	12.0	39.0	8.0	0	540	1.0
pepperoni:							
(*Jack's Pizza Bursts*), 3 oz.	260	8.0	25.0	15.0	15	550	1.0
uncured (*Van's*), 4.3 oz.	330	10.0	32.0	17.0	15	400	1.0
sausage (*Hot Pockets*)	330	10.0	36.0	16.0	20	630	2.0
sausage/pepperoni:							
(*Jack's Pizza Bursts*), 3 oz.	250	8.0	25.0	13.0	10	470	1.0
spinach (*Amy's* Pocket)	280	13.0	37.0	9.0	15	460	3.0
supreme (*Jack's Pizza Bursts*), 3 oz.	260	8.0	25.0	14.0	15	490	1.0
Pizza appetizer, see "Pizza snacks"							
Pizza crust, refrigerated (*Pillsbury All Ready*), ⅙ pkg.	160	5.0	31.0	2.0	0	470	<1.0
Pizza crust mix:							
(*Arrowhead Mills Organic*), ⅙ crust .	150	7.0	30.0	.5	0	115	1.0
(*"Jiffy"*), ⅕ pkg.	140	3.0	26.0	2.5	0	280	<1.0

Food and Measure	cal.	prot. (gms)	carbo. (gms)	fat (gms)	chol. (mgs)	sod. (mgs)	fiber (gms)
Pizza crust mix *(cont.)*							
(*Martha White* Deep							
Pan), ⅕ pkg.	140	5.0	28.0	1.0	0	320	<1.0
white (*Watkins* Deep							
Dish), ⅛ pkg.	180	6.0	36.0	1.0	0	60	2.0
whole wheat (*Watkins*							
Thin), ⅛ pkg.	90	3.0	18.0	1.0	0	75	2.0
Pizza Hut, ⅛ pie,							
except as noted:							
Fit 'N Delicious, 12"							
chicken/onion/pepper	170	9.0	23.0	4.5	15	520	1.0
chicken/mushroom	160	9.0	22.0	4.5	15	730	1.0
ham/mushroom or							
ham/pineapple . .	160	8.0	23.0	4.5	15	580	1.0
pepper/onion	150	6.0	23.0	4.0	10	420	1.0
tomato/mushroom .	150	6.0	22.0	4.0	10	630	1.0
Fit 'N Delicious, 14"							
chicken/mushroom	230	13.0	30.0	6.0	25	1010	2.0
chicken/onion/pepper	230	13.0	32.0	6.0	25	730	2.0
ham/mushroom . . .	230	11.0	31.0	7.0	20	820	2.0
ham/pineapple	230	11.0	32.0	6.0	20	830	1.0
pepper/onion	210	8.0	32.0	6.0	10	580	2.0
tomato/mushroom .	210	9.0	31.0	6.0	10	870	2.0
hand-tossed, 12":							
cheese only	230	12.0	25.0	10.0	25	620	1.0
ham/pineapple	220	10.0	26.0	8.0	20	620	1.0
Meat Lover's	340	17.0	25.0	19.0	45	1040	1.0
pepperoni	240	12.0	24.0	11.0	25	690	1.0
pepperoni/mushroom	230	11.0	25.0	9.0	20	610	1.0
sausage/onion	260	12.0	26.0	12.0	30	670	1.0
supreme	270	13.0	26.0	13.0	30	780	2.0
Veggie Lover's	210	10.0	26.0	8.0	15	580	2.0
hand-tossed, 14":							
cheese only	340	17.0	36.0	14.0	35	900	2.0
ham/pineapple	310	15.0	38.0	11.0	30	900	2.0
Meat Lover's	490	24.0	37.0	27.0	65	1510	2.0
pepperoni	360	17.0	35.0	16.0	40	1010	2.0
pepperoni/mushroom	330	16.0	36.0	14.0	30	890	2.0
sausage/onion	370	17.0	38.0	17.0	40	960	2.0
supreme	390	19.0	37.0	18.0	40	1130	2.0
Veggie Lover's	310	14.0	37.0	12.0	25	840	2.0
pan pizza, 12":							
cheese only	270	11.0	27.0	13.0	25	570	1.0
ham/pineapple	250	10.0	28.0	11.0	20	560	1.0

Food and Measure	cal.	prot. (gms)	carbo. (gms)	fat (gms)	chol. (mgs)	sod. (mgs)	fiber (gms)
Meat Lover's	370	17.0	28.0	22.0	45	990	2.0
pepperoni	280	12.0	27.0	14.0	25	640	1.0
pepperoni/mushroom	260	11.0	27.0	13.0	20	560	1.0
sausage/onion	300	12.0	28.0	15.0	30	610	1.0
supreme	310	13.0	28.0	16.0	30	720	2.0
Veggie Lover's	250	10.0	28.0	11.0	15	530	2.0
pan pizza, 14":							
cheese only	390	16.0	38.0	19.0	35	800	2.0
ham/pineapple	360	14.0	39.0	16.0	30	790	2.0
Meat Lover's	530	23.0	39.0	31.0	65	1400	2.0
pepperoni	400	16.0	37.0	21.0	40	900	2.0
pepperoni/mushroom	380	15.0	37.0	18.0	30	790	2.0
sausage/onion	420	17.0	39.0	22.0	40	860	2.0
supreme	440	18.0	39.0	23.0	40	1020	2.0
Veggie Lover's	350	14.0	39.0	16.0	25	730	2.0
personal pan pizza, whole 6" pie:							
cheese only	620	28.0	69.0	26.0	60	1370	3.0
ham/pineapple	570	25.0	70.0	21.0	50	1360	3.0
Meat Lover's	890	41.0	70.0	49.0	115	2460	4.0
pepperoni	640	28.0	67.0	29.0	65	1530	3.0
pepperoni/mushroom	600	26.0	68.0	25.0	55	1350	3.0
sausage/onion	690	29.0	71.0	33.0	70	1530	4.0
supreme	710	32.0	70.0	34.0	70	1800	4.0
Veggie Lover's	560	24.0	70.0	22.0	40	1250	4.0
stuffed crust, 14":							
cheese only	360	18.0	37.0	16.0	40	1050	2.0
ham/pineapple	350	17.0	39.0	14.0	40	1090	2.0
Meat Lover's	520	26.0	38.0	29.0	75	1690	2.0
pepperoni	390	19.0	37.0	19.0	50	1200	2.0
pepperoni/mushroom	360	18.0	37.0	16.0	40	1090	2.0
sausage/onion	410	19.0	39.0	20.0	50	1160	2.0
supreme	420	21.0	39.0	21.0	50	1320	2.0
Veggie Lover's	340	16.0	38.0	14.0	35	1030	2.0
thin 'n crispy, 12":							
cheese only	200	10.0	21.0	8.0	25	570	1.0
ham/pineapple	180	9.0	23.0	6.0	20	570	1.0
Meat Lover's	310	15.0	22.0	19.0	45	1010	1.0
pepperoni	210	10.0	21.0	10.0	25	640	1.0
pepperoni/mushroom	190	9.0	21.0	8.0	20	560	1.0
sausage/onion	230	10.0	23.0	11.0	30	620	1.0
supreme	230	11.0	22.0	11.0	30	730	1.0
Veggie Lover's	180	8.0	23.0	7.0	15	550	1.0

Food and Measure	cal.	prot. (gms)	carbo. (gms)	fat (gms)	chol. (mgs)	sod. (mgs)	fiber (gms)
Pizza Hut (cont.)							
thin 'n crispy, 14":							
cheese only	280	14.0	30.0	12.0	35	810	1.0
ham/pineapple	260	12.0	32.0	9.0	30	810	1.0
Meat Lover's	430	21.0	31.0	25.0	65	1430	2.0
pepperoni	300	14.0	29.0	14.0	40	920	1.0
pepperoni/mushroom	270	13.0	30.0	12.0	30	800	1.0
sausage/onion	320	14.0	32.0	15.0	40	870	2.0
supreme	330	16.0	31.0	16.0	40	1040	2.0
Veggie Lover's	260	12.0	31.0	10.0	25	770	2.0
XL Full House Pizza,							
1/12 of pie:							
cheese only	280	12.0	30.0	12.0	30	690	2.0
ham/pineapple	260	11.0	32.0	10.0	20	680	2.0
Meat Lover's	370	17.0	31.0	20.0	45	1090	2.0
pepperoni	280	12.0	30.0	13.0	30	750	2.0
pepperoni/mushroom	270	11.0	30.0	11.0	25	670	2.0
sausage/onion	300	12.0	32.0	14.0	30	720	2.0
supreme	310	13.0	31.0	14.0	30	830	2.0
Veggie Lover's	260	10.0	31.0	10.0	20	650	2.0
appetizers:							
breadsticks, 1 pc.:							
regular	150	4.0	20.0	6.0	0	230	1.0
cheese	200	7.0	21.0	10.0	15	370	1.0
dipping sauce ...	40	1.0	8.0	0	0	270	0
wings, hot, 2 pcs. .	120	11.0	1.0	7.0	65	500	0
wings, mild, 2 pcs.	110	11.0	2.0	7.0	65	390	0
wings dipping sauce:							
blue cheese	220	1.0	3.0	23.0	15	400	0
ranch	220	1.0	3.0	23.0	20	400	0
desserts:							
apple pizza, slice ..	260	4.0	52.0	5.0	0	290	1.0
cherry pizza, slice .	260	4.0	47.0	4.5	0	280	1.0
cinnamon sticks, 2 .	170	4.0	27.0	5.0	0	180	1.0
icing dipping ...	190	0	47.0	0	0	0	0
Pizza mix (*Chef Boyar-*							
dee Kit), 1/4 pkg.:							
cheese	260	10.0	45.0	4.5	10	760	2.0
cheese, two	250	9.0	45.0	4.0	5	730	2.0
pepperoni	290	11.0	44.0	8.0	15	740	2.0
Pizza pocket, see							
"Pizza, stuffed/							
pocket"							

Food and Measure	cal.	prot. (gms)	carbo. (gms)	fat (gms)	chol. (mgs)	sod. (mgs)	fiber (gms)
Pizza rolls, see "Pizza snack"							
Pizza sauce, ¼ cup, except as noted:							
(*Contadina* Original/ Squeeze)	30	1.0	6.0	0	0	340	1.0
(*Eden* Organic Pizza/ Pasta), ½ cup	65	2.0	9.0	2.5	0	300	5.0
(*Furmano's*)	25	1.0	4.0	.5	0	190	1.0
(*Muir Glen* Organic) . .	40	1.0	6.0	1.0	0	230	2.0
w/cheese, four (*Contadina*)	30	<1.0	6.0	.5	0	390	<1.0
chunky, deep dish (*Furmano's*)	15	1.0	3.0	0	0	190	1.0
pepperoni flavor (*Contadina*)	35	1.0	5.0	1.0	0	390	<1.0
Pizza snacks (see also "Pizza, stuffed/ pocket"), frozen:							
(*Cedarlane* Mini Bistro), 3 pcs., 4 oz.	280	10.0	27.0	15.0	25	660	2.0
cheese:							
(*Amy's*), ½ of 6-oz. pkg., 5-6 pcs.	190	9.0	22.0	7.0	10	390	2.0
(*Jack's Pizza Bursts* Supercheese), 3 oz.	250	9.0	25.0	13.0	20	440	1.0
double (*Pizza Mini's*), 5 pcs., 3 oz.	240	5.0	30.0	11.0	10	410	2.0
cheeseburger (*Michelina's Zap'ems*), 5.5-oz. pkg.	430	13.0	43.0	23.0	25	690	2.0
chicken, pesto, w/moz- zarella (*Alexia Pizza Snacks*), 6 pcs., 3 oz.	220	9.0	23.0	10.0	10	310	1.0
pepperoni:							
(*Jack's Pizza Bursts*), 3 oz.	260	8.0	25.0	15.0	15	550	1.0
(*Ristorante* Antipasto), 3 pcs., 3 oz.	240	9.0	20.0	14.0	25	720	1.0
pepperoni/cheese:							
(*Michelina's Budget Gourmet*), 5-oz. pkg.	380	12.0	39.0	20.0	20	770	3.0

Food and Measure	cal.	prot. (gms)	carbo. (gms)	fat (gms)	chol. (mgs)	sod. (mgs)	fiber (gms)
Pizza snacks, pepperoni/cheese *(cont.)*							
(*Michelina's Lean Gourmet*), 11 pcs., 3 oz.	200	8.0	24.0	8.0	10	290	2.0
(*Michelina's Zap'ems*), 5.5-oz. pkg.	420	13.0	42.0	21.0	25	850	3.0
pepperoni/sausage (*Jack's Pizza Bursts*), 3 oz.	250	8.0	25.0	13.0	10	470	1.0
rolls, 3 pcs., 3.3 oz.:							
combo (*Totino's Mega Ultimate*) .	200	8.0	25.0	8.0	10	480	1.0
pepperoni (*Totino's Mega Ultimate*) .	230	9.0	25.0	11.0	15	580	1.0
rolls, 6 pcs., 3 oz.:							
cheese (*Michelina's*)	210	8.0	23.0	10.0	15	410	1.0
cheese (*Totino's*) . .	190	8.0	26.0	6.0	5	480	1.0
cheesy taco (*Totino's*)	210	7.0	23.0	10.0	20	440	1.0
combo (*Totino's*) . .	220	8.0	24.0	11.0	10	470	1.0
hamburger (*Totino's*)	210	8.0	24.0	9.0	10	490	1.0
meat, 4 (*Michelina's*)	230	9.0	23.0	12.0	15	410	1.0
meat, 3 (*Totino's*) . .	210	8.0	24.0	9.0	10	470	1.0
pepperoni (*Michelina's*)	230	8.0	24.0	11.0	10	460	1.0
pepperoni (*Totino's*)	210	8.0	25.0	10.0	10	480	1.0
sausage (*Totino's*) .	210	8.0	46.0	10.0	10	410	1.0
sausage/pepperoni (*Michelina's*) . . .	220	7.0	24.0	10.0	10	420	1.0
supreme (*Totino's*) .	210	7.0	25.0	9.0	10	390	2.0
sausage:							
and pepperoni (*Pizza Mini's*), 5 pcs., 3 oz.	230	6.0	29.0	10.0	10	440	2.0
roasted peppers, Parmesan (*Alexia Pizza Snacks*), 6 pcs., 3 oz.	210	7.0	23.0	10.0	10	210	1.0
spinach:							
(*Amy's*), ½ of 6-oz. pkg., 5-6 pcs. . . .	200	8.0	26.0	7.0	15	420	1.0
(*Ristorante* Antipasto), 3 pcs., 3 oz.	180	6.0	20.0	8.0	10	660	0
supreme (*Jack's Pizza Bursts*), 3 oz.	260	8.0	25.0	14.0	15	490	1.0

Food and Measure	cal.	prot. (gms)	carbo. (gms)	fat (gms)	chol. (mgs)	sod. (mgs)	fiber (gms)
Plantain, fresh:							
raw:							
(*Frieda's*), 3 oz. ...	100	1.0	27.0	0	0	0	2.0
1 medium, 6.3 oz. .	218	2.3	57.1	.6	0	7	4.1
mashed (*Dole*), 1 cup	232	2.0	62.0	0	0	10	5.0
sliced, ½ cup	91	1.0	23.6	.3	0	3	1.7
cooked, sliced, ½ cup	89	.6	24.0	.1	0	4	1.8
Plantain chips:							
(*El Isleno*), 1 oz......	150	<1.0	17.0	9.0	0	35	2.0
(*Goya*), 1 oz.	150	<1.0	19.0	8.0	0	85	1.0
Plum, fresh:							
(*Del Monte*), 2 medium, 4.7 oz.	80	1.0	19.0	1.0	0	0	2.0
(*Dole*), 1 medium, 2.3 oz.	40	0	10.0	0	0	0	1.0
Japanese or hybrid, 2⅛" fruit	36	.5	8.6	.4	0	tr.	<1.0
sliced, ½ cup	46	.7	10.7	.5	0	1	1.2
Plum, can/jar, purple:							
in juice:							
½ cup	73	.7	19.1	<.1	0	2	1.3
3 plums and 2 tbsp. liquid	55	.5	14.4	<.1	0	1	1.0
in light syrup:							
½ cup	79	.5	20.5	.1	0	25	1.3
3 plums and 2¾ tbsp. liquid	83	.5	21.7	.1	0	26	1.3
in heavy syrup:							
½ cup	115	.5	30.0	.1	0	25	1.3
purple, whole (*Oregon*), ½ cup	100	1.0	25.0	0	0	15	2.0
Plum, dried (prune):							
(*Del Monte*), 5 pcs., 1.5 oz.	110	1.0	26.0	0	0	0	3.0
(*Dole*), ¼ cup, 1.4 oz.	110	1.0	26.0	0	0	5	2.0
(*Earthbound Farm* Organic), 5 pcs., 1.5 oz.	110	1.0	25.0	0	0	0	3.0
(*Sunsweet*), 1.4 oz. ...	100	1.0	24.0	0	0	5	3.0
pitted:							
(*Shiloh Farms/Shiloh Farms* Organic), 5 pcs., 1.4 oz. ..	124	1.0	29.0	0	0	6	3.0
(*Sun•Maid*), ¼ cup, 1.4 oz.	100	1.0	26.0	0	0	0	3.0

Food and Measure	cal.	prot. (gms)	carbo. (gms)	fat (gms)	chol. (mgs)	sod. (mgs)	fiber (gms)
Plum, dried, pitted (cont.)							
bite size (*Sunsweet*), 7 pcs., 1.4 oz. ...	100	1.0	24.0	0	0	5	3.0
cherry, lemon, or orange essence (*Sunsweet*), 5 pcs., 1.4 oz.	100	1.0	24.0	0	0	5	3.0
cooked, w/pits:							
(*Sunsweet* Ready to Serve), ⅔ cup ..	150	2.0	37.0	0	0	15	3.0
unsweetened, ½ cup	113	1.2	29.8	.2	0	2	7.0
puree, 1 oz.	73	.6	18.5	.1	0	7	.9
Plum, dried, canned, in heavy syrup:							
← pitted (*Oregon* Italian Prunes), ½ cup ...	130	2.0	28.0	.5	0	20	7.0
pitted, 4 oz.	119	1.0	31.5	.2	0	3	4.3
½ cup	123	1.0	32.5	.2	0	3	4.4
5 pcs., 2 tbsp. liquid .	90	.8	23.9	.2	0	2	3.3
Plum, pickled, see "Umeboshi plum"							
Plum drink, 8 fl. oz.:							
(*Sunsweet PlumSmart* Light)	60	0	15.0	0	0	20	3.0
red (*Nantucket Nectars*)	120	0	30.0	0	0	25	0
Plum juice (see also "Prune juice")							
(*Sunsweet Plum-Smart*), 8 fl. oz. ...	160	0	36.0	0	0	55	3.0
Plum pudding (*Crosse & Blackwell*), ⅓ of 14-oz. pkg.	460	6.0	87.0	10.0	0	240	5.0
Plum sauce:							
(*Ka•Me*), 2 tbsp......	70	0	16.0	0	0	360	0
(*Roland*), 1 tbsp.	45	0	11.0	0	0	420	0
Poi, ½ cup	134	.5	32.7	.2	0	14	.5
Pokeberry shoots:							
raw, ½ cup	18	2.1	3.0	.3	0	18	1.4
boiled, drained, ½ cup	16	1.9	2.5	.3	0	15	1.2
Pole beans, see "Green beans"							
Polenta (see also "Cornmeal"):							
(*Roland*), 2 tbsp.	80	2.0	18.0	0	0	0	2.0

Food and Measure	cal.	prot. (gms)	carbo. (gms)	fat (gms)	chol. (mgs)	sod. (mgs)	fiber (gms)
(*Shiloh Farms* Organic), ¼ cup	110	3.0	22.0	1.5	0	10	1.0
Polenta, refrigerated, prepared (*Frieda's* Organic Traditional), 2 slices, ½", 3.5 oz.	70	2.0	15.0	0	0	310	1.0
Polish sausage (see also "Kielbasa"), 1 link:							
(*Farmer John*), 2 oz.	170	8.0	1.0	16.0	30	520	0
(*Farmland*), 2.7 oz.	240	10.0	2.0	22.0	50	760	0
beef (*Hebrew National*), 3 oz.	240	11.0	2.0	22.0	45	680	0
smoked (*Johnsonville*), 2.7 oz.	240	9.0	2.0	21.0	60	640	0
Pollock, meat only:							
Atlantic, 4 oz.:							
raw	104	22.1	0	1.1	80	98	0
baked or broiled	134	28.3	0	1.4	103	125	0
walleye, 4 oz.:							
raw	91	19.5	0	.9	81	112	0
baked or broiled	128	26.7	0	1.3	109	132	0
Pollock entree, frozen, breaded (*Schooner*), 3.5-oz. fillet	170	7.0	21.0	6.0	25	90	1.0
Pomegranate:							
(*Frieda's*), 5 oz.	100	1.0	24.0	0	0	0	1.0
w/peel, 9.7-oz. fruit	104	1.5	26.4	.5	0	5	.9
Pomegranate drink (*Langers* Cocktail), 8 fl. oz.	140	0	34.0	0	0	15	0
Pomegranate drink blend, 8 fl. oz.:							
blueberry:							
(*Apple & Eve*)	130	0	33.0	0	0	10	0
(*Honest Ade* Organic)	48	0	12.0	0	0	5	0
cranberry (*SoBe Elixer 3C*)	100	0	26.0	0	0	25	0
lemonade (*Odwalla PomaGrand*)	110	0	28.0	0	0	10	0
limeade (*Odwalla PomaGrand*)	120	0	30.0	0	0	10	0
pear (*Nantucket Nectars*)	110	0	28.0	0	0	25	0

Food and Measure	cal.	prot. (gms)	carbo. (gms)	fat (gms)	chol. (mgs)	sod. (mgs)	fiber (gms)
Pomegranate juice, 8 fl. oz.:							
(*Apple & Eve Organics*)	130	0	33.0	0	0	25	0
(*Frutzzo*)	140	<1.0	35.0	0	0	10	0
(*Langers* All Pomegranate)	140	0	34.0	0	0	15	0
(*Pom* 100%)	160	0	40.0	0	0	10	0
(*R.W. Knudsen* Nectar Organic)	120	0	30.0	0	0	15	0
(*R.W. Knudsen Just Pomegranate/Just Pomegranate Organic*)	150	<1.0	38.0	0	0	20	0
(*R.W. Knudsen Simply Nutritious Vita Pomegranate*)	130	0	33.0	0	0	10	0
sparkling (*Langers*) . .	150	0	37.0	0	0	15	0
Pomegranate juice blend, 8 fl. oz.:							
acai (*Frutzzo*)	140	<1.0	34.0	0	0	10	0
berry (*Odwalla Poma-Grand*)	160	0	40.0	0	0	30	0
blueberry:							
(*Frutzzo*)	130	<1.0	32.0	0	0	5	0
(*Minute Maid*)	120	0	31.0	.5	0	20	0
(*Pom*)	160	0	39.0	0	0	20	0
blueberry or cranberry (*Langers*)	140	0	34.0	0	0	15	0
cherry:							
(*Frutzzo*)	140	<1.0	34.0	0	0	5	0
(*Nantucket Nectars*)	120	0	29.0	0	0	30	0
(*Pom*)	150	<1.0	38.0	0	0	20	0
cranberry (*Apple & Eve*)	140	0	34.0	0	0	25	0
mango:							
(*Odwalla Poma-Grand*)	160	0	39.0	0	0	20	0
(*Pom*)	140	0	36.0	0	0	10	0
raspberry (*Frutzzo*) . .	130	<1.0	32.0	0	0	5	0
tangerine (*Pom*)	140	<1.0	34.0	0	0	20	0
Pomegranate juice concentrate:							
(*R.W. Knudsen*), 8 fl. oz.*	150	1.0	37.0	0	0	10	0
(*Tree of Life*), 8 tsp. . .	110	2.0	31.0	0	0	5	0

Food and Measure	cal.	prot. (gms)	carbo. (gms)	fat (gms)	chol. (mgs)	sod. (mgs)	fiber (gms)
Pomegranate syrup, see "Grenadine"							
Pompano, Florida, meat only:							
raw, 4 oz.	186	21.0	0	10.7	57	74	0
baked or broiled, 4 oz.	239	26.4	0	13.8	73	86	0
Ponzu sauce (*Eden* Organic), 1 tbsp. . . .	5	0	1.0	0	0	340	0
Popcorn, unpopped, 2 tbsp., except as noted:							
(*Act II* Kettle Corn) . . .	170	4.0	16.0	11.0	0	210	3.0
(*Garden of Eatin'* Organic No Oil), ¼ cup	110	4.0	23.0	1.5	0	90	4.0
(*Jolly Time* Crispy 'n White)	150	3.0	16.0	10.0	0	410	6.0
(*Jolly Time* Crispy 'n White Light)	120	3.0	20.0	5.0	0	320	7.0
(*Jolly Time* Mallow Magic)	170	1.0	16.0	12.0	0	170	3.0
(*Jolly Time* Healthy Pop Kettle Corn Regular/ Minis)	90	3.0	23.0	2.0	0	280	8.0
(*Jolly Time* KettleMania)	150	2.0	15.0	11.0	0	230	3.0
(*Newman's Own* Natural), 1.1 oz.	130	2.0	18.0	5.0	0	200	3.0
(*Newman's Own* 94% Fat Free), 1.1 oz. . .	110	3.0	20.0	1.5	0	250	4.0
(*Orville Redenbacher's* Corn on the Cob) . .	180	2.0	15.0	13.0	0	280	3.0
(*Orville Redenbacher's* Movie Theater Pour Over)	170	2.0	14.0	14.0	0	330	3.0
(*Orville Redenbacher's* Natural)	160	3.0	17.0	11.0	0	480	3.0
(*Orville Redenbacher's* Natural Light)	120	3.0	19.0	4.5	0	340	3.0
(*Popweaver* Kettle) . . .	120	2.0	17.0	4.5	0	240	3.0
(*Popweaver* Natural) .	140	2.0	17.0	7.0	0	300	3.0
(*Smart Balance* Movie Style)	170	3.0	16.0	11.0	0	420	3.0
(*Smart Balance* Smart 'n Healthy), 3 tbsp.	120	4.0	24.0	2.0	0	85	5.0

Food and Measure	cal.	prot. (gms)	carbo. (gms)	fat (gms)	chol. (mgs)	sod. (mgs)	fiber (gms)
Popcorn, unpopped *(cont.)*							
butter flavor:							
(*Act II*)	160	3.0	18.0	10.0	0	350	3.0
(*Act II* 94% Fat Free), 3 tbsp.	130	4.0	28.0	2.5	0	310	5.0
(*Act II* Butter Lover's)	170	2.0	16.0	12.0	0	460	3.0
(*Act II* Buttery Kettle Corn)	170	2.0	17.0	12.0	0	200	3.0
(*Act II* Extreme) . . .	180	2.0	15.0	13.0	0	410	3.0
(*Act II* Light)	110	3.0	19.0	4.5	0	400	3.0
(*Act II* Movie Theater)	170	2.0	16.0	12.0	0	430	3.0
(*Act II* Zesty)	170	3.0	18.0	11.0	0	470	3.0
(*Garden of Eatin'* Organic), ¼ cup .	150	3.0	21.0	6.0	0	180	2.0
(*Jiffy Pop*)	140	3.0	19.0	7.0	0	220	3.0
(*Jolly Time* White & Buttery)	150	3.0	17.0	10.0	0	300	4.0
(*Jolly Time Better Butter*)	160	3.0	18.0	10.0	0	350	5.0
(*Jolly Time Blast O Butter*)	150	3.0	19.0	12.0	0	340	9.0
(*Jolly Time Blast O Butter* Light)	130	3.0	21.0	6.0	0	340	6.0
(*Jolly Time Butter• Licious*)	150	2.0	16.0	10.0	0	390	5.0
(*Jolly Time Butter• Licious* Light) . . .	130	4.0	22.0	5.0	0	230	4.0
(*Newman's Own*), 1.1 oz.	130	2.0	18.0	5.0	0	180	3.0
(*Newman's Own* Butter Boom), 1.1 oz.	130	2.0	18.0	5.0	0	290	3.0
(*Newman's Own* Light), 1.1 oz. . .	120	3.0	19.0	4.0	0	170	4.0
(*Orville Redenbacher's*)	170	2.0	17.0	12.0	0	380	3.0
(*Orville Redenbacher's* Kettle Korn)	180	2.0	16.0	13.0	<5	190	3.0
(*Orville Redenbacher's* Light)	120	3.0	19.0	5.0	0	320	3.0
(*Orville Redenbacher's* Movie Theater) . .	170	2.0	16.0	12.0	0	360	3.0
(*Orville Redenbacher's* Movie Theater Light)	120	3.0	19.0	4.5	0	310	3.0

Food and Measure	cal.	prot. (gms)	carbo. (gms)	fat (gms)	chol. (mgs)	sod. (mgs)	fiber (gms)
(*Orville Redenbacher's* Movie Theater Pour Over)	170	2.0	14.0	14.0	0	330	3.0
(*Orville Redenbacher's* Old Fashioned) ..	160	2.0	17.0	11.0	0	330	3.0
(*Orville Redenbacher's* Organic)	170	2.0	17.0	12.0	0	330	3.0
(*Orville Redenbacher's* Smart Pop! Organic), 3 tbsp.	120	4.0	26.0	2.0	0	280	5.0
(*Orville Redenbacher's* Sweet 'n Buttery) ..	180	2.0	15.0	14.0	1	240	3.0
(*Orville Redenbacher's* Ultimate)	160	2.0	15.0	12.0	0	430	3.0
(*Popweaver*)	150	2.0	17.0	8.0	0	380	3.0
(*Popweaver* Light) .	120	2.0	17.0	4.0	0	230	3.0
(*Smart Balance* Light)	120	3.0	18.0	4.5	0	290	4.0
extra (*Popweaver*) .	170	2.0	17.0	10.0	0	460	3.0
caramel: (*Orville Redenbacher's*)	160	1.0	24.0	8.0	0	45	1.0
apple (*Jolly Time Healthy Pop*) ...	100	4.0	23.0	2.0	0	260	7.0
cheddar (*Orville Redenbacher's* Pour Over)	150	2.0	12.0	12.0	0	280	2.0
cheese (*Jolly Time The Big Cheez*)	160	2.0	17.0	11.0	0	340	6.0
honey butter (*Orville Redenbacher's*) ...	180	2.0	16.0	12.0	0	170	3.0
salsa (*Jolly Time* Sassy Salsa)	160	2.0	16.0	11.0	0	320	3.0
yellow: (*Eden* Organic)	80	2.0	20.0	1.0	0	0	5.0
or white (*Jolly Time*)	100	4.0	24.0	1.0	0	0	6.0
white (*Newman's Own*), 1.1 oz.	130	2.0	18.0	5.0	0	200	3.0
Popcorn, popped:							
(*Bachman*), 1.1 oz. ..	170	2.0	15.0	11.0	0	240	6.0
(*Bachman* Lite), 1.1 oz.	120	4.0	23.0	1.5	0	115	4.0
(*Herr's*), 1 oz.	140	2.0	11.0	10.0	0	250	3.0
(*Herr's* Light), 1 oz. ...	120	2.0	19.0	4.0	0	80	3.0
butter/butter flavor: (*Gibble's*), 1 oz. ...	160	2.0	14.0	11.0	0	230	3.0
(*Snyder's*), ⅝ oz. ..	110	1.0	6.0	8.0	0	150	1.0
(*Wise*), 1 oz.	150	1.0	14.0	10.0	0	280	3.0

Food and Measure	cal.	prot. (gms)	carbo. (gms)	fat (gms)	chol. (mgs)	sod. (mgs)	fiber (gms)
Popcorn, popped *(cont.)*							
caramel (*Crunch 'n Munch*), ⅔ cup ...	150	2.0	23.0	6.0	10	100	<1.0
caramel nut:							
(*Cracker Jack*), 1 oz.	120	2.0	23.0	2.0	0	70	1.0
(*Fiddle Faddle*), 1.1 oz.	120	1.0	22.0	3.5	5	230	<1.0
cheddar (*Chester's*), 1 oz.............	160	2.0	15.0	10.0	0	200	3.0
cheddar, white:							
(*Bachman*), 1 oz. ..	160	3.0	16.0	9.0	4	340	3.0
(*Cape Cod*), 1 oz. .	160	4.0	12.0	11.0	0	250	2.0
(*Smartfood*), 1 oz. .	160	3.0	14.0	10.0	<5	290	2.0
(*Wise*), 1 oz.	150	3.0	13.0	10.0	5	400	2.0
ranch (*Herr's*), 1 oz.	140	2.0	16.0	9.0	0	310	3.0
cheese:							
(*Bachman*), 1.1 oz.	160	3.0	17.0	9.0	<5	220	4.0
(*Herr's* Regular or Hot), 1 oz.	140	2.0	13.0	8.0	0	240	3.0
hot (*Wise*), 1 oz. ...	150	2.0	14.0	10.0	<5	280	2.0
hot (*Chester's Flamin' Hot*), 1 oz. ...	160	3.0	11.0	9.0	0	330	3.0
toffee, butter (*Crunch 'n Munch*), ⅔ cup .	140	2.0	23.0	5.0	<5	160	1.0
Popcorn cake:							
plain (*Hain*), .3-oz. pc.	35	1.0	8.0	0	0	55	<1.0
butter (*Orville Redenbacher's*), 2 pcs., .6 oz.	60	2.0	14.0	1.0	0	65	2.0
butter, mini:							
(*Hain*), 6 pcs., .5 oz.	60	1.0	10.0	1.0	0	85	<1.0
(*Orville Redenbacher's*), 9 pcs., .5 oz. ...	60	2.0	12.0	1.0	0	65	2.0
caramel:							
(*Hain*), .45-oz. pc. .	50	1.0	8.0	0	0	20	<1.0
(*Orville Redenbacher's*), .4-oz. pc.	45	<1.0	11.0	0	0	20	1.0
caramel, mini:							
(*Hain*), 6 pcs., .5 oz.	60	1.0	13.0	0	0	15	<1.0
(*Orville Redenbacher's*), 6 pcs., .5 oz. ...	60	1.0	13.0	0	0	30	1.0
cheddar, mild, mini (*Hain*), 6 pcs., .5 oz. .	60	2.0	11.0	1.0	0	160	<1.0

Food and Measure	cal.	prot. (gms)	carbo. (gms)	fat (gms)	chol. (mgs)	sod. (mgs)	fiber (gms)
cheddar, white:							
(*Orville Redenbacher's*),							
2 pcs., .6 oz. ...	60	2.0	14.0	1.0	0	65	2.0
mini (*Hain*), 6 pcs.,							
.5 oz.	60	2.0	11.0	1.0	0	170	<1.0
peanut/caramel, mini							
(*Orville Redenbacher's*),							
6 pcs., .5 oz.	60	1.0	12.0	.5	0	30	1.0
and rice, see "Rice cake"							
sour cream/onion, mini							
(*Orville Redenbacher's*),							
9 pcs., .5 oz.	60	2.0	12.0	0	0	85	2.0
Popcorn seasoning:							
butter flavor:							
(*Jolly Time* Buttery),							
¼ tsp.	0	4.0	0	0	0	610	0
(*Kernel Season's*),							
¼ tsp.	3	0	1.0	0	0	80	0
cheddar flavor (*Fanci Food*), ½ tsp.	5	0	<1.0	0	0	125	0
Parmesan garlic (*Kernel Season's*), ¼ tsp. ...	2	0	0	0	0	56	0
Popeye's, 1 serving:							
chicken, mild:							
breast, breaded ...	350	33.0	8.0	20.0	179	1130	0
no skin/breading	120	24.0	0	2.0	120	540	0
leg, breaded	110	11.0	3.0	7.0	92	280	0
no skin/breading	50	9.0	0	2.0	85	190	0
thigh, breaded	280	16.0	7.0	20.0	135	710	0
no skin/breading	80	11.0	0	4.0	98	230	0
wing, breaded	150	9.0	5.0	10.0	59	690	0
no skin/breading	40	7.0	0	1.5	58	400	<1.0
strips, breaded,							
2 pcs.	250	22.0	16.0	10.0	55	1080	1.0
no skin/breading	130	25.0	3.0	2.5	50	620	0
chicken, spicy:							
breast, breaded ...	360	31.0	8.0	22.0	170	760	1.0
no skin/breading	120	25.0	<1.0	2.0	112	380	<1.0
leg, breaded	100	9.0	3.0	5.0	71	230	0
no skin/breading	50	9.0	0	1.5	60	135	0
thigh, breaded	300	15.0	7.0	24.0	131	490	0
no skin/breading	80	12.0	2.0	3.0	98	170	0
wing, breaded	140	8.0	5.0	9.0	79	290	0
no skin/breading	40	6.0	0	2.0	66	125	<1.0

Food and Measure	cal.	prot. (gms)	carbo. (gms)	fat (gms)	chol. (mgs)	sod. (mgs)	fiber (gms)
***Popeye's*, chicken, spicy** *(cont.)*							
strips, breaded, 2 pc.	270	22.0	21.0	11.0	55	1430	<1.0
no skin/breading	150	23.0	5.0	4.0	55	820	0
Cajun wings, 6 pcs. . .	595	34.0	19.0	43.0	260	1274	0
Louisiana legends:							
chicken/sausage							
jambalaya	660	30.0	60.0	33.0	96	2280	3.0
chicken, smothered	630	30.0	72.0	24.0	69	2229	3.0
etouffee, chicken . .	480	36.0	18.0	30.0	60	2610	6.0
etouffee, crawfish .	540	21.0	75.0	15.0	144	1920	6.0
popcorn shrimp	280	12.0	22.0	16.0	95	1110	<1.0
sandwich, deluxe	630	35.0	53.0	31.0	71	1480	3.0
w/out mayo	480	33.0	54.0	15.0	55	1290	3.0
sides:							
biscuit	240	4.00	26.0	13.0	0	490	1.0
chicken, smothered	210	10.0	24.0	8.0	23	743	1.0
coleslaw	260	<1.0	14.0	23.0	15	260	9.0
corn on cob	190	6.0	37.0	2.0	0	0	4.0
etouffee, chicken . .	160	12.0	6.0	10.0	20	870	2.0
etouffee, crawfish .	180	7.0	25.0	5.0	48	640	2.0
french fries	310	4.0	35.0	17.0	7	660	3.0
green beans	70	2.0	14.0	1.0	5	400	2.0
jambalaya	220	10.0	20.0	11.0	32	760	1.0
mashed potatoes . .	100	1.0	17.0	3.0	0	380	<1.0
w/gravy	130	3.0	18.0	4.0	5	580	2.0
red beans, rice	320	10.0	31.0	19.0	20	710	17.0
rice, Cajun	170	8.0	22.0	6.0	60	530	2.0
Poppy seeds:							
(*Shiloh Farms* Organic),							
1 tsp.	20	1.0	1.0	2.0	0	0	1.0
1 tsp.	15	.5	.7	1.3	0	1	.8
Porgy, see "Scup"							
Pork (see also "Pork,							
refrigerated"), meat							
only, 4 oz.:							
back ribs, roasted, lean							
w/fat	420	27.5	0	33.5	134	115	0
ground, cooked	337	29.1	0	23.6	107	83	0
leg, see "Ham"							
loin, whole:							
braised, lean w/fat .	271	30.9	0	15.4	90	54	0
braised, lean only . .	231	32.4	0	10.3	90	57	0
broiled, lean w/fat .	274	30.9	0	15.8	90	70	0
broiled, lean only . .	238	32.4	0	11.1	90	73	0

Food and Measure	cal.	prot. (gms)	carbo. (gms)	fat (gms)	chol. (mgs)	sod. (mgs)	fiber (gms)
roasted, lean w/fat .	281	30.7	0	16.6	93	67	0
roasted, lean only .	237	32.5	0	10.9	92	66	0
loin, blade:							
braised, lean w/fat .	366	24.8	0	28.8	96	62	0
braised, lean only . .	255	28.4	0	14.8	94	70	0
broiled, lean w/fat .	363	25.5	0	28.2	98	79	0
broiled, lean only . .	265	28.8	0	15.8	95	91	0
roasted, lean w/fat .	366	26.9	0	27.9	106	34	0
roasted, lean only .	280	30.2	0	16.8	106	33	0
loin, center:							
braised, lean w/fat .	280	31.7	0	16.0	98	67	0
braised, lean only . .	229	33.8	0	9.4	96	70	0
broiled, lean w/fat .	272	32.6	0	14.8	93	66	0
broiled, lean only. . .	229	34.2	0	9.2	93	68	0
panfried, lean w/fat .	314	33.9	0	18.8	104	91	0
panfried, lean only .	263	36.5	0	11.9	104	97	0
roasted, lean w/fat .	265	29.8	0	15.3	91	71	0
roasted, lean only .	226	31.2	0	10.2	90	75	0
loin, center rib:							
braised, lean w/fat .	284	30.2	0	17.1	83	45	0
braised, lean only . .	234	32.1	0	10.7	81	47	0
broiled, lean w/fat .	298	32.6	0	17.6	93	70	0
broiled, lean only . .	248	34.9	0	11.0	92	74	0
roasted, lean w/fat .	289	31.1	0	17.3	83	52	0
roasted, lean only .	253	32.6	0	12.6	81	53	0
loin, top, bone-in:							
braised, lean w/fat .	264	31.5	0	14.4	85	48	0
braised, lean only . .	229	33.0	0	9.7	83	48	0
broiled, lean w/fat .	260	34.0	0	12.7	92	71	0
broiled, lean only . .	230	35.3	0	8.8	91	74	0
roasted, lean w/fat .	256	31.9	0	13.0	89	50	0
roasted, lean only .	220	34.3	0	8.2	89	51	0
loin, top, boneless:							
panfried, lean w/fat	291	32.9	0	16.8	89	62	0
panfried, lean only .	255	34.6	0	11.9	87	65	0
ribs, country-style:							
braised, lean w/fat .	336	27.1	0	24.4	99	67	0
braised, lean only . .	265	29.5	0	15.4	98	71	0
roasted, lean w/fat .	372	26.5	0	28.7	104	59	0
roasted, lean only. .	280	30.2	0	16.8	106	33	0
shoulder, whole:							
roasted, lean w/fat .	331	26.4	0	24.3	102	77	0
roasted, lean only .	261	28.7	0	15.4	102	85	0

Food and Measure	cal.	prot. (gms)	carbo. (gms)	fat (gms)	chol. (mgs)	sod. (mgs)	fiber (gms)
Pork (cont.)							
shoulder, arm (picnic):							
braised, lean w/fat .	374	31.7	0	26.3	124	100	0
braised, lean only . .	281	36.6	0	13.8	129	116	0
roasted, lean w/fat .	360	26.6	0	27.2	107	79	0
roasted, lean only .	259	30.3	0	14.3	108	91	0
shoulder, Boston blade:							
braised, lean w/fat .	362	32.5	0	24.7	128	79	0
braised, lean only . .	310	35.3	0	17.6	132	85	0
broiled, lean w/fat .	294	29.0	0	18.8	108	78	0
broiled, lean only . .	257	30.3	0	14.2	107	84	0
roasted, lean w/fat .	305	26.2	0	21.4	98	76	0
roasted, lean only .	263	27.5	0	16.2	96	100	0
sirloin, bone-in:							
braised, lean w/fat .	278	28.8	0	17.1	93	58	0
braised, lean only . .	223	30.6	0	10.2	92	60	0
broiled, lean w/fat .	294	30.2	0	18.2	98	77	0
broiled, lean only . .	242	32.3	0	11.5	96	82	0
roasted, lean w/fat .	296	30.9	0	28.2	99	68	0
roasted, lean only .	245	32.7	0	11.7	98	71	0
sirloin, boneless:							
braised, lean w/fat .	214	30.1	0	9.5	92	52	0
braised, lean only . .	198	30.6	0	7.5	92	52	0
broiled, lean w/fat .	236	34.6	0	9.8	103	64	0
broiled, lean only . .	219	35.3	0	7.6	104	64	0
roasted, lean w/fat .	235	32.3	0	10.7	98	64	0
roasted, lean only .	225	32.7	0	9.4	98	64	0
spareribs, lean w/fat,							
braised	450	33.0	0	34.4	137	106	0
tenderloin:							
broiled, lean w/fat .	228	33.9	0	9.2	107	73	0
roasted, lean w/fat .	196	31.5	0	6.9	90	62	0
roasted, lean only .	186	31.9	0	5.5	90	64	0
Pork, cured:							
arm (picnic), roasted:							
lean w/fat, 4 oz. . . .	318	23.2	0	24.2	66	1216	0
lean w/fat, chopped							
or diced, 1 cup . .	392	28.6	0	29.9	81	1501	0
lean only, 4 oz.	193	28.3	0	8.0	54	1396	0
lean only, chopped							
or diced, 1 cup . .	238	34.9	0	9.9	67	1723	0
blade roll, lean w/fat,							
roasted, 4 oz.	325	19.6	.4	26.6	76	1103	0
leg, see "Ham"							

Food and Measure	cal.	prot. (gms)	carbo. (gms)	fat (gms)	chol. (mgs)	sod. (mgs)	fiber (gms)
Pork, frozen/refrigerated, raw, 4 oz., except as noted:							
bacon-wrapped fillet (*Farmland Extra Tender*), 5 oz.	290	38.0	1.0	14.0	115	610	0
butt (*Always Tender*) .	250	18.0	0	20.0	65	330	0
chop (see also "loin, below"):							
(*Tyson*)	200	20.0	0	13.0	45	290	0
boneless, center cut (*Farmland Nutrition Wise*), ½ chop or 1 thin chop, 4 oz.	130	22.0	1.0	3.0	60	230	0
chop, boneless:							
peppercorn rub (*Farmland Nutrition Wise*), ½ chop, 4 oz.	130	22.0	1.0	3.0	60	260	0
sirloin (*Hatfield Simply Tender*), 6.2-oz. pc.	220	35.0	0	8.0	100	490	0
chop, marinated, center cut (*Hatfield*):							
Italian	140	20.0	3.0	5.0	55	900	0
Jamaican jerk	140	20.0	4.0	5.0	55	790	0
oven-roasted	140	21.0	2.0	5.0	60	640	0
peppercorn	140	20.0	4.0	5.0	55	730	0
crown roast (*Always Tender*)	190	21.0	0	12.0	60	350	0
fillet (*Always Tender Original*)	130	19.0	1.0	5.0	45	360	0
ground:							
(*Farmland*)	230	20.0	0	16.0	75	80	0
(*Farmland* All Natural)	250	16.0	0	19.0	70	55	0
(*Farmland* All Natural Burgers)	320	18.0	0	28.0	80	45	0
(*Organic Prairie*) ..	300	19.0	0	24.0	80	65	0
(*Tyson* Reduced Fat)	260	18.0	0	20.0	65	320	0
leg, steamship:							
(*Farmland* All Natural)	140	24.0	0	4.5	75	65	0
(*Farmland Extra Tender*)	230	18.0	1.0	17.0	75	220	0

Food and Measure	cal.	prot. (gms)	carbo. (gms)	fat (gms)	chol. (mgs)	sod. (mgs)	fiber (gms)
Pork, frozen/refrigerated, raw *(cont.)*							
loin, bone-in:							
(*Always Tender*),							
3.5 oz.	189	18.0	0	12.0	53	299	0
(*Farmland Extra*							
Tender)	130	21.0	1.0	4.5	60	280	0
center cut (*Farmland*							
All Natural)	130	26.0	0	2.0	70	60	0
center cut (*Tyson*) .	190	20.0	0	13.0	45	330	0
loin, boneless:							
(*Farmland Nutrition*							
Wise)	130	22.0	1.0	3.0	60	230	0
(*Hatfield* Natural . . .	270	30.0	0	15.0	90	55	0
(*Hatfield Simply*							
Tender)	130	21.0	2.0	5.0	60	610	0
half loin (*Tyson*) . . .	190	20.0	0	12.0	45	330	0
roast (*Tyson*)	190	20.0	0	12.0	45	290	0
roast, rib eye (*Tyson*)	200	20.0	0	13.0	45	290	0
loin, boneless, center							
cut:							
(*Always Tender*) . . .	170	21.0	0	9.0	60	330	0
(*Farmland* All Natu-							
ral), 3 oz.	140	26.0	0	3.0	70	55	0
(*Farmland* All Natural							
Extra Lean for							
Chops)	117	23.1	0	2.0	62	56	0
(*Farmland Extra*							
Tender)	160	22.0	0	8.0	65	190	0
(*Farmland Nutrition*							
Wise)	130	22.0	1.0	3.0	60	230	0
(*Hatfield Simply*							
Tender Roast) . .	120	21.0	2.0	3.0	65	600	0
chop, assorted or							
butterfly (*Tyson*)	190	20.0	0	13.0	45	330	0
roast (*Farmland*							
Extra Tender) . . .	230	19.0	1.0	16.0	65	270	0
roast (*Farmland*							
Nutrition Wise) . .	130	21.0	1.0	4.5	60	280	0
loin fillet, seasoned:							
Asian 5-spice or							
chipotle barbecue							
rub (*Farmland*							
Nutrition Wise) . .	130	22.0	1.0	3.0	60	360	0
barbecue (*Hatfield*)	140	20.0	5.0	5.0	55	950	0

Food and Measure	cal.	prot. (gms)	carbo. (gms)	fat (gms)	chol. (mgs)	sod. (mgs)	fiber (gms)
citrus, center cut (*Always Tender*) .	140	21.0	3.0	5.0	45	360	0
honey mustard (*Always Tender*) .	140	20.0	4.0	5.0	45	510	0
horseradish black pepper (*Always Tender*)	120	20.0	3.0	3.5	40	420	0
Italian (*Hatfield*) . . .	140	20.0	3.0	5.0	55	900	0
mojo criollo (*Always Tender*)	140	20.0	3.0	5.0	45	570	0
mushroom (*Hatfield*)	140	20.0	3.0	5.0	55	760	0
oven roasted (*Hatfield*)	140	21.0	2.0	5.0	60	640	0
Parmesan (*Always Tender*)	120	20.0	1.0	4.0	45	390	0
sun-dried tomato, center cut (*Always Tender*)	130	19.0	2.0	4.0	45	440	0
tarragon mustard (*Always Tender*) .	130	20.0	4.0	3.5	35	480	0
medallions, all varieties (*Always Tender*), 6 oz.	240	32.0	4.0	11.0	90	750	0
picnic: (*Always Tender*)	240	19.0	0	18.0	70	350	0
rib ends, boneless (*Always Tender*) . . .	160	20.0	0	9.0	60	330	0
ribs/spareribs: (*Always Tender* Spareribs)	280	17.0	0	23.0	80	330	0
(*Farmland Extra Tender* Spareribs)	290	17.0	0	24.0	80	230	0
(*Hatfield* Natural) . .	320	19.0	0	26.0	85	85	0
(*Tyson* Ribs)	200	20.0	0	13.0	45	290	0
(*Tyson* Spareribs) .	290	16.0	0	24.0	80	330	0
baby back (*Always Tender*)	250	18.0	0	20.0	80	330	0
baby back (*Hatfield* Natural)	320	18.0	0	26.0	90	85	0
baby back, Buffalo (*Tyson*)	300	16.0	4.0	24.0	80	1080	0
baby back, w/garlic or teriyaki (*Always Tender*)	240	18.0	2.0	18.0	80	530	0

Food and Measure	cal.	prot. (gms)	carbo. (gms)	fat (gms)	chol. (mgs)	sod. (mgs)	fiber (gms)
Pork, frozen/refrigerated, raw, ribs/spareribs *(cont.)*							
baby back, pepper rub (*Tyson*)	290	16.0	0	24.0	85	390	0
baby back, Southwest (*Tyson*)	290	16.0	2.0	23.0	80	730	0
baby back, teriyaki (*Always Tender*) .	240	18.0	2.0	18.0	80	530	0
loin (*Farmland*) ...	320	18.0	0	26.0	90	85	0
loin back (*Farmland Extra Tender*) ...	290	17.0	1.0	24.0	80	340	0
loin back (*Tyson*) ..	250	17.0	0	20.0	70	360	0
loin, country style (*Tyson*)	180	20.0	0	12.0	45	330	0
roast, fresh:							
(*Always Tender*) ...	170	20.0	0	10.0	60	330	0
(*Farmland* Natural) .	160	22.0	0	7.0	75	90	0
(*Tyson*)	130	21.0	0	4.5	65	300	0
roast, seasoned:							
garden herb (*Hatfield*)	150	18.0	3.0	7.0	60	820	0
Italian (*Hatfield*) ...	150	18.0	3.0	7.0	60	910	0
onion garlic (*Always Tender*)	170	18.0	1.0	10.0	60	550	0
oven-roasted (*Hatfield*)	140	21.0	2.0	5.0	60	640	0
roast flavor (*Always Tender*)	170	18.0	1.0	10.0	60	480	0
sirloin, peppercorn (*Hatfield*)	140	20.0	4.0	5.0	55	730	0
sirloin, teriyaki (*Hatfield*)	140	20.0	4.0	5.0	55	870	0
round, top, roast, boneless (*Farmland Nutrition Wise*)	130	21.0	1.0	4.5	60	220	0
shoulder roast:							
(*Always Tender*)	170	18.0	1.0	10.0	60	480	0
(*Farmland Extra Tender* Bone-In) .	230	19.0	1.0	16.0	65	270	0
onion garlic (*Always Tender*)	170	18.0	1.0	10.0	60	550	0
shoulder steak (*Tyson*)	260	17.0	0	21.0	70	320	0
sirloin:							
(*Farmland* All Natural Boneless)	114	22.2	0	2.1	68	58	0
roast (*Tyson*)	140	21.0	0	6.0	65	300	0

Food and Measure	cal.	prot. (gms)	carbo. (gms)	fat (gms)	chol. (mgs)	sod. (mgs)	fiber (gms)
for strips (*Farmland Extra Tender*) ...	130	20.0	1.0	5.0	60	280	0
tip (*Farmland* All Natural)	113	20.6	0	2.8	57	50	0
tip (*Farmland Nutrition Wise*)	120	23.0	1.0	2.0	70	230	0
stew (*Tyson*)	130	21.0	0	4.5	65	300	0
tenderloin (see also "loin," above):							
(*Always Tender*) ...	120	22.0	0	3.5	60	330	0
(*Farmland* All Natural)	109	22.1	0	1.6	59	53	0
(*Farmland Nutrition Wise*)	120	21.0	1.0	3.0	60	220	0
(*Hatfield* Natural) ..	130	24.0	0	4.0	75	55	0
(*Hatfield Simply Tender*)	120	20.0	2.0	3.0	60	600	0
(*Tyson*)	120	21.0	0	3.5	65	300	0
tips (*Farmland Nutrition Wise*)	120	23.0	1.0	3.0	60	230	0
tenderloin, seasoned:							
(*Always Tender* Original)	120	19.0	1.0	4.0	50	400	0
apple bourbon (*Always Tender*) .	140	19.0	5.0	4.0	50	500	0
citrus ginger rub (*Farmland Nutrition Wise*)	130	23.0	1.0	3.0	65	310	0
garlic (*Always Tender*)	130	19.0	1.0	5.0	45	600	0
honey mustard (*Hatfield*)	150	18.0	9.0	4.0	55	900	0
Italian (*Hatfield*) ...	120	19.0	3.0	3.0	60	890	0
mesquite (*Always Tender*)	120	19.0	2.0	4.0	45	550	0
peppercorn (*Hatfield*)	120	19.0	4.0	3.0	60	710	0
peppercorn (*Always Tender*)	120	18.0	2.0	4.0	50	630	0
peppercorn rub (*Farmland Nutrition Wise*)	130	23.0	1.0	3.0	65	310	0
raspberry chipotle (*Always Tender*) .	130	18.0	5.0	4.0	50	320	0
teriyaki (*Hatfield*) ..	120	19.0	4.0	3.0	60	850	0
teriyaki (*Always Tender*)	130	19.0	5.0	4.0	50	500	0

Food and Measure	cal.	prot. (gms)	carbo. (gms)	fat (gms)	chol. (mgs)	sod. (mgs)	fiber (gms)
Pork, frozen/refrigerated, cooked:							
w/barbecue sauce:							
pulled (*Curley's* Bold & Spicy), ¼ cup, 2.1 oz.	100	9.0	10.0	3.0	30	410	2.0
pulled (*Hormel*), 2 oz.	90	8.0	10.0	2.5	25	510	0
shanks, bone-in (*Farmland* KC Wild Wings), 5 oz.	190	21.0	13.0	5.0	70	1120	0
shanks, bone-in, hot (*Farmland* KC Wild Wings), 5 oz.	170	23.0	6.0	6.0	75	1780	0
shredded, honey hickory sauce w/ (*Lloyd's*), ¼ cup .	80	7.0	10.0	1.5	15	440	0
shredded, original sauce w/ (*Lloyd's*), ¼ cup	90	7.0	11.0	1.5	15	400	0
breaded (*Goya* Pasteles, 5.6-oz. pc.	300	7.0	31.0	17.0	60	960	3.0
chop:							
braised (*Organic Prairie*), 3.3 oz. .	220	26.0	0	13.0	80	55	0
w/gravy (*Hormel*), 5 oz.	150	20.0	3.0	6.0	55	750	0
pulled, see "w/barbecue sauce," above							
ribs, barbecue sauce:							
baby back (*Lloyd's*), 2 ribs w/honey hickory sauce, 4.8 oz.	340	21.0	19.0	20.0	85	810	0
baby back (*Lloyd's*), 2 ribs w/original sauce, 4.8 oz.	290	14.0	20.0	17.0	70	850	1.0
spareribs (*Lloyd's*), 2 ribs w/original sauce, 5 oz.	350	18.0	25.0	20.0	70	1020	<1.0
roast, 5 oz.:							
(*Hormel*)	180	28.0	1.0	7.0	85	600	0
in gravy (*Tyson*) ...	190	19.0	5.0	10.0	55	590	0

Food and Measure	cal.	prot. (gms)	carbo. (gms)	fat (gms)	chol. (mgs)	sod. (mgs)	fiber (gms)
sweet and sour (*Simply Simmered*), 5 oz...	150	14.0	21.0	1.5	5	840	5.0
teriyaki sauce, shanks, bone-in (*Farmland* KC Wild Wings), 5 oz. .	190	22	16.0	5.0	70	970	0
Pork, ground, see "Pork, frozen/refrigerated, raw"							
Pork, pickled (see also "Pig's feet"), hocks or tidbits (*Hormel*), 2 oz.	100	8.0	0	8.0	45	690	0
"Pork," vegetarian, frozen (*Gardenburger* BBQ Riblets), 5 oz. w/sauce	240	17.0	33.0	4.5	0	580	5.0
Pork back fat, 1 oz. . .	230	2.6	0	25.3	16	3	0
Pork belly, raw, 1 oz. .	147	2.7	0	15.0	20	9	0
Pork coating mix (see also "Chicken coating mix"), seasoned, ⅛ pkg., except as noted:							
(*Oven Fry* Extra Crispy)	60	2.0	11.0	1.5	0	340	0
(*Shake 'n Bake* Original), 1 tbsp.	45	1.0	8.0	.5	0	230	0
(*Shake 'n Bake* Original 2 Pack w/Bag), 1 tbsp.	40	1.0	8.0	0	0	240	0
chops (*McCormick Bag 'n Season*), 2 tsp...	15	0	4.0	0	0	590	0
tenderloin, herb-roasted (*McCormick Bag 'n Season*)	5	0	0	0	0	180	0
Pork dinner, frozen, boneless (*Swanson Hungry-Man*), 1-lb. pkg.	930	24.0	106.0	49.0	85	1940	4.0
Pork entree, frozen (see also "Pork, frozen/refrigerated, cooked"), 1 pkg., except as noted:							
cutlet, boneless (*Stouffer's*), 10 oz. .	370	13.0	31.0	21.0	25	1110	3.0

Food and Measure	cal.	prot. (gms)	carbo. (gms)	fat (gms)	chol. (mgs)	sod. (mgs)	fiber (gms)
Pork entree, frozen *(cont.)*							
roast:							
(*Lean Cuisine*), 9.5 oz.	250	16.0	38.0	3.5	35	660	3.0
w/vegetables (*Tyson Kit*), ⅛ of 32-oz. pkg.	190	21.0	18.0	3.5	60	190	2.0
savory (*South Beach Living*), 9.4 oz.	230	22.0	13.0	9.0	55	680	4.0
stir-fry (*Lean Cuisine Spa Cuisine*), 8.25 oz.	280	19.0	39.0	5.0	30	680	5.0
Pork entree mix, chops w/herb stuffing (*Campbell's Supper Bakes* Savory), ⅙ pkg. mix	160	5.0	30.0	2.0	<5	780	1.0
Pork fat, roasted, 1 oz.	167	2.2	0	17.5	24	177	0
Pork gravy, can or jar, ¼ cup:							
(*Heinz Home Style*) . .	20	1.0	3.0	.5	0	250	0
golden (*Campbell's*) . .	45	1.0	3.0	3.0	5	310	0
Pork gravy mix (*Mc-Cormick*), ¼ cup* .	20	0	4.0	0	0	370	0
Pork lunch meat (see also "Ham lunch meat"), 2 oz.:							
(*Boar's Head* Porketta)	80	15.0	0	2.0	35	540	0
barbecue flavor (*Dietz & Watson*)	50	11.0	0	1.0	30	390	0
honey barbecue (*Black Bear*)	60	9.0	3.0	1.0	30	290	0
Italian style (*Dietz & Watson*)	50	11.0	0	1.0	30	390	0
roast:							
(*Hatfield Deli Choice*)	60	10.0	0	2.0	20	320	0
sirloin (*Dietz & Watson*)	50	11.0	0	1.0	30	390	0
seasoned (*Boar's Head Fresh Ham*)	80	14.0	0	3.0	35	310	0
Pork rind snack, .5 oz., except as noted:							
(*Baken-ets* Fried Skins)	80	7.0	0	5.0	20	310	0
(*Herr's* Original)	80	9.0	0	5.0	20	270	0
(*Wise* Original)	80	8.0	0	5.0	20	300	0

Food and Measure	cal.	prot. (gms)	carbo. (gms)	fat (gms)	chol. (mgs)	sod. (mgs)	fiber (gms)
barbecue:							
(*Herr's* BBQ)	80	8.0	0	5.0	20	400	0
(*Wise* Hot & Spicy)	70	8.0	1.0	4.5	20	430	0
(*Wise* Sweet & Mild)	90	8.0	<1.0	6.0	15	270	0
hot:							
(*Baken-ets* Hot 'n							
Spicy Skins)	80	7.0	<1.0	5.0	20	470	<1.0
(*Herr's*), 1 oz.	140	1.0	17.0	7.0	0	400	1.0
salt and vinegar							
(*Baken-ets* Skins) . .	70	7.0	<1.0	4.5	15	320	<1.0
Pot pie, see specific							
entree listings							
Pot roast, see "Beef							
dinner, frozen" and							
"Beef entree, frozen"							
Pot stickers entrée							
(see also "Chicken							
entree, frozen"),							
Asian style (*Lean*							
Cuisine), 9-oz. pkg.	260	9.0	47.0	4.0	15	530	3.0
Potato:							
raw:							
(*Del Monte*),							
1 medium, 5.2 oz.	100	4.0	26.0	0	0	0	3.0
(*Frieda's* Assorted							
Fingerling Bag),							
4 pcs., 5.2 oz. . .	100	4.0	25.0	0	0	0	3.0
(*Frieda's* Baby/Finger-							
ling/Red/Purple/Yukon							
Gold/YellowFinnish),							
½ cup, 3 oz.	70	2.0	15.0	0	0	5	1.0
unpeeled:							
1 large, 6.5 oz. . .	145	3.8	33.1	.2	0	11	2.9
1 long, 7.1 oz. . .	160	4.2	36.3	.2	0	12	3.2
peeled, 2½" potato .	88	2.3	20.1	.1	0	7	1.8
peeled, diced, ½ cup	59	1.6	13.5	.1	0	5	1.2
baked:							
in skin, 4¾" x 2⅓" .	220	4.7	51.0	.2	0	16	4.8
w/out skin, 2⅓" . . .	145	3.1	33.6	.2	0	8	2.3
w/out skin, ½ cup .	57	1.2	13.2	.1	0	3	.9
skin only, 1 oz.	56	1.2	13.1	0	0	6	2.2
boiled in skin, peeled:							
2½" potato, 4.8 oz.	118	2.5	27.4	.1	0	6	2.4
½ cup	68	1.5	15.7	.1	0	3	1.4

Food and Measure	cal.	prot. (gms)	carbo. (gms)	fat (gms)	chol. (mgs)	sod. (mgs)	fiber (gms)
Potato *(cont.)*							
boiled w/out skin:							
2½" potato	116	2.3	27.0	.1	0	7	2.4
½ cup	67	1.3	15.6	.1	0	4	1.4
microwaved in skin:							
w/skin, 4¾" x 2⅓"							
potato	212	4.9	48.7	.2	0	16	4.7
peeled, ½ cup	78	1.6	18.2	.1	0	5	1.2
skin only, 2 oz.	75	2.5	16.8	.1	0	9	3.2
mashed, w/whole milk:							
½ cup	81	2.0	18.4	.6	2	318	2.1
w/butter, ½ cup . . .	111	2.0	17.5	4.4	13	309	2.1
w/margarine, ½ cup	111	2.0	17.5	4.4	2	309	2.1
Potato, can/jar:							
whole:							
(*Butterfield* New),							
3½ pcs.	90	2.0	20.0	0	0	330	2.0
(*Del Monte* New),							
2 pcs.	60	1.0	13.0	0	0	360	2.0
(*Sunshine*), 3 pcs. .	90	2.0	20.0	0	0	330	2.0
(*S&W* Small), 2 pcs.	60	1.0	13.0	0	0	360	2.0
diced, new potato:							
(*Butterfield*), ⅔ cup	100	2.0	22.0	0	0	350	3.0
(*Del Monte*),½ cup	45	1.0	11.0	0	0	280	<1.0
sliced, new potato:							
(*Butterfield*), ½ cup	100	2.0	22.0	0	0	390	4.0
(*Del Monte*), ⅔ cup	60	1.0	13.0	0	0	360	2.0
Potato, dried, see							
"Potato dish, mix"							
Potato, frozen/refriger-							
ated (see also "Po-							
tato dish, frozen"),							
3 oz., except as noted:							
diced, w/onion (*Simply*							
Potatoes), ⅔ cup . .	60	1.0	13.0	0	0	220	1.0
fried/fries:							
(*Inland Valley* Stix) .	170	2.0	19.0	10.0	0	360	2.0
(*Inland Valley* Criss-							
Cut)	160	2.0	22.0	7.0	0	300	2.0
(*Inland Valley* Fajita							
Fries)	170	3.0	22.0	8.0	0	400	2.0
(*Inland Valley* Long							
Branch)	160	2.0	21.0	7.0	0	360	2.0

Food and Measure	cal.	prot. (gms)	carbo. (gms)	fat (gms)	chol. (mgs)	sod. (mgs)	fiber (gms)
(Inland Valley Santa Fe Corn Fries) ..	190	2.0	25.0	9.0	0	540	2.0
(McCain Classic Cut)	120	2.0	20.0	4.0	0	360	2.0
(McCain Smiles) ...	160	2.0	24.0	6.0	0	390	2.0
beer batter (McCain)	170	2.0	19.0	10.0	0	290	2.0
cross cut, seasoned, (Inland Valley CrissCut)	190	2.0	21.0	11.0	0	540	2.0
cross cut, seasoned, w/skin (McCain) .	170	2.0	21.0	9.0	0	490	2.0
French (Inland Valley)	130	2.0	21.0	4.0	0	310	2.0
French (Inland Valley Crispy Classics) .	180	2.0	28.0	7.0	0	230	3.0
julienne (Alexia Yukon Gold Organic) ...	130	2.0	22.0	3.5	0	180	2.0
olive oil, Parmesan/ garlic or sun-dried tomato/pesto (Alexia Oven Reds)	120	3.0	19.0	3.5	0	270	2.0
olive oil/rosemary/ garlic (Alexia Oven Fries)	120	2.0	22.0	3.5	0	240	2.0
olive oil/sea salt (Alexia Oven Fries)	120	2.0	21.0	3.5	0	180	2.0
olive oil/sun-dried tomato/pesto (Alexia Oven Reds)	120	2.0	22.0	3.5	0	240	2.0
spirals (Inland Valley Curly QQQ's) ...	180	2.0	25.0	8.0	0	390	2.0
spirals, seasoned (Inland Valley QQQ's)	190	2.0	25.0	9.0	0	390	2.0
spirals, seasoned (McCain Golden Crisp)	140	2.0	18.0	7.0	0	390	2.0
steak (Inland Valley)	110	2.0	18.0	3.0	0	310	2.0
steak (McCain)	120	2.0	21.0	3.0	0	330	2.0
straight cut (Cascadian Farm Organic)	130	2.0	21.0	4.0	0	15	2.0
straight cut (McCain)	120	2.0	20.0	4.0	0	360	2.0
straight cut (McCain Golden Crisp) ...	140	2.0	23.0	5.0	0	380	2.0

Food and Measure	cal.	prot. (gms)	carbo. (gms)	fat (gms)	chol. (mgs)	sod. (mgs)	fiber (gms)
Potato, frozen/refrigerated, fried/fries *(cont.)*							
waffle, w/seasoned salt (*Alexia Waffle Fries*)	170	2.0	21.,0	9.0	0	440	2.0
wedge cut (*Cascadian Farm* Organic Oven Fries)	110	2.0	21.0	3.0	0	15	2.0
wedges (*Inland Valley Tater Babies*) . . .	130	2.0	19.0	5.0	0	360	2.0
wedges (*McCain Route 66* Classic)	170	2.0	20.0	9.0	0	630	2.0
wedges, seasoned, w/skin (*McCain*) .	120	2.0	17.0	5.0	0	390	2.0
fries, crinkle cut:							
(*Alexia Oven Crinkles* Organic)	120	2.0	19.0	4.0	0	330	3.0
(*Cascadian Farm* Organic)	130	2.0	21.0	4.0	0	15	2.0
(*Inland Valley*)	150	2.0	25.0	5.0	0	330	2.0
(*Inland Valley* 64 oz.)	130	2.0	22.0	4.0	5	25	2.0
(*Inland Valley Crispy Classics*)	180	2.0	25.0	8.0	0	300	3.0
(*Kineret*)	120	2.0	20.0	4.0	0	25	2.0
(*McCain*)	130	2.0	21.0	4.0	0	320	2.0
(*McCain Golden Crisp*)	150	2.0	23.0	6.0	0	380	2.0
onion/garlic or salt/ pepper (*Alexia Oven Crinkles* Organic)	120	2.0	19.0	4.0	0	330	3.0
seasoned (*McCain*)	130	2.0	20.0	5.0	0	410	2.0
fries, shoestring:							
(*Cascadian Farm* Organic)	140	2.0	21.0	5.0	0	15	2.0
(*McCain*)	140	2.0	21.0	5.0	0	290	2.0
(*McCain* 5-Minute Fries!)	210	2.0	22.0	8.0	0	340	3.0
(*McCain Golden Crisp* Fast Food) .	150	2.0	20.0	7.0	0	400	2.0
hash browns:							
(*Cascadian Farm* Organic)	60	2.0	14.0	0	0	10	1.0
(*Inland Valley Simply Shreds*)	70	2.0	15.0	0	0	330	2.0
(*Mr. Dell's* Original Shredded), 1 cup	60	2.0	12.0	0	0	0	1.0

Food and Measure	cal.	prot. (gms)	carbo. (gms)	fat (gms)	chol. (mgs)	sod. (mgs)	fiber (gms)
(*Simply Potatoes Shredded*), ½ cup	70	1.0	16.0	0	0	55	2.0
O'Brien (*Inland Valley Simply Shreds*) .	60	2.0	14.0	0	0	180	2.0
O'Brien (*Mr. Dell's*), 1 cup	60	2.0	14.0	0	0	0	2.0
Southern style (*Inland Valley*) ..	70	2.0	16.0	0	0	15	2.0
Southern style (*Mr. Dell's*), ¾ cup ...	70	2.0	14.0	0	0	0	2.0
Southwest (*Simply Potatoes*), ⅔ cup	60	2.0	13.0	0	0	310	1.0
Yukon gold, seasoned salt (*Alexia Hash Browns* Organic)	80	2.0	17.0	0	0	300	2.0
mashed, ⅔ cup, except as noted:							
(*Inland Valley* Homestyle Micro)	160	3.0	22.0	6.0	5	500	3.0
(*Shedd's Country Crock* Homestyle)	180	2.0	23.0	9.0	15	470	2.0
(*Simply Potatoes*) .	110	2.0	15.0	5.0	10	500	3.0
(*Simply Potatoes* Country Style) ..	110	3.0	20.0	2.0	5	105	3.0
garlic (*Shedd's Country Crock*) .	160	2.0	22.0	7.0	10	430	2.0
garlic (*Simply Potatoes*)	130	3.0	16.0	6.0	15	450	2.0
loaded (*Shedd's Country Crock*) .	200	4.0	22.0	11.0	25	410	2.0
red, w/garlic, Parmesan (*Alexia Mashed Potatoes*), ½ cup	150	3.0	20.0	6.0	15	115	2.0
scalloped (*Shedd's Country Crock*) .	210	4.0	21.0	11.0	25	680	2.0
sour cream/chive (*Simply Potatoes*)	130	3.0	18.0	5.0	15	380	3.0
Yukon gold, w/sea salt (*Alexia Mashed Potatoes*), ½ cup	150	3.0	20.0	6.0	20	80	2.0
w/onions, peppers (*Cascadian Farm* Organic Country Style)	50	1.0	12.0	0	0	10	1.0

Food and Measure	cal.	prot. (gms)	carbo. (gms)	fat (gms)	chol. (mgs)	sod. (mgs)	fiber (gms)
Potato, frozen/refrigerated (cont.)							
patties (*Inland Valley Home Browns*),							
2.25-oz. patty	130	2.0	15.0	7.0	0	250	2.0
popcorn (*McCain*) ...	220	2.0	20.0	15.0	0	430	2.0
puffs/nuggets:							
(*Cascadian Farm Spud Puppies Organic*)	160	2.0	23.0	7.0	0	400	2.0
(*Inland Valley Tater Puffs*)	160	2.0	20.0	7.0	0	310	2.0
(*Inland Valley Stars & Stix*)	170	2.0	23.0	7.0	0	420	2.0
(*McCain Mash-Bites*)	170	2.0	24.0	7.0	0	430	2.0
(*McCain Tasti Tater*)	160	2.0	20.0	7.0	0	410	3.0
stuffed, w/cheese (*Inland Valley Stuffed Spudz*) ..	210	7.0	20.0	11.0	20	570	2.0
Yukon gold (*Alexia Potato Nuggets*) .	150	2.0	18.0	8.0	0	340	1.0
roasted, seasoned:							
(*McCain Roasters All-American*) ...	120	2.0	21.0	3.0	0	370	2.0
grilled garlic, onion (*McCain Roasters*)	120	2.0	22.0	3.0	0	370	2.0
onion, French (*McCain Roasters*) ..	110	2.0	20.0	3.0	0	310	2.0
slices (*Simply Potatoes Homestyle*), ⅔ cup	70	2.0	16.0	0	0	135	1.0
wedges, red, ½ cup:							
(*Simply Potatoes*) .	50	2.0	10.0	0	0	85	2.0
rosemary/garlic (*Simply Potatoes*)	80	2.0	16.0	0	0	360	3.0
Potato, mix, see "Potato dish, mix"							
Potato, sweet, see "Sweet potato"							
Potato chips/crisps (see also "Potato soy crisps," "Potato sticks" and "Sweet potato chips"), 1 oz.:							
(*Bachman* Golden Crisp)	150	2.0	16.0	9.0	0	115	0

Food and Measure	cal.	prot. (gms)	carbo. (gms)	fat (gms)	chol. (mgs)	sod. (mgs)	fiber (gms)
(*Bachman Golden Ridges*)	160	2.0	15.0	10.0	<5	140	0
(*Bachman Golden Wavy*)	150	2.0	16.0	8.0	0	95	1.0
(*Barbara's/Barbara's Ripple*)	150	2.0	15.0	10.0	0	180	1.0
(*Cape Cod* Classic/Wavy)	150	2.0	17.0	8.0	0	110	1.0
(*Cape Cod* 40% Reduced Fat)	130	2.0	18.0	6.0	0	110	1.0
(*Cape Cod* Robust Russet)	150	2.0	16.0	8.0	0	150	1.0
(*Garden of Eatin'*) ...	150	2.0	16.0	9.0	0	140	1.0
(*Gibble's*)	150	2.0	14.0	9.0	5	130	1.0
(*Herr's* Kettle)	160	2.0	14.0	10.0	0	180	1.0
(*Herr's* Kettle Reduced Fat)	135	2.0	18.0	6.0	0	180	1.0
(*Herr's* Kettle Russet) .	140	2.0	16.0	8.0	0	180	1.0
(*Herr's* Lightly Salted)	140	2.0	16.0	8.0	0	90	1.0
(*Herr's* Old Bay)	150	2.0	14.0	10.0	0	360	1.0
(*Herr's* Old Fashioned)	180	1.0	11.0	10.0	5	200	<1.0
(*Herr's* Original/Rippled)	140	2.0	16.0	8.0	0	180	1.0
(*Kettle* Bakes Lightly Salted)	120	3.0	21.0	3.0	0	115	2.0
(*Kettle* Organic Lightly Salted)	150	2.0	15.0	9.0	0	110	2.0
(*Kettle/Kettle* Krinkle Cut Lightly Salted) .	150	2.0	15.0	9.0	0	110	2.0
(*Lay's* Classic/Wavy) .	150	2.0	15.0	10.0	0	180	1.0
(*Lay's* Kettle)	150	2.0	18.0	8.0	0	110	1.0
(*Lay's* Kettle Reduced Fat)	140	2.0	19.0	6.0	0	160	2.0
(*Lay's* Lightly Salted) .	150	2.0	15.0	10.0	0	90	1.0
(*Lay's* Original Baked!)	110	2.0	23.0	1.5	0	150	2.0
(*Lay's* Original Light) .	75	2.0	17.0	0	0	200	1.0
(*Lay's Stax* Original) ..	150	2.0	16.0	9.0	0	160	1.0
(*Maui Style*)	150	2.0	16.0	9.0	0	150	1.0
(*Munchos* Crisps) ...	160	1.0	16.0	10.0	0	230	1.0
(*Pringles* Original) ...	160	1.0	14.0	11.0	0	170	<1.0
(*Pringles* Original Minis)	120	1.0	13.0	7.0	0	140	<1.0
(*Ruffles* Original)	160	2.0	14.0	10.0	0	160	1.0
(*Ruffles* Original Baked!)	120	2.0	21.0	3.0	0	200	2.0
(*Ruffles* Original Light)	70	2.0	17.0	0	0	190	1.0
(*Ruffles* Reduced Fat)	140	2.0	18.0	7.0	0	180	1.0
(*Snyder's* Original) ...	150	2.0	19.0	7.0	0	90	3.0
(*Snyder's* Ripple)	140	2.0	18.0	6.0	0	100	4.0

Food and Measure	cal.	prot. (gms)	carbo. (gms)	fat (gms)	chol. (mgs)	sod. (mgs)	fiber (gms)
Potato chips/crisps *(cont.)*							
(*Terra* Au Naturel) ...	150	2.0	15.0	9.0	0	0	2.0
(*Terra* Golds)	130	2.0	19.0	5.0	0	80	0
(*Terra* Blues)	130	2.0	19.0	6.0	0	115	3.0
(*Terra* Red Bliss)	140	1.0	18.0	7.0	0	110	2.0
(*Wise* Kettle)	150	2.0	15.0	9.0	0	170	1.0
(*Wise* Kettle Reduced Fat)	130	2.0	18.0	6.0	0	160	1.0
(*Wise* Lightly Salted) .	150	2.0	14.0	10.0	0	80	1.0
(*Wise* Original/Wavy) .	150	2.0	14.0	10.0	0	160	1.0
(*Wise New York Deli* Kettle)	150	2.0	15.0	9.0	0	170	1.0
(*Wise* Ridgies)	150	2.0	14.0	10.0	0	160	1.0
au gratin (*Lay's* Wavy)	150	2.0	14.0	10.0	<5	200	1.0
baked potato, loaded (*Pringles*)	150	1.0	14.0	10.0	0	170	<1.0
barbecue:							
(*Bachman Golden Ridges* Bar-B-Q) .	150	2.0	15.0	9.0	<5	320	0
(*Cape Cod* Beachside BBQ)	150	2.0	17.0	8.0	0	160	1.0
(*Gibble's* BBQ)	150	2.0	15.0	8.0	5	260	1.0
(*Gibble's* Krinkle Kut BBQ)	140	2.0	16.0	8.0	5	370	3.0
(*Herr's* BBQ)	150	2.0	14.0	10.0	0	240	1.0
(*Kettle Chipotle Chili Barbecue* Organic)	150	2.0	15.0	9.0	0	160	2.0
(*Kettle Krinkle Cut* Classic)	150	2.0	16.0	9.0	0	170	2.0
(*Lay's*)	150	2.0	15.0	10.0	0	200	1.0
(*Lay's* Baked!)	120	2.0	23.0	3.0	0	210	2.0
(*Lay's* Light)	75	2.0	17.0	0	0	250	1.0
(*Lay's Natural Thick Cut Country*) ...	150	2.0	15.0	9.0	0	150	1.0
(*Moore's*)	150	2.0	14.0	10.0	0	220	1.0
(*Snyder's*)	150	2.0	20.0	6.0	0	300	4.0
(*Wise*)	150	2.0	15.0	10.0	0	210	1.0
hickory (*Lay's* Wavy)	150	2.0	16.0	9.0	0	210	1.0
hickory (*Terra*)	150	2.0	15.0	9.0	0	5	1.0
hickory honey (*Kettle Bakes*)	120	3.0	21.0	3.0	0	160	2.0
honey (*Herr's* BBQ)	150	2.0	14.0	10.0	0	280	1.0
honey (*Wise*)	150	2.0	15.0	10.0	0	190	1.0
hot/spicy (*Lay's*) ..	150	2.0	15.0	10.0	0	200	1.0

Food and Measure	cal.	prot. (gms)	carbo. (gms)	fat (gms)	chol. (mgs)	sod. (mgs)	fiber (gms)
hot/spicy or mesquite (*Lay's Stax*)	150	1.0	15.0	9.0	0	190	1.0
mesquite (*Lay's* Kettle)	140	2.0	16.0	8.0	0	210	1.0
Southwest (*Pringles* Select Bold Crunch)	140	1.0	16.0	8.0	0	210	1.0
sweet (*Eatsmart*) ..	150	2.0	19.0	7.0	0	290	3.0
blend (*Terra Potpourri*)	140	2.0	17.0	7.0	0	110	4.0
Buffalo:							
bleu (*Kettle Krinkle Cut*)	150	2.0	16.0	9.0	0	150	2.0
wing (*Herr's* Kettle)	160	2.0	16.0	8.0	0	300	1.0
wing (*Pringles* Extreme)	150	1.0	14.0	10.0	0	280	1.0
wing, hot (*Snyder's*)	150	2.0	19.0	7.0	0	340	4.0
cheddar:							
(*Kettle* Beer)	150	2.0	15.0	9.0	0	180	1.0
(*Lay's Stax*)	150	1.0	15.0	10.0	0	190	1.0
(*Pringles*)	150	1.0	14.0	11.0	0	210	<1.0
(*Pringles* Extreme) .	150	1.0	14.0	11.0	0	190	1.0
(*Pringles* Minis) ...	120	1.0	12.0	7.0	0	220	<1.0
Jack (*Pringles* Select Bold Crunch) ...	130	1.0	16.0	8.0	0	160	1.0
white, aged (*Kettle* Bakes)	120	3.0	20.0	3.0	0	170	2.0
cheddar/sour cream:							
(*Herr's*)	150	2.0	14.0	10.0	0	310	1.0
(*Lay's*)	150	2.0	15.0	10.0	0	230	1.0
(*Lay's* Baked!)	120	2.0	21.0	3.5	0	210	2.0
(*Ruffles*)	160	2.0	14.0	10.0	0	230	1.0
(*Ruffles* Baked!) ...	140	2.0	25.0	4.0	0	250	2.0
(*Ruffles* Light)	75	3.0	16.0	0	0	230	1.0
(*Wise Ridgies*)	150	2.0	15.0	9.0	0	190	1.0
cheese, four (*Lay's* Kettle)	150	2.0	17.0	8.0	0	170	1.0
chili cheese (*Pringles*)	150	1.0	14.0	10.0	0	230	<1.0
chili limón (*Lay's*) ...	150	2.0	14.0	10.0	0	210	1.0
dill pickle:							
(*Lay's*)	160	2.0	13.0	10.0	0	360	1.0
(*Pringles* Extreme) .	150	1.0	14.0	10.0	0	110	1.0
(*Snyder's* Kosher) .	140	2.0	20.0	6.0	0	360	4.0
dill and sour cream (*Kettle Krinkle Cut*)	150	2.0	16.0	9.0	0	170	2.0

Food and Measure	cal.	prot. (gms)	carbo. (gms)	fat (gms)	chol. (mgs)	sod. (mgs)	fiber (gms)
Potato chips/crisps *(cont.)*							
garlic, roasted, and Parmesan (*Terra Red Bliss*)	140	2.0	16.0	7.0	0	115	2.0
herb, fine (*Terra Red Bliss*)	140	2.0	18.0	7.0	0	70	3.0
honey Dijon (*Kettle*) ..	150	2.0	16.0	9.0	0	150	1.0
hot:							
(*Bachman Golden Ridges Hot!*) ...	150	2.0	15.0	9.0	0	230	1.0
(*Gibble's* Red Hot) .	140	2.0	16.0	8.0	5	290	1.0
(*Herr's* Red Hot) ...	150	2.0	14.0	10.0	0	300	1.0
(*Lay's Flamin' Hot*)	160	2.0	15.0	10.0	0	330	1.0
jalapeño:							
(*Herr's* Kettle)	160	2.0	14.0	10.0	0	300	1.0
(*Lay's* Kettle)	140	2.0	16.0	8.0	0	170	1.0
(*Pringles*)	150	1.0	14.0	10.0	0	190	<1.0
(*Snyder's*)	150	2.0	20.0	6.0	0	330	4.0
(*Wise New York Deli Kettle*)	140	2.0	16.0	8.0	0	210	1.0
cheddar (*Cape Cod*)	140	2.0	16.0	8.0	0	260	2.0
jerk (*Kettle Krinkle Cut Island Jerk*)	150	2.0	16.0	9.0	0	150	2.0
ketchup (*Herr's Heinz*)	150	2.0	15.0	10.0	0	300	1.0
lemon pepper (*Terra Unsalted*)	150	2.0	15.0	10.0	0	5	1.0
lime (*Lay's Limón*) ...	150	2.0	15.0	10.0	0	370	1.0
onion:							
(*Lay's Kettle Maui*) .	150	2.0	17.0	8.0	0	170	1.0
(*Maui Style*)	150	2.0	16.0	9.0	0	200	1.0
French (*Eatsmart*) .	150	2.0	19.0	7.0	0	190	3.0
onion and garlic:							
(*Terra Golds*)	130	2.0	19.0	5.0	0	65	1.0
(*Wise*)	150	2.0	14.0	10.0	0	310	1.0
pizza flavor:							
(*Pringles*)	150	1.0	14.0	10.0	0	190	<1.0
(*Pringles* Minis) ...	120	1.0	13.0	7.0	0	170	<1.0
ranch:							
(*Lay's Wavy*)	150	2.0	16.0	9.0	0	200	1.0
(*Lay's Stax*)	150	1.0	15.0	9.0	0	180	1.0
(*Pringles*)	150	2.0	14.0	10.0	0	190	<1.0
jalapeño (*Pringles Select Bold Crunch*)	130	1.0	16.0	8.0	0	160	<1.0

Food and Measure	cal.	prot. (gms)	carbo. (gms)	fat (gms)	chol. (mgs)	sod. (mgs)	fiber (gms)
red pepper, roasted, w/goat cheese (*Kettle*)	150	2.0	16.0	9.0	0	180	1.0
salt and pepper:							
(*Herr's*)	150	2.0	14.0	10.0	0	420	1.0
(*Terra Golds*)	130	2.0	19.0	5.0	0	120	1.0
fresh ground (*Kettle Krinkle Cut*)	150	2.0	16.0	9.0	0	200	2.0
sea salt (*Terra* Kettles Krinkle Cut Blends)	140	2.0	18.0	6.0	0	65	<1.0
sea salt/black pepper (*Kettle* Organic) .	150	2.0	16.0	9.0	0	210	2.0
sea salt/cracked pepper (*Cape Cod*)	140	2.0	16.0	7.0	0	160	1.0
sea salt/spice (*Terra Frites*)	150	2.0	18.0	8.0	0	160	3.0
salt and vinegar:							
(*Herr's*)	150	2.0	14.0	10.0	0	340	1.0
(*Herr's* Kettle Cooked Boardwalk)	140	2.0	16.0	8.0	0	300	1.0
(*Lay's*)	150	2.0	15.0	10.0	0	380	1.0
(*Lay's Stax*)	150	1.0	14.0	9.0	0	230	1.0
(*Maui Style*)	150	2.0	15.0	8.0	0	220	1.0
(*Pringles*)	150	1.0	14.0	10.0	0	180	<1.0
(*Snyder's*)	140	2.0	19.0	6.0	0	250	4.0
(*Terra Golds*)	130	2.0	20.0	5.0	0	110	2.0
(*Wise*)	150	2.0	14.0	10.0	0	290	1.0
sea salt (*Cape Cod*)	150	2.0	17.0	8.0	0	130	1.0
sea salt (*Kettle*) ...	150	2.0	16.0	9.0	0	160	1.0
sea salt (*Lay's* Kettle)	140	2.0	17.0	7.0	0	260	1.0
sea salt/malt vinegar (*Terra Frites*) ...	150	2.0	18.0	8.0	0	200	3.0
salsa, fire-roasted (*Snyder's*)	150	2.0	20.0	6.0	0	240	4.0
sea salt:							
(*Ruffles* Natural Reduced Fat) ...	140	2.0	17.0	7.0	0	160	1.0
w/blue potato (*Terra* Kettles Krinkle Cut Blends)	140	2.0	18.0	6.0	0	90	<1.0
w/sweet potato (*Terra* Kettles Krinkle Cut Blends)	140	2.0	18.0	7.0	0	120	<1.0
shoestring (*Jays*)	150	1.0	16.0	9.0	0	190	1.0

Food and Measure	cal.	prot. (gms)	carbo. (gms)	fat (gms)	chol. (mgs)	sod. (mgs)	fiber (gms)
Potato chips/crisps *(cont.)*							
sour cream/onion:							
(*Herr's*)	150	2.0	14.0	10.0	0	310	1.0
(*Herr's* Kettle)	140	2.0	16.0	8.0	0	310	1.0
(*Lay's*)	160	2.0	15.0	10.0	0	210	1.0
(*Lay's* Baked!)	120	2.0	21.0	3.0	0	210	2.0
(*Moore's Ridgies*) .	150	2.0	14.0	10.0	0	210	1.0
(*Pringles*)	150	1.0	14.0	10.0	0	180	<1.0
(*Pringles* Minis) . . .	120	1.0	13.0	7.0	0	140	<1.0
(*Ruffles*)	160	2.0	14.0	10.0	0	190	1.0
(*Snyder's*)	150	2.0	20.0	6.0	0	210	4.0
(*Wise Ridgies*)	150	2.0	14.0	10.0	0	220	1.0
steak and Worcestershire (*Herr's*)	160	2.0	16.0	10.0	0	360	1.0
sun-dried tomato/ balsamic vinegar (*Terra Red Bliss*) . .	140	2.0	18.0	7.0	0	85	3.0
Thai, spicy (*Kettle*) . . .	150	2.0	15.0	9.0	0	180	1.0
vinegar (*Bachman Golden Ridges*) . . .	150	1.0	15.0	10.0	<5	240	0
yogurt/green onion:							
(*Barbara's*)	150	2.0	15.0	9.0	0	240	1.0
(*Kettle*)	150	2.0	15.0	9.0	0	190	1.0
Potato dish, can or microwave:							
au gratin: (*Del Monte Savory Sides*), ½ cup	80	2.0	13.0	2.5	0	470	1.0
w/chickpeas, tomato (*Tasty Bite* Bombay), ½ of 10-oz. pkg. . .	105	5.0	13.0	4.0	0	412	3.0
scalloped (*Glory*), ½ cup	70	2.0	14.0	1.0	0	330	1.0
scalloped, and ham:							
(*Dinty Moore* Big Bowl), 1 cup . . .	280	10.0	23.0	16.0	40	920	0
(*Dinty Moore* Micro Cup), 7.5 oz. . . .	240	9.0	20.0	13.0	35	1020	2.0
Potato dish, frozen (see also "Potato, frozen/refrigerated"):							
au gratin (*Health is Wealth*), ½ of 10-oz. pkg.	220	9.0	20.0	12.0	40	380	2.0
baby, and vegetable blend (*Birds Eye*), ¾ cup .	40	1.0	8.0	0	0	20	1.0

Food and Measure	cal.	prot. (gms)	carbo. (gms)	fat (gms)	chol. (mgs)	sod. (mgs)	fiber (gms)
baked, twice, 1 pc.:							
(*Inland Valley Gourmet*), 5.2 oz.	230	8.0	23.0	12.0	30	310	2.0
broccoli/cheese (*Health is Wealth*)	210	6.0	34.0	6.0	10	380	5.0
cheddar (*Health is Wealth*)	200	4.0	25.0	10.0	10	340	2.0
cheese, triple (*Inland Valley* 4 Pack), 5.2 oz.	250	7.0	33.0	10.0	20	410	3.0
cheese, triple (*Inland Valley* 8 Pack), 8 oz.	400	10.0	51.0	17.0	35	690	5.0
sour cream/bacon/ chive (*Inland Valley*), 5.2 oz. . . .	240	5.0	36.0	8.0	10	330	3.0
sour cream/chive (*Health is Wealth*)	180	4.0	24.0	8.0	20	380	2.0
cheddar:							
(*Lean Cuisine One Dish Favorites Deluxe*), 10⅜ oz.	260	14.0	35.0	7.0	20	620	4.0
bacon bake (*Stouffer's*), ½ of 10-oz. pkg.	270	9.0	21.0	17.0	20	500	2.0
broccoli (*Michelina's Signature*), 9.5 oz.	310	13.0	33.0	15.0	35	1160	4.0
mashed (*Larry's*), 5 oz.:							
bacon/cheddar	200	5.0	23.0	10.0	10	650	1.0
bacon/onion/tomato	180	3.0	25.0	8.0	5	650	2.0
broccoli/cheddar . .	180	3.0	22.0	8.0	5	390	2.0
butter, old-fashioned	190	3.0	25.0	9.0	10	370	2.0
cheddar	190	4.0	25.0	8.0	5	460	2.0
cheddar/sour cream	200	4.0	24.0	9.0	10	450	2.0
garlic, roasted	200	3.0	25.0	10.0	15	160	2.0
sour cream/chives .	180	3.0	25.0	8.0	5	440	2.0
pancakes, see "Potato pancakes"							
puffs, w/roasted garlic (*The Fillo Factory Organic*), ½ of 10-oz. pkg.	330	8.0	43.0	14.0	20	450	2.0
roasted, w/broccoli, cheese sauce:							
(*Birds Eye*), ⅔ cup	100	2.0	15.0	4.0	0	470	1.0

Food and Measure	cal.	prot. (gms)	carbo. (gms)	fat (gms)	chol. (mgs)	sod. (mgs)	fiber (gms)
Potato dish, frozen, roasted w/broccoli *(cont.)*							
(*Green Giant* Bag), 1 cup	120	4.0	20.0	2.0	<5	620	2.0
(*Green Giant* Box), ¾ cup	110	3.0	18.0	3.0	5	490	2.0
(*Lean Cuisine One Dish Favorites*), 10.25-oz. pkg. ..	220	11.0	33.0	5.0	15	620	5.0
cheese (*Smart Ones*), 10-oz. pkg.	220	9.0	34.0	6.0	15	480	5.0
roasted, w/garlic and herbs (*Green Giant*), 1¼ cups	200	3.0	33.0	7.0	0	420	2.0
Potato dish, mix (see also "Potato seasoning mix"), ½ cup*, except as noted:							
(*Betty Crocker Seasoned Skillet* Traditional) .	180	2.0	22.0	9.0	0	500	2.0
au gratin:							
(*Betty Crocker*), ⅔ cup*	150	3.0	22.0	6.0	<5	660	1.0
(*Betty Crocker* Deluxe Loaded)	140	4.0	23.0	4.5	5	610	1.0
(*Dr. Oetker/Sherriff*), ⅙ pkg.	100	2.0	19.0	1.0	0	540	0
(*Hungry Jack*), 1 oz.	100	2.0	21.0	1.0	n.a.	570	2.0
(*Idahoan*), ⅔ cup ..	110	3.0	20.0	1.5	0	690	2.0
cheesy (*Velveeta*), ⅕ pkg.	180	5.0	26.0	6.0	10	780	2.0
cheesy cheddar (*Betty Crocker* Deluxe) .	180	4.0	22.0	9.0	5	650	1.0
casserole, roasted garlic and oil (*Betty Crocker*), ¾ cup* .	160	3.0	27.0	6.0	0	650	2.0
cheese, four (*Hungry Jack*), 1 oz.	150	2.0	21.0	1.0	n.a.	570	2.0
cheddar and bacon:							
(*Betty Crocker*), ⅔ cup*	130	3.0	21.0	4.0	<5	690	1.0
(*Hungry Jack*), 1 oz.	150	2.0	21.0	1.0	n.a.	570	2.0
cheese, three (*Betty Crocker*), ⅔ cup* .	130	3.0	22.0	4.0	<5	600	2.0

Food and Measure	cal.	prot. (gms)	carbo. (gms)	fat (gms)	chol. (mgs)	sod. (mgs)	fiber (gms)
garlic, roasted:							
(Betty Crocker) ...	120	2.0	20.0	4.0	0	530	1.0
and herb (Betty Crocker Seasoned Skillets)	170	3.0	22.0	9.0	0	440	2.0
hash browns:							
(Betty Crocker Seasoned Skillets)	120	2.0	19.0	4.0	0	450	2.0
(Idahoan), ⅓ cup ..	90	2.0	18.0	.5	0	110	1.0
cheesy (Idahoan Club Pack), ½ cup	120	2.0	23.0	2.0	0	450	2.0
julienne (Betty Crocker), ⅔ cup*	110	2.0	20.0	3.5	<5	660	1.0
mashed:							
(Dr. Oetker/Sherriff), ⅓ cup mix	70	1.0	14.0	0	0	10	1.0
(Hungry Jack Original), ⅓ cup mix .	80	2.0	19.0	0	0	20	1.0
(Idahoan Original), ⅓ cup mix	80	2.0	18.0	0	0	15	2.0
(Martha White Instant Spud), ⅓ cup flakes	80	2.0	17.0	0	0	20	2.0
all varieties (Hungry Jack Easy Mash'd), ¼ cup mix	150	2.0	17.0	1.5	n.a.	430	2.0
butter, creamy (Betty Crocker Homestyle)	160	3.0	21.0	7.0	5	430	2.0
butter herb (Betty Crocker) .	160	3.0	20.0	8.0	<5	460	1.0
butter herb (Idahoan), ¼ cup	110	2.0	20.0	2.5	0	560	1.0
buttery (Idahoan Homestyle), ¼ cup	110	2.0	20.0	2.5	0	450	1.0
cheese, 4 (Betty Crocker)	160	3.0	21.0	7.0	<5	550	1.0
cheese, 4 (Idahoan), ¼ cup	100	2.0	19.0	2.5	0	550	1.0
cheese, 3 (Betty Crocker Deluxe), ⅔ cup*	190	4.0	24.0	9.0	5	720	1.0
cheesy (Velveeta), ⅛ pkg.	140	4.0	19.0	5.0	10	460	1.0

Food and Measure	cal.	prot. (gms)	carbo. (gms)	fat (gms)	chol. (mgs)	sod. (mgs)	fiber (gms)
Potato dish, mix, mashed *(cont.)*							
garlic, roasted (*Betty Crocker*)	160	3.0	20.0	8.0	5	410	1.0
garlic, roasted (*Idahoan*), ¼ cup	110	2.0	20.0	2.5	0	600	1.0
garlic, roasted, and cheddar (*Betty Crocker*)	160	3.0	20.0	8.0	5	480	1.0
loaded, baked (*Idahoan*), ¼ cup	110	2.0	19.0	2.5	0	450	2.0
sour cream and chive (*Betty Crocker*) .	150	3.0	21.0	7.0	5	410	1.0
Southwest (*Idahoan*), ¼ cup	110	2.0	20.0	2.5	0	520	2.0
onion, creamy, w/chives or sour cream/chives (*Hungry Jack*), 1 oz.	150	2.0	21.0	1.0	n.a.	570	2.0
scalloped:							
(*Betty Crocker*) ...	130	3.0	22.0	4.0	<5	630	1.0
(*Dr. Oetker/Sherriff*), ⅙ pkg.	100	2.0	19.0	1.0	0	540	0
(*Idahoan*), ⅔ cup ..	100	2.0	21.0	1.5	0	610	1.0
cheesy (*Betty Crocker* Homestyle)	150	4.0	22.0	6.0	<5	620	2.0
cheesy (*Hungry Jack*), 1 oz.	100	2.0	20.0	1.5	n.a.	580	2.0
cheesy bacon (*Velveeta*), ⅕ pkg. ..	190	6.0	26.0	7.0	15	850	2.0
creamy (*Betty Crocker* Deluxe), ⅔ cup*	140	3.0	23.0	4.5	5	740	1.0
creamy (*Hungry Jack*), 1 oz.	150	2.0	21.0	1.0	n.a.	570	2.0
garlic, roasted, creamy (*Betty Crocker* Deluxe), ⅔ cup*	160	4.0	25.0	6.0	5	720	1.0
sour cream and chive (*Betty Crocker*), ⅔ cup*	120	2.0	21.0	4.0	<5	690	1.0
Potato entree, see "Potato dish"							
Potato flour:							
(*Shiloh Farms*), ¼ cup	100	2.0	23.0	0	0	10	2.0
1 cup	571	11.0	132.9	.5	0	88	9.4

Food and Measure	cal.	prot. (gms)	carbo. (gms)	fat (gms)	chol. (mgs)	sod. (mgs)	fiber (gms)
Potato pancake (see also "Sweet potato dish"), frozen/refrigerated, 1 pc., except as noted:							
(*Dr. Praeger's*), 2.25 oz.	100	2.0	13.0	4.0	15	190	3.0
(*Empire Kosher*), 2 oz.	120	1.0	19.0	5.0	0	260	1.0
(*Golden*), 1.3 oz.	70	2.0	10.0	3.0	<5	190	1.0
(*Inland Valley*), 2 oz.	120	2.0	12.0	8.0	20	310	2.0
(*Kineret*), 1.5 oz.	70	1.0	9.0	3.0	0	100	1.0
(*Old Fashioned Kitchen*), 2.5 oz.	130	4.0	18.0	6.0	8	350	2.0
mini:							
(*Kineret* Latkas), 11 pcs., 3 oz.	170	2.0	21.0	8.0	0	320	2.0
(*McCain Homestyle BabyCakes*), 4 pcs., 2.6 oz.	150	1.0	17.0	9.0	0	440	2.0
(*Old Fashioned Kitchen*), 4 pcs., 3 oz.	160	5.0	22.0	7.0	10	420	2.0
Potato pancake mix:							
(*Carmel*), 3 tbsp.	80	2.0	18.0	1.0	0	500	2.0
(*Hungry Jack*), 2 tbsp.	70	2.0	15.0	0	0	360	1.0
(*Manischewitz*), 3 tbsp.	80	2.0	18.0	1.0	0	500	2.0
Potato salad, refrigerated (*Blue Ridge Farm*), 4 oz.	200	1.0	19.0	14.0	15	480	1.0
Potato salad seasoning (*Watkins*), ¼ tsp.	0	0	0	0	0	135	0
Potato seasoning mix:							
cheese, four (*McCormick*), 1 tbsp.	30	1.0	3.0	1.0	5	280	0
herb, Italian (*McCormick* Potato Steamers), 2 tsp.	30	0	4.0	1.0	0	590	0
roasted garlic and rosemary (*McCormick* Potato Steamers), 1 tbsp.	30	0	4.0	1.9	0	560	0
toasted onion and garlic (*McCormick*), 1 tbsp.	20	0	4.0	0	5	570	0
Potato soy crisps, 1 oz.:							
(*Genisoy Soytato* Chips Lightly Salted)	120	8.0	15.0	3.0	0	210	2.0

Food and Measure	cal.	prot. (gms)	carbo. (gms)	fat (gms)	chol. (mgs)	sod. (mgs)	fiber (gms)
Potato soy crisps *(cont.)*							
barbecue:							
(*GeniSoy*)	120	6.0	17.0	3.0	0	410	2.0
(*Genisoy* Soytato Chips)	120	7.0	16.0	3.0	0	250	2.0
Parmesan garlic or ranch (*GeniSoy*) . .	120	6.0	16.0	3.0	0	440	2.0
sea salt/black pepper (*GeniSoy*)	90	6.0	16.0	3.0	0	220	2.0
sour cream/onion (*Genisoy* Soytato Chips)	120	8.0	15.0	3.0	0	240	2.0
Potato starch (*Manischewitz*), 1 tbsp. . .	30	0	8.0	0	0	0	0
Potato sticks, canned, shoestring:							
(*Butterfield*), ⅔ cup .	150	2.0	16.0	9.0	0	90	2.0
(*Butterfield* Single Serve), 1 cup	250	3.0	26.0	15.0	0	150	3.0
Poultry seasoning (see also "Chicken seasoning"), 1 tsp. .	5	.1	1.0	.1	0	tr.	.2
Pout, ocean, meat only:							
raw, 4 oz.	90	18.9	0	1.0	59	69	0
baked or broiled, 4 oz.	116	24.2	0	1.3	76	88	0
Pretzel, 1 oz.:							
(*Herr's* Circle H Mini) .	170	3.0	32.0	3.0	0	675	2.0
(*Herr's* Extra Dark Specials)	110	3.0	21.0	1.0	0	450	2.0
(*Snyder's* Snaps)	110	3.0	24.0	1.0	0	340	<1.0
Buffalo wing, hot (*Snyder's* Pieces) . .	140	2.0	17.0	7.0	0	380	<1.0
butter:							
(*Snyder's* Snaps) . .	120	3.0	25.0	1.0	0	270	1.0
sesame, sticks (*Snyder's*)	120	3.0	22.0	2.0	0	250	2.0
sticks (*Bachman*) . .	100	2.0	20.0	1.0	0	520	1.0
sticks, tiny (*Snyder's*)	120	3.0	25.0	0	0	360	<1.0
twists (*Bachman*) . .	110	3.0	23.0	1.0	0	820	1.0
twists, braided (*Quinlan*)	110	3.0	23.0	1.0	0	240	1.0
buttermilk ranch (*Snyder's* Pieces) . .	140	2.0	19.0	6.0	0	230	1.0

Food and Measure	cal.	prot. (gms)	carbo. (gms)	fat (gms)	chol. (mgs)	sod. (mgs)	fiber (gms)
w/cheese (*Handi-Snacks Mister Salty*)	90	3.0	12.0	3.5	5	380	0
cheddar:							
(*Rold Gold* Baked Mini Sticks)	140	0	10.0	7.0	0	230	1.0
(*Rold Gold* Tiny Twists)	110	3.0	22.0	1.0	0	370	1.0
(*Snyder's* Pieces) ..	130	2.0	18.0	6.0	0	260	<1.0
twists, savory (*Pepperidge Farm* Baked Natural Thins), 11 pcs., 1.1 oz. .	140	2.0	26.0	3.0	0	600	1.0
cheese filled:							
cheddar (*Combos*) .	130	3.0	19.0	4.5	0	310	0
nacho (*Combos*) ..	130	3.0	19.0	4.5	0	320	1.0
chocolate coated, see "Candy"							
crackers, see "Cracker"							
crisps, 11 pcs., 1 oz.:							
(*Pretzel Crisps* Original)	110	3.0	23.0	0	0	330	1.0
Buffalo wing (*Pretzel Crisps*)	110	3.0	22.0	1.5	0	540	1.0
everything (*Pretzel Crisps*)	110	3.0	23.0	.5	0	170	1.0
garlic (*Pretzel Crisps*)	110	3.0	23.0	0	0	230	1.0
honey mustard onion (*Pretzel Crisps*) .	110	3.0	22.0	1.5	0	450	1.0
garlic bread:							
(*Snyder's* Nibblers)	130	2.0	24.0	3.0	0	180	<1.0
(*Snyder's* Pieces) ..	140	3.0	18.0	7.0	0	160	1.0
hard (*Snyder's* Unsalted)	100	3.0	22.0	0	0	90	<1.0
honey mustard: (*Rold Gold* Tiny Twists) ..	110	3.0	23.0	1.0	0	430	1.0
honey mustard onion:							
(*Rold Gold* Mini Sticks)	140	2.0	19.0	6.0	0	120	1.0
(*Snyder's* Multigrain Nibblers), 1.1 oz.	140	3.0	20.0	5.0	0	150	3.0
(*Snyder's* Nibblers)	130	3.0	23.0	3.0	0	95	<1.0
(*Snyder's* Pieces) ..	140	2.0	18.0	7.0	0	240	<1.0
honey wheat:							
(*Bachman* Wheat & Honey)	110	3.0	23.0	1.0	0	190	1.0

Pretzel, honey wheat *(cont.)*

Food and Measure	cal.	prot. (gms)	carbo. (gms)	fat (gms)	chol. (mgs)	sod. (mgs)	fiber (gms)
(*Herr's*)	110	3.0	21.0	2.0	0	300	2.0
sticks (*Snyder's*) ..	120	3.0	24.0	2.0	0	230	2.0
sticks (*Snyder's* Organic)	130	3.0	24.0	2.0	0	210	1.0
twists, braided (*Rold Gold*)	110	2.0	23.0	1.0	0	230	1.0
twists, braided (*Quinlan*)	110	2.0	24.0	1.0	0	200	1.0
jalapeño (*Snyder's* Pieces)	140	2.0	20.0	5.0	0	370	<1.0
multigrain, 5, sticks (*Snyder's*)	120	3.0	23.0	2.0	0	160	1.0
mustard, deli-style (*Gardetto's* Mix), ½ cup, 1.1 oz.	130	3.0	24.0	2.0	0	220	1.0
nuggets (*Bachman Nutzels*)	110	3.0	23.0	1.0	0	100	1.0
oat bran:							
(*Shiloh Farms*)	110	3.0	21.0	1.0	0	260	2.0
(*Shiloh Farms* No Salt)	110	3.0	21.0	1.0	0	60	2.0
sticks (*Snyder's* Organic)	120	3.0	25.0	0	0	320	2.0
onion (*Snyder's* Steak-house Pieces)	140	2.0	18.0	7.0	0	220	0
peanut butter filled:							
(*Bachman*)	160	8.0	15.0	8.0	0	250	1.0
(*Herr's*), 1.1 oz. ...	160	8.0	15.0	8.0	0	250	1.0
(*Tree of Life* Natural), 8 pcs., 1.4 oz. ..	200	4.0	26.0	9.0	0	160	<1.0
pizza flavor filled (*Combos* Pizzeria) .	130	2.0	20.0	4.5	0	310	1.0
pumpernickel onion:							
sticks (*Snyder's*) ..	120	3.0	23.0	2.0	0	280	2.0
sticks (*Snyder's* Organic)	120	3.0	24.0	1.5	0	225	1.0
rods:							
(*Bachman* Caddy) .	110	3.0	23.0	1.0	0	600	1.0
(*Bachman* "Rolled")	110	3.0	24.0	.5	0	260	1.0
(*Rold Gold* Classic)	110	3.0	22.0	1.0	0	610	1.0
(*Snyder's*)	120	3.0	24.0	1.0	0	290	1.0
sandwich:							
cheddar (*Snyder's*) .	150	3.0	16.0	8.0	<5	200	<1.0

Food and Measure	cal.	prot. (gms)	carbo. (gms)	fat (gms)	chol. (mgs)	sod. (mgs)	fiber (gms)
jalapeño cheddar (*Snyder's*)	140	3.0	17.0	7.0	<5	190	1.0
peanut butter (*Snyder's*)	140	4.0	16.0	7.0	0	140	<1.0
shapes (*Bachman Kidzels*)	120	2.0	23.0	1.5	0	95	1.0
sourdough:							
(*Herr's* Specials), 1.5 oz.	170	4.0	31.0	0	0	675	2.0
bite size (*Snyder's* Nibblers)	120	3.0	25.0	0	0	200	<1.0
hard (*Bachman*) ...	110	3.0	22.0	1.0	0	420	1.0
hard (*Herr's*)	100	3.0	23.0	0	0	450	2.0
hard (*Rold Gold*) ..	100	3.0	21.0	.5	0	500	1.0
hard (*Snyder's*) ...	100	3.0	22.0	0	0	240	1.0
hard (*Snyder's* Unsalted)	100	3.0	22.0	0	0	90	1.0
hard, bite size (*Herr's*), 1.1 oz. .	100	3.0	23.0	0	0	450	2.0
nuggets (*Bachman* Bites)	110	3.0	22.0	1.0	0	240	1.0
twists (*Bachman* Specials)	110	3.0	22.0	1.0	0	240	1.0
spelt:							
(*VitaSpelt*)	110	4.0	21.0	1.5	0	260	<1.0
(*VitaSpelt* Low Sodium)	110	4.0	21.0	1.5	0	90	<1.0
sourdough (*Vita-Spelt* Organic) ..	110	3.0	23.0	.5	0	350	3.0
sticks:							
(*Bachman*)	100	2.0	20.0	1.0	0	520	1.0
(*Herr's* Stix)	115	3.0	21.0	2.0	0	450	2.0
(*Rold Gold* Classic)	100	2.0	23.0	0	0	580	1.0
(*Snyder's* Dipping Stix)	120	3.0	24.0	1.0	0	240	1.0
(*Snyder's* Multigrain Lightly Salted), 1.1 oz.	120	3.0	23.0	2.0	0	160	3.0
(*Snyder's* Olde Tyme)	120	3.0	23.0	1.5	0	200	<1.0
sesame (*Snyder's* Old Fashioned) ..	120	3.0	23.0	2.0	0	200	<1.0
whole grain (*Herr's*), 1.1 oz.	110	3.0	22.0	1.0	0	300	4.0

Food and Measure	cal.	prot. (gms)	carbo. (gms)	fat (gms)	chol. (mgs)	sod. (mgs)	fiber (gms)
Pretzel *(cont.)*							
twists:							
(*Bachman* Classic) .	100	3.0	22.0	1.0	0	650	1.0
(*Bachman* Fat Free							
Thins)	110	3.0	23.0	0	0	125	1.0
(*Bachman* Thin 'n							
Right)	120	3.0	23.0	1.0	0	125	1.0
(*Gibble's* Thin)	110	2.0	22.0	2.0	0	640	1.0
(*Herr's* Extra Thin) .	100	3.0	22.0	1.0	0	450	2.0
(*Herr's* Extra Thin							
No Salt)	100	3.0	24.0	0	0	100	2.0
(*Pepperidge Farm*							
Baked Natural							
Thins), 11 pcs.,							
1.1 oz.	110	2.0	21.0	0	0	340	1.0
(*Rold Gold* Braided)	110	2.0	22.0	1.0	0	410	1.0
(*Rold Gold* Tiny) . .	110	2.0	23.0	1.0	0	450	1.0
(*Rold Gold* Tiny Fat							
Free)	100	3.0	23.0	0	0	420	1.0
(*Snyder's* Homestyle)	120	3.0	25.0	1.0	0	230	1.0
(*Snyder's* Multigrain							
Olde Tyme), 1.1 oz.	120	3.0	22.0	2.0	0	170	2.0
(*Snyder's* Olde Tyme)	120	3.0	24.0	1.0	0	120	1.0
mini (*Bachman* Low							
Sodium Petite) . .	110	3.0	25.0	0	0	50	<1.0
mini (*Gibble's*)	110	2.0	22.0	1.5	0	580	1.0
mini (*Jays*)	110	3.0	24.0	0	0	300	<1.0
mini (*Quinlan*)	110	2.0	23.0	1.0	0	420	<1.0
mini (*Snyder's*) . . .	110	3.0	25.0	0	0	250	<1.0
mini (*Snyder's*							
Unsalted)	110	3.0	25.0	0	0	75	<1.0
mini, baked							
(*Bachman*)	110	3.0	25.0	0	0	190	1.0
thins (*Quinlan*)	110	2.0	23.0	1.0	0	550	<1.0
thins (*Rold Gold*) . .	110	2.0	23.0	1.0	0	560	1.0
thins (*Snyder's*) . . .	110	3.0	23.0	0	0	330	<1.0
whole wheat:							
(*Shiloh Farms*)	90	2.0	20.0	.5	0	260	3.0
(*Shiloh Farms* No Salt)	90	2.0	18.0	0	0	30	3.0
Pretzel, soft, frozen:							
(*SuperPretzel*),							
2.25-oz. pc.:							
no salt added	160	5.0	34.0	1.0	0	130	1.0
w/salt added	160	5.0	34.0	1.0	0	920	1.0

Food and Measure	cal.	prot. (gms)	carbo. (gms)	fat (gms)	chol. (mgs)	sod. (mgs)	fiber (gms)
(*SuperPretzel*), 2.5-oz. pc.:							
no salt added	190	6.0	40.0	1.0	0	160	2.0
w/salt added	190	6.0	40.0	1.0	0	930	2.0
(*SuperPretzel Soft Pretzel Bites*), 5 pcs., 1.9 oz.:							
no salt added	150	3.0	32.0	.5	0	115	1.0
w/salt added	150	3.0	32.0	.5	0	900	1.0
filled, 2 pcs.:							
cheddar (*SuperPretzel Softstix*) .	130	4.0	22.0	3.0	10	260	1.0
mozzarella (*SuperPretzel Pretzelfils*)	130	6.0	20.0	3.5	5	420	1.0
pepperjack (*SuperPretzel Pretzelfils*)	130	5.0	21.0	3.5	5	400	1.0
pizza (*SuperPretzel Pretzelfils*)	130	5.0	22.0	2.0	5	180	1.0
Prickly pear:							
(*Andy Boy* Cactus Pear), 1 large, trimmed, 3.6 oz.	40	1.0	8.0	1.0	0	25	2.0
(*Frieda's* Cactus Pear), 5 oz.	60	1.0	13.0	.5	0	5	5.0
4.8-oz. fruit, 3.6 oz. trimmed	42	.8	9.9	.5	0	5	3.7
1 cup	61	1.1	14.3	.8	0	7	5.4
Prosciutto, 1 oz., except as noted:							
(*Applegate Farms*) ...	70	2.0	0	4.0	25	570	0
(*Black Bear*)	60	8.0	1.0	3.0	15	500	0
(*Boar's Head* Riserva Stradolce)	60	8.0	0	3.0	15	750	0
(*Carando*)	70	7.0	1.0	4.0	25	510	0
(*Di Lusso* Parma), 2 oz.	170	15.0	0	12.0	50	1060	0
(*Dietz & Watson*)	60	8.0	1.0	3.0	15	500	0
(*Dietz & Watson* Classico)	50	2.0	0	4.5	10	230	0
ham (*Di Lusso*), 2 oz.	120	15.0	0	7.0	50	1100	0
Prune, see "Plum, dried"							
Prune juice, 8 fl. oz.:							
(*L&A*)	180	0	41.0	0	0	10	3.0
(*Langers* Plus)	180	0	41.0	0	0	10	1.0
(*R.W. Knudsen* Organic)	170	1.0	46.0	0	0	20	3.0
(*Sunsweet*)	180	2.0	43.0	0	0	30	3.0

Food and Measure	cal.	prot. (gms)	carbo. (gms)	fat (gms)	chol. (mgs)	sod. (mgs)	fiber (gms)
Prune juice *(cont.)*							
(*Tree of Life Pure Fruit*)	180	1.0	43.0	0	0	0	2.0
canned	182	1.6	44.7	.1	0	10	2.6
Psyllium husk (*Shiloh Farms*), 2 tbsp. . . .	30	0	8.0	0	0	5	8.0
Pudding (see also "Rice pudding"), 3.5-oz. cont., except as noted:							
banana:							
(*Handi-Snacks*) . . .	90	1.0	20.0	1.0	0	160	0
(*Hunt's Snack Pack*)	110	1.0	19.0	3.5	0	150	0
cream (*Swiss Miss Pie Lovers*)	130	2.0	23.0	3.5	<5	170	0
cream pie (*Hunt's Snack Pack*)	110	1.0	19.0	3.5	0	150	0
creamy (*Kozy Shack*), ½ cup	130	3.0	22.0	3.0	15	150	0
split (*Handi-Snacks*)	100	1.0	21.0	1.0	0	170	0
berry, mixed (*Jell-O Smoothie*), 4 oz. . .	100	1.0	18.0	2.5	10	40	0
butterscotch:							
(*Handi-Snacks*) . . .	90	1.0	21.0	1.0	0	160	0
(*Hunt's Snack Pack*)	120	1.0	21.0	3.5	0	150	0
(*Kozy Shack*), ½ cup	130	3.0	23.0	3.5	15	135	0
(*Kozy Shack* No Sugar), ½ cup . .	80	3.0	9.0	3.0	10	120	4.0
(*Swiss Miss*)	130	2.0	22.0	3.5	0	180	0
caramel cream:							
(*Hunt's Snack Pack*)	120	1.0	21.0	3.5	0	160	0
(*Jell-O Creamy Sugar Free*), 3.75 oz. . .	60	1.0	13.0	1.0	0	200	1.0
cheesecake, strawberry (*Jell-O*)	130	1.0	16.0	2.0	0	100	1.0
chocolate:							
(*Handi-Snacks* 14 oz.)	100	1.0	23.0	1.0	0	150	1.0
(*Handi-Snacks* 21 oz.)	90	1.0	23.0	1.0	0	150	1.0
(*Handi-Snacks* Fat Free)	90	2.0	21.0	0	0	170	1.0
(*Hunt's Snack Pack*)	120	2.0	21.0	3.5	0	135	<1.0
(*Hunt's Snack Pack Chocolate Lovers Family*), 1/12 pkg. .	120	2.0	22.0	3.5	0	135	0
(*Hunt's Snack Pack Fat Free*)	90	2.0	20.0	0	0	140	0

Food and Measure	cal.	prot. (gms)	carbo. (gms)	fat (gms)	chol. (mgs)	sod. (mgs)	fiber (gms)
(*Hunt's Snack Pack No Sugar*)	60	1.0	8.0	3.0	0	110	<1.0
(*Jell-O*), 4 oz.	140	2.0	27.0	4.0	0	190	1.0
(*Jell-O* Fat Free), 4 oz.	100	2.0	23.0	0	0	180	1.0
(*Jell-O* Sugar Free), 3.75 oz.	60	2.0	14.0	1.5	0	180	1.0
(*Kozy Shack* Real), ½ cup	140	4.0	24.0	3.5	15	140	<1.0
(*Kozy Shack* No Sugar), ½ cup ..	90	4.0	10.0	3.0	10	120	4.0
(*Swiss Miss* Dream)	150	3.0	26.0	4.0	<5	170	<1.0
w/chocolate topping (*Jell-O Sundae Toppers*), 3.75 oz.	110	2.0	23.0	1.5	0	170	1.0
cream (*Swiss Miss Pie Lovers*)	150	3.0	26.0	4.0	<5	170	<1.0
milk (*Hunt's Snack Pack* Variety Triples)	120	2.0	22.0	3.5	0	135	<1.0
milk (*Swiss Miss*) .	150	3.0	27.0	3.5	0	190	0
milk (*Swiss Miss* Low Fat)	130	3.0	26.0	2.0	0	180	0
chocolate butterscotch (*Hunt's Snack Pack* Family), 1/12 pkg....	130	2.0	22.0	4.5	0	180	0
chocolate caramel (*Hunt's Snack* Pack Triples)	120	2.0	22.0	3.5	0	140	0
chocolate chip cookie (*Handi-Snacks* Doubles)	100	1.0	22.0	1.0	0	150	1.0
chocolate fudge sundae (*Jell-O*), 4 oz.	140	2.0	25.0	3.5	0	170	0
chocolate/vanilla: (*Handi-Snacks* Doubles)	100	1.0	22.0	1.0	0	160	0
(*Hunt's Snack Pack* Family), 1/12 pkg. .	120	2.0	21.0	3.5	0	135	0
(*Hunt's Snack Pack* Fat Free Family), 1/12 pkg.	80	2.0	20.0	0	0	140	0
(*Hunt's Snack* Pack Triples)	120	2.0	21.0	3.5	0	130	0

Food and Measure	cal.	prot. (gms)	carbo. (gms)	fat (gms)	chol. (mgs)	sod. (mgs)	fiber (gms)
Pudding *(cont.)*							
chocolate/vanilla swirl:							
(*Jell-O*), 4 oz.	140	2.0	26.0	4.0	0	170	1.0
(*Jell-O* Fat Free), 4 oz.	100	2.0	23.0	0	0	200	1.0
(*Jell-O* Sugar Free),							
3.75 oz.	60	2.0	13.0	1.5	0	180	1.0
(*Swiss Miss*)	140	2.0	27.0	3.5	0	160	0
coffee, creamy (*Kozy*							
Shack), ½ cup	120	3.0	21.0	2.5	10	115	0
w/cookies (*Jell-O Oreo*),							
4 oz.	120	2.0	25.0	1.5	0	200	1.0
devil's food/chocolate							
(*Jell-O* Fat Free), 4 oz.	100	2.0	22.0	0	0	190	1.0
flan:							
(*Kozy Shack* Restau-							
rant Style), ½ cup	190	5.0	28.0	6.0	50	235	0
crème caramel (*Kozy*							
Shack), ½ cup . .	150	4.0	27.0	3.5	35	85	0
mango sauce (*Kozy*							
Shack), ½ cup . .	140	4.0	24.0	4.0	40	100	0
fudge rocky road							
(*Handi-Snacks*							
Doubles)	100	1.0	23.0	1.0	0	130	1.0
ice cream sandwich							
(*Hunt's Snack Pack*							
Triples)	120	2.0	21.0	3.5	0	135	0
lemon:							
(*Hunt's Snack Pack*)	120	0	25.0	2.5	0	65	0
meringue (*Hunt's*							
Snack Pack)	120	0	25.0	2.5	0	60	0
meringue (*Swiss*							
Miss Pie Lovers)	140	0	28.0	3.0	0	600	0
s'mores (*Hunt's Snack*							
Pack Triples)	120	1.0	22.0	3.5	0	115	0
strawberries and cream							
swirl (*Jell-O Crème*							
Savers), 4 oz.	130	2.0	25.0	3.0	10	85	0
strawberry banana (*Jell-O*							
Smoothie), 4 oz. . .	100	1.0	18.0	2.5	10	40	0
tapioca:							
(*Hunt's Snack Pack*)	120	1.0	20.0	3.5	0	140	0
(*Hunt's Snack Pack*							
Fat Free)	80	1.0	19.0	0	0	150	0
(*Jell-O*), 4 oz.	130	1.0	25.0	3.0	0	150	0

Food and Measure	cal.	prot. (gms)	carbo. (gms)	fat (gms)	chol. (mgs)	sod. (mgs)	fiber (gms)
(*Jell-O* Fat Free), 4 oz.	100	1.0	23.0	0	0	230	0
(*Kozy Shack* Old Fashioned), ½ cup	130	3.0	23.0	3.0	15	140	0
(*Kozy Shack* No Sugar), ½ cup . .	90	3.0	11.0	3.0	15	140	4.0
(*Swiss Miss*)	140	2.0	24.0	3.5	0	180	0
vanilla:							
(*Handi-Snacks*) . . .	90	1.0	20.0	0	0	160	0
(*Hunt's Snack Pack*)	120	1.0	20.0	3.5	0	130	0
(*Hunt's Snack Pack* No Sugar)	60	<1.0	8.0	3.5	0	115	0
(*Jell-O*), 4 oz.	130	1.0	24.0	3.5	0	160	0
(*Jell-O* Sugar Free), 3.75 oz.	60	1.0	13.0	1.0	0	190	0
(*Kozy Shack* Natural), ½ cup	130	3.0	22.0	3.0	15	150	0
(*Swiss Miss*)	140	2.0	24.0	3.5	0	180	0
caramel sundae (*Jell-O* Fat Free), 4 oz.	100	1.0	23.0	0	0	230	0
w/caramel or chocolate topping (*Jell-O* Sundae Toppers), 3.75 oz.	110	1.0	23.0	1.0	0	160	0
vanilla/chocolate (*Jell-O* Fat Free), 4 oz.	100	1.0	24.0	0	0	210	0
Pudding bar, frozen, assorted (*Jell-O* Pops), 1.65-fl.-oz. bar	90	2.0	15.0	3.0	0	40	0
Pudding and pie filling mix (see also "Mousse mix"), dry, ¼ pkg. or 1 serving, except as noted:							
almond (*Dr. Oetker*) . .	40	0	10.0	0	0	30	0
banana:							
(*Shirriff*)	110	0	27.0	0	0	140	0
cream (*Jell-O* Cook & Serve 3 oz.) . .	80	0	20.0	0	0	180	0
cream (*Jell-O* Instant)	90	0	23.0	0	0	360	0
cream (*Jell-O* Sugar/ Fat Free)	25	0	6.0	0	0	320	0

Food and Measure	cal.	prot. (gms)	carbo. (gms)	fat (gms)	chol. (mgs)	sod. (mgs)	fiber (gms)
Pudding and pie filling mix *(cont.)*							
butterscotch:							
(*Jell-O* Cook & Serve)	100	0	24.0	0	0	130	0
(*Jell-O* Instant)	90	0	23.0	0	0	390	0
(*Jell-O* Instant Sugar/							
Fat Free)	25	0	6.0	0	0	320	0
(*Shirriff*)	110	0	28.0	0	0	130	0
cheesecake:							
(*Jell-O* Instant)	100	0	24.0	0	0	360	0
(*Jell-O* Instant Sugar/							
Fat Free)	25	0	6.0	0	0	310	0
chocolate:							
(*Dr. Oetker*)	40	0	10.0	0	0	30	0
(*Dr. Oetker* Organic)	120	.4	30.0	.3	0	100	0
(*Jell-O* Cook & Serve)	90	1.0	22.0	0	0	110	1.0
(*Jell-O* Cook & Serve							
Sugar Free)	30	1.0	7.0	0	0	110	1.0
(*Jell-O* Instant)	100	0	25.0	0	0	420	1.0
(*Jell-O* Instant Sugar/							
Fat Free)	35	1.0	8.0	0	0	300	1.0
(*Mori Nu Mates*) . .	110	0	22.0	2.0	0	5	1.0
(*My*T*Fine*)	80	0	20.0	0	0	130	<1.0
(*Shirriff*)	110	1.0	27.0	.4	0	100	0
white (*Jell-O* Instant)	90	0	23.0	0	0	350	0
white (*Jell-O* Instant							
Sugar/Fat Free) .	25	0	6.0	0	0	320	0
chocolate fudge:							
(*Jell-O* Cook & Serve)	90	1.0	22.0	0	0	115	1.0
(*Jell-O* Instant)	100	1.0	25.0	0	0	380	1.0
(*Jell-O* Instant Sugar/							
Fat Free)	35	1.0	8.0	0	0	310	1.0
coconut:							
(*Dr. Oetker* Organic)	100	.3	22.0	1.5	0	100	0
(*Shirriff*)	120	.1	27.0	1.5	0	130	0
cream (*Jell-O* Cook							
& Serve)	90	1.0	18.0	2.5	0	150	1.0
cream (*Jell-O* Instant)	100	0	21.0	2.5	0	270	1.0
cookies and cream							
(*Jell-O Oreo* Instant)	120	0	28.0	1.0	0	390	0
cream (*Dr. Oetker*) . . .	40	0	10.0	0	0	30	0
crème brûlée:							
(*Dr.Oetker*)	110	1.0	23.0	1.5	10	90	0
milk chocolate (*Dr. Oetker*)	110	1.0	24.0	1.5	35	100	0

Food and Measure	cal.	prot. (gms)	carbo. (gms)	fat (gms)	chol. (mgs)	sod. (mgs)	fiber (gms)
crème caramel (*Dr. Oetker/Shirriff*) ...	100	.3	23.0	.3	15	45	0
devil's food (*Jell-O Instant*)	140	0	25.0	0	0	360	1.0
flan (*Roland*)	70	0	17.0	0	0	90	0
lemon:							
(*Dr. Oetker*)	40	0	10.0	0	0	30	0
(*Jell-O* Cook & Serve 2.9 oz.)	50	0	12.0	0	0	70	0
(*Jell-O* Cook & Serve 4.3 oz.)	60	0	14.0	0	0	80	0
(*Jell-O* Instant)	90	0	24.0	0	0	310	0
(*My*T*Fine*), ⅙ pkg.	50	0	12.0	0	0	120	0
(*Shirriff* Light)	45	0	11.0	0	0	50	0
(*Shirriff* Original) ..	90	0	23.0	0	0	60	0
crème (*Mori Nu Mates*)	120	0	22.0	3.0	0	5	0
lime, key (*Shirriff*) ...	90	0	23.0	0	0	60	0
panna cotta (*Dr. Oetker*)	120	1.0	29.0	0	0	25	0
pistachio:							
(*Jell-O* Instant)	100	0	23.0	.5	0	360	0
(*Jell-O* Instant Sugar/Fat Free) .	30	0	6.0	0	0	300	0
pumpkin spice (*Jell-O Instant*)	90	0	23.0	0	0	340	0
raspberry (*Dr. Oetker*)	40	0	10.0	0	0	30	0
tapioca (*Jell-O* Cook & Serve)	90	0	22.0	0	0	120	0
vanilla:							
(*Dr. Oetker*)	40	0	10.0	0	0	45	0
(*Dr. Oetker* Organic)	100	0	26.0	0	0	100	0
(*Jell-O* Cook & Serve 3 oz.)	80	0	20.0	0	0	135	0
(*Jell-O* Cook & Serve 4.6 oz.)	80	0	21.0	0	0	135	0
(*Jell-O* Cook & Serve Sugar Free)	20	0	5.0	0	0	115	0
(*Jell-O* Instant)	90	0	23.0	0	0	350	0
(*Jell-O* Instant Sugar/ Fat Free)	25	0	6.0	0	0	300	0
(*Mori Nu Mates*) ..	110	0	23.0	2.0	0	5	0
(*My*T*Fine*)	70	0	18.0	0	0	120	0
(*Shirriff*)	100	0	26.0	0	0	100	0
French (*Jell-O* Instant)	90	0	23.0	0	0	350	0

Food and Measure	cal.	prot. (gms)	carbo. (gms)	fat (gms)	chol. (mgs)	sod. (mgs)	fiber (gms)
Puff pastry, see "Pastry, puff"							
Pummelo (see also "Melogold"):							
(*Frieda's*), 5 oz.	50	1.0	13.0	0	0	0	1.0
1 lb. 3 oz. fruit w/out rind	231	4.6	58.6	.2	0	6	6.1
sections, 1 cup	72	1.4	18.3	.1	0	2	1.9
Pumpkin, fresh:							
mini (*Frieda's* Orange/ White), ¾ cup, 3 oz.	20	1.0	6.0	0	0	0	1.0
pulp, ½ cup:							
raw, 1" cubes	15	.6	3.8	.1	0	1	1.0
boiled, drained, mashed	24	.9	6.0	.1	0	2	1.0
Pumpkin, canned, ½ cup:							
(*Libby's* 100% Pure) .	40	2.0	9.0	.5	0	5	5.0
puree (*Tree of Life* Organic)	50	1.0	10.0	0	0	5	4.0
w/ or w/out winter squash	41	1.3	9.9	.3	0	6	3.4
Pumpkin flower:							
raw, ½ cup	3	.2	.5	<.1	0	1	<1.0
boiled, drained, ½ cup	10	.7	2.2	.1	0	4	.6
Pumpkin leaf:							
raw, ½ cup	4	.6	.5	.1	0	2	<1.0
boiled, drained, ½ cup	7	1.0	1.2	.1	0	3	.9
Pumpkin pie mix, see "Pie filling"							
Pumpkin pie spice, 1 tsp.	6	.1	1.2	.2	0	1	.3
Pumpkin seeds:							
in shell, roasted:							
1 oz. or 85 seeds ..	127	5.3	15.3	5.5	0	5	n.a.
1 cup	285	11.9	34.4	12.4	0	12	n.a.
salted, 1 oz.	127	5.3	15.3	5.5	0	163	n.a.
in shell, dry-roasted:							
(*Eden* Organic), ¼ cup	200	10.0	5.0	16.0	0	100	5.0
spicy (*New England Natural*), ¼ cup, 1.2 oz.	140	6.0	17.0	6.0	0	115	11.0

Food and Measure	cal.	prot. (gms)	carbo. (gms)	fat (gms)	chol. (mgs)	sod. (mgs)	fiber (gms)
spicy, w/tamari (*Eden* Organic), ¼ cup .	200	10.0	5.0	16.0	0	75	5.0
shelled:							
(*Tree of Life*), 1 oz.	180	9.0	4.0	14.0	0	5	<3.0
raw (*SunRidge Farms* Natural/Organic), ¼ cup, 1.1 oz. . .	160	7.0	5.0	14.0	0	5	1.0
1 oz., 142 kernels .	154	7.0	5.1	13.0	0	5	n.a.
shelled, roasted:							
(*Tree of Life* Organic Salted), 1 oz. . . .	160	<9.0	4.0	12.0	0	100	<1.0
(*Tree of Life* Salted), ¼ cup, 2 oz.	300	13.0	8.0	24.0	0	330	4.0
1 oz.	148	9.4	3.8	12.0	0	5	1.8
salted, 1 oz.	148	9.4	3.8	12.0	0	163	1.8
tamari (*SunRidge Farms*), 1.1 oz.	150	7.0	5.0	13.0	0	95	1.0
Purslane, ½ cup:							
raw	4	.3	.7	<.1	0	10	<1.0
boiled, drained	10	.9	2.1	.1	0	26	<1.0
Pussycat drink mixer, dry (*Bar-Tender's*), 2 pouches	70	0	17.0	0	0	40	0

Q

Food and Measure	cal.	prot. (gms)	carbo. (gms)	fat (gms)	chol. (mgs)	sod. (mgs)	fiber (gms)
Quail:							
raw, meat w/skin, (4.3 oz. quail w/bone), 3.8 oz.	210	21.4	0	13.1	83	58	0
raw, meat only (4.3 oz. quail w/bone, skin), 3.2 oz.	123	20.0	0	4.2	64	47	0
raw, breast meat only: 1 breast, 2 oz.	69	12.7	0	1.8	32	31	0
cooked, meat w/skin, 1 oz.	66	7.1	0	4.0	25	15	0
Quail egg, see "Egg, quail"							
Quesadilla, frozen:							
cheese, three (*Cedarlane*), 3-oz. pc.	250	10.0	27.0	11.0	25	420	0
cheese, beans, vegetables (*Smart Ones* Fiesta), 8-oz. pkg. .	220	10.0	32.0	5.0	10	630	14.0
chicken: (*Tyson* Meal Kit), 3.9-oz. pc.*	250	15.0	26.0	10.0	35	430	3.0
grilled (*José Olé* Minis), 3 pcs., 3.3 oz.	240	9.0	32.0	8.0	20	650	3.0
chicken/cheese: (*El Monterey*), 2 pcs., 6-oz.	380	17.0	43.0	15.0	35	930	2.0
(*Smart Ones*), 8-oz. pkg.	220	12.0	26.0	7.0	20	620	5.0
grilled, three cheese (*El Monterey*), 3.5-oz. pc.	260	13.0	20.0	14.0	35	420	1.0

Food and Measure	cal.	prot. (gms)	carbo. (gms)	fat (gms)	chol. (mgs)	sod. (mgs)	fiber (gms)
grilled, three cheese, batter fried (*El Monterey Cruncheros*), 2 pcs., 6 oz.	450	19.0	34.0	26.0	55	840	1.0
steak, shredded, cheese (*El Monterrey*), 2 pcs., 6 oz.	400	21.0	42.0	15.0	55	860	1.0
Quince:							
(*Frieda's*), 5 oz.	80	1.0	21.0	0	0	5	3.0
1 medium, 5.3 oz.	53	.4	14.1	.1	0	4	1.7
peeled, seeded, 1 oz. .	16	.1	4.3	<.1	0	1	.5
Quinoa, dry, ¼ cup, except as noted:							
(*Arrowhead Mills*), ⅓ cup	160	6.0	30.0	2.5	0	10	3.0
(*Eden* Organic)	180	7.0	29.0	3.5	0	10	11.0
white or red (*Shiloh Farms* Organic) ...	170	6.0	27.0	2.5	0	30	4.0
Quinoa dish mix (*Seeds of Change* Organic), 1 cup*:							
cilantro, zesty	290	9.0	56.0	3.5	0	700	3.0
herb, French	290	8.0	56.0	3.5	0	860	3.0
tomato basil	290	9.0	55.0	3.5	0	720	4.0
Quinoa flakes (*Shiloh Farms* Organic), ⅓ cup	134	4.0	23.0	2.0	0	2	2.0
Quinoa flour (*Shiloh Farms* Organic), ¼ cup	150	5.0	27.0	2.5	0	25	4.0
Quinoa seeds (*Arrowhead* Mills), ¼ cup .	140	5.0	25.0	2.0	0	0	4.0
Quiznos:							
breakfast sandwich:							
bacon/egg/cheddar	440	25.0	36.0	25.5	190	1120	4.0
egg/cheddar	350	19.0	36.0	20.0	175	720	3.0
ham/egg/cheddar ..	350	23.0	37.0	16.5	180	1100	4.0
steak/cheddar	390	30.0	36.0	17.5	195	1040	3.0
vegetable/cheddar .	310	17.0	38.0	15.5	160	630	4.0
subs, chicken, regular:							
Baja, w/bacon	890	63.0	74.0	43.0	130	2595	7.0
carbonara w/bacon	1030	57.0	74.0	55.5	150	2540	4.0
honey bourbon	640	51.0	88.0	9.5	100	1960	8.0

Food and Measure	cal.	prot. (gms)	carbo. (gms)	fat (gms)	chol. (mgs)	sod. (mgs)	fiber (gms)
***Quiznos*, subs, chicken, regular** *(cont.)*							
honey mustard							
w/bacon	1000	54.0	75.0	55.0	135	2166	8.0
subs, classic, regular:							
club w/bacon	890	42.0	66.0	51.0	120	2545	8.0
honey bacon club . .	930	45.0	89.0	43.0	85	2900	8.0
Italian	1020	39.0	70.0	57.5	105	3070	8.0
steakhouse beef dip	730	31.0	68.0	38.0	50	1875	6.0
traditional	770	35.0	68.0	38.0	80	2195	8.0
veggie	870	26.0	75.0	51.0	35	2290	11.0
subs, deli favorites,							
regular:							
honey ham/Swiss . .	940	39.0	66.0	58.0	105	2195	8.0
roast beef/cheddar .	880	29.0	63.0	59.0	95	1165	7.0
tuna melt	1420	31.0	63.0	118.0	150	1535	7.0
turkey/cheddar	910	34.0	67.0	58.0	110	2285	8.0
subs, prime rib,							
regular:							
cheesesteak	1220	58.0	71.0	78.0	150	1985	7.0
ranchero	1080	51.0	68.0	66.0	140	2130	7.0
peppercorn	1100	52.0	73.0	67.5	145	2070	7.0
sub, steak, black angus,							
regular	910	66.0	97.0	26.5	140	2730	4.0
subs, turkey, regular:							
bacon guacamole . .	940	45.0	78.0	50.5	95	3120	10.0
ranch and Swiss . .	740	36.0	70.0	35.0	60	2175	10.0
Tuscan	760	45.0	79.0	32.0	65	2065	6.0
sammies, flatbread:							
The Champ	310	12.0	26.0	18.0	35	810	1.0
chicken, Alpine	310	17.0	26.0	16.0	35	615	1.0
chicken, balsamic .	190	11.0	28.0	3.5	15	580	1.0
Cowboy Club	370	16.0	27.0	22.0	40	760	1.0
Italiano	325	14.0	24.0	18.5	35	860	1.0
steak, black angus .	200	11.0	28.0	4.0	15	650	1.0
steak melt, bistro . .	320	14.0	26.0	18.0	35	700	1.0
turkey, Sonoma . . .	300	11.0	26.0	18.0	35	815	1.0
soup/bread bowls:							
broccoli cheese:							
bowl	260	11.0	17.0	16.0	45	1330	3.0
cup	150	7.0	10.0	10.0	25	800	2.0
broccoli cheese,							
French country							
bread bowl	720	28.0	100.0	23.0	45	1730	5.0

Food and Measure	cal.	prot. (gms)	carbo. (gms)	fat (gms)	chol. (mgs)	sod. (mgs)	fiber (gms)
chicken noodle:							
bowl	260	11.0	37.0	6.0	55	2580	0
cup	130	6.0	18.0	3.0	30	1290	0
chili, bowl	290	18.0	24.0	13.0	55	1230	8.0
chili, cup	140	9.0	12.0	7.0	30	620	4.0
chili bread bowl ...	730	31.0	104.0	22.0	50	1680	8.0
green chili bisque:							
bowl	240	10.0	8.0	18.0	35	1140	2.0
cup	150	6.0	5.0	11.0	20	680	1.0
mushroom bisque:							
bowl	220	4.0	9.0	18.0	15	1110	2.0
cup	130	2.0	5.0	11.0	10	670	1.0
salad, chopped, w/flat-bread, dressing:							
black and bleu	720	42.0	84.0	23.5	80	2860	6.0
chicken, raspberry chipotle	830	42.0	96.0	32.0	90	1970	9.0
chicken, roasted, honey mustard ..	1110	43.0	70.0	74.0	145	2030	6.0
chicken Caesar	1000	45.0	63.0	64.0	140	2380	7.0
cobb, classic	960	39.0	62.0	62.0	215	2070	6.0
side salad, no dressing	15	1.0	3.0	0	0	5	1.0
dessert cookie:							
chocolate chip, double	370	5.0	58.0	15.0	0	230	3.0
chocolate chunk, dark	380	5.0	58.0	15.0	25	300	1.0
oatmeal raisin	340	5.0	59.0	11.0	25	290	2.0
Snickerdoodle	400	3.0	59.0	16.0	20	280	0

R

Food and Measure	cal.	prot. (gms)	carbo. (gms)	fat (gms)	chol. (mgs)	sod. (mgs)	fiber (gms)
Rabbit, domesticated, meat only:							
roasted, 4 oz.	223	33.0	0	9.1	93	53	0
stewed, 4 oz.	234	34.5	0	9.6	98	42	0
stewed, diced, 1 cup .	288	42.5	0	11.8	120	52	0
Rabbit, wild, meat only, stewed:							
4 oz.	196	37.4	0	4.0	139	51	0
diced, 1 cup	242	46.2	0	4.9	172	63	0
Raccoon, meat only, roasted, 4 oz.	289	33.1	0	16.4	109	90	0
Radiatore pasta mix, basil/herb (*Near East*), 1 cup*	240	8.0	41.0	6.0	0	440	2.0
Radicchio, fresh:							
(*Frieda's*), 3 oz.	20	1.0	4.0	0	0	20	1.0
3 oz.	20	1.2	3.8	.2	0	19	.8
1 medium leaf, .3 oz. .	2	.1	.4	<.1	0	2	0
shredded, 1 cup	9	.6	1.8	.1	0	8	.4
Radish:							
(*Del Monte*), 3 oz. . . .	15	1.0	3.0	0	0	25	1.0
10 medium, ¾"–1" . . .	7	.3	1.6	.2	0	11	.7
sliced, ½ cup	12	.4	2.1	.3	0	14	.9
Radish, black (*Frieda's*), ¾ cup, 3 oz.	15	1.0	3.0	0	0	20	1.0
Radish, Oriental:							
(*Frieda's* Chinese Lo Bok), ⅔ cup, 3 oz. . .	25	1.0	5.0	0	0	55	2.0
(*Frieda's* Daikon), ½ cup, 1.1 oz.	15	1.0	1.0	1.0	0	0	0
(*Frieda's* Korean Moo), ⅔ cup, 3 oz.	15	1.0	3.0	0	0	20	1.0
7" pc., 11.9 oz.	61	2.0	12.8	.3	0	71	5.4

Food and Measure	cal.	prot. (gms)	carbo. (gms)	fat (gms)	chol. (mgs)	sod. (mgs)	fiber (gms)
sliced, ½ cup	8	.3	1.8	<.1	0	9	.7
boiled, drained, sliced, ½ cup	12	.5	2.5	.2	0	10	1.2
Radish, Oriental, dried:							
daikon, shredded (*Eden Organic*), 2 tbsp. . .	45	1.0	9.0	0	0	20	3.0
½ cup, .5 oz.	157	4.6	36.8	.8	0	161	4.8
Radish, pickled, see "Daikon, picked"							
Radish, white-icicle:							
1 medium, .6 oz.	2	.2	.5	<.1	0	3	.2
sliced, ½ cup	7	.6	1.3	.1	0	8	.7
Raisins, ¼ cup, except as noted:							
seeded, not packed . .	107	.9	28.5	.2	0	11	2.5
seedless:							
(*Del Monte*)	130	1.0	31.0	0	0	10	2.0
(*Dole*)	130	1.0	31.0	0	0	10	2.0
(*Earthbound Farm Organic Thompson*)	120	1.0	32.0	0	0	0	2.0
(*Sun•Maid*), 1-oz. box	90	1.0	22.0	0	0	5	2.0
(*Sun•Maid* Baking) .	110	1.0	27.0	0	0	5	2.0
(*Sun•Maid/Sun•Maid* Jumbo/Golden) .	130	1.0	31.0	0	0	10	2.0
(*Sunsweet* Jumbo Red)	130	1.0	31.0	0	0	10	2.0
golden, not packed	110	1.3	28.9	.2	0	5	1.5
golden, w/cherries (*Sun•Maid*)	130	1.0	31.0	0	0	5	2.0
not packed	109	1.2	28.7	.2	0	5	1.5
vine-dried (*Frieda's* Raisins on the Vine), 4 oz.	316	3.0	77.0	1.0	0	20	6.0
coated, see "Candy"							
fruit flavored, all flavors (*Amazin' Raisins*), 1 oz.	84	1.0	22.0	0	0	4	2.0
Rambuten, canned, in syrup, ½ cup	62	.5	15.7	.2	0	17	1.4
Ranch dip, 2 tbsp:							
(*Litehouse*)	130	0	3.0	13.0	10	230	0
(*Litehouse* Lite)	70	1.0	3.0	7.0	10	125	0

Food and Measure	cal.	prot. (gms)	carbo. (gms)	fat (gms)	chol. (mgs)	sod. (mgs)	fiber (gms)
Ranch dip *(cont.)*							
(*Litehouse* Organic) . .	130	1.0	2.0	13.0	10	200	0
(*Marie's* Homestyle) . .	80	1.0	2.0	7.0	15	200	0
(*Marzetti's*)	120	1.0	2.0	12.0	20	210	0
(*Marzetti's* Light)	60	0	2.0	6.0	5	240	0
(*Marzetti's* Nonfat) . . .	30	2.0	6.0	0	0	330	0
(*Marzetti's* Organic) . .	130	1.0	3.0	13.0	15	290	0
Buffalo (*Marzetti's*) . .	110	1.0	2.0	12.0	20	310	0
buttermilk:							
(*Marie's*)	100	1.0	2.0	9.0	15	230	0
(*Marie's* Lite)	60	3.0	3.0	5.0	10	310	0
creamy:							
(*Kraft*)	60	1.0	3.0	4.5	0	190	0
(*Lay's*)	60	1.0	1.0	5.0	<5	240	<1.0
Southwest:							
(*Litehouse*)	120	0	2.0	13.0	10	220	0
(*Marzetti's*)	120	1.0	2.0	12.0	20	170	0
(*Marzetti's* Nonfat) .	30	1.0	6.0	0	0	270	0
Ranch dip mix:							
(*Lay's*), 2 tbsp.*	60	1.0	3.0	6.0	15	220	0
(*McCormick*), ¾ tsp. .	5	0	0	0	0	300	0
Raspberry, fresh:							
(*Del Monte*), 1 cup . . .	50	1.0	17.0	0	0	0	8.0
½ cup	31	.6	7.1	.3	0	<1	4.2
Raspberry, canned, red, in heavy syrup (*Oregon*),							
½ cup	120	<1.0	30.0	0	0	10	5.0
Raspberry, dried:							
(*Frieda's*), ⅓ cup, 1.4 oz.	145	1.0	36.0	.5	0	0	6.0
(*Fruit Additions*), .9-oz. pkg.	90	2.0	21.0	1.0	0	0	6.0
(*Shiloh Farms* Organic), ⅓ cup	130	1.0	32.0	.5	0	0	7.0
Raspberry, frozen:							
(*Cascadian Farm* Organic), 1¼ cup . .	60	1.0	17.0	0	0	0	6.0
(*C&W* Ultimate), thawed, ¾ cup	70	2.0	15.0	0	0	0	7.0
(*Dole*), 1 cup	70	0	16.0	0	0	0	5.0
(*Tree of Life* Red Organic), ⅔ cup	50	0	12.0	0	0	0	2.0
sweetened, ½ cup . . .	129	.9	32.7	.2	0	1	5.5

Food and Measure	cal.	prot. (gms)	carbo. (gms)	fat (gms)	chol. (mgs)	sod. (mgs)	fiber (gms)
Raspberry drink, 8 fl. oz.:							
(*Newman's Own* Razz-Ma-Tazz)	120	0	28.0	0	0	5	0
peach (*Snapple*)	120	0	29.0	0	0	10	0
Raspberry juice, frozen:							
(*Cascadian Farm* Organic), 8 fl. oz.*	120	0	30.0	0	0	10	0
(*Dole* Country), ¼ cup	140	<1.0	34.0	0	0	10	0
Ravioli, frozen/ refrigerated:							
beef:							
(*Buitoni* Classic), 1¼ cups	350	15.0	49.0	10.0	60	500	3.0
(*Celentano*), 3 pcs., 3 oz.	210	9.0	28.0	7.0	45	300	2.0
cheese:							
(*Celentano* 13 oz.), 4 pcs., 4.3 oz.	260	13.0	40.0	5.0	35	320	2.0
(*Celentano* 26/33 oz.), 4 pcs., 4.3 oz.	230	11.0	36.0	3.5	30	270	2.0
(*Celentano* Light), 4 pcs., 4.3 oz.	200	10.0	34.0	2.5	20	290	2.0
mini (*Celentano*), 12 pcs., 4 oz.	210	10.0	35.0	3.5	25	200	2.0
mini (*Celentano* 26 oz.), 12 pcs., 4 oz.	220	10.0	36.0	2.5	25	190	2.0
cheese, four:							
(*Buitoni*), 1¼ cups	330	14.0	45.0	10.0	60	550	3.0
(*Buitoni* Family Size), 1⅓ cups	330	14.0	45.0	10.0	60	550	3.0
(*Buitoni* Light), 1¼ cups	260	13.0	41.0	4.5	45	460	2.0
cheese, three, mini (*Buitoni* Ravioletti), 1 cup	270	12.0	43.0	5.0	30	340	2.0
chicken/roasted garlic (*Buitoni*), 1¼ cups	330	14.0	47.0	10.0	50	530	3.0
whole wheat pasta:							
cheese, four (*Buitoni*), 1¼ cups	320	15.0	40.0	11.0	70	700	5.0
chicken, roasted/sun-dried tomato (*Monterrey*), 1 cup	230	15.0	34.0	5.0	40	180	4.0

Food and Measure	cal.	prot. (gms)	carbo. (gms)	fat (gms)	chol. (mgs)	sod. (mgs)	fiber (gms)
Ravioli, frozen/refrigerated *(cont.)*							
tomato/basil/mozzarella (*Monterrey*), 1 cup	250	12.0	34.0	7.0	35	250	4.0
vegetable/cheese (*Monterey*), 1 cup	240	12.0	35.0	6.0	25	340	4.0
Ravioli entree, canned, 1 cup:							
(*Chef Boyardee* Mini)	250	8.0	35.0	9.0	15	950	3.0
beef:							
(*Chef Boyardee* Mini Bites)	280	10.0	31.0	13.0	25	890	3.0
(*Chef Boyardee* Overstuffed)	270	11.0	42.0	6.0	20	950	3.0
beef, meat sauce:							
(*SpaghettiOs RavioliOs*)	270	11.0	38.0	8.0	20	1090	4.0
mini (*Campbell's*) . .	260	11.0	43.0	4.5	10	1060	5.0
cheese, tomato sauce:							
(*Annie's* Organic Cheesy)	180	6.0	31.0	3.5	5	730	3.0
(*Chef Boyardee*) . . .	200	8.0	31.0	4.5	10	790	2.0
cheesy burger (*Chef Boyardee*)	250	11.0	38.0	6.0	10	950	3.0
Ravioli entree, frozen, 1 pkg.:							
(*Ethnic Gourmet* Chile Relleno), 10 oz. . . .	290	13.0	49.0	5.0	20	510	4.0
beef (*Michelina's Authentico* Bellisio), 8 oz.	220	9.0	28.0	7.0	15	720	3.0
butternut squash:							
(*Ethnic Gourmet*), 10 oz.	380	11.0	54.0	14.0	15	610	3.0
(*Lean Cuisine Spa Cuisine*), 9.8 oz. .	350	13.0	56.0	9.0	35	660	6.0
cheese:							
(*Amy's*), 9.5 oz. . . .	380	14.0	55.0	12.0	25	680	4.0
(*Cedarlane Dr. Sears Zone*), 9.3 oz. . . .	340	24.0	36.0	12.0	40	710	3.0
(*Lean Cuisine One Dish Favorites*), 8.5 oz.	240	11.0	38.0	6.0	40	600	3.0
Alfredo (*Michelina's Authentico*), 8 oz.	450	16.0	57.0	17.0	65	890	2.0

Food and Measure	cal.	prot. (gms)	carbo. (gms)	fat (gms)	chol. (mgs)	sod. (mgs)	fiber (gms)
three (*Stouffer's Family*), ⅙ of 53-oz. pkg.	310	14.0	36.0	12.0	40	1030	3.0
Florentine (*Smart Ones*), 8.5 oz.	250	11.0	40.0	5.0	30	720	4.0
meatless (*Hain Vegetarian Classics*), 10 oz.	220	14.0	40.0	3.0	0	200	8.0
portobello (*Contessa*):							
w/sauce, 6.7 oz.	360	14.0	39.0	17.0	65	640	2.0
w/out sauce, 4.5 oz.	230	12.0	36.0	5.0	35	280	2.0
Red bean (see also "Kidney beans"), canned, ½ cup:							
(*Allens*)	100	6.0	19.0	.5	0	310	9.0
(*Bush's*)	110	6.0	19.0	.5	0	460	6.0
(*Eden* Organic Small) .	100	6.0	17.0	.5	0	25	5.0
seasoned:							
(*Glory* New Orleans)	110	7.0	20.0	.5	0	540	5.0
(*Glory* Sensibly) . . .	100	6.0	18.0	0	0	250	4.0
(*S&W* Louisiana) . .	80	6.0	20.0	0	0	480	5.0
w/rice (*Glory*)	90	5.0	18.0	.5	0	680	3.0
Red bean entree, frozen (*Moosewood* Organic Chilaquile), 10-oz. pkg.	410	15.0	49.0	17.0	25	760	8.0
Red bean seasoning (*Zatarain's*), 1 tsp. . .	15	0	3.0	0	0	370	0
Red kuri squash (*Frieda's*), ¾ cup, 3 oz.	30	1.0	7.0	0	0	0	1.0
Red snapper, see "Snapper"							
Redfish, see "Ocean perch"							
Refried beans, canned, ½ cup:							
(*Allens*)	150	7.0	24.0	2.5	0	360	11.0
(*Amy's* Organic)	140	7.0	21.0	3.0	0	390	6.0
(*Bearito's* Organic) . . .	150	8.0	23.0	3.0	0	630	6.0
(*Bearito's* Organic Nonfat)	100	6.0	17.0	0	0	530	4.0
(*Bush's*)	150	9.0	24.0	3.0	0	490	7.0
(*Bush's* Nonfat)	130	9.0	24.0	0	0	490	7.0
(*Las Palmas*)	150	8.0	23.0	3.0	0	540	9.0
(*Old El Paso*)	100	6.0	17.0	.5	0	570	6.0

Food and Measure	cal.	prot. (gms)	carbo. (gms)	fat (gms)	chol. (mgs)	sod. (mgs)	fiber (gms)
Refried beans *(cont.)*							
(*Old El Paso* Nonfat) .	100	6.0	18.0	0	0	580	6.0
(*Rosarita*)	120	7.0	18.0	2.0	0	310	6.0
(*Rosarita* Nonfat)	100	7.0	19.0	0	0	510	6.0
(*Rosarita* Vegetarian) .	120	7.0	19.0	2.0	0	540	7.0
(*Taco Bell* Nonfat) . . .	100	6.0	18.0	0	0	540	4.0
(*Taco Bell* Vegetarian)	120	7.0	20.0	1.0	0	610	6.0
(*Zapata*)	130	8.0	22.0	0	0	290	7.0
bayo or black bean							
(*Sabores Aztecas*) .	90	10.0	28.0	2.5	0	420	8.0
black bean:							
(*Allens* Nonfat)	120	7.0	23.0	0	0	500	8.0
(*Amy's* Organic) . . .	140	7.0	20.0	3.0	0	440	6.0
(*Bearito's* Organic) .	130	8.0	22.0	1.0	0	530	5.0
(*Bearito's* Organic							
Nonfat)	90	6.0	17.0	0	0	530	4.0
(*Eden* Organic)	110	6.0	18.0	1.5	0	180	7.0
(*Rosarita* Nonfat) . .	110	7.0	19.0	0	0	320	8.0
(*Zapata*)	120	8.0	20.0	0	0	290	5.0
spicy (*Eden* Organic)	110	6.0	18.0	1.5	0	180	7.0
blacksoy and black							
beans (*Eden* Organic)	90	8.0	13.0	3.0	0	170	6.0
w/green chiles:							
(*Amy's* Organic) . . .	130	7.0	20.0	3.0	0	440	6.0
(*Bearito's* Organic							
Nonfat)	120	8.0	22.0	0	0	630	5.0
(*Old El Paso*)	100	6.0	19.0	.5	<5	580	6.0
(*Rosarita* Nonfat) . .	100	7.0	18.0	0	0	310	7.0
kidney bean (*Eden*							
Organic)	80	7.0	15.0	1.0	0	180	6.0
pinto bean, regular or							
spicy (*Eden* Organic)	90	6.0	19.0	1.0	0	180	7.0
w/salsa:							
(*Pace*)	70	4.0	14.0	0	0	590	4.0
(*Rosarita* Nonfat) . .	100	7.0	18.0	0	0	320	6.0
spicy:							
(*Bearito's*)	150	8.0	23.0	3.0	0	630	6.0
(*Old El Paso* Nonfat)	100	6.0	18.0	0	0	570	6.0
(*Rosarita*)	120	7.0	19.0	2.0	0	320	7.0
(*Zapata*)	130	8.0	24.0	0	0	370	8.0
jalapeño (*Pace*) . . .	70	5.0	14.0	0	0	590	5.0
Refried beans mix,							
instant (*Fantastic*),							
¼ cup	130	7.0	21.0	2.0	0	270	7.0

Food and Measure	cal.	prot. (gms)	carbo. (gms)	fat (gms)	chol. (mgs)	sod. (mgs)	fiber (gms)
Relish, see "Pickle relish" and specific listings							
Rémoulade sauce:							
(*Boar's Head* Cajun Style), 2 tbsp.	90	0	2.0	9.0	5	180	0
(*Crosse & Blackwell*), 2 tbsp.	60	0	9.0	3.0	5	440	0
(*Louisiana* New Orleans), 1 tbsp.	80	0	2.0	7.0	0	100	0
Rhubarb, fresh:							
1 stalk	11	.5	2.3	.1	0	2	.9
diced, ½ cup	13	.6	2.8	.1	0	2	1.1
Rhubard, frozen, sweetened, cooked, ½ cup	139	.5	37.4	.1	0	2	2.4
Rice (see also "Wild rice"), dry, ¼ cup, except as noted:							
Arborio:							
(*Fantastic*)	160	3.0	36.0	0	0	0	>1.0
(*Lundberg* Organic/ Eco-Farmed) ...	160	6.0	34.0	1.0	0	0	1.0
(*RiceSelect* Risotto)	150	3.0	37.0	0	0	0	0
(*S&W* Italian)	160	3.0	37.0	0	0	0	<1.0
(*Vigo*), ⅓ cup	150	3.0	35.0	0	0	0	0
or carnaroli (*Roland*)	170	4.0	38.0	.5	0	0	2.0
basmati, brown:							
(*Arrowhead Mills* Organic)	140	3.0	31.0	1.5	0	0	2.0
(*Lundberg* Eco-Farmed)	170	4.0	38.0	2.0	0	0	2.0
(*Lundberg* Organic)	160	4.0	34.0	1.5	0	0	2.0
basmati, white:							
(*Arrowhead Mills* Organic)	150	3.0	33.0	.5	0	0	<1.0
(*Carolina/Mahatma*)	160	3.0	36.0	0	0	0	0
(*Casbah*)	170	3.0	39.0	0	0	0	1.0
(*Fantastic*)	160	3.0	36.0	0	0	0	>1.0
(*Lundberg* Eco-Farmed)	180	4.0	41.0	.5	0	0	0
(*Lundberg* Organic)	170	4.0	38.0	.5	0	0	1.0
(*RiceSelect* Kasmati)	150	3.0	34.0	.5	0	0	.5
(*Roland*)	180	4.0	40.0	0	0	0	<1.0
(*S&W*)	160	3.0	35.0	0	0	0	0

Food and Measure	cal.	prot. (gms)	carbo. (gms)	fat (gms)	chol. (mgs)	sod. (mgs)	fiber (gms)
Rice (cont.)							
blends:							
(*Lundberg Black Japonica*)	170	5.0	38.0	2.0	0	0	3.0
(*Lundberg Countrywild*)	150	3.0	35.0	1.5	0	0	3.0
(*Lundberg Jubilee*) .	170	4.0	39.0	1.5	0	0	3.0
(*Lundberg Wild Blend*)	150	4.0	35.0	1.5	0	0	3.0
white, long grain, and wild (*S&W*) .	140	3.0	31.0	0	0	0	1.0
white/brown/red (*RiceSelect Royal Blend Texmati*) ..	160	4.0	34.0	.5	0	0	2.0
wild/basmati (*Lundberg* Organic) ...	160	4.0	34.0	.5	0	0	2.0
wild/*Whani* (*Lundberg* Organic) ...	160	4.0	35.0	1.0	0	0	2.0
brown:							
(*Lundberg* Sweet Organic)	180	4.0	40.0	1.5	0	0	2.0
(*Lundberg Golden Rose* Organic) ..	160	3.0	34.0	1.0	0	0	1.0
(*Lundberg Wehani* Organic)	170	4.0	37.0	1.5	0	0	3.0
(*RiceSelect Texmati*)	170	4.0	35.0	1.0	0	0	2.0
(*Success* Boil-in-Bag), ½ cup	150	4.0	33.0	1.0	0	0	2.0
(*Uncle Ben's* Natural Whole Grain) ...	170	5.0	35.0	1.5	0	0	2.0
(*Uncle Ben's Fast & Natural* Instant) .	170	4.0	36.0	1.0	0	20	2.0
brown, light (*Rice Select Texmati*) ...	160	4.0	33.0	1.0	0	0	1.0
brown, long grain:							
(*Arrowhead Mills* Organic)	160	6.0	32.0	1.0	0	0	1.0
(*Carolina/Mahatma*)	150	3.0	32.0	1.0	0	0	1.0
(*Lundberg* Eco-Farmed)	170	3.0	37.0	2.0	0	0	3.0
(*Lundberg* Organic)	170	4.0	38.0	1.5	0	0	3.0
(*S&W*)	150	3.0	32.0	1.0	0	0	1.0
brown, short grain:							
(*Arrowhead Mills* Organic)	180	4.0	38.0	1.0	0	0	2.0

Food and Measure	cal.	prot. (gms)	carbo. (gms)	fat (gms)	chol. (mgs)	sod. (mgs)	fiber (gms)
(*Lundberg* Eco-Farmed)	170	3.0	40.0	1.5	0	0	3.0
(*Lundberg* Organic)	180	3.0	40.0	1.5	0	0	3.0
glutinous or sweet ...	171	3.2	37.8	.3	0	3	1.3
gold, parboiled							
(*Carolina/Mahatma*)	160	3.0	37.0	0	0	0	<1.0
jasmine:							
(*Carolina/Mahatma*)	160	3.0	36.0	0	0	0	0
(*Fantastic*)	160	3.0	36.0	0	0	0	>1.0
(*RiceSelect Jasmati*)	150	3.0	34.0	0	0	0	.5
(*Success* Boil-in-Bag)	150	3.0	36.0	0	0	0	0
(*A Taste of Thai*) ..	160	3.0	36.0	0	0	0	0
(*Vigo*), 1/3 cup	160	0	36.0	0	0	0	1.0
brown (*Lundberg* Organic)	160	4.0	34.0	2.0	0	0	2.0
white (*Lundberg* Eco-Farmed) ...	160	3.0	36.0	.5	0	0	0
white (*Lundberg* Organic)	160	3.0	36.0	.5	0	0	1.0
sushi:							
(*Lundberg* Organic)	160	3.0	36.0	.5	0	0	1.0
(*RiceSelect*)	190	3.0	45.0	0	0	0	0
white, long grain:							
(*Carolina/Mahatma*)	150	3.0	35.0	0	0	0	0
(*Lundberg* Organic)	160	4.0	36.0	0	0	0	0
(*S&W* Organic) ...	150	3.0	35.0	0	0	0	1.0
(*Uncle Ben's* Instant), 1/2 cup	190	3.0	43.0	.5	0	15	1.0
(*Uncle Ben's Original Converted*)	170	4.0	38.0	0	0	0	0
(*Vigo*), 1/3 cup	160	3.0	35.0	.5	0	0	0
parboiled (*Zatarain's*)	170	4.0	37.0	0	0	0	0
white, medium grain:							
(*River*)	160	3.0	37.0	0	0	0	1.0
(*Water Maid*)	160	3.0	36.0	0	0	0	1.0
white, short grain (*Mahatma* Valencia)	160	3.0	36.0	0	0	0	<1.0
Rice, precooked, plain:							
(*Uncle Ben's* Boil-in-Bag), 1/3 cup	190	4.0	44.0	.5	0	0	1.0
(*Uncle Ben's Ready Rice*):							
brown, 1 cup	220	5.0	41.0	4.0	0	5	2.0
white, 1 cup	230	4.0	44.0	3.5	0	0	1.0

Food and Measure	cal.	prot. (gms)	carbo. (gms)	fat (gms)	chol. (mgs)	sod. (mgs)	fiber (gms)
Rice and beans, canned *(Eden* Organic), ½ cup:							
Cajun small red	110	3.0	23.0	1.0	0	115	3.0
Caribbean black	120	4.0	23.0	1.0	0	100	4.0
garbanzos	110	3.0	23.0	1.0	0	135	2.0
kidney beans	110	3.0	23.0	1.0	0	135	3.0
pinto beans	120	4.0	24.0	1.0	0	140	3.0
Rice and beans entree, see "Rice entree, frozen" and "Rice entree, microwave"							
Rice and beans mix, see "Rice dish, mix"							
Rice beverage (see also "Rice-soy beverage"), 8 fl. oz.:							
(AmaZake Gimme Green)	190	5.0	37.0	2.5	0	35	0
(AmaZake Go Go Green)	210	5.0	36.0	6.0	0	40	0
(AmaZake Oh So Original)	150	3.0	34.0	0	0	20	0
(AmaZake Rice Nog) .	190	3.0	39.0	2.0	0	65	0
(Pacific Low Fat)	130	1.0	27.0	2.0	0	75	0
(Rice Dream)	120	1.0	24.0	2.5	0	100	0
(Rice Dream Heartwise)	130	1.0	27.0	2.0	0	80	3.0
(Rice Dream Organic)	120	1.0	23.0	2.5	0	100	0
(Rice Dream Refrigerated)	120	1.0	23.0	2.5	0	80	0
almond *(AmaZake)* ...	200	4.0	36.0	4.0	0	20	0
banana *(AmaZake)* ...	160	3.0	35.0	0	0	20	0
carob *(Rice Dream)* ..	150	1.0	30.0	2.5	0	80	<1.0
chai *(AmaZake* Tiger) .	170	3.0	35.0	2.0	0	20	0
chocolate:							
(AmaZake Chimp) .	190	9.0	35.0	2.0	0	20	0
(Rice Dream)	160	2.0	34.0	3.0	0	90	<1.0
almond *(AmaZake)* .	200	4.0	36.0	4.0	0	20	0
chocolate chai *(Rice Dream)*	160	1.0	35.0	3.0	0	70	1.0
cinnamon vanilla *(Rice Dream* Horchata) ..	130	7.0	16.0	4.0	0	150	2.0
coconut *(AmaZake* Cool)	200	4.0	36.0	6.0	0	25	0
hazelnut *(AmaZake)* ..	200	4.0	36.0	4.0	0	20	0
mango *(AmaZake)* ...	170	2.0	35.0	0	0	40	0
mocha java *(AmaZake)*	180	3.0	37.0	2.0	0	20	0

Food and Measure	cal.	prot. (gms)	carbo. (gms)	fat (gms)	chol. (mgs)	sod. (mgs)	fiber (gms)
vanilla:							
(*AmaZake* Gorilla)	190	9.0	35.0	2.0	0	20	0
(*Pacific* Low Fat)	130	1.0	27.0	2.0	0	75	0
(*Rice Dream* Classic)	130	1.0	27.0	2.5	0	105	0
(*Rice Dream* Enriched)	130	1.0	26.0	2.5	0	105	0
(*Rice Dream* Heartwise)	140	1.0	30.0	2.0	0	80	3.0
(*Rice Dream* Refrigerated)	130	1.0	26.0	2.5	0	80	0
vanilla hazelnut (*Rice Dream*)	140	1.0	29.0	2.5	0	65	0
vanilla pecan pie (*AmaZake*)	200	4.0	36.0	4.0	0	20	0
Rice bran (*Shiloh Farms* Organic), ¼ cup	110	11.0	27.0	0	0	25	11.0
Rice cake, brown rice, 1 pc., except as noted:							
(*Quaker/Mother's* Lightly Salted), .3 oz.	35	1.0	7.0	0	0	15	0
plain:							
(*Lundberg* Organic/ Eco-Farmed), .65 oz.	70	1.0	15.0	0	0	55	1.0
mini (*Hain* Munchies), 14 pcs., .6 oz.	60	1.0	13.0	.5	0	115	<1.0
apple cinnamon:							
(*Hain*), .5 oz.	50	1.0	9.0	0	0	10	0
(*Quaker/Mother's*), .5 oz.	50	1.0	11.0	0	0	0	0
or buttery caramel (*Lundberg* Eco-Farmed), .75 oz.	80	2.0	18.0	.5	0	0	1.0
mini (*Hain* Munchies), 9 pcs., .6 oz.	60	1.0	14.0	.5	0	<5	<1.0
mini (*Quaker Quakes*), 8 pcs., .56 oz.	60	1.0	15.0	0	0	50	0
barbecue, mini (*Quaker Quakes*), 10 pcs., .56 oz.	70	1.0	12.0	2.5	0	150	0
butter, popped corn (*Mother's/Quaker*), .3 oz.	35	1.0	8.0	0	0	45	0
butter toffee (*Quaker Cracker Jack*), .5 oz.	60	1.0	13.0	.5	0	70	0

Food and Measure	cal.	prot. (gms)	carbo. (gms)	fat (gms)	chol. (mgs)	sod. (mgs)	fiber (gms)
Rice cake *(cont.)*							
caramel corn:							
(*Lundberg* Organic),							
.75 oz.	80	1.0	18.0	.5	0	40	1.0
(*Mother's*), .45 oz. .	50	1.0	11.0	0	0	35	0
(*Quaker*), .45 oz. . .	50	1.0	11.0	0	0	30	0
mini (*Quaker Quakes*),							
7 pcs., .5 oz.	60	1.0	13.0	0	0	150	0
cheddar, mini (*Quaker*							
Quakes), 9 pcs., .5 oz.	70	1.0	11.0	2.5	0	230	0
cheddar, white:							
(*Quaker*), .4 oz. . . .	45	1.0	8.0	.5	0	160	0
popcorn (*Mother's*),							
.35 oz.	40	1.0	8.0	0	0	90	0
cheese, nacho, mini							
(*Quaker Quakes*),							
9 pcs., .5 oz.	70	1.0	11.0	2.5	0	200	0
chocolate:							
crunch (*Quaker*),							
.5 oz.	60	1.0	12.0	1.0	0	35	0
mini (*Quaker Quakes*),							
7 pcs., 5 oz.	60	1.0	13.0	1.0	0	45	0
cinnamon toast (*Lund-*							
berg Organic), .75 oz.	80	1.0	18.0	.5	0	0	1.0
w/corn and oats, all							
varieties:							
(*Quaker* Multigrain							
Cakes), .5 oz. . . .	50	1.0	12.0	1.0	0	85	1.0
(*Quaker* Multigrain							
Minis), 9 pcs., .5 oz.	60	1.0	12.0	1.0	0	90	1.0
green tea, sweet,							
w/lemon (*Lundberg*							
Organic), .75 oz. . .	80	1.0	17.0	0	0	0	1.0
honey nut:							
(*Hain*), .5 oz.	50	1.0	10.0	.5	0	20	0
(*Lundberg* Eco-							
Farmed), .75 oz. . .	80	2.0	18.0	.5	0	5	1.0
mini (*Hain* Munchies),							
9 pcs., .6 oz. . . .	60	1.0	14.0	.5	0	25	<1.0
koku seaweed (*Lund-*							
berg Organic), .75 oz.	80	2.0	16.0	0	0	90	1.0
mini (*Quaker Quakes*							
Kettle Corn), 7 pcs.,							
.5 oz.	60	1.0	13.0	.5	0	120	0

Food and Measure	cal.	prot. (gms)	carbo. (gms)	fat (gms)	chol. (mgs)	sod. (mgs)	fiber (gms)
mochi sweet (*Lundberg Organic*), .7 oz. ...	70	1.0	15.0	0	0	55	1.0
peanut butter chocolate chip (*Quaker*), .5 oz.	60	1.0	12.0	1.0	0	70	0
w/popcorn (*Lundberg Organic*), .7 oz. ...	70	1.0	16.0	0	0	55	1.0
ranch, mini (*Quaker Quakes*), 10 pcs., .56 oz.	70	1.0	12.0	2.5	0	210	0
sesame, toasted (*Lundberg Eco-Farmed*), .7 oz.	70	2.0	15.0	0	0	65	1.0
sour cream/onion, mini (*Quaker Quakes*), 10 pcs., .56 oz. ...	70	1.0	12.0	2.5	0	200	0
tamari:							
flax w/ (*Lundberg Organic*), .7 oz. .	70	2.0	16.0	.5	0	120	2.0
w/seaweed (*Lundberg Organic*), .65 oz. .	70	1.0	15.0	0	0	125	1.0
sesame (*Lundberg Eco-Farmed/ Organic*), .7 oz. .	70	2.0	16.0	.5	0	120	2.0
Rice chips/crisps, 1 oz., except as noted:							
(*Eden* Organic Chips), 1.1 oz.	150	2.0	19.0	7.0	0	100	0
barbecue (*Lundberg Santa Fe*)	140	2.0	18.0	7.0	0	110	<1.0
cheese, nacho (*Lundberg*)	140	2.0	18.0	7.0	0	140	1.0
honey Dijon (*Lundberg*)	140	1.0	18.0	7.0	0	260	1.0
lime (*Lundberg Fiesta*)	140	2.0	18.0	7.0	0	270	1.0
Oriental (*Tree of Life Snacks*), 1.1 oz. ...	110	2.0	25.0	0	0	170	0
pico de gallo (*Lundberg*)	140	2.0	18.0	7.0	0	230	<1.0
puffs, five-flavor arare (*Eden* Organic), 1.1 oz.	110	3.0	24.0	0	0	160	2.0
sea salt (*Lundberg*) ..	140	2.0	18.0	7.0	0	110	<1.0
sesame seaweed (*Lundberg*)	140	2.0	18.0	7.0	0	90	<1.0
wasabi:							
(*Lundberg*)	140	2.0	18.0	7.0	0	270	1.0
(*Sunbird Snacks*) ..	110	2.0	26.0	0	0	190	n.a.

Food and Measure	cal.	prot. (gms)	carbo. (gms)	fat (gms)	chol. (mgs)	sod. (mgs)	fiber (gms)
Rice dinner mix, ⅙ of 12-oz. pkg., except as noted:							
rice and cuttlefish (*Vigo* Calamares) . .	300	9.0	46.0	8.0	150	890	0
yellow rice and:							
chicken (*Vigo*)	230	8.0	44.0	2.5	15	620	1.0
cod fish (*Vigo* Bacala)	270	9.0	44.0	6.0	30	900	0
seafood (*Vigo* Paella), ⅙ of 19-oz. pkg.	330	10.0	47.0	11.0	110	660	0
Rice dish, canned:							
Creole (*Glory* New Orleans), ½ cup . . .	80	2.0	18.0	0	5	500	1.0
dirty (*Glory* Southern Style), ½ cup	90	3.0	17.0	1.5	5	510	1.0
Spanish (*Zapata*), ⅔ cup	100	2.0	21.0	1.0	0	320	3.0
Rice dish, frozen/ refrigerated (see also "Rice entree, frozen"):							
cheddar broccoli (*Shedd's Country Crock*), 1 cup	270	8.0	35.0	11.0	20	790	1.0
cheesy, and broccoli (*Green Giant*), ½ cup	100	2.0	18.0	2.0	0	340	<1.0
w/peas, mushrooms (*Green Giant* Medley), ½ cup	90	2.0	17.0	1.5	0	300	1.0
pilaf (*Green Giant*), ½ cup	70	2.0	14.0	1.0	0	380	1.0
Southwestern (*Shedd's Country Crock*), 1 cup	250	7.0	44.0	6.0	0	680	5.0
white and wild (*Green Giant*), ½ cup	90	2.0	17.0	2.0	0	450	<1.0
Rice dish, microwave (see also "Rice entree, microwave"), 1 cup, except as noted:							
basmati (*Patak's*), 1 pouch	430	9.0	87.0	5.0	0	440	2.0
beans, red, and (*Zata-rain's*)	270	8.0	58.0	5.0	0	1350	3.0

Food and Measure	cal.	prot. (gms)	carbo. (gms)	fat (gms)	chol. (mgs)	sod. (mgs)	fiber (gms)
beef:							
(*Lundberg Rice-Xpress*), ½ of 8.45-oz. pkg.	240	6.0	47.0	3.5	0	650	5.0
(*Rice-a-Roni* Express Hearty)	270	7.0	51.0	6.0	0	1040	1.0
brown and wild (*Uncle Ben's Ready Whole Grain Medley*)	220	6.0	40.0	4.5	0	720	2.0
butter/garlic (*Uncle Ben's Ready Rice*) .	190	4.0	47.0	4.5	0	850	1.0
Cajun (*Uncle Ben's Ready Rice*)	210	6.0	42.0	2.0	0	980	3.0
Caribbean (*Zatarain's*)	320	5.0	61.0	6.0	0	1250	1.0
cheese, four (*Uncle Ben's Ready Rice*) .	250	5.0	42.0	6.0	5	890	1.0
w/chicken (*Chef Boyardee*), 1 bowl	230	6.0	30.0	9.0	20	720	2.0
chicken flavor:							
(*Rice-A-Roni* Express Golden)	270	6.0	51.0	6.0	0	1010	1.0
(*Uncle Ben's Ready Whole Grain Rice*)	230	5.0	41.0	4.5	0	800	2.0
herb (*Lundberg RiceXpress*), ½ of 8.45-oz. pkg.	250	4.0	47.0	4.5	0	670	6.0
roasted (*Uncle Ben's Ready Rice*)	230	5.0	44.0	4.0	0	960	1.0
Southern (*Zatarain's*)	300	6.0	58.0	4.5	0	800	1.0
coconut (*Patak's*), 1 pouch	500	10.0	87.0	12.0	0	880	4.0
fried, Asian (*Rice-A-Roni* Express)	280	6.0	51.0	6.0	0	710	2.0
garlic and cilantro (*Patak's*), 1 pouch .	420	9.0	86.0	4.5	0	880	3.0
garlic herb white/wild (*Rice-A-Roni* Express)	280	6.0	51.0	6.0	0	790	2.0
jambalaya (*Zatarain's*)	300	7.0	57.0	5.0	5	1340	2.0
long grain and wild (*Uncle Ben's Ready Rice*) .	240	5.0	44.0	3.5	0	500	1.0
Mexican:							
(*Rice-A-Roni* Express)	280	6.0	51.0	6.0	0	710	1.0
pesto pilaf (*Tasty Bite*), 5 oz.	229	4.0	39.0	7.0	0	440	3.0

Food and Measure	cal.	prot. (gms)	carbo. (gms)	fat (gms)	chol. (mgs)	sod. (mgs)	fiber (gms)
Rice dish, microwave, Mexican *(cont.)*							
pilaf (*Rice-A-Roni* Express Savory) .	270	7.0	50.0	6.0	0	1100	1.0
pilaf (*Tasty Bite* Fiesta), 5 oz. . . .	185	3.0	38.0	2.0	0	423	1.0
Santa Fe:							
(*Uncle Ben's Ready Whole Grain Medley*)	240	7.0	45.0	4.0	0	690	6.0
grill (*Lundberg RiceXpress*), ½ of 8.45-oz. pkg. . . .	260	5.0	50.0	4.5	0	472	3.0
sesame teriyaki (*Lundberg RiceXpress*), ½ 8.45-oz. pkg. . .	270	5.0	50.0	4.5	0	786	2.0
Spanish style (*Uncle Ben's Ready Rice*) .	240	5.0	44.0	3.5	0	500	1.0
stir-fry (*Zatarain's*) . . .	260	6.0	53.0	3.0	0	1420	1.0
tandoori pilaf (*Tasty Bite*), 5 oz.	183	3.0	37.0	3.0	0	458	1.0
teriyaki (*Uncle Ben's Ready Rice*)	190	5.0	51.0	4.0	0	730	1.0
Thai lime pilaf (*Tasty Bite*), 5 oz. pkg. . . .	212	8.0	38.9	6.0	0	230	1.0
vegetable:							
garden (*Uncle Ben's Ready Rice*)	220	4.0	43.0	3.5	0	770	<1.0
harvest (*Uncle Ben's Ready Whole Grain Medley*) . .	220	6.0	42.0	3.5	0	660	5.0
yellow:							
(*Patak's*), 1 pouch .	440	10.0	89.0	5.0	0	1140	2.0
(*Zatarain's*)	280	5.0	55.0	4.0	0	1290	1.0
Rice dish, mix (see also "Grains, mixed, dish"), 1 cup*, except as noted:							
almond, toasted, pilaf (*Near East*)	230	6.0	40.0	6.0	10	670	2.0
and beans:							
(*Seeds of Change* Organic Tuscan) .	180	4.0	40.0	1.0	0	670	2.0
(*Vigo* Santa Fe), ⅓ cup	200	8.0	38.0	2.0	0	950	3.0
black (*Carolina*), 2 oz.	200	7.0	39.0	1.5	0	930	5.0

Food and Measure	cal.	prot. (gms)	carbo. (gms)	fat (gms)	chol. (mgs)	sod. (mgs)	fiber (gms)
black (*Vigo*), ⅓ cup	190	7.0	39.0	1.0	2	950	5.0
black (*Zatarain's*) ..	230	8.0	47.0	.5	0	1480	6.0
red (*Carolina/ Mahatma*), 2 oz. ..	190	7.0	41.0	.5	0	890	3.0
red (*Rice-A-Roni*) .	290	8.0	51.0	7.0	0	1170	5.0
red (*Vigo*), ⅓ cup .	190	7.0	40.0	1.0	0	730	4.0
red (*Zatarain's*), 3 tbsp.	190	8.0	40.0	0	0	1190	5.0
white (*Zatarain's*), 3 tbsp.	220	8.0	47.0	.5	0	1410	7.0
beef/beef favor:							
(*Knorr Lipton Rice Sides*), ½ cup ..	240	6.0	48.0	2.0	0	930	1,9
(*Rice-A-Roni*)	310	7.0	51.0	9.0	0	1110	2.0
(*Rice-a-Roni* Lower Sodium)	270	7.0	51.0	5.0	0	740	2.0
biryani:							
(*Neera's*)	132	3.0	29.0	1.0	0	4	1.0
w/lentils (*Baji's*), ½ of 9-oz. pkg.....	210	5.0	35.0	6.0	0	600	2.0
black-eyed peas (*Zatarain's*)	220	9.0	46.0	.5	0	1330	4.0
broccoli and cheese:							
(*Carolina*), 2 oz. ...	200	5.0	39.0	3.0	5	820	1.0
(*Mahatma*), 2 oz. ..	230	6.0	43.0	3.5	5	930	1.0
(*Riceland*), ¼ cup .	270	6.0	48.0	6.0	5	860	1.0
(*Vigo* Risotto con Broccoli), ⅓ cup	190	6.0	39.0	1.0	8	900	1.0
broccoli au gratin:							
(*Rice-A-Roni*)	360	7.0	46.0	17.0	5	1000	2.0
(*Uncle Ben's Country Inn*)	200	4.0	43.0	2.0	5	790	1.0
(*Zatarain's*)	220	6.0	44.0	1.5	5	1130	1.0
butter herb pilaf (*Marrakesh Express*), 2 oz.	200	5.0	43.0	.5	0	840	0
cheddar (*Rice-a-Roni*)	370	8.0	49.0	17.0	10	1080	2.0
cheddar broccoli:							
(*Knorr Lipton Rice Sides*), ½ cup ..	260	7.0	50.0	2.5	0	940	2.0
and carrots (*Knorr Lipton Sides Plus*), ⅔ cup	250	8.0	50	2.0	<5	710	4.0
pilaf (*Marrakesh Express*), 2 oz.	200	5.0	40.0	2.0	0	790	0

Food and Measure	cal.	prot. (gms)	carbo. (gms)	fat (gms)	chol. (mgs)	sod. (mgs)	fiber (gms)
Rice dish, mix *(cont.)*							
cheese:							
four, creamy (*Rice-A-Roni*)	280	6.0	37.0	12.0	5	810	1.0
Italian, and herb (*Rice-A-Roni Nature's Way*) . .	340	7.0	52.0	12.0	5	740	1.0
chicken flavor:							
(*Carolina*), 2 oz. . . .	190	5.0	42.0	0	0	970	<1.0
(*Knorr Lipton Cajun Sides* New Orleans Style), ½ cup . . .	240	7.0	51.0	1.0	0	760	2.0
(*Knorr Lipton Rice Sides*), ½ cup . .	250	6.0	48.0	3.0	5	900	1.0
(*Mahatma*), 2 oz. . .	190	5.0	42.0	.5	0	930	1.0
(*Rice-A-Roni*)	310	7.0	51.0	9.0	0	1160	2.0
(*Rice-A-Roni* Lower Sodium)	270	7.0	51.0	5.0	0	730	2.0
(*Riceland*), ¼ cup .	190	5.0	42.0	1.0	0	960	1.0
(*Uncle Ben's Country Inn*)	200	6.0	41.0	1.0	0	940	1.0
(*Zatarain's*)	210	5.0	44.0	1.0	5	900	1.0
broccoli (*Knorr Lipton Rice Sides*), ½ cup	240	7.0	48.0	2.0	<5	870	1.0
broccoli (*Knorr Lipton Rice Sides Whole Grain*), ⅔ cup	270	7.0	45.0	2.0	5	830	3.0
broccoli (*Rice-A-Roni*)	230	6.0	40.0	5.0	0	1020	2.0
broccoli (*Uncle Ben's Country Inn*) . . .	190	5.0	42.0	1.0	0	910	1.0
creamy (*Knorr Lipton Rice Sides*), ½ cup	270	7.0	49.0	5.0	0	840	1.0
garlic (*Rice-a-Roni*)	260	5.0	41.0	8.0	0	820	1.0
mushroom (*Rice-A-Roni*)	350	8.0	51.0	13.0	5	1430	2.0
Parmesan (*Rice-A-Roni*)	370	8.0	51.0	15.0	5	1360	3.0
pilaf (*Near East*) . . .	220	5.0	43.0	4.0	10	830	2.0
sesame (*Knorr Lipton Rice Sides*), ½ cup	300	7.0	51.0	4.0	0	820	3.0
smothered (*Zatarain's*)	130	3.0	28.0	0	0	760	1.0
teriyaki (*Rice-A-Roni*)	250	5.0	41.0	8.0	0	820	1.0

Food and Measure	cal.	prot. (gms)	carbo. (gms)	fat (gms)	chol. (mgs)	sod. (mgs)	fiber (gms)
vegetable (*Uncle Ben's Country Inn*)	200	5.0	41.0	1.5	0	720	1.0
wild rice (*Uncle Ben's Country Inn*)	200	5.0	42.0	1.0	0	800	1.0
chicken, roasted, garlic pilaf (*Near East*) ...	200	5.0	44.0	3.0	5	600	2.0
chipotle (*Knorr Lipton Fiesta Sides*), ½ cup	260	7.0	55.0	1.5	0	760	2.0
coconut ginger (*A Taste of Thai*), ¾ cup*	190	5.0	42.0	2.0	0	430	2.0
Creole (*Luzianne* Dinner), ¼ cup	150	3.0	34.0	1.0	5	810	1.0
curry:							
(*Baji's* Nasi Goreng), ½ of 9-oz. pkg. ..	230	5.0	42.0	5.0	0	370	3.0
pilaf (*Near East*) ...	220	4.0	44.0	3.5	10	710	2.0
yellow (*A Taste of Thai*), ¾ cup* ..	180	3.0	39.0	1.5	0	480	1.0
dirty rice:							
(*Knorr Lipton Cajun Sides*), ½ cup ..	250	8.0	50.0	1.5	5	830	2.0
(*Luzianne* Cajun Creole), ¼ cup ..	160	4.0	35.0	1.0	0	680	0
(*Neera's* Jamaican)	175	3.0	28.0	6.0	0	5	2.0
(*Zatarain's*), ⅓ cup	130	3.0	29.0	0	0	620	1.0
brown (*Zatarain's*), 3 tbsp.	140	3.0	30.0	1.0	0	780	2.0
w/cheese (*Zatarain's*)	170	4.0	32.0	3.0	5	1040	1.0
wild and (*Zatarain's Mossy Oak*)	130	3.0	29.0	0	0	680	0
etouffee (*Luzianne* Dinner), ⅓ cup .	200	5.0	42.0	1.0	0	1030	1.0
fried:							
(*Rice-A-Roni*)	320	7.0	49.0	11.0	0	1490	2.0
chicken (*Knorr Lipton Asian Sides*), ½ cup	290	7.0	49.0	1.5	0	870	1.0
Oriental (*Uncle Ben's Country Inn*) ...	200	6.0	42.0	1.0	0	580	1.0
garlic, roasted, herb (*Zatarain's*)	160	4.0	34.0	1.5	5	670	1.0
garlic basil coconut (*A Taste of Thai*), ¾ cup*	180	3.0	37.0	2.0	0	380	1.0

Food and Measure	cal.	prot. (gms)	carbo. (gms)	fat (gms)	chol. (mgs)	sod. (mgs)	fiber (gms)
Rice dish, mix *(cont.)*							
garlic butter (*Knorr Lipton Cajun Sides*), ½ cup	250	7.0	49.0	4.0	10	710	1.0
garlic herb pilaf (*Near East*)	220	5.0	43.0	3.5	0	680	1.0
gravy and (*Zatarain's*)	200	5.0	45.0	.5	0	1200	1.0
gumbo (*Luzianne* Cajun Creole), ¼ cup	160	4.0	33.0	1.0	0	760	1.0
herb and butter:							
(*Knorr Lipton Rice Sides*), ½ cup ..	250	6.0	46.0	4.0	10	840	1.0
(*Rice-A-Roni*)	310	5.0	52.0	9.0	0	1160	1.0
jambalaya:							
(*Baji's*), ½ of 9-oz. pkg.	270	7.0	49.0	5.0	5	420	5.0
(*Luzianne* Cajun Creole), ⅓ cup ..	200	5.0	43.0	1.0	0	690	1.0
(*Vigo* Cajun), ⅓ cup	200	5.0	41.0	1.5	0	660	2.0
(*Zatarain's* Reduced Sodium), 1.3 oz.	130	3.0	29.0	0	0	360	1.0
(*Zatarian's Mossy Oak*)	130	3.0	29.0	0	0	460	0
lemon grass basil (*Baji's*), ½ of 9-oz. pkg.	290	5.0	35.0	15.0	0	470	4.0
lentil pilaf:							
(*Near East*)	200	11.0	36.0	3.5	10	680	8.0
(*Seeds of Change* Organic Moroccan)	180	5.0	38.0	1.0	0	750	3.0
(*Vigo*), ⅓ cup	190	7.0	40.0	.5	0	810	4.0
long grain and wild:							
(*Carolina/Mahatma*), 2 oz.	200	5.0	43.0	.5	0	550	2.0
(*Rice-A-Roni*)	240	5.0	42.0	6.0	0	910	2.0
(*Rice-A-Roni Nature's Way*)	250	5.0	43.0	7.0	0	760	1.0
(*Riceland*), ¼ cup .	190	5.0	41.0	.5	0	740	2.0
(*Uncle Ben's* Fast Cook)	190	5.0	41.0	.5	0	680	1.0
(*Uncle Ben's* Original)	200	6.0	44.0	0	0	670	1.0
(*Vigo*), ⅓ cup	190	5.0	42.0	0	3	800	0
(*Zatarain's*), 2½ tbsp.	230	6.0	49.0	1.0	0	1000	2.0
butter/herb (*Uncle Ben's* Fast Cook)	190	5.0	40.0	1.0	0	810	1.0

Food and Measure	cal.	prot. (gms)	carbo. (gms)	fat (gms)	chol. (mgs)	sod. (mgs)	fiber (gms)
chicken, herb-roasted (*Uncle Ben's*) ...	190	5.0	39.0	1.0	0	640	3.0
garlic, roasted, and olive oil (*Uncle Ben's*)	180	5.0	39.0	1.0	0	590	3.0
garlic herb (*Near East*)	220	5.0	43.0	4.0	10	720	2.0
pilaf (*Near East*) ...	220	5.0	43.0	4.0	10	830	2.0
tomato, sun-dried, Florentine (*Uncle Ben's*)	180	6.0	39.0	1.0	0	580	3.0
vegetable, roasted, and chicken (*Near East*)	220	5.0	42.0	4.0	10	770	2.0
vegetable pilaf (*Uncle Ben's*) ...	180	5.0	40.0	1.0	0	610	3.0
Masala, and lentils (*A Taste of India*)	270	5.0	47.0	6.0	0	680	3.0
medley (*Knorr Lipton Rice Sides*), ½ cup	230	7.0	46.0	2.0	0	840	1.0
Mexican:							
(*Knorr Lipton Fiesta Sides*), ½ cup ..	250	7.0	52.0	1.0	0	940	2.0
(*Rice-A-Roni*)	250	6.0	40.0	8.0	0	820	2.0
(*Uncle Ben's Country Inn* Fiesta)	200	5.0	42.0	1.0	0	680	1.0
(*Vigo*), ⅓ cup	190	5.0	42.0	0	10	600	1.0
cheesy (*Old El Paso*), ⅔ cup*	290	4.0	55.0	6.0	<5	820	2.0
mushroom:							
(*Knorr Lipton Rice Sides*), ½ cup ..	220	7.0	51.0	1.0	0	980	1.0
brown and wild (*Uncle Ben's*) ...	200	6.0	42.0	1.5	0	570	3.0
wild, and herb pilaf (*Near East*)	220	5.0	43.0	3.5	10	570	1.0
nutted pilaf (*Casbah*), ¼ cup	170	5.0	35.0	2.5	0	440	1.0
paella (*Baji's*), ½ of 9-oz. pkg.	200	4.0	31.0	7.0	<5	440	3.0
Parmesan:							
pilaf (*Marrakesh Express*), 2 oz. ...	200	5.0	42.0	1.0	0	870	1.0

Food and Measure	cal.	prot. (gms)	carbo. (gms)	fat (gms)	chol. (mgs)	sod. (mgs)	fiber (gms)
Rice dish, mix, Parmesan *(cont.)*							
Romano (*Rice-A-Roni Nature's Way*)	280	7.0	42.0	9.0	10	770	1.0
and pasta (*Vigo* Stars & Strips), ⅓ cup ..	190	6.0	41.0	0	0	560	0
pilaf (see also specific listings):							
(*Carolina/Mahatma* Classic), 2 oz. ..	190	5.0	43.0	.5	0	790	1.0
(*Casbah*), ¼ cup ..	160	9.0	35.0	.5	0	580	1.0
(*Knorr Lipton Rice Sides*), ½ cup ..	220	6.0	46.0	1.0	0	880	1.0
(*Near East*)	220	4.0	43.0	4.0	10	810	1.0
(*Rice-A-Roni*)	310	7.0	51.0	9.0	0	1200	2.0
(*Uncle Ben's Country Inn*)	200	5.0	43.0	.5	0	640	1.0
(*Vigo*), ⅓ cup	190	6.0	41.0	0	0	560	0
(*Zatarain's*)	210	5.0	45.0	1.0	0	690	1.0
pilau (*Neera's* Shahi) .	286	6.0	48.0	8.0	0	6	2.0
risotto (see also specific listings):							
Alfredo (*Lundberg* Organic), ½ cup*	140	3.0	31.0	0	0	410	1.0
asparagus/mushrooms (*Roland*), ¼ cup	150	4.0	32.0	.5	10	770	1.0
butternut squash (*Lundberg* Eco-Farmed), ½ cup*	143	4.0	31.0	1.0	0	496	1.0
cheddar broccoli (*Lundberg* Eco-Farmed), ½ cup*	146	4.0	30.0	1.0	2	516	1.0
garlic primavera (*Lundberg* Eco-Farmed), ½ cup*	140	4.0	29.0	1.0	0	520	1.0
Italian herb (*Lundberg* Eco-Farmed), ½ cup*	140	4.0	28.0	1.0	0	530	1.0
Milanese (*Alessi*), ⅓ cup	190	4.0	42.0	0	0	710	1.0
mushroom, wild (*Marrakesh Express*), 2 oz.	190	5.0	42.0	.5	0	720	1.0

Food and Measure	cal.	prot. (gms)	carbo. (gms)	fat (gms)	chol. (mgs)	sod. (mgs)	fiber (gms)
Parmesan (*Marrakesh Express*), 2 oz.	200	5.0	42.0	1.0	0	760	1.0
Parmesan (*Roland*), ¼ cup	150	5.0	30.0	1.5	10	520	1.0
Parmesan, creamy (*Lundberg* Eco-Farmed), ½ cup*	140	5.0	27.0	1.5	5	490	1.0
porcini mushroom (*Alessi*), ⅓ cup .	190	3.0	44.0	0	0	810	1.0
porcini mushroom (*Roland*), ¼ cup	150	4.0	32.0	.5	10	770	1.0
porcini mushroom, wild (*Lundberg* Organic), ½ cup*	143	4.0	31.0	0	0	535	1.0
red pepper, roasted (*Marrakesh Express*), 2 oz.	200	4.0	43.0	1.0	0	610	1.0
w/saffron (*Roland*), ¼ cup	150	4.0	32.0	1.0	10	520	1.0
sun-dried tomato (*Alessi*), ⅓ cup .	190	4.0	42.0	0	0	600	1.0
sun-dried tomato (*Roland*), ¼ cup	150	4.0	32.0	1.0	10	790	1.0
sun-dried tomato herb (*Marrakesh Express*), 2 oz. . .	190	5.0	42.0	0	0	500	1.0
Tuscan (*Lundberg* Organic), ½ cup*	140	3.0	31.0	0	0	735	1.0
vegetable primavera (*Roland*), ¼ cup	150	4.0	32.0	1.0	10	770	1.0
saffron, see "yellow," below							
sesame ginger (*Near East*)	270	5.0	55.0	4.5	5	540	1.0
Spanish:							
(*Carolina/Mahatma* Authentic), 2 oz. .	180	4.0	42.0	0	0	650	1.0
(*Casbah*), ¼ cup . .	160	4.0	36.0	.5	0	480	1.0
(*Knorr Lipton Fiesta Sides*), ½ cup . .	240	6.0	51.0	1.0	0	880	2.0
(*Old El Paso*), ⅓ pkg.*	290	5.0	55.0	4.5	0	890	2.0
(*Rice-A-Roni*)	260	6.0	44.0	7.0	0	1340	2.0
(*Zatarain's*), 2 tbsp.	180	4.0	41.0	0	0	750	1.0
pilaf (*Near East*) . . .	310	5.0	54.0	8.0	20	1090	2.0

Food and Measure	cal.	prot. (gms)	carbo. (gms)	fat (gms)	chol. (mgs)	sod. (mgs)	fiber (gms)
Rice dish, mix *(cont.)*							
spiced, w/raisins (*A Taste of India*)	340	4.0	52.0	13.0	0	790	3.0
sweet and sour (*A Taste of China*)	270	2.0	60.0	2.0	0	470	3.0
taco (*Knorr Lipton Fiesta Sides*), ½ cup	250	7.0	52.0	1.0	0	760	2.0
teriyaki (*Knorr Lipton Asian Sides*), ½ cup	240	6.0	50.0	1.0	0	800	1.0
tomato, sun-dried, and basil (*Near East*) ..	290	6.0	54.0	7.0	0	1140	2.0
tomato basil pilaf: (*Marrakesh Express*), 2 oz.	190	6.0	41.0	0	0	570	0
vegetable:							
fire-roasted (*Zatarain's*)	170	4.0	38.0	0	0	800	1.0
garden (*Rice-A-Roni*)	270	6.0	41.0	10.0	0	910	2.0
white and wild, see "long grain and wild," above							
yellow:							
(*Carolina/Mahatma Saffron*), 2 oz. ..	190	4.0	43.0	0	0	970	<1.0
(*Riceland Saffron*), ¼ cup	180	4.0	42.0	0	0	960	1.0
(*Vigo*), ⅓ cup	190	5.0	43.0	0	0	730	.5
(*Vigo 2 lb.*), ⅓ cup	190	5.0	43.0	0	0	685	.5
jasmine (*Casbah Saffroned*), ¼ cup	170	4.0	39.0	0	0	390	0
Spanish style (*Vigo Saffron*), ⅓ cup .	190	5.0	43.0	0	0	730	.5
spicy (*Carolina*), 2 oz.	180	4.0	41.0	.5	0	1150	<1.0
spicy (*Mahatma*), 2 oz.	190	4.0	42.0	.5	0	1010	1.0
Rice entree, frozen, 1 pkg., except as noted:							
and beans, Santa Fe: (*Lean Cuisine One Dish Favorites*), 10⅜ oz.	290	10.0	49.0	6.0	15	590	5.0
(*Michelina's Lean Gourmet*), 9 oz. .	330	8.0	55.0	15.0	15	710	4.0
(*Smart Ones*), 10 oz.	310	10.0	51.0	7.0	15	660	4.0

Food and Measure	cal.	prot. (gms)	carbo. (gms)	fat (gms)	chol. (mgs)	sod. (mgs)	fiber (gms)
and beans, vegetables (*Seeds of Change* Organic Spicy Yucatan Frijoles), 10 oz.	340	14.0	54.0	5.0	0	680	10.0
beans, red, w/sausage (*Zatarain's* New Orleans), 12 oz. ...	510	16.0	68.0	20.0	30	1200	5.0
brown, and vegetables (*Amy's* Bowls):10 oz.	260	9.0	36.0	9.0	0	550	5.0
light sodium, 10 oz.	260	9.0	36.0	9.0	0	270	5.0
black-eyed peas, 9 oz.	290	11.0	38.0	11.0	0	580	8.0
teriyaki, 9.5 oz. ...	290	10.0	52.0	4.5	0	780	4.0
w/cheese (*Ethnic Gourmet* Shahi Paneer), 11 oz.	560	22.0	49.0	30.0	60	400	7.0
chicken and, see "Chicken entree, frozen"							
curry, w/tofu (*Helen's Kitchen*), 9 oz.:							
Indian	300	14.0	63.0	8.0	0	300	5.3
Thai, w/vegetables .	280	12.0	30.0	4.8	0	390	2.0
dirty, w/beef and pork (*Zatarain's* New Orleans), 10 oz. ...	470	15.0	61.0	18.0	35	930	2.0
fried rice:							
chicken (*Contessa*):							
w/sauce, 8 oz. ..	250	15.0	39.0	3.5	45	640	3.0
w/out sauce, 7 oz.	220	14.0	34.0	3.5	45	240	3.0
chicken (*Lean Cuisine* Café Classics), 10 oz.	280	17.0	39.0	6.0	50	690	3.0
chicken (*Michelina's Yu Sing*), 8 oz. ...	410	12.0	64.0	11.0	40	1100	2.0
pork and shrimp (*Michelina's Yu Sing*), 8 oz.	410	11.0	63.0	11.0	35	860	2.0
shrimp (*Gorton's* Bowl), 10.5 oz. ...	350	13.0	68.0	2.5	65	1100	1.0
shrimp (*Michelina's Yu Sing*), 8 oz. ...	340	9.0	62.0	6.0	40	780	2.0
pilaf, vegetable: (*Michelina's Lean Gourmet*), 8 oz. ..	220	5.0	39.0	5.0	10	600	4.0

Food and Measure	cal.	prot. (gms)	carbo. (gms)	fat (gms)	chol. (mgs)	sod. (mgs)	fiber (gms)
Rice entree, frozen, pilaf, vegetable *(cont.)*							
(*Rice Expressions* Organic), ¼ of 20-oz. pkg.	165	4.0	30.0	3.0	0	470	3.5
herb butter sauce (*Birds Eye*), 1 cup	190	4.0	34.0	4.0	10	450	1.0
wild rice (*Michelina's Budget Gourmet*), 8 oz.	320	7.0	59.0	6.0	10	630	2.0
portobello risotto (*Seeds of Change Organic di Milano*), 10 oz.	320	11.0	61.0	3.5	5	750	3.0
risotto Parmigiano (*Michelina's Authentico*), 8 oz.	400	14.0	37.0	21.0	50	610	1.0
Tex-Mex (*Rice Expressions* Organic), ¼ of 20-oz. pkg. . . .	190	3.5	40.0	1.5	0	540	<1.0
Thai stir-fry (*Amy's*), 9.5 oz.	310	8.0	45.0	11.0	0	420	5.0
and vegetables:							
stir-fry (*Michelina's Budget Gourmet/ Zap'ems*), 8 oz. .	450	7.0	60.0	20.0	10	700	2.0
teriyaki stir-fry (*Seeds of Change Organic*), 10 oz. .	310	9.0	49.0	2.0	0	630	4.0
Rice entree, microwave, 1 cont.:							
and beans:							
black, Southwest (*Hormel*), 7.5 oz.	160	4.0	27.0	3.5	0	1130	3.0
red, w/sausage (*Zatarain's* Complete), 6.5 oz. . . .	350	13.0	57.0	7.0	15	1430	6.0
cheddar broccoli (*Bowl Appétit!*)	290	8.0	51.0	7.0	10	950	2.0
w/chicken (*Dinty Moore* Micro), 7.5 oz.	190	7.0	23.0	8.0	20	1150	1.0
dirty, w/pork (*Zatarain's* Complete), 1 cup . .	280	6.0	54.0	4.5	0	1360	2.0
sweet and sour (*Hormel Compleats*), 10 oz.	290	13.0	54.0	2.0	35	960	3.0

Food and Measure	cal.	prot. (gms)	carbo. (gms)	fat (gms)	chol. (mgs)	sod. (mgs)	fiber (gms)
teriyaki (*Bowl Appétit!*)	260	7.0	54.0	3.0	0	1160	2.0
vegetable, herb chicken flavor (*Bowl Appétit!*)	260	7.0	49.0	5.0	15	780	2.0
Rice flakes (see also "Cereal"), dry (*Shiloh Farms* Organic), ½ cup	200	4.0	44.0	1.0	0	0	1.0
Rice flour:							
brown:							
(*Arrowhead Mills* Organic), ⅓ cup .	130	3.0	27.0	1.0	0	0	2.0
(*Hodgson Mill*), <¼ cup	110	3.0	23.0	1.0	0	0	1.0
(*Lundberg* Organic/ Eco-Farmed), ¼ cup	110	2.0	22.0	1.5	0	0	2.0
white (*Arrowhead Mills* Organic), ⅓ cup ...	120	2.0	28.0	0	0	0	<1.0
Rice pasta, see "Pasta"							
Rice pasta dish mix, and cheddar (*Annie's*), 2.5 oz. ..	270	6.0	52.0	3.5	10	390	1.0
Rice pudding, ready-to-eat, ½ cup, except as noted:							
(*Handi-Snacks*), 3.5 oz.	140	3.0	19.0	6.0	0	130	0
(*Kozy Shack* European)	130	4.0	22.0	3.5	25	130	0
(*Kozy Shack* No Sugar)	90	4.0	14.0	3.0	15	115	0
(*Kozy Shack* Original)	130	4.0	22.0	3.0	20	135	0
cinnamon raisin (*Kozy Shack*)	140	4.0	24.0	3.0	20	130	0
Rice pudding mix:							
(*Jell-O* Americana), ¼ pkg.	80	1.0	23.0	0	0	100	0
(*Watkins*), 1½ tbsp. ...	50	1.0	12.0	0	0	190	0
(*Zatarain's*), ½ cup*	120	1.0	26.0	1.0	10	130	1.0
Rice seasoning, Mexican (*Lawry's*), 1⅓ tbsp.	30	<1.0	6.0	0	0	620	0
Rice syrup, brown (*Lundberg Sweet Dreams* Organic/ Eco-Farmed), 2 tbsp.	150	0	36.0	0	0	70	0
Rice-soy beverage (*EdenBlend* Organic), 8 fl. oz.	120	7.0	18.0	3.0	0	90	<1.0

Food and Measure	cal.	prot. (gms)	carbo. (gms)	fat (gms)	chol. (mgs)	sod. (mgs)	fiber (gms)
Rigatoni pasta entree, frozen, 1 pkg.:							
w/broccoli and chicken:							
(*Healthy Choice*), 8.5 oz.	250	14.0	30.0	7.0	25	600	5.0
(*Michelina's Budget Gourmet*), 8 oz. . .	290	11.0	43.0	9.0	25	570	3.0
creamy (*Smart Ones*), 9 oz.	240	16.0	39.0	3.5	25	780	4.0
cheese stuffed:							
(*Michelina's Lean Gourmet*), 8 oz. . .	220	8.0	33.0	6.0	30	510	3.0
marinara (*Michelina's Authentico*), 8.5 oz.	280	11.0	40.0	8.0	40	750	4.0
three cheese (*Lean Cuisine*), 10 oz. . .	240	12.0	35.0	6.0	20	660	4.0
w/chicken and broccoli (*Smart Ones*), 9 oz.	290	20.0	33.0	8.0	55	630	2.0
w/meatballs (*Lean Cuisine Dinnertime Selects*), 15.375 oz.	390	23.0	56.0	8.0	35	830	7.0
Risotto, see "Rice dish, mix"							
Rockfish, meat only:							
raw, 4 oz.	107	21.3	0	1.8	39	68	0
baked or broiled, 4 oz.	137	27.3	0	2.3	50	87	0
Roe (see also "Caviar"), mixed species:							
raw, 1 oz., 2 tbsp. . . .	40	6.3	.4	1.8	106	26	0
baked or broiled, 1 oz.	58	8.1	.5	2.3	135	33	0
Roll (see also "Biscuit"), 1 roll, except as noted:							
brown and serve (*Cobblestone Mill* Pistolettes)	90	4.0	19.0	1.0	0	125	1.0
club (*Pepperidge Farm* Hot & Crusty)	130	4.0	24.0	1.5	0	250	1.0
dinner:							
(*Pepperidge Farm* Parker House) . .	80	3.0	14.0	2.0	0	95	<1.0
potato (*Martin's*) . .	90	4.0	17.0	1.0	0	130	2.0
soft (*Pepperidge Farm* Country Style)	90	3.0	17.0	1.5	0	150	1.0
egg, 2 oz.	174	5.4	29.5	3.6	28	309	2.1

Food and Measure	cal.	prot. (gms)	carbo. (gms)	fat (gms)	chol. (mgs)	sod. (mgs)	fiber (gms)
French:							
(*Pepperidge Farm* Hot & Crusty) . . .	100	3.0	19.0	1.0	0	180	1.0
7-grain (*Pepperidge Farm* Hot & Crusty)	110	4.0	21.0	2.0	0	200	2.0
hamburger:							
(*Nature's Own White-wheat*)	100	5.0	21.0	2.0	0	230	5.0
(*Pepperidge Farm* Classic)	120	5.0	22.0	2.0	0	180	1.0
(*Pepperidge Farm* Premium)	210	8.0	35.0	4.5	0	390	<1.0
potato (*Cobblestone Mill*)	140	5.0	30.0	1.5	0	220	3.0
w/sesame seeds (*Pepperidge Farm* Premium)	220	8.0	36.0	5.0	<5	370	5.0
wheat, whole (*Pepperidge Farm* 100% Classic) . .	120	6.0	18.0	2.0	0	190	2.0
whole grain wheat (*Cobblestone Mill*)	130	7.0	24.0	1.5	0	240	4.0
whole grain white (*Pepperidge Farm* Classic)	100	6.0	18.0	1.0	0	190	2.0
hoagie:							
(*Cobblestone Mill* Philly Style)	180	7.0	36.0	2.5	0	340	2.0
honey wheat (*Cobblestone* Mill) . . .	170	8.0	33.0	2.0	0	340	3.0
w/sesame seeds (*Martin's*)	230	11.0	42.0	7.0	0	470	12.0
w/sesame seeds (*Pepperidge Farm*)	210	7.0	35.0	6.0	0	350	2.0
unseeded (*Martin's*)	220	10.0	44.0	3.0	0	460	7.0
hot dog:							
(*Arnold Select*)	120	4.0	23.0	1.5	0	230	1.0
(*Cobblestone Mill*) .	120	5.0	22.0	2.5	0	200	1.0
(*Country Kitchen*) .	120	4.0	23.0	1.5	0	220	1.0
(*Nature's Own White-wheat*)	80	5.0	18.0	1.5	0	190	4.0
(*Pepperidge Farm* Classic)	140	5.0	26.0	2.5	0	190	<1.0

Food and Measure	cal.	prot. (gms)	carbo. (gms)	fat (gms)	chol. (mgs)	sod. (mgs)	fiber (gms)
Roll, hot dog *(cont.)*							
potato (*Cobblestone Mill*)	130	5.0	28.0	1.5	0	210	3.0
wheat, whole grain (*Country Kitchen*)	130	5.0	25.0	1.5	0	230	3.0
whole grain wheat (*Cobblestone Mill*)	100	6.0	20.0	1.5	0	190	3.0
whole grain white (*Pepperidge Farm* Classic)	110	6.0	21.0	1.0	0	220	2.0
kaiser or hard (*Cobblestone Mill* Gourmet Kaiser)	230	8.0	44.0	04.0	0	470	2.0
oat bran, 2 oz.	134	5.4	22.8	2.6	0	234	2.3
onion:							
(*Cobblestone Mill*) .	170	6.0	31.0	2.5	0	290	1.0
(*Kasanof's*)	210	7.0	31.0	4.0	35	290	1.0
party rolls, 3 pcs.:							
(*Pepperidge Farm*) .	130	5.0	26.0	2.0	0	190	1.0
potato (*Martin's*) ..	130	6.0	26.0	1.5	0	190	3.0
po' boy, long (*Cobblestone Mill*) .	240	9.0	48.0	3.0	0	450	2.0
potato, long (*Martin's*)	130	6.0	26.0	1.5	0	200	4.0
rye, 2 oz.	162	5.8	30.1	1.9	0	506	2.8
sandwich:							
(*Nature's Own* Butter Buns)	120	5.0	23.0	2.0	5	115	1.0
onion, w/poppy seeds (*Pepperidge Farm* Classic)	150	6.0	28.0	2.5	0	230	1.0
seeded (*Cobblestone Mill*)	200	8.0	34.0	4.0	0	350	1.0
sesame seed (*Pepperidge Farm*)	130	5.0	22.0	3.0	0	220	1.0
sandwich, potato:							
(*Martin's*)	130	6.0	25.0	1.5	0	200	3.0
(*Martin's* Sliced) ...	90	4.0	16.0	1.0	0	130	2.0
(*Martin's* Big Marty's)	170	9.0	32.0	3.0	0	280	6.0
whole wheat (*Martin's*)	80	6.0	15.0	1.0	0	135	4.0
sourdough (*Pepperidge Farm* Hot & Crusty)	100	4.0	21.0	1.0	0	190	1.0
sub:							
12-grain (*Cobblestone Mill*)	210	12.0	38.0	4.0	0	380	6.0

Food and Measure	cal.	prot. (gms)	carbo. (gms)	fat (gms)	chol. (mgs)	sod. (mgs)	fiber (gms)
wheat (*Cobblestone Mill*)	220	8.0	44.0	2.5	0	460	4.0
white (*Cobblestone Mill*)	170	6.0	34.0	1.5	0	360	2.0
wheat:							
(*Nature's Own* Double Fiber)	80	6.0	15.0	1.5	0	160	5.0
(*Pepperidge Farm*) .	220	8.0	36.0	4.5	0	310	1.0
honey (*Nature's Own*)	180	8.0	35.0	2.0	0	310	1.0
whole grain (*Nature's Own* Sugar Free)	110	6.0	23.0	1.5	0	240	4.0
Roll, frozen/refrigerated (see also "Biscuit, frozen/refrigerated"), 1 pc., except as noted:							
(*Alexia Biscuit*), 2 oz. .	170	3.0	20.0	9.0	0	450	<1.0
cheddar (*Sister Schubert's*), 2 pcs.	230	6.0	23.0	12.0	35	350	1.0
ciabatta, w/rosemary, olive oil (*Alexia Artisan*), 1.5 oz. . . .	100	3.0	19.0	1.5	0	220	1.0
crescent:							
(*Pillsbury* Big & Buttery)	170	3.0	20.0	10.0	0	370	<1.0
(*Pillsbury* Big & Flaky)	180	3.0	20.0	10.0	0	370	<1.0
(*Pillsbury* Original/ Butter Flake)	110	2.0	11.0	6.0	0	220	0
(*Pillsbury* Reduced Fat)	110	2.0	12.0	4.5	0	220	0
garlic butter (*Pillsbury*)	110	2.0	11.0	7.0	0	260	0
dinner:							
(*Pillsbury* Oven Baked Butterflake)	160	4.0	21.0	7.0	0	370	0
(*Pillsbury* Traditional)	110	3.0	20.0	2.0	0	280	<1.0
(*Sister Schubert's* Pre-Baked)	140	3.0	23.0	4.0	10	240	1.0
cheese garlic (*Mamma Bella*) .	140	3.0	18.0	6.0	0	250	1.0
French, crusty (*Pillsbury*)	90	3.0	15.0	1.0	0	190	<1.0
garlic (*Pillsbury*) . .	140	3.0	17.0	6.0	0	220	<1.0
sourdough, crusty (*Pillsbury*)	90	4.0	17.0	1.0	0	200	<1.0

Food and Measure	cal.	prot. (gms)	carbo. (gms)	fat (gms)	chol. (mgs)	sod. (mgs)	fiber (gms)
Roll, frozen/refrigerated, dinner *(cont.)*							
wheat *(Sister Schubert's)*	140	3.0	22.0	4.0	10	240	2.0
white, soft *(Pillsbury)*	110	3.0	17.0	4.0	0	190	<1.0
whole wheat *(Pillsbury)*	90	4.0	17.0	1.0	0	170	3.0
egg twists *(Kineret Chall-Ettes)*	160	6.0	27.0	4.0	20	240	<1.0
focaccia, 3-cheese *(Alexia Artisan)*	110	4.0	19.0	2.0	0	230	1.0
French *(Alexia Classic Artisan)*	100	4.0	20.0	0	0	230	1.0
garlic or jalapeño knots *(Papa Ciro's)*	90	3.0	14.0	2.0	0	140	1.0
Parker House style *(Sister Schubert's)*, 3 pcs.	220	4.0	31.0	8.0	25	350	1.0
sausage wrap *(Sister Schubert's)*	110	3.0	13.0	5.0	15	210	0
wheat *(Pepperidge Farm Artisan Hearth Fired)*	120	5.0	25.0	.5	0	180	2.0
whole grain w/flax *(Alexia Artisan)*	90	4.0	19.0	1.0	0	220	3.0
Roll, sweet, see "Bun, sweet"							
Roman beans, canned *(Goya)*, ½ cup	90	7.0	19.0	0	0	370	6.0
Roseapple, 1 oz.	7	.2	1.6	.1	0	<1	<1.0
Roselle, 1 oz., ½ cup	14	.3	3.2	.2	0	2	<1.0
Rosemary, fresh, 1 oz.	37	.9	5.9	1.7	0	7	4.0
Rosemary, dried, 1 tsp.	4	.1	.8	.2	0	1	.2
Rotelle pasta dish, frozen, and vegetables, herb butter sauce *(Birds Eye)*, 1 cup	160	5.0	26.0	4.0	0	240	1.0
Rotini pasta dish mix:							
cheddar, white, w/broccoli *(Kraft Deluxe)*, ½ of 9.4-oz. pkg.	390	16.0	48.0	15.0	25	1470	2.0
cheesy cheddar *(Knorr Lipton Pasta Sides)*, ½ of 4.2-oz. pkg.	220	8.0	41.0	2.0	<5	670	1.0

Food and Measure	cal.	prot. (gms)	carbo. (gms)	fat (gms)	chol. (mgs)	sod. (mgs)	fiber (gms)
Rotini pasta entree, frozen, 1 pkg.:							
proscuitto and basil (*Michelina's Lean Gourmet*), 8 oz.	310	12.0	44.0	9.0	30	430	2.0
w/vegetables, tofu, cheese (*Amy's*), 9.5 oz.	400	15.0	41.0	19.0	20	690	4.0
Rotini pasta mix:							
cheese brocolli (*Velveeta*), ½ pkg.	400	15.0	49.0	16.0	25	1230	2.0
four cheese sauce (*Annie's*), 2.5 oz. ..	260	11.0	47.0	3.5	5	520	1.0
white cheddar sauce (*Annie's Deluxe*), 3.4 oz., 1 cup*	300	13.0	44.0	9.0	25	720	2.0
Roughy, orange, meat only:							
raw, 4 oz.	78	16.7	0	.8	23	72	0
baked or broiled, 4 oz.	101	21.4	0	1.0	29	92	0
Rowal, ½ cup, 4 oz. .	127	2.6	27.2	2.0	0	5	7.1
Rubs, dry:							
chicken:							
(*Emeril's*), ½ tsp. ...	0	0	0	0	0	80	0
(*Grill Mates*), 2 tsp.	15	0	2.0	0	0	260	0
cinnamon chipotle (*Grill Mates*), 2 tsp.	15	0	3.0	0	0	500	0
jerk (*Neera's* Jamaican), 1 tsp.	5	0	2.0	0	0	185	0
pork (*Grill Mates*), 2 tsp.	15	0	2.0	0	0	220	0
ribs (*Emeril's*), ½ tsp.	0	0	0	0	0	160	0
roasting, herb, ½ tsp.:							
cracked peppercorn (*McCormick*) ...	5	0	0	0	0	250	0
French (*McCormick*)	10	0	1.0	0	0	300	0
savory (*McCormick*)	5	0	0	0	0	190	0
seafood:							
(*Grill Mates*), 2 tsp.	15	0	3.0	0	0	190	0
(*Old Bay*), ¾ tsp. ..	5	0	0	0	0	210	0
herb w/lemon (*McCormick*), 2 tsp. ..	15	0	2.0	0	0	300	0
steak:							
(*Emeril's*), ½ tsp. ...	0	0	0	0	0	220	0
(*Grill Mates*), 2 tsp.	15	0	2.0	0	0	440	0

Food and Measure	cal.	prot. (gms)	carbo. (gms)	fat (gms)	chol. (mgs)	sod. (mgs)	fiber (gms)
Rubs (cont.)							
turkey (*McCormick*),							
½ tsp.	0	0	0	0	0	190	0
Rum runner, drink							
mixer, frozen							
(*Bacardi*), 2 fl. oz. .	120	0	32.0	0	0	5	0
Rutabaga, fresh:							
1 large, 1.7 lbs.	278	9.3	62.8	1.5	0	154	19.3
cubed:							
raw (*Glory*), 1 cup .	50	2.0	11.0	0	0	30	4.0
raw, ½ cup	25	.8	5.7	.1	0	14	1.8
boiled, drained	33	1.1	7.4	.2	0	17	1.5
boiled, drained, mashed,							
½ cup	47	1.6	10.5	.3	0	25	2.2
Rutabaga, canned							
(*Sunshine*),							
½ cup	30	<1.0	7.0	0	0	220	1.0
Rye, whole grain:							
(*Shiloh Farms* Organic),							
¼ cup	160	6.0	34.0	1.0	0	0	6.0
1 cup	567	25.0	117.9	4.2	0	10	24.7
Rye flakes (*Shiloh*							
Farms Organic),							
⅓ cup	110	4.0	34.0	.5	0	0	4.0
Rye flour:							
(*Arrowhead Mills*							
Organic), ¼ cup ...	110	3.0	23.0	.5	0	0	4.0
(*Hodgson Mill* Regular/							
Organic), <¼ cup ..	90	3.0	22.0	1.0	0	0	5.0
dark, 1 cup	415	18.0	88.0	3.4	0	2	28.9
light, 1 cup	374	8.6	81.8	1.4	0	2	14.9
medium, 1 cup	361	9.9	79.0	1.8	0	3	14.9
Rye malt, see "Malt							
syrup"							

S

Food and Measure	cal.	prot. (gms)	carbo. (gms)	fat (gms)	chol. (mgs)	sod. (mgs)	fiber (gms)
Sablefish, meat only:							
raw, 4 oz.	222	15.2	0	17.4	56	64	0
baked or broiled, 4 oz.	284	19.5	0	22.2	71	82	0
Sablefish, smoked:							
(*Acme/Blue Hill Bay*							
Alaskan Black Cod),							
2 oz.	150	8.0	0	13.0	35	370	0
4 oz.	291	20.0	0	22.8	73	836	0
Safflower kernels,							
dried, 1 oz.	147	4.6	9.7	10.9	0	<1	1.0
Safflower meal, par-							
tially defatted, 1 oz.	97	10.1	13.8	.7	0	n.a.	<3.0
Saffron, 1 tsp.	2	.1	.5	<.1	0	1	0
Sage, ground, 1 tsp. .	2	.1	.4	.1	0	<1	0
Sake, see "Wine"							
Salad blend (see also							
"Lettuce"), fresh,							
3 oz., except as							
noted:							
(*Dole American*/Italian/							
Greener Selection) .	15	1.0	3.0	0	0	10	1.0
(*Dole European*)	15	1.0	3.0	0	0	15	1.0
(*Dole Very Veggie*) . . .	20	1.0	4.0	0	0	15	1.0
(*Fresh Express*							
American)	15	1.0	3.0	0	0	10	1.0
(*Fresh Express* Italian)	15	1.0	2.0	0	0	10	1.0
(*Fresh Express* Italian							
Organic)	15	1.0	3.0	0	0	5	1.0
(*Fresh Express* Rivera)	10	1.0	2.0	0	0	5	1.0
(*Ready Pac* All							
American)	15	1.0	3.0	0	0	15	1.0
(*Ready Pac Lafayette*)	10	1.0	3.0	0	0	5	<1.0
arugula blend (*Earth-*							
bound Farm Organic)	10	2.0	3.0	0	0	25	1.0

Food and Measure	cal.	prot. (gms)	carbo. (gms)	fat (gms)	chol. (mgs)	sod. (mgs)	fiber (gms)
Salad blend (cont.)							
baby blends:							
(*Earthbound Farm* Organic Lettuces)	15	1.0	3.0	0	0	60	1.0
(*Earthbound Farm* Organic Mixed) .	15	2.0	4.0	0	0	70	2.0
(*Fresh Express* Spring Mix)	15	1.0	3.0	0	0	40	2.0
(*Fresh Express* Sweet Greens) ..	10	1.0	2.0	0	0	10	1.0
(*Fresh Express* Veggie Spring Mix) .	20	2.0	5.0	0	0	35	2.0
(*Fresh Express* 50/50 Mix)	10	2.0	5.0	0	0	65	4.0
butter/red leaf (*Dole*) .	10	1.0	3.0	0	0	10	1.0
cole slaw:							
(*Dole* Angel Hair) ..	25	1.0	5.0	0	0	20	2.0
(*Dole* Classic)	25	1.0	5.0	0	0	25	2.0
(*Fresh Express* Angel Hair/3-Color) .	20	1.0	5.0	0	0	15	2.0
(*Fresh Express* Old Fashioned)	25	1.0	5.0	0	0	15	2.0
field greens:							
(*Dole*)	15	1.0	4.0	0	0	30	2.0
(*Fresh Express*) ...	20	1.0	3.0	0	0	15	2.0
herb salad (*Earthbound Farm* Organic)	15	2.0	4.0	0	0	70	2.0
iceberg blend (*Dole Iceberg Butter Crunch*)	15	1.0	3.0	0	0	10	1.0
iceberg/carrots/cabbage:							
(*Dole* Classic Iceberg)	15	1.0	4.0	0	0	15	1.0
(*Fresh Express* Iceberg Garden) ...	15	1.0	3.0	0	0	10	4.0
iceberg and romaine:							
(*Fresh Express* Green & Crisp)	15	1.0	3.0	0	0	10	1.0
w/carrots, double (*Fresh Express*) .	20	1.0	4.0	0	0	10	1.0
w/cheese (*Dole* Say Cheese), 3.5 oz. .	80	5.0	3.0	6.0	20	n.a.	1.0
lettuce:							
five (*Fresh Express*)	15	1.0	1.0	0	0	20	1.0
trio (*Fresh Express*)	15	1.0	3.0	0	0	10	1.0

Food and Measure	cal.	prot. (gms)	carbo. (gms)	fat (gms)	chol. (mgs)	sod. (mgs)	fiber (gms)
mâche blend (*Earthbound Farm* Organic)	25	2.0	5.0	0	0	25	2.0
romaine blend:							
(*Dole* Leafy)	15	1.0	3.0	0	0	15	1.0
(*Dole Hearts Delight*)	15	1.0	3.0	0	0	10	1.0
carrots, red cabbage (*Dole* Classic) ...	15	1.0	4.0	0	0	10	1.0
carrots/red cabbage (*Fresh Express* Premium)	15	1.0	3.0	0	0	10	2.0
iceberg (*Dole Just Lettuce*)	15	1.0	3.0	0	0	10	1.0
spinach plus carrots (*Fresh Express*) ...	25	2.0	4.0	0	0	65	2.0
spring mix (*Earthbound Farm* Organic)	15	2.0	4.0	0	0	70	2.0
Salad blend kit, fresh, w/dressing, 3.5 oz., except as noted:							
(*Dole* Winter Medley) .	190	0	11.0	16.0	0	300	3.0
(*Dole* Asian Crunch) ..	120	2.0	12.0	6.0	0	230	2.0
(*Dole Bacon Lettuce Toss*)	130	3.0	8.0	9.0	10	300	1.0
(*Dole Fall Harvest*) ...	150	2.0	10.0	11.0	0	220	2.0
(*Dole Spring Garden*), 3 oz.	140	2.0	11.0	11.0	0	390	2.0
(*Fresh Express Asian Supreme*), ¼ pkg. .	170	3.0	17.0	10.0	0	380	2.0
(*Fresh Express Mediterranean Supreme*), ½ pkg.	150	4.0	16.0	10.0	5	350	5.0
(*Fresh Express Pacifica! Veggie Supreme*) ..	220	4.0	18.0	15.0	10	340	2.0
(*Fresh Express Salsa! Ensalada Supreme*), 1/4 pkg.	120	3.0	10.0	8.0	10	280	2.0
Asian:							
(*Ready Pac*)	120	2.0	14.0	7.0	0	270	1.0
(*Ready Pac* Grand) .	130	3.0	19.0	6.0	0	260	2.0
baby greens (*Earthbound Farm* Organic)	220	3.0	3.0	23.0	0	260	2.0
blue cheese (*Ready Pac* American)	110	2.0	8.0	8.0	10	250	1.0
Caesar:							
(*Dole*)	170	3.0	8.0	15.0	10	440	2.0

Food and Measure	cal.	prot. (gms)	carbo. (gms)	fat (gms)	chol. (mgs)	sod. (mgs)	fiber (gms)
Salad blend kit, Caesar *(cont.)*							
(*Dole* Light)	100	3.0	8.0	7.0	10	370	1.0
(*Earthbound Farm* Organic), 5.6 oz.	230	4.0	7.0	20.0	10	420	2.0
(*Fresh Express*), ⅓ pkg.	150	2.0	8.0	13.0	10	370	2.0
(*Fresh Express* B.L.T.), ⅓ pkg.	170	4.0	8.0	14.0	15	460	2.0
(*Fresh Express* Caesar Lite), ⅓ pkg.	100	2.0	8.0	7.0	10	360	2.0
(*Fresh Express* Supreme), ⅓ pkg.	170	3.0	8.0	14.0	10	430	1.0
(*Ready Pac* Classic)	190	5.0	8.0	15.0	10	390	1.0
(*Ready Pac* Santa Fe)	150	3.0	7.0	12.0	10	250	1.0
garlic (*Dole*), 3 oz. . .	180	3.0	8.0	15.0	5	420	1.0
cole slaw (*Ready Pac*)	130	1.0	13.0	9.0	5	160	2.0
Parisian (*Ready Pac*) .	140	3.0	11.0	11.0	5	190	2.0
ranch, sunflower (*Dole*), 3 oz.	160	2.0	5.0	16.0	5	220	2.0
Romano (*Dole*), 3 oz. .	150	3.0	9.0	12.0	5	570	2.0
spinach, baby (*Earthbound Farm* Organic)	130	5.0	12.0	1.0	0	330	6.0
taco (*Dole Taco Toss*)	130	2.0	9.0	10.0	5	370	2.0
Salad bowl, fresh (see also "Salad entree kit"), w/dressing (*Ready Pac Bistro*), 1 cont.:							
Caesar, Santa Fe	320	13.0	17.0	23.0	35	640	2.0
chef salad	320	19.0	13.0	23.0	70	1120	2.0
chicken, Asian style ..	230	13.0	19.0	11.0	30	820	2.0
chicken, Caesar	360	18.0	6.0	30.0	65	1040	1.0
chicken/cranberry/ walnut	300	14.0	26.0	17.0	35	680	2.0
cobb salad	350	19.0	6.0	28.0	170	1470	2.0
Greek salad	400	8.0	8.0	37.0	20	960	3.0
spinach bacon	300	20.0	24.0	15.0	150	1240	3.0
Salad dressing, 2 tbsp., except as noted:							
(*Annie's Naturals* Goddess)	130	1.0	2.0	13.0	0	320	0
(*Annie's Naturals* Organic Goddess) .	120	0	1.0	13.0	0	250	0
(*Wish-Bone Western* Original)	160	0	11.0	12.0	0	250	0

Food and Measure	cal.	prot. (gms)	carbo. (gms)	fat (gms)	chol. (mgs)	sod. (mgs)	fiber (gms)
(Wish-Bone Western Light!)	70	0	13.0	2.0	0	270	0
artichoke Parmesan (Annie's Naturals) .	130	1.0	1.0	13.0	<5	250	0
asiago peppercorn:							
(Marzetti)	130	1.0	2.0	16.0	15	220	0
(T. Marzetti)	160	1.0	1.0	14.0	10	230	0
(Teresa's)	130	1.0	2.0	14.0	0	230	0
bacon flavor (Wish-Bone Western)	140	0	10.0	11.0	0	240	0
bacon vinaigrette (Emeril's)	110	0	4.0	10.0	0	150	0
basil Parmesan (Bernstein's)	100	1.0	2.0	10.0	5	400	0
balsamic vinaigrette:							
(Annie's Naturals Natural/Organic) .	100	0	3.0	10	0	75	0
(Girard's)	90	0	3.0	9.0	0	330	0
(Girard's Nonfat) ..	25	0	6.0	0	0	390	0
(Good Seasons) ...	90	0	4.0	8.0	0	320	0
(Ken's)	110	0	1.0	12.0	0	290	0
(La Martinique) ...	120	0	0	12.0	0	700	0
(Litehouse)	80	0	4.0	7.0	0	135	0
(Litehouse Organic)	130	0	4.0	13.0	0	135	0
(Marie's)	50	0	3.0	4.5	0	220	0
(Marzetti)	100	0	4.0	9.0	0	340	0
(Marzetti Light) ...	50	0	5.0	3.0	0	210	0
(Newman's Own) ..	90	0	3.0	9.0	0	350	0
(Newman's Own Lighten Up!/ Organic Light) ..	45	0	2.0	4.0	0	470	0
(Pfeiffer)	100	0	4.0	9.0	0	330	0
(Teresa's)	100	0	4.0	9.0	0	340	0
(T. Marzetti Light) .	45	0	5.0	3.0	0	350	0
(T. Marzetti Organic)	90	0	3.0	9.0	0	360	0
(Wish-Bone)	50	0	3.0	5.0	0	280	0
(Wish-Bone Light) .	60	0	3.0	5.0	0	290	0
cheese, three (Newman's Own)	100	0	2.0	11.0	0	380	0
Italian (Wish-Bone)	70	0	4.0	6.0	0	370	0
white (Girard's) ...	110	0	5.0	9.0	0	240	0
white (Marzetti) ...	100	0	5.0	9.0	0	220	0
blackberry poppy seed (Teresa's)	130	0	6.0	11.0	0	160	0

Food and Measure	cal.	prot. (gms)	carbo. (gms)	fat (gms)	chol. (mgs)	sod. (mgs)	fiber (gms)
Salad dressing (cont.)							
blue cheese:							
(*Emeril's*)	110	<1.0	<1.0	12.0	0	280	0
(*Kraft Roka Light*							
Done Right)	70	1.0	3.0	6.0	5	290	0
(*Litehouse* Big Bleu)	160	1.0	1.0	17.0	15	230	0
(*Litehouse* Chunky/							
Original)	150	1.0	1.0	16.0	15	220	0
(*Marie's* Super) . . .	160	2.0	1.0	17.0	20	210	0
(*Pfeiffer*)	150	1.0	1.0	16.0	10	280	0
(*T. Marzetti* Bistro) .	180	1.0	1.0	19.0	15	210	0
(*T. Marzetti* French)	160	1.0	11.0	13.0	0	270	0
(*T. Marzetti* Organic)	130	1.0	1.0	14.0	10	300	0
(*T. Marzetti* The Ulti-							
mate)	160	1.0	1.0	17.0	15	250	0
(*Wish-Bone* Light) .	50	<1.0	6.0	2.0	0	310	0
bacon (*Litehouse*) .	150	1.0	1.0	16.0	15	240	0
w/gorgonzola (*Wish-*							
Bone)	140	0	1.0	15.0	<5	300	0
blue cheese, chunky:							
(*Bernstein's*)	120	1.0	2.0	13.0	5	180	0
(*Ken's*)	140	0	1.0	16.0	0	320	<1.0
(*Ken's* Lite)	80	1.0	4.0	7.0	0	350	0
(*Marie's*)	160	1.0	0	17.0	15	170	0
(*Marie's* Lite)	80	1.0	7.0	6.0	5	280	0
(*T. Marzetti*)	150	1.0	1.0	15.0	15	320	0
(*T. Marzetti* Light) .	80	1.0	4.0	7.0	15	340	1.0
(*Wish-Bone*)	150	0	2.0	15.0	5	260	0
(*Wish-Bone* Nonfat)	35	<1.0	7.0	0	0	270	<1.0
blue cheese vinaigrette:							
(*Girard's*)	100	1.0	3.0	10.0	5	500	0
(*La Martinique*) . . .	160	2.0	0	17.0	5	450	0
(*Litehouse*)	130	1.0	3.0	13.0	5	210	0
(*Marie's*)	120	2.0	4.0	11.0	5	200	0
Italian (*T. Marzetti*)	90	0	2.0	9.0	0	530	0
buttermilk (*Annie's*							
Naturals Organic) . .	70	<1.0	1.0	7.0	10	210	0
Caesar:							
(*Annie's* Naturals							
Organic)	120	1.0	1.0	12.0	<5	170	0
(*Cardini's* Light) . . .	80	1.0	5.0	7.0	30	250	0
(*Cardini's* Nonfat) . .	40	0	9.0	0	0	510	0
(*Cardini's* Original) .	160	1.0	1.0	17.0	30	240	0
(*Cardini's* Southwest)	140	1.0	3.0	14.0	10	380	0

Food and Measure	cal.	prot. (gms)	carbo. (gms)	fat (gms)	chol. (mgs)	sod. (mgs)	fiber (gms)
(*Emeril's*)	130	0	2.0	14.0	10	190	0
(*Girard's*)	140	1.0	1.0	15.0	10	360	0
(*Girard's Lite*)	90	1.0	5.0	8.0	10	370	0
(*Girard's Nonfat*) ..	40	0	9.0	0	0	510	0
(*Ken's*)	160	0	1.0	18.0	0	430	0
(*Ken's Lite*)	70	1.0	3.0	6.0	0	620	0
(*Kraft Light Done Right*)	60	1.0	3.0	4.5	10	320	0
(*Litehouse* Caesar Caesar)	130	1.0	2.0	13.0	15	250	0
(*Litehouse* Organic)	110	0	2.0	12.0	0	250	0
(*Marie's*)	170	1.0	1.0	19.0	15	170	0
(*Marzetti*)	120	1.0	2.0	12.0	5	310	0
(*Newman's Own*) ..	150	1.0	1.0	16.0	0	420	0
(*Newman's Own Lighten Up!*)	70	1.0	3.0	6.0	5	520	0
(*Pfeiffer*)	120	1.0	2.0	12.0	5	310	0
(*T. Marzetti* Organic)	150	0	1.0	16.0	5	250	0
(*T. Marzetti* Supreme)	140	1.0	1.0	15.0	10	320	0
(*T. Marzetti* Supreme Light)	70	1.0	2.0	7.0	10	330	0
asiago, creamy (*Brianna's*)	140	1.0	1.0	15.0	20	280	0
cilantro pepita (*El Torito*)	140	1.0	1.0	14.0	10	260	0
garlic (*Litehouse*) ..	150	0	1.0	16.0	5	90	0
Italian, w/oregano (*Kraft* Special Collection)	100	1.0	2.0	10.0	0	470	0
vinaigrette (*T. Marzetti* Light)	70	1.0	2.0	6.0	5	420	0
vinaigrette w/ Parmesan (*Kraft* Special Collection)	60	1.0	1.0	5.0	5	440	0
Caesar, creamy:							
(*Bernstein's*)	120	0	1.0	13.0	15	200	0
(*Ken's*)	160	1.0	0	18.0	10	280	0
(*Ken's Lite*)	90	1.0	4.0	8.0	5	320	<1.0
(*Marie's*)	120	1.0	1.0	13.0	30	240	0
(*Marzetti*)	160	1.0	1.0	17.0	30	240	0
(*Newman's Own*) ..	150	1.0	1.0	16.0	<5	450	0
(*Wish-Bone*)	170	<1.0	1.0	18.0	10	300	0
(*Wish-Bone* Light) .	50	<1.0	7.0	2.0	10	310	0

Food and Measure	cal.	prot. (gms)	carbo. (gms)	fat (gms)	chol. (mgs)	sod. (mgs)	fiber (gms)
Salad dressing, Caesar *(cont.)*							
w/aged Parmesan							
(*Good Seasons*) .	100	1.0	3.0	9.0	5	240	0
Champagne:							
(*Girard's*)	150	0	1.0	16.0	0	490	0
(*Girard's* Light)	60	0	2.0	5.0	0	500	0
cheese:							
(*Bernstein's*							
Fantastico)	100	1.0	2.0	10.0	5	400	0
(*Bernstein's* Light							
Fantastico)	25	1.0	3.0	1.5	5	370	0
blend, Italian (*Marie's*)	170	1.0	1.0	18.0	15	160	0
chicken salad, Chinese							
(*Girard's*)	120	0	6.0	11.0	0	350	0
coleslaw/slaw:							
(*Kraft* Coleslaw Maker)	110	0	7.0	9.0	0	230	0
(*Litehouse*)	100	0	8.0	8.0	5	120	0
(*Marie's*)	150	0	8.0	13.0	0	170	0
(*Marzetti*)	160	0	6.0	14.0	20	380	0
(*Marzetti* Low Fat) .	60	0	12.0	1.5	15	370	0
(*Marzetti* Southern							
Recipe)	150	0	14.0	11.0	15	210	0
(*Marzetti/T. Marzetti*							
Light)	100	0	10.0	7.0	20	380	0
(*Pfeiffer*)	140	0	6.0	13.0	15	340	0
(*Teresa's* Asian) . . .	140	0	7.0	13.0	15	320	0
cranberry vinaigrette							
(*Litehouse* Nonfat) .	25	0	5.0	0	0	95	0
cranberry walnut							
(*Newman's Own*							
Lighten Up!)	70	1.0	8.0	4.0	0	230	0
Dijon, sweet, vinaigrette							
(*Seeds of Change*							
Organic)	60	0	6.0	4.0	0	160	0
feta:							
chunky (*Marie's*) . .	160	1.0	1.0	17.0	15	160	0
vinaigrette, Greek							
(*Seeds of Change*							
Organic)	60	1.0	5.0	4.5	0	270	0
French:							
(*Annie's Naturals*							
Organic)	90	0	3.0	9.0	0	170	0
(*Emeril's* Kicked Up)	80	0	8.0	5.0	0	200	0
(*Girard's* Original) .	120	0	0	16.0	0	410	0

Food and Measure	cal.	prot. (gms)	carbo. (gms)	fat (gms)	chol. (mgs)	sod. (mgs)	fiber (gms)
(*Kraft* Nonfat)	45	0	11.0	0	0	290	0
(*Marie's* Tangy) . . .	130	0	7.0	12.0	0	270	0
(*Marzetti* California)	140	0	9.0	11.0	0	230	0
(*Marzetti* Country) .	160	0	7.0	14.0	5	180	0
(*Pfeiffer*)	150	0	7.0	13.0	5	220	0
(*Pfeiffer* California) .	140	0	9.0	11.0	0	230	0
(*Wish-Bone* Deluxe)	120	0	5.0	11.0	0	170	0
(*Wish-Bone* Deluxe Light)	50	0	7.0	2.0	0	250	<1.0
creamy (*Ken's*)	130	0	6.0	12.0	0	150	0
creamy (*Ken's* Lite)	70	0	5.0	5.0	0	130	0
creamy (*Kraft Light Done Right*)	80	0	9.0	4.5	0	280	0
herb garden (*Bernstein's*)	130	0	6.0	12.0	0	260	0
honey (*T. Marzetti*)	170	0	11.0	14.0	15	240	0
honey (*T. Marzetti* Light)	80	0	12.0	3.5	0	260	0
sweet (*Litehouse*) .	90	0	4.0	8.0	0	280	0
sweet honey (*Kraft Catalina* Special Collection)	130	0	8.0	11.0	0	320	0
sweet and spicy (*Wish-Bone*)	130	0	6.0	12.0	0	330	0
sweet and spicy (*Wish-Bone* Light)	50	0	9.0	2.0	0	250	0
w/vermouth honey (*Ken's* Country) .	150	0	10.0	12.0	0	220	0
w/vermouth honey (*Ken's* Country Lite)	100	0	11.0	6.0	0	230	0
vinaigrette (*La Martinique* True)	170	0	0	19.0	0	430	0
garlic, green (*Annie's Naturals* Organic) . .	90	<1.0	2.0	9.0	0	140	0
garlic, roasted: (*Cardini's*)	130	0	1.0	14.0	5	310	0
balsamic (*Bernstein's* Light Fantastic) .	45	0	3.0	3.5	0	320	0
vinaigrette (*Pfeiffer*)	130	0	9.0	10.0	0	330	0
vinaigrette (*Teresa's*)	130	0	2.0	13.0	0	370	0
ginger: (*Makoto*)	80	1.0	2.0	7.0	0	440	0
(*Marzetti* Asian) . . .	120	0	4.0	12.0	0	220	0

Food and Measure	cal.	prot. (gms)	carbo. (gms)	fat (gms)	chol. (mgs)	sod. (mgs)	fiber (gms)
Salad dressing, ginger *(cont.)*							
(*Spectrum* Organic Omega-3 Asian) .	140	0	3.0	14.0	10	280	0
(*Teresa's* Asian) ...	120	0	4.0	12.0	0	210	0
vinaigrette (*Annie's Naturals* Gingerly)	40	1.0	4.0	2.0	0	270	0
ginger mango vinai- grette (*T. Marzetti*) .	120	0	8.0	9.0	0	310	0
gorgonzola (*T. Marzetti*)	150	1.0	2.0	16.0	15	290	0
green goddess:							
(*Annie's Naturals* Organic)	130	<1.0	2.0	13.0	<5	380	0
(*Seven Seas*)	130	0	1.0	13.0	0	260	0
Greek, w/imported olive oil (*Ken's*) ...	100	0	2.0	11.0	0	220	0
Greek vinaigrette:							
(*Girard's*)	100	0	2.0	11.0	0	300	0
(*Kraft*)	110	0	2.0	11.0	0	320	0
w/oregano and feta (*Good Seasons Athenos* Light) ..	60	0	2.0	5.0	0	350	0
herb vinaigrette (*Emeril's* House) ..	100	0	1.0	10.0	0	70	0
honey balsamic:							
(*Marzetti*)	120	0	5.0	11.0	0	250	0
(*T. Marzetti*)	120	0	5.0	11.0	0	240	0
honey Dijon:							
(*Good Seasons Grey Poupon* Light) ..	60	0	6.0	3.5	0	280	0
(*Kraft*)	110	0	6.0	10.0	0	210	0
(*Kraft* Nonfat)	50	1.0	10.0	0	0	340	1.0
(*Marie's*)	130	0	5.0	12.0	10	200	0
(*Marzetti*)	130	0	6.0	12.0	10	180	0
(*Marzetti* Nonfat) ..	50	0	12.0	0	0	290	0
(*Pfeiffer*)	130	0	6.0	12.0	10	180	0
(*Teresa's* Nonfat) ..	50	0	12.0	0	0	290	0
(*T. Marzetti*)	140	0	6.0	12.0	10	160	0
(*T. Marzetti* Light) .	90	0	8.0	6.0	10	180	0
(*Wish-Bone* Light) .	50	0	8.0	2.0	0	250	<1.0
peppercorn (*Girard's*)	140	0	7.0	13.0	10	240	0
honey mustard:							
(*Cardini's*)	140	0	5.0	13.0	0	220	0
(*Emeril's*)	100	0	3.0	9.0	0	250	0
(*Ken's*)	130	0	7.0	11.0	15	210	0

Food and Measure	cal.	prot. (gms)	carbo. (gms)	fat (gms)	chol. (mgs)	sod. (mgs)	fiber (gms)
(*Ken's* Lite)	90	0	10.0	5.0	5	190	0
(*Litehouse*)	140	0	3.0	14.0	10	160	0
(*Marie's*)	140	0	6.0	13.0	10	220	0
(*Newman's Own* Lighten Up!)	70	0	7.0	4.0	0	290	0
vinaigrette (*Annie's Naturals* Low Fat)	45	0	6.0	2.0	0	200	0
huckleberry vinaigrette (*Litehouse* Nonfat) .	20	0	4.0	0	0	90	0
Italian:							
(*Annie's Naturals* Light)	60	0	2.0	6.0	0	250	0
(*Annie's Naturals* Tuscany)	80	0	5.0	7.0	0	240	0
(*Bernstein's* Dressing & Marinade)	110	0	1.0	12.0	0	330	0
(*Bernstein's* Restaurant Recipe)	120	1.0	1.0	12.0	5	360	0
(*Cardini's*)	120	0	1.0	13.0	0	220	0
(*Girard's* Olde Venice)	130	0	2.0	13.0	0	510	0
(*Ken's* Dressing & Marinade)	150	0	1.0	17.0	0	450	0
(*Ken's* Dressing & Marinade Lite) . .	50	0	2.0	5.0	0	440	0
(*Ken's* Dressing & Marinade Nonfat)	25	0	5.0	0	0	380	0
(*Ken's* Zesty)	90	0	5.0	8.0	0	530	0
(*Kraft* Fat Free)	15	0	4.0	0	0	430	0
(*Kraft* Special Collection Classic) . .	50	0	4.0	4.0	0	420	0
(*Marzetti*)	100	0	3.0	10.0	0	590	0
(*Marzetti* House) . .	120	0	2.0	13.0	0	370	0
(*Marzetti* Nonfat) . .	15	0	4.0	0	0	290	0
(*Marzetti* Venice) . .	120	0	2.0	12.0	0	390	0
(*Newman's Own* Family Recipe) . .	120	1.0	1.0	13.0	0	400	0
(*Newman's Own* Tuscan Organic) .	100	0	1.0	11.0	0	380	0
(*Newman's Own* Lighten Up!)	60	0	0	6.0	0	260	0
(*Pfeiffer*)	100	0	4.0	10.0	0	590	0
(*Pfeiffer* Light)	50	0	3.0	4.5	0	300	0
(*Pfeiffer* Nonfat) . . .	20	0	4.0	0	0	290	0
(*Pfeiffer* Tuscan) . .	110	0	1.0	12.0	0	420	0

Food and Measure	cal.	prot. (gms)	carbo. (gms)	fat (gms)	chol. (mgs)	sod. (mgs)	fiber (gms)
Salad dressing, Italian *(cont.)*							
(*Seven Seas Viva*)	90	0	2.0	9.0	0	380	0
(*Seven Seas Viva* Nonfat)	15	0	2.0	0	0	480	0
(*Seven Seas Viva* Reduced Fat)	45	0	2.0	4.0	0	370	0
(*Seven Seas Viva* Robust)	90	0	2.0	9.0	0	380	0
(*Wish-Bone*)	90	0	3.0	8.0	0	490	0
(*Wish-Bone* House)	100	0	3.0	10.0	5	260	0
(*Wish-Bone* Light)	35	0	4.0	2.0	0	350	0
(*Wish-Bone* Light Country)	30	0	3.0	1.5	0	300	0
(*Wish-Bone* Nonfat)	35	<1.0	7.0	0	0	270	<1.0
(*Wish-Bone* Robusto)	90	0	3.0	8.0	0	530	0
balsamic (*Bernstein's*)	110	0	2.0	11.0	0	270	0
w/basil and Romano (*Ken's* Northern Lite)	50	0	1.0	5.0	0	330	0
w/blue cheese crumbles (*Cardini's*)	130	0	2.0	13.0	5	480	0
w/blue cheese crumbles (*Marzetti*)	130	1.0	2.0	13.0	5	180	0
cheese, three (*Ken's*)	110	1.0	4.0	11.0	0	340	0
cheese, three (*Kraft*)	130	1.0	1.0	14.0	0	310	.0
cheese, three (*Marzetti*)	150	0	2.0	16.0	10	280	0
cheese/garlic (*Bernstein's*)	110	1.0	2.0	11.0	0	340	0
cheese/garlic (*Bernstein's* Nonfat)	10	0	2.0	0	0	380	0
creamy (*Ken's*)	120	0	3.0	13.0	0	300	0
creamy (*Ken's* Lite)	80	0	5.0	6.0	0	320	0
creamy (*Kraft*)	110	0	2.0	11.0	0	250	0
creamy (*Marzetti*)	140	0	2.0	14.0	10	220	0
creamy (*Newman's Own*)	140	1.0	2.0	14.0	10	270	0
creamy (*Pfeiffer*)	160	1.0	1.0	17.0	10	230	0
creamy (*Seven Seas*)	110	0	2.0	12.0	0	510	0
creamy (*Wish-Bone*)	110	<1.0	4.0	10.0	0	240	0
garlic (*Pfeiffer* Zesty)	100	0	4.0	10.0	0	600	0
garlic, creamy (*Marie's*)	180	1.0	1.0	19.0	15	135	0

Food and Measure	cal.	prot. (gms)	carbo. (gms)	fat (gms)	chol. (mgs)	sod. (mgs)	fiber (gms)
garlic, roasted, vinaigrette (*T. Marzetti*)	130	0	2.0	13.0	0	530	0
herb, sweet (*Bernstein's*)	130	0	8.0	11.0	0	380	0
pesto (*Kraft* Special Collection)	70	1.0	5.0	5.0	0	270	0
red wine and garlic (*Bernstein's*)	110	0	2.0	11.0	0	250	0
w/Romano (*Ken's*) .	110	0	1.0	12.0	0	300	0
Romano cheese (*Girard's*)	130	1.0	2.0	13.0	0	500	0
sweet (*T. Marzetti*) .	150	0	8.0	14.0	0	250	0
vinaigrette (*Good Seasons*)	60	0	3.0	4.5	0	300	0
vinaigrette (*Marie's*)	80	0	3.0	8.0	0	350	0
lemon:							
chive (Annie's Naturals)	150	0	1.0	16.0	0	150	0
herb (*Cardini's*) ...	80	0	2.0	8.0	0	230	0
sesame (*Spectrum* Organic Omega-3)	120	0	2.0	12.0	5	280	0
lime (*Newman's Own Lighten Up!*)	60	0	4.0	5.0	0	280	0
maple ginger (*Annie's Naturals* Organic) ..	100	0	3.0	10.0	0	120	0
oil and vinegar w/balsamic vinegar (*Annie's Naturals* Organic)	140	0	1.0	16.0	0	110	0
olive oil vinaigrette:							
(*Ken's* Lite)	60	0	3.0	6.0	0	240	0
(*Wish-Bone*)	60	0	4.0	5.0	0	250	0
olive oil and vinegar (*Newman's Own*) ..	150	0	1.0	16.0	0	150	0
onion, Vidalia:							
sweet (*Ken's*)	120	0	10.0	9.0	0	115	0
sweet (*Ken's* Lite) .	80	0	11.0	4.5	0	120	0
sweet (*Marzetti*) ..	130	0	8.0	11.0	10	300	0
Oriental (*Bernstein's* Light Fantastic) ...	60	0	10.0	1.5	0	310	0
papaya poppy seed (*Annie's Naturals* Organic)	120	0	4.0	11.0	0	200	0

Food and Measure	cal.	prot. (gms)	carbo. (gms)	fat (gms)	chol. (mgs)	sod. (mgs)	fiber (gms)
Salad dressing *(cont.)*							
Parmesan:							
creamy, w/cracked							
peppercorn (*Ken's*)	180	1.0	2.0	18.0	10	300	0
creamy, w/cracked							
peppercorn							
(*Ken's* Lite)	110	1.0	3.0	9.0	10	290	0
peppercorn (*Girard's*)	160	1.0	2.0	17.0	10	260	0
and roasted garlic							
(*Newman's Own*)	110	0	2.0	11.0	0	250	0
Parmesan Romano							
(*Kraft* Special							
Collection)	140	1.0	1.0	14.0	10	310	0
pear vinaigrette							
(*Cardini's*)	100	0	6.0	9.0	0	150	0
peppercorn vinaigrette							
(*Marzetti*)	140	0	5.0	13.0	0	300	0
pomegranate:							
blueberry vinaigrette							
(*Litehouse* Organic)	20	0	5.0	0	0	115	0
chipotle (*Spectrum*							
Organic Omega-3)	130	1.0	2.0	13.0	5	210	0
poppy seed:							
(*La Martinique*) . . .	170	0	8.0	15.0	0	330	0
(*Marie's*)	150	0	8.0	13.0	10	170	0
(*Marzetti*)	160	0	11.0	13.0	0	310	0
(*Pfeiffer*)	160	0	11.0	13.0	10	310	0
(*T. Marzetti*)	150	0	8.0	13.0	0	190	0
shallots (*Cardini's*) .	160	0	8.0	14.0	0	170	0
potato salad (*Marzetti*)	160	0	6.0	15.0	20	340	0
ranch:							
(*Annie's Naturals*							
Cowgirl)	120	1.0	3.0	11.0	10	260	0
(*Bernstein's* Light							
Fantastic)	45	1.0	5.0	2.0	0	240	0
(*Ken's*)	140	0	2.0	15.0	10	310	0
(*Ken's* Lite)	80	0	6.0	6.0	10	310	0
(*Litehouse*)	120	1.0	2.0	12.0	10	190	0
(*Litehouse* Lite) . . .	70	0	2.0	6.0	5	220	0
(*Litehouse* Organic)	130	1.0	2.0	13.0	10	200	0
(*Marzetti*)	130	0	2.0	13.0	10	240	0
(*Newman's Own*) . .	140	0	2.0	15.0	10	250	0
(*Pfeiffer*)	130	1.0	2.0	13.0	10	240	0
(*Pfeiffer* Light)	90	1.0	6.0	7.0	10	370	1.0

Food and Measure	cal.	prot. (gms)	carbo. (gms)	fat (gms)	chol. (mgs)	sod. (mgs)	fiber (gms)
(*Pfeiffer* Nonfat) . . .	25	0	7.0	0	0	390	1.0
(*T. Marzetti* Baja) . .	150	0	2.0	15.0	5	280	0
(*T. Marzetti* Classic)	160	1.0	1.0	17.0	10	200	0
(*T. Marzetti* Classic Light)	80	1.0	2.0	8.0	10	250	0
(*Wish-Bone*)	120	0	2.0	13.0	5	250	0
(*Wish-Bone* Classic)	140	0	2.0	15.0	10	230	0
(*Wish-Bone* Light) .	40	0	5.0	2.0	0	290	0
(*Wish-Bone* Nonfat)	30	0	7.0	0	0	280	<1.0
bacon (*Ken's*)	140	0	2.0	15.0	10	320	0
buttermilk (*Ken's*) .	180	0	1.0	20.0	5	280	0
buttermilk (*Marie's*)	150	0	1.0	16.0	5	260	0
buttermilk (*Marzetti*)	160	1.0	1.0	17.0	10	200	0
chipotle, smoky (*Bernstein's*)	120	1.0	3.0	12.0	5	410	0
creamy (*Marie's*) . .	170	1.0	1.0	19.0	15	150	0
creamy (*Marie's* Lite)	90	1.0	6.0	6.0	5	240	0
garlic (*Kraft*)	180	0	1.0	19.0	10	270	0
garlic (*Wish-Bone*) .	140	0	2.0	15.0	0	310	0
jalapeño (*Litehouse*)	120	0	2.0	12.0	10	220	0
jalapeño (*Marie's*) .	160	1.0	1.0	17.0	10	220	0
onion, spring (*Wish-Bone*)	130	0	2.0	14.0	0	310	0
Parmesan (*Marie's*)	170	1.0	1.0	19.0	15	160	0
Parmesan (*T. Marzetti* Organic) . . .	140	1.0	2.0	14.0	5	310	0
Parmesan, aged (*Cardini's*)	150	1.0	2.0	15.0	10	290	0
Parmesan, aged (*Marzetti*)	140	1.0	2.0	14.0	10	290	0
Parmesan garlic (*Bernstein's* Light Fantastic)	50	1.0	6.0	2.5	5	330	0
peppercorn (*Ken's*)	180	0	1.0	19.0	5	280	0
peppercorn (*Pfeiffer*)	170	1.0	2.0	18.0	10	220	0
salsa (*Litehouse* Lite)	60	0	2.0	5.0	5	200	0
raspberry: (*Girard's*)	120	0	9.0	10.0	0	65	0
(*Girard's* Nonfat) . .	60	0	14.0	0	0	210	0
pecan (*Ken's* Nonfat)	50	0	12.0	0	0	280	0
walnut (*Newman's Own Lighten Up!*)	70	0	7.0	5.0	0	120	0
raspberry vinaigrette: (*Annie's Naturals*) .	35	0	5.0	1.5	0	75	0

Food and Measure	cal.	prot. (gms)	carbo. (gms)	fat (gms)	chol. (mgs)	sod. (mgs)	fiber (gms)
Salad dressing, raspberry vinaigrette *(cont.)*							
(*Marie's*)	40	0	8.0	.5	0	60	0
cabarnet (*T. Marzetti Light*)	70	0	7.0	4.5	0	200	0
hazelnut (*Wish-Bone*)	80	0	9.0	5.0	0	260	0
lime (*Litehouse Organic*)	40	0	5.0	2.0	0	55	0
pomegranate (*Cardini's*)	100	0	5.0	8.0	0	150	0
red, w/poppyseeds (*Good Seasons*) .	60	0	5.0	4.0	0	290	0
walnut (*Ken's Lite*) .	80	0	7.0	6.0	0	120	0
walnut (*Wish-Bone Light*)	80	0	7.0	5.0	0	260	0
raspberry white balsamic (*Teresa's*) . . .	100	0	4.0	9.0	0	190	0
red pepper, roasted, vinaigrette (*Annie's Naturals*)	70	0	3.0	6.0	0	240	0
red wine vinaigrette:							
(*Marie's*)	60	0	6.0	4.5	0	210	0
(*Girard's* Nonfat) . .	20	0	5.0	0	0	590	0
(*Kraft Light Done Right*)	45	0	3.0	4.0	0	310	0
(*Pfeiffer*)	90	0	3.0	9.0	0	450	0
(*Seven Seas*)	90	0	2.0	9.0	0	480	0
(*Seven Seas* Reduced Fat)	45	0	3.0	4.0	0	320	0
(*Wish-Bone*)	80	0	9.0	5.0	0	240	0
(*Wish-Bone* Nonfat)	30	0	7.0	0	0	230	0
olive oil (*Annie's Naturals* Organic)	160	0	1.0	17.0	0	120	0
olive oil (*Litehouse*)	130	0	2.0	14.0	0	125	0
red wine vinegar/oil:							
(*Ken's*)	120	0	2.0	12.0	0	360	0
(*Ken's* Lite)	50	0	2.0	5.0	0	280	0
(*Newman's Own Lighten Up!*)	50	0	2.0	4.5	0	390	0
Romano (*Emeril's*) . . .	110	<1.0	2.0	12.0	0	370	0
Romano basil vinaigrette (*Wish-Bone*)	60	0	2.0	5.0	0	390	0
Russian:							
(*Ken's*)	140	0	5.0	14.0	15	280	0
(*Pfeiffer*)	140	0	5.0	14.0	15	240	0

Food and Measure	cal.	prot. (gms)	carbo. (gms)	fat (gms)	chol. (mgs)	sod. (mgs)	fiber (gms)
(*Wish-Bone*)	120	0	14.0	6.0	0	360	0
sesame, Asian:							
(*Annie's Naturals* Organic)	140	0	4.0	14.0	0	210	0
(*Ken's* Lite)	70	0	8.0	4.0	0	450	0
(*Teresa's* Oriental) .	110	0	8.0	9.0	0	290*	0
roasted (*Cardini's*) .	120	1.0	6.0	10.0	0	360	0
vinaigrette (*Wish-Bone* Light)	70	0	6.0	5.0	0	290	0
sesame ginger:							
(*Good Seasons*) ...	110	0	7.0	9.0	0	300	0
(*Litehouse* Nonfat) .	35	0	8.0	0	0	230	0
(*Marie's*)	100	0	7.0	8.0	0	250	0
(*Marzetti*)	110	1.0	6.0	9.0	0	330	0
(*Newman's Own* Lighten Up!*)	35	0	5.0	1.5	0	390	0
vinaigrette, w/chamomile (*Annie's Naturals* Organic)	100	1.0	4.0	9.0	0	240	0
shiitake sesame (*Annie's Naturals*) .	120	0	1.0	13.0	0	250	0
spinach:							
(*Girard's*)	70	1.0	14.0	2.0	0	250	0
(*T. Marzetti*)	70	0	13.0	1.5	0	250	0
salad (*Litehouse*) ..	50	1.0	11.0	0	0	260	0
salad (*Marie's*)	70	1.0	13.0	1.5	0	230	0
strawberry:							
Chardonnay (*Marzetti/T. Marzetti*) .	110	0	7.0	9.0	0	150	0
Chardonnay (*Teresa's*)	120	0	7.0	10.0	0	150	0
vinaigrette (*T. Marzetti*)	110	0	6.0	10.0	0	150	0
sweet and sour:							
(*Marzetti*)	160	0	11.0	13.0	0	220	0
(*Marzetti* Nonfat) ..	45	0	11.0	0	0	290	0
(*Old Dutch*)	50	0	13.0	0	0	480	0
(*Pfeiffer*)	160	0	10.0	13.0	0	220	0
tamari:							
ginger (*San-J*)	25	<1.0	5.0	0	0	500	0
mustard (*San-J*) ..	25	<1.0	5.0	0	0	150	0
peanut (*San-J*)	70	3.0	9.0	2.0	0	230	<1.0
sesame (*San-J*) ...	45	1.0	4.0	2.5	0	600	<1.0
Thousand Island:							
(*Annie's Naturals* Organic)	90	<1.0	5.0	7.0	<5	140	0

Food and Measure	cal.	prot. (gms)	carbo. (gms)	fat (gms)	chol. (mgs)	sod. (mgs)	fiber (gms)
Salad dressing, Thousand Island *(cont.)*							
(*Ken's* Squeezable) .	140	0	4.0	13.0	15	300	0
(*Litehouse*)	130	0	3.0	13.0	10	250	0
(*Marie's*)	150	0	4.0	15.0	15	210	0
(*Marzetti*)	140	0	4.0	14.0	15	260	0
(*Newman's Own* Two Thousand)	140	0	4.0	14.0	10	260	0
(*Pfeiffer*)	140	0	4.0	14.0	10	240	0
(*Pfeiffer* Light)	70	0	6.0	5.0	15	360	0
(*T. Marzetti*)	150	0	5.0	15.0	15	250	0
(*Wish-Bone*)	130	0	6.0	12.0	10	300	0
(*Wish-Bone* Light) .	50	0	9.0	2.0	5	290	0
tomato, sun-dried:							
(*Kraft* Special Collection)	60	0	4.0	5.0	0	340	0
(*Newman's Own* Lighten Up!)	60	0	5.0	4.0	0	380	0
vinaigrette (*Teresa's*)	120	0	6.0	11.0	0	320	0
vinaigrette, w/roasted red pepper (*Good Seasons*)	60	0	4.0	5.0	0	340	0
tomato bacon:							
(*Ken's*)	150	0	3.0	15.0	5	310	0
(*Kraft* Special Collection Tangy)	130	1.0	8.0	10.0	0	410	0
wasabi ginger vinaigrette (*Girard's*) . . .	100	0	4.0	9.0	0	320	0
Salad dressing mix (*Good Seasons*), ⅛ pkt. mix:							
Caesar, gourmet	15	0	2.0	0	0	300	0
cheese garlic	5	0	1.0	0	0	330	0
garlic and herb	5	0	1.0	0	0	340	0
Italian, cruet kit	5	0	1.0	0	0	320	0
Italian, fat free	10	0	3.0	0	0	290	0
Italian, mild	10	0	2.0	0	0	370	0
Italian, zesty	5	0	1.0	0	0	220	0
sesame, Asian	15	0	3.0	0	0	350	0
Salad entree kit, fresh (*Hillshire Farms Entree Salads*), w/out lettuce, 1 pkg.:							
chicken bacon club . .	300	24.0	17.0	16.0	60	1440	1.0
w/out dressing	250	24.0	13.0	12.0	60	1140	0

Food and Measure	cal.	prot. (gms)	carbo. (gms)	fat (gms)	chol. (mgs)	sod. (mgs)	fiber (gms)
chicken Caesar	420	27.0	16.0	35.0	90	1630	0
w/out dressing	240	24.0	13.0	10.0	55	1120	0
turkey/cranberry/ham	270	17.0	29.0	8.0	50	1210	2.0
w/out dressing	210	17.0	13.0	8.0	55	960	1.0
turkey/ham chef	420	21.0	16.0	29.0	80	1370	0
w/out dressing	260	20.0	13.0	12.0	60	1150	0
Salad seasoning (*McCormick Salad Supreme*), 1/4 tsp. . .	0	0	0	0	0	60	0
Salad toppers (see also specific listings): (*McCormick Salad Toppins*), 1⅓ tbsp.	35	1.0	2.0	1.5	0	90	0
bacon almond crunch (*Marzetti's* Salad Accents), 1 tbsp. . .	35	1.0	3.0	2.5	0	55	1.0
fruit and nut (*Marzetti's* Salad Accents), 1 tbsp. . . .	45	1.0	5.0	2.0	0	25	1.0
garden vegetable (*McCormick Salad Toppins*), 1⅓ tbsp.	35	1.0	3.0	2.0	0	60	0
sesame, Asian (*Marzetti's* Salad Accents), 1 tbsp. . .	40	1.0	3.0	2.5	0	55	1.0
Salami, 2 oz., except as noted: beef:							
(*Boar's Head*)	120	10.0	0	9.0	25	470	0
(*Hansel 'n Gretel*) .	170	7.0	4.0	14.0	35	660	0
(*Hebrew National*) .	160	8.0	0	15.0	25	450	0
(*Hebrew National* Presliced), 3 pcs., 1.9 oz.	150	7.0	0	14.0	25	430	0
(*Oscar Mayer* Deli Thin), 1.8 oz. . . .	150	8.0	1.0	13.0	40	640	0
lean (*Hebrew National*)	90	9.0	1.0	5.0	25	480	0
cooked:							
(*Boar's Head*)	130	8.0	0	11.0	40	550	0
(*Dietz & Watson*) . .	130	8.0	2.0	10.0	30	530	0
(*Farmland*), 1.3-oz. slice	100	5.0	2.0	8.0	35	440	0
regular or hot (*Hansel 'n Gretel*)	160	7.0	4.0	12.0	40	770	0

Food and Measure	cal.	prot. (gms)	carbo. (gms)	fat (gms)	chol. (mgs)	sod. (mgs)	fiber (gms)
Salami *(cont.)*							
cotto:							
(*Farmer John*)	140	7.0	3.0	11.0	45	470	0
(*Oscar Mayer*), 1 oz.	70	3.0	1.0	5.0	25	280	0
beef (*Oscar Mayer*),							
1 oz.	60	4.0	1.0	4.5	20	360	0
dry, Italian, 1 oz.:							
(*Boar's Head Bianco*							
D'Oro)	110	7.0	1.0	8.0	25	470	0
(*Di Lusso*)	110	6.0	1.0	9.0	30	480	0
(*Hormel*)	110	6.0	1.0	9.0	30	480	0
Genoa:							
(*Applegate Farms*),							
1 oz.	100	8.0	0	7.0	15	540	0
(*Applegate Farms*							
Deli Counter),							
1 oz.	120	8.0	0	10.0	10	630	0
(*Applegate Farms*							
Organic), 1 oz. . .	100	7.0	1.0	7.0	25	400	0
(*Black Bear*), 1 oz. .	90	8.0	1.0	7.0	23	500	0
(*Boar's Head*)	190	12.0	1.0	15.0	50	920	0
(*Carando*), 1 oz. . .	110	5.0	0	10.0	25	450	0
(*Carando* Cubes/							
Sticks), 1 oz. . . .	110	5.0	0	10.0	25	460	0
(*Di Lusso*)	210	12.0	0	18.0	50	940	0
(*Di Lusso* Natural							
Casing)	170	15.0	0	12.0	50	1060	0
(*Farmland*), 1 oz. . .	110	5.0	0	10.0	25	460	0
(*Hansel 'n Gretel*) .	220	11.0	3.0	18.0	50	980	0
(*Hormel San Remo*							
Brand)	210	12.0	0	18.0	50	940	0
hot (*Applegate*							
Farms), 1 oz.	100	8.0	0	7.0	15	540	0
hard:							
(*Black Bear*), 1 oz. .	110	6.0	1.0	10.0	30	450	0
(*Boar's Head*), 1 oz.	110	6.0	<1.0	9.0	30	490	0
(*Carando* Cubes/							
Sliced), 1 oz. . . .	120	5.0	0	11.0	30	480	0
(*Carando* Stick), 1 oz.	120	5.0	0	10.0	25	480	0
(*Di Lusso*)	220	10.0	0	20.0	70	900	0
(*Dietz & Watson*),							
1 oz.	110	6.0	1.0	10.0	30	440	0
(*Farmland*), 1 oz. . .	120	5.0	0	10.0	25	480	0

Food and Measure	cal.	prot. (gms)	carbo. (gms)	fat (gms)	chol. (mgs)	sod. (mgs)	fiber (gms)
(*Hansel 'n Gretel*) .	230	12.0	2.0	20.0	50	920	0
(*Hormel Homeland*), 1 oz.	110	6.0	0	10.0	30	450	0
(*Oscar Mayer*), 1 oz.	100	7.0	1.0	8.0	25	510	0
uncured (*Hormel Natural Choice*), 1 oz.	110	6.0	0	14.0	35	510	0
"Salami," vegetarian (*Yves*), 4 slices, 2.2 oz.	80	15.0	4.0	0	0	480	0
Salisbury steak, see "Beef dinner" and "Beef entree"							
Salmon , meat only:							
Atlantic, farmed, 4 oz.:							
raw	207	22.6	0	12.3	67	66	0
baked or broiled . . .	234	25.0	0	14.0	71	69	0
Atlantic, wild, 4 oz.:							
raw	161	22.5	0	7.2	62	50	0
baked or broiled . . .	206	28.8	0	9.2	81	64	0
Chinook, 4 oz.:							
raw	204	22.8	0	11.9	75	53	0
baked or broiled . . .	262	29.2	0	15.2	96	68	0
chum, 4 oz.:							
raw	136	22.8	0	4.3	84	112	0
baked or broiled . . .	175	29.3	0	5.5	108	73	0
coho, farmed, 4 oz.:							
raw	182	24.1	0	8.7	58	53	0
baked or broiled . . .	202	27.6	0	9.3	71	59	0
coho, wild, 4 oz.:							
raw	165	25.0	0	6.7	51	53	0
baked or broiled . . .	158	26.6	0	4.9	62	66	0
boiled, poached, or steamed	209	31.0	0	8.5	65	60	0
pink, 4 oz.:							
raw	132	22.6	0	3.9	59	76	0
baked or broiled . . .	169	29.0	0	5.0	76	98	0
sockeye, 4 oz.:							
raw	191	24.2	0	9.7	70	53	0
baked or broiled . . .	245	31.0	0	12.4	99	75	0
Salmon, baked (*Acme/Blue Hill Bay*), 2 oz.	130	11.0	1.0	9.0	30	420	0

Food and Measure	cal.	prot. (gms)	carbo. (gms)	fat (gms)	chol. (mgs)	sod. (mgs)	fiber (gms)
Salmon, can or pkg., in water, ¼ cup, except as noted:							
Atlantic (*Bumble Bee Prime Fillet*)	80	12.0	0	3.0	10	170	0
chum, drained, 4 oz. .	160	24.3	0	6.2	44	552	0
keta (*Bumble Bee*) . . .	90	13.0	0	4.0	40	270	0
pink:							
(*Bumble Bee*)	90	12.0	0	5.0	40	270	0
(*Chicken of the Sea*)	90	12.0	0	5.0	40	270	0
(*Roland*)	90	12.0	0	5.0	40	270	0
wild Alaskan (*Miramonte*)	90	12.0	0	5.0	40	60	0
pink, skin/boneless:							
(*Bumble Bee*)	50	11.0	0	1.0	20	150	0
(*Chicken of the Sea*)	60	10.0	0	2.0	20	280	0
(*Chicken of the Sea*), 3-oz. can	80	14.0	0	2.0	30	390	0
(*Chicken of the Sea Premium*), 3-oz. pouch	90	15.0	0	3.0	30	420	0
red:							
(*Bumble Bee/Bumble Bee* Blueback) . .	110	13.0	0	7.0	40	270	0
(*Bumble Bee* Coho Medium)	90	12.0	0	5.0	40	270	0
(*Chicken of the Sea*)	110	13.0	0	7.0	40	270	0
(*Roland* Sockeye) . .	110	13.0	0	7.0	40	270	0
(*Rubinstein's* Blueback)	110	13.0	0	7.0	40	270	0
skin/boneless (*Genova*)	60	10.0	0	2.0	20	280	0
red sockeye, drained, w/bone, 4 oz.	174	23.2	0	8.3	50	611	0
Salmon, frozen/refriger-ated, wild Alaska (*Peter Pan*), 4 oz.:							
chum	136	23.0	0	4.3	84	57	0
choco/silver	165	24.4	0	6.6	51	52	0
sockeye/red	190	24.0	0	9.7	70	53	0
Salmon, marinated (*Spence & Co.* Gravlax), 2 oz.	120	13.0	<1.0	7.0	30	910	<1.0

Food and Measure	cal.	prot. (gms)	carbo. (gms)	fat (gms)	chol. (mgs)	sod. (mgs)	fiber (gms)
Salmon, seasoned, pouch:							
pink, 4 oz.:							
(*Bumble Bee Prime Fillet*)	150	25.0	2.0	4.5	45	600	0
teriyaki (*Bumble Bee Prime Fillet*)	160	24.0	8.0	3.0	45	690	0
steak (*Chicken of the Sea*), 5.25 oz.:							
honey barbecue sauce	200	25.0	18.0	3.0	40	920	0
mandarin orange glaze	170	25.0	14.0	1.5	40	470	0
roasted garlic marinade	150	25.0	8.0	2.0	40	720	0
wild sockeye, 3.5 oz.:							
ginger (*SeaBear*) ..	132	24.0	0	4.0	15	260	0
Thai chili (*SeaBear*)	142	24.0	3.0	4.0	15	300	0
Salmon, smoked, 2 oz.:							
(*Acme/Blue Hill Bay*) .	70	13.0	0	2.5	30	790	0
(*Echo Falls*)	100	13.0	2.0	4.0	40	720	0
Chinook.	66	10.4	0	2.4	13	445	0
barbecue style (*Cracovia*)	140	14.0	0	9.0	20	360	0
Nova style, king, wild (*SeaBear*)	60	12.0	0	1.5	20	660	0
pastrami style:							
(*A&B Famous*), 2 oz.	110	10.0	1.0	7.0	20	880	0
(*Spence & Co.*) ...	120	13.0	<1.0	7.0	30	910	<1.0
sockeye, wild:							
(*SeaBear*)	110	14.0	0	6.0	80	340	0
Nova style (*SeaBear*)	90	14.0	1.0	3.0	20	560	0
Salmon, smoked, can or pkg.:							
in oil, drained (*Bumble Bee* 3.75 oz.), 3 oz.	150	16.0	0	9.0	55	400	0
Pacific (*Chicken of the Sea*), 3-oz. pouch ..	120	21.0	1.0	3.5	45	490	0
Salmon, smoked, spread:							
(*SeaBear*), 8-oz. cont.	578	22.3	6.5	51.4	186	459	.5
cheese, w/dill (*Goldy's*), 2 tbsp.	90	2.0	1.0	8.0	30	160	0
pâté (*Trois Petits Cochons*), 2 oz.	110	5.0	2.0	9.0	35	250	0

Food and Measure	cal.	prot. (gms)	carbo. (gms)	fat (gms)	chol. (mgs)	sod. (mgs)	fiber (gms)
Salmon appetizer, frozen, and cheese, in mini fillo shells, (*Athens*), 2 pcs., 1 oz.	70	3.0	5.0	4.0	5	115	0
Salmon cake, frozen, breaded (*Dr. Praeger's*), 2.9-oz. pc. . .	190	10.0	15.0	10.0	15	350	3.0
Salmon cake mix:							
(*Old Bay Salmon Classic*), 1²/₃ tbsp.	35	1.0	4.0	1.0	45	90	0
(*Zatarain's*), 4 tbsp. . .	110	4.0	23.0	1.0	0	440	2.0
Salmon entree, frozen, 1 pkg., except as noted:							
w/basil (*Lean Cuisine Spa Cuisine*), 9.5 oz.	220	18.0	24.0	6.0	20	660	4.0
dill, creamy (Healthy Choice Café Steamers), 9.8 oz. .	240	19.0	26.0	6.0	15.0	600	5.0
grilled, 3.1-oz. fillet:							
(*Gorton's* Classic) .	100	15.0	2.0	3.0	35	270	0
lemon butter (*Gorton's*)	100	17.0	1.0	3.0	40	300	0
w/lemon dill sauce (*Lean Cuisine Spa Cuisine*), 8.625 oz. .	240	16.0	30.0	6.0	30	690	4.0
Mediterranean (*Lean Cuisine Spa Cuisine*), 8.625 oz.	230	18.0	30.0	4.0	25	660	3.0
Salmon franks, see "Frankfurters"							
Salmon gefilte fish, see "Gefilte fish, frozen"							
Salmon oil, see "Oil"							
Salmon pâté, see "Salmon, smoked, spread"							
Salmon salami (*A&B Famous*), 2 oz.	120	8.0	2.0	9.0	20	470	0
Salsa (see also "Picante sauce"), 2 tbsp., except as noted:							
(*Chi-Chi's* Garden) . . .	15	0	3.0	0	0	130	0
(*Emeril's* Kicked Up Chunky)	15	0	3.0	0	0	160	0

Food and Measure	cal.	prot. (gms)	carbo. (gms)	fat (gms)	chol. (mgs)	sod. (mgs)	fiber (gms)
(*Emeril's* Original) ...	10	0	3.0	0	0	190	0
(*Herdez* Ranchera) ...	15	0	1.0	0	0	220	0
(*Herdez* Taquera)	10	0	2.0	0	0	280	0
(*Herdez* Verde)	10	0	1.0	0	0	310	0
(*La Victoria* Salsa Victoria)	10	0	2.0	0	0	115	0
(*Pace* Salsa Verde) ...	15	0	2.0	.5	0	230	0
(*Pace* Thick & Chunky)	10	0	2.0	0	0	230	<1.0
(*Tostitos* Restaurant Style)	15	<1.0	3.0	0	0	210	<1.0
(*Watkins* Tropical) ...	60	0	14.0	0	0	210	0
all varieties:							
(*Bravo*)	10	1.0	2.0	0	0	180	0
(*Old El Paso* Thick 'n Chunky)	10	0	3.0	0	0	230	0
(*Tostitos* All Natural)	15	2.0	3.0	0	0	260	1.0
artichoke garlic (*Jose Goldstein*) ......>	15	0	2.0	0	0	135	0
black bean (*Mrs. Renfro's*)	15	1.0	3.0	0	0	230	0
black bean and corn:							
(*Amy's* Organic) ...	15	1.0	3.0	0	0	170	<1.0
(*Fiesta*)	10	0	2.0	0	0	60	0
(*Muir Glen* Organic)	20	<1.0	4.0	0	0	135	<1.0
(*Newman's Own*) ..	20	1.0	5.0	0	0	140	2.0
(*Pace*)	25	1.0	5.0	0	0	150	1.0
(*Walnut Acres* Organic Midnight Sun)	15	1.0	3.0	0	0	125	1.0
cheese (salsa con queso), see "Cheese dip":							
chipotle:							
(*Muir Glen* Organic)	10	0	2.0	0	0	140	0
(*Pace* Chunky)	10	0	2.0	0	0	230	<1.0
corn (*Mrs. Renfro's*)	15	0	3.0	0	0	230	0
spicy (*Amy's* Organic)	10	0	2.0	0	0	160	0
cilantro:							
(*Pace* Chunky)	10	0	2.0	0	0	270	<1.0
(*Walnut Acres* Fiesta)	10	0	2.0	0	0	135	0
mild or medium (*La Victoria*)	5	0	2.0	0	0	180	0
w/corn and kidney beans (*Cape Cod*) .	15	1.0	3.0	0	0	210	1.0

Food and Measure	cal.	prot. (gms)	carbo. (gms)	fat (gms)	chol. (mgs)	sod. (mgs)	fiber (gms)
Salsa *(cont.)*							
fire-roasted tomato:							
mild or medium							
(*Zapata* Verde) ..	10	0	2.0	0	0	100	0
mild, medium, or hot							
(*Zapata* Roja) ...	10	0	2.0	0	0	130	0
fruit (*Neera's* Caribbean),							
1 tbsp.	25	0	7.0	0	0	60	0
garlic:							
(*Emeril's* Gaaahlic							
Lovers)	15	0	3.0	0	0	200	0
(*Mrs. Renfro's*) ...	10	0	2.0	0	0	220	0
(*Jose Goldstein* XXX)	10	0	2.0	0	0	160	0
cactus (*Jose*							
Goldstein)	10	0	2.0	0	0	230	0
chipotle (*Jose*							
Goldstein)	5	0	2.0	.5	0	140	0
cilantro (*Muir Glen*							
Organic)	10	0	2.0	0	0	130	0
garlic, roasted:							
chunky (*Newman's*							
Own)	10	1.0	2.0	0	0	150	1.0
medium (*Ortega*) ..	10	0	2.0	0	0	240	<1.0
and olive (*Jose*							
Goldstein)	10	0	1.0	1.0	0	115	0
green chili (*Ortega*) ..	10	0	2.0	0	0	200	0
habanero:							
(*Frontier Traders* Wild							
& Hot)	10	0	2.0	0	0	110	0
garlic (*Pain is Good*)	15	0	2.0	0	0	160	0
hot:							
(*Chi-Chi's/Chi-Chi's*							
Fiesta)	10	0	2.0	0	0	220	0
(*Herdez/Herdez*							
Casera)	10	0	1.0	0	0	240	0
(*La Victoria* Ran-							
chera 16 oz.) ...	10	0	2.0	0	0	125	0
(*La Victoria* Ran-							
chera 24 oz.) ...	10	0	2.0	0	0	160	0
(*La Victoria* Thick 'n							
Chunky)	10	0	2.0	0	0	220	0
(*Mrs. Renfro's*) ...	15	0	3.0	0	0	310	0
jalapeño:							
green (*Mrs. Renfro's*)	10	0	2.0	0	0	390	0

Food and Measure	cal.	prot. (gms)	carbo. (gms)	fat (gms)	chol. (mgs)	sod. (mgs)	fiber (gms)
green, extra hot (*La Victoria*)	10	0	2.0	0	0	150	0
red, extra hot (*La Victoria*)	10	0	2.0	0	0	95	0
smoked (*Fiesta*) . . .	15	0	2.0	0	0	240	0
smoked (*Frontier Traders* Wild & Medium)	10	0	2.0	0	0	240	0
smoked (*Pain is Good*)	15	4.0	3.0	1.0	0	200	0
lime and garlic (*Pace* Chunky)	15	0	3.0	0	0	210	<1.0
mango (*Newman's Own*)	20	1.0	5.0	0	0	140	2.0
medium:							
(*La Victoria* Suprema 12 oz.)	5	0	1.0	0	0	135	0
(*La Victoria* Suprema 16/24 oz.)	10	0	1.0	0	0	135	0
(*La Victoria* Thick 'n Chunky)	10	0	2.0	0	0	200	0
(*La Victoria* Thick 'n Chunky Verde) . .	10	0	2.0	0	0	140	0
(*Mrs. Renfro's*) . . .	15	0	3.0	0	0	280	0
(*Ortega* Homestyle)	10	<1.0	2.0	0	0	220	<1.0
(*Ortega* Restaurant Chunky)	10	0	2.0	0	0	230	0
(*Ortega* Thick & Chunky)	10	0	2.0	0	0	180	<1.0
medium or mild :							
(*Amy's* Organic) . . .	10	0	2.0	0	0	190	0
(*Chi-Chi's*)	10	0	2.0	0	0	150	0
(*Herdez* Casera) . . .	10	0	1.0	0	0	270	0
(*Muir Glen* Organic)	10	0	3.0	0	0	130	0
(*Taco Bell* Thick 'n Chunky)	15	1.0	3.0	0	0	210	0
mild:							
(*La Victoria* Suprema 16/24 oz.)	10	0	2.0	0	0	105	0
(*La Victoria* Thick 'n Chunky 16 oz.) . .	10	0	2.0	0	0	220	0
(*La Victoria* Thick 'n Chunky 24 oz.) . .	10	0	2.0	0	0	190	0
(*La Victoria* Thick 'n Chunky Verde) . .	10	0	2.0	0	0	180	0

Food and Measure	cal.	prot. (gms)	carbo. (gms)	fat (gms)	chol. (mgs)	sod. (mgs)	fiber (gms)
Salsa, mild *(cont.)*							
(*Mrs. Renfro's*) ...	15	0	3.0	0	0	240	0
(*Ortega* Homestyle)	10	<1.0	2.0	0	0	220	<1.0
(*Ortega* Mexican) ..	15	1.0	3.0	0	0	180	1.0
(*Ortega* Thick & Chunky)	10	<1.0	2.0	0	0	210	<1.0
mild, medium, or hot:							
(*El Torito* Original) .	10	0	2.0	0	0	180	0
(*Newman's Own*) ..	10	0	2.0	0	0	105	1.0
peach:							
(*Frontier Traders* Wild & Mild) ...	15	0	4.0	0	0	100	0
(*Mrs. Renfro's*) ...	10	0	3.0	0	0	170	0
chunky (*Newman's Own*)	25	0	6.0	0	0	90	<1.0
Southwest, sweet (*Walnut Acres* Organic)	20	0	5.0	0	0	85	0
peanut chipotle (*Fiesta*)	25	1.0	3.0	1.5	0	190	1.0
pepper, triple (*Pace*) ..	15	<1.0	3.0	0	0	190	1.0
pico de gallo (*Pace*) ..	10	0	3.0	0	0	150	0
pineapple:							
(*Newman's Own*) ..	15	0	3.0	0	0	90	1.0
Jamaican (*Pain is Good*)	15	0	3.0	0	0	110	0
raspberry:							
(*Frontier Traders* Wild & Mild) ...	15	0	4.0	0	0	70	0
chipotle (*Mrs. Renfro's*)	15	0	4.0	0	0	70	0
red pepper, roasted, and garlic (*Pace* Chunky)	10	0	2.0	0	0	230	<1.0
roasted (*Mrs. Renfro's*)	10	0	2.0	0	0	220	0
Southwest:							
(*Emeril's*)	15	0	4.0	0	0	105	0
Tex-Mex (*Frontier Traders*)	10	0	2.0	0	0	110	0
sweet (*Eatsmart* Garden Style)	20	0	5.0	0	0	95	0
tequila lime:							
(*Newman's Own*) ..	15	0	3.0	0	0	170	0
(*Pace*)	15	0	3.0	0	0	190	0

Food and Measure	cal.	prot. (gms)	carbo. (gms)	fat (gms)	chol. (mgs)	sod. (mgs)	fiber (gms)
tomato, fire-roasted (*El Torito*)	10	0	2.0	0	0	170	0
vegetable, fire-roasted (*Amy's*)	10	0	3.0	0	0	200	0
Salsa, refrigerated, 2 tbsp.:							
(*Emerald Valley* Organic Fiesta)	20	<1.0	4.0	0	0	125	<1.0
garlic, roasted (*Cedar's* Mexicana Gold) ...	30	1.0	6.0	0	0	520	1.0
green (*Emerald Valley* Organic)	10	0	2.0	0	0	110	<1.0
hot (*Cedar's* Mexicana Gold)	25	1.0	6.0	0	0	540	2.0
hot or medium (*Cedar's* Mexicana Gold) ...	25	1.0	6.0	0	0	540	2.0
hot, medium, or mild (*Emerald Valley* Organic)	10	0	2.0	0	0	140	0
mild (*Cedar's* Mexicana Gold)	30	1.0	6.0	0	0	530	1.0
pineapple mango (*Cedar's* Mexicana Gold)	10	0	2.0	0	0	340	<1.0
Salsa dip (see also "Cheese dip") (*Bison*), 2 tbsp. ...	60	1.0	3.0	5.0	20	220	0
Salsa seasoning: (*McCormick*), ¼ tsp. ..	5	0	1.0	0	0	120	0
and sour cream dip (*Watkins*), 1 tsp. ...	10	0	2.0	0	0	160	0
Salsify:							
raw:							
(*Frieda's*), 3 oz. ...	70	3.0	16.0	0	0	15	3.0
untrimmed, 1 lb..	325	13.0	73.4	.8	0	79	13.0
sliced, ½ cup	55	2.2	12.5	.1	0	13	2.2
boiled, drained, sliced, ½ cup	46	1.9	10.5	.1	0	11	2.1
Salsify, canned, cut (*Roland*), ½ cup ..	35	1.0	7.0	0	0	280	3.0
Salt, ¼ tsp.:							
(*Morton*)	0	0	0	0	0	590	0
(*Shiloh Farms* Himalayan Pink)	0	0	0	0	0	400	0

Food and Measure	cal.	prot. (gms)	carbo. (gms)	fat (gms)	chol. (mgs)	sod. (mgs)	fiber (gms)
Salt *(cont.)*							
all varieties (*Roland*)	0	0	0	0	0	400	0
sea salt:							
(*Hain*)	0	0	0	0	0	590	0
(*McCormick* Grinder)	0	0	0	0	0	400	0
(*Shiloh Farms*)	0	0	0	0	0	420	0
French (*Eden*)	0	0	0	0	0	390	0
Portuguese (*Eden*) .	0	0	0	0	0	410	0
Salt, seasoned (see also specific listings), ¼ tsp.:							
(*Lawry's*)	0	0	0	0	0	380	0
(*McCormick Season-All*)	0	0	0	0	0	350	0
(*McCormick Season-All* Less Sodium) . .	0	0	0	0	0	240	0
black pepper (*Lawry's*)	0	0	0	0	0	170	0
peppered (*McCormick Season-All*)	0	0	0	0	0	110	0
spicy (*McCormick Season-All*)	0	0	0	0	0	250	0
Salt, substitute, ¼ tsp.	0	0	0	0	0	0	0
Salt pork:							
dry (*Farmer John*), 2 oz.	250	7.0	1.0	24.0	35	1560	0
raw, 1 oz.	212	1.4	0	22.8	25	404	0
Sandwich relish (*Wickles* Hoagie & Sub), 1 tbsp.	10	0	2.0	0	0	270	0
Sandwich sauce, canned, ¼ cup, except as noted:							
(*Hormel Not-So-Sloppy-Joe*)	60	1.0	13.0	.5	0	700	1.0
sloppy Joe:							
(*Del Monte*)	50	1.0	11.0	0	0	620	0
(*Manwich* Original)	40	<1.0	9.0	0	0	410	2.0
hickory flavor (*Del Monte*)	60	1.0	14.0	0	0	660	0
Sandwich sauce, refrigerated (*Manwich* Heat and Serve), ¼ cup	70	5.0	6.0	3.0	5	310	2.0
Sandwich sauce mix (*Fantastic* Sloppy Joe), ¼ cup	80	9.0	11.0	.5	0	510	3.0

Food and Measure	cal.	prot. (gms)	carbo. (gms)	fat (gms)	chol. (mgs)	sod. (mgs)	fiber (gms)
Sandwich sauce seasoning mix, see "Sloppy Joe seasoning"							
Sandwich spread (see also "Meat spread," and specific listings), mayonnaise style:							
(*Cains*), 1 tbsp.	70	0	2.0	7.0	5	130	0
(*Dietz & Watson*), 1 tsp.	50	0	3.0	4.0	<5	105	0
(*Hellmann's/Best Foods*), 1 tbsp.	60	0	2.0	5.0	<5	200	0
(*Kraft* Burger), 2 tbsp.	150	0	4.0	15.0	15	210	0
Sandwiches, see "Panini," "Wraps, filled," and specific listings							
Sapodilla:							
(*Frieda's*), 3-oz. fruit .	70	0	17.0	1.0	0	10	5.0
1 medium, 3" x 2½" . .	140	.7	33.9	1.9	0	20	9.0
½ cup	100	.5	24.1	1.3	0	15	6.4
Sapote:							
(*Frieda's*), 5 oz.	190	3.0	47.0	1.0	0	15	4.0
11.2-oz. fruit, 7.9 oz. trimmed	301	4.8	76.0	1.4	0	23	5.9
trimmed, 1 oz.	38	.6	9.6	.2	0	3	.7
Sardine, fresh, see "Herring"							
Sardine, canned (see also "Herring, canned"), 3.75-oz. can, except as noted:							
Atlantic, in oil:							
drained, 2 oz.	118	14.8	0	6.5	81	286	0
2 medium, 3" long .	50	5.9	0	2.8	34	121	0
in hot sauce:							
(*Beach Cliff* Louisiana)	140	17.0	2.0	8.0	100	420	0
(*Bela*), ¼ cup	110	13.0	0	7.0	20	120	0
(*Bumble Bee*)	170	15.0	1.0	12.0	60	470	0
(*Chicken of the Sea*)	130	17.0	2.0	6.0	60	490	2.0
in lemon/oil:							
(*Bela*), ¼ cup	130	12.0	0	9.0	20	115	0
(*Vigo*), 3 pcs.	125	11.0	0	8.0	20	250	0
in mustard sauce:							
(*Beach Cliff*)	140	17.0	2.0	8.0	100	460	0
(*Bumble Bee*)	130	15.0	2.0	6.0	40	490	1.0

Food and Measure	cal.	prot. (gms)	carbo. (gms)	fat (gms)	chol. (mgs)	sod. (mgs)	fiber (gms)
Sardine, canned, in mustard sauce *(cont.)*							
(*Chicken of the Sea*)	150	17.0	2.0	8.0	60	490	2.0
(*Yankee Clipper*), ¼ cup	90	10.0	1.0	5.0	35	260	0
and dill (*Brunswick*)	150	16.0	3.0	8.0	100	580	0
in olive oil, drained:							
(*Bela*), ¼ cup	120	13.0	0	7.0	20	130	0
(*Brunswick*), 3.25 oz.	190	20.0	0	13.0	110	250	0
(*Roland*), 2 pcs., approx. ½ can ..	100	13.0	1.0	5.0	35	260	0
skin/boneless (*Granadaisa*), ¼ cup ..	120	13.0	0	7.0	24	280	0
skin/boneless (*Roland*), 3 pcs.	120	13.0	1.0	7.0	20	350	0
in oil, drained:							
(*Beach Cliff* 3.75 oz.), 3.2 oz.	190	20.0	1.0	13.0	110	250	0
(*Beach Cliff* Small Size 3.75 oz.), 3.4 oz.	200	20.0	0	13.0	115	260	0
(*Bumble Bee* 3.75 oz.), 2.65 oz. ...	130	13.0	0	9.0	35	340	0
w/chili peppers (*Roland*), ¼ cup	110	13.0	0	6.0	40	370	0
w/hot green chilies (*Beach Cliff* 3.75 oz.), 3.2 oz.	190	19.0	1.0	12.0	100	270	0
w/hot tabasco pepper (*Brunswick* 3.75 oz.), 3.3 oz.	190	20.0	0	12.0	110	280	0
lightly smoked (*Chicken of the Sea*)	190	12.0	2.0	14.0	45	430	0
lightly smoked (*Roland*), 3 pcs.	110	13.0	0	6.0	40	370	0
lightly smoked (*Yankee Clipper*), ¼ cup	120	14.0	0	7.0	40	110	0
plain or hot spiced (*Vigo*), 2 pcs.	130	11.0	0	9.0	20	250	0
skin/boneless (*Roland*), 3 pcs.	120	13.0	0	7.0	25	280	0
skin/boneless (*Vigo*), 3 pcs.	130	14.0	1.0	8.0	20	250	0
spiced (*Roland*) ...	120	14.0	0	8.0	10	110	0

Food and Measure	cal.	prot. (gms)	carbo. (gms)	fat (gms)	chol. (mgs)	sod. (mgs)	fiber (gms)
in tomato sauce:							
(*Beach Cliff*)	140	16.0	2.0	7.0	100	420	0
(*Bela*), ¼ cup	120	11.0	0	9.0	25	135	0
(*Chicken of the Sea*)	130	17.0	2.0	6.0	60	490	2.0
(*Chicken of the Sea*), 2 oz.	90	10.0	1.0	5.0	35	260	1.0
(*Consul*), 3 pcs.	80	10.0	1.0	4.0	35	170	1.0
(*Roland*), ¼ cup ..	90	10.0	1.0	5.0	40	220	0
(*Vigo*), ½ of 4⅜-oz. can	100	9.0	0	7.0	20	250	0
(*Yankee Clipper*), ¼ cup	90	10.0	1.0	5.0	40	220	0
and basil (*Brunswick*)	150	16.0	3.0	8.0	100	530	0
Pacific, 2 oz.	101	9.3	n.a.	6.8	35	235	<1.0
w/chili (*Roland*), ¼ cup	50	9.0	1.0	1.0	45	280	0
in water, drained:							
(*Beach Cliff* 3.75 oz.), 3.2 oz.	150	19.0	0	8.0	115	230	0
(*Bumble Bee* 3.75-oz.), 2.65 oz.	120	13.0	0	7.0	35	340	0
(*Brunswick* No Salt 3.75 oz.), 3.25 oz.	140	19.0	0	7.0	100	200	0
all varieties (*Roland* Low Sodium), ¼ cup	90	12.0	0	5.0	25	35	0
Sardine oil, see "Oil"							
Satsuma, see "Tangerine"							
Sauce, see "Finishing sauce" and specific sauce listings							
Sauerkraut, 2 tbsp., except as noted:							
(*Boar's Head*)	5	0	1.0	0	0	180	<1.0
(*Del Monte*)	0	0	<1.0	0	0	180	<1.0
(*Del Monte* Bavarian) .	15	0	4.0	0	0	180	0
(*Eden* Organic), ½ cup	25	2.0	4.0	0	0	580	3.0
(*Hebrew National*) ...	5	0	1.0	0	0	180	1.0
(*S&W*)	0	0	1.0	0	0	180	<1.0
chopped or shredded (*Bush's*)	5	0	1.0	0	0	180	1.0
Sauerkraut dish, canned, ½ cup:							
w/apples (*Glory*)	45	1.0	11.0	0	0	560	1.0

Food and Measure	cal.	prot. (gms)	carbo. (gms)	fat (gms)	chol. (mgs)	sod. (mgs)	fiber (gms)
Sauerkraut dish *(cont.)* country style *(Glory Savory)*	30	1.0	7.0	0	0	510	2.0
Sausage (see also specific listings), cooked, except as noted: beef, breakfast, 2 links, 1.6 oz.:							
(Hebrew National) .	140	5.0	1.0	13.0	15	480	0
(Hebrew National Reduced Fat) ...	120	6.0	2.0	10.0	20	540	0
maple *(Hebrew National)*	140	5.0	1.0	13.0	15	490	0
beef, smoked, 1 link: *(Hatfield Phillies)*, 3.2 oz.	230	11.0	2.0	19.0	60	1110	0
(Johnsonville Smokies), 6 links, 2 oz. ...	180	6.0	2.0	16.0	35	540	0
(Oscar Mayer Smokies), 1.75 oz.	150	6.0	1.0	13.0	30	490	0
mild *(Hatfield)*, 3.2 oz.	280	12.0	2.0	23.0	65	1090	0
chicken, 1 link: Andouille, Cajun *(Bilinski)*, 2 oz. .	80	9.0	1.0	4.0	60	300	0
and apple *(Applegate Farms* Organic), 3 oz.	140	14.0	6.0	6.0	65	500	1.0
apple, smoked *(Aidells)*, 3.5 oz. .	210	16.0	1.0	16.0	90	730	0
apple, smoked, minis *(Aidells)*, 5 links, 2 oz.	100	16.0	1.0	8.0	50	370	0
apple, sweet *(Al Fresco)*, 3 oz. ...	160	14.0	10.0	7.0	60	480	0
apple, sweet *(Bilinski* Organic), 3 oz. ..	110	15.0	5.0	3.0	60	490	<1.0
apple, sweet, cinnamon *(Empire Kosher)*, 2.5 oz. .	80	13.0	3.0	2.0	45	610	0
apple Chardonnay *(Bilinski)*, 2 oz. .	70	10.0	2.5	5.5	60	350	0
Buffalo style *(Al Fresco)*, 3 oz.	130	13.0	4.0	6.0	60	620	0

Food and Measure	cal.	prot. (gms)	carbo. (gms)	fat (gms)	chol. (mgs)	sod. (mgs)	fiber (gms)
cilantro and bell pepper (*Bilinski*), 2 oz.	70	9.0	1.0	3.5	40	270	1.0
garlic, roasted (*Al Fresco*), 3 oz.	140	15.0	3.0	7.0	70	480	0
Italian, sweet (*Al Fresco*), 3 oz.	130	15.0	1.0	7.0	65	480	0
Italian, sweet (*Bilinski* Organic), 3 oz.	110	18.0	0	3.5	70	540	0
jalapeño, spicy (*Al Fresco*), 3 oz.	130	15.0	2.0	7.0	65	480	0
jalapeño, spicy (*Bilinski*), 2 oz.	70	9.0	0	4.0	55	270	0
lemon, smoked (*Aidells*), 3.5 oz.	210	15.0	1.0	16.0	90	700	0
mango (*Aidells*), 3.5 oz.	210	17.0	6.0	13.0	65	740	0
mushroom garlic (*Empire Kosher*), 2.5 oz.	80	13.0	3.0	2.0	45	610	0
peppers and onions, Italian style (*Bilinski*), 2 oz.	70	9.0	1.0	3.5	60	270	0
pesto Romano (*Bilinski*), 2 oz.	90	10.0	0	5.0	40	320	0
porcini mushroom (*Bilinski* Organic), 3 oz.	100	17.0	1.0	3.0	65	410	0
spinach and garlic (*Bilinski*), 2 oz.	70	9.0	1.0	3.5	40	270	1.0
sun-dried tomato (*Bilinski*), 2 oz.	70	10.0	2.0	3.5	40	280	0
sun-dried tomato basil (*Al Fresco*) 3 oz.	140	15.0	2.0	7.0	70	480	0
sun-dried tomato basil (*Empire Kosher*), 2.5 oz.	80	13.0	3.0	2.0	45	650	0
teriyaki ginger (*Al Fresco*), 3 oz.	140	15.0	5.0	7.0	65	610	0
chicken, breakfast (*Al Fresco*), 1.2-oz. link: plain	70	6.0	4.0	3.0	30	170	0

Food and Measure	cal.	prot. (gms)	carbo. (gms)	fat (gms)	chol. (mgs)	sod. (mgs)	fiber (gms)
Sausage, chicken, breakfast (cont.)							
blueberry, wild	70	6.0	5.0	3.0	30	170	0
country style	60	7.0	0	3.5	30	190	0
chicken, breakfast (Applegate Farms), 3 links, 3 oz.:							
and apple	160	16.0	4.0	8.0	85	480	0
and maple	150	14.0	4.0	8.0	65	510	0
and sage	140	15.0	1.0	8.0	70	520	0
chicken, raw, I link, 3.2 oz. except as noted:							
apple, sweet (Al Fresco)	170	20.0	9.0	6.0	50	630	0
Buffalo style (Al Fresco)	120	15.0	2.0	6.0	70	610	0
cranberry orange (Al Fresco)	170	21.0	9.0	6.0	50	640	0
Italian (Organic Prairie), 3 oz. ...	150	14.0	1.0	10.0	65	580	0
Italian, sweet (Al Fresco)	130	15.0	1.0	7.0	70	480	0
Italian herb (Al Fresco)	170	21.0	8.0	6.0	50	580	0
mango chipotle (Al Fresco)	170	21.0	8.0	6.0	50	670	0
tequila lime (Al Fresco)	160	21.0	5.0	6.0	55	730	0
chicken/turkey, see "turkey/chicken," below							
duck, smoked (Aidells), 3.5-oz. link	220	17.0	1.0	16.0	60	700	0
garlic (Trois Petits Cochons Saucisson a l'Ail), 2 oz.	80	11.0	1.0	3.5	35	430	0
pepper and onion (Dietz & Watson), 2 oz.	150	8.0	1.0	13.0	30	460	0
pork:							
(Hatfield Pennsylvania Dutch), 2 oz.	140	11.0	2.0	10.0	35	530	0
link, raw, 1 oz.	118	3.3	.3	11.4	19	189	0
link, cooked, .5 oz. .	105	6.6	.6	22.8	39	378	0
patty, raw, 2-oz. patty	286	6.6	.6	22.8	39	378	0

Food and Measure	cal.	prot. (gms)	carbo. (gms)	fat (gms)	chol. (mgs)	sod. (mgs)	fiber (gms)
pork, breakfast chub/ roll, 2 oz.:							
(*Hatfield*)	170	8.0	1.0	15.0	35	430	0
w/apple, raw (*Farmland* Cider House)	280	10.0	4.0	25.0	60	500	0
and bacon, panfried (*Farmland*)	230	9.0	1.0	21.0	50	640	0
honey maple, panfried (*Farmland*)	230	9.3	.8	21.3	45	650	0
hot, panfried (*Farmland* Hot & Zesty)	250	8.0	1.0	25.0	60	560	0
panfried (*Farmland* Original)	230	9.0	1.0	21.0	45	610	0
raw (*Farmland* Special Select Premium)	270	11.0	0	24.0	45	540	0
pork, breakfast chub, raw (*Organic Prairie*), 4 oz.	280	18.0	1.0	23.0	75	930	0
pork, breakfast links, 3 links, except as noted:							
(*Farmer John*), 2 links	150	10.0	1.0	12.0	45	560	0
(*Farmer John* Lower Fat), 2 links	100	6.0	1.0	8.0	25	340	0
(*Farmland* Lower Sodium)	220	10.0	0	21.0	50	420	0
(*Farmland* Original), 2 links	260	11.0	1.0	23.0	40	610	0
(*Farmland* Precooked), 2 links	170	6.0	<1.0	15.0	30	260	0
(*Farmland* Special Select)	200	11.4	.3	16.6	35	685	0
(*Farmland* Simply Natural*), 1.5 oz. ..	180	8.0	0	17.0	45	380	0
(*Hatfield*)	260	13.0	2.0	22.0	55	650	0
(*Hatfield* Jumbo), 1 link	170	8.0	1.0	15.0	35	430	0
(*Jimmy Dean*)	150	8.0	1.0	13.0	40	310	0
(*Johnsonville*)	180	11.0	2.0	14.0	35	610	0
(*Little Sizzlers*)	200	8.0	0	19.0	40	580	0
(*Little Sizzlers* Heat & Serve)	200	8.0	0	19.0	40	620	0
(*Organic Prairie* Brown & Serve), 2 links	150	9.0	0	13.0	40	500	0

Food and Measure	cal.	prot. (gms)	carbo. (gms)	fat (gms)	chol. (mgs)	sod. (mgs)	fiber (gms)
Sausage, pork, breakfast links (cont.)							
(*Oscar Mayer* Ready to Serve), 2 links	130	7.0	1.0	11.0	35	350	0
w/apple (*Farmland* Cider House) ...	270	10.0	4.0	23.0	60	500	0
and bacon (*Farmland*)	230	10.0	1.0	21.0	50	640	0
brown sugar honey (*Johnsonville*) ..	170	8.0	4.0	13.0	35	480	0
honey maple (*Farmland*), 5 links ...	260	10.0	3.0	23.0	40	520	0
honey maple (*Farmland* Special Select)	200	11.0	3.0	16.0	35	460	0
hot (*Farmland* Hot & Zesty)	250	12.0	2,0	22.0	40	380	0
maple (*Johnsonville* Vermont)	180	11.0	2.0	14.0	35	610	0
maple (*Little Sizzlers*)	210	8.0	2.0	19.0	40	580	0
pork, breakfast patty, 2 pcs., except as noted:							
(*Farmland* Precooked)	220	7.0	0	21.0	35	350	0
(*Johnsonville* Homestyle), 1 pc.	140	8.0	0	11.0	30	410	0
(*Johnsonville* Original)	180	10.0	1.0	15.0	40	450	0
(*Jones Dairy Farm* Golden Brown Precooked), 1 pc.	120	4.0	0	12.0	25	220	0
(*Little Sizzlers*)	200	8.0	0	19.0	40	580	0
(*Oscar Mayer* Ready to Serve)	180	9.0	2.0	15.0	40	620	0
honey maple (*Farmland* Special Select)	200	11.0	0	17.0	35	690	0
maple (*Johnsonville* Vermont)	210	12.0	2.0	17.0	45	590	0
pork, Italian:							
(*Johnsonville* Heat & Serve), 2.7-oz. link	280	12.0	3.0	24.0	55	980	0
hot (*Hatfield* Burger), 3-oz. patty	210	16.0	3.0	14.0	45	650	0
hot (*Hatfield* Link), 2 oz.	210	15.0	3.0	15.0	45	760	0
hot (*Hatfield* Rope), 2 oz.	140	10.0	2.0	10.0	30	510	0

Food and Measure	cal.	prot. (gms)	carbo. (gms)	fat (gms)	chol. (mgs)	sod. (mgs)	fiber (gms)
hot (*Johnsonville* All Natural Ground), 2 oz.	170	10.0	1.0	13.0	40	400	0
hot, mild, or sweet (*Johnsonville* Links), 3 oz.	270	15.0	3.0	22.0	60	710	0
mild or sweet (*Johnsonville* All Natural Ground), 2 oz.	170	10.0	1.0	13.0	40	480	0
sweet (*Hatfield* Burger), 3-oz. patty .	210	16.0	2.0	14.0	50	780	0
sweet (*Hatfield* Link), 2 oz.	210	16.0	3.0	15.0	45	710	0
sweet (*Hatfield* Rope), 2 oz.	140	10.0	2.0	10.0	30	480	0
pork, Italian, flavored: cheese and basil (*Premio*), 2 oz. . . .	150	10.0	1.0	11.0	35	380	0
fennel (*Premio* Sweet Luganiga), 2 oz. .	150	10.0	2.0	11.0	35	400	0
peppers, onion, mushroom (*Premio*), 2 oz.	150	10.0	1.0	11.0	35	410	0
red pepper onion (*Hatfield*), 1 link	180	13.0	3.0	12.0	40	640	0
sweet basil (*Premio*), 2.5-oz. link	190	13.0	2.0	14.0	45	570	0
tomato, garlic, rosemary (*Premio*), 2.5-oz. link	150	10.0	1.0	11.0	35	400	0
pork, Italian, raw (*Organic Prairie*), 3-oz. link	200	13.0	1.0	18.0	55	580	0
pork, smoked, 1 link, except as noted: (*Boar's Head* Natural Casing), 4 oz. . . .	310	15.0	2.0	27.0	65	920	0
(*Farmland* Deli Style), 2 oz.	180	7.0	2.0	16.0	35	570	0
(*Farmland/Farmland* Grillable), 2.7 oz.	240	9.0	2.0	22.0	50	790	0
(*Hatfield* Loop), 2 oz.	140	7.0	3.0	11.0	30	430	0

Food and Measure	cal.	prot. (gms)	carbo. (gms)	fat (gms)	chol. (mgs)	sod. (mgs)	fiber (gms)
Sausage, pork, smoked *(cont.)*							
(*Oscar Mayer* Little Smokies), 6 links, 2 oz.	170	7.0	1.0	15.0	35	570	0
(*Oscar Mayer* Smokies), 1.75 oz.	150	6.0	1.0	13.0	30	500	0
Andouille (*Aidells* Cajun), 3.5 oz. . .	220	16.0	1.0	17.0	55	770	0
Andouille (*Applegate Farms* Organic), 3 oz.	200	12.0	2.0	15.0	50	510	1.0
Andouille (*Johnsonville* New Orleans), 2.7 oz.	230	9.0	2.0	20.0	40	630	0
bacon cheddar (*Farmland*), 2.7 oz.	240	11.0	<1.0	21.0	55	820	0
cheddar (*Hatfield*), 3.2 oz.	230	13.0	4.0	19.0	50	780	0
cheddar (*Johnsonville* Bedder with Cheddar), 2.7 oz.	240	9.0	2.0	21.0	60	640	0
cheddar (*Johnsonville* Bedder with Cheddar Natural Casing), 2.8 oz. .	250	10.0	2.0	23.0	50	650	0
cheese (*Farmland*), 2.7 oz.	240	10.0	2.0	22.0	50	920	0
cheese (*Oscar Mayer* Little Smokies), 6 links, 2 oz. . . .	190	7.0	2.0	17.0	35	750	0
hot (*Boar's Head*), 3.2 oz.	250	12.0	1.0	22.0	55	740	0
hot (*Farmland*), 2.7 oz.	250	10.0	2.0	22.0	50	870	0
hot (*Hatfield*), 3.2 oz.	230	11.0	5.0	18.0	45	700	0
hot, Creole (*Aidells*), 3.5 oz.	220	17.0	2.0	16.0	55	600	0
pork/beef, raw, .5 oz. .	112	3.9	.8	10.3	20	228	0
summer, see "Summer sausage"							
turkey, breakfast:							
(*Shady Brook Farms*), 2 links	120	13.0	1.0	2.0	45	470	0

Food and Measure	cal.	prot. (gms)	carbo. (gms)	fat (gms)	chol. (mgs)	sod. (mgs)	fiber (gms)
roll (*Shady Brook Farms*), ⅙ pkg. .	100	12.0	0	5.0	40	320	0
turkey, breakfast, raw:							
(*Jennie-O* Links), 2 oz.	140	9.0	0	11.0	45	360	0
(*Jennie-O* Patties), 2.25 oz.	160	10.0	0	13.0	50	420	0
(*Jennie-O Breakfast Lover's* links), 2 oz.	130	9.0	0	11.0	45	330	0
(*Perdue*), 2 oz.	80	9.0	0	5.0	30	350	0
(*Shady Brook Farms*), 2 links, 2.6 oz. . .	130	13.0	2.0	7.0	45	480	0
(*Wampler*), 4 oz. . .	230	17.0	1.0	17.0	100	880	0
Italian, sweet (*Perdue*), 2 oz.	90	9.0	2.0	5.0	40	270	0
maple (*Jennie-O* Links), 2 oz.	140	8.0	2.0	11.0	40	370	0
roll (*Shady Brook Farms*), ⅙ pkg. .	100	13.0	1.0	4.5	40	350	0
turkey, Italian, 1 link:							
hot (*Shady Brook Farms*), 3.3 oz. . .	140	15.0	2.0	8.0	50	570	0
hot, lean, raw (*Jennie-O*), 3.8 oz.	160	17.0	0	10.0	65	850	0
sweet (*Perdue* 3.2 oz. raw), 2.8 oz.	150	15.0	4.0	8.0	70	440	0
sweet, lean, raw (*Jennie-O*), 3.8 oz.	160	17.0	0	10.0	65	650	0
turkey, smoked:							
(*Jennie-O Turkey Store* Lean), 2 oz.	70	9.0	1.0	3.0	35.0	550	0
(*Johnsonville*), 2.25-oz. link	110	10.0	4.0	6.0	45	710	0
cheddar (*Johnsonville*), 2.25-oz. link	120	10.0	4.0	6.0	45	740	0
turkey/beef/pork, smoked (*Healthy Choice*), 2 oz.	80	7.0	6.0	2.5	25	480	0
turkey/chicken, 3.5-oz. link, except as noted:							
Andouille (*Applegate Farms* Organic), 3-oz. link	120	13.0	3.0	6.0	60	620	1.0

Food and Measure	cal.	prot. (gms)	carbo. (gms)	fat (gms)	chol. (mgs)	sod. (mgs)	fiber (gms)
Sausage, turkey/chicken (cont.)							
Andouille, Cajun, minis (*Aidells*), 5 links, 2 oz. . . .	80	11.0	1.0	3.0	45	490	0
artichoke and garlic, smoked (*Aidells*)	160	16.0	3.0	10.0	90	650	0
habanero green chili, smoked (*Aidells*)	170	16.0	2.0	11.0	55	600	0
Italian, sweet (*Applegate* Farms Organic), 3-oz. link	130	15.0	2.0	7.0	70	500	1.0
pesto, smoked (*Aidells*)	220	18.0	2.0	16.0	75	780	0
portobello mushroom (*Aidells*)	160	15.0	3.0	9.0	85	700	0
roasted red pepper (*Applegate Farms* Organic), 3-oz. link	120	14.0	2.0	6.0	65	500	1.0
roasted red pepper w/corn (*Aidells*) .	120	18.0	2.0	4.0	70	800	0
smoked (*Aidells* New Mexico) . . .	210	15.0	2.0	16.0	80	600	0
and smoked bacon (*Aidells* Breakfast), 2 links, 2 oz. . . .	170	9.0	3.0	7.0	40	420	0
spinach and feta (*Applegate Farms* Organic), 3-oz. link	120	13.0	2.0	7.0	60	470	0
sun-dried tomato, smoked (*Aidells*)	210	19.0	1.0	14.0	80	730	0
sun-dried tomato, smoked, minis (*Aidells*), 5 links, 2 oz.	110	11.0	1.0	7.0	45	370	0
Sausage, canned, Vienna (*Libby's*), 3 links	140	5.0	4.0	12.0	40	430	1.0
"Sausage," vegetarian, canned (see also specific listings):							
(*Loma Linda* Little Links), 2 pcs., 1.6 oz.	90	8.0	3.0	5.0	0	250	2.0
(*Loma Linda* Linkettes), 1.2-oz. pc.	70	7.0	1.0	4.0	0	160	1.0

Food and Measure	cal.	prot. (gms)	carbo. (gms)	fat (gms)	chol. (mgs)	sod. (mgs)	fiber (gms)
(*Loma Linda Veja-Links*), 1.1-oz. pc.	50	5.0	1.0	3.0	0	180	0
(*Loma Linda Veja-Links Low Fat*), 1.1-oz. pc.	45	5.0	3.0	1.5	0	220	0
(*Worthington* Super-Links), 1.7-oz. pc .	110	7.0	2.0	8.0	0	350	1.0
(*Worthington Saucettes*), 1.3-oz. pc.	90	6.0	1.0	6.0	0	200	1.0
"Sausage," vegetarian, frozen (see also specific listings):							
burger, breakfast, on wheat bun (*Nate's mitey-bites*), 4.5-oz. pc.	350	22.0	34.0	13.0	0	800	6.0
links:							
(*Boca* Breakfast), 2 links, 1.6 oz. . .	70	8.0	5.0	3.0	0	330	2.0
(*Boca* Breakfast Organic), 2 pcs., 1.6 oz.	90	10.0	5.0	3.0	0	370	2.0
(*Morningstar Farms*), 2 links, 1.6 oz. . .	80	9.0	3.0	3.0	0	300	2.0
(*Tofurky* Breakfast), 1.6-oz. link	130	11.0	6.0	6.0	0	330	4.0
(*Worthington Prosage*), 2 links, 1.6 oz.	80	9.0	3.0	3.0	0	320	2.0
apple, spiced (*Veggie Patch*), 2-oz. link	110	7.0	7.0	6.0	0	300	0
Italian (*Boca*), 2.5-oz. link	130	13.0	6.0	6.0	0	650	1.0
Italian, sweet (*Tofurky*), 3.5 oz.	280	29.0	12.0	13.0	0	620	8.0
jalapeño cheddar (*Veggie Patch*), 2-oz. link	100	8.0	3.0	6.0	5	440	<1.0
smoked (*Boca*), 2.5-oz. link	130	14.0	6.0	6.0	0	680	1.0
sun-dried tomato artichoke (*Veggie Patch*), 2-oz. link	100	8.0	5.0	6.0	0	340	1.0
patties, 1.3-oz. pc., except as noted:							
(*Amy's* Breakfast) . .	110	4.0	12.0	6.0	0	280	3.0

Food and Measure	cal.	prot. (gms)	carbo. (gms)	fat (gms)	chol. (mgs)	sod. (mgs)	fiber (gms)
"Sausage," vegetarian, frozen, patties *(cont.)*							
(*Boca* Breakfast) ..	60	7.0	5.0	2.5	0	280	2.0
(*Boca* Breakfast Organic)	70	8.0	5.0	2.5	0	310	2.0
(*Gardenburger*), 1.5 oz.	45	5.0	4.0	2.5	0	270	2.0
(*Morningstar Farms*)	80	10.0	3.0	3.0	0	260	1.0
(*Morningstar Farms* w/Organic Soy) .	80	8.0	4.0	3.0	0	240	1.0
(*Yves*), 2 pcs., 2 oz.	80	11.0	4.0	2.0	0	350	2.0
Sausage entree, frozen, jambalaya (*Zatarain's*), 12-oz. pkg.	480	13.0	77.0	14.0	25	1380	3.0
Sausage entree, microwave, and chicken gumbo (*Zatarain's*), 8-oz. pkg.	150	7.0	16.0	7.0	20	1000	1.0
Sausage seasoning (*Tone's*), 1 tsp.	12	.4	2.7	.3	0	1	.7
Sausage stick (see also "Beef jerky") (*Applegate Farms Joy Stick*), 1-oz. pc.	100	9.0	0	7.0	25	700	<1.0
Savory, ground, 1 tsp.	4	.1	1.0	.1	0	<1	<1.0
Scallion, see "Onion, green"							
Scallop, meat only:							
raw, 4 oz.	100	19.0	2.7	.9	38	183	0
raw, 2 large or 5 small, 1.1 oz.	26	5.0	.7	.2	10	48	0
steamed, 4 oz.	127	26.3	0	1.6	60	301	0
"Scallop," imitation, from surimi, 4 oz. .	112	14.5	12.1	.5	25	902	0
"Scallop," vegetarian, canned (*Worthington Skallops*), ½ cup, 3 oz.	90	17.0	4.0	0	0	390	3.0
Scallop dish, frozen: bacon wrapped:							
(*Original Rangoon*), 4 pcs.	190	16.0	1.0	14.0	45	440	0
jumbo, stuffed (*Original Rangoon*), 1 pc.	120	12.0	5.0	6.0	30	330	0

Food and Measure	cal.	prot. (gms)	carbo. (gms)	fat (gms)	chol. (mgs)	sod. (mgs)	fiber (gms)
breaded, fried (*Mrs. Paul's*), 13 pcs., 3.5 oz.	260	12.0	28.0	11.0	25	700	<1.0
Scallop squash (see also "Sunburst Squash"), ½ cup:							
raw, sliced	12	.8	2.5	.1	0	1	1.2
boiled, drained, sliced	14	.9	3.0	.2	0	1	1.1
boiled, drained, mashed	19	1.2	4.0	.2	0	1	1.4
Scampi sauce, see "Seafood sauce"							
Scrapple, 2 oz.:							
(*Dietz & Watson* Philadelphia)	120	6.0	7.0	8.0	40	320	0
(*Scrapple*)	90	5.0	5.0	5.0	35	310	0
beef (*Hatfield*)	90	4.0	7.0	5.0	15	320	0
Scrod, fresh, see "Cod, Atlantic"							
Scup, meat only:							
raw, 4 oz.	119	21.4	0	3.1	59	48	0
baked or broiled, 4 oz.	153	27.5	0	4.0	76	61	0
Sea bass, meat only:							
raw, 4 oz.	110	20.9	0	2.3	47	77	0
baked or broiled, 4 oz.	141	26.8	0	2.9	60	99	0
Sea trout, meat only:							
raw, 4 oz.	118	19.0	0	4.1	94	66	0
baked or broiled, 4 oz.	151	24.3	0	5.3	120	84	0
Sea vegetables, see "Seaweed"							
Seafood, see specific listings							
Seafood antipasto, mixed, in sauce:							
(*Roland*), ⅓ cup	120	5.0	2.0	10.0	10	550	0
(*Vigo*), ¼ of 9.25-oz. can	110	12.0	3.0	6.0	15	250	0
Seafood appetizer, mixed, frozen, breaded (*Matlaw's* Party Pack):							
calamari, 2 oz.	200	7.0	25.0	10.0	70	600	2.0
crab bites, 2 oz.	90	5.0	5.0	3.0	10	400	0
shrimp, 2 oz.	145	7.0	12.0	8.0	30	450	1.0
dipping sauce, 2 tbsp.	80	0	21.0	0	0	240	1.0

Food and Measure	cal.	prot. (gms)	carbo. (gms)	fat (gms)	chol. (mgs)	sod. (mgs)	fiber (gms)
Seafood appetizer *(cont.)*							
puff pastry (*Matlaw's*):							
crab, 1.1 oz.	60	3.0	7.0	2.5	15	170	1.0
shrimp Alfredo,							
1.1 oz.	70	4.0	7.0	3.0	25	140	1.0
smoked salmon/four							
cheese, 1.1 oz. . .	80	3.0	7.0	4.0	15	160	1.0
Seafood coating mix							
(see also "Batter/							
breading mix"):							
(*Golden Dipt* Fish Fry							
Seafood Fry Mix),							
2 tbsp.	60	1.0	13.0	0	0	450	0
(*Golden Dipt* Seafood							
Fry Mix), 2 tbsp. . .	60	1.0	13.0	0	0	570	0
(*Oven Fry* Fish), 1 tbsp.	45	1.0	9.0	.5	0	290	0
(*Zatarain's Fish-Fri*							
Crispy Southern),							
2 tbsp.	50	1.0	11.0	0	0	520	1.0
(*Zatarain's Wonderful*							
Fish-Fri), 1½ tbsp. .	45	1.0	10.0	0	0	0	0
beer batter (*Golden*							
Dipt), ¼ cup	100	1.0	20.0	0	0	730	0
Cajun:							
(*Golden Dipt* Fry Mix),							
2 tbsp.	60	1.0	13.0	0	0	490	0
(*Luzianne*), 2 tbsp. .	100	2.0	22.0	1.0	0	1200	1.0
(*Oven Easy*), ¼ cup	90	2.0	13.0	3.0	0	540	0
cracker meal (*Golden							
Dipt* Seafood Fry),							
¼ cup	130	3.0	24.0	1.0	0	10	0
fish and chips:							
(*Don's Chuck Wagon*),							
¼ cup	100	3.0	21.0	0	0	740	1.0
(*Golden Dipt* Seafood							
Batter), ¼ cup . .	100	1.0	21.0	0	0	840	0
fish mix, batter (*Don's							
Chuck Wagon*),							
¼ cup	95	4.0	21.0	0	0	710	1.0
garlic (*Zatarian's Fish-							
Fri*), 1½ tbsp.	40	1.0	9.0	0	0	580	0
garlic butter (*McCormick*							
Seafood Steamers),							
1 tbsp.	40	0	2.0	2.5	10	380	0

Food and Measure	cal.	prot. (gms)	carbo. (gms)	fat (gms)	chol. (mgs)	sod. (mgs)	fiber (gms)
lemon garlic (*McCormick* Seafood Steamers), 1 tbsp.	25	0	4.0	.5	0	400	0
lemon pepper:							
(*Oven Easy*), ¼ cup	90	2.0	13.0	3.0	0	540	0
(*Zatarain's Fish-Fri*), 1½ tbsp.	40	1.0	9.0	0	0	830	0
shrimp (Zatarain's Shrimp-Fri), 1½ tbsp.	40	1.0	9.0	0	0	460	0
Seafood entree, frozen:							
(*Contessa* Vera Cruz), 2 cups	220	18.0	34.0	1.5	45	910	5.0
scampi (*Stouffer's*), 14-oz. pkg.	410	16.0	56.0	12.0	85	960	5.0
Seafood salad kit, w/crab, crackers (*Bumble Bee*),							
2.75-oz. can salad .	90	4.0	15.0	1.0	10	550	1.0
6 crackers, .6 oz. . .	90	2.0	12.0	4.5	0	180	0
Seafood sauce (see also "Marinade," "Tartar sauce" and specific listings):							
(*McCormick* Santa Fe Style), 2 tbsp.	50	0	6.0	2.0	0	440	0
Asian (*McCormick*), 2 tbsp.	50	0	7.0	1.5	0	470	0
Cajun (*McCormick*), 2 tbsp.	15	0	3.0	0	0	370	0
cocktail, ¼ cup:							
(*Crosse & Blackwell*)	100	1.0	23.0	0	0	710	0
(*Del Monte*)	100	1.0	24.0	0	0	910	0
(*Golden Dipt*)	100	0	18.0	0	0	1280	0
(*Heinz*)	60	1.0	15.0	0	0	690	1.0
(*Kraft*)	60	1.0	11.0	.5	0	880	1.0
(*Marzetti*)	140	1.0	25.0	4.0	0	650	0
(*McCormick*)	100	0	18.0	0	0	1280	0
(*Old Bay*)	110	0	18.0	.5	0	960	0
(*Zatarain's*)	70	1.0	17.0	0	0	950	0
hot (*McCormick* Extra)	100	0	18.0	0	0	1300	0
hot and spicy (*Kraft*)	60	1.0	11.0	.5	0	900	1.0
Creole (*Crosse & Blackwell*), ¼ cup .	45	1.0	9.0	0	0	410	1.0

Food and Measure	cal.	prot. (gms)	carbo. (gms)	fat (gms)	chol. (mgs)	sod. (mgs)	fiber (gms)
Seafood sauce (cont.)							
lemon butter dill:							
(*McCormick*), 2 tbsp.	100	0	4.0	9.0	5	190	0
(*McCormick* Fat							
Free), 2 tbsp. ...	30	0	7.0	0	0	190	0
lemon dill (*Crosse &*							
Blackwell), ¼ cup .	130	0	33.0	0	0	15	0
lemon herb							
(*McCormick*), 2 tbsp.	140	0	1.0	15.0	0	220	0
Mediterranean							
(*McCormick*), 2 tbsp.	20	0	4.0	0	0	380	0
scampi:							
(*Crosse & Blackwell*),							
¼ cup	260	1.0	7.0	2.5	0	450	0
(*McCormick*), 2 tbsp.	160	0	0	17.0	0	190	0
Seafood seasoning							
(see also "Rubs,"							
"Seafood coating mix"							
and specific listings):							
(*Old Bay*), ¼ tsp.	0	0	0	0	0	160	0
(*Old Bay* 30% Less							
Sodium)	0	0	0	0	0	95	0
(*Old Bay* Seafood							
Steamers), 2 tsp. ...	15	0	2.0	0	0	640	0
blackened (*Old Bay*),							
½ tsp.	0	0	0	0	0	95	0
w/garlic and herb							
(*Old Bay*), ¼ tsp. ...	0	0	0	0	0	100	0
w/lemon and herb							
(*Old Bay*), ¼ tsp. ...	0	0	0	0	0	150	0
Seasoning, see speci-							
fic listings							
Seaweed:							
agar:							
(*Eden* Organic Agar							
Agar), .25-oz. bar	25	0	5.0	0	0	0	5.0
dried, 1 oz.	87	1.8	22.9	.1	0	29	2.2
flakes (*Eden* Organic							
Agar Agar), 1 tbsp.	0	0	1.0	0	0	10	1.0
raw, 2 tbsp.	3	.5	.7	0	0	1	<.1
strips, white (*Ro-*							
land), ½ cup .	20	0	5.0	0	0	15	0
arame, wild (*Eden*							
Organic), ½ cup .	30	1.0	7.0	0	0	120	7.0

Food and Measure	cal.	prot. (gms)	carbo. (gms)	fat (gms)	chol. (mgs)	sod. (mgs)	fiber (gms)
dulse flakes (*Eden* Organic), 1 tsp.	3	0	0	0	0	15	0
hiziki, wild (*Eden* Organic), ½ cup	30	0	6.0	0	0	160	6.0
hodai, dried (*Roland*), 2 pcs., .5 oz.	50	1.0	11.0	0	0	410	5.0
Irish moss, raw, 1 oz.	14	.4	3.5	<.1	0	19	.4
kelp, raw, 1 oz.	12	.5	2.7	.2	0	66	.4
kombu, wild (*Eden* Organic), ½ of 7" pc.	5	0	1.0	0	0	90	1.0
laver, raw, 1 oz.	10	1.6	1.4	.1	0	1	4.1
mekabu (*Eden* Organic), 1 tsp.	0	0	0	0	0	35	0
nori, 1 sheet, except as noted:							
(*Eden* Organic)	10	1.0	0	0	0	5	1.0
(*Eden* Organic Sushi)	5	1.0	0	0	0	5	1.0
(*Eden* Organic Sushi 50-sheet Pkg.)	10	1.0	<1.0	0	0	5	<1.0
(*Roland*)	10	1.0	1.0	0	0	0	1.0
krinkles, toasted (*Eden* Organic), ½ cup	10	1.0	1.0	0	0	5	1.0
spicy strips (*Eden* Organic 5-sheet Pkg.)	0	<1.0	<1.0	0	0	20	<1.0
spirulina, 1 oz.:							
raw	8	1.7	.7	.1	0	28	n.a.
dried	82	16.3	6.8	2.2	0	297	1.0
wakame:							
(*Eden* Organic), ½ cup	25	2.0	4.0	0	0	660	4.0
flakes (*Eden* Organic), 1 tsp.	0	0	0	0	0	90	0
raw, 1 oz.	13	.9	2.6	.2	0	247	.1
Seaweed chips (*Eden* Organic Sea Vegetable), 25 pcs., 1.1 oz.	140	<1.0	23.0	5.0	0	220	0
Seitan, 3 oz.:							
(*White Wave* Traditional)	90	18.0	3.0	1.0	0	380	1.0
chicken style (*White Wave* Meat of Wheat	130	24.0	9.0	0	0	270	3.0

Food and Measure	cal.	prot. (gms)	carbo. (gms)	fat (gms)	chol. (mgs)	sod. (mgs)	fiber (gms)
Seitan *(cont.)*							
stir-fry strips, vegetarian (*White Wave*)	110	22.0	2.0	1.5	0	420	1.0
Semolina, whole grain, 1 cup	601	21.2	121.6	1.8	0	2	6.5
Semolina flour (*Hodgson Mill* Pasta), <¼ cup	105	4.0	21.0	0	0	0	1.0
Sesame flour, 1 oz.:							
high fat	149	8.7	7.6	10.5	0	12	1.8
partially defatted	108	11.4	10.0	3.4	0	12	1.7
low fat	95	14.2	10.1	.5	0	11	1.4
Sesame ginger dip (*Marzetti's*), 2 tbsp.	120	1.0	2.0	12.0	20	190	0
Sesame meal, partially defatted, 1 oz.	161	4.8	7.4	13.6	0	11	1.1
Sesame nut mix (*Planters*), 1 oz. ...	160	5.0	9.0	13.0	0	240	2.0
Sesame paste (see also "Tahini"), from whole seeds, 1 tbsp.	95	2.9	4.1	8.1	0	2	.9
Sesame seed condiment, ½ tsp.:							
(*Eden Shake* Organic Furikake)	5	0	1.0	0	0	25	1.0
salt, regular, garlic, or seaweed (*Eden* Organic Gomasio) ...	15	<1.0	<1.0	1.5	0	80	0
Sesame seeds:							
whole:							
(*Arrowhead Mills* Organic), ¼ cup .	190	6.0	8.0	17.0	0	0	4.0
black (*Shiloh Farms* Organic), ¼ cup .	160	5.0	6.0	14.0	0	3	3.1
dried, 1 tbsp.	52	1.6	2.1	4.5	0	1	1.1
roasted, toasted, 1 oz.	160	4.8	7.3	13.6	0	3	4.0
kernels:							
(*Arrowhead Mills* Organic), ¼ cup .	210	9.0	3.0	19.0	0	15	1.0
dried, 1 tsp.	16	.7	.3	1.5	0	1	<1.0
toasted, 1 oz.	161	4.8	7.4	13.6	0	11	4.8
Sesame seeds, flavored (*Roland*), 1 tsp.:							
bamboo charcoal	30	1.0	2.0	2.0	0	40	0

Food and Measure	cal.	prot. (gms)	carbo. (gms)	fat (gms)	chol. (mgs)	sod. (mgs)	fiber (gms)
garlic or wasabi	30	1.0	2.0	2.0	0	45	0
plum	30	1.0	2.0	2.0	0	70	0
soy sauce	30	1.0	2.0	2.0	0	100	0
Sesame spread, see "Sesame butter"							
Sesame stick snack:							
(*SunRidge Farms*), ¼ cup, 1.1 oz.	170	3.0	14.0	12.0	0	440	<1.0
(*Tree of Life*), 1.1 oz. .	180	3.0	12.0	12.0	0	310	2.0
spelt, 1 oz.:							
(*Shiloh Farms*)	150	3.0	14.0	9.0	0	220	2.0
Cajun (*VitaSpelt*) . .	150	3.0	15.0	9.0	0	240	1.0
garlic (*VitaSpelt*) . .	150	3.0	15.0	9.0	0	220	2.0
sour cream/onion (*VitaSpelt*)	150	3.0	15.0	9.0	0	270	1.0
Sesbania flower:							
raw, 1 cup	5	.3	1.4	<.1	0	3	n.a.
steamed, ½ cup	11	.6	2.7	<.1	0	6	n.a.
Shad, meat only:							
raw, 4 oz.	223	19.2	0	15.6	85	58	0
baked or broiled, 4 oz.	286	24.6	0	20.0	109	74	0
Shallot, fresh:							
minced (*Frieda's*), 1 tbsp., 1.1 oz.	20	1.0	5.0	0	0	0	0
peeled, 1 oz.	20	.7	4.8	<.1	0	3	<1.0
chopped, 1 tbsp.	7	.3	1.7	<.1	0	1	<1.0
Shallot, freeze-dried, 1 tbsp.	3	.1	.7	tr.	0	1	<1.0
Shark, meat only, raw, 4 oz.	148	23.8	0	5.1	58	90	0
Sheepshead, meat only:							
raw, 4 oz.	123	22.9	0	2.7	56	81	0
baked or broiled, 4 oz.	143	29.5	0	1.8	73	83	0
Shellie beans, canned w/liquid, ½ cup . . .	37	2.1	7.6	.2	0	408	4.1
Shells, pasta, entree, frozen, 1 pkg., except as noted:							
and cheese, jalapeños (*Michelina's Zap'ems*), 8 oz.	340	13.0	47.0	11.0	20	690	2.0
cheese stuffed, sauce:							
(*Amy's*), 10 oz.	310	19.0	30.0	13.0	30	740	5.0
(*Celentano*), 10 oz. .	420	17.0	53.0	14.0	30	1000	7.0

Food and Measure	cal.	prot. (gms)	carbo. (gms)	fat (gms)	chol. (mgs)	sod. (mgs)	fiber (gms)
Shells, pasta, entree, cheese stuffed, sauce *(cont.)*							
(*Celentano*), ½ of 14-oz. pkg.	320	14.0	42.0	10.0	25	690	4.0
(*Celentano* Light), 10 oz.	340	17.0	53.0	6.0	20	800	7.0
w/broccoli (*Celentano* Light), 10 oz. . . .	330	16.0	53.0	5.0	15	630	8.0
cheese stuffed, w/out sauce (*Celentano*), ½ of 12.5-oz. pkg. . .	330	18.0	42.0	9.0	40	680	2.0
spinach and broccoli (Celentano Organic Vegetarian), 10 oz. . .	320	19.0	47.0	7.0	0	680	8.0
vegetables and, garlic butter sauce (*Birds Eye*), 9 oz.	270	6.0	32.0	13.0	15	430	3.0
Shells, pasta, mix, 2.5 oz. mix, except as noted:							
Alfredo (*Annie's* Organic)	260	10.0	46.0	3.5	10	670	2.0
cheddar, rice pasta (*DeBoles*), ¼ pkg. .	100	3.0	19.0	1.5	5	100	0
cheddar, white:							
(*Annie's*)	270	10.0	47.0	4.0	10	530	2.0
(*Annie's* Family Size)	270	10.0	48.0	4.5	10	550	1.0
(*Annie's* Organic) . .	280	11.0	47.0	5.0	15	530	1.0
(*Annie's* Organic Family Size)	270	12.0	46.0	4.5	10	570	2.0
(*Annie's Simply Organic*)	240	10.0	48.0	2.0	5	790	2.0
(*Kraft* Organic), ½ of 6-oz. pkg.	240	10.0	49.0	2.5	5	630	2.0
(*Pasta Roni*), 1 cup*	290	8.0	38.0	12.0	5	710	2.0
whole wheat shells (*Annie's* Organic)	270	11.0	46.0	5.0	15	530	5.0
whole wheat, extra cheesy (*Annie's* Deluxe), 3 oz., 1 cup*	260	9.0	37.0	9.0	25	620	5.0
cheddar, Wisconsin:							
(*Annie's*)	270	10.0	46.0	4.0	10	530	2.0
(*Annie's* Deluxe), 3.6 oz., 1 cup* . .	320	14.0	46.0	10.0	25	760	2.0
(*Annie's* Organic) . .	270	12.0	46.0	4.5	10	570	2.0

Food and Measure	cal.	prot. (gms)	carbo. (gms)	fat (gms)	chol. (mgs)	sod. (mgs)	fiber (gms)
cheese (*Kraft* Organic), ½ of 6-oz. pkg.	290	12.0	58.0	2.5	5	750	2.0
cheese, 4 oz. mix:							
(*Velveeta* Light 2% Milk)	330	14.0	58.0	4.5	25	990	2.0
(*Velveeta* Original) .	360	13.0	49.0	12.0	20	940	2.0
bacon (*Velveeta*) ..	360	14.0	45.0	14.0	25	1120	1.0
garlic, creamy (*Knorr Lipton Italian Sides*), ⅔ cup	270	8.0	47.0	5.0	10	740	1.0
Shepherd's pie, frozen:							
beef, see "Beef entree, frozen"							
meatless (*Amy's*), 8-oz. pkg.	160	5.0	27.0	4.0	0	490	5.0
Sherbet (see also "Sorbet"), ½ cup:							
berry rainbow (*Dreyer's/ Edy's*)	130	1.0	29.0	1.5	5	35	0
cherry (*Turkey Hill* Orchard)	120	1.0	28.0	1.0	5	15	0
lime:							
(*Blue Bunny*)	110	0	25.0	0	0	30	0
key (*Dreyer's/Edy's*)	130	1.0	28.0	1.5	5	35	0
orange:							
(*Blue Bunny*)	110	0	25.0	0	0	30	0
(*Good Humor*)	130	1.0	28.0	1.0	5	30	0
(*Land O Lakes*) ...	130	2.0	28.0	1.5	5	35	0
(*Turkey Hill* Grove) .	120	1.0	26.0	1.0	5	20	0
Swiss (*Dreyer's/Edy's*)	150	1.0	30.0	3.0	5	40	0
orange, w/vanilla ice cream:							
(*Blue Bunny* Orange Dream)	130	2.0	19.0	5.0	20	45	0
(*Breyer's* Natural) ..	130	2.0	21.0	4.0	10	35	0
(*Dreyer's/Edy's*) ...	120	1.0	23.0	2.0	10	40	0
(*Good Humor* Orange Cream) ..	120	2.0	19.0	3.5	10	35	0
swirl (*Turkey Hill*) .	130	2.0	19.0	6.0	20	35	0
pineapple (*Blue Bunny*)	100	0	25.0	0	0	25	0
rainbow, fruit:							
(*Blue Bunny*)	110	0	25.0	0	0	30	0
(*Good Humor*)	130	1.0	28.0	1.0	5	30	0
(*Turkey Hill*)	120	1.0	26.0	1.0	5	15	0

Food and Measure	cal.	prot. (gms)	carbo. (gms)	fat (gms)	chol. (mgs)	sod. (mgs)	fiber (gms)
Sherbet *(cont.)*							
raspberry:							
(*Blue Bunny*)	110	0	26.0	0	0	30	0
(*Dreyer's/Edy's*) . . .	130	1.0	28.0	1.0	4	35	0
black (*New England*							
Creamery)	110	<1.0	28.0	0	0	30	0
tropical rainbow							
(*Dreyer's/Edy's*) . . .	130	1.0	29.0	1.0	5	35	0
Sherbet bar, see "Iced							
confection bar"							
Shiso leaf powder							
(*Eden* Organic), 1 tsp.	0	0	0	0	0	200	0
Shortening, all varieties							
(*Crisco*), 1 tbsp. . . .	110	0	0	12.0	0	0	0
Shrimp, meat only:							
raw, 4 oz.	120	23.0	1.0	2.0	173	168	0
raw, 4 large, 1 oz.	30	5.7	.3	.5	43	42	0
boiled or steamed:							
4 oz.	112	23.7	0	1.2	221	254	0
4 large, .8 oz.	22	4.6	0	.2	43	49	0
Shrimp, can or pkg.:							
(*Chicken of the Sea*							
Pouch), 2.5 oz. . . .	55	12.0	1.0	.5	180	500	0
all varieties, 2 oz.:							
(*Bumble Bee*)	40	10.0	0	0	115	430	0
(*Chicken of the Sea*)	45	10.0	1.0	.5	145	400	0
canned, 1 cup	154	29.6	1.3	2.5	222	216	0
Shrimp, frozen (see							
also "Shrimp entree"):							
barbecue:							
(*Contessa*), 4 pcs.:							
w/sauce	150	17.0	6.0	7.0	135	960	0
w/out sauce	120	17.0	3.0	4.0	140	490	0
bacon wrapped							
(*Original Rangoon*							
Rangoons), 3 pcs.	140	15.0	3.0	8.0	40	470	0
battered:							
beer (*Gorton's Shrimp*							
Temptations),							
5 pcs., 3.5 oz. . .	240	7.0	25.0	12.0	40	670	0
beer (*Mrs. Paul's/*							
Van de Kamp's),							
6 pcs., 4 oz.	200	14.0	22.0	6.0	90	750	1.0

Food and Measure	cal.	prot. (gms)	carbo. (gms)	fat (gms)	chol. (mgs)	sod. (mgs)	fiber (gms)
tempura (*Blue Horizon Organic*), 3.5 oz.	160	15.0	21.0	1.5	85	290	1.0
tempura (*Tiger Thai*):							
shrimp, 1-oz. pc.	70	3.0	7.0	3.0	15	50	<1.0
sauce, 1 oz.	30	<1.0	7.0	0	0	670	0
breaded:							
(*Matlaw's* Torpedo):							
shrimp, 4 oz. ...	180	16.0	24.0	2.5	95	370	3.0
sauce, ½ cup ...	80	2.0	20.0	0	0	1010	1.0
(*Schooner* Crunchies), 6 pcs., 3.2 oz. ..	210	7.0	28.0	7.0	30	420	1.0
garlic (*Blue Horizon Organic*), 3.5 oz.	160	15.0	21.0	2.0	80	360	1.0
breaded, butterfly:							
(*Gorton's Shrimp Temptations*), 5 pcs., 3.5 oz. ..	250	11.0	27.0	11.0	55	430	4.0
(*Mrs. Paul's/Van de Kamp's*), 7 pcs., 4 oz.	250	12.0	27.0	11.0	65	540	1.0
cocktail (*.Margaritaville* Paradise), ½ pkg.:							
shrimp, 3 oz.	60	12.0	0	0	130	340	0
sauce, 2 tbsp.	26	0	6.0	0	0	391	<1.0
coconut:							
(*Contessa*), 5 pcs.:							
w/sauce	270	9.0	29.0	14.0	75	440	3.0
w/out sauce	230	8.0	18.0	14.0	75	390	1.0
(*Margaritaville* Calypso), ½ pkg.:							
shrimp, 4 oz. ...	300	12.0	25.0	17.0	70	530	0
sauce, 2 tbsp. ..	50	0	14.0	0	0	160	0
curry, Thai (*Contessa*), 5 pcs.:							
w/sauce	290	7.0	34.0	14.0	65	1070	1.0
w/out sauce	210	7.0	15.0	14.0	60	790	1.0
w/jalapeño, asiago cheese (*Original Rangoon*), 3 pcs. ...	150	18.0	2.0	8.0	90	470	0
jerk (*Margaritaville* Jammin'), ½ of 8-oz. pkg.	140	16.0	4.0	7.0	145	1040	0

Food and Measure	cal.	prot. (gms)	carbo. (gms)	fat (gms)	chol. (mgs)	sod. (mgs)	fiber (gms)
Shrimp, frozen *(cont.)*							
lemon butter sauced (*Gorton's Shrimp Temptations*), 4 oz.	120	8.0	8.0	6.0	65	740	0
lime (*Margaritaville Island*), ½ of 8-oz. pkg.	130	16.0	2.0	7.0	155	720	0
Marsala (*Contessa*), 10 pcs.:							
w/sauce	230	11.0	28.0	7.0	105	560	1.0
w/out sauce	130	11.0	17.0	1.5	100	440	1.0
orange (*Contessa*), 10 pcs.:							
w/sauce	180	11.0	29.0	2.0	100	750	2.0
w/out sauce	130	11.0	17.0	1.5	100	440	1.0
panko (*Blue Horizon Organic*), 3.5 oz. . .	160	15.0	22.0	1.5	80	360	1.0
Parmesan garlic butter (*Matlaw's* Natural), 2 pcs., 2 oz.	140	9.0	3.0	10.0	90	270	0
popcorn, breaded:							
(*Blue Horizon Organic*), 3.5 oz.	160	15.0	21.0	2.0	80	360	1.0
(*Gorton's*), 20 pcs., 3.2 oz.	240	8.0	24.0	12.0	55	630	0
(*Mrs. Paul's/Van de Kamp's*), 20 pcs., 4 oz.	260	11.0	30.0	11.0	80	750	2.0
(*Schooner*), 12 pcs., 3.5 oz.	150	7.0	14.0	7.0	15	80	1.0
scampi:							
(*Contessa*), 8 pcs., 4 oz.	240	10.0	6.0	19.0	105	540	1.0
(*Margaritaville* Sunset), ½ of 8-oz. pkg.	270	12.0	10.0	20.0	130	460	0
sauced (*Gorton's Shrimp Temptations*), 4 oz.	120	10.0	8.0	6.0	65	630	<1.0
skewers (*Margaritaville* Sunset), ⅓ pkg.:							
shrimp, 4 oz.	80	14.0	5.0	1.0	150	840	0
sauce, 2 tbsp.	25	0	6.0	0	35	35	0
stuffed w/crab (*Matlaw's*), 1.5-oz. pc. . .	70	7.0	3.0	3.0	.65	180	0

Food and Measure	cal.	prot. (gms)	carbo. (gms)	fat (gms)	chol. (mgs)	sod. (mgs)	fiber (gms)
whiskey Jack (*Contessa*), 8 pcs., 4 oz.	210	9.0	4.0	18.0	70	670	1.0
wontons (*Original Rangoon Rangoons*), 3 pcs.	220	12.0	29.0	5.0	25	580	<1.0
Shrimp coating, see "Seafood coating mix"							
Shrimp cocktail, see "Shrimp, frozen"							
Shrimp dinner, frozen, garlic (*Healthy Choice*), 11.5-oz. pkg.	280	13.0	44.0	5.0	25	600	5.0
Shrimp entree, frozen (see also "Shrimp, frozen"), 1 pkg. except as noted:							
Alfredo:							
(*Gorton's* Shrimp Bowl), 10.5 oz. . . .	250	13.0	39.0	5.0	75	1230	4.0
(*Lean Cuisine* Café Classics), 9 oz. . . .	260	18.0	36.0	5.0	60	590	3.0
(*Michelina's Signature*), 8 oz.	300	15.0	35.0	11.0	90	430	2.0
penne (*Blue Horizon Organic*), ½ of 10-oz. pkg.	430	17.0	39.0	22.0	115	380	2.0
and angel-hair pasta (*Lean Cuisine* Café Classics), 10 oz.	220	14.0	32.0	4.0	50	590	2.0
fajita (*Contessa*), seasoned, 2 pcs., 8 oz.	290	16.0	46.0	4.0	50	760	4.0
fried rice, see "Rice entree, frozen"							
garlic (*Birds Eye Voila!*), 1 cup	220	9.0	27.0	8.0	10	510	2.0
garlic butter (*Gorton's* Bowl), 10.5 oz.	260	13.0	38.0	6.0	65	910	2.0
General Tsao (*Contessa*):							
w/sauce, 8.7 oz. . . .	280	11.0	55.0	1.5	55	750	3.0
w/out sauce, 7.4 oz.	200	10.0	37.0	1.0	55	270	3.0
kung pao (*Contessa*):							
w/sauce, 8 oz.	200	10.0	30.0	3.5	45	760	3.0
w/out sauce, 6.7 oz.	160	9.0	24.0	3.5	45	240	3.0

Food and Measure	cal.	prot. (gms)	carbo. (gms)	fat (gms)	chol. (mgs)	sod. (mgs)	fiber (gms)
Shrimp entree *(cont.)*							
lemon garlic (*Lean Cuisine Dinnertime Selects*), 12 oz. . . .	350	18.0	54.0	7.0	75	830	5.0
lime cilantro (*Kashi*), 10 oz.	250	12.0	33.0	8.0	10	690	6.0
lo mein:							
(*Contessa*):							
w/sauce, 8 oz. . .	250	13.0	39.0	4.0	40	750	3.0
w/out sauce, 7 oz.	190	12.0	29.0	2.5	40	290	3.0
(*Smart Ones* Dragon), 9.25 oz.	240	14.0	36.0	4.0	75	690	3.0
marinara, w/linguine (*Smart Ones*), 9 oz.	180	9.0	30.0	1.5	20	750	4.0
Mediterranean:							
(*Contessa*):							
w/sauce, 10 oz. .	400	23.0	63.0	5.0	35	750	6.0
w/out sauce, 8.5 oz.	320	22.0	46.0	5.0	35	330	6.0
(*Contessa* le Menu):							
w/sauce, 8 oz.	190	12.0	29.0	2.5	35	570	3.0
w/out sauce, 7 oz.	140	10.0	24.0	.5	35	170	2.0
pasta, lemon and garlic (*Cedarlane Dr. Sears Zone*), 11 oz.	340	24.0	34.0	12.0	95	730	4.0
w/pasta, vegetables (*Michelina's Lean Gourmet*), 8 oz.	260	11.0	39.0	6.0	45	520	2.0
penne vodka w/ (*Blue Horizon Organic*), ½ of 10-oz. pkg. . .	270	17.0	38.0	6.0	75	280	3.0
pesto farfalle w/ (*Blue Horizon Organic*), ½ of 10-oz. pkg. . .	280	17.0	38.0	6.0	70	430	3.0
primavera (*Contessa* le Menu):							
w/sauce, 7 oz.	280	12.0	32.0	11.0	35	590	3.0
w/out sauce, 6 oz. .	180	12.0	29.0	1.0	35	180	3.0
primavera or Santa Fe (*Contessa*):							
w/sauce, 7 oz.	260	12.0	26.0	12.0	75	640	2.0
w/out sauce, 6 oz. .	160	11.0	24.0	2.0	75	240	2.0
scampi:							
(*Birds Eye Voila!*), 1 cup*	190	11.0	31.0	2.5	60	540	3.0

Food and Measure	cal.	prot. (gms)	carbo. (gms)	fat (gms)	chol. (mgs)	sod. (mgs)	fiber (gms)
(*Michelina's Lean Gourmet*), 8 oz. .	290	10.0	45.0	6.0	30	630	2.0
(*Stouffer's Corner Bistro*), 14 oz. . . .	410	21.0	57.0	11.0	80	990	6.0
rotini w/ (*Blue Horizon Organic*), ½ of 10-oz. pkg.	270	17.0	38.0	6.0	75	280	3.0
Spanish (*Contessa*):							
w/sauce, 10 oz. . . .	250	15.0	34.0	5.0	70	950	4.0
w/out sauce, 8.4 oz.	200	15.0	30.0	2.0	60	570	3.0
stir-fry:							
(*Contessa*):							
w/sauce, 10 oz. .	230	18.0	32.0	2.0	40	740	4.0
w/out sauce, 8.4 oz.	150	17.0	14.0	2.0	40	270	4.0
(*Contessa* le Menu):							
w/sauce, 8 oz. . .	140	8.0	24.0	.5	35	540	4.0
w/out sauce, 6 oz.	80	7.0	10.0	0	35	180	4.0
Szechuan, w/ (*Lean Cuisine Spa Cuisine*), 9 oz.	230	13.0	39.0	2.5	60	680	5.0
sweet/sour (*Contessa*):							
w/sauce, 10 oz. . . .	250	14.0	46.0	.5	65	490	4.0
w/out sauce, 8.6 oz.	200	13.0	34.0	0	65	310	3.0
teriyaki (*Gorton's* Bowl), 10.5 oz.	320	10.0	57.0	6.0	45	1250	2.0
Sloppy Joe sauce, see "Sandwich sauce"							
Sloppy Joe seasoning:							
(*Lawry's*), 2 tsp.	20	0	5.0	0	0	480	0
(*McCormick*), 1 tsp. . . .	20	0	3.0	0	0	300	0
Smelt, rainbow, meat only:							
raw, 4 oz.	110	20.0	0	2.8	80	68	0
baked or broiled, 4 oz.	141	25.6	0	3.5	102	87	0
Snack chips/crisps (see also "Snack mix" and specific listings), 1 oz., except as noted:							
(*Ritz* Toasted)	130	2.0	21.0	4.5	0	290	1.0
all varieties (*Wheat Thins* Toasted)	120	2.0	20.0	4.0	0	290	1.0
apple cinnamon (*Garden Harvest* Toasted)	120	2.0	22.0	3.0	0	65	3.0

Food and Measure	cal.	prot. (gms)	carbo. (gms)	fat (gms)	chol. (mgs)	sod. (mgs)	fiber (gms)
Snack chips/crisps *(cont.)*							
banana (*Garden Harvest* Toasted)	120	2.0	22.0	3.0	0	60	3.0
bruschetta bread crisps (*Gardetto's*), 1.1 oz.	110	3.0	17.0	3.0	0	330	2.0
cheddar:							
(*Ritz* Toasted)	130	2.0	19.0	6.0	0	290	1.0
aged (*Snyder's* Multi-Grain Puffs), 1.1 oz.	130	2.0	18.0	6.0	0	280	2.0
baked (*Snyder's* MultiGrain Crunchies)	130	2.0	18.0	6.0	0	280	2.0
white (*Snyder's* MultiGrain Puffs), 1.1 oz.	130	2.0	18.0	6.0	0	230	3.0
chili and lime (*Sabritones*)	150	2.0	13.0	10.0	0	690	1.0
garlic, roasted, rye (*Gardetto's* Special Request), 1.1 oz.	160	2.0	16.0	10.0	0	340	1.0
ranch, Southwest (*Ritz* Toasted)	130	2.0	19.0	6.0	0	260	1.0
rosemary olive oil bread chips (*Gardetto's* Special Request), 1.1 oz.	140	4.0	19.0	5.0	0	300	0
sour cream/onion (*Ritz* Toasted)	130	2.0	19.0	6.0	0	270	0
tomato basil (*Garden Harvest* Toasted)	120	2.0	20.0	4.0	0	220	3.0
vegetable (*Garden Harvest* Toasted)	120	2.0	20.0	3.5	0	240	3.0
Snack mix (see also "Trail mix"):							
(*Beer Nuts* Bar Mix), 1 oz.	160	4.0	18.0	9.0	0	290	2.0
(*Cheerios* Original), 2/3 cup	110	3.0	20.0	3.0	0	300	1.0
(*Cheez-It* Party Mix), 1/2 cup	120	3.0	21.0	4.5	0	290	1.0
(*Chex Mix* Bold Party Blend), 1/2 cup	140	3.0	20.0	6.0	0	390	<1.0
(*Chex Mix* Traditional), 2/3 cup	130	2.0	22.0	4.0	0	380	1.0

Food and Measure	cal.	prot. (gms)	carbo. (gms)	fat (gms)	chol. (mgs)	sod. (mgs)	fiber (gms)
(*Gardetto's* Original), ½ cup	150	3.0	20.0	6.0	0	310	1.0
(*Gardetto's* Reduced Fat), ½ cup	130	3.0	20.0	4.0	0	320	1.0
(*Hershey's Snacksters*), .7-oz. pkg.	100	1.0	15.0	3.5	<5	60	1.0
(*Munchies Flamin' Hot*), 1 oz., ¾ cup	140	2.0	18.0	7.0	0	200	1.0
(*Nabisco* Traditional), 1.1 oz.	130	2.0	21.0	5.0	0	360	1.0
(*Nabisco Mixers*), 1 oz.	130	2.0	19.0	4.5	0	340	1.0
(*Quaker* Traditional), ½ cup	130	2.0	19.0	5.0	0	220	1.0
(*Reese's Snacksters*), .7-oz. pkg.	100	2.0	13.0	4.0	0	65	<1.0
(*SunRidge Farms* Zen Party Mix), ¼ cup, 1.1 oz.	160	5.0	11.0	11.0	0	190	2.0
cheddar:							
(*Cheerios*), ⅔ cup	120	3.0	21.0	3.0	0	310	1.0
(*Chex Simply*), ⅔ cup	130	3.0	22.0	4.0	0	380	1.0
(*Chex Mix*), ⅔ cup	130	2.0	22.0	4.0	0	330	<1.0
(*Quaker* Baked), ½ cup	130	2.0	19.0	4.5	0	230	1.0
cheese:							
(*Munchies* Cheese Fix), ¾ cup	140	2.0	18.0	7.0	0	250	1.0
Italian blend (*Gardetto's*), ½ cup	140	3.0	20.0	5.0	0	320	<1.0
chocolate, dark (*Chex Mix*), ⅔ cup	140	2.0	23.0	4.5	0	170	<1.0
chocolate peanut butter (*Chex Mix*), ⅔ cup	150	3.0	24.0	5.0	0	190	<1.0
chocolate turtle (*Chex Mix*), ⅔ cup	150	2.0	24.0	5.0	<5	230	<1.0
cinnamon crunch (*Quaker*), ½ cup	130	2.0	20.0	5.0	0	80	2.0
fruit/nut, ⅔ cup:							
apple cinnamon walnut (*Chex Mix*)	130	1.0	24.0	3.5	0	180	<1.0
tropical, w/almond (*Chex Mix*)	140	1.0	24.0	5.0	0	160	<1.0
honey graham (*Quaker*), ½ cup	140	2.0	19.0	6.0	0	120	2.0

Food and Measure	cal.	prot. (gms)	carbo. (gms)	fat (gms)	chol. (mgs)	sod. (mgs)	fiber (gms)
Snack mix *(cont.)*							
hot and spicy (*Chex Mix*),							
⅔ cup	130	2.0	20.0	4.0	0	420	1.0
Italian recipe							
(*Gardetto's*), ½ cup	150	3.0	20.0	6.0	0	290	<1.0
multigrain (*SunChips*),							
1 oz.:							
original	140	2.0	18.0	6.0	0	120	2.0
cheddar or salsa	140	2.0	19.0	6.0	0	160	2.0
onion, French	140	2.0	18.0	6.0	0	130	2.0
Oriental, ¼ cup:							
cracker mix (*Sun-*							
Ridge Farms)	110	2.0	27.0	0	0	200	0
party mix (*SunRidge*							
Farms)	160	5.0	12.0	11.0	0	200	2.0
peanut lovers (*Chex*							
Mix), ½ cup	140	3.0	19.0	5.0	0	340	1.0
ranch (*Chex Mix*							
Summer), ⅔ cup	120	3.0	21.0	3.0	0	430	<1.0
ranch (*Munchies*							
Totally), ¾ cup	140	2.0	19.0	6.0	0	250	1.0
sweet and salty (*Chex*							
Mix), ½ cup:							
caramel crunch	130	2.0	23.0	3.5	0	250	1.0
honey nut	130	2.0	22.0	4.0	0	280	<1.0
trail mix	140	2.0	22.0	4.5	0	230	1.0
wasabi:							
(*Sunbird Snacks*),							
⅔ cup	150	5.0	17.0	7.0	0	300	1.0
(*SunRidge Farms*							
Samurai), ¼ cup	130	4.0	18.0	5.0	0	125	1.0
Snail, fresh, raw, 1 oz.	26	4.6	<.1	.4	14	20	0
Snail, canned:							
(*Fanci Food* Very Large),							
6 pcs.	25	5.0	0	.5	65	85	0
(*Roland* Extra Large),							
½ cup	50	10.0	1.0	1.0	135	150	1.0
Snail, sea, see							
"Whelk"							
Snapper, meat only:							
raw, 4 oz.	113	23.3	0	1.5	42	73	0
baked or broiled, 4 oz.	145	30.0	0	2.0	53	65	0
Snow peas, see "Peas,							
edible-podded"							

Food and Measure	cal.	prot. (gms)	carbo. (gms)	fat (gms)	chol. (mgs)	sod. (mgs)	fiber (gms)
Soft drinks, carbonated, 12 fl. oz., except as noted:							
(*Blue Sky* Dr. Becker) .	140	0	38.0	0	0	10	0
apple:							
(*Goya*)	150	0	37.0	0	0	10	0
(*Izze*)	138	0	34.0	0	0	10	0
(*R.W. Knudsen* Spritzer Organic)	170	0	44.0	0	0	35	
(*Sidra Mundet*), 8 fl. oz.	130	0	31.0	0	0	40	0
blackberry (*Izze*)	100	1.0	23.0	0	0	10	0
boysenberry (*R.W. Knudsen* Spritzer) .	160	<1.0	40.0	0	0	20	<1.0
cherry (*Santa Cruz Organic*)	140	0	34.0	0	0	20	0
cherry, black:							
(*Blue Sky* Natural) . .	140	0	37.0	0	0	10	0
(*Blue Sky* Organic Cherish)	150	0	37.0	0	0	10	0
(*IBC*)	180	0	48.0	0	0	55	0
(*R.W. Knudsen* Spritzer)	180	<1.0	46.0	0	0	30	0
(*R.W. Knudsen* Spritzer Light) . .	100	0	26.0	0	0	30	0
cherry vanilla crème (*Blue Sky*)	170	0	46.0	0	0	10	0
Clementine (*Izze*)	100	0	23.0	0	0	10	0
coconut (*Goya*)	200	0	45.0	0	0	65	0
cola:							
(*Blue Sky* Natural) . .	160	0	42.0	0	0	10	0
(*Blue Sky* Organic) .	160	0	40.0	0	0	10	0
(*Coca-Cola* Classic)	140	0	39.0	0	0	50	0
(*Dr Pepper/Dr Pepper Free*), 8 fl. oz.	100	0	27.0	0	0	35	0
(*Goya* Champagne) .	200	0	47.0	0	0	60	0
(*Pepsi/Pepsi* Free) .	150	0	41.0	0	0	30	0
cherry (*R.W. Knudsen* Spritzer)	170	<1.0	41.0	0	0	25	0
cherry, wild (*Pepsi*) .	160	0	42.0	0	0	30	0
cherry vanilla (*Dr Pepper*), 8 fl. oz.	100	0	26.0	0	0	40	0
citrus, 8 fl. oz.:							
(*Mountain Dew*) . . .	110	0	31.0	0	0	40	0

Food and Measure	cal.	prot. (gms)	carbo. (gms)	fat (gms)	chol. (mgs)	sod. (mgs)	fiber (gms)
Soft drinks, citrus *(cont.)*							
(*Mountain Dew Code Red*)	110	0	31.0	0	0	50	0
(*7Up/7Up Cherry*) .	100	0	26.0	0	0	25	0
(*Sun Drop*)	130	0	34.0	0	0	20	0
cranberry (*R.W. Knudsen* Spritzer) .	190	1.0	46.0	0	0	65	0
cream:							
(*A&W*), 8 fl. oz. . . .	120	0	31.0	0	0	30	0
(*Blue Sky*)	140	0	38.0	0	0	10	0
(*IBC*)	180	0	48.0	0	0	75	0
(*Mug*)	180	0	47.0	0	0	60	0
vanilla crème (*R.W. Knudsen* Spritzer)	160	<1.0	38.0	0	0	25	0
vanilla crème (*Santa Cruz Organic*) . . .	160	0	40.0	0	0	10	0
fruit punch:							
(*Goya*)	190	0	49.0	0	0	40	0
(*Jarritos* Tutti Frutti), 8 fl. oz.	120	0	29.0	0	0	50	0
ginger ale:							
(*Blue Sky* Jamaican)	140	0	37.0	0	0	10	0
(*Blue Sky* Organic) .	150	0	39.0	0	0	10	0
(*Canada Dry*)	120	0	33.0	0	0	40	0
(*R.W. Knudsen* Spritzer)	160	<1.0	39.0	0	0	20	0
(*Santa Cruz Organic*)	150	0	37.0	0	0	10	0
(*Schweppes*)	120	0	34.0	0	0	60	0
ginger beer:							
(*Goya*)	190	0	43.0	0	0	30	0
(*Reed's* Jamaican Brew Premium/ Extra Ginger) . . .	145	0	37.4	0	0	5	0
golden (*Goya* El Dorado)	160	0	39.0	0	0	30	0
grape:							
(*Blue Sky*)	130	0	36.0	0	0	10	0
(*Goya*)	230	0	57.0	0	0	5	0
(*R.W. Knudsen* Spritzer)	180	<1.0	45.0	0	0	20	0
(*Tropicana Twister*)	190	0	50.0	0	0	65	0
Concord (*Santa Cruz Organic*)	150	0	36.0	0	0	15	0

Food and Measure	cal.	prot. (gms)	carbo. (gms)	fat (gms)	chol. (mgs)	sod. (mgs)	fiber (gms)
grapefruit:							
(*Blue Sky*)	140	0	38.0	0	0	10	0
(*Goya*)	180	0	46.0	0	0	35	0
(*Izze*)	150	2.0	37.0	0	0	15	0
(*Jarritos* Toronja),							
13.5 fl. oz.	190	0	47.0	0	0	80	0
pink (*Mirinda*)	160	0	43.0	0	0	65	0
guava:							
(*Goya*)	170	0	42.0	0	0	30	0
(*Jarritos* Guayaba),							
13.5 fl. oz.	190	0	48.0	0	0	60	0
guarana (*Goya*)	160	0	39.0	0	0	0	0
lemon (*Izze*)	150	1.0	36.0	0	0	15	0
lemon lime:							
(*Blue Sky* Natural) .	130	0	35.0	0	0	10	0
(*Blue Sky* Organic) .	160	0	40.0	0	0	10	0
(*Goya*)	170	0	42.0	0	0	35	0
(*R.W. Knudsen*							
Spritzer)	170	1.0	41.0	0	0	25	0
(*Santa Cruz Organic*)	140	0	36.0	0	0	10	0
(*Sierra Mist*)	140	0	39.0	0	0	35	0
(*Sprite/Sprite*							
Remix)	140	0	38.0	0	0	70	0
lemonade (see also							
"Lemonade"):							
(*R.W. Knudsen*							
Spritzer Light) ..	90	<1.0	22.0	0	0	20	0
(*Santa Cruz Organic*)	150	0	38.0	0	0	0	0
Jamaican (*R.W.*							
Knudsen Spritzer)	160	<1.0	40.0	0	0	20	0
raspberry (*Santa*							
Cruz Organic) ...	120	0	29.0	0	0	10	0
lime (*Jarritos* Limon),							
13.5 fl. oz.	190	0	48.0	0	0	65	0
mandarin (*R.W.*							
Knudsen Spritzer) .	170	1.0	40.0	0	0	30	0
mango:							
(*R.W. Knudsen*							
Spritzer)	170	<1.0	42.0	0	0	20	0
(*R.W. Knudsen*							
Spritzer Light) ..	110	<1.0	27.0	0	0	20	0
(*R.W. Knudsen*							
Spritzer Fandango)	170	1.0	42.0	0	0	20	0

Food and Measure	cal.	prot. (gms)	carbo. (gms)	fat (gms)	chol. (mgs)	sod. (mgs)	fiber (gms)
Soft drinks *(cont.)*							
orange:							
(*Blue Sky* Natural Truly)	140	0	38.0	0	0	10	0
(*Blue Sky* Organic Divine)	180	0	44.0	0	0	10	0
(*Goya* Mandarin) ..	170	0	44.0	0	0	35	0
(*Jarritos* Mandarin), 13.5 fl. oz.	200	0	50.0	0	0	65	0
(*Mirinda*)	180	0	48.0	0	0	35	0
(*Tropicana Twister*)	190	0	52.0	0	0	35	0
crème (*Blue Sky*) ..	160	0	44.0	0	0	10	0
orange passion fruit (*R.W. Knudsen* Spritzer)	160	<1.0	42.0	0	0	20	0
peach (*R.W. Knudsen* Spritzer)	160	2.0	39.0	0	0	25	0
pear (*Izze*)	130	1.0	33.0	0	0	15	0
pineapple:							
(*Goya*)	170	0	43.0	0	0	40	0
(*Jarritos* Pina), 13.5 fl. oz.	190	0	48.0	0	0	65	0
pomegranate (*Izze*) ..	120	0	34.0	0	0	15	0
raspberry:							
(*Blue Sky*)	170	0	45.0	0	0	10	0
(*R.W. Knudsen* Spritzer Bottle) ..	200	<1.0	46.0	0	0	25	0
(*R.W. Knudsen* Spritzer Can) ...	170	0	38.0	0	0	25	0
(*R.W. Knudsen* Spritzer Light) ..	110	<1.0	26.0	0	0	20	0
root beer:							
(*A&W*), 8 fl. oz. ...	120	0	31.0	0	0	30	0
(*Barq's*), 8 fl. oz. ..	110	0	30.0	0	0	50	0
(*Blue Sky* Natural) .	160	0	43.0	0	0	10	0
(*Blue Sky* Organic Encore)	170	0	43.0	0	0	10	0
(*IBC*)	160	0	43.0	0	0	55	0
(*Mug*)	160	0	43.0	0	0	65	0
(*Santa Cruz Organic*)	150	0	36.0	0	0	0	0
sangria (*Senorial*) ...	180	0	44.0	0	0	70	0
strawberry:							
(*Jarritos Fresa*), 13.5 fl. oz.	190	0	48.0	0	0	60	0

Food and Measure	cal.	prot. (gms)	carbo. (gms)	fat (gms)	chol. (mgs)	sod. (mgs)	fiber (gms)
(*Mirinda*)	160	0	43.0	0	0	65	0
(*R.W. Knudsen* Spritzer)	160	<1.0	39.0	0	0	20	0
(*Tropicana Twister*)	160	0	43.0	0	0	50	0
tamarind (*Jarritos*), 13.5 fl. oz.	200	0	50.0	0	0	65	0
tangerine:							
(*R.W. Knudsen* Spritzer)	200	<1.0	48.0	0	0	25	0
(*R.W. Knudsen* Spritzer Light) ..	90	<1.0	22.0	0	0	20	0
(*Santa Cruz Organic*)	160	0	39.0	0	0	15	0
tonic (*Schweppes*) ...	130	0	35.0	0	0	55	0
vanilla crème, see "cream," above							
Sofrito, in jars (*Goya*), 1 tsp.	0	0	0	0	0	45	0
Sole, see "Flatfish"							
Sole entree, frozen, stuffed (*Oven Poppers*), 5-oz. pc., except as noted:							
crabmeat	240	17.0	15.0	13.0	35	400	0
crabmeat, lump	200	18.0	9.0	10.0	80	430	0
crabmeat mini, 2 oz. .	120	6.0	8.0	7.0	25	140	0
w/garlic, shrimp, and almonds	260	16.0	16.0	14.0	60	380	0
w/shrimp, lobster, in Newberg sauce ...	170	21.0	6.0	6.0	130	540	0
w/spinach, cheese ...	210	15.0	13.0	10.0	55	270	0
Sopressata, 1 oz.:							
(*Di Lusso*)	110	7.0	0	9.0	30	400	0
hot (*Dietz & Watson*) .	90	8.0	1.0	7.0	22	500	0
hot or sweet:							
(*Applegate Farms*) .	100	8.0	0	7.0	15	540	0
(*Boar's Head*)	100	8.0	0	7.0	25	500	0
sweet (*Dietz & Watson*)	90	5.0	1.0	6.0	14	500	0
Sorbet (see also "Sherbet"), ½ cup:							
acai berry (*Häagen-Dazs Reserve* Brazilian) .	120	0	25.0	2.0	0	0	1.0
berries, mixed (*Sharon's*)	110	0	24.0	0	0	11	1.0
blackberry cabernet (*Ciao Bella*)	111	0	27.0	0	0	0	2.0

Food and Measure	cal.	prot. (gms)	carbo. (gms)	fat (gms)	chol. (mgs)	sod. (mgs)	fiber (gms)
Sorbet *(cont.)*							
blueberry:(*Sharon's*)	80	0	21.0	0	0	0	1.0
w/blackberry (*Ben & Jerry's Berried Treasure*)	110	0	29.0	0	0	5	1.0
chocolate:							
(*Ciao Bella*)	157	2.0	43.0	<1.0	0	25	3.0
(*Häagen-Dazs*)	130	2.0	28.0	.5	0	70	2.0
(*Sharon's* Dutch)	150	0	27.0	0	0	20	>1.0
coconut:							
(*Ciao Bella*)	180	1.0	27.0	9.0	0	15	0
(*Häagen-Dazs*)	170	1.0	26.0	7.0	0	26	0
(*Palapa Azul*)	110	1.0	15.0	6.0	0	15	0
(*Sharon's*)	180	<1.0	24.0	8.0	0	30	0
hibiscus flower (*Palapa Azul*)	110	1.0	28.0	0	0	0	0
lemon:							
(*Ciao Bella*)	140	0	36.0	0	0	0	0
(*Häagen-Dazs Zesty*)	110	0	28.0	0	0	25	<1.0
(*Sharon's*)	130	0	32.0	0	0	0	0
mango:							
(*Ciao Bella*)	107	<1.0	27.0	0	0	0	1.0
(*Häagen-Dazs*)	120	0	37.0	0	0	10	0
(*Palapa Azul*)	80	0	21.0	0	0	0	0
(*Sharon's*)	100	0	25.0	0	0	0	<1.0
orange, blood (*Ciao Bella*)	98	0	24.0	0	0	5	3.0
passion fruit:							
(*Ciao Bella*)	92	1.0	22.0	0	0	4	0
(*Sharon's*)	120	<1.0	30.0	0	0	100	0
peach (*Häagen-Dazs Orchard*)	130	0	33.0	0	0	0	<1.0
pineapple, w/passion fruit (*Ben & Jerry's Jamaican Me Crazy*)	130	0	33.0	0	0	10	1.0
raspberry:							
(*Ciao Bella*)	100	0	25.0	0	0	0	1.0
(*Häagen-Dazs*)	120	0	30.0	0	0	0	2.0
(*Sharon's*)	110	0	26.0	0	0	8	>1.0
strawberry:							
(*Häagen-Dazs*)	120	0	31.0	0	0	10	1.0
(*Sharon's*)	110	0	23.0	0	0	0	1.0
strawberry Chardonnay (*Ciao Bella*)	170	0	36.0	0	0	0	1.0

Food and Measure	cal.	prot. (gms)	carbo. (gms)	fat (gms)	chol. (mgs)	sod. (mgs)	fiber (gms)
strawberry kiwi (*Ben & Jerry's*)	110	0	29.0	0	0	10	1.0
tropical (*Häagen-Dazs*)	150	0	38.0	0	0	25	0
Sorbet bar (see also "Fruit bar"), 1 bar:							
orange or raspberry, vanilla ice cream: (*Healthy Choice*) ..	90	1.0	17.0	1.0	5	35	1.0
raspberry w/vanilla yogurt (*Häagen-Dazs*)	100	2.0	21.0	0	0	12	<1.0
Sorghum, whole grain: (*Shiloh Farms* Organic),							
½ cup	339	11.0	66.0	3.0	0	6	10.0
1 cup	650	21.7	143.3	6.3	0	12	n.a.
Sorghum syrup:							
½ cup	479	0	123.7	0	0	13	0
1 tbsp.	61	0	15.7	0	0	2	0
Sorrel, see "Dock"							
Soup, ready-to-serve, 1 cup, except as noted:							
acorn squash and mango, creamy (*Imagine* Organic) .	70	1.0	14.0	1.5	0	430	2.0
alphabet (*Amy's* Organic)	80	3.0	16.0	0	0	580	2.0
bean:							
(*Amy's* Tuscan Organic)	160	5.0	25.0	4.5	0	680	5.0
(*Dominique's* U.S. Senate)	170	11.0	29.0	1.5	0	800	9.0
and ham (*Campbell's Chunky* Hearty) .	180	11.0	30.0	2.0	10	780	8.0
and ham (*Healthy Choice*)	180	11.0	29.0	2.0	5	480	10.0
bean, black:							
(*Imagine Bistro* Organic Cuban) .	170	8.0	30.0	3.5	0	480	6.0
(*Muir Glen* Organic Southwest)	130	7.0	25.0	<1.0	0	680	8.0
w/bacon (*Progresso*)	160	8.0	29.0	1.0	<5	760	8.0
w/chicken sausage, spicy (*Pacific* Organic)	170	11.0	28.0	3.0	10	650	8.0

Food and Measure	cal.	prot. (gms)	carbo. (gms)	fat (gms)	chol. (mgs)	sod. (mgs)	fiber (gms)
Soup, bean, black, *(cont.)*							
red pepper, blended (*Campbell's Select*)	120	3.0	23.0	1.5	<5	820	4.0
vegetable (*Amy's Organic*)	130	6.0	25.0	1.5	0	430	5.0
bean, white:							
w/roasted ham (*Campbell's Select Savory*)	170	9.0	30.0	1.0	5	680	7.0
w/smoked bacon (*Pacific Organic*)	240	13.0	27.0	9.0	10	790	7.0
beef:							
Burgundy (*Campbell's Chunky*)	160	14.0	18.0	3.0	25	800	4.0
mushroom (*Progresso*)	100	7.0	13.0	.5	15	960	1.0
pot roast (*Healthy Choice* Micro) . .	110	7.0	18.0	1.0	0	480	5.0
pot roast w/vegetables (*Progresso*)	130	8.0	20.0	2.0	15	830	2.0
and potato, baked (*Progresso*)	100	6.0	15.0	2.5	15	930	1.0
rib roast, w/potato, herbs (*Campbell's Chunky*)	110	8.0	17.0	1.0	10	890	3.0
w/rice, white/wild (*Campbell's Chunky*)	150	8.0	24.0	2.0	10	990	3.0
slow-roasted, w/mushrooms (*Campbell's Chunky*)	120	7.0	18.0	1.5	15	830	3.0
slow-roasted, and vegetables (*Campbell's Select*)	100	6.0	16.0	1.5	10	910	2.0
steak and fusilli (*Pacific Organic*)	110	6.0	14.0	4.0	20	590	1.0
stew (*Campbell's Chunky* Fully Loaded)	160	10.0	20.0	4.0	20	810	3.0
Stroganoff (*Campbell's Chunky* Fully Loaded)	250	12.0	18.0	14.0	40	810	4.0

Food and Measure	cal.	prot. (gms)	carbo. (gms)	fat (gms)	chol. (mgs)	sod. (mgs)	fiber (gms)
and vegetable (*Muir Glen* Organic) . . .	90	5.0	12.0	3.0	10	890	2.0
vegetable (*Progresso* Micro)	100	8.0	15.0	1.5	15	820	2.0
vegetable (*Progresso* Traditional)	100	7.0	17.0	1.0	15	850	2.0
w/vegetables, country (*Campbell's Chunky*)	150	10.0	21.0	2.5	15	890	4.0
w/vegetables, country (*Campbell's Chunky* Micro) . .	150	10.0	21.0	3.0	20	900	5.0
beef barley:							
(*Campbell's Chunky*)	170	10.0	26.0	2.5	10	890	4.0
(*Campbell's Healthy Request Chunky*)	140	9.0	21.0	2.0	15	480	5.0
(*Progresso*)	140	9.0	15.0	3.5	15	650	2.0
(*Progresso* 99% Fat Free)	120	7.0	20.0	1.5	10	720	4.0
roasted (*Campbell's Select*)	130	9.0	22.0	1.0	10	920	2.0
vegetable (*Progresso*)	130	9.0	22.0	1.0	15	970	3.0
beef broth:							
(*College Inn*)	25	4.0	0	1.0	0	900	0
(*College Inn* French Onion Style)	15	4.0	0	0	0	850	0
(*Imagine* Organic) .	20	2.0	1.0	1.0	5	700	0
(*Pacific*)	20	4.0	1.0	0	0	570	0
(*Pacific* Organic) . .	25	3.0	1.0	1.0	5	570	0
(*Swanson*)	15	2.0	1.0	0	0	890	0
(*Swanson* Lower Sodium)	15	3.0	1.0	0	0	440	0
(*Swanson* Organic)	15	2.0	1.0	.5	0	550	0
w/onion (*Swanson*)	20	2.0	2.0	.5	5	830	0
stock (*Imagine* Organic)	15	3.0	1.0	0	0	630	0
broccoli:							
cream of (*Campbell's Soup at Hand*), 1 cont.	150	3.0	17.0	7.0	5	890	7.0
creamy (*Imagine* Organic)	60	3.0	10.0	1.5	0	470	2.0

Food and Measure	cal.	prot. (gms)	carbo. (gms)	fat (gms)	chol. (mgs)	sod. (mgs)	fiber (gms)
Soup, *(cont.)*							
butternut squash:							
(*Amy's* Organic) . . .	100	2.0	20.0	2.5	0	580	2.0
(*Amy's* Organic Light Sodium)	100	2.0	20.0	2.5	0	290	2.0
creamy (*Imagine* Organic)	90	0	18.0	2.0	0	460	2.0
creamy (*Pacific* Organic)	90	2.0	17.0	2.0	0	550	3.0
creamy (*Pacific* Organic Low Sodium)	90	2.0	17.0	2.0	0	280	3.0
golden (*Campbell's Select*)	90	2.0	18.0	1.5	5	810	3.0
golden (*Campbell's Select* Organic) .	110	2.0	21.0	1.5	5	850	4.0
carrot, creamy:							
cashew ginger (*Pacific*)	120	1.0	19.0	5.0	0	650	3.0
roasted (*Pacific*) . . .	100	3.0	18.0	1.0	0	780	2.0
celery, cream of (*Health Valley* Organic)	90	2.0	11.0	5.0	0	680	0
chicken:							
(*Healthy Choice* Hearty)	130	9.0	20.0	2.0	20	480	3.0
(*Progresso* Homestyle)	100	6.0	14.0	2.0	10	800	1.0
Alfredo (*Campbell's Select*)	180	10.0	18.0	7.0	10	930	2.0
barley (*Progresso*) .	100	6.0	16.0	2.5	15	900	3.0
broccoli, cheese and potato (*Campbell's Chunky*)	200	7.0	14.0	11.0	15	910	1.0
cheese enchilada (*Progresso Carb Monitor*)	170	8.0	8.0	12.0	25	970	<1.0
corn chowder (*Campbell's Chunky*) . .	190	8.0	20.0	9.0	25	850	3.0
corn chowder (*Progresso*)	210	7.0	23.0	9.0	15	790	2.0
creamy (*Campbell's Soup at Hand*), 1 cont.	130	4.0	13.0	9.0	5	890	4.0
creamy (*Imagine* Organic)	70	3.0	12.0	1.5	5	680	1.0

Food and Measure	cal.	prot. (gms)	carbo. (gms)	fat (gms)	chol. (mgs)	sod. (mgs)	fiber (gms)
and dumplings (Campbell's Chunky) ..	180	9.0	19.0	7.0	30	890	4.0
and dumplings (Campbell's Chunky Micro Bowl)	190	8.0	18.0	9.0	25	890	3.0
and dumplings (Healthy Choice)	140	9.0	21.0	2.5	20	480	3.0
and dumplings, herb (Progresso)	100	5.0	14.0	2.5	30	790	<1.0
fajita, w/rice, beans (Campbells Chunky)	140	9.0	23.0	1.5	15	850	4.0
fajita, spicy (Pacific Organic)	150	8.0	24.0	2.5	5	770	5.0
gumbo (Healthy Choice Zesty) ...	100	6.0	16.0	2.0	20	480	4.0
gumbo (Progresso Less Sodium) ...	110	7.0	18.0	1.5	15	450	2.0
meatballs (Progresso Chickarina)	130	8.0	12.0	5.0	15	920	<1.0
mushroom chowder (Campbell's Chunky) ......:	210	7.0	19.0	12.0	10	910	3.0
w/penne (Pacific Organic)	100	6.0	16.0	1.0	20	790	1.0
pot pie (Progresso)	170	8.0	21.0	6.0	15	940	2.0
rotini (Progresso) .	100	7.0	13.0	2.0	15	960	1.0
Southwestern (Progresso)	120	6.0	19.0	2.5	10	780	2.0
and stars (Campbell's Soup at Hand), 1 cont.	60	3.0	10.0	1.5	5	890	2.0
chicken, grilled, w/vegetables, pasta (Campbell's Chunky)	110	8.0	15.0	2.0	15	880	2.0
chicken, roasted:							
(Progresso Italiano)	70	6.0	10.0	1.0	15	940	<1.0
garlic (Progresso) .	100	7.0	13.0	2.0	20	950	1.0
rotini (Progresso) .	80	6.0	11.0	2.5	10	980	<1.0
w/rotini and penne (Campbell's Select)	100	8.0	16.0	.5	10	860	2.0
chicken broth:							
(Campbell's Low Sodium), 1 can .	25	4.0	1.0	.5	5	140	0
(College Inn)	15	1.0	0	1.0	0	930	0

Soup, chicken broth, *(cont.)*

Food and Measure	cal.	prot. (gms)	carbo. (gms)	fat (gms)	chol. (mgs)	sod. (mgs)	fiber (gms)
(*College Inn* Light & Fat Free)	5	1.0	0	0	0	450	0
(*Imagine* Organic Cooking Stock) .	15	3.0	1.0	0	0	610	0
(*Imagine* Organic Free Range)	10	1.0	1.0	0	0	570	0
(*Imagine* Organic Free Range Low Sodium)	20	1.0	1.0	1.0	5	95	0
(*Pacific* Free Range/ Free Range Organic)	10	1.0	1.0	0	0	570	0
(*Pacific* Organic Low Sodium)	15	2.0	1.0	0	0	70	0
(*Swanson*)	10	1.0	1.0	.5	5	960	0
(*Swanson* Organic)	15	1.0	1.0	.5	0	550	0
(*Swanson Natural Goodness*)	15	3.0	1.0	0	0	570	0
(*Valley Fresh*)	30	2.0	1.0	2.0	<5	1000	0
(*Valley Fresh* 40% Less Sodium) . . .	15	2.0	1.0	0	<5	600	0
w/lemon and herbs (*College Inn*) . . .	15	1.0	0	1.0	0	715	0
w/roasted garlic (*College Inn*) . . .	20	1.0	3.0	0	0	1000	0
w/roasted garlic (*Swanson*)	20	1.0	2.0	1.0	<5	950	0
w/roasted vegetables, herbs (*College Inn*)	20	1.0	3.0	0	0	1060	0
chicken flavor broth (*Imagine* Organic No-Chicken)	10	1.0	2.0	0	0	450	0
chicken noodle:							
(*Annie Chun's* Micro Bowl), 5.5 oz. . . .	260	8.0	52.0	2.0	0	990	2.0
(*Campbell's* Micro) .	70	4.0	10.0	2.0	15	870	<1.0
(*Campbell's* Low Sodium), 1 can .	160	12.0	17.0	4.5	30	140	2.0
(*Campbell's Chunky* Classic)	110	8.0	15.0	2.5	20	890	2.0
(*Campbell's Chunky* Micro)	110	8.0	14.0	2.0	25	840	2.0

Food and Measure	cal.	prot. (gms)	carbo. (gms)	fat (gms)	chol. (mgs)	sod. (mgs)	fiber (gms)
(*Campbell's Healthy Request Chunky*)	120	7.0	15.0	2.5	20	480	1.0
(*Campbell's Healthy Request Chunky* Classic Micro) ..	110	7.0	15.0	3.0	20	480	1.0
(*Muir Glen* Organic)	70	4.0	10.0	2.0	10	800	1.0
(*Progresso*)	100	7.0	12.0	2.5	25	950	1.0
(*Progresso 50% Less Sodium*) ...	90	7.0	12.0	1.5	20	470	1.0
(*Progresso 99% Fat Free*)	100	6.0	12.0	2.0	20	950	1.0
(*Progresso Homestyle*)	110	8.0	14.0	2.0	25	920	1.0
(*Progresso* Micro) .	80	6.0	10.0	2.0	20	890	1.0
egg noodles (*Campbell's Healthy Request Select*) .	100	7.0	13.0	2.5	15	480	2.0
egg noodles (*Campbell's Select*) ...	110	9.0	14.0	1.5	15	990	1.0
egg noodles (*Campbell's Select* Micro)	90	8.0	12.0	1.5	20	960	2.0
mini noodles (*Campbell's Soup at Hand*), 1 cont. ...	80	4.0	11.0	2.0	10	980	2.0
mini noodles (*Campbell's Soup at Hand 25% Less Sodium*), 1 cont.	80	4.0	11.0	2.0	10	730	2.0
chicken rice:							
(*Healthy Choice*) ..	110	7.0	17.0	1.5	10	480	3.0
(*Healthy Choice Fiesta*)	120	6.0	20.0	2.0	15	480	3.0
(*Healthy Choice* Micro)	90	6.0	13.0	1.5	15	440	2.0
long grain (*Campbell's Healthy Request Select*) .	110	7.0	18.0	1.5	10	480	2.0
long grain (*Campbell's Select*) ...	100	7.0	18.0	.5	15	980	2.0
long grain (*Campbell's Select* Micro)	90	7.0	15.0	.5	10	970	1.0
white/wild, savory (*Campbell's Chunky*)	110	7.0	18.0	2.0	10	810	2.0
wild (*Muir Glen* Organic)	70	4.0	10.0	2.0	10	710	1.0

Food and Measure	cal.	prot. (gms)	carbo. (gms)	fat (gms)	chol. (mgs)	sod. (mgs)	fiber (gms)
Soup, chicken rice *(cont.)*							
wild *(Progresso)* ..	100	6.0	15.0	1.5	15	870	1.0
wild *(Progresso Micro)*	100	5.0	16.0	1.5	15	900	1.0
wild, creamy *(Progresso)*	150	6.0	13.0	8.0	15	900	<1.0
wild, savory *(Pacific Organic)*	90	5.0	17.0	.5	5	790	1.0
w/vegetables *(Progresso)*	100	5.0	16.0	1.0	15	870	<1.0
chicken sausage gumbo:							
(Progresso)	130	6.0	18.0	4.0	15	900	1.0
grilled *(Campbell's Chunky)*	140	8.0	21.0	2.5	15	850	3.0
grilled *(Campbell's Chunky* Micro*)* ..	120	7.0	18.0	2.5	15	780	3.0
grilled *(Campbell's Healthy Request Chunky)*	140	8.0	21.0	2.5	15	480	3.0
grilled *(Campbell's Healthy Request Chunky* Micro*)* ..	130	8.0	20.0	2.5	15	480	3.0
chicken tortilla:							
(Campbell's Healthy Request Select Micro)	130	8.0	19.0	2.5	10	480	3.0
(Campbell's Select)	130	8.0	19.0	2.5	10	850	3.0
(Campbell's Select Micro)	130	8.0	18.0	2.5	10	820	2.0
(Healthy Choice) ..	160	10.0	25.0	2.0	15	470	4.0
chicken vegetable:							
(Campbell's Chunky Hearty)	90	7.0	13.0	1.5	15	790	2.0
(Campbell's Select)	110	7.0	19.0	.5	10	870	2.0
(Progresso Carb Monitor)	70	6.0	7.0	2.0	20	840	7.0
herbed, roasted vegetables *(Campbell's Select)* ...	100	8.0	15.0	.5	15	890	2.0
chili, see "Chili"							
clam chowder, Manhattan:							
(Bahr's)	120	9.0	15.0	2.5	20	810	2.0
(Campbell's Chunky)	120	5.0	19.0	3.5	5	830	3.0

Food and Measure	cal.	prot. (gms)	carbo. (gms)	fat (gms)	chol. (mgs)	sod. (mgs)	fiber (gms)
(*Dominique's*)	80	5.0	11.0	1.5	0	760	3.0
(*Progresso*)	100	3.0	17.0	2.0	10	910	2.0
clam chowder, New England:							
(*Campbell's Chunky*)	210	7.0	25.0	9.0	10	890	5.0
(*Campbell's Chunky Micro*)	180	6.0	20.0	8.0	10	870	4.0
(*Campbell's Healthy Request Chunky*)	120	6.0	20.0	2.0	10	480	3.0
(*Campbell's Select*)	160	6.0	15.0	8.0	10	870	2.0
(*Campbell's Select 98% Fat Free Micro*)	110	6.0	16.0	2.0	10	870	3.0
(*Campbell's Soup at Hand*), 1 cont. ...	160	4.0	13.0	10.0	5	890	5.0
(*Dominique's*)	200	7.0	13.0	14.0	15	970	4.0
(*Healthy Choice*) ..	110	5.0	19.0	1.0	10	480	2.0
(*Progresso*)	190	6.0	20.0	10.0	10	890	2.0
(*Progresso 99% Fat Free*)	120	5.0	21.0	2.0	5	720	2.0
(*Progresso Rich & Hearty*)	190	6.0	22.0	9.0	10	840	2.0
clam stock (*Kitchen Basics*)	20	3.0	0	0	0	600	0
coconut, Thai (*Amy's*)	220	4.0	10.0	13.0	0	580	2.0
corn:							
chipotle bisque (*Imagine Bistro Organic*)	100	3.0	22.0	1.0	0	590	2.0
creamy buttery sweet (*Pacific*)	120	3.0	20.0	2.0	5	750	2.0
creamy sweet (*Imagine*)	120	4.0	20.0	3.0	0	450	3.0
Southwest (*Campbell's Select*) ...	190	3.0	26.0	8.0	5	610	4.0
corn chowder:							
(*Amy's* Organic) ...	190	3.0	25.0	10.0	25	580	3.0
Southwest (*Campbell's Select* Organic) .	190	3.0	26.0	8.0	5	790	4.0
Southwestern (*Progresso*)	190	4.0	28.0	7.0	0	730	3.0
ham, honey-roasted w/potatoes (*Campbell's Chunky*)	130	8.0	20.0	2.5	15	810	3.0

Food and Measure	cal.	prot. (gms)	carbo. (gms)	fat (gms)	chol. (mgs)	sod. (mgs)	fiber (gms)
Soup *(cont.)*							
ham stock (*Kitchen Basics*)	20	3.0	0	0	0	480	0
hot and sour, noodle (*Annie Chun's* Micro), 5.5 oz.	280	8.0	55.0	2.5	0	910	2.0
Italian style wedding:							
(*Campbell's Healthy Request Select*) .	120	7.0	15.0	2.5	10	480	2.0
(*Campbell's Healthy Request Select Micro*)	120	7.0	15.0	3.0	15	480	2.0
(*Campbell's Select*)	120	7.0	15.0	3.0	15	840	2.0
(*Campbell's Select Micro*)	110	7.0	15.0	2.5	15	790	2.0
(*Campbell's Soup at Hand*), 1 cont. ...	90	3.0	10.0	4.5	10	860	2.0
(*Healthy Choice*) ..	130	10.0	17.0	2.5	10	440	4.0
(*Progresso*)	130	6.0	15.0	5.0	15	940	1.0
(*Progresso* Micro) .	120	6.0	14.0	4.0	10	940	1.0
Korean kimchi noodle (*Annie Chun's* Micro), ½ of 6-oz. bowl ...	140	6.0	28.0	1.5	0	720	1.0
lentil:							
(*Amy's Organic*) ...	150	8.0	19.0	4.5	0	590	9.0
(*Amy's Organic Light Sodium*)	150	8.0	20.0	4.5	0	290	5.0
(*Muir Glen Organic Savory*)	130	6.0	23.0	2.0	0	950	3.0
(*Progresso*)	150	9.0	28.0	2.0	0	870	5.0
(*Progresso 99% Fat Free*)	150	9.0	28.0	2.0	0	870	5.0
(*Progresso* Micro) .	130	7.0	21.0	3.0	0	840	3.0
curried red (*Pacific*)	140	5.0	19.0	4.5	0	750	5.0
vegetable (*Amy's Organic*)	150	7.0	23.0	4.0	0	680	6.0
vegetable (*Amy's Organic Light Sodium*)	150	7.0	23.0	4.0	0	340	6.0
lobster bisque:							
(*Baxter's*)	120	5.0	10.0	6.0	60	740	1.0
(*Dominique's*)	130	4.0	11.0	8.0	30	950	<1.0
macaroni and bean (*Progresso*)	160	7.0	25.0	3.5	0	890	6.0

Food and Measure	cal.	prot. (gms)	carbo. (gms)	fat (gms)	chol. (mgs)	sod. (mgs)	fiber (gms)
meatball:							
(*Progresso Carb Monitor* Tuscan)	100	5.0	9.0	5.0	15	840	1.0
w/bow-ties (*Campbell's Select* Mediterranean)	120	7.0	14.0	3.5	15	800	3.0
and rice (*Campbell's Select* Azteca)	110	5.0	17.0	3.0	10	800	2.0
minestrone:							
(*Amy's* Organic)	90	3.0	17.0	1.5	0	580	3.0
(*Amy's* Organic Light Sodium)	90	3.0	17.0	1.5	0	290	3.0
(*Campbell's Select*)	100	5.0	20.0	0	0	950	3.0
(*Campbell's Select* Micro)	100	4.0	19.0	.5	5	900	4.0
(*Healthy Choice* Micro)	200	7.0	40.0	2.0	5	470	5.0
(*Muir Glen* Organic Classic)	110	4.0	19.0	2.0	0	960	5.0
(*Progresso*)	110	4.0	19.0	2.0	0	980	4.0
(*Progresso* 50% Less Sodium)	120	5.0	24.0	2.0	0	470	4.0
(*Progresso* 99% Fat Free)	100	5.0	19.0	1.0	0	630	4.0
(*Progresso* Micro)	90	4.0	17.0	1.5	0	930	4.0
beef steak (*Pacific* Organic)	100	5.0	12.0	3.0	15	790	2.0
chicken (*Progresso*)	120	6.0	16.0	3.5	15	870	3.0
miso noodle (*Annie Chun's* Micro), 5.5 oz.	230	6.0	45.0	2.5	0	890	2.0
mushroom, cream of:							
(*Amy's* Organic)	140	3.0	13.0	9.0	5	590	2.0
(*Campbell's* Low Sodium), 1 can	160	3.0	10.0	8.0	10	60	3.0
mushroom, creamy:							
(*Progresso*)	130	2.0	9.0	10.0	10	820	1.0
portobello (*Campbell's Select*)	100	3.0	14.0	4.0	10	790	2.0
portobello (*Imagine*)	80	3.0	10.0	3.0	0	390	3.0
mushroom broth (*Pacific* Organic)	5	0	1.0	0	0	530	0
noodle:							
(*Amy's* No Chicken)	90	5.0	12.0	3.0	0	540	2.0

Food and Measure	cal.	prot. (gms)	carbo. (gms)	fat (gms)	chol. (mgs)	sod. (mgs)	fiber (gms)
Soup, noodle *(cont.)*							
Thai (*Annie Chun's* Tom Yum Micro), ½ of 6-oz. bowl .	150	5.0	30.0	1.5	0	730	1.0
udon (*Annie Chun's* Micro), 5.3 oz. ...	220	6.0	45.0	1.5	0	920	1.0
onion, French:							
(*Baxter's*)	70	2.0	15.0	0	0	570	2.0
(*Pacific* Organic) ..	35	1.0	6.0	0	0	600	<1.0
(*Progresso*)	50	1.0	8.0	1.5	<5	850	<1.0
pasta and 3-bean (*Amy's* Organic) ...	130	5.0	19.0	5.0	0	680	4.0
pea, split:							
(*Amy's* Organic) ...	100	7.0	19.0	0	0	670	3.0
(*Amy's* Organic Light Sodium)	100	7.0	19.0	0	0	280	4.0
(*Muir Glen* Organic Homestyle)	170	10.0	35.0	1.0	0	900	5.0
green, w/bacon (*Progresso*) :...	170	9.0	28.0	1.0	<5	910	5.0
w/ham (*Campbell's Chunky*)	180	12.0	27.0	2.5	10	780	4.0
w/ham (*Healthy Choice*)	170	9.0	22.0	2.0	5	480	3.0
w/ham (*Progresso*)	150	9.0	25.0	1.0	10	730	4.0
w/ham, roasted (*Campbell's Select*)	160	10.0	29.0	1.0	5	830	5.0
w/ham and Swiss (*Pacific* Organic)	250	14.0	28.0	10.0	25	660	11.0
pea, sweet, creamy (*Imagine* Organic) .	80	4.0	14.0	1.5	0	570	3.0
penne, in chicken broth (*Progresso*)	.80	4.0	14.0	1.0	0	940	1.0
pepper steak (*Campbell's Chunky*)	120	8.0	18.0	1.5	15	800	3.0
pork:							
(*Campbell's Chunky* BBQ)	170	12.0	22.0	3.5	15	920	5.0
roast, w/carrots, potato (*Campbell's Chunky*)	120	8.0	16.0	3.0	15	890	3.0
pork stock (*Kitchen Basics*)	20	3.0	0	0	0	480	0

Food and Measure	cal.	prot. (gms)	carbo. (gms)	fat (gms)	chol. (mgs)	sod. (mgs)	fiber (gms)
pot roast (*Campbell's Chunky* Savory) ...	120	8.0	18.0	1.5	15	880	3.0
potato:							
(*Campbell's Soup at Hand* Velvety), 1 cont.	160	2.0	21.0	7.0	<5	870	4.0
broccoli cheese (*Campbell's Select*)	120	3.0	18.0	4.0	<5	890	4.0
broccoli cheese chowder (*Progresso*) .	180	5.0	18.0	10.0	10	920	2.0
creamy, w/roasted garlic (*Campbell's Select*)	180	3.0	20.0	10.0	10	770	2.0
potato, baked:							
w/cheddar, bacon (*Campbell's Chunky*)	160	4.0	23.0	6.0	<5	870	2.0
w/steak, cheese (*Campbell's Chunky*)	210	9.0	21.0	10.0	15	940	3.0
potato ham chowder (*Campbell's Chunky* Old Fashioned)	190	6.0	17.0	11.0	15	800	2.0
potato leek:							
(*Amy's* Organic) ...	180	2.0	21.0	10.0	30	580	2.0
(*Baxter's*)	120	2.0	24.0	2.0	0	620	3.0
creamy (*Imagine* Organic)	110	2.0	18.0	3.0	0	550	3.0
red pepper, roasted, tomato, creamy:							
(*Pacific* Organic) ..	110	5.0	16.0	2.0	10	720	1.0
(*Pacific* Organic Light Sodium) ..	110	5.0	16.0	2.0	10	360	1.0
rigatoni and meatballs (*Campbell's Chunky* Fully Loaded)	220	13.0	24.0	8.0	20	800	6.0
Salisbury steak, mushrooms, onions (*Campbell's Chunky*)	150	9.0	19.0	4.5	15	890	5.0
sausage, Italian, w/pasta, pepperoni:							
(*Campbell's Select*)	150	7.0	18.0	6.0	15	870	3.0
(*Campbell's Select* Micro)	130	7.0	15.0	6.0	15	870	2.0

Food and Measure	cal.	prot. (gms)	carbo. (gms)	fat (gms)	chol. (mgs)	sod. (mgs)	fiber (gms)
Soup *(cont.)*							
seafood stock (*Kitchen Basics*)	10	3.0	0	0	0	420	0
sirloin burger, w/vegetables:							
(*Campbell's Chunky*)	180	10.0	20.0	7.0	15	900	4.0
(*Campbell's Chunky* Micro)	160	10.0	18.0	4.0	15	870	4.0
sirloin steak:							
grilled, w/vegetables (*Campbell's Chunky* Hearty)	130	8.0	19.0	2.0	10	890	4.0
and vegetables (*Progresso*)	130	8.0	21.0	2.0	15	870	2.0
steak:							
grilled, w/vegetables, penne (*Progresso*)	120	8.0	16.0	2.0	20	990	1.0
and noodles (*Healthy Choice* Micro) ..	140	13.0	14.0	3.0	20	460	2.5
and noodles (*Progresso* Homestyle)	110	9.0	16.0	2.0	25	830	1.0
and potato (*Campbell's Chunky*) ..	130	10.0	18.0	2.0	15	920	2.0
and roasted russet potato (*Progresso*)	140	8.0	23.0	1.5	15	990	2.0
and sautéed mushrooms (*Progresso*)	110	7.0	18.0	2.0	10	930	1.0
sweet potato (*Imagine* Organic)	110	2.0	23.0	1.5	0	400	1.0
tomato:							
(*Campbell's* Micro) .	110	3.0	24.0	0	0	790	3.0
(*Campbell's Soup at Hand* Classic), 1 cont.	120	3.0	31.0	0	0	890	2.0
(*Campbell's Soup at Hand* Classic 25% Less Sodium), 1 cont.	120	3.0	27.0	0	0	660	2.0
(*Muir Glen* Organic)	130	5.0	25.0	2.0	0	880	2.0
(*Progresso* Hearty)	110	2.0	23.0	1.0	0	980	3.0
basil (*Campbell's Select* Harvest) .	80	1.0	18.0	0	0	750	1.0
basil (*Progresso*) ..	160	2.0	30.0	3.0	0	960	1.0

Food and Measure	cal.	prot. (gms)	carbo. (gms)	fat (gms)	chol. (mgs)	sod. (mgs)	fiber (gms)
garden (*Campbell's Select*)	100	3.0	21.0	.5	5	700	2.0
fire-roasted (*Imagine Bistro* Organic) ..	120	2.0	24.0	2.5	0	670	2.0
Italian, w/basil, garlic (*Campbell's Select* Gold Label)	90	3.0	19.0	0	0	770	3.0
Italian, w/basil, garlic (*Campbell's Select* Gold Label Organic)	80	2.0	19.0	0	0	770	3.0
rotini (*Progresso*) .	140	4.0	29.0	1.0	0	950	3.0
tomato, cream of:							
(*Amy's* Organic) ...	100	2.0	17.0	2.0	10	690	3.0
(*Amy's* Organic Light Sodium)	100	2.0	17.0	2.5	10	340	3.0
tomato, creamy:							
(*Baxter's*)	160	2.0	23.0	7.0	10	630	1.0
(*Campbell's* Micro) .	160	3.0	25.0	5.0	5	750	3.0
(*Campbell's Soup at Hand*), 1 cont. ...	190	4.0	34.0	4.0	<5	940	4.0
(*Imagine* Organic) .	80	2.0	15.0	1.0	0	620	2.0
(*Muir Glen* Organic)	170	4.0	26.0	6.0	15	840	2.0
(*Pacific* Organic) ..	100	5.0	16.0	2.0	10	750	1.0
(*Pacific* Organic Light Sodium) ..	100	5.0	16.0	2.0	10	380	1.0
(*Progresso*)	190	4.0	30.0	6.0	15	900	1.0
(*Walnut Acres* Organic)	100	3.0	17.0	2.5	10	600	<1.0
basil (*Imagine* Organic)	90	3.0	17.0	1.5	0	430	2.0
Parmesan (*Campbell's Select* Gold Label)	200	5.0	25.0	9.0	25	890	4.0
tomato bisque, chunky:							
(*Amy's* Organic) ...	120	2.0	21.0	3.5	10	680	2.0
(*Amy's* Organic Light Sodium)	120	2.0	21.0	3.5	10	340	2.0
turkey:							
broth (*College Inn*) .	20	2.0	0	1.0	0	950	0
noodle (*Progresso*)	80	5.0	12.0	1.5	15	930	1.0
pot pie (*Campbell's Chunky*)	200	11.0	21.0	8.0	35	800	4.0
turtle (Dominique's Snapper)	100	6.0	15.0	2.0	0	1130	1.0

Food and Measure	cal.	prot. (gms)	carbo. (gms)	fat (gms)	chol. (mgs)	sod. (mgs)	fiber (gms)
Soup *(cont.)*							
vegetable:							
(*Amy's* Chunky Organic)	60	3.0	13.0	0	0	680	3.0
(*Campbell's* Micro) .	110	4.0	22.0	.5	<5	800	3.0
(*Campbell's Chunky* Savory)	110	3.0	22.0	1.0	0	770	4.0
(*Campbell's Healthy Request* Chunky)	120	4.0	24.0	1.0	0	480	4.0
(*Campbell's Select*)	100	3.0	21.0	.5	0	900	3.0
(*Campbell's Soup at Hand* Blended Medley), 1 cont.	100	3.0	19.0	1.5	<5	890	4.0
(*Healthy Choice* Country Can) . . .	110	5.0	19.0	1.0	5	480	4.0
(*Healthy Choice* Country Micro) .	100	4.0	21.0	.5	0	480	5.0
(*Progresso*)	80	3.0	16.0	.5	0	950	2.0
(*Progresso* Italiano)	100	2.0	18.0	2.0	0	1050	3.0
(*Progresso* Micro) .	80	3.0	17.0	.5	0	970	2.0
barley (*Amy's* Organic)	70	2.0	13.0	1.0	0	580	3.0
barley (*Progresso* Light Savory) . . .	60	2.0	14.0	0	0	740	4.0
w/barley, vegetarian (*Progresso*)	100	3.0	20.0	.5	0	980	4.0
fire-roasted, South-western (*Amy's* Organic)	140	4.0	23.0	4.5	0	680	4.0
garden (*Healthy Choice*)	120	5.0	24.0	.5	5	480	5.0
garden (*Muir Glen* Organic)	80	3.0	16.0	1.0	0	960	3.0
garden (*Progresso*)	90	3.0	20.0	0	0	940	3.0
garden (*Progresso* 50% Less Sodium)	100	3.0	22.0	0	0	450	3.0
herb and rotini (*Progresso*)	100	4.0	19.0	1.0	0	1100	5.0
Italian style (*Progresso* Light) . . .	60	2.0	14.0	0	0	820	4.0
and noodle (*Progresso* Light) . . .	60	2.0	13.0	.5	5	860	4.0
w/pasta (*Campbell's Chunky* Hearty) .	120	4.0	23.0	2.0	5	870	4.0

Food and Measure	cal.	prot. (gms)	carbo. (gms)	fat (gms)	chol. (mgs)	sod. (mgs)	fiber (gms)
and rice (*Progresso* Light Homestyle)	60	7.0	18.0	1.5	15	450	2.0
Southwestern (*Progresso* Light)	60	3.0	12.0	0	0	840	4.0
vegetable beef:							
(*Campbell's* Micro) .	80	5.0	15.0	.5	10	880	3.0
(*Campbell's Chunky* Old Fashioned) . .	110	9.0	13.0	1.5	15	880	3.0
(*Campbell's Healthy Request Chunky* Old Fashioned) . .	110	7.0	17.0	2.0	10	480	3.0
(*Campbell's Soup at Hand*), 1 cont. . . .	60	3.0	10.0	1.0	5	930	1.0
(*Healthy Choice*) . .	130	9.0	22.0	1.0	15	480	4.0
slow cooked (*Progresso*)	120	8.0	20.0	1.0	15	840	3.0
vegetable broth:							
(*College Inn* Garden)	25	0	6.0	0	0	590	0
(*Imagine* Organic) .	20	2.0	2.0	0	0	550	0
(*Imagine* Organic Low Sodium) . . .	20	0	3.0	0	0	140	<1.0
(*Pacific* Organic) . .	15	0	3.0	0	0	530	1.0
(*Pacific* Organic Low Sodium)	15	0	3.0	0	0	140	1.0
(*Swanson*)	15	0	3.0	0	0	940	0
(*Swanson* Organic)	15	0	3.0	0	0	550	0
vegetable stock:							
(*Imagine* Organic) .	30	1.0	6.0	0	0	580	0
(*Kitchen Basics*) . . .	20	0	0	0	0	330	0
(*Pacific*)	15	0	3.0	0	0	530	0
Soup, condensed, undiluted, ½ cup:							
asparagus, cream of (*Campbell's*)	110	2.0	9.0	7.0	5	830	3.0
bean, w/bacon: (*Campbell's*)	170	8.0	25.0	4.0	5	860	8.0
beef, w/vegetables and barley (*Campbell's*)	90	5.0	15.0	1.5	10	890	3.0
beef broth (*Campbell's*)	15	3.0	1.0	0	0	860	0
beef consommé (*Campbell's*)	20	4.0	1.0	0	0	810	0
beef noodle (*Campbell's*)	70	4.0	8.0	2.0	10	820	<1.0
broccoli cream of: (*Campbell's*)	90	2.0	12.0	3.5	5	750	1.0

Food and Measure	cal.	prot. (gms)	carbo. (gms)	fat (gms)	chol. (mgs)	sod. (mgs)	fiber (gms)
Soup, condensed, broccoli cream of *(cont.)*							
(*Campbell's* 98% Fat Free)	60	2.0	10.0	2.0	<5	700	2.0
broccoli cheese:							
(*Campbell's*)	100	2.0	12.0	4.5	5	820	0
(*Campbell's* 98% Fat Free)	70	3.0	12.0	1.5	5	790	1.0
celery, cream of:							
(*Campbell's*)	90	1.0	9.0	6.0	<5	860	3.0
(*Campbell's* 98% Fat Free)	60	1.0	8.0	3.0	5	580	1.0
(*Campbell's Healthy Request*)	70	1.0	12.0	2.0	<5	480	1.0
cheddar cheese							
(*Campbell's*)	110	2.0	12.0	5.0	5	890	1.0
cheese, nacho (*Campbell's Fiesta*)	120	3.0	10.0	8.0	10	790	1.0
chicken:							
alphabet (*Campbell's*)	70	4.0	11.0	1.5	10	660	1.0
dumplings (*Campbell's*)	70	3.0	10.0	2.5	10	760	1.0
gumbo (*Campbell's*)	60	2.0	10.0	1.0	5	870	1.0
stars (*Campbell's*) .	70	3.0	10.0	2.0	5	640	1.0
vegetable (*Campbell's*)	80	3.0	15.0	1.0	5	890	2.0
vegetable (*Campbell's Southwest*)	110	5.0	21.0	1.0	5	830	4.0
wonton (*Campbell's*)	60	4.0	8.0	1.0	10	870	0
chicken, cream of:							
(*Campbell's*)	120	3.0	10.0	8.0	10	870	2.0
(*Campbell's* 98% Fat Free)	70	2.0	10.0	2.5	10	590	1.0
(*Campbell's Healthy Request*)	80	2.0	12.0	2.5	5	460	1.0
w/herbs (*Campbell's*)	80	2.0	9.0	3.5	5	810	2.0
and mushrooms (*Campbell's*)	80	3.0	7.0	6.0	10	830	4.0
chicken broth (*Campbell's*)	20	1.0	1.0	1.0	<5	770	0
chicken mushroom barley (*Campbell's*)	90	4.0	16.0	1.5	5	720	3.0
chicken noodle:							
(*Campbell's*)	60	3.0	8.0	2.0	15	890	<1.0

Food and Measure	cal.	prot. (gms)	carbo. (gms)	fat (gms)	chol. (mgs)	sod. (mgs)	fiber (gms)
(*Campbell's 25%* Less Sodium)	60	3.0	8.0	2.0	15	660	1.0
(*Campbell's* Home-style)	70	4.0	9.0	2.0	10	700	2.0
(*Campbell's Healthy Request*)	60	3.0	8.0	2.0	10	470	1.0
(*Campbell's Healthy Request* Homestyle)	60	3.0	8.0	2.0	10	480	1.0
(*Campbell's Noodle O's*)	80	4.0	12.0	2.5	10	620	1.0
creamy (*Campbell's*)	120	4.0	11.0	7.0	15	870	4.0
chicken w/rice:							
(*Campbell's*)	70	2.0	13.0	1.5	5	820	1.0
(*Campbell's Healthy Request*)	70	2.0	13.0	1.5	5	480	1.0
white and wild (*Campbell's*)	70	3.0	12.0	1.5	5	820	1.0
clam bisque (*Chincoteague*)	100	8.0	13.0	2.0	15	990	1.0
clam chowder, Manhattan:							
(*Campbell's*)	70	2.0	12.0	.5	<5	880	2.0
(*Chincoteague*)	100	8.0	13.0	2.0	15	990	1.0
clam chowder, New England:							
(*Campbell's*)	90	4.0	13.0	2.5	5	880	1.0
(*Chincoteague*)	80	5.0	10.0	2.5	10	590	<1.0
(*Chincoteague* 99% Fat Free)	70	2.0	12.0	1.0	5	610	<1.0
corn chowder (*Chincoteague*)	100	2.0	16.0	3.5	0	890	1.0
crab:							
(*Chincoteague* She)	70	4.0	7.0	3.0	20	770	0
and cheddar (*Chincoteague*)	90	4.0	10.0	3.5	20	590	0
cream of (*Chincoteague*)	200	11.0	23.0	6.0	35	830	0
red, vegetable (*Chincoteague*)	90	5.0	12.0	2.5	15	880	2.0
Italian style wedding (*Campbell's*)	90	4.0	12.0	2.5	10	810	3.0
lentil (*Campbell's*)	140	9.0	24.0	1.0	0	800	6.0
lobster bisque:							
(*Bahr's*)	70	2.0	9.0	2.0	5	980	0

Food and Measure	cal.	prot. (gms)	carbo. (gms)	fat (gms)	chol. (mgs)	sod. (mgs)	fiber (gms)
Soup, condensed, lobster bisque *(cont.)*							
(*Chincoteague*)	90	4.0	10.0	4.0	15	650	0
cheddar							
(*Chincoteague*) ..	110	4.0	10.0	6.0	20	610	0
minestrone:							
(*Campbell's*)	90	4.0	17.0	1.0	<5	960	3.0
(*Campbell's Healthy Request*)	80	3.0	15.0	.5	0	460	3.0
mushroom:							
beefy (*Campbell's*) .	50	3.0	6.0	2.0	5	890	0
golden (*Campbell's*)	80	2.0	10.0	3.5	5	890	1.0
mushroom, cream of:							
(*Campbell's*)	100	1.0	9.0	6.0	5	870	2.0
(*Campbell's 25% Less Sodium*) ...	110	2.0	8.0	8.0	5	650	2.0
(*Campbell's 98% Fat Free*)	70	2.0	9.0	2.5	<5	630	1.0
(*Campbell's Healthy Request*)	70	2.0	10.0	2.0	5	470	1.0
w/roasted garlic (*Campbell's*)	70	2.0	11.0	2.5	0	710	2.0
noodle:							
in chicken broth (*Campbell's Double Noodle*) .	100	4.0	17.0	1.5	10	620	2.0
curly (*Campbell's*) .	80	4.0	11.0	2.0	15	630	1.0
mega, in chicken broth (*Campbell's*)	90	4.0	14.0	2.0	15	600	2.0
onion:							
cream of (*Campbell's*)	100	1.0	10.0	6.0	5	800	3.0
French (*Campbell's*)	45	2.0	6.0	1.5	<5	900	1.0
oyster stew:							
(*Bahr's*)	80	3.0	11.0	3.5	25	680	0
(*Campbell's*)	80	2.0	5.0	6.0	20	910	0
(*Chincoteague*)	80	3.0	11.0	3.5	25	680	0
pasta, in chicken broth:							
w/chicken (*Campbell's Goldfish*) ..	70	3.0	11.0	1.5	10	600	2.0
w/meatballs (*Campbell's Goldfish*) ..	80	4.0	11.0	2.5	10	560	2.0
pea:							
green (*Campbell's*) .	180	9.0	28.0	3.0	0	870	4.0
split, w/ham, bacon (*Campbell's*)	180	10.0	27.0	3.5	5	850	5.0

Food and Measure	cal.	prot. (gms)	carbo. (gms)	fat (gms)	chol. (mgs)	sod. (mgs)	fiber (gms)
pepper jack (*Campbell's* Southwest)	110	2.0	13.0	6.0	5	880	4.0
pepper pot (*Campbell's*)	90	5.0	9.0	4.0	25	980	1.0
potato, cream of (*Campbell's*)	100	2.0	15.0	2.0	5	800	2.0
Scotch broth (*Campbell's*)	70	3.0	9.0	1.0	5	880	2.0
shrimp, cream of (*Campbell's*)	90	2.0	8.0	5.0	10	860	1.0
shrimp bisque (*Chincoteague*)	80	2.0	10.0	3.0	20	590	0
tomato:							
(*Campbell's*)	90	2.0	20.0	0	0	710	1.0
(*Campbell's* 25% Less Sodium) . . .	90	2.0	20.0	0	0	530	1.0
(*Campbell's Healthy Request*)	90	2.0	17.0	1.5	0	470	1.0
bisque (*Campbell's*)	130	2.0	23.0	3.5	5	880	1.0
rice (*Campbell's* Old Fashioned)	110	1.0	23.0	2.0	<5	770	1.0
vegetable:							
(*Campbell's*)	100	4.0	20.0	.5	5	890	3.0
(*Campbell's* Old Fashioned)	80	3.0	14.0	1.5	5	920	2.0
(*Campbell's Healthy Request*)	100	4.0	19.0	1.0	0	480	3.0
beef (*Campbell's*) . .	80	5.0	15.0	1.0	5	890	3.0
beef (*Campbell's Healthy Request*)	90	5.0	15.0	1.0	5	480	3.0
vegetarian (*Campbell's*)	90	3.0	18.0	.5	0	790	2.0
Soup, frozen/refrigerated, 1 cup, except as noted:							
bean:							
black (*Tabatchnik*), 7.5 oz.	230	13.0	39.0	2.5	0	420	9.0
white, vegetables (*Moosewood Organic Tuscan*) .	130	6.0	24.0	2.0	0	760	5.0
Southwest (*Tabatchnik*), 7.5 oz.	220	11.0	35.0	5.0	0	440	9.0
Yankee (*Tabatchnik*), 7.5 oz.	180	1.0	33.0	1.5	0	340	10.0

Soup, frozen/refrigerated *(cont.)*

Food and Measure	cal.	prot. (gms)	carbo. (gms)	fat (gms)	chol. (mgs)	sod. (mgs)	fiber (gms)
broccoli and cheese, creamy (*Moosewood* Organic)	160	5.0	17.0	6.0	20	800	3.0
cabbage (*Tabatchnik*), 7.5 oz.	90	2.0	21.0	1.0	0	160	1.0
chicken broth w/noodles, dumplings (*Tabatchnik*), 7.25 oz.	150	5.0	19.0	6.0	65	740	<1.0
chicken broth w/noodles, vegetables (*Tabatchnik*), 7.25 oz.	70	3.0	13.0	1.0	15	460	0
chicken noodle (*Organic Classics*)	110	7.0	15.0	3.0	15	760	2.0
clam chowder (*Phillips*)	180	19.0	18.0	8.0	30	860	0
crab (*Phillips*)	120	6.0	19.0	2.0	15	670	4.0
crab and corn (*Phillips*)	310	7.0	18.0	23.0	30	500	0
lentil:							
(*Tabatchnik* Tuscan), 7.5 oz.	160	11.0	29.0	0	0	360	8.0
curried (*Moosewood* Organic Tibetan)	130	6.0	19.0	4.0	0	320	7.0
lobster bisque (*Phillips*)	330	9.0	19.0	25.0	135	800	1.0
minestrone (*Tabatchnik*), 7.5 oz.	100	5.0	18.9	1.5	0	320	4.0
mushroom barley:							
(*Moosewood* Organic)	90	3.0	14.0	2.0	0	720	3.0
(*Tabatchnik*), 7.5 oz.	80	3.0	17.0	1.0	0	420	3.0
onion, French, w/croutons (*Organic Classics*)	140	3.0	17.0	6.0	0	790	2.0
potato (*Tabatchnik* Old Fashion), 7.5 oz. ..	100	3.0	21.0	1.5	0	330	2.0
potato corn chowder, creamy (*Moosewood* Organic)	170	5.0	28.0	6.0	15	410	3.0
seafood chowder:							
(*Organic Classics*) .	160	11.0	17.0	6.0	50	800	1.0
(*Tabatchnik* Rock Island), 7.5 oz. ...	130	5.0	15.0	6.0	25	440	<1.0
sweet potato bisque (*Moosewood* Organic Savannah)	200	6.0	20.0	11.0	20	580	2.0

Food and Measure	cal.	prot. (gms)	carbo. (gms)	fat (gms)	chol. (mgs)	sod. (mgs)	fiber (gms)
tomato and rice (*Moosewood* Organic Mediterranean)	100	3.0	18.0	3.0	0	510	2.0
vegetable:							
(*Tabatchnik*), 7.5 oz.	90	3.0	17.0	1.5	0	350	4.0
(*Tabatchnik* Low Sodium), 7.5 oz.	90	4.0	17.0	1.5	0	45	4.0
noodle (*Moosewood* Organic Hungarian)	80	2.0	13.0	1.5	0	480	2.0
Soup, mix, dry, 1 cont. or pkg., except as noted:							
bean:							
(*Alessi* Neapolitan), ¼ of 6-oz. pkg. . .	140	6.0	29.0	.5	0	680	6.0
(*Alessi* Tuscan), ¼ of 6-oz. pkg.	150	7.0	28.0	.5	0	660	7.0
chili (*Fantastic* Buckaroo)	160	12.0	33.0	2.0	0	720	10.0
chili (*Fantastic* Cha Cha), 1 cup* . . .	110	6.0	20.0	1.5	0	580	7.0
and ham (*Hormel* Micro)	190	9.0	29.0	4.0	10	720	7.0
bean, black:							
(*Fantastic* Baja) . . .	130	8.0	31.0	.5	0	740	9.0
(*Nile Spice*)	170	12.0	36.0	1.5	0	640	12.0
(*Vigo*), ¼ of 6-oz. pkg.	150	8.0	28.0	0	0	750	9.0
chicken (*Comida Loca*), 1 cup* . . .	90	5.0	15.0	1.5	0	610	3.0
w/couscous, spicy (*Health Valley* Cup), ⅓ cup	130	6.0	29.0	0	0	290	5.0
w/rice (*Health Valley* Cup Zesty), ⅓ cup	100	5.0	22.0	0	0	240	4.0
bean, garbanzo (*Vigo* Spanish), ¼ of 6-oz. pkg.	150	6.0	30.0	1.0	0	660	8.0
bean, red, and rice (*Nile Spice*)	170	10.0	35.0	1.0	0	590	10.0
beef vegetable (*Hormel* Micro) . . .	90	6.0	16.0	1.0	10	790	1.0
broccoli cheddar (*Fantastic* Great Lakes) .	100	4.0	15.0	3.0	10	590	3.0

Food and Measure	cal.	prot. (gms)	carbo. (gms)	fat (gms)	chol. (mgs)	sod. (mgs)	fiber (gms)
Soup, mix *(cont.)*							
chicken, cream of							
(*Cup-a-Soup*)	70	1.0	14.0	1.5	0	730	0
chicken noodle:							
(*Alessi* Sicilian), ¼							
of 6-oz. pkg. ...	70	3.0	14.0	0	10	750	2.0
(*Cup-a-Soup*)	80	2.0	17.0	.5	<5	920	0
(*Hormel* Micro) ...	100	7.0	12.0	2.5	25	790	0
w/vegetables							
(*Health Valley*							
Fat Free), 1 cup*	110	5.0	24.0	0	0	290	3.0
"chicken" noodle,							
vegetarian:							
(*Fantastic*)	90	5.0	17.0	1.0	0	770	2.0
(*Fantastic* New							
England), 1 cup*	90	7.0	14.0	1.0	0	700	1.0
chicken rice (*Hormel*							
Micro)	110	4.0	18.0	3.0	10	850	1.0
chili, green (*Comida*							
Loca), 1 cup*	70	2.0	15.0	.5	0	770	2.0
clam chowder, New En-							
gland (*Hormel* Micro)	140	5.0	18.0	5.0	20	800	1.0
coconut ginger (*A*							
Taste of Thai), 1 tsp.	15	0	2.0	1.0	0	620	0
collard greens (*Vigo*),							
¼ of 6-oz. pkg. ...	160	8.0	26.0	2.5	0	680	n.a.
corn chowder:							
(*Nile* Spice Sweet) .	110	3.0	22.0	2.0	5	400	3.0
green chili (*Comida*							
Loca), ⅙ pkg. ..	100	3.0	18.0	2.0	0	500	1.0
couscous (*Nile Spice*):							
lentil curry	200	10.0	36.0	1.5	0	730	4.0
minestrone	180	8.0	34.0	1.5	0	590	2.0
Parmesan	200	8.0	34.0	3.0	10	570	2.0
hot and sour:							
(*Fantastic*)	170	6.0	33.0	2.0	0	780	3.0
(*Fantastic* New Year),							
1 cup*	70	0	15.0	.5	0	580	0
lentil:							
(*Alessi* Sicilian),							
⅓ cup	150	8.0	27.0	0	0	690	5.0
(*Nile Spice*)	170	11.0	34.0	1.5	0	540	11.0
w/couscous (*Health*							
Valley Cup), ⅓ cup	130	7.0	28.0	0	0	310	5.0

Food and Measure	cal.	prot. (gms)	carbo. (gms)	fat (gms)	chol. (mgs)	sod. (mgs)	fiber (gms)
minestrone:							
(*Fantastic* Mamma's)	160	9.0	30.0	2.5	5	710	6.0
(*Nile Spice*)	140	8.0	30.0	1.0	0	590	8.0
miso:							
dark (*San-J*)	40	4.0	3.0	1.5	0	1150	1.0
green onion, w/tofu							
(*Fantastic*)	140	6.0	26.0	1.5	0	770	2.0
mild (*San-J*)	45	3.0	5.0	1.5	0	1360	<1.0
red (*Westbrae Natural* Instant)	35	2.0	3.0	1.5	0	750	0
sesame (*Fantastic*) .	140	5.0	27.0	2.0	0	730	2.0
white (*San-J*)	40	3.0	3.0	1.5	0	860	0
white (*Westbrae Natural* Instant) .	35	2.0	3.0	1.5	0	780	0
noodle, ramen (*Roland*):	460	8.0	62.0	20.0	0	1830	4.0
w/beef	460	8.0	62.0	20.0	0	1830	4.0
w/chicken	460	9.0	62.0	20.0	0	1600	4.0
w/crab	470	9.0	62.0	20.0	0	1750	4.0
w/mushroom	470	0	82.0	20.0	0	1620	4.0
w/pork	470	9.0	62.0	20.0	0	1810	4.0
w/shrimp	470	9.0	62.0	20.0	0	1730	4.0
onion:							
French (*Fantastic* Classic)	90	3.0	15.0	2.5	0	690	2.0
three, noodle (*Fantastic*)	180	7.0	36.0	2.0	5	900	3.0
pea, split:							
(*Alessi* Sicilian), ¼ of 6-oz. pkg. .	120	7.0	24.0	.5	0	740	5.0
(*Fantastic*)	140	10.0	28.0	.5	0	410	5.0
(*Fantastic* Dutch), 1 cup*	120	8.0	15.0	1.0	0	580	5.0
(*Nile Spice*)	200	13.0	35.0	1.0	0	600	8.0
potato w/broccoli, creamy (*Health Valley* Cup), ⅓ cup	80	4.0	17.0	0	0	390	3.0
potato leek:							
(*Nile Spice*)	110	4.0	19.0	3.0	10	570	3.0
creamy (*Fantastic*) .	120	4.0	22.0	2.5	10	620	2.0
Thai, spicy (*Fantastic*)	150	5.0	32.0	.5	0	720	2.0
tomato:							
w/croutons (*Cup-a-Soup*)	90	1.0	16.0	2.5	0	870	<1.0

Food and Measure	cal.	prot. (gms)	carbo. (gms)	fat (gms)	chol. (mgs)	sod. (mgs)	fiber (gms)
Soup, mix, tomato, *(cont.)*							
and shells *(Fantastic*							
Tuscan)	140	6.0	31.0	1.0	0	730	6.0
tortilla:							
(Chi-Chi's Fiesta),							
⅛ pkg.	80	3.0	14.0	1.5	0	820	1.0
bean *(Fantastic*							
Southwest)	170	8.0	34.0	3.5	0	630	8.0
vegetable:							
chicken flavored							
(Nile Spice)	110	4.0	21.0	1.5	5	670	2.0
rice *(Fantastic*							
Summer)	110	4.0	25.0	.5	0	630	4.0
wakame *(San-J)*	50	<1.0	11.0	0	0	960	<1.0
Sour cream, see							
"Cream, sour"							
Sour drink mixer,							
whiskey, 4 fl. oz.:							
(Holland House)	130	0	31.0	0	0	80	0
(Mr & Mrs T)	90	0	22.0	0	0	45	0
Soursop, ½ cup	75	1.1	18.9	.3	0	16	3.7
Soy, cultured, see							
"Yogurt," soy"							
Soy bean, see							
"Soybean"							
Soy beverage (see also							
"Rice-soy beverage"),							
8 fl. oz., except as							
noted:							
(Edensoy Organic Extra							
Original)	130	11.0	13.0	4.0	0	100	<1.0
(Edensoy Organic Extra							
Original), 8.45 fl. oz.	140	11.0	14.0	4.0	0	105	<1.0
(Edensoy Organic Light							
Original)	100	5.0	15.0	2.0	0	90	0
(Edensoy Organic							
Original)	140	11.0	14.0	5.0	0	105	<1.0
(Edensoy Organic							
Unsweetened)	120	12.0	5.0	6.0	0	5	<1.0
(8th Continent Original)	80	6.0	7.0	3.0	0	100	0
(8th Continent Original							
Fat Free)	60	6.0	8.0	0	0	100	0
(8th Continent Original							
Light)	50	6.0	2.0	2.0	0	115	0

Food and Measure	cal.	prot. (gms)	carbo. (gms)	fat (gms)	chol. (mgs)	sod. (mgs)	fiber (gms)
(*Organic Valley* Original)	110	7.0	11.0	4.0	0	100	3.0
(*Organic Valley* Unsweetened)	80	7.0	3.0	4.0	0	110	1.0
(*Pacific* Organic Unsweetened)	90	9.0	4.0	4.5	0	15	2.0
(*Pacific* Select Low Fat)	70	5.0	9.0	2.5	0	115	1.0
(*Pacific* Ultra)	120	10.0	12.0	4.0	0	150	1.0
(*Silk*)	100	7.0	8.0	4.0	0	120	1.0
(*Silk* Light)	70	6.0	8.0	2.0	0	120	1.0
(*Silk* Plus Bone Health)	100	6.0	11.0	3.5	0	95	2.0
(*Silk* Plus DHA Omega-3)	110	7.0	8.0	5.0	0	120	1.0
(*Silk* Unsweetened) ..	80	7.0	4.0	4.0	0	85	1.0
(*Soy Dream* Organic Original Classic Refrigerated)	130	7.0	16.0	4.0	0	150	2.0
(*Soy Dream* Organic Original Enriched) .	100	7.0	8.0	4.0	0	135	2.0
(*Soy Dream* Organic Original Enriched Refrigerated)	100	8.0	9.0	3.5	0	140	2.0
(*WestSoy* Lite)	70	4.0	10.0	2.0	0	95	<1.0
(*WestSoy* Low Fat) ..	110	1.0	20.0	2.5	0	105	0
(*WestSoy* Nonfat) ...	70	6.0	10.0	0	0	105	<1.0
(*WestSoy* Organic Original)	130	8.0	18.0	3.5	0	125	3.0
(*WestSoy* Plus)	100	7.0	10.0	4.0	0	135	<1.0
(*WestSoy* Soy Slender)	60	6.0	3.0	3.0	0	105	3.0
(*WestSoy* Unsweetened)	90	9.0	5.0	4.5	0	30	4.0
almond (*WestSoy* Unsweetened)	90	9.0	5.0	4.5	0	30	4.0
cappucino (*WestSoy* Soy Slender)	70	7.0	4.0	3.0	0	125	3.0
carob (*Edensoy* Organic)	170	7.0	28.0	4.0	0	95	<1.0
chai:							
(*Odwalla Soy Smart*)	150	6.0	22.0	4.0	0	30	0
(*Silk*)	130	6.0	19.0	3.5	0	100	0
chocolate:							
(*Edensoy* Organic) .	180	8.0	28.0	4.0	0	105	<1.0
(*8th Continent*) ...	140	7.0	22.0	3.0	0	125	1.0
(*8th Continent* Light)	90	7.0	12.0	1.5	0	120	<1.0
(*Odwalla Soy Smart*)	160	6.0	24.0	4.5	0	60	0
(*Organic Valley*) ...	130	5.0	20.0	3.0	0	160	3.0
(*Silk*)	140	5.0	23.0	3.5	0	100	2.0

Food and Measure	cal.	prot. (gms)	carbo. (gms)	fat (gms)	chol. (mgs)	sod. (mgs)	fiber (gms)
Soy beverage , chocolate *(cont.)*							
(*Silk* Aseptic), 8¼ oz.	150	5.0	25.0	3.5	0	100	2.0
(*Silk* Light)	120	5.0	22.0	1.5	0	100	2.0
(*Soy Dream* Organic Enriched)	150	7.0	21.0	4.0	0	125	3.0
(*WestSoy* Shake) . .	170	7.0	30.0	3.5	0	130	4.0
(*WestSoy* Soy Slender)	70	7.0	5.0	3.0	0	125	4.0
(*WestSoy* Unsweetened) . .	100	9.0	6.0	4.5	0	30	5.0
chocolate banana (*Odwalla Super Protein*)	170	10.0	24.0	3.5	0	240	0
coffee (*Silk*)	150	5.0	25.0	3.5	0	100	0
mocha (*Silk*)	140	5.0	22.0	3.5	0	100	0
nog (*Silk*)	90	3.0	15.0	2.0	0	75	0
spice (*Silk*), 11 fl. oz. . .	190	8.0	27.0	5.0	0	160	1.0
vanilla:							
(*Edensoy* Organic) .	150	7.0	24.0	3.0	0	85	<1.0
(*Edensoy* Organic Extra)	150	7.0	23.0	3.0	0	90	<1.0
(*Edensoy* Organic Light)	110	4.0	22.0	1.0	0	110	0
(*8th Continent*) . . .	100	6.0	11.0	3.0	0	105	0
(*8th Continent* Nonfat)	70	6.0	11.0	0	0	100	0
(*8th Continent* Light)	60	6.0	5.0	2.0	0	110	0
(*Odwalla Soy Smart*)	120	6.0	16.0	3.5	0	55	0
(*Organic Valley*) . . .	110	6.0	14.0	3.0	0	100	2.0
(*Pacific* Select Low Fat)	80	5.0	9.0	2.5	0	115	<1.0
(*Pacific* Ultra)	130	10.0	14.0	4.0	0	150	1.0
(*Silk*)	100	6.0	10.0	3.5	0	95	1.0
(*Silk* Light)	80	6.0	10.0	2.0	0	95	1.0
(*Silk* Plus Fiber) . . .	100	6.0	14.0	3.5	0	95	5.0
(*Silk* Very Vanilla) .	130	6.0	19.0	4.0	0	140	1.0
(*Soy Dream* Organic Classic)	140	7.0	18.0	4.0	0	135	2.0
(*Soy Dream* Organic Enriched)	120	7.0	14.0	4.0	0	135	2.0
(*Soy Dream* Organic Enriched Refrigerated) . . .	120	8.0	14.0	3.5	0	130	2.0
(*WestSoy* Lite)	90	5.0	14.0	2.0	0	75	<1.0
(*WestSoy* Low Fat)	120	4.0	21.0	1.5	0	90	2.0

Food and Measure	cal.	prot. (gms)	carbo. (gms)	fat (gms)	chol. (mgs)	sod. (mgs)	fiber (gms)
(*WestSoy* Nonfat)	80	6.0	12.0	0	0	105	<1.0
(*WestSoy* Plus)	130	7.0	16.0	4.0	0	135	<1.0
(*WestSoy* Shake)	170	7.0	28.0	3.0	0	125	3.0
(*WestSoy* Soy Slender)	70	6.0	4.0	3.0	0	125	3.0
(*WestSoy* Unsweetened)	100	9.0	5.0	4.5	0	30	4.0
vanilla almond (*Odwalla*)	190	10.0	25.0	6.0	0	80	3.0
vanilla chai tea (*Bolthouse Farms Perfectly Protein*)	160	10.0	25.0	3.0	0	60	0
Soy butter, see "Soy spread"							
Soy chips/crisps (see also "Potato soy crisps"), 1 oz.:							
(*Genisoy* Crispy Dippers Lightly Salted)	120	8.0	16.0	3.0	0	220	2.0
(*Genisoy* Smart Hearts Lightly Salted)	120	7.0	17.0	3.0	0	270	2.0
(*Stacy's* Sticky Bun)	130	6.0	15.0	5.0	0	180	3.0
apple cinnamon (*GeniSoy* Crisps)	110	7.0	17.0	2.0	0	160	2.0
barbecue:							
(*GeniSoy* Crisps)	120	7.0	17.0	3.0	0	270	2.0
(*Quaker* Crisps)	110	6.0	15.0	4.0	0	400	2.0
(*Stacy's* Sweet)	120	6.0	16.0	4.5	0	390	3.0
cheddar (*GeniSoy* Crisps)	110	7.0	14.0	3.0	0	270	2.0
cheddar, white:							
(*Genisoy* Crispy Dippers)	120	7.0	16.0	2.5	0	270	2.0
(*Genisoy* Smart Hearts)	120	7.0	16.0	3.0	0	270	2.0
(*Quaker* Crisps)	120	7.0	14.0	4.5	5	270	2.0
cheese:							
(*Stacy's* Simply Cheese)	130	7.0	13.0	6.0	0	230	3.0
nacho (*GeniSoy* Crisps)	110	7.0	15.0	2.0	0	170	2.0
garlic, roasted, onion (*GeniSoy* Crisps)	100	7.0	14.0	2.0	0	280	2.0
Parmesan, garlic, olive oil (*Eatsmart* Crisps)	160	8.0	11.0	9.0	0	290	5.0
ranch (*GeniSoy* Crisps)	120	7.0	15.0	3.0	0	270	2.0

Food and Measure	cal.	prot. (gms)	carbo. (gms)	fat (gms)	chol. (mgs)	sod. (mgs)	fiber (gms)
Soy chips/crisps *(cont.)*							
salt and vinegar (*Geni-Soy* Crisps)	100	7.0	14.0	2.0	0	290	2.0
sea salted (*GeniSoy* Crisps)	110	7.0	14.0	3.0	0	270	2.0
tomato/Romano/olive oil (*Eatsmart* Crisps)	150	7.0	11.0	9.0	0	360	5.0
tortilla chips:							
(*Genisoy* Lightly Salted)	110	8.0	14.0	3.0	0	280	2.0
nacho (*Genisoy*) . .	110	8.0	13.0	3.0	0	260	2.0
Soy flour, see "Soybean flour"							
Soy meal, defatted, raw, 1 cup	414	54.8	49.0	2.9	0	3	14.0
Soy milk, see "Soy beverage"							
Soy nuts, roasted:							
(*Amport Foods* Lightly Salted), 3 tbsp., 1.1 oz.	140	10.0	10.0	7.0	0	90	5.0
(*Frieda's* Salted), ⅓ cup, 1.1 oz.	140	11.0	9.0	7.0	0	50	1.0
(*GeniSoy* Unsalted), 1 oz.	120	11.0	10.0	5.0	0	10	5.0
(*SunRidge Farms* Organic). ¼ cup, 1.1 oz.	150	11.0	9.0	8.0	0	95	5.0
(*Tree of Life*), 1.3 oz. .	150	12.0	9.0	7.0	0	80	3.0
(*Tree of Life* Organic), 1 oz.	130	<11.0	9.0	6.0	0	90	<2.0
apple, crispy (*Amport Foods*), 3 tbsp., 1.1 oz.	140	9.0	11.0	8.0	0	20	7.0
barbecue:							
(*Amport Foods*), 3 tbsp., 1 oz. . . .	130	9.0	10.0	7.0	0	210	5.0
(*GeniSoy*), 1 oz. . . .	120	10.0	11.0	4.0	0	230	7.0
barbecue, honey, or wasabi (*Frieda's*), ¼ cup	140	10.0	11.0	7.0	0	110	5.0
hickory smoked (*Geni-Soy*), 1 oz.	120	10.0	11.0	5.0	0	290	6.0

Food and Measure	cal.	prot. (gms)	carbo. (gms)	fat (gms)	chol. (mgs)	sod. (mgs)	fiber (gms)
honey (*Amport Foods*), 3 tbsp., 1.1 oz.	140	10.0	11.0	6.0	0	66	1.0
sea salted (*GeniSoy*), 1 oz.	120	10.0	11.0	4.0	0	230	7.0
toasted:							
1 oz. or 95 kernels .	129	10.5	8.7	6.8	0	1	1.0
whole, 1 cup	490	40.0	33.0	25.9	0	4	3.9
Soy protein, concentrate, 1 oz.:							
w/alcohol	94	16.5	8.8	.1	0	1	<2.0
acid/water wash	94	16.5	8.8	.1	0	255	<2.0
Soy sauce, 1 tbsp.:							
(*House of Tsang* Less Sodium)	5	0	0	0	0	300	0
(*La Choy*)	10	1.0	1.0	0	0	1160	0
(*La Choy* Lite)	15	1.0	2.0	0	0	550	0
(*World Harbors Angostura*)	10	1.0	1.0	0	0	670	0
(*World Harbors Angostura Lite*) ...	10	1.0	2.0	0	0	390	0
citrus seasoned (*Mitsukan* Ajipon) .	10	0	1.0	0	0	580	0
ginger flavor:							
(*House of Tsang*) ..	20	0	4.0	0	0	760	0
(*House of Tsang.* Less Sodium) ...	10	0	2.0	0	0	320	0
shoyu:							
(*Eden* Imported) ...	15	2.0	2.0	0	0	1010	0
(*Eden* Organic)	15	2.0	2.0	0	0	1040	0
(*Eden* Organic Imported Reduced Sodium)	10	2.0	2.0	0	0	500	0
(*San-J* Organic) ...	10	2.0	1.0	0	0	960	0
(*Tree of Life* Organic)	15	2.0	0	0	0	960	0
tamari:							
(*Eden* Organic)	15	2.0	2.0	0	0	860	0
(*Eden* Organic Imported)	10	2.0	2.0	0	0	990	0
(*San-J* Organic Wheat Free)	10	2.0	<1.0	0	0	940	0
(*San-J* Premium) ..	15	2.0	1.0	0	0	960	0
(*San-J* Premium/ Organic Wheat Free/Reduced Sodium)	15	2.0	1.0	0	0	700	0

Food and Measure	cal.	prot. (gms)	carbo. (gms)	fat (gms)	chol. (mgs)	sod. (mgs)	fiber (gms)
Soy sauce, tamari *(cont.)*							
(*Tree of Life* Organic Wheat Free)	15	2.0	0	0	0	940	0
Soy spread, creamy or crunchy (*Soy Wonder*), 2 tbsp. ..	170	8.0	10.0	11.0	0	170	1.0
Soybean, fresh (see also "Edamame"):							
raw, shelled, ½ cup ..	188	16.6	14.1	8.7	0	19	5.4
boiled, drained, ½ cup	127	11.1	10.0	5.8	0	13	3.8
Soybean, canned, ½ cup:							
(*Westbrae Natural* Organic)	150	13.0	11.0	7.0	0	140	3.0
black (*Eden* Organic Blacksoy)	120	11.0	8.0	6.0	0	30	7.0
Soybean, dried:							
dry, ¼ cup:							
(*Arrowhead Mills* Organic)	160	14.0	11.0	8.0	0	0	4.0
black or yellow (*Shiloh Farms* Organic)	170	15.0	14.0	8.0	0	0	10.0
dry-roasted	194	17.0	14.1	9.3	0	1	3.5
roasted	202	15.2	14.5	10.9	0	70	3.5
boiled, ½ cup	149	14.3	8.5	7.7	0	1	5.2
Soybean, frozen, see "Edamame, frozen"							
Soybean curd, see "Tofu"							
Soybean flakes (*Shiloh Farms* Organic), ¼ cup	120	12.0	8.0	5.0	0	0	3.0
Soybean flour, ¼ cup:							
(*Arrowhead Mills* Organic)	100	7.0	9.0	4.5	0	0	4.0
(*Hodgson Mill*), <¼ cup	80	14.0	10.0	0	0	0	6.0
(*Hodgson Mill* Organic), <¼ cup	120	10.0	10.0	6.0	0	0	6.0
stirred:							
full fat, raw	93	7.4	7.5	4.4	0	3	2.1
defatted	82	11.8	9.6	.3	0	5	4.4
low fat	72	10.2	8.4	.6	0	4	2.3

Food and Measure	cal.	prot. (gms)	carbo. (gms)	fat (gms)	chol. (mgs)	sod. (mgs)	fiber (gms)
Soybean kernels, roasted, see "Soy nuts"							
Soybean sprouts, steamed, ½ cup ...	38	4.0	3.1	2.1	0	5	.4
Spaghetti, see "Pasta"							
Spaghetti entree, canned, 1 cup:							
w/meatballs (*Chef Boyardee* Mini)	250	10.0	30.0	10.0	10	900	3.0
tomato cheese sauce (*Campbell's*)	200	7.0	40.0	1.5	5	950	3.0
Spaghetti entree, frozen, 1 pkg.:							
Bolognese (*Smart Ones*), 11.5 oz.	310	16.0	48.0	6.0	15	580	5.0
cheesy (*Stouffer's Bake*), 12 oz.	460	21.0	39.0	24.0	120	950	4.0
marinara, 8 oz.:							
(*Michelina's Budget Gourmet*)	270	9.0	49.0	3.5	0	620	3.0
(*Michelina's Zap'ems*)	250	8.0	47.0	2.0	0	430	3.0
w/meat sauce:							
(*Healthy Choice*), 9 oz.	220	10.0	36.0	3.5	10	510	5.0
(*Lean Cuisine One Dish Favorites*), 11.5 oz.	290	15.0	47.0	4.5	15	600	4.0
(*Michelina's Authentico*), 8.5 oz.	300	11.0	46.0	7.0	10	750	4.0
(*Michelina's Lean Gourmet*), 8.5 oz.	300	11.0	46.0	6.0	10	540	3.0
(*Michelina's Signature*), 11.5 oz. ..	370	17.0	59.0	7.0	20	570	4.0
(*Stouffer's*), 12 oz. .	350	17.0	44.0	12.0	30	660	5.0
w/meatballs:							
(*Lean Cuisine One Dish Favorites*), 9.5 oz.	260	18.0	35.0	5.0	25	560	5.0
(*Michelina's Authentico*), 9 oz.	320	14.0	41.0	10.0	20	800	4.0
(*Michelina's Zap'ems*), 8 oz.	270	12.0	37.0	8.0	15	710	3.0
(*Stouffer's*), 12⅝ oz.	360	19.0	45.0	12.0	35	850	6.0

Food and Measure	cal.	prot. (gms)	carbo. (gms)	fat (gms)	chol. (mgs)	sod. (mgs)	fiber (gms)
Spaghetti entree, frozen *(cont.)*							
roasted red pepper (*Michelina's Lean Gourmet*), 8 oz. . .	270	9.0	46.0	6.0	5	500	3.0
Sicilian (*Michelina's Signature*), 8 oz. . . .	290	13.0	38.0	8.0	25	850	3.0
Spaghetti entree, microwave, meat sauce.:							
(*Hormel* Micro Meal), 7.5 oz.	210	14.0	31.0	5.0	15	750	3.0
(*Hormel Compleats*), 10 oz.	280	15.0	36.0	8.0	25	1300	4.0
Spaghetti entree mix, ¼ pkg.:							
Italian, tangy (*Kraft Spaghetti Classics*)	200	8.0	38.0	1.5	0	600	1.0
w/meat sauce (*Kraft Spaghetti Classics*)	330	12.0	46.0	11.0	15	830	3.0
Spaghetti sauce, see "Pasta sauce"							
Spaghetti squash:							
raw (*Frieda's*), 3 oz. . . .	30	1.0	6.0	0	0	15	1.0
baked or boiled, drained, ½ cup	23	.5	5.0	.2	0	14	1.1
Spanakopita, see "Spinach appetizer" and "Spinach entree"							
Spareribs, see "Pork" and "Pork, frozen/ refrigerated"							
Spelt, grain, ¼ cup:							
(*Shiloh Farms* Organic)	130	7.0	32.0	1.0	0	0	8.0
(*VitaSpelt* Berries Organic)	160	6.0	34.0	1.0	0	0	7.0
(*VitaSpelt* Kernels) . . .	180	7.0	32.0	<1.0	0	0	<8.0
(*VitaSpelt* Kernels Organic)	130	7.0	32.0	1.0	0	0	8.0
Spelt bran (*Shiloh Farms* Organic), ¼ cup . . .	30	2.0	10.0	0	0	<1	7.0
Spelt flakes (see also "Cereal, ready-to-eat"), ¼ cup:							
(*Shiloh Farms* Organic)	140	6.0	28.0	.5	0	0	4.0
toasted (*VitaSpelt*) . . .	93	3.5	20.0	.5	0	1	3.0

Food and Measure	cal.	prot. (gms)	carbo. (gms)	fat (gms)	chol. (mgs)	sod. (mgs)	fiber (gms)
Spelt flour:							
(*Arrowhead Mills* Organic), ⅓ cup ...	130	4.0	25.0	1.0	0	0	4.0
(*Hodgson Mill* Organic), <¼ cup	85	5.0	21.0	1.0	0	0	5.0
(*Shiloh Farms* Organic), ¼ cup	110	5.0	23.0	1.0	0	0	2.0
sprouted (*Shiloh Farms* Organic), ¼ cup ...	90	4.0	20.0	1.0	0	0	3.0
white (*VitaSpelt* Organic), ¼ cup	100	4.0	21.0	<1.0	0	0	<1.0
whole grain (*VitaSpelt* Organic), ¼ cup ...	110	5.0	23.0	1.0	0	0	2.0
Spinach, fresh:							
raw:							
(*Del Monte*), 1½ cups	40	2.0	10.0	0	0	160	5.0
(*Dole/Dole* Baby), 3 oz.	20	2.0	3.0	0	0	65	2.0
(*Fresh Express/ Fresh Express* Baby), 3 oz.	20	2.0	3.0	0	0	65	2.0
baby (*Ready Pac*), 4 cups, 3 oz. ...	20	2.0	3.0	0	0	65	2.0
flat leaf (*Fresh Express*), 1½ cups, 3 oz.	40	2.0	10.0	0	0	160	5.0
cooked, boiled, drained, ½ cup	21	2.7	3.4	.2	0	63	2.2
Spinach, canned, ½ cup:							
leaf:							
(*Popeye* No Salt) ..	40	4.0	5.0	.5	0	30	2.0
(*S&W*)	30	2.0	4.0	0	0	360	2.0
cut (*Freshlike*)	45	5.0	5.0	1.0	0	200	3.0
leaf or chopped:							
(*Del Monte*)	30	2.0	4.0	0	0	360	2.0
(*Popeye*)	30	3.0	4.0	0	0	190	2.0
seasoned (*Glory*)	20	2.0	4.0	0	0	510	2.0
drained	25	3.0	3.6	.5	0	29	2.6
Spinach, frozen (see also "Spinach dish"):							
leaf or chopped (*Birds Eye/C&W*), ⅓ cup .	30	2.0	3.0	0	0	125	1.0

Food and Measure	cal.	prot. (gms)	carbo. (gms)	fat (gms)	chol. (mgs)	sod. (mgs)	fiber (gms)
Spinach, frozen (cont.)							
cut leaf:							
(*Birds Eye*), 1 cup .	30	2.0	3.0	0	0	120	1.0
(*Cascadian Farm* Organic), ⅓ cup .	20	2.0	3.0	0	0	130	3.0
(*Tree of Life* Organic), 1 cup	20	2.0	2.0	1.0	0	110	2.0
cut leaf or chopped (*Seabrook Farms*), ⅓ cup	20	2.0	2.0	0	0	115	2.0
chopped:							
(*C&W* Baby/Organic), 1 cup	30	2.0	3.0	0	0	120	1.0
(*Green Giant* No Sauce), ½ cup . .	25	2.0	3.0	0	0	200	1.0
chopped or leaf, drained, ½ cup	27	3.0	5.1	.2	0	82	2.6
in butter sauce, cut leaf (*Green Giant*), ½ cup	30	2.0	4.0	1.0	<5	330	2.0
Spinach, malabar, cooked, 1 cup	10	1.3	1.2	.4	0	24	.9
Spinach, New Zealand, chopped:							
raw, ½ cup, 1 oz.	4	.4	.7	.1	0	37	n.a.
boiled, drained, ½ cup	11	1.2	2.0	.2	0	97	n.a.
Spinach appetizer (see also "Spinach dip"), frozen/refrigerated:							
w/feta:							
(*Amy's*), 5–6 pcs. . .	170	7.0	24.0	6.0	15	430	2.0
(*Athens/Apollo* Spanikopita), 2 pcs., 2 oz.	160	4.0	17.0	8.0	20	240	1.0
(*The Fillo Factory* Organic Spanako- pita), 4 pcs., 3.3 oz.	210	7.0	26.0	9.0	10	340	2.0
triangles (*The Fillo Factory* Spanako- pita), 3 pcs., 3 oz.	190	6.0	20.0	10.0	20	280	1.0
nuggets/rolls, breaded:							
(*Veggie Patch* Nug- gets, 4 pcs., 3 oz.	150	6.0	19.0	7.0	0	390	3.0

Food and Measure	cal.	prot. (gms)	carbo. (gms)	fat (gms)	chol. (mgs)	sod. (mgs)	fiber (gms)
w/artichoke (*Morning-star Farms* Veggie Bites), 3 pcs., 3 oz.	190	9.0	16.0	10.0	10	570	2.0
w/artichoke, cheese (*Veggie Patch Bistro Au Naturel*), 3 pcs., 2.6 oz. . .	170	4.0	16.0	11.0	10	380	1.0
w/cheese (*Kineret*), 3½ pcs., 2.8 oz. . .	180	8.0	19.0	8.0	5	620	6.0
with cheese, three (*Veggie Patch* Bites), 3 pcs., 2.6 oz.	150	6.0	16.0	8.0	10	350	3.0
pâté w/Roquefort (*Les Trois Petits Cochons*), 2 oz.	100	5.0	3.0	8.0	80	310	1.0
Spinach dip, 2 tbsp.:							
(*Marzetti's*)	130	1.0	2.0	13.0	20	250	0
artichoke (*Fiesta*)	60	3.0	12.0	.5	0	390	0
Parmesan (*Marie's*) . .	90	2.0	2.0	9.0	15	200	0
Spinach dip, frozen, w/cheese, artichoke, Alfredo (*T.G.I. Friday's*), 2 tbsp. . .	45	2.0	2.0	3.5	10	115	<1.0
Spinach dip mix, dry (*McCormick*), 1 tsp. .	10	0	1.0	0	0	100	0
Spinach dish, frozen, ½ cup, except as noted:							
creamed:							
(*Birds Eye* Real) . . .	100	3.0	7.0	7.0	35	630	1.0
(*C&W*)	100	4.0	6.0	7.0	20	410	4.0
(*Green Giant*)	70	3.0	9.0	2.5	0	520	1.0
(*Seabrook Farms*) .	120	4.0	10.0	6.0	15	450	3.0
(*Stouffer's*), ½ of 9-oz. pkg.	200	5.0	8.0	16.0	25	490	2.0
pancake (*Dr. Praeger's*), 2-oz. cake	80	2.0	9.0	4.0	0	190	2.0
Spinach entree, frozen, 1 pkg., except as noted:							
w/cheese, palak paneer:							
(*Amy's*), 10 oz.	320	8.0	36.0	18.0	20	550	5.0
(*Ethnic Gourmet*), 11 oz.	240	13.0	23.0	11.0	35	810	4.0

Food and Measure	cal.	prot. (gms)	carbo. (gms)	fat (gms)	chol. (mgs)	sod. (mgs)	fiber (gms)
Spinach entree, frozen *(cont.)*							
cheese pie (*The Fillo Factory*), ⅛ of 24-oz. pkg.	240	10.0	27.0	11.0	20	490	2.0
and feta pie:							
(*Cedarlane* Organic Spanakopita), ½ of 10-oz. pkg.	260	12.0	38.0	8.0	20	650	2.0
(*The Fillo Factory* Organic), ½ of 10-oz. pkg.	300	11.0	34.0	14.0	20	470	3.0
Spinach entree, pkg.:							
w/cheese:							
(*Tamarind Tree* Palak Paneer), 9.25-oz. pkg.	380	14.0	46.0	15.0	35	640	6.0
(*Tasty Bite* Kashmir), ½ of 10-oz. pkg. .	133	6.0	8.0	8.0	0	693	3.0
w/garbanzos (*Tamarind Tree* Saag Chole), 9.25-oz. pkg.	370	14.0	55.0	10.0	0	800	13.0
w/lentils (*Tasty Bite* Dal), ½ of 10-oz. pkg. . .	115	5.0	13.0	5.0	0	534	4.0
w/soy (*Tasty Bite*), ½ of 10-oz. pkg. . .	110	5.0	10.0	7.0	0	450	3.0
Spinach snack rolls/ nuggets, see "Spinach appetizer"							
Spinach pocket sandwich, frozen, 1 pc.:							
and feta:							
(*Amy's*), 4.5 oz. . . .	260	11.0	34.0	9.0	20	590	3.0
(*Aunt Trudy's*), 5 oz.	270	11.0	31.0	12.0	20	510	3.0
and potato (*Aunt Trudy's* Organic), 5 oz.	250	6.0	40.0	9.0	0	380	4.0
Spiny lobster, meat only:							
raw, 4 oz.	127	23.4	2.8	1.7	80	201	0
boiled or steamed:							
2 lbs. in shell	233	43.1	5.1	3.2	146	370	0
4 oz.	138	29.9	3.5	2.2	102	257	0
Spleen, braised:							
beef, 4 oz.	164	28.5	0	4.8	394	65	0
lamb, 4 oz.	177	30.0	0	5.4	437	66	0

Food and Measure	cal.	prot. (gms)	carbo. (gms)	fat (gms)	chol. (mgs)	sod. (mgs)	fiber (gms)
pork, 4 oz.	169	32.0	0	3.6	572	121	0
veal, 4 oz.	146	27.3	0	3.3	507	66	0
Split peas:							
dry, green, ¼ cup:							
(*Arrowhead Mills*							
Organic)	160	12.0	24.0	1.0	0	10	4.0
or yellow (*Shiloh*							
Farms Organic) .	110	11.0	27.0	0	0	25	11.0
boiled, ½ cup	116	8.2	20.7	.4	0	2	8.1
Sports drink, all flavors,							
8 fl. oz.:							
(*Blue Sport*)	45	0	12.0	0	0	130	0
(*Gatorade*)	50	0	14.0	0	0	110	0
(*Recharge*)	70	0	18.0	0	0	25	0
Spot, meat only:							
raw, 4 oz.	140	21.0	0	5.6	68	33	0
baked or broiled, 4 oz.	179	26.9	0	7.1	87	42	0
Sprats, smoked, canned							
(*Roland*), ¼ cup . . .	165	12.0	0	19.0	85	360	0
Spring roll (see also							
"Egg roll"), frozen:							
chicken and cheese							
(*Original Rangoon*),							
1-oz. pc.	80	6.0	5.0	4.0	20	160	0
shrimp:							
(*Matlaw's* Party							
Pack), 4 oz.	190	13.0	25.0	6.0	70	630	3.0
Chinese or Thai style							
(*Blue Horizon Or-*							
ganic), 3 pcs.,							
2.1 oz.	130	3.0	15.0	4.0	0	250	1.0
steak/cheese (*Original*							
Rangoon), 2-oz. pc.	225	11.0	40.0	12.0	40	470	0
vegetable:							
Chinese or Thai style							
(*Blue Horizon Or-*							
ganic), 3 pcs.,							
2.1 oz.	110	3.0	16.0	4.0	0	210	1.0
Indian style (*Blue*							
Horizon Organic),							
3 pcs., 2.1 oz. . . .	110	3.0	15.0	4.0	0	250	1.0
SpriteMelon (*Frieda's*),							
10.6-oz. melon	115	0	29.0	0	0	190	2.0

Food and Measure	cal.	prot. (gms)	carbo. (gms)	fat (gms)	chol. (mgs)	sod. (mgs)	fiber (gms)
Sprouts, see "Bean sprouts" and specific listings							
Squab, fresh, raw:							
meat w/skin, 4 oz. ...	333	20.9	0	27.0	108	61	0
breast meat only, 4 oz.	161	19.8	0	8.5	102	62	0
Squash, see specific listings							
Squash puree, cinnamon spiced, frozen (*Green Giant*), ½ cup	80	1.0	19.0	0	0	110	1.0
Squid, fresh, meat only, raw, 4 oz.	104	17.7	3.5	1.6	265	50	0
Squid, canned, see "Cuttlefish"							
Squirrel, meat only, roasted, 4 oz.	196	34.9	0	5.3	137	135	0
Star fruit, see "Carambola"							
Star spangled squash (*Frieda's*), 3 oz. ...	20	2.0	3.0	0	0	0	1.0
Starbucks, drinks[1]:							
Classics, grande, no cream/topping:							
caramel apple cider	310	0	74.0	0	0	25	0
chocolate milk	350	18.0	52.0	11.0	35	190	2.0
chocolate milk, nonfat	280	18.0	53.0	2.5	10	190	2.0
cinnamon dulce crème	280	12.0	40.0	7.0	30	150	0
honey crème	270	12.0	39.0	7.0	30	160	0
hot chocolate	300	14.0	47.0	9.0	25	140	2.0
pumpkin spice crème	320	15.0	50.0	7.0	30	230	0
vanilla crème	260	12.0	36.0	7.0	30	150	0
white hot chocolate	410	16.0	61.0	12.0	30	260	0
coffee, 16 oz. grande:							
caffé misto/café au lait	110	7.0	10.0	4.0	15	90	0
iced, shaken	90	0	21.0	0	0	5	0

[1]*Unless otherwise noted, data are for 16 fl. oz. grande, prepared with 2% reduced fat milk; for whipped cream and toppings values, see "drink extras."*

Food and Measure	cal.	prot. (gms)	carbo. (gms)	fat (gms)	chol. (mgs)	sod. (mgs)	fiber (gms)
espresso, hot, 1 fl. oz.:							
plain	5	0	1.0	0	0	0	0
con panna	30	0	2.0	2.5	10	0	0
macchiato, 2%	10	0	1.0	0	0	0	0
espresso, hot, grande, no cream/topping:							
caffé Americano ...	15	1.0	3.0	0	0	10	0
caffé latte	190	12.0	18.0	7.0	30	150	0
caffé mocha	260	13.0	41.0	8.0	25	125	2.0
cappuccino	120	8.0	12.0	4.0	15	85	0
caramel macchiato .	240	10.0	34.0	7.0	25	130	0
cinnamon dolce latte	260	11.0	40.0	6.0	25	135	0
w/no sugar syrup	180	12.0	18.0	6.0	25	150	0
honey latte	260	11.0	38.0	6.0	25	135	0
peppermint white chocolate mocha	460	14.0	78.0	11.0	25	230	0
pumpkin spice latte	310	14.0	49.0	6.0	25	210	0
vanilla or syrup flavored latte ...	250	12.0	36.0	6.0	25	135	0
white chocolate mocha	400	15.0	61.0	11.0	25	240	0
espresso, iced, grande, no cream/topping:							
caffé Americano ...	15	1.0	3.0	0	0	10	0
caffé latte	130	8.0	13.0	4.5	20	100	0
caffé mocha	200	9.0	35.0	6.0	15	75	2.0
caramel macchiato .	230	10.0	33.0	6.0	25	125	0
honey latte	190	7.0	32.0	4.0	15	90	0
peppermint white chocolate latte ..	400	9.0	72.0	9.0	15	180	0
pumpkin spice latte	250	10.0	44.0	4.0	15	160	0
vanilla or syrup flavored latte ...	190	7.0	30.0	4.0	15	90	0
white chocolate mocha	340	10.0	55.0	9.0	15	190	0
espresso, skinny, non- fat milk, grande:							
hot, all varieties ...	130	12.0	19.0	0	5	170	0
iced, all varieties ..	80	7.0	12.0	0	5	105	0
Frappuccino coffee, grande, no cream/ topping:							
caffé vanilla	310	5.0	67.0	3.0	15	230	0
caramel	270	5.0	53.0	3.5	15	230	0

Food and Measure	cal.	prot. (gms)	carbo. (gms)	fat (gms)	chol. (mgs)	sod. (mgs)	fiber (gms)
Starbucks, Frappuccino coffee, grande, no cream/topping *(cont.)*							
cinnamon dolce ...	260	5.0	52.0	3.0	15	220	0
coffee	240	5.0	48.0	3.0	15	220	0
espresso	190	4.0	38.0	2.5	10	170	0
honey	260	5.0	54.0	3.0	15	220	0
java chip	340	7.0	64.0	8.0	15	230	2.0
mocha	260	6.0	54.0	3.5	15	230	0
pumpkin spice	290	6.0	59.0	3.5	15	260	0
white chocolate mocha	300	6.0	59.0	4.5	15	250	0
Frappuccino coffee, light, grande, no cream/topping:							
caffé vanilla	190	6.0	42.0	1.0	0	240	3.0
caramel	160	5.0	30.0	1.5	5	230	3.0
cinnamon dolce ...	140	5.0	29.0	.5	0	230	3.0
coffee	130	5.0	25.0	.5	0	230	3.0
espresso	110	6.0	29.0	1.0	0	230	3.0
honey	150	5.0	31.0	.5	0	230	3.0
java chip	200	6.0	36.0	4.5	0	220	4.0
mocha	140	6.0	29.0	1.0	0	230	3.0
pumpkin spice	150	6.0	31.0	.5	0	240	3.0
white chocolate mocha	180	6.0	34.0	2.0	0	260	3.0
Frappuccino crème, grande, no cream/ topping:							
double chocolate chip	400	13.0	75.0	8.0	5	290	2.0
honey	310	10.0	63.0	1.0	5	300	1.0
pumpkin spice	360	12.0	71.0	2.5	5	350	0
strawberries/créme	440	12.0	92.0	2.5	5	320	1.0
Tazo chai	330	10.0	67.0	2.0	5	290	1.0
Tazo green tea	380	11.0	78.0	2.5	5	290	1.0
vanilla bean	350	11.0	72.0	2.5	5	310	0
Tazo tea, grande[1]:							
chai latte, hot or iced	240	7.0	44.0	4.0	15	95	0
green tea latte	240	8.0	41.0	4.5	15	85	1.0
green tea latte, iced	270	10.0	44.0	5.0	20	115	1.0
iced, all teas	80	0	21.0	0	0	10	0
iced, tea lemonade, all teas	130	0	33.0	0	0	10	0

[1]Data are for 16 fl. oz. grande; lattes are prepared with 2% reduced fat milk.

Food and Measure	cal.	prot. (gms)	carbo. (gms)	fat (gms)	chol. (mgs)	sod. (mgs)	fiber (gms)
drink extras:							
syrup, 2 pumps:							
flavored	40	0	10.0	0	0	0	0
mocha	50	1.0	12.0	1.0	0	0	<1.0
sugar free	0	0	0	0	0	0	0
toppings:							
caramel	15	0	2.0	.5	0	5	0
chocolate	5	0	1.0	0	0	0	0
sprinkles	0	0	0	0	0	0	0
whipped cream, for 16 fl. oz. grande:							
cold drinks	110	1.0	3.0	11.0	40	10	0
hot drinks	70	0	2.0	7.0	25	5	0
Steak sauce (see also "Marinade"), 1 tbsp., except as noted:							
(*A.1.*)	15	0	3.0	0	0	280	0
(*A.1.* Bold & Spicy w/*Tabasco*)	20	0	5.0	0	0	260	0
(*A.1.* Carb Well)	5	0	1.0	0	0	230	0
(*A.1.* Thick & Hearty) .	25	0	6.0	0	0	290	0
(*Buccaneer Blends* Pirates Original) ...	20	0	4.0	0	0	115	0
(*Canadian Club*)	15	0	3.0	0	0	125	0
(*Emeril's*)	20	0	4.0	0	0	200	0
(*HP*)	15	0	4.0	0	0	140	0
(*London Pub* Steak & Chop)	15	0	3.0	0	0	80	0
(*Newman's Own*)	20	0	4.0	.5	0	85	0
(*Rio Grande*)	30	0	7.0	0	0	115	0
(*San-J* Japanese)	15	2.0	2.0	0	0	940	0
(*Smith & Wollensky* Pepper Steak)	30	2.0	2.0	1.0	<5	280	0
(*Watkins*)	20	0	4.0	0	0	200	0
(*World Harbors* Prairie Fire Steakhouse) ..	35	0	7.0	0	0	135	0
cracked pepper (*A.1.*)	15	0	0	0	0	230	0
and burger (*TryMe* Bullfighter)	15	0	4.0	0	0	220	0
garlic, roasted (*A.1.*) .	20	0	5.0	0	0	170	0
hickory, sweet (*A.1.* w/*Bull's Eye* BBQ Sauce)	20	0	4.0	0	0	210	0

Food and Measure	cal.	prot. (gms)	carbo. (gms)	fat (gms)	chol. (mgs)	sod. (mgs)	fiber (gms)
Steak sauce *(cont.)*							
Jamaican *(Pickapeppa)*,							
1 tsp.	5	0	1.0	0	0	40	0
mesquite, smoky *(A.1.)*	30	0	8.0	0	0	240	0
spicy:							
(Buccaneer Blends							
Swashbucklin') . .	20	0	4.0	0	0	110	0
(London Pub)	19	0	4.0	0	0	120	0
teriyaki *(A.1.)*	20	0	4.0	0	0	280	0
Steak sauce, cooking,							
see "Grilling sauce"							
Steak seasoning,							
¼ tsp.:							
(Grill Mates Montreal)	0	0	0	0	0	120	0
(McCormick Steak-							
house Grinder)	0	0	0	0	0	70	0
broiled *(McCormick)* .	0	0	0	0	0	230	0
Stir-fry sauce (see also							
"Marinade," and spe-							
cific sauces) *(House*							
of Tsang), 1 tbsp.:							
Bangkok Padang	45	1.0	4.0	2.5	0	250	0
General Tsao	45	0	10.0	.5	0	230	0
oyster flavor	30	0	7.0	0	0	600	0
Saigon Sizzle	45	0	7.0	2.0	0	380	0
soy, Imperial citrus . .	25	0	5.0	0	0	170	0
sweet and sour	35	0	9.0	0	0	75	0
Szechuan, spicy	25	0	4.0	1.0	0	500	0
teriyaki, Korean	35	0	5.0	1.5	0	460	0
Stomach, pork, raw,							
1 oz.	44	4.7	0	2.7	55	15	0
Strawberry, fresh:							
(Dole), 8 medium	45	1.0	12.0	0	0	0	4.0
halves, ½ cup	23	.5	5.3	.3	0	1	1.8
pureed, ½ cup	35	.7	8.1	.4	0	1	2.7
Strawberry, canned,							
½ cup:							
in light syrup *(Oregon)*	100	1.0	23.0	0	0	5	2.0
in heavy syrup	117	.7	29.9	.3	0	5	2.2
Strawberry, dried:							
(Frieda's), ½ cup,							
1.4 oz.	150	1.0	34.0	0	0	0	3.0
(Fruit Additions),							
.8-oz. pkg.	80	1.0	20.0	0	0	0	0

Food and Measure	cal.	prot. (gms)	carbo. (gms)	fat (gms)	chol. (mgs)	sod. (mgs)	fiber (gms)
(*Shiloh Farms* Organic), ⅓ cup, 1.4 oz.	130	1.0	33.0	.5	0	0	2.0
Strawberry, frozen:							
whole:							
(*Cascadian Farm* Organic), 1 cup .	45	<1.0	13.0	0	0	0	3.0
(*Dole*), 1 cup	50	0	13.0	0	0	0	3.0
(*Tree of Life* Organic), ¾ cup	50	0	13.0	0	0	0	2.0
whole or sliced (*C&W* Ultimate), ⅔ cup ..	50	0	12.0	0	0	5	1.0
sliced:							
(*Dole*), 1 cup	50	0	13.0	0	0	0	3.0
(*Dole* Sugar Tub), ½ cup	150	0	38.0	0	0	0	2.0
unsweetened, ½ cup .	39	.5	10.1	.1	0	2	2.3
Strawberry drink, sparkling (*R.W. Knudsen*), 8 fl. oz. .	110	<1.0	27.0	0	0	15	0
Strawberry drink blend, 8 fl. oz., except as noted:							
all varieties (*Langers*)	120	0	30.0	0	0	10	0
banana:							
(*SoBe Lizard Fuel*) .	120	0	30.0	0	0	25	0
(*Tropicana* Smoothie), 11 fl. oz.	220	2.0	53.0	0	0	35	2.0
(*V8 Splash* Smoothie)	90	3.0	20.0	0	0	70	0
daiquiri (*SoBe Lizard Lava*)	130	0	31.0	0	0	20	0
kiwi:							
(*Capri Sun*)	120	0	32.0	0	0	20	0
(*Hi-C Blast*)	120	0	31.0	0	0	140	0
(*V8 Splash*)	70	0	18.0	0	0	50	0
raspberry (*Minute Maid*)	120	0	33.0	0	0	20	0
Strawberry drink mix (*Nesquik*), 2 tbsp. ..	60	0	15.0	0	0	0	0
Strawberry glaze:							
(*Litehouse*), 3 tbsp. ..	70	0	17.0	0	0	50	0
(*Litehouse* Sugar Free), 3 tbsp.	35	0	8.0	0	0	55	0
(*Marie's*), 2 tbsp.	40	0	10.0	0	0	40	0
(*Marzetti's*), 3 tbsp. ..	60	0	16	0	0	65	0

Food and Measure	cal.	prot. (gms)	carbo. (gms)	fat (gms)	chol. (mgs)	sod. (mgs)	fiber (gms)
Strawberry glaze *(cont.)*							
(*Marzetti's* Fat Free),							
3 tbsp.	10	0	3.0	0	0	60	0
Strawberry juice blend,							
8 fl. oz., except as							
noted:							
(*Odwalla Strawberry*							
C Monster)	160	2.0	38.0	0	0	20	0
banana:							
(*Bolthouse Farms*) .	124	1.0	29.0	0	0	10	<1.0
(*Odwalla* Smoothie)	130	1.0	31.0	0	0	5	0
kiwi (*Apple & Eve*),							
6.75 fl. oz.	100	0	24.0	0	0	20	0
lime (*Snapple*),							
11.5 fl. oz	180	0	45.0	0	0	15	0
mango (*Apple & Eve*							
Passion)	120	0	30.0	0	0	25	0
orange (*Tropicana*) . . .	140	<1.0	34.0	0	0	10	0
Strawberry milk, see							
"Milk, flavored"							
Strawberry syrup, 2 tbsp.:							
(*Hershey's*)	100	0	26.0	0	0	10	0
(*Hershey's* Sugar Free)	10	0	4.0	0	0	55	0
(*Nesquik*)	110	0	27.0	0	0	0	0
(*Smucker's Sundae*							
Syrup)	110	0	26.0	0	0	5	0
Strawberry topping,							
2 tbsp.:							
(*Smucker's*)	100	0	24.0	0	0	0	0
(*Smucker's* Sugar Free)	25	0	9.0	0	0	0	0
Strawberry kiwi drink							
mix (*Special K₂O*							
Protein Water),							
.5-oz. pkt.	30	5.0	6.0	0	0	40	5.0
String bean, see "Green							
bean"							
Strudel, see "Apple							
pastry, fillo" and "Cake"							
Stuffing, refrigerated,							
½ cup:							
(*Shedd's Spread Country*							
Crock Homestyle) .	150	5.0	22.0	5.0	5	450	1.0
corn bread (*Shedd's*							
Spread Country Crock)	150	4.0	22.0	5.0	5	470	1.0

Food and Measure	cal.	prot. (gms)	carbo. (gms)	fat (gms)	chol. (mgs)	sod. (mgs)	fiber (gms)
Stuffing mix, dry, except as noted:							
(*Kellogg's*), 1 cup mix	120	4.0	25.0	1.0	0	330	1.0
(*Kellogg's*), 1 cup* . . .	240	5.0	26.0	13.0	0	800	1.0
chicken:							
(*Pepperidge Farm* One-Step), ½ cup	160	5.0	25.0	4.0	0	520	2.0
(*Stove Top*), ⅙ of 6-oz. pkg.	110	3.0	21.0	1.0	0	430	1.0
(*Stove Top* Lower Sodium), ⅙ of 6-oz. pkg.	110	3.0	22.0	1.0	0	250	1.0
(*Stove Top* One Step), ⅛ of 8-oz. pkg. . .	120	3.0	19.0	3.0	0	460	1.0
Creole (*Zatarain's*), ½ cup*	100	3.0	20.0	1.0	0	530	1.0
w/whole wheat (*Stove Top*), ⅕ of 5-oz. pkg. . .	100	5.0	18.0	1.5	0	480	3.0
corn bread:							
(*Mrs. Cubbison's*), ¾ cup	120	4.0	24.0	1.0	0	340	2.0
(*Pepperidge Farm*), ¾ cup	170	4.0	33.0	2.0	0	480	2.0
(*Stove Top*), ⅙ of 6-oz. pkg.	100	3.0	22.0	1.0	0	500	1.0
(*Zatarain's*), ½ cup*	100	3.0	21.0	.5	0	450	1.0
cranberry and herb (*Chatham Village*), ¾ cup	150	5.0	32.0	.5	0	700	1.0
herb:							
(*Arrowhead Mills* Organic), ½ cup .	120	3.0	20.0	3.0	0	240	1.0
(*Chatham Village* Traditional), ¾ cup	150	5.0	30.0	.5	0	760	1.0
(*Stove Top* Home-style), ⅛ of 8-oz. cont.	110	3.0	20.0	2.5	0	440	1.0
garden (*Pepperidge Farm* One-Step), ½ cup	160	5.0	24.0	5.0	0	500	2.0
seasoned (*Mrs. Cubbison's* Cube), ¾ cup	120	3.0	24.0	1.0	0	340	1.0

Food and Measure	cal.	prot. (gms)	carbo. (gms)	fat (gms)	chol. (mgs)	sod. (mgs)	fiber (gms)
Stuffing mix, herb *(cont.)*							
seasoned (*Pep-peridge Farm*), ¾ cup	170	5.0	33.0	2.0	0	600	3.0
pork (*Stove Top*), ⅛ of 6-oz. pkg.	110	3.0	21.0	1.0	0	430	1.0
sage and onion (*Pep-peridge Farm*), ¾ cup	140	5.0	26.0	1.0	0	540	3.0
seasoned, ¾ cup:							
(*Mrs. Cubbison's Dressing*)	120	4.0	24.0	1.0	0	340	2.0
(*Pepperidge Farm Country Style*)	140	5.0	27.0	1.0	0	380	2.0
(*Pepperidge Farm Cube*)	140	4.0	28.0	1.0	0	530	2.0
turkey:							
(*Pepperidge Farm One-Step*), ½ cup	170	4.0	23.0	7.0	0	540	1.0
(*Stove Top*), ⅛ of 6-oz. pkg.	110	3.0	21.0	1.0	0	460	1.0
Sturgeon, meat only:							
raw, 4 oz.	120	18.3	0	4.6	68	61	0
baked or broiled, 4 oz.	153	23.5	0	5.9	87	78	0
smoked, 4 oz.	196	35.4	0	5.0	91	838	0
Subway:							
breakfast sandwich, 6" bread:							
cheese	420	23.0	44.0	18.0	190	1010	5.0
chipotle steak/cheese	600	34.0	49.0	32.0	220	1470	6.0
double bacon/cheese	510	30.0	45.0	25.0	210	1380	5.0
honey mustard ham/ cheese	470	28.0	52.0	19.0	200	1500	5.0
Western w/cheese	450	28.0	46.0	19.0	200	1390	5.0
breakfast wrap:							
cheese	520	25.0	55.0	23.0	190	1260	2.0
chipotle steak/cheese	700	35.0	60.0	37.0	220	1720	3.0
double bacon/cheese	610	30.0	56.0	30.0	210	1630	2.0
honey mustard ham/ cheese	580	30.0	64.0	25.0	200	1750	2.0
Western w/cheese	550	30.0	58.0	24.0	200	1640	2.0
6" sub:							
chicken/bacon ranch	580	36.0	47.0	30.0	99	1390	6.0
cold cut combo	410	21.0	47.0	17.0	60	1530	5.0
Italian, spicy	480	21.0	45.0	25.0	55	1660	5.0

Food and Measure	cal.	prot. (gms)	carbo. (gms)	fat (gms)	chol. (mgs)	sod. (mgs)	fiber (gms)
Italian BMT	450	23.0	47.0	21.0	55	1770	5.0
meatball marinara .	560	24.0	63.0	24.0	45	1590	8.0
steak and cheese ...	400	29.0	48.0	12.0	60	1110	6.0
Subway Melt	380	25.0	48.0	12.0	45	1600	5.0
tuna	530	22.0	44.0	31.0	45	1010	5.0
6" sub, 6 grams fat or less:							
chicken, roasted ...	310	24.0	48.0	5.0	25	830	6.0
chicken teriyaki ...	370	26.0	59.0	5.0	50	1200	5.0
ham, Black Forest .	290	18.0	47.0	5.0	25	1260	5.0
roast beef	290	19.0	45.0	5.0	20	900	5.0
Subway Club	320	24.0	47.0	6.0	35	1290	5.0
turkey breast	280	18.0	46.0	4.5	20	1000	5.0
turkey/ham	290	20.0	47.0	5.0	25	1210	5.0
Veggie Delite	230	9.0	44.0	3.0	0	500	5.0
6" double meat:							
chicken, roasted ...	400	38.0	51.0	8.0	45	1160	6.0
chicken/bacon ranch	710	55.0	48.0	35.0	160	1890	6.0
chicken teriyaki ...	480	43.0	65.0	7.0	100	1820	6.0
cold cut combo ...	550	31.0	49.0	28.0	110	2360	5.0
ham	350	28.0	49.0	7.0	50	2020	5.0
Italian BMT	630	34.0	49.0	35.0	100	2850	5.0
meatball marinara .	860	37.0	82.0	42.0	85	2480	11.0
roast beef	360	29.0	46.0	7.0	40	1300	5.0
steak and cheese ..	540	46.0	52.0	18.0	105	1510	7.0
Subway Club	420	39.0	50.0	8.0	65	2080	5.0
Subway Melt	490	40.0	51.0	17.0	80	2500	5.0
turkey breast	330	28.0	48.0	5.0	40	1500	5.0
turkey/ham	360	31.0	50.0	7.0	50	1930	5.0
footlong low fat sub:							
chicken, roasted ...	630	47.0	95.0	11.0	45	1660	11.0
chicken teriyaki ...	750	52.0	118.0	10.0	100	2400	11.0
ham, Black Forest .	570	37.0	93.0	10.0	50	2520	11.0
roast beef	580	38.0	90.0	10.0	40	1800	11.0
Subway Club	640	48.0	94.0	12.0	65	2580	11.0
turkey breast	560	37.0	92.0	9.0	40	2000	11.0
turkey/ham	580	40.0	93.0	10.0	50	2420	11.0
Veggie Delite	450	18.0	88.0	6.0	0	1000	11.0
4" *Subway* minis:							
ham, Black Forest .	180	11.0	30.0	3.0	10	710	4.0
roast beef	190	13.0	30.0	3.5	15	600	4.0
tuna w/cheese	320	13.0	30.0	18.0	30	690	4.0
turkey breast	190	12.0	30.0	3.0	15	670	4.0

Food and Measure	cal.	prot. (gms)	carbo. (gms)	fat (gms)	chol. (mgs)	sod. (mgs)	fiber (gms)
Subway *(cont.)*							
6" sub, regional/limited offer:							
barbecue chicken ..	310	16.0	52.0	6.0	35	1090	6.0
barbecue rib patty .	420	20.0	47.0	19.0	50	810	5.0
Buffalo chicken ...	380	25.0	46.0	18.0	55	1490	5.0
The Feast	590	44.0	52.0	25.0	105	3120	5.0
pastrami, double meat	580	33.0	48.0	30.0	14	1860	5.0
Philly cheesesteak, double meat	520	40.0	50.0	19.0	100	1390	6.0
Subway seafood ...	450	16.0	51.0	22.0	25	1130	6.0
veggie patty	390	24.0	56.0	8.0	10	1080	8.0
salads, no dressing:							
chicken, roasted ...	140	19.0	11.0	2.5	50	390	4.0
chicken teriyaki ...	210	20.0	26.0	3.0	50	780	4.0
ham, Black Forest .	120	12.0	14.0	3.0	25	840	4.0
roast beef	120	13.0	12.0	3.0	20	480	4.0
Subway Club	150	18.0	14.0	4.0	35	870	4.0
turkey breast	110	12.0	13.0	2.5	20	580	4.0
turkey/ham	120	14.0	14.0	3.0	25	790	4.0
Veggie Delite	60	3.0	11.0	1.0	0	80	4.0
salad dressing:							
Italian, fat free	35	1.0	7.0	0	0	720	0
ranch	320	0	3.0	35.0	30	560	0
8" pizza, regional:							
cheese	680	32.0	96.0	22.0	40	1070	4.0
cheese/veggies	740	36.0	100.0	25.0	50	1210	5.0
pepperoni	790	38.0	96.0	32.0	60	1350	4.0
sausage	830	40.0	97.0	35.0	71	1310	4.0
soup, 10-oz. bowl, regional:							
broccoli, cream of .	160	6.0	18.0	7.0	10	1010	5.0
broccoli/cheese ...	200	5.0	17.0	12.0	25	1180	3.0
chicken/dumpling ..	170	8.0	23.0	5.0	35	1390	2.0
chicken noodle	80	6.0	11.0	2.0	15	1240	1.0
chicken rice	100	6.0	17.0	2.0	10	1300	1.0
chili con carne	290	19.0	35.0	8.0	25	990	12.0
clam chowder	150	6.0	20.0	5.0	10	990	4.0
minestrone	80	4.0	15.0	1.0	<5	1125	4.0
potato w/bacon ...	240	5.0	26.0	13.0	15	1050	3.0
tomato/vegetable w/rotini	90	3.0	20.0	0	0	1140	2.0

Food and Measure	cal.	prot. (gms)	carbo. (gms)	fat (gms)	chol. (mgs)	sod. (mgs)	fiber (gms)
vegetable beef	100	6.0	15.0	2.0	10	1450	3.0
wild rice w/chicken	210	6.0	21.0	11.0	25	1250	2.0
condiments/extras:							
American cheese ..	40	2.0	1.0	3/5	10	200	0
bacon, 2 slices	45	3.0	0	3.5	10	190	0
cheddar, natural ...	60	4.0	0	5.0	15	95	0
chipotle sauce	96	0	1.0	10.0	8	215	0
honey mustard sauce	30	0	7.0	0	0	115	0
mayo, 1 tbsp.	110	0	0	12.0	10	80	0
mayo, light, 1 tbsp.	50	0	<1.0	5.0	5	100	0
mustard, 2 tsp. ...	5	0	<1.0	0	0	115	0
olive oil blend, 1 tsp.	45	0	0	5.0	0	0	0
onion sauce, sweet	40	0	9.0	0	0	85	0
pepper Jack cheese	50	3.0	0	4.0	15	140	0
provolone	50	4.0	0	4.0	10	125	0
ranch dressing	120	0	1.0	13.0	10	210	0
red wine vinaigrette	29	0	6.0	0	1	340	0
Swiss cheese	50	4.0	0	4.5	15	30	0
Fruzie Express, small:							
berry lishus	110	1.0	28.0	0	0	30	1.0
w/banana	140	1.0	35.0	0	0	30	2.0
peach pizzazz	100	0	26.0	0	0	25	0
pineapple delight ..	130	1.0	33.0	0	0	25	1.0
w/banana	160	1.0	40.0	0	0	25	2.0
sunrise refresher ..	120	1.0	29.0	0	0	20	1.0
Succotash, canned							
cream-style, ½ cup	103	3.5	23.4	.7	0	325	4.0
Succotash, frozen							
boiled, drained,							
½ cup	79	3.7	17.0	.8	0	38	4.6
Sucker, white, meat only:							
raw, 4 oz.	105	19.0	0	2.6	47	45	0
baked or broiled, 4 oz.	135	24.4	0	3.4	60	58	0
Sugar, beet or cane:							
brown:							
1 oz.	107	0	27.6	0	0	11	0
1 cup, not packed .	546	0	141.0	0	0	57	0
1 cup, packed	828	0	214.0	0	0	86	0
cubes, rough cut, white							
or Demerara (*Roland*),							
1 cube	20	0	5.0	0	0	0	0
granulated:							
(*Hain* Organic), 1 tsp.	10	0	3.0	0	0	0	0

Food and Measure	cal.	prot. (gms)	carbo. (gms)	fat (gms)	chol. (mgs)	sod. (mgs)	fiber (gms)
Sugar beet or cane, granulated *(cont.)*							
1 oz.	110	0	28.3	0	0	<1	0
1 cup	773	0	199.8	0	0	<1	0
1 tbsp.	46	0	12.0	0	0	<1	0
1 tsp.	15	0	4.0	0	0	<1	0
powder/confectioner's:							
1 cup, sifted	389	0	99.5	0	0	1	0
1 tbsp., unsifted . . .	31	0	8.0	0	0	<1	0
Sugar, date (*Tree of Life*), 1 tsp.	10	0	3.0	0	0	0	0
Sugar, maple, 1 oz. . .	99	0	25.5	0	0	4	0
Sugar, substitute (see also "Fructose"):							
(*Equal*), 1 pkt.	4	0	<1.0	0	0	0	0
(*NutraSweet*), 1 tsp. .	2	0	<1.0	0	0	0	0
(*Splenda*), 1 pkt.	0	0	<1.0	0	0	0	0
(*Sweet'n Low*), 1 pkt. .	4	0	1.0	0	0	0	0
Sugar, turbinado (*Tree of Life*), 1 tsp.	15	0	4.0	0	0	0	0
Sugar apple:							
1 medium, 9.9 oz. . . .	146	3.2	36.6	.5	0	15	6.8
½ cup	118	2.6	29.6	.4	0	12	5.5
Sugar snap peas, see "Peas, edible-podded"							
Summer sausage, 2 oz., except as noted:							
(*Farmland*)	190	9.0	1.0	17.0	40	800	0
(*Old Smokehouse*) . . .	200	8.0	2.0	18.0	55	970	0
(*Oscar Mayer*), 1.6 oz.	140	7.0	0	12.0	40	660	0
all varieties (*Johnsonville*)	170	9.0	1.0	15.0	45	680	0
beef:							
(*Di Lusso*)	210	9.0	0	19.0	60	860	0
(*Farmland*)	150	16.0	0	10.0	50	610	0
(*Oscar Mayer*), 1 oz.	90	4.0	1.0	7.0	20	400	0
hickory smoked (*Di Lusso*)	210	10.0	0	18.0	60	940	0
Summer squash (see also specific listings), all varieties:							
raw:							
(*Del Monte*), ½ medium, 3.5 oz. .	20	1.0	4.0	0	0	0	2.0
sliced, 1 cup	23	1.3	4.9	.2	0	2	2.2

Food and Measure	cal.	prot. (gms)	carbo. (gms)	fat (gms)	chol. (mgs)	sod. (mgs)	fiber (gms)
boiled, drained, sliced, 1 cup	36	1.6	7.8	.6	0	2	2.5
Sun choke, see "Jerusalem artichoke"							
Sunburst squash, baby (*Frieda's*), ⅔ cup, 3 oz.	15	1.0	3.0	0	0	0	1.0
Sunfish, pumpkinseed, meat only:							
raw, 4 oz.	101	22.0	0	.8	76	91	0
baked or broiled, 4 oz.	129	28.2	0	1.0	98	117	0
Sunflower butter, 1 tbsp.	93	3.2	4.4	7.6	0	1	.8
Sunflower chips, all varieties (*Snyder's* MultiGrain), 1 oz. ..	140	2.0	20.0	6.0	0	190	2.0
Sunflower seed flour, partially defatted, 1 cup	261	38.5	28.7	1.3	0	2	4.2
Sunflower seeds:							
(*Arrowhead Mills* Organic), ¼ cup ...	170	7.0	6.0	15.0	0	0	3.0
(*Frito-Lay*), 3 tbsp., 1 oz.	180	6.0	4.0	14.0	0	130	2.0
(*Shiloh Farms* Raw-in-Shell), ½ cup, 1 oz.	130	6.0	5.0	14.0	0	0	3.0
raw, kernels:							
(*Shiloh Farms* Organic), ¼ cup, 1.1 oz.	180	8.0	6.0	14.0	0	10	2.0
(*SunRidge Farms* Organic), ¼ cup, 1.1 oz.	170	7.0	.0	15.0	0	0	3.0
(*Tree of Life*), ¼ cup	210	8.0	7.0	18.0	0	15	2.0
(*Tree of Life* Organic), 1 oz.	170	<6.0	5.0	15.0	0	0	<3.0
unsalted:							
dry-roasted, 1 oz. .	165	5.5	6.8	14.1	0	1	3.2
oil-roasted, 1 oz. ..	174	6.1	4.2	16.3	0	1	4.2
toasted, 1 oz.	176	4.9	5.8	16.1	0	1	3.3
dry-roasted (*Planters*), 1.1 oz.	180	7.0	6.0	15.0	0	260	3.0
roasted (*SunRidge Farms*), 1.1 oz.	170	7.0	6.0	15.0	0	0	3.0

Food and Measure	cal.	prot. (gms)	carbo. (gms)	fat (gms)	chol. (mgs)	sod. (mgs)	fiber (gms)
Sunflower seeds *(cont.)*							
roasted, salted:							
(*Amport Foods*),							
¼ cup, 1.1 oz. . .	190	8.0	5.0	15.0	0	330	2.0
(*Planters*), 1 oz.	180	7.0	5.0	15.0	0	120	2.0
(*Planters*), ½ of							
2.25-oz. pkg. . . .	190	6.0	8.0	16.0	0	140	4.0
(*Planters*), 3-oz. pkg.	280	10.0	8.0	23.0	0	180	4.0
(*Planters* Kernels),							
1 oz.	160	7.0	5.0	14.0	0	150	4.0
(*SunRidge Farms*),							
¼ cup, 1.1 oz. . .	180	7.0	6.0	15.0	0	105	3.0
(*Tree of Life* Organic),							
1 oz.	180	<6.0	4.0	16.0	0	170	<2.0
salted in shell							
(*Amport Foods*),							
¼ cup, 1.1 oz. . .	190	8.0	5.0	15.0	0	240	2.0
barbecue (*Frito-Lay*),							
1 pkg.	230	7.0	7.0	17.0	0	230	3.0
hot (*Frito-Lay Flamin'*							
Hot), 1 pkg.	210	7.0	6.0	17.0	0	430	3.0
ranch (*Frito-Lay*), 1 pkg.	200	5.0	7.0	17.0	0	140	3.0
tamari (*New England*							
Naturals), ¼ cup,							
1.2 oz.	190	8.0	7.0	15.0	0	115	5.0
Surimi, pollock, 4 oz.	112	17.2	7.8	1.0	34	162	0
Sushi wrapper, colored							
(*Frieda's*), .14-oz. pc.	15	2.0	0	0	0	25	0
Swamp cabbage:							
raw, .6-oz. shoot	2	.3	.4	<.1	0	15	.3
boiled, drained, chopped,							
½ cup	10	1.0	1.8	.1	0	60	.9
Sweet dumpling							
squash (*Frieda's*),							
¾ cup, 3 oz.	30	1.0	7.0	0	0	0	1.0
Sweet peas, see "Peas,							
green"							
Sweet potato:							
raw:							
(*Del Monte*), 1							
medium, 4.6 oz. . .	130	2.0	33.0	0	0	45	4.0
5" x 2" potato	136	2.1	31.6	.4	0	17	3.9
cubed (*Glory*), 4.9 oz.	140	2.0	36.0	0	0	50	4.0

Food and Measure	cal.	prot. (gms)	carbo. (gms)	fat (gms)	chol. (mgs)	sod. (mgs)	fiber (gms)
baked in skin:							
5" x 2" potato	118	2.0	27.7	.1	0	12	3.4
mashed, ½ cup ...	103	1.7	24.3	.1	0	10	3.0
boiled w/out skin:							
4 oz.	86	1.6	20.1	.2	0	31	2.8
mashed, ½ cup ...	125	2.5	31.7	.3	0	48	4.5
Sweet potato, canned, ½ cup, except as noted:							
candied:							
(*Glory* Yams)	210	1.0	52.0	0	0	240	1.0
(*Royal Prince*)	210	1.0	50.0	0	0	30	2.0
(*S&W* Yams)	170	2.0	46.0	0	0	360	4.0
casserole (*Glory* Southern Style) ...	180	2.0	43.0	0	0	250	2.0
cut (*Princella/Sugary Sam*), ⅔ cup	160	0	39.0	0	0	35	3.0
mashed (*Princella/ Sugary Sam*), ⅔ cup	120	1.0	28.0	0	0	30	3.0
puree (*Tree of Life* Organic)	130	3.0	30.0	0	0	100	2.0
in syrup:							
light syrup (*Glory Sweet Traditions*), ⅔ cup	160	3.0	37.0	0	0	300	2.0
whole (*Royal Prince/ Trappey's* 1.7-oz.), 3 pcs.	200	1.0	48.0	0	0	40	4.0
whole, in heavy syrup (*Trappey's* 15.75-oz.) 4 pcs.	200	1.0	48.0	0	0	40	4.0
w/liquid	101	1.1	23.9	.2	0	50	2.8
drained	106	1.3	24.9	.3	0	38	2.9
orange pineapple (*Royal Prince*)	210	1.0	50.0	0	0	30	3.0
Sweet potato, frozen/ refrigerated (see also "Sweet potato dish"):							
baked, cubed, ½ cup .	88	1.5	20.6	.1	0	7	2.6
candied:							
(*Green Giant*), ¾ cup	240	2.0	41.0	7.0	0	430	3.0
(*Mrs. Paul's*), 5 oz.	300	1.0	73.0	1.0	0	130	3.0

Food and Measure	cal.	prot. (gms)	carbo. (gms)	fat (gms)	chol. (mgs)	sod. (mgs)	fiber (gms)
Sweet potato, frozen/refrigerated *(cont.)*							
casserole, ½ cup:							
(*Glory* Savory Accents)	170	1.0	37.0	2.0	0	210	0
(*Green Giant*)	200	3.0	30.0	9.0	0	360	3.0
fries, 3 oz.:							
crinkle cut (*McCain*)	120	0	22.0	3.0	0	180	2.0
julienne (*Alexia Sweet Potato*) . .	150	2.0	24.0	6.0	0	140	3.0
mashed:							
(*Shedd's Country Crock*), ⅔ cup . .	200	2.0	36.0	6.0	10	260	2.0
(*Simply Potatoes*), ⅔ cup	100	2.0	21.0	1.0	0	115	3.0
w/brown sugar (*Larry's*), 4 oz.	140	2.0	27.0	3.5	10	530	2.0
Sweet potato chips, 1 oz.:							
(*Terra* Chips)	160	1.0	15.0	11.0	0	10	3.0
w/beets (*Terra* Sweets & Beets)	150	2.0	15.0	9.0	0	5	1.0
honey chipotle barbecue (*Pringles*)	140	1.0	16.0	8.0	0	210	1.0
spiced (*Terra*)	160	1.0	14.0	11.0	0	150	2.0
Sweet potato dish, frozen/refrigerated:							
nuggets:							
(*Dr. Praeger's* Bites), 2 pcs., 2 oz.	110	3.0	20.0	2.5	0	180	1.0
(*Dr. Praeger's* Littles), 2 pcs., 1.3 oz. . .	60	<1.0	9.0	2.0	0	85	<1.0
pancake:							
(*Dr. Praeger's*), 2-oz. pc.	80	2.0	12.0	2.0	0	140	3.0
(*Golden*), 1.3-oz. pc.	80	1.0	10.0	4.0	0	20	0
mini (*Old Fashioned Kitchen*), 4 pcs., 3 oz.	170	3.0	23.0	8.0	0	40	<1.0
Southern (*Health is Wealth*), ½ of 10-oz. pkg.	190	2.0	26.0	5.0	15	260	2.0
Sweet potato dish mix:							
casserole (*Betty Crocker*), ½ cup*	280	3.0	42.0	11.0	<5	410	2.0
pancakes (*Manischewitz*), 3 tbsp.	80	2.0	18.0	1.0	0	500	2.0

Food and Measure	cal.	prot. (gms)	carbo. (gms)	fat (gms)	chol. (mgs)	sod. (mgs)	fiber (gms)
Sweet potato leaf:							
raw, chopped, ½ cup .	6	.7	1.1	.1	0	2	<1.0
steamed, ½ cup	11	.7	2.3	.1	0	4	.6
Sweet and sour drink							
mixer (*Angostura*),							
2 fl. oz.	70	0	18.0	0	0	5	0
Sweet and sour sauce,							
2 tbsp., except as							
noted:							
(*Acadia Naturals*)	60	0	15.0	0	0	210	0
(*Ah-So/China Pride*							
Sweet & Pungent) .	80	0	19.0	0	0	260	1.0
(*Contadina*), 1 tbsp. ..	40	0	8.0	1.0	0	115	0
(*Crosse & Blackwell*) .	90	0	23.0	0	0	30	0
(*La Choy*)	60	0	14.0	0	0	110	0
(*House of Tsang*),							
1 tbsp.	35	0	8.0	0	0	50	0
(*Kraft*)	60	0	13.0	0	0	130	0
(*Polynesian* Golden							
Chicken Nugget) ..	70	0	18.0	0	0	270	0
(*Polynesian* Sparerib)	80	0	19.0	0	0	260	1.0
(*San-J* Sweet & Spicy)	50	<1.0	13.0	0	0	350	0
(*World Harbors Maui*							
Mountain)	60	0	14.0	0	0	250	0
duck sauce:							
(*Ah-So*)	50	0	13.0	0	0	15	0
(*Mee Tu*)	80	0	19.0	0	0	260	1.0
(*Roland*)	70	0	17.0	0	0	300	0
(*Saucy Susan*)	80	0	19.0	0	0	260	1.0
tangerine (*Heaven and*							
Earth), 1 tbsp.	25	<1.0	6.0	0	0	5	0
Sweetbreads, see							
"Pancreas" and							
"Thymus"							
Swiss chard, fresh:							
raw (*Frieda's*), 3 oz. ..	15	2.0	3.0	0	0	180	1.0
raw, chopped, ½ cup .	3	.3	.7	<.1	0	38	.3
boiled, drained,							
chopped, ½ cup ...	18	1.7	3.6	.1	0	158	1.8
Swordfish, fresh, meat							
only:							
raw, 4 oz.	137	22.5	0	4.6	45	102	0
baked or broiled, 4 oz.	176	28.8	0	5.8	57	130	0

Food and Measure	cal.	prot. (gms)	carbo. (gms)	fat (gms)	chol. (mgs)	sod. (mgs)	fiber (gms)
Syrup, see specific listings							
Szechuan paste (*Roland*), 1 tsp.	5	0	1.0	0	0	180	0
Szechuan sauce (see also "Stir-fry sauce"), (*San-J*), 1 tsp.	5	0	<1.0	0	0	180	0

T

Food and Measure	cal.	prot. (gms)	carbo. (gms)	fat (gms)	chol. (mgs)	sod. (mgs)	fiber (gms)
Tabouli salad (*Cedar's*), 2 tbsp.	30	1.0	4.0	1.5	0	95	<1.0
Tabouli salad mix:							
(*Casbah*), ⅓ cup	110	4.0	23.0	.5	0	390	1.0
(*Fantastic*), ⅓ cup . . .	150	5.0	33.0	1.0	0	550	6.0
(*Near East*), 1 oz.	80	3.0	21.0	0	0	270	5.0
(*Near East*), ⅔ cup* .	120	4.0	23.0	3.0	0	270	5.0
Taco, frozen:							
beef and cheese:							
(*José Olé* Minis), 4 pcs., 3 oz.	200	7.0	19.0	11.0	20	350	3.0
(*José Olé* Soft), 5 oz.	280	14.0	31.0	11.0	25	850	1.0
vegetarian (*Nate's* Rolled), 2-oz. pc.:							
bean/soy cheese . .	130	5.0	26.0	.5	0	95	1.0
green chile/tomatillos	120	6.0	23.0	0	0	90	0
red chile/soy cheese	130	7.0	23.0	.5	0	150	<1.0
***Taco Bell*:**							
Big Bell Value Menu:							
burrito:							
beef combo	440	21.0	51.0	18.0	45	1630	4.0
beef/potato	530	15.0	66.0	23.0	30	1720	6.0
cheesy bean/rice	470	13.0	58.0	20.0	15	1400	6.0
chicken, spicy . .	400	14.0	48.0	17.0	30	1190	3.0
caramel apple empanada	290	3.0	37.0	14.0	5	300	1.0
cheesy potatoes . . .	290	4.0	29.0	17.0	15	830	2.0
Double Decker taco	320	14.0	38.0	13.0	25	810	6.0
taco, soft:							
chicken, spicy . .	170	10.0	20.0	6.0	25	580	2.0
soft, grande	430	19.0	43.0	20.0	45	1440	5.0
burritos:							
bean	350	13.0	54.0	9.0	5	1190	8.0

Food and Measure	cal.	prot. (gms)	carbo. (gms)	fat (gms)	chol. (mgs)	sod. (mgs)	fiber (gms)
Taco Bell, burritos *(cont.)*							
Burrito Supreme:							
beef	420	17.0	51.0	17.0	40	1340	7.0
chicken	400	20.0	49.0	13.0	45	1360	6.0
steak	390	18.0	49.0	14.0	40	1250	6.0
Fiesta:							
beef	370	14.0	49.0	13.0	25	1200	4.0
chicken	350	18.0	47.0	10.0	30	1220	3.0
steak	340	15.0	47.0	11.0	25	1110	3.0
Grilled Stuft:							
beef	680	27.0	76.0	30.0	55	2120	9.0
chicken	640	34.0	73.0	23.0	65	2160	7.0
steak	630	30.0	72.0	25.0	55	1930	7.0
7-layer	490	17.0	65.0	18.0	25	1350	9.0
chalupas:							
bacon club	490	23.0	28.0	31.0	45	970	2.0
Baja, beef	410	13.0	30.0	27.0	35	780	4.0
Baja, chicken	390	17.0	29.0	23.0	40	800	3.0
Baja, steak	390	15.0	28.0	24.0	35	690	3.0
nacho cheese, beef	370	12.0	32.0	22.0	20	770	3.0
nacho cheese, chicken	350	16.0	30.0	18.0	25	790	2.0
nacho cheese, steak	340	14.0	30.0	19.0	20	680	2.0
supreme, beef	380	14.0	30.0	23.0	40	620	3.0
supreme, chicken . .	360	17.0	29.0	20.0	45	650	2.0
supreme, steak . . .	360	15.0	28.0	21.0	40	530	2.0
gorditas:							
Gordita Baja:							
beef	340	13.0	29.0	19.0	35	780	4.0
chicken	320	17.0	28.0	16.0	40	800	3.0
steak	320	15.0	27.0	17.0	35	690	3.0
Gordita Supreme:							
beef	310	14.0	29.0	16.0	40	620	3.0
chicken	290	17.0	28.0	12.0	45	650	2.0
steak	290	15.0	28.0	13.0	40	530	2.0
nacho cheese, beef	300	12.0	31.0	14.0	25	770	3.0
nacho cheese, chicken	280	16.0	29.0	11.0	25	800	2.0
nacho cheese, steak	270	14.0	29.0	12.0	20	680	2.0
taco, crunchy:							
regular	170	8.0	13.0	10.0	25	350	3.0
Taco Supreme	210	9.0	15.0	13.0	40	370	3.0
Taco Supreme Double Decker . .	370	14.0	40.0	17.0	40	820	7.0

Food and Measure	cal.	prot. (gms)	carbo. (gms)	fat (gms)	chol. (mgs)	sod. (mgs)	fiber (gms)
taco, soft:							
beef, *Taco Supreme*	250	11.0	23.0	13.0	40	650	3.0
chicken, Ranchero .	270	14.0	21.0	14.0	35	820	2.0
steak, grilled	270	12.0	20.0	16.0	35	660	2.0
Fresco Menu:							
burrito, bean	330	12.0	54.0	7.0	0	1200	9.0
burrito, chicken							
fiesta	330	16.0	48.0	8.0	25	1240	3.0
Burrito Supreme:							
chicken	330	18.0	49.0	8.0	25	1360	7.0
steak	330	16.0	48.0	8.0	20	1250	7.0
chicken *Border Bowl,*							
no dressing	350	19.0	51.0	8.0	25	1600	10.0
taco, crunchy	150	7.0	13.0	8.0	20	370	3.0
taco, soft, beef	180	8.0	21.0	7.0	20	650	3.0
grilled steak	160	10.0	20.0	4.5	2[	550	2.0
chicken, ranchero .	170	12.0	21.0	4.0	25	730	3.0
steak, grilled ...	160	10.0	20.0	4.5	20	550	2.0
specialties:							
Border Bowl, chicken	640	22.0	60.0	35.0	30	1800	10.0
no dressing	440	21.0	57.0	15.0	30	1540	10.0
Border Bowl, steak .	600	28.0	68.0	24.0	55	2120	9.0
Crunchwrap Supreme	560	17.0	68.0	24.0	35	1430	5.0
Crunchwrap Supreme,							
spicy chicken ...	540	19.0	67.0	23.0	40	1360	4.0
Enchirito, beef	360	18.0	34.0	17.0	50	1420	7.0
Enchirito, chicken .	340	22.0	33.0	13.0	50	1450	6.0
Enchirito, steak ...	330	20.0	33.0	14.0	45	1330	6.0
Mexican pizza	530	20.0	46.0	30.0	40	1000	6.0
MexiMelt	280	15.0	22.0	14.0	40	860	3.0
quesadilla, cheese .	470	19.0	39.0	26.0	50	1100	2.0
quesadilla, chicken .	520	28.0	40.0	28.0	75	1420	3.0
quesadilla, steak ..	520	26.0	39.0	28.0	70	1370	3.0
taco salad, *Express*	610	25.0	56.0	32.0	65	1420	14.0
taco salad, fiesta ..	840	30.0	65.0	45.0	65	1780	15.0
w/out shell	470	23.0	41.0	24.0	65	1510	13.0
taco salad, chicken							
fiesta	790	37.0	77.0	38.0	75	1830	13.0
w/out shell	430	30.0	38.0	18.0	75	1560	11.0
taquitos, chicken ..	310	18.0	37.0	11.0	40	980	2.0
taquitos, steak	310	16.0	36.0	11.0	35	870	2.0
tostada	240	11.0	27.0	10.0	15	730	7.0
nachos/sides:							
cinnamon twists ...	170	1.0	26.0	7.0	0	200	1.0

Food and Measure	cal.	prot. (gms)	carbo. (gms)	fat (gms)	chol. (mgs)	sod. (mgs)	fiber (gms)
***Taco Bell*, nachos/sides** *(cont.)*							
guacamole, 1.5 oz.	70	1.0	5.0	5.0	0	180	2.0
Mexican rice	180	6.0	23.0	7.0	15	790	1.0
nachos	330	4.0	32.0	21.0	5	530	2.0
nachos *BellGrande*	770	19.0	77.0	44.0	35	1280	12.0
nachos supreme	440	12.0	41.0	26.0	35	800	7.0
pintos 'n cheese	160	9.0	19.0	6.0	15	670	7.0
salsa, 1.5 oz.	15	0	3.0	0	0	160	0
sour cream, 1.5 oz.	80	1.0	3.0	7.0	25	30	0
Taco entree kit, mix only:							
(*Las Palmas*), ¼ pkg.	170	3.0	25.0	7.0	0	910	3.0
(*Old El Paso* Dinner Kit), ⅙ pkg.	130	2.0	18.0	5.0	0	750	1.0
(*Old El Paso* Gordita Dinner Kit), ⅛ pkg.	240	4.0	33.0	10.0	0	830	1.0
(*Old El Paso* Hard & Soft Dinner Kit):							
hard, ⅓ pkg.	130	2.0	19.0	4.5	0	770	1.0
soft, ⅓ pkg.	180	4.0	32.0	5.0	0	1050	1.0
(*Old El Paso* Soft Dinner Kit), ⅕ pkg.	190	4.0	32.0	5.0	0	1170	1.0
(*Old El Paso* Soft Taco Bake), ¼ pkg.	200	4.0	30.0	7.0	5	930	1.0
(*Old El Paso Stand 'n Stuff* Dinner Kit), ⅕ pkg.	160	3.0	23.0	6.0	0	900	2.0
(*Ortega*), ⅙ pkg.	160	2.0	22.0	7.0	0	640	3.0
(*Ortega*), ⅑ of 16.7-oz. pkg.	150	2.0	21.0	6.0	0	770	2.0
(*Ortega* Hard & Soft), w/2 tacos	120	2.0	16.0	6.0	0	170	2.0
(*Ortega* Hard & Soft), w/2 tortillas	210	5.0	35.0	4.5	0	590	<1.0
(*Ortega* Soft), ⅕ pkg.	240	5.0	41.0	5.0	0	1230	<1.0
(*Taco Bell* Dinner), ⅙ pkg.	130	2.0	19.0	4.5	0	510	2.0
(*Taco Bell* Dinner Cheesy Double Decker), ⅙ pkg.	230	5.0	30.0	9.0	5	960	2.0
(*Taco Bell* Soft Dinner Kit), ⅕ pkg.	230	6.0	40.0	5.0	0	980	2.0
chicken, soft (*Old El Paso* Dinner Kit), ⅕ pkg.	190	4.0	32.0	5.0	0	960	1.0

Food and Measure	cal.	prot. (gms)	carbo. (gms)	fat (gms)	chol. (mgs)	sod. (mgs)	fiber (gms)
blue or yellow corn (*Garden of Eatin'* Dinner Kit), ⅛ pkg.	150	2.0	20.0	6.0	0	600	1.0
Taco filling mix (*Fantastic*), ¼ cup .	90	12.0	12.0	1.0	0	450	4.0
Taco sauce, 1 tbsp., except as noted:							
(*Ortega*)	10	0	1.0	0	0	60	0
chipotle (*La Victoria*) .	5	0	1.0	0	0	120	0
green (*Pace*)	5	0	1.0	0	0	100	0
hot (*Old El Paso*)	5	0	1.0	0	0	340	0
medium or mild:							
(*Old El Paso*)	5	0	1.0	0	0	90	0
(*Taco Bell*), 2 tbsp.	10	0	2.0	0	0	210	0
mild (*Old El Paso Taco Toppers*), 2 tbsp. . .	15	0	3.0	0	0	190	0
ranch, zesty (*Old El Paso Taco Toppers*), 2 tbsp.	70	0	2.0	6.0	<5	330	0
red (*Pace*), 2 tbsp. . . .	10	0	2.0	0	0	130	0
Taco seasoning mix, 2 tsp., except as noted:							
(*Chi-Chi's* Fiesta), ⅛ pkg.	15	0	3.0	0	0	240	0
(*Lawry's*)	15	0	3.0	0	0	340	<1.0
(*McCormick*)	20	0	3.0	0	0	430	0
(*McCormick* 30% Less Sodium)	20	0	3.0	0	0	300	0
(*Old El Paso*)	15	0	4.0	0	0	560	0
(*Old El Paso* Less Sodium)	15	0	4.0	0	0	330	0
(*Ortega*), 1 tbsp.	20	0	4.0	0	0	430	0
(*Pace*)	10	0	3.0	0	0	430	1.0
(*Taco Bell*)	20	1.0	3.0	0	0	370	1.0
(*Wick Fowler's*)	20	0	3.0	1.0	0	510	0
cheesy:							
(*McCormick*)	20	0	3.0	1.0	0	390	0
(*Old El Paso*)	20	0	4.0	.5	0	400	0
chicken (*Lawry's*)	20	0	5.0	0	0	440	<1.0
chipotle (*Taco Bell*) . .	20	1.0	3.0	0	0	370	1.0
hot:							
(*Lawry's*)	15	0	3.0	0	0	370	<1.0
(*McCormick*)	20	0	3.0	0	0	430	0
(*Ortega*), 1½ tsp. . . .	20	0	4.0	0	0	350	0

Food and Measure	cal.	prot. (gms)	carbo. (gms)	fat (gms)	chol. (mgs)	sod. (mgs)	fiber (gms)
Taco seasoning mix *(cont.)*							
hot and spicy *(Old El Paso)*	20	0	4.0	0	0	560	0
mild:							
(McCormick)	20	1.0	4.0	0	0	460	0
(Old El Paso)	15	0	4.0	0	0	360	0
Taco shell (see also "Tostada shell"):							
(Old El Paso), 3 pcs. ..	150	2.0	20.0	7.0	0	135	1.0
(Old El Paso Super Stuffer), 2 pcs.	170	3.0	23.0	8.0	0	150	2.0
(Old El Paso Stand 'n Stuff), 2 pcs.	130	2.0	16.0	6.0	0	110	1.0
(Taco Bell), 3 pcs. ...	150	2.0	22.0	6.0	0	.5	2.0
(Zapata), 2 pcs.	110	2.0	14.0	5.0	0	5	1.0
blue or yellow corn:							
(Bearito's), 2 pcs...	140	2.0	17.0	7.0	0	5	1.0
(Garden of Eatin'), 2 pcs., 1 oz.	140	2.0	17.0	7.0	0	5	1.0
(Zapata), 2 pcs. ...	140	2.0	17.0	7.0	0	5	1.0
soft, see "Tortilla"							
white corn *(Old El Paso)*, 3 pcs.	150	2.0	20.0	6.0	0	140	1.0
white or yellow corn *(Ortega)*, 2 pcs., 1 oz.	120	2.0	16.0	6.0	0	170	2.0
yellow corn *(Las Palmas)*, 2 pcs., 1 oz.	120	2.0	16.0	6.0	0	170	2.0
Taco snack, frozen, beef/cheese *(Michelina's Zap'ems)*, 5.5-oz. pkg.	340	11.0	33.0	17.0	20	830	2.0
Tahini, sesame, 2 tbsp.:							
(Arrowhead Mills Organic)	190	8.0	3.0	18.0	0	10	<1.0
(Cedar's Paste)	210	6.0	5.0	19.0	0	5	3.0
(MaraNatha Natural Raw)	190	6.0	9.0	16.0	0	110	2.0
(MaraNatha Natural Roasted)	210	6.0	10.0	16.0	0	110	3.0
(Roland)	180	7.0	3.0	16.0	0	70	1.0
(Tree of Life Organic) .	180	5.0	8.0	15.0	0	10	5.0
Tamale, canned, beef, 2 pcs.:							
(Hormel Jumbo)	190	6.0	21.0	10.0	25	980	3.0

Food and Measure	cal.	prot. (gms)	carbo. (gms)	fat (gms)	chol. (mgs)	sod. (mgs)	fiber (gms)
(*Hormel/Hormel* Hot-Spicy)	140	4.0	15.0	7.0	15	710	2.0
Tamale, frozen, 1 pc.:							
beef, shredded (*El Monterey*), 4.5 oz. .	310	9.0	27.0	19.0	30	660	3.0
chicken (*El Monterey*), 4.5 oz.	240	8.0	27.0	12.0	25	750	2.0
pork (*Goya*), 4 oz. . . .	350	10.0	42.0	16.0	25	250	5.0
Tamale entree, frozen, 1 pkg.:							
black bean (*Amy's* Verde), 10.25 oz. . .	330	7.0	5.0	10.0	0	780	8.0
cheese (*Amy's* Verde), 10.25 oz.	360	10.0	45.0	16.0	20	780	5.0
Monterey Jack (*Cedarlane* Organic), 9 oz.:							
green chili	290	9.0	39.0	11.0	20	700	4.0
mushroom	280	11.0	41.0	9.0	15	730	4.0
spinach	320	12.0	40.0	13.0	25	760	5.0
pie, meatless (*Amy's* Mexican), 8 oz. . . .	150	5.0	27.0	3.0	0	590	4.0
Tamari sauce, see "Soy sauce"							
Tamarillo, red or gold (*Frieda's*), 2 pcs., 4.2 oz.	40	2.0	9.0	0	0	0	4.0
Tamarind:							
1 fruit, 3" x 1"	5	.1	1.3	<.1	0	1	.1
pulp, ½ cup	144	1.7	37.5	.4	0	17	3.1
Tamarind sauce:							
(*Neera's* Asian), 2 tsp.	61	0	16.0	0	0	110	0
dipping (*Neera's*), 1 tsp.	15	0	3.0	0	0	98	0
Tamarindo (*Frieda's*), 1.1-oz. pod	70	1.0	19.0	0	0	10	2.0
Tandoori paste, see "Curry paste"							
Tangerine, fresh:							
(*Chiquita*), 3.8-oz. pc.	50	1.0	15.0	.5	0	0	3.0
(*Del Monte* Satsuma), 3.8-oz. pc.	50	1.0	15.0	0	0	0	3.0
(*Frieda's* Delite/Pixie Mandarin), 1 cup, 5 oz.	60	0	16.0	0	0	0	3.0

Food and Measure	cal.	prot. (gms)	carbo. (gms)	fat (gms)	chol. (mgs)	sod. (mgs)	fiber (gms)
Tangerine, fresh *(cont.)*							
(*Frieda's* Page Mandarin), 1 cup, 5 oz.	60	0	12.0	0	0	0	3.0
(*Frieda's* Satsuma Mandarin), 1 cup, 5 oz.	60	1.0	16.0	0	0	0	3.0
clementine, 2.6 oz. . .	35	.6	8.9	.1	0	1	1.3
1 large 2½" diam., 3.5 oz.	43	.6	11.0	.2	0	1	2.3
sections, 1 cup	86	1.2	21.8	.4	0	2	4.5
Tangerine, can/jar (mandarin orange), ½ cup, except as noted:							
in juice, w/liquid	46	.8	11.9	<.1	0	6	.9
in light syrup:							
(*Del Monte*)	80	0	19.0	0	0	15	<1.0
(*Dole*)	80	0	19.0	0	0	15	<1.0
(*Fanci Food*), ⅓ cup	80	1.0	19.0	0	0	10	1.0
(*Roland*)	70	1.0	17.0	0	0	10	1.0
(*SunFresh*)	80	0	19.0	0	0	15	<1.0
w/liquid, ½ cup . . .	77	.6	20.4	.1	0	8	.9
in orange gelatin:							
(*Del Monte* Lite), 4.5-oz. cup	60	0	14.0	0	0	40	0
(*Dole*), 4.3-oz. cup .	90	<1.0	23.0	0	0	25	<1.0
in water (*Roland*), ½ cup	45	1.0	10.0	0	0	15	1.0
Tangerine drink:							
sparkling (*Santa Cruz Organic*), 8 fl. oz. . .	110	0	26.0	0	0	10	0
tropical (*Tropicana Fruit Squeeze*), 15.2 fl. oz.	35	0	9.0	0	0	50	0
Tangerine juice, 8 fl. oz.:							
(*Odwalla*)	110	1.0	25.0	0	0	0	0
fresh	106	1.2	25.0	1.2	0	2	.5
canned, sweetened . .	125	1.3	29.9	.5	0	2	.5
frozen*	111	1.0	26.7	.3	0	2	.5
Tapenade, see "Olive spread"							

Food and Measure	cal.	prot. (gms)	carbo. (gms)	fat (gms)	chol. (mgs)	sod. (mgs)	fiber (gms)
Tapioca (*Reese* Pearls), 1 tbsp.	35	0	9.0	0	0	0	0
Tapioca pudding, see "Pudding"							
Tapioca flour (*Shiloh Farms*), ¼ cup	150	0	27.0	.5	0	0	0
Taquito, frozen:							
corn wrap, 3 pcs.:							
chicken (*El Monterey*), 4.5 oz.	290	13.0	30.0	13.0	30	430	2.0
chicken (*José Olé*), 3 oz.	190	7.0	26.0	8.0	10	370	3.0
steak, shredded (*El Monterey*), 4.5 oz.	300	11.0	31.0	13.0	40	560	1.0
steak, shredded (*José Olé*), 3 oz. ..	190	8.0	25.0	7.0	<5	440	3.0
corn wrap, vegetarian (*Nate's* Organic), 1.1-oz. pc.:							
beef style	90	3.0	9.0	4.5	0	210	1.0
black bean/soy cheese	80	2.0	10.0	3.0	0	200	1.0
chicken style	90	3.0	10.0	4.0	0	210	1.0
flour wrap:							
chicken breast, char-broiled (*El Monterey* Mexican Grill), 3 pcs., 5 oz.	380	15.0	36.0	19.0	35	670	1.0
chicken/cheese (*El Monterey*), 3 pcs., 4.5 oz.	350	10.0	36.0	18.0	15	650	2.0
chicken/cheese (*José Olé*), 2 pcs., 3 oz.	240	8.0	28.0	10.0	15	500	3.0
chicken, seasoned batter (*El Monterey* Southwest), 2 pcs., 2.8 oz.	170	6.0	20.0	8.0	10	330	1.0
steak/cheese (*José Olé*), 2 pcs., 3 oz.	230	9.0	28.0	10.0	10	510	3.0
steak/cheese (*José Olé* Minis), 4 pcs., 3 oz.	190	7.0	24.0	9.0	5	390	3.0
steak/cheese, shredded (*El Monterey*), 3 pcs., 4.5 oz. ..	350	11.0	36.0	17.0	20	650	1.0

Food and Measure	cal.	prot. (gms)	carbo. (gms)	fat (gms)	chol. (mgs)	sod. (mgs)	fiber (gms)
Taquito *(cont.)*							
flour, batter fried *(El Monterey Cruncheros)*, 4 pcs., 5.6 oz.:							
beef, taco/cheese ..	460	12.0	38.0	29.0	40	1040	2.0
chicken, Southwest	400	14.0	52.0	17.0	25	880	2.0
chicken/cheese	390	12.0	40.0	20.0	25	790	1.0
Taquito, breakfast, egg/bacon/cheese *(El Monterey)*, 3 pcs., 4.5 oz.	360	11.0	36.0	20.0	85	650	1.0
Taramosalata *(Krinos)*, 1 tbsp.	90	1.0	0	10.0	15	115	0
Taro, fresh:							
raw:							
(Frieda's Root), 3 oz.	90	1.0	22.0	0	0	10	3.0
sliced, ½ cup	56	.8	13.8	.1	0	6	2.1
cooked, sliced, ½ cup	94	.3	22.8	.1	0	10	3.4
Tahitian, ½ cup:							
raw, sliced	25	1.7	4.3	.6	0	31	n.a.
cooked, sliced	30	2.8	4.7	.5	0	37	n.a.
Taro chips/crisps (see also "Vegetable chips/crisps"), 1 oz.:							
(Terra Chips)	140	1.0	19.0	6.0	0	110	4.0
spiced *(Terra Chips)* ..	130	1.0	20.0	5.0	0	170	2.0
Taro leaf:							
raw, ½ cup	6	.7	.9	.1	0	1	.5
steamed, ½ cup	17	2.0	2.9	.3	0	1	1.5
Taro shoots, ½ cup:							
raw, sliced	5	.4	1.0	<.1	0	<1	n.a.
cooked, sliced	10	.5	2.2	.1	0	1	n.a.
Tarragon, ground, 1 tsp.	5	.4	.8	.1	0	1	.1
Tart shell, see "Pastry shell" and "Fillo dough"							
Tartar sauce, 2 tbsp.:							
(Crosse & Blackwell) .	80	0	7.0	9.0	10	270	0
(Hellmann's/Best Foods)	80	0	4.0	7.0	10	330	0
(Kraft)	60	0	4.0	4.5	5	230	0
(Kraft Fat Free)	25	0	5.0	0	0	200	0
(Marzetti)	120	0	3.0	12.0	10	160	0
(McCormick)	160	0	3.0	15.0	25	220	0
(McCormick Fat Free)	30	0	7.0	0	0	250	0

Food and Measure	cal.	prot. (gms)	carbo. (gms)	fat (gms)	chol. (mgs)	sod. (mgs)	fiber (gms)
(Old Bay)	130	0	3.0	12.0	15	210	0
hot and spicy (Kraft) .	70	0	4.0	6.0	5	240	0
lemon herb (Kraft) ...	150	0	1.0	16.0	15	170	0
Tea, plain, regular or instant, all varieties, 1 bag or tsp.	0	0	0	0	0	0	0
Tea, iced, 8 fl. oz., except as noted:							
(AriZona Sweet)	90	0	23.0	0	0	20	0
(Lipton PureLeaf Extra Sweet)	110	0	28.0	0	0	0	0
(Lipton PureLeaf Sweetened)	60	0	16.0	0	0	0	0
(Snapple Decaf)	100	0	25.0	0	0	10	0
(SoBe Dragon 3G) ...	110	0	30.0	0	0	15	0
(SoBe Zen Tea 3G) ...	100	0	28.0	0	0	10	0
(Turkey Hill)	90	0	22.0	0	0	15	0
(Turkey Hill Sweet Southern Brew) ...	90	0	21.0	0	0	10	0
all varieties (AriZona Diet)	0	0	0	0	0	20	0
berry: (Snapple Mixed-Up)	80	0	22.0	0	0	110	0
(Snapple Out of the Blue)	90	0	25.0	0	0	15	0
black tea: (Honest Tea Organic Assam)	17	0	5.0	0	0	5	0
(Pacific Organic) ..	60	0	16.0	0	0	10	0
(Snapple Earl Grey/ Orange Pekoe) ..	35	0	8.0	0	0	0	0
(Snapple English Breakfast)	40	0	10.0	0	0	0	0
ginseng (AriZona) .	60	0	15.0	0	0	20	0
w/ginseng, herbs (SoBe 3G)	90	0	22.0	0	0	15	0
black and white tea (AriZona)	50	0	14.0	0	0	10	0
green tea: (AriZona)	70	0	18.0	0	0	20	0
(AriZona Extra Sweet)	90	0	23.0	0	0	10	0
(Honest Tea Organic)	17	0	5.0	0	0	5	0
(Lipton Brisk)	80	0	23.0	0	0	65	0
(Snapple Original) .	60	0	15.0	0	0	15	0

Food and Measure	cal.	prot. (gms)	carbo. (gms)	fat (gms)	chol. (mgs)	sod. (mgs)	fiber (gms)
Tea, iced, green tea *(cont.)*							
(*SoBe* 3G)	100	0	25.0	0	0	10	0
(*Turkey Hill*)	70	0	17.0	0	0	20	0
all varieties (*AriZona* Diet)	5	0	2.0	0	0	20	0
apple or peach (*AriZona*)	70	0	18.0	0	0	10	0
w/citrus (*Lipton Brisk*)	80	0	21.0	0	0	70	0
citrus fusion (*Snapple*)	80	0	23.0	0	0	110	0
hibiscus (*Pom* Light)	35	0	16.0	0	0	0	0
w/honey (*Honest Tea* Organic)	30	0	8.0	0	0	5	0
w/honey (*Lipton PureLeaf*)	60	0	16.0	0	0	0	0
lemonade (*AriZona*)	50	0	14.0	0	0	25	0
lime (*Snapple*)	100	0	25.0	0	0	10	0
mango (*Turkey Hill*)	90	0	21.0	0	0	10	0
mango or Asian pear (*Snapple*)	60	0	15.0	0	0	0	0
mint (*Honest Tea Organic Moroccan*)	17	0	5.0	0	0	5	0
orange, mandarin (*AriZona*)	70	0	19.0	0	0	20	0
passion fruit (*Honest Tea* Organic Green Dragon)	30	0	8.0	0	0	5	0
passion fruit (*Lipton PureLeaf*)	60	0	16.0	0	0	0	0
plum, Asian (*AriZona*)	70	0	18.0	0	0	20	0
pomegranate (*AriZona*)	70	0	19.0	0	0	10	0
pomegranate lychee (*Pom*)	70	0	18.0	0	0	15	0
green tea/juice blend:							
apple or pomegranate (*AriZona*)	80	0	20.0	0	0	10	0
white grape (*AriZona*)	80	0	21.0	0	0	10	0
herbal (*AriZona* Rx):							
Energy	120	0	31.0	0	0	25	0
Stress	60	0	16.0	0	0	20	0
lemon:							
(*AriZona*)	90	0	25.0	0	0	20	0
(*Honest Tea* Organic Lori's)	30	0	8.0	0	0	5	0
(*Lipton*)	60	0	16.0	0	0	65	0

Food and Measure	cal.	prot. (gms)	carbo. (gms)	fat (gms)	chol. (mgs)	sod. (mgs)	fiber (gms)
(*Lipton* Brisk)	80	0	22.0	0	0	65	0
(*Lipton* PureLeaf) .	60	0	15.0	0	0	0	0
(*Nantucket Nectars* Squeezed)	80	0	22.0	0	0	25	0
(*Newman's Own* Virgin Lemon-Aided)	110	0	27.0	0	0	40	0
(*Pacific* Organic) . .	70	0	17.0	0	0	10	0
(*Snapple*)	100	0	25.0	0	0	10	0
lemonade:							
(*AriZona* Arnold Palmer)	50	0	14.0	0	0	25	0
(*Nantucket Nectars* Squeezed Half and Half	90	0	22.0	0	0	25	0
(*Snapple*)	110	0	28.0	0	0	10	0
(*Turkey Hill*)	100	0	24.0	0	0	10	0
oolong:							
(*SoBe* 3G)	90	0	24.0	0	0	10	0
blueberry (*Turkey Hill*)	100	0	24.0	0	0	10	0
w/peach (*Honest Tea* Organic Oo-la-long)	30	0	8.0	0	0	5	0
orange (*Turkey Hill*) . .	100	0	25.0	0	0	10	0
peach:							
(*AriZona*)	70	0	18.0	0	0	20	0
(*Lipton*)	70	0	19.0	0	0	70	0
(*Lipton* PureLeaf) .	60	0	15.0	0	0	0	0
(*Pacific* Organic) . .	70	0	17.0	0	0	10	0
(*Snapple*)	100	0	26.0	0	0	10	0
(*Turkey Hill*)	110	0	28.0	0	0	10	0
peppermint (*Honest Tea* Organic First Nation)	17	0	5.0	0	0	5	0
pomegranate:							
(*Pom*)	70	0	17.0	0	0	15	0
blackberry (*Pom*) . .	80	0	20.0	0	0	10	0
raspberry:							
(*AriZona*)	90	0	25.0	0	0	20	0
(*Lipton* Brisk)	90	0	23.0	0	0	50	0
(*Lipton* PureLeaf) .	60	0	16.0	0	0	0	0
(*Pacific* Organic) . .	70	0	18.0	0	0	10	0
(*Snapple*)	100	0	26.0	0	0	10	0
(*Turkey Hill*)	110	0	28.0	0	0	10	0

Food and Measure	cal.	prot. (gms)	carbo. (gms)	fat (gms)	chol. (mgs)	sod. (mgs)	fiber (gms)
Tea, iced *(cont.)*							
red tea:							
all varieties (*Snapple*)	40	0	7.0	0	0	0	0
orange blossom (*Pom* Light)	35	0	14.0	0	0	0	0
pomegranate w/goji berry (*Honest Tea* Organic)	40	0	10.0	0	0	5	0
white tea:							
(*Honest Tea* Organic Perfect)	35	0	9.5	0	0	5	0
all varieties (*Snapple*)	60	0	15.0	0	0	15	0
blueberry (*AriZona*)	70	0	19.0	0	0	10	0
mango acai (*Honest Tea* Organic)	35	0	10.0	0	0	5	0
pomegranate w/acai (*Honest Tea* Organic)	35	0	9.5	0	0	5	0
pomegranate, peach, passion fruit (*Pom*)	70	0	19.0	0	0	15	0
raspberry (*Lipton*) .	60	0	16.0	0	0	65	0
tangerine (*Lipton PureLeaf*)	60	0	16.0	0	0	0	0
tangerine (*Turkey Hill*)	70	0	17.0	0	0	10	0
wildberry (*Pom* Light)	35	0	16.0	0	0	5	0
Tea, iced, mix, dry:							
(*Special K₂O* Protein Water), .5-oz. pkt. .	30	5.0	7.0	0	0	35	5.0
chai latte (*General Foods International Coffee*), 1⅓ tbsp. . . .	70	0	12.0	2.0	0	60	0
lemonade, classic or raspberry (*Country Time*), 2 tbsp.	90	0	22.0	0	0	10	0
Teff, grain (*Shiloh Farms*), ¼ cup	160	5.0	32.0	1.0	0	5	6.0
Teff flour (*Shiloh Farms*), ¼ cup	113	4.0	22.0	1.0	0	5	4.0
Tekka (*Eden* Organic), 1 tsp.	5	<1.0	<1.0	0	0	70	0
Tempeh:							
five grain:							
(*Turtle Island Foods* Organic), 3 oz. . .	190	11.0	20.0	6.0	0	10	6.0

Food and Measure	cal.	prot. (gms)	carbo. (gms)	fat (gms)	chol. (mgs)	sod. (mgs)	fiber (gms)
(*White Wave*), ⅓ block, 2.7 oz. . .	160	12.0	15.0	6.0	0	10	7.0
soy:							
(*Turtle Island Foods* Organic), 3 oz. . . .	160	13.0	20.0	3.5	0	10	7.0
(*White Wave* Original), ⅓ block, 2.7 oz. .	180	16.0	12.0	8.0	0	10	7.0
spicy veggie (*Turtle Island Foods* Organic), 3 oz.	145	13.0	20.0	3.5	0	25	7.0
1 oz.	55	5.3	2.7	3.1	0	3	n.a.
½ cup	160	15.4	7.8	9.0	0	7	n.a.
Temptation melon (*Frieda's*), 1/10 melon, 4.7 oz.	55	1.0	14.0	0	0	45	1.0
Tempura batter mix see "Batter/breading mix"							
Tenderizer, see "Meat tenderizer"							
Teriyaki sauce (see also "Marinade"), 1 tbsp.:							
(*Annie Chun's*)	25	1.0	5.0	0	0	350	0
(*La Choy*)	40	<1.0	10.0	0	0	570	0
(*San-J*)	15	1.0	2.0	0	0	460	0
(*World Harbors* Angosutra)	20	0	4.0	0	0	350	0
(*Yamasa*)	20	1.0	3.0	0	0	460	0
Texas toast, see "Bread, frozen/ refrigerated"							
Thai sauce (see also "Chili sauce, Asian," "Peanut sauce," and specific listings):							
(*Neera's* Sauce & Marinade), 1 tsp. . .	29	0	8.0	1.0	0	164	0
(*World Harbors* East Asian), 2 tbsp.	40	0	8.0	0	0	350	0
pad Thai (*A Taste of Thai*), 2 tbsp.	90	1.0	20.0	1.0	0	790	1.0
Thyme, ground, 1 tsp.	4	.1	.9	.1	0	1	.3

Food and Measure	cal.	prot. (gms)	carbo. (gms)	fat (gms)	chol. (mgs)	sod. (mgs)	fiber (gms)
Thymus, 4 oz.:							
beef, braised	362	24.8	0	28.3	333	132	0
veal, braised	197	35.8	0	4.9	532	75	0
Tilapia, fresh:							
raw, 4 oz.	109	22.8	0	1.9	57	59	0
baked or broiled, 4 oz.	145	29.6	0	3.0	64	63	0
Tilapia, frozen, raw							
(*Matlaw's*), 4 oz. ..	97	21.0	1.0	1.0	57	40	0
Tilapia entree, frozen:							
breaded fillet, 1 pc.:							
(*Gorton's*), 4 oz.	250	12.0	23.0	12.0	25	480	1.0
(*Gorton's Five Star*),							
3.1 oz.	80	14.0	<1.0	2.5	50	150	0
(*Matlaw's*), 4 oz. ..	260	15.0	26.0	10.0	30	790	0
(*Mrs. Paul's/Van de*							
Kamp's), 4 oz. ..	240	16.0	17.0	11.0	35	280	<1.0
stuffed fillet (*Oven*							
Poppers), 5 oz.:							
ginger teriyaki sauce	250	18.0	11.0	15.0	60	260	0
lemon garlic sauce .	240	19.0	4.0	16.0	55	240	0
sun-dried tomato,							
shrimp, lobster .	180	19.0	8.0	8.0	80	320	0
Tilefish, meat only:							
raw, 4 oz.	109	19.9	0	2.6	57	60	0
baked or broiled, 4 oz.	167	27.8	0	5.3	73	67	0
***T. J. Cinnamons*:**							
chocolate twist	250	4.0	34.0	12.0	5	110	2.0
cinnamon twist	260	3.0	33.0	14.0	5	190	1.0
mocha chill	306	11.0	48.0	7.0	29	214	1.0
Original Gourmet							
Cinnamon Roll	507	10.0	73.0	10.0	7	373	4.0
pecan sticky bun	688	12.0	91.0	22.0	7	420	5.0
TJ icing	117	1.0	18.0	5.0	8	50	0
Toaster pastry and							
muffins (see also							
"Breakfast sandwich/							
pastry"), 1 pc.:							
apple (*Amy's* Toaster							
Pops)	140	4.0	26.0	3.5	0	110	1.0
apple cinnamon:							
(*Nature's Path*							
Organic)	210	3.0	40.0	4.5	0	150	1.0
(*Pop•Tarts*)	210	2.0	37.0	6.0	0	180	<1.0

Food and Measure	cal.	prot. (gms)	carbo. (gms)	fat (gms)	chol. (mgs)	sod. (mgs)	fiber (gms)
frosted (*Nature's Path* Organic) ...	210	2.0	39.0	4.5	0	130	1.0
apple strudel (*Pop•Tarts*)	200	2.0	35.0	6.0	0	170	<1.0
berry:							
double, frosted (*Pop•Tarts*)	200	2.0	36.0	5.0	0	160	<1.0
frosted (*Pop•Tarts* Wild! Berry)	210	2.0	39.0	5.0	0	170	<1.0
wild (*Toaster Strudel*)	190	3.0	25.0	9.0	5	190	<1.0
blueberry:							
(*Nature's Path* Organic)	210	3.0	40.0	4.5	0	150	1.0
(*Pop•Tarts*)	210	2.0	37.0	6.0	0	180	<1.0
(*Toaster Strudel*) ..	190	3.0	26.0	9.0	5	190	<1.0
frosted (*Nature's Path* Organic) ...	200	2.0	38.0	4.0	0	125	1.0
frosted (*Pop•Tarts*)	200	2.0	37.0	5.0	0	170	<1.0
streusel muffin top (*Awrey's*), 3 oz. .	290	4.0	39.0	14.0	30	250	<1.0
brown sugar cinnamon:							
(*Pop•Tarts*)	210	2.0	33.0	8.0	0	190	<1.0
(*Toaster Strudel*) ..	200	3.0	28.0	9.0	5	210	1.0
frosted (*Pop•Tarts*)	210	2.0	34.0	7.0	0	170	<1.0
frosted (*Pop•Tarts* Low Fat)	190	2.0	38.0	3.0	0	210	<1.0
maple (*Nature's Path* Organic) ...	210	3.0	37.0	5.0	0	135	1.0
maple, frosted (*Nature's Path* Organic)	210	3.0	39.0	4.5	0	125	1.0
whole grain (*Pop• Tarts*)	200	3.0	34.0	7.0	0	170	3.0
caramel chocolate, frosted (*Pop•Tarts*)	200	2.0	35.0	5.0	0	230	<1.0
cherry:							
(*Toaster Strudel*) ..	190	3.0	25.0	8.0	5	190	<1.0
frosted (*Pop•Tarts*)	200	2.0	37.0	5.0	0	160	<1.0
cherry pomegranate, frosted (*Nature's Path Pomegran* Organic)	200	3.0	37.0	4.5	0	150	1.0
chocolate, frosted:							
(*Nature's Path* Organic)	210	3.0	38.0	5.0	0	130	1.0

Food and Measure	cal.	prot. (gms)	carbo. (gms)	fat (gms)	chol. (mgs)	sod. (mgs)	fiber (gms)
Toaster pastry and muffins, chocolate, frosted *(cont.)*							
hot (*Pop•Tarts*) ...	200	2.0	34.0	6.0	0	200	<1.0
chocolate chip:							
(*Pop•Tarts*)	220	3.0	36.0	7.0	0	240	<1.0
cookie dough (*Pop•Tarts*)	200	3.0	35.0	5.0	0	190	<1.0
chocolate fudge, frosted (*Pop•Tarts*)	200	3.0	37.0	5.0	0	210	<1.0
chocolate vanilla:							
(*Pop•Tarts Splitz*) ..	200	2.0	35.0	6.0	0	200	<1.0
crème, frosted (*Pop•Tarts*)	200	2.0	37.0	5.0	0	210	<1.0
cinnamon roll (*Pop•Tarts*)	210	2.0	34.0	7.0	0	160	<1.0
cookies and cream, frosted (*Pop•Tarts*)	200	2.0	35.0	5.0	0	260	<1.0
cranberry orange:							
(*Awrey's* Toaster Rounds)	150	2.0	19.0	7.0	20	140	0
muffin top (*Awrey's*)	290	4.0	38.0	14.0	45	280	<1.0
cream cheese:							
(*Toaster Strudel*) ..	200	3.0	23.0	11.0	10	220	<1.0
strawberry (*Amy's* Toaster Pops) ...	150	4.0	26.0	3.5	0	110	1.0
and strawberry (*Toaster Strudel*)	200	3.0	24.0	10.0	10	210	<1.0
corn muffin top (*Awrey's*)	350	5.0	43.0	18.0	60	240	0
corn bread (*Awrey's* Toaster Rounds) ..	180	2.0	22.0	9.0	30	150	0
gingerbread (*Pop•Tarts*)	200	2.0	36.0	5.0	0	220	1.0
hot fudge sundae (*Pop•Tarts*)	200	2.0	37.0	5.0	0	220	<1.0
lemon poppyseed:							
(*Awrey's* Toaster Rounds)	160	2.0	21.0	8.0	25	160	0
muffin top (*Awrey's*)	330	5.0	41.0	16.0	50	310	0
mint chocolate chip (*Pop•Tarts*)	200	2.0	36.0	5.0	0	210	<1.0
raspberry:							
(*Toaster Strudel*) ..	190	3.0	26.0	9.0	5	190	<1.0
frosted (*Nature's Path* Organic) ...	210	3.0	39.0	5.0	0	150	1.0
frosted (*Pop•Tarts*)	210	2.0	38.0	5.0	0	160	<1.0

Food and Measure	cal.	prot. (gms)	carbo. (gms)	fat (gms)	chol. (mgs)	sod. (mgs)	fiber (gms)
s'mores, frosted (*Pop•Tarts*)	200	3.0	36.0	5.0	0	210	<1.0
strawberry:							
(*Nature's Path Organic*)	210	3.0	40.0	4.5	0	150	1.0
(*Pop•Tarts*)	210	2.0	37.0	6.0	0	180	<1.0
(*Toaster Strudel*) ..	190	3.0	26.0	9.0	5	190	<1.0
frosted (*Nature's Path Organic*) ...	210	3.0	40.0	4.0	0	140	1.0
frosted (*Pop•Tarts*)	200	2.0	37.0	5.0	0	170	<1.0
frosted (*Pop•Tarts Low Fat*)	190	2.0	39.0	3.0	0	210	<1.0
milk shake, frosted (*Pop•Tarts*)	200	2.0	35.0	6.0	0	190	<1.0
whole grain (*Pop•Tarts*)	190	2.0	35.0	5.0	0	160	3.0
strawberry banana (*Toaster Strudel*) ..	180	2.0	24.0	9.0	5	180	0
strawberry blueberry (*Pop•Tarts Splitz*) ..	200	2.0	36.0	5.0	0	180	<1.0
strawberry cheese danish (*Pop•Tarts*) .	200	2.0	35.0	6.0	0	180	<1.0
wildberry acai, frosted (*Nature's Path Organic*)	210	3.0	39.0	5.0	0	130	1.0
Toffee, see "Candy"							
Toffee baking chips (*Hershey's Heath Bits 'O Brickle* Bits), 1 tbsp., .5 oz.	80	<1.0	9.0	5.0	5	80	0
Toffee syrup (*Heath Sundae*), 2 tbsp. ..	100	0	24.0	0	0	130	0
Toffee topping (*Heath Shell*), 2 tbsp.	210	<1.0	17.0	17.0	0	40	1.0
Tofu (see also "Seitan" and "Tempeh"), fresh, except as noted:							
cubed, 2.8 oz.:							
super firm (*Azumaya*)	100	10.0	3.0	5.0	0	0	2.0
super firm (*Nasoya*)	100	10.0	3.0	5.0	0	0	<2.0
extra firm:							
(*Azumaya*), 2.8 oz. ..	70	7.0	2.0	4.0	0	0	1.0
(*Azumaya* Lite), 2.8 oz.	60	7.0	3.0	2.0	0	30	1.0

Food and Measure	cal.	prot. (gms)	carbo. (gms)	fat (gms)	chol. (mgs)	sod. (mgs)	fiber (gms)
Tofu, extra firm *(cont.)*							
(*Frieda's*), 3 oz. ...	90	10.0	10.0	5.0	0	10	0
(*Frieda's* Organic),							
3 oz.	70	7.0	2.0	4.0	0	10	0
(*Nasoya*), 2.8 oz. ...	80	8.0	2.0	4.0	0	0	1.0
(*White Mountain*							
Organic), 3.2 oz.	90	10.0	1.0	6.0	0	10	1.0
(*White Wave/White*							
Wave Organic),							
3 oz.	110	11.0	3.0	6.0	0	5	1.0
firm:							
(*Azumaya*), 2.8 oz. .	70	7.0	2.0	4.0	0	0	<1.0
(*Frieda's*), 3 oz. ...	60	6.0	2.0	3.0	0	10	0
(*Frieda's* Organic),							
3 oz.	70	7.0	1.0	4.0	0	10	0
(*Nasoya*), 2.8 oz. ..	70	7.0	2.0	3.0	0	0	<1.0
(*Nasoya* Lite), 2.8 oz.	40	7.0	1.0	1.5	0	25	<1.0
(*Tree of Life*), 3.2 oz.	110	11.0	4.0	5.0	0	5	2.0
(*Tree of Life* Reduced							
Fat), 3.2 oz.	90	10.0	4.0	4.0	0	5	2.0
(*Tree of Life* Water							
Pack), 3.2 oz. ...	100	9.0	2.0	5.0	0	5	0
(*White Wave*), ⅛ of							
1-lb. box.	110	11.0	3.0	6.0	0	5	1.0
½ cup	183	19.9	5.4	11.0	0	17	2.9
silken:							
(*Azumaya*), 2.8 oz. :	70	7.0	2.0	4.0	0	0	<1.0
(*Azumaya* Lite),							
3.2 oz.	40	5.0	3.0	1.0	0	45	0
(*Nasoya*), 3.2 oz. ..	45	4.0	1.0	2.0	0	0	0
(*Nasoya* Lite), 3.2 oz.	30	6.0	0	1.0	0	65	0
soft:							
(*Frieda's*), 3 oz. ...	45	5.0	1.0	2.5	0	15	0
(*Frieda's* Organic),							
3 oz.	50	5.0	2.0	2.5	0	10	0
(*Nasoya*), 2.8 oz. ..	60	6.0	1.0	3.0	0	0	<1.0
(*White Wave* Organic),							
⅛ of 1-lb. pkg. ...	110	10.0	3.0	6.0	0	5	1.0
baked (*Frieda's*), 3 oz.:							
garlic herb	120	10.0	8.0	6.0	0	240	1.0
sesame garlic	130	10.0	10.0	6.0	0	210	1.0
baked (*White Wave*),							
2-oz. pc.:							
garlic herb Italian ..	90	9.0	2.0	5.0	0	240	1.0

Food and Measure	cal.	prot. (gms)	carbo. (gms)	fat (gms)	chol. (mgs)	sod. (mgs)	fiber (gms)
lemon pepper	90	9.0	3.0	5.0	0	200	1.0
teriyaki, Oriental ...	100	9.0	4.0	5.0	0	240	2.0
sesame peanut, Thai	90	9.0	2.0	5.0	0	280	1.0
tomato basil, Roma	90	9.0	3.0	5.0	0	240	1.0
dried (*Eden* Organic), .4-oz. pc.	50	5.0	0	2.5	0	0	2.0
salted and fermented (fuyu), 1 oz.	33	2.3	1.5	2.3	0	814	<1.0
seasoned, 3 oz.:							
Chinese spice (*Nasoya*)	90	8.0	3.0	5.0	0	220	1.0
garlic onion (*Azumaya* Zesty)	90	8.0	3.0	5.0	0	250	1.0
garlic onion (*Nasoya*)	90	8.0	3.0	5.0	0	250	1.0
Oriental spice (*Azumaya*)	90	8.0	3.0	5.0	0	220	1.0
smoked, all varieties (*Tree of Life*), 3 oz.	120	18.0	3.0	5.0	0	120	0
Tofu, canned, in water (*Roland*), 4 pcs. ...	59	6.0	2.0	3.0	0	290	1.0
Tofu breakfast, frozen, 9-oz. pkg.:							
Rancheros (*Amy's*) ..	380	21.0	37.0	17.0	15	580	7.0
scramble (*Amy's*)	320	19.0	19.0	19.0	0	580	4.0
Tofu dessert, peach mango (*Frieda's*), 3 oz.	60	2.0	9.0	1.5	0	0	0
Tofu dip, 4 oz.:							
hot (*White Mountain*) .	135	11.0	0	8.0	0	640	0
onion (*White Mountain*)	160	14.0	0	10.0	0	535	0
Tofu dish (*TofuTown Tofu Tenders*), ½ of 10-oz. pkg.:							
black bean, Havana ..	210	15.0	18.0	8.0	0	690	2.0
sesame ginger teriyaki	240	15.0	24.0	9.0	0	680	3.0
tahini, Mediterranean .	240	15.0	16.0	13.0	0	640	3.0
tamari, light	120	14.0	15.0	7.0	0	640	2.0
Tofu salad:							
(*White Mountain* Original), 4 oz.	100	14.0	0	5.0	0	420	0
"egg" (*White Mountain* No-Egg), 4 oz.	120	14.0	0	7.0	0	430	0
Tofu scrambler mix (*Fantastic*), 1 tbsp. ..	35	1.0	7.0	0	0	260	1.0

Food and Measure	cal.	prot. (gms)	carbo. (gms)	fat (gms)	chol. (mgs)	sod. (mgs)	fiber (gms)
Tomatillo, fresh:							
(*Frieda's*), ⅔ cup, 3 oz.	25	1.0	5.0	1.0	0	0	2.0
1 medium, 1⅝" diam.	11	.3	2.0	.4	0	tr.	.6
chopped, ½ cup	21	.6	3.8	.7	0	1	1.3
Tomatillo, canned:							
(*Sabores Aztecas*), 4.5 oz.	20	2.0	3.0	0	0	240	2.0
crushed (*Las Palmas*), ½ cup	45	1.0	7.0	1.5	0	n.a.	2.0
Tomato, fresh, ripe:							
raw:							
(*Del Monte*), 1 medium, 5.2 oz.	35	1.0	7.0	.5	0	0	1.0
(*Frieda's* Baby Roma/ Teardrop), ⅔ cup, 3 oz.	20	1.0	4.0	0	0	10	1.0
2⅜" tomato	26	1.0	5.7	.4	0	11	1.4
chopped, 1 cup . . .	38	1.5	8.4	.6	0	16	2.0
boiled:							
2 medium, 8.8 oz. . .	66	2.6	14.3	1.0	0	27	2.5
1 cup	65	2.6	14.0	1.0	0	27	2.4
orange:							
3.9-oz. tomato	18	1.3	3.5	.2	0	47	1.0
chopped, 1 cup . . .	25	1.8	5.0	.3	0	66	1.4
yellow:							
7.8-oz. tomato	32	2.1	6.3	.6	0	49	1.5
chopped, 1 cup . . .	21	1.4	4.1	.4	0	32	1.0
Tomato, can/jar (see also "Tomato paste," "Tomato puree," and "Tomato sauce"), ½ cup, except as noted:							
(*Alessi* Prima Passata)	25	2.0	4.0	0	0	170	2.0
whole, peeled:							
(*Eden* Organic)	30	1.0	4.0	0	0	10	1.0
(*Hunt's*)	20	1.0	4.0	0	0	190	1.0
(*Hunt's* No Salt) . . .	20	<1.0	4.0	0	0	25	1.0
(*Muir Glen* Organic/ Organic Plum) . .	25	1.0	5.0	0	0	260	1.0
(*S&W*)	25	1.0	6.0	0	0	250	2.0
w/basil (*Eden* Organic)	30	1.0	4.0	0	0	10	1.0
w/basil (*Muir Glen* Organic)	25	1.0	5.0	0	0	260	1.0

Food and Measure	cal.	prot. (gms)	carbo. (gms)	fat (gms)	chol. (mgs)	sod. (mgs)	fiber (gms)
w/basil (*Progresso*)	20	1.0	4.0	0	0	260	1.0
fire-roasted (*Muir Glen* Organic) . . .	25	1.0	5.0	0	0	290	1.0
wedges (*Del Monte*) . .	35	1.0	9.0	0	0	380	2.0
chunky, w/green chili (*Ro*Tel*)	20	<1.0	4.0	0	0	520	1.0
diced:							
(*Contadina* Recipe Ready)	30	<1.0	6.0	0	0	200	1.0
(*Del Monte/Del Monte* Petite) . . .	25	1.0	6.0	0	0	250	2.0
(*Del Monte* No Salt)	25	1.0	6.0	0	0	50	2.0
(*Eden* Organic)	30	1.0	6.0	0	0	5	2.0
(*Hunt's* Original) . . .	20	1.0	5.0	0	0	380	<1.0
(*Hunt's* Petite)	20	1.0	5.0	0	0	330	1.0
(*Muir Glen* Organic)	30	1.0	6.0	0	0	290	1.0
(*Muir Glen* Organic No Salt)	30	1.0	6.0	0	0	15	1.0
(*Pacific* Organic) . .	30	<1.0	6.0	0	0	200	<1.0
(*Progresso*)	25	1.0	5.0	0	0	250	1.0
(*Ro*Tel*)	25	<1.0	5.0	0	0	520	1.0
(*S&W* Petite-Cut Rich Juice)	25	1.0	6.0	0	0	250	2.0
(*S&W* Ready-Cut) .	25	1.0	6.0	0	0	250	2.0
(*S&W* Ready-Cut No Salt)	25	1.0	6.0	0	0	50	2.0
chili style, zesty (*Del Monte*)	30	1.0	8.0	0	0	600	2.0
chunky, pasta style (*Del Monte*)	45	1.0	11.0	0	0	560	2.0
w/balsamic vinegar/ basil/oil (*Hunt's*) .	60	1.0	8.0	3.0	0	460	1.0
w/basil or roasted onion (*Eden* Organic)	30	1.0	6.0	0	0	5	2.0
w/basil/garlic or garlic/onion (*Muir Glen* Organic) . . .	30	1.0	6.0	0	0	290	1.0
w/basil/garlic/ oregano (*Del Monte*)	50	2.0	11.0	0	0	650	<1.0
w/basil/garlic/ oregano (*Hunt's*)	25	<1.0	6.0	0	0	520	1.0

Food and Measure	cal.	prot. (gms)	carbo. (gms)	fat (gms)	chol. (mgs)	sod. (mgs)	fiber (gms)
Tomato, can/jar, diced *(cont.)*							
w/cilantro/lime (*Furmano's* Petite)	30	1.0	6.0	.5	0	240	1.0
fire-roasted (*Muir Glen* Organic) ...	30	1.0	6.0	0	0	290	1.0
fire-roasted, w/green chili (*Muir Glen* Organic)	30	1.0	6.0	0	0	420	1.0
w/garlic, roasted (*Hunt's*)	30	1.0	6.0	0	0	460	1.0
w/garlic, roasted (*S&W Ready-Cut*)	30	2.0	5.0	.5	0	240	<1.0
w/garlic and olive oil (*Del Monte* Petite)	45	1.0	10.0	.5	0	620	1.0
w/garlic/onion (*Del Monte*)	40	2.0	8.0	.5	0	610	<1.0
w/green chili (*Eden* Organic)	30	2.0	5.0	0	0	35	2.0
w/green chili (*Fanci Food*)	25	1.0	5.0	0	0	340	1.0
w/green chili (*Furmano's* Petite) ..	25	1.0	5.0	0	0	260	2.0
w/green chili (*Hunt's*)	30	2.0	6.0	0	0	360	2.0
w/green chili (*Ro*Tel*)	20	<1.0	4.0	0	0	520	1.0
w/green chili (*S&W Ready-Cut*)	30	1.0	6.0	0	0	500	1.0
w/green chili, mild (*Del Monte*)	30	1.0	6.0	0	0	500	1.0
w/green pepper/ celery/onion (*Hunt's*)	45	1.0	9.0	0	0	340	1.0
w/green pepper/ onion (*Del Monte*)	40	1.0	9.0	0	0	480	2.0
w/green pepper/ onion (*Furmano's*)	30	1.0	7.0	.5	0	250	2.0
hot (*Ro*Tel*)	20	<1.0	4.0	0	0	520	1.0
Italian (*Fanci Food*)	30	1.0	5.0	0	0	330	1.0
Italian (*Furmano's*) .	40	1.0	8.0	0	0	340	1.0
Italian (*Ro*Tel*) ...	30	1.0	6.0	0	0	520	1.0
Italian (*S&W Ready-Cut*)	25	1.0	4.0	0	0	190	<1.0
w/Italian herbs (*Contadina* Recipe Ready)	45	1.0	10.0	0	0	470	<1.0

Food and Measure	cal.	prot. (gms)	carbo. (gms)	fat (gms)	chol. (mgs)	sod. (mgs)	fiber (gms)
w/Italian herbs (*Muir Glen* Organic) ...	30	1.0	6.0	0	0	350	1.0
w/Italian herbs (*Progresso*)	40	1.0	8.0	0	0	330	1.0
w/jalapeño (*Del Monte* Petite Cut)	30	1.0	6.0	0	0	500	1.0
w/jalapeño (*S&W Petite-Cut*)	30	1.0	7.0	0	0	380	2.0
marinara (*Contadina Recipe Ready*) ..	70	1.0	13.0	1.5	0	600	2.0
Mexican (*Ro*Tel*) .	30	<1.0	6.0	0	0	540	1.0
w/mushrooms/garlic (*Del Monte*)	45	1.0	10.0	0	0	590	1.0
w/onion, sweet (*Hunt's*)	45	1.0	10.0	0	0	490	<1.0
w/onion, sweet (*S&W Petite-Cut*)	45	1.0	10.0	0	0	550	1.0
w/onion/green pepper (*S&W Ready-Cut*)	40	1.0	9.0	0	0	480	2.0
primavera (*Contadina* Recipe Ready)	60	1.0	13.0	0	0	560	2.0
w/red pepper, roasted (*Contadina* Recipe Ready)	60	1.0	13.0	0	0	550	2.0
in sauce (*Hunt's*) ..	30	1.0	7.0	0	0	430	1.0
seasoned, for chili (*Hunt's* Family Favorites)	25	1.0	5.0	0	0	400	1.0
crushed, ¼ cup, except as noted:							
(*Contadina* Recipe Ready)	20	<1.0	4.0	0	0	150	1.0
(*Hunt's*), ½ cup ...	30	2.0	7.0	0	0	350	2.0
(*Progresso*)	20	1.0	3.0	0	0	95	0
(*Eden* Organic)	20	1.0	3.0	0	0	0	1.0
(*Pacific* Organic) ..	20	<1.0	4.0	0	0	150	1.0
w/basil (*Muir Glen* Organic)	25	1.0	5.0	0	0	190	1.0
w/basil or onion/ garlic (*Eden* Organic)	20	1.0	3.0	0	0	0	1.0
fire-roasted (*Muir Glen* Organic) ...	20	<1.0	4.0	0	0	160	1.0

Food and Measure	cal.	prot. (gms)	carbo. (gms)	fat (gms)	chol. (mgs)	sod. (mgs)	fiber (gms)
Tomato, can/jar, crushed *(cont.)*							
w/garlic, roasted (*Contadina* Recipe Ready)	20	<1.0	3.0	0	0	150	1.0
Italian (*S&W*)	20	1.0	4.0	0	0	95	1.0
Italian herbs (*Contadina* Recipe Ready)	20	<1.0	3.0	0	0	150	<1.0
in puree (*S&W*) ...	20	1.0	4.0	0	0	125	1.0
and okra, seasoned:							
(*Glory Sensibly*) ...	30	1.0	2.0	0	0	170	2.0
and corn (*Glory Sensibly*)	35	1.0	8.0	0	0	150	2.0
stewed:							
(*Contadina*)	35	1.0	9.0	0	0	220	1.0
(*Del Monte*)	35	1.0	9.0	0	0	360	2.0
(*Del Monte* No Salt)	35	1.0	9.0	0	0	50	2.0
(*Furmano's*)	45	1.0	10.0	0	0	270	2.0
(*Hunt's*)	30	1.0	7.0	0	0	450	1.0
(*Hunt's* No Salt) ...	40	1.0	9.0	0	0	30	1.0
(*S&W*)	35	1.0	7.0	0	0	270	2.0
(*S&W* No Salt)	35	1.0	9.0	0	0	50	2.0
Cajun (*Del Monte*) .	35	1.0	9.0	0	0	460	2.0
Italian (*Contadina*) .	35	1.0	8.0	0	0	260	1.0
Italian (*Del Monte*) .	30	1.0	8.0	0	0	420	2.0
Italian (*Furmano's*) .	40	1.0	8.0	0	0	370	2.0
Italian or Mexican (*S&W*)	35	1.0	7.0	0	0	270	2.0
Mexican (*Del Monte*)	35	1.0	9.0	0	0	400	2.0
Tomato, dried:							
(*Aessi* Pkg.), 2 pcs. ..	20	1.0	4.0	0	0	45	1.0
(*Roland* Pkg.), 1 pc. ..	10	0	2.0	0	0	60	0
1 oz.	73	4.0	15.8	.8	0	594	3.5
1 pc., 32 pcs. per cup	5	.3	1.1	.1	0	42	.3
½ cup	70	3.8	15.3	.8	0	566	3.3
chopped or halves (*Frieda's*), ⅓ cup, 1.1 oz.	100	2.0	19.0	1.0	0	10	2.0
yellow, chopped or halves (*Frieda's*), ½ cup, 3 oz.	220	12.0	47.0	2.5	0	1780	10.0
marinated, in oil:							
(*Alessi*), 1 pc.	35	1.0	3.0	2.0	0	450	1.0

Food and Measure	cal.	prot. (gms)	carbo. (gms)	fat (gms)	chol. (mgs)	sod. (mgs)	fiber (gms)
(*Roland* 3 oz.), 2 halves	35	0	0	4.0	0	80	0
(*Roland* 10 oz.), 2 halves	25	1.0	3.0	1.5	0	40	1.0
drained, ½ cup . . .	117	2.8	12.8	7.7	0	146	3.2
Tomato, dried, blend, seasoned (*Frieda's* Tomato Toss), ½ cup, 1.1 oz.	100	6.0	19.0	0	0	105	4.0
Tomato, green, raw, 1 large, 6.4 oz.	44	2.2	9.3	.4	0	24	2.0
Tomato, pickled:							
(*Ba-Tampte*), ½ pc., 1.5 oz.	5	0	1.0	0	0	310	0
wedges, sweet, w/onion, peppers (*Mrs. Renfro's*), 1 oz. . . .	25	0	6.0	0	0	75	0
Tomato, sun-dried, see "Tomato, dried"							
Tomato chutney, see "Chutney"							
Tomato dip, 1 oz.:							
Moroccan, spicy (*Sabra* Matbucha) .	20	0	3.0	1.0	0	95	0
Turkish (*Sabra* Salad)	80	1.0	3.0	2.0	0	150	1.0
Tomato dip seasoning, and horseradish (*Watkins*), 1 tsp. . .	10	0	2.0	0	0	85	0
Tomato juice, 8 fl. oz., except as noted:							
(*Campbell's*)	50	2.0	10.0	0	0	680	2.0
(*Campbell's*), 5.5 fl. oz.	30	1.0	6.0	0	0	520	1.0
(*Campbell's* Low Sodium)	50	2.0	10.0	0	0	140	2.0
(*Campbell's* Organic) .	50	2.0	10.0	0	0	680	2.0
(*Campbell's* Healthy Request)	50	2.0	10.0	0	0	480	2.0
(*Del Monte*)	50	2.0	10.0	0	0	760	1.0
(*R.W. Knudsen* Organic)	60	2.0	14.0	0	0	390	0
(*Tree of Life Pure Fruit*)	50	1.0	10.0	0	0	480	0
Tomato okra corn casserole, frozen (*Glory* Savory Accents), ½ cup . .	110	4.0	14.0	4.5	5	460	2.0

Food and Measure	cal.	prot. (gms)	carbo. (gms)	fat (gms)	chol. (mgs)	sod. (mgs)	fiber (gms)
Tomato paste, 2 tbsp.:							
(*Contadina*)	30	2.0	6.0	0	0	20	1.0
(*Hunt's*)	25	1.0	6.0	0	0	95	2.0
(*Hunt's* No Salt)	30	1.0	6.0	0	0	15	2.0
(*Muir Glen* Organic) ..	30	2.0	6.0	0	0	20	1.0
(*S&W*)	30	2.0	6.0	0	0	20	1.0
w/basil, garlic, oregano							
(*Hunt's*)	25	1.0	6.0	0	0	260	2.0
w/Italian seasoning							
(*Contadina*)	35	1.0	7.0	.5	0	290	1.0
w/pesto (*Contadina*) ..	35	1.0	5.0	.5	0	300	<1.0
w/roasted garlic							
(*Contadina*)	35	1.0	6.0	.5	0	300	1.0
Tomato powder							
(*AlpineAire*), ⅔ oz.	90	0	22.0	0	0	40	0
Tomato puree, ¼ cup:							
(*Contadina*)	20	<1.0	4.0	0	0	15	<1.0
(*Furmano's*)	20	1.0	4.0	0	0	40	1.0
(*Muir Glen* Organic) ..	20	1.0	5.0	0	0	20	1.0
(*Progresso*)	25	1.0	5.0	0	0	15	1.0
(*S&W*)	30	1.0	6.0	0	0	15	2.0
Tomato relish, 1 tbsp.,							
except as noted:							
(*B&G* Piccalilli)	20	0	5.0	0	0	120	0
hot (*Mrs. Renfro's*) ..	10	0	3.0	0	0	40	0
mild (*Mrs. Renfro's*) .	10	0	3.0	0	0	45	0
sun-dried (*Peloponnese*)	25	0	2.0	1.5	0	200	0
Tomato sauce (see							
also "Pasta sauce"							
and "Tomato,							
canned"), ¼ cup:							
(*Contadina*)	15	<1.0	3.0	0	0	280	<1.0
(*Contadina* Extra Thick							
& Zesty)	20	1.0	3.0	0	0	340	1.0
(*Del Monte*)	20	1.0	4.0	0	0	340	<1.0
(*Furmano's*)	20	1.0	4.0	0	0	270	1.0
(*Hunt's*)	15	<1.0	3.0	0	0	360	1.0
(*Hunt's* No Salt)	15	<1.0	4.0	0	0	15	1.0
(*Muir Glen* Organic) ..	20	<1.0	5.0	0	0	310	1.0
(*Muir Glen* Organic							
Chunky)	20	<1.0	4.0	0	0	160	1.0
(*Muir Glen* Organic No							
Salt)	20	<1.0	5.0	0	0	30	1.0
(*Pacific* Organic)	15	<1.0	3.0	0	0	280	1.0

Food and Measure	cal.	prot. (gms)	carbo. (gms)	fat (gms)	chol. (mgs)	sod. (mgs)	fiber (gms)
(S&W Homestyle) ...	20	1.0	4.0	0	0	260	1.0
w/basil, garlic, oregano (Hunt's)	15	<1.0	3.0	0	0	350	<1.0
w/garlic, roasted (Hunt's)	15	<1.0	3.0	0	0	380	<1.0
w/garlic and onion (Contadina)	20	<1.0	4.0	0	0	270	<1.0
Italian style (Contadina)	15	<1.0	4.0	0	0	320	1.0
for lasagna (Hunt's Family Favorites) ..	30	1.0	6.0	0	0	330	1.0
for meat loaf (Hunt's Family Favorites) ..	30	1.0	7.0	0	0	390	2.0
for pizza, see "Pizza sauce"							
seasoned (Hunt's Family Favorites) ..	25	1.0	5.0	0	0	270	1.0
Tongue, braised:							
beef, 4 oz.	321	25.1	.4	23.5	121	68	0
lamb, 4 oz.	312	24.5	0	23.0	214	76	0
pork, 4 oz.	307	27.3	0	21.1	166	124	0
veal (calves), 4 oz. ...	229	29.3	0	11.5	270	73	0
Tongue lunch meat, beef, 2 oz.	120	10.0	0	9.0	50	330	0
Topping, dessert (see also specific flavors), 2 tbsp.:							
(Smucker's Magic Shell Turtle Delight)	210	1.0	17.0	15.0	0	30	1.0
(Smucker's Magic Shell Twix)	210	1.0	18.0	15.0	0	35	1.0
(Smucker's Milky Way)	140	1.0	24.0	4.5	5	50	0
(Smucker's Sunday Syrup 3 Musketeers)	110	1.0	23.0	2.0	0	60	0
Tortellini (see also "Tortelloni"), frozen or refrigerated, 1 cup, except as noted:							
cheese:							
(Celentano)	240	9.0	45.0	2.5	25	490	2.0
mixed (Buitoni) ...	320	15.0	49.0	7.0	45	530	3.0
three (Buitoni)	320	15.0	50.0	7.0	40	480	3.0
three, whole wheat pasta (Buitoni) ..	340	16.0	44.0	11.0	65	480	8.0
whole wheat pasta (Monterey Classic)	290	13.0	48.0	6.0	35	290	5.0

Food and Measure	cal.	prot. (gms)	carbo. (gms)	fat (gms)	chol. (mgs)	sod. (mgs)	fiber (gms)
Tortellini *(cont.)*							
herb chicken (*Buitoni*)	350	13.0	52.0	10.0	40	380	2.0
olive, Sicilian, lemon							
(*Cafferata* Olota Olive)	218	7.0	43.0	2.0	0	320	1.0
spinach and cheese							
(*Buitoni*)	320	15.0	49.0	7.0	55	510	3.0
Tortellini entree,							
frozen, 1 pkg.:							
Alfredo (*Michelina's*							
Authentico), 8 oz...	280	12.0	26.0	15.0	50	1460	1.0
pesto (*Amy's* Bowls),							
9.5 oz.	430	20.0	45.0	19.0	40	640	3.0
Tortelloni, frozen or							
refrigerated (see							
also "Tortellini"),							
1 cup:							
cheese and roasted							
garlic (*Buitoni*)	270	12.0	37.0	8.0	35	360	2.0
chicken and proscuitto							
(*Buitoni*)	330	15.0	46.0	9.0	40	650	2.0
mozzarella and herb							
(*Buitoni*)	330	14.0	47.0	9.0	40	440	2.0
portobello mushroom							
and cheese (*Buitoni*)	290	10.0	49.0	6.0	25	400	3.0
sausage, sweet Italian							
(*Buitoni*)	330	12.0	48.0	10.0	35	300	3.0
Tortilla (see also							
"Wraps"), 1 pc.,							
except as noted:							
corn (*Chi-Chi's* 6"),							
2 pcs., 1.2 oz.	130	3.0	26.0	1.5	0	15	0
flour:							
(*Chi-Chi's* 6"), 1.2 oz.	110	2.0	17.0	2.5	0	260	0
(*Chi-Chi's* 8"), 1.7 oz.	150	3.0	25.0	4.0	0	380	0
(*Chi-Chi's* 10"), 2.5 oz.	220	5.0	36.0	6.0	0	540	0
(*Old El Paso*), 2 pcs.,							
1.75 oz.	160	4.0	26.0	4.5	0	370	1.0
flour, for burritos:							
(*Chi-Chi's* 9"), 2.1 oz.	170	4.0	31.0	3.5	0	450	1.8
(*Old El Paso*), 1.4 oz.	130	3.0	20.0	4.0	0	300	0
flour, for fajitas (*Chi-*							
Chi's 6"), 1 pc.	80	2.0	14.0	1.5	0	260	1.8
flour, for soft tacos:							
(*Chi-Chi's* 8"), 2 oz.	160	4.0	29.0	3.5	0	510	1.8

ood and Measure	cal.	prot. (gms)	carbo. (gms)	fat (gms)	chol. (mgs)	sod. (mgs)	fiber (gms)
(Old El Paso), 1.8 oz.	160	4.0	26.0	4.5	0	370	1.0
(Taco Bell), 2 pcs., 2.1 oz.	200	4.0	35.0	5.0	0	380	1.0
ortilla black bean casserole, frozen (Amy's Bowls), 9.5-oz. pkg.	390	17.0	41.0	18.0	25	780	7.0
ortilla chips, see "Corn chips/crisps"							
ortilla chips, multi-grain, 1 oz.:							
Snyder's MultiGrain Lightly Salted)	130	2.0	20.0	5.0	0	110	3.0
ax gold (Snyder's MultiGrain)	140	2.0	18.0	7.0	0	230	3.0
alapeño red or savory blue (Snyder's MultiGrain)	140	2.0	17.0	7.0	0	190	3.0
ostada shell (see also "Taco shell"):							
Old El Paso), 3 pcs. .	160	2.0	19.0	10.0	0	115	2.0
Ortega), 2 pcs.	120	2.0	16.0	6.0	0	170	2.0
Zapata), 2 pcs.	110	2.0	14.0	5.0	0	5	1.0
lue or yellow corn (Bearito's), 2 pcs. . .	140	2.0	17.0	7.0	0	5	1.0
rail mix:							
Amport Foods Berry Trails), 1.1 oz.	140	4.0	15.0	8.0	0	60	1.0
Amport Foods Rain-bow Munch), 1.1 oz.	130	3.0	17.0	7.0	0	60	1.0
Amport Foods Santa Fe Trail), 1.1 oz. . . .	140	4.0	15.0	8.0	0	280	1.0
Amport Foods Trail Mix), 1.1 oz.	150	5.0	12.0	10.0	0	160	1.0
Cape Cod Cranberry Trail Mix), ¼ cup . .	150	4.0	17.0	9.0	0	0	3.0
Chocolate Crunch Trail Mix), 1 oz. . . .	130	4.0	11.0	9.0	0	20	2.0
Eden Organic All Mixed Up), 1.1 oz. . .	160	8.0	7.0	12.0	0	70	4.0
Eden Organic All Mixed Up Too), 3 tbsp., 1.1 oz.	140	5.0	10.0	11.0	0	15	4.0

Food and Measure	cal.	prot. (gms)	carbo. (gms)	fat (gms)	chol. (mgs)	sod. (mgs)	fiber (gms)
Trail mix *(cont.)*							
(Frito-Lay Original), 3 tbsp.	160	4.0	14.0	9.0	0	45	2.0
(Happy Trails Mix), ¼ cup, 1.2 oz.	150	4.0	16.0	9.0	0	20	3.0
(Kettle Camping Mix), 1 oz.	140	4.0	11.0	8.0	0	10	2.0
(Kettle Chocolate Lovers Mix), 1 oz.	130	3.0	15.0	7.0	0	10	2.0
(Kettle Honey Cranberry Mix), 1 oz.	120	3.0	16.0	6.0	0	40	2.0
(Kettle Honey Roasted Harvest Mix), 1 oz.	130	3.0	16.0	6.0	0	20	2.0
(Kettle Natural Chocolate Lovers Mix), 1 oz.	120	3.0	16.0	7.0	0	5	2.0
(Kettle Sporting Mix), 1 oz.	140	5.0	10.0	10.0	0	0	2.0
(Kettle X-Treme Trail Mix), 1 oz.	150	5.0	9.0	11.0	0	0	2.0
(Organic Chocolate Trail Mix), 1 oz.	140	4.0	14.0	9.0	0	20	2.0
(Organic Harvest Trail Mix), ¼ cup	120	2.0	16.0	6.0	0	5	2.0
(Planters Energy Mix), 1.5-oz. pkg.	240	6.0	14.0	19.0	0	135	3.0
(Planters Golden Nut Crunch), 1.1 oz. ...	160	5.0	12.0	11.0	0	90	2.0
(Planters Sweet & Nutty/ Nut-rition), 1.1 oz. .	160	5.0	12.0	11.0	0	90	2.0
(Raisin Conscious Nuts), 3 tbsp.	120	4.0	10.0	8.0	0	55	2.0
(Really Nuts! Hershey's), .5-oz. pkg.	70	2.0	6.0	5.0	0	35	<1.0
(Really Nuts! Mauna Loa), 1.7-oz. pkg...	260	4.0	25.0	17.0	0	80	1.0
(Really Nuts! Reese's), 1.8-oz. pkg.	280	10.0	18.0	20.0	0	220	3.0
(SunRidge Farms Cocono Deluxe), ¼ cup .	160	5.0	10.0	12.0	0	20	2.0
(SunRidge Farms Deluxe Organic), ¼ cup	130	4.0	4.0	6.0	0	15	2.0
(SunRidge Farms Hit the Trail Organic), ¼ cup, 1.1 oz.	150	6.0	11.0	11.0	0	20	2.0

Food and Measure	cal.	prot. (gms)	carbo. (gms)	fat (gms)	chol. (mgs)	sod. (mgs)	fiber (gms)
(*SunRidge Farms* Super Deluxe), ¼ cup ...	150	5.0	11.0	11.0	0	50	2.0
(*Tex-Mex Mix*), ¼ cup	150	5.0	12.0	10.0	0	220	3.0
(*Tree of Life* Athletic Mix), 1 oz.	200	<8.0	11.0	14.0	0	95	<3.0
(*Tree of Life* Everyday), 1.1 oz.	150	4.0	14.0	10.0	0	120	2.0
(*Tree of Life* Golden Mix Organic). 1 oz.	150	<4.0	8.0	12.0	0	0	<2.0
(*Tree of Life* High Life Mix Organic), 1 oz.	168	<4.0	13.0	12.0	0	80	<2.0
(*Tree of Life* Hawaiian Mix Organic), 1 oz.	110	<1.0	11.0	7.0	0	0	<2.0
(*Tree of Life* Just Nuts), 1.1 oz.	180	6.0	.5	17.0	0	0	2.0
(*Tree of Life* Organic), ¼ cup, 1.1 oz.	130	4.0	14.0	8.0	0	0	2.0
banana/date/walnut (*Fruit Additions*), ¼ cup, 1.1 oz.	130	2.0	18.0	6.0	0	0	2.0
berry, wild, mix (*Eden* Organic), 3 tbsp., 1.1 oz.	150	5.0	13.0	8.0	0	10	4.0
cinnamon apple/raisin/ almond (*Fruit Additions*), 1.1 oz.	110	2.0	21.0	3.0	0	35	1.0
cranberry mix: (*SunRidge Farms* Harvest Organic/ Jubilee), 1.1 oz. .	140	4.0	13.0	9.0	0	15	2.0
(*Tree of Life* Organic), 1 oz.	120	<2.0	11.0	5.0	0	0	<2.0
and chocolate (*Craisins*), 1.75 oz.	230	5.0	26.0	13.0	0	170	n.a.
fruit and nut (*Craisins*), 1.75 oz.	230	3.0	31.0	10.0	0	60	n.a.
fruit and nut: (*Planters*), 1 oz.	140	4.0	14.0	9.0	0	10	2.0
(*Planters* 9 oz.), .95 oz.	120	3.0	14.0	7.0	0	10	2.0
ginger (*SunRidge Farms* Wild Harvest), ¼ cup, 1.1 oz.	120	2.0	19.0	5.0	0	25	3.0

Food and Measure	cal.	prot. (gms)	carbo. (gms)	fat (gms)	chol. (mgs)	sod. (mgs)	fiber (gms)
Trail mix *(cont.)*							
macadamia/fruit (*Mauna Loa* Island/ Tropical), 1.1 oz. ...	160	2.0	16.0	10.0	0	25	2.0
nuts and:							
chocolate (*Planters* 9 oz.), 1.2 oz.	170	4.0	16.0	11.0	0	15	2.0
chocolate (*Planters* Snack Pack), 1.2-oz. pkg.	180	4.0	17.0	11.0	0	20	2.0
honey, and caramel (*Planters*), 1.1 oz.	160	4.0	16.0	10.0	0	150	1.0
honey-roasted and fruit (*Kettle*), 1 oz.	120	3.0	16.0	6.0	0	15	1.0
raisins (*Planters*), 1 oz.	150	5.0	10.0	11.0	0	15	2.0
seeds and raisins (*Planters*), 1.1 oz.	160	6.0	11.0	12.0	0	15	2.0
spicy, and Cajun sticks (*Planters*), 1 oz.	150	5.0	13.0	10.0	0	270	2.0
pineapple mix (*Tree of Life* Organic), 1 oz.	120	<3.0	4.0	12.0	0	0	<2.0
tropical mix:							
(*SunRidge Farms*), ¼ cup, 1.1 oz. ...	140	4.0	13.0	9.0	0	15	3.0
(*Tree of Life* Organic), 1 oz.	120	<2.0	12.0	8.0	0	0	<2.0
Trail mix bar, see "Granola/cereal bar"							
Tree fern, cooked, chopped, ½ cup ...	28	.2	7.8	.1	0	3	2.6
Triple sec (*Angostura*), 1 tsp.	15	0	0	0	0	5	0
Triticale, whole-grain, 1 cup	646	25.1	138.5	4.0	0	10	34.8
Triticale flour, whole-grain, 1 cup	440	17.1	95.1	2.4	0	3	19.0
Trout, meat only:							
mixed species, 4 oz.:							
raw	168	23.6	0	7.5	66	59	0
baked or broiled ...	215	30.2	0	9.6	84	76	0

Food and Measure	cal.	prot. (gms)	carbo. (gms)	fat (gms)	chol. (mgs)	sod. (mgs)	fiber (gms)
rainbow, farmed, 4 oz.:							
raw	156	23.7	0	6.1	67	40	0
baked or broiled . . .	192	27.5	0	8.2	77	48	0
rainbow, wild, 4 oz.:							
raw	135	23.2	0	3.9	67	35	0
baked or broiled . . .	170	26.0	0	6.6	78	64	0
sea, see "Sea trout"							
Trout, smoked:							
canned, in olive oil							
(*Roland*), ¼ cup . .	130	14.0	0	8.0	45	300	0
refrigerated, peppered							
(*Spence & Co.*),							
2 oz.	100	14.0	0	5.0	30	430	0
Truffle cream, 1 tbsp.:							
black (*Roland*)	20	0	1.0	2.0	0	100	0
white (*Roland*)	60	1.0	1.0	6.0	25	10	0
Truffles, black (*Roland*),							
¼ cup	10	0	1.0	0	0	50	1.0
Tuna, meat only:							
bluefin, 4 oz.:							
raw	163	26.5	0	5.6	43	44	0
baked or broiled . . .	209	33.9	0	7.1	56	57	0
skipjack, 4 oz.:							
raw	117	25.0	0	1.2	53	42	0
baked or broiled . . .	150	32.0	0	1.5	68	53	0
yellowfin, 4 oz.:							
raw	123	26.5	0	1.1	51	42	0
baked or broiled . . .	158	34.0	0	1.4	66	53	0
Tuna, can or pouch,							
drained, 2 oz. or							
¼ cup, except as							
noted:							
chunk light, in oil:							
(*Bumble Bee*)	110	13.0	0	6.0	30	250	0
(*Bumble Bee/Coral*							
3 oz.), 2.6 oz. . . .	140	15.0	0	8.0	40	350	0
(*Chicken of the Sea*)	110	13.0	0	6.0	30	250	0
(*Chicken of the Sea*							
3 oz.), 2.7 oz. . . .	140	17.0	0	8.0	40	350	0
(*Coral*)	110	13.0	0	6.0	30	290	0
chunk light, in water:							
(*Bumble Bee*)	60	13.0	0	.5	30	250	0
(*Bumble Bee* 3 oz.),							
2.6 oz.	70	15.0	0	1.0	40	350	0

Food and Measure	cal.	prot. (gms)	carbo. (gms)	fat (gms)	chol. (mgs)	sod. (mgs)	fiber (gms)
Tuna, can or pouch, chunk light, in water *(cont.)*							
(*Bumble Bee "Touch of Lemon"*)	60	13.0	0	.5	30	250	0
(*Chicken of the Sea*)	60	13.0	0	.5	30	250	0
(*Chicken of the Sea*), 3 oz. can	80	18.0	0	1.0	40	350	0
(*Chicken of the Sea 50% Less Salt*) .	60	13.0	0	.5	30	125	0
(*Chicken of the Sea Low Sodium*) . . .	60	14.0	0	.5	30	90	0
(*Chicken of the Sea Tongol/Yellowfin*)	60	13.0	0	.5	30	250	0
(*Coral*)	60	13.0	0	.5	30	290	0
(*Roland Tongol Low Sodium*)	50	12.0	0	0	25	10	0
chunk white, in oil:							
(*Bumble Bee Albacore*)	100	13.0	0	5.0	25	250	0
(*Bumble Bee Albacore 3 oz.*), 2.6 oz.	140	16.0	0	8.0	35	350	0
chunk white, in water:							
(*Bumble Bee Albacore*)	60	13.0	0	1.0	25	250	0
(*Bumble Bee Albacore 3 oz.*), 2.6 oz.	70	16.0	0	1.0	35	350	0
(*Bumble Bee Albacore Very Low Sodium*) . . .	70	15.0	0	1.0	25	35	0
(*Chicken of the Sea*)	60	13.0	0	1.0	25	250	0
(*Chicken of the Sea Low Sodium*) . . .	80	18.0	0	1.0	35	50	0
(*Chicken of the Sea Very Low Sodium*)	60	14.0	0	.5	25	35	0
light, in water, premium pouch:							
(*Bumble Bee*)	60	13.0	0	.5	30	250	0
(*Chicken of the Sea*)	60	13.0	0	.5	30	250	0
solid light, in olive oil:							
(*Bumble Bee Tonno*)	120	15.0	0	6.0	35	330	0
(*Genova Tonno*) . . .	130	14.0	0	8.0	30	250	0
(*Genova Tonno*), 3-oz. can	190	19.0	0	12.0	40	350	0
(*Progresso*)	120	15.0	0	6.0	35	330	0

Food and Measure	cal.	prot. (gms)	carbo. (gms)	fat (gms)	chol. (mgs)	sod. (mgs)	fiber (gms)
solid light, in water:							
(*Chicken of the Sea* Yellowfin)	70	15.0	0	1.0	30	250	0
(*Genova* Tonno) ...	70	14.0	0	1.0	30	250	0
solid white, in olive oil:							
(*Genova* Tonno) ...	110	14.0	0	6.0	25	250	0
(*Progresso* Albacore)	90	16.0	0	3.0	20	330	0
solid white, in oil, albacore:							
(*Bumble Bee*)	90	14.0	0	3.0	25	250	0
(*Bumble Bee* 3 oz.), 2.7 oz.	130	19.0	0	5.0	35	350	0
(*Chicken of the Sea*)	90	14.0	0	3.0	25	250	0
solid white, in water							
(*Genova* Tonno) ...	70	15.0	0	1.0	25	250	0
solid white, in water, Albacore:							
(*Bumble Bee*)	70	15.0	0	1.0	25	250	0
(*Bumble Bee* 3 oz.), 2.7 oz.	90	20.0	0	1.0	35	350	0
(*Bumble Bee* Premium), 3-oz. pouch	90	19.0	0	1.5	40	380	0
(*Bumble Bee* Premium Pouch)	60	13.0	0	1.0	25	250	0
(*Bumble Bee* Prime Fillet)	70	16.0	0	1.0	25	250	0
(*Chicken of the Sea*)	70	15.0	0	1.0	25	250	0
(*Chicken of the Sea* Pouch)	60	13.0	0	1.0	25	250	0
(*Chicken of the Sea*), 3-oz. can	100	21.0	0	1.0	35	350	0
(*Chicken of the Sea*), 3-oz. pouch	100	20.0	0	1.5	40	380	0
(*Roland*)	50	12.0	0	0	10	90	0
Tuna, seasoned, can or pouch (see also "Tuna salad lunch kit"), 1 can or pkg.:							
albacore steak (*Bumble Bee* Prime Fillet*), 4-oz. pouch:							
ginger soy	170	34.0	3.0	2.5	40	1030	0
lemon and cracked pepper	160	36.0	0	1.0	50	370	0
mesquite grilled ...	150	35.0	0	1.5	40	370	0

Food and Measure	cal.	prot. (gms)	carbo. (gms)	fat (gms)	chol. (mgs)	sod. (mgs)	fiber (gms)
Tuna, seasoned, can or pouch *(cont.)*							
(Bumble Bee Sensations),							
5-oz. can:							
lemon and cracked							
pepper	130	21.0	2.0	4.0	30	410	0
spicy Thai chili	190	17.0	11.0	8.0	45	550	1.0
sun-dried tomato							
basil	130	18.0	2.0	5.0	30	360	0
(Bumble Bee Sensations							
Medley), w/crackers							
3-oz. pkg. w/out							
crackers:							
lemon pepper ...	110	18.0	2.0	3.0	25	350	0
sun-dried tomato							
and basil	110	16.0	2.0	4.0	25	300	0
spicy Thai chili ..	160	15.0	9.0	7.0	35	470	1.0
crackers only, 6 pcs.	90	1.0	11.0	4.5	0	110	0
Tuna, smoked *(Acme/*							
Blue Hill Bay), 2 oz.	70	13.0	2.0	1.0	20	1	0
Tuna cake mix *(Old*							
Bay Tuna Classic),							
1⅓ tbsp.	30	1.0	3.0	1.0	35	90	0
Tuna entree, microwave,							
casserole, w/pasta,							
vegetables *(Hormel*							
Compleats), 10 oz. .	240	17.0	26.0	7.0	35	880	1.0
Tuna entree mix,							
1 cup*:							
broccoli, creamy *(Tuna*							
Helper)	310	14.0	38.0	12.0	15	900	1.0
fettuccine Alfredo *(Tuna*							
Helper)	300	12.0	32.0	13.0	15	1000	1.0
melt *(Tuna Helper)* ...	300	14.0	37.0	11.0	15	1060	1.0
Parmesan, creamy							
(Tuna Helper)	290	15.0	31.0	9.0	15	890	1.0
pasta:							
cheesy *(Tuna Helper)*	290	13.0	34.0	12.0	15	950	1.0
creamy *(Tuna Helper)*	320	14.0	32.0	13.0	15	880	1.0
spirals, creamy *(Annie's*							
Organic Skillet Meal)	260	18.0	30.0	7.0	80	650	1.0
tetrazzini *(Tuna Helper)*	290	15.0	33.0	11.0	15	980	1.0
Tuna jerky *(Seafood*							
Importers, Inc.),							
1-oz. pkg.	90	14.0	8.0	0	15	370	2.0

Food and Measure	cal.	prot. (gms)	carbo. (gms)	fat (gms)	chol. (mgs)	sod. (mgs)	fiber (gms)
Tuna salad, ⅓ cup:							
(*Wampler*)	180	6.0	9.0	12.0	20	450	1.0
chunky (*Wampler*) ...	180	8.0	8.0	13.0	20	380	1.0
Tuna salad dressing							
(*Kraft Tuna Salad Maker*), 1 tbsp.	35	0	2.0	2.5	5	135	0
Tuna salad kit,							
w/crackers, 1 pkg.:							
(*Bumble Bee* Original):							
2.9-oz. can salad ..	190	8.0	6.0	16.0	15	270	1.0
6 crackers, .6 oz. ..	90	1.0	11.0	4.5	0	110	0
(*Bumble Bee* Fat Free):							
2.9-oz. can salad ..	70	7.0	10.0	0	20	450	0
6 crackers, .6 oz. ..	80	2.0	14.0	1.5	0	310	1.0
(*Bumble Bee*), w/mayo:							
2.9-oz can chunk							
light tuna	70	15.0	0	1.0	40	358	0
6 crackers, .6 oz. ..	90	2.0	12.0	4.5	0	180	0
mayo (*Hellmann's*), 3.7-oz. pkt.	260	17.0	12.0	17.0	45	610	0
(*Bumble Bee Lunch on the Run*), kit components:							
tuna salad, 2.9 oz. .	230	8.0	7.0	19.0	25	250	1.0
crackers, 6 pcs., .6 oz.	90	1.0	12.0	4.5	0	190	0
diced peaches, 4 oz.	80	0	19.0	0	0	15	1.0
cookie, .67 oz.	160	2.0	21.0	7.0	10	120	0
(*Bumble Bee Lunch on the Run*), total kit, 8.2 oz.	560	11.0	59.0	30.5	35	575	2.0
Turban squash (*Frieda's*), ¾ cup, 3 oz.	30	1.0	7.0	0	0	0	1.0
Turbot, European, meat only:							
raw, 4 oz.	108	18.2	0	3.4	54	170	0
baked or broiled, 4 oz.	138	23.3	0	4.3	70	218	0
Turkey (see also "Turkey, frozen/ refrigerated"), fresh, roasted:							
meat w/skin, 4 oz. ...	236	31.9	0	11.0	93	77	0
meat only:							
4 oz.	193	3.2	0	5.6	86	79	0
diced, 1 cup	238	41.0	0	7.0	107	99	0

Food and Measure	cal.	prot. (gms)	carbo. (gms)	fat (gms)	chol. (mgs)	sod. (mgs)	fiber (gms)
Turkey, fresh, roasted (cont.)							
skin only, 1 oz.	125	5.6	0	11.2	32	15	0
dark meat:							
w/skin, 4 oz.	251	31.2	0	13.1	101	86	0
meat only, 4 oz. . . .	212	32.4	0	8.2	96	90	0
meat only, diced,							
1 cup	262	40.0	0	10.1	119	110	0
light meat:							
w/skin, 4 oz.	223	32.4	0	9.4	86	71	0
meat only, 4 oz.	178	33.9	0	3.7	78	73	0
meat only, diced,							
1 cup	219	41.9	0	4.5	97	89	0
breast, meat w/skin:							
½ breast, 1.9 lb.,							
(4.2 lbs. raw							
w/bone)	1637	248.1	0	64.1	643	541	0
4 oz.	214	32.6	0	8.4	84	71	0
ground, see "Turkey							
ground"							
leg, meat w/skin:							
1.2 lb. (1.5 lbs. raw							
w/bone)	1133	152.2	0	53.6	466	420	0
4 oz. . . . . , .	236	31.6	0	11.1	96	87	0
wing, meat w/skin:							
6.6 oz. (9.9 oz. raw							
w/bone)	426	50.9	0	23.1	150	114	0
4 oz.	260	31.0	0	14.1	92	69	0
Turkey, canned, chunk,							
white (*Valley Fresh*),							
2 oz.	80	16.0	0	1.5	55	150	0
Turkey, frozen/re-							
frigerated, raw,							
4 oz., except as							
noted:							
whole:							
(*Empire Kosher*) . .	180	23.0	0	9.0	75	210	0
(*Empire Kosher*							
Frozen)	180	21.0	0	10.0	65	220	0
(*Organic Prairie*) . .	190	23.0	0	10.0	70	70	0
whole, seasoned:							
(*Jennie-O Oven Ready*							
Homestyle)	160	20.0	0	9.0	70	370	0
(*Shady Brook Farms*							
Simply Done) . . .	160	20.0	1.0	8.0	65	510	0

Food and Measure	cal.	prot. (gms)	carbo. (gms)	fat (gms)	chol. (mgs)	sod. (mgs)	fiber (gms)
butter, garlic, herb (*Jennie-O Oven Ready*)	150	21.0	0	7.0	70	350	0
breast, bone-in:							
(*Shady Brook Farms Fresh*)	190	24.0	0	9.0	70	60	0
(*Shady Brook Farms Frozen*)	160	21.0	0	7.0	65	340	0
seasoned (*Shady Brook Farms Simply Done*) . . .	170	21.0	1.0	8.0	60	500	0
breast, bone-in, split:							
lemon garlic (*Shady Brook Farms Simply Done*) . . .	170	24.0	1.0	8.0	60	480	0
mesquite or rotisserie (*Shady Brook Farms Simply Done*) . . .	170	21.0	1.0	8.0	60	480	0
seasoned (*Jennie-O Oven Ready*) . . .	130	22.0	0	4.0	55	420	0
breast, boneless roast:							
marinated (*Foster Farms Savory Selections*)	110	22.0	0	2.5	55	600	0
rotisserie (*Shady Brook Farms*) . . .	130	22.0	4.0	3.5	55	380	0
rotisserie, Italian herb (*Shady Brook Farms*) . . .	170	19.0	3.0	8.0	55	680	0
seasoned (*Jennie-O Oven Ready*) . . .	100	23.0	1.0	1.0	40	460	0
breast, bone/skinless:							
(*Perdue/Perdue Fit & Easy*)	120	27.0	0	1.0	60	55	0
chops (*Shady Brook Farms*)	110	25.0	0	.5	65	250	0
cutlet (*Jennie-O*) . .	120	26.0	0	1.0	45	75	0
cutlet or scallopini (*Shady Brook Farms*)	110	25.0	0	.5	60	240	0
London broil (*Shady Brook Farms*) . . .	130	28.0	0	.5	70	55	0
thin (*Perdue Fit & Easy*), 3.3-oz. pc.	100	23.0	0	1.0	50	45	0

Food and Measure	cal.	prot. (gms)	carbo. (gms)	fat (gms)	chol. (mgs)	sod. (mgs)	fiber (gms)
Turkey, frozen/refrigerated, raw (cont.)							
breast, carved, oven roasted (Perdue Short Cuts), ½ cup	90	20.0	2.0	1.0	45	420	0
breast, w/gravy (Perdue Mealtime Starters), ½ cup ..	140	16.0	7.0	5.0	45	710	0
breast strips (Jennie-O)	120	26.0	0	1.0	45	75	0
breast tenderloin:							
(Jennie-O)	120	26.0	0	1.0	45	75	0
(Perdue Fit & Easy)	120	27.0	0	1.0	60	55	0
(Shady Brook Farms)	130	28.0	0	.5	70	55	0
breast tenderloin, marinated:							
(Jennie-O)	110	21.0	4.0	1.0	50	840	0
applewood smoked (Jennie-O)	110	22.0	2.0	1.0	45	660	0
barbecue (Foster Farms Savory Servings)	120	22.0	4.0	1.5	30	430	0
Dijon, creamy (Shady Brook Farms) ...	140	21.0	4.0	4.0	50	500	0
Italian herb (Shady Brook Farms) ...	130	21.0	4.0	3.5	50	490	0
lemon garlic (Jennie-O)	120	22.0	1.0	2.0	40	580	0
lemon garlic (Shady Brook Farms) ...	130	21.0	2.0	.5	55	500	0
lemon pepper (Foster Farms Savory Servings)	120	22.0	2.0	2.0	35	310	0
pepper, seasoned (Jennie-O) .....:	100	22.0	2.0	1.0	45	650	0
rotisserie (Shady Brook Farms) ...	130	21.0	2.0	.5	50	630	0
tequila lime (Jennie-O)	110	20.0	4.0	1.0	40	800	0
teriyaki (Foster Farms Savory Servings)	120	22.0	4.0	1.5	25	460	0
ground, see "Turkey, ground"							
strips, marinated:							
Asian grill (Shady Brook Farms) ...	160	17.0	8.0	7.0	55	490	0
chipotle citrus (Shady Brook Farms) ...	130	17.0	6.0	4.0	60	500	0

Food and Measure	cal.	prot. (gms)	carbo. (gms)	fat (gms)	chol. (mgs)	sod. (mgs)	fiber (gms)
herb, mild (*Shady Brook Farms*) ...	130	18.0	6.0	4.0	60	450	0
thighs, skinless chops (*Empire Kosher*) ..	140	23.0	0	5.0	85	200	0
Turkey, frozen/refrigerated, cooked, 3 oz., except as noted:							
whole, unseasoned:							
dark (*Perdue*)	190	21.0	0	11.0	90	70	0
white (*Perdue*)	150	23.0	0	7.0	65	50	0
breast, bone/skinless: (*Perdue Fit & Easy*)	110	26.0	0	.5	60	40	0
breast, in gravy, home-style, or sliced (*Jennie-O So-Easy*), 5 oz.	110	20.0	4.0	1.0	40	680	0
breast, rotisserie, bone-in (*Jennie-O*) .	130	23.0	0	4.0	55	240	0
breast, stuffed (*Jenny-O*), 6 oz.:							
cheddar/broccoli ..	230	34.0	3.0	9.0	80	980	0
herb stuffing	260	35.0	13.0	7.0	65	730	0
pepper cheese/rice .	260	33.0	12.0	7.0	75	1000	0
Swiss cheese/ham .	270	39.0	2.0	12.0	95	1150	0
drums, smoked (*Jennie-O*)	140	18.0	0	8.0	80	620	0
drumsticks (*Perdue*) .	130	22.0	0	5.0	85	70	0
and gravy (*Hormel*), 5.7 oz.	130	21.0	4.0	3.0	50	1150	4.0
meatballs, see "Meatballs"							
wings:							
(*Perdue*)	160	22.0	0	8.0	90	65	0
(*Perdue* Drummettes), 3.3-oz. pc.	180	24.0	0	9.0	95	70	0
Turkey, ground:							
raw, 4 oz.:							
(*Applegate Farms Organic*)	170	24.0	0	8.0	85	65	0
(*Empire Kosher Fresh*)	180	22.0	0	10.0	85	200	0
(*Jennie-O*)	220	20.0	0	17.0	85	85	0
(*Organic Prairie*) ..	180	23.0	0	9.0	70	75	0
(*Perdue*)	230	18.0	0	17.0	100	75	0
(*Shady Brook Farms* 15% Fat)	240	20.0	0	17.0	85	75	0

Food and Measure	cal.	prot. (gms)	carbo. (gms)	fat (gms)	chol. (mgs)	sod. (mgs)	fiber (gms)
Turkey, ground (cont.)							
(Shady Brook Farms 7% Fat)	160	22.0	0	8.0	80	85	0
(Wampler)	210	18.0	0	15.0	100	30	0
breast (Perdue Fit & Easy)	120	27.0	0	1.5	65	60	0
breast (Shady Brook Farms 99% Fat Free)	120	28.0	0	1.0	70	55	0
lean (Jennie-O) ...	160	23.0	0	8.0	80	80	0
lean (Perdue)	160	24.0	0	8.0	105	95	0
lean, extra (Jennie-O)	120	26.0	0	1.0	45	80	0
seasoned, Italian (Shady Brook Farms 7% Fat) ..	160	22.0	1.0	8.0	80	580	0
seasoned, savory (Jennie-O)	160	20.0	0	9.0	95	280	0
white (Empire)	140	23.0	0	5.0	60	210	0
raw, patties, 4 oz.:							
(Jennie-O All Natural Burger)	160	19.0	0	9.0	100	90	0
(Jennie-O Burger) .	220	18.0	0	17.0	80	220	0
(Perdue)	160	21.0	0	8.0	90	75	0
(Wampler Burger) .	210	18.0	0	15.0	100	30	0
barbecue flavor (Wampler)	220	18.0	3.0	15.0	100	280	0
char-grilled flavor (Perdue)	180	21.0	1.0	10.0	90	660	0
lean (Jennie-O Burger)	160	22.0	0	8.0	75	550	0
seasoned (Wampler)	180	21.0	1.0	11.0	75	400	0
seasoned, Italian (Jennie-O Burger)	160	20.0	0	8.0	80	680	0
cooked, 3 oz.:							
(Perdue)	190	19.0	0	13.0	95	55	0
breast (Perdue Fit & Easy)	110	25.0	0	1.0	50	40	0
lean (Perdue)	140	21.0	0	7.0	90	85	0
patties (Perdue) ...	160	20.0	0	8.0	85	65	0
"Turkey," vegetarian, canned (Worthington Turkee Slices), 3 slices, 3.3 oz.	110	14.0	5.0	12.0	0	530	0

Food and Measure	cal.	prot. (gms)	carbo. (gms)	fat (gms)	chol. (mgs)	sod. (mgs)	fiber (gms)
frozen:							
(*Tofurky* Original), 5 slices, 1.8 oz.	100	13.0	6.0	3.0	0	300	3.0
(*Yves*), 4 slices, 2.2 oz.	100	16.0	5.0	1.5	0	340	0
peppered (*Tofurky*), 5 slices, 1.8 oz.	100	12.0	6.0	3.0	0	300	3.0
smoked (*Worthington*), 3 slices, 2 oz.	140	10.0	4.0	9.0	0	450	0
smoked, hickory (*Tofurky*), 5 slices, 1.8 oz.	100	13.0	6.0	3.0	0	250	3.0
Turkey bacon:							
(*Applegate Farms*), 1-oz. slice	35	6.0	0	1.0	15	210	0
(*Applegate Farms* Organic), 1-oz. slice	30	5.0	0	1.0	15	210	0
extra lean (*Jennie-O*), .5 oz.	20	3.0	0	0	10	140	0
Turkey bologna:							
(*Applegate Farms*), 2 oz.	70	11.0	0	2.0	30	360	0
(*Empire Kosher*), 2 slices, 1.6 oz.	80	5.0	.5	6.0	35	420	0
(*Foster Farms*), 1-oz. slice	70	4.0	0	6.0	25	300	0
(*Jennie-O*), 2 oz.	110	8.0	2.0	9.0	45	670	0
(*Louis Rich/Oscar Mayer* 50% Less Fat), 1 oz.	50	3.0	1.0	4.0	20	270	0
Turkey burger, see "Turkey, ground"							
Turkey dinner, frozen, breast, 1 pkg.:							
grilled (*Healthy Choice* Complete), 10.8 oz.	270	19.0	42.0	3.0	30	380	5.0
roasted:							
(*Healthy Choice* Traditional Complete), 10.5 oz.	300	21.0	42.0	4.0	25	550	6.0
breast (*Stouffer's*), 16 oz.	390	21.0	48.0	13.0	40	1290	6.0
Turkey entree, canned, stew (*Dinty Moore*), 1 cup	140	10.0	19.0	3.0	20	910	2.0

Food and Measure	cal.	prot. (gms)	carbo. (gms)	fat (gms)	chol. (mgs)	sod. (mgs)	fiber (gms)
Turkey entree, frozen, (see also "Turkey, frozen/refrigerated, cooked"), 1 pkg., except as noted:							
breast and gravy, w/corn bread dressing (*Glory Savory Singles*), 11 oz.	440	18.0	49.0	18.0	30	1380	2.0
breast medallions, w/potato, gravy (*Boston Market*), 15 oz.	360	24.0	35.0	14.0	55	1570	5.0
cream sauce, w/pasta (*Michelina's Budget Gourmet*), 8 oz.	240	9.0	38.0	6.0	20	500	2.0
glazed tenderloins (*Lean Cuisine*), 9 oz.	260	13.0	41.0	5.0	25	670	4.0
meat balls, w/spaghetti (*Empire Kosher*), 13 oz.	400	23.0	48.0	13.0	75	970	4.0
meat loaf (*Empire Kosher*), 11 oz.	330	20.0	31.0	14.0	70	890	6.0
medallions, 9 oz.:							
cranberry (*Smart Ones Fruit Inspirations*)	350	18.0	59.0	4.5	25	560	4.0
mushroom gravy (*Smart Ones*)	200	18.0	11.0	10.0	35	660	3.0
pie/pot pie:							
(*Blake's* Natural), 8 oz.	370	15.0	40.0	16.0	20	380	3.0
(*Empire Kosher*), 8 oz.	460	21.0	43.0	23.0	25	820	10.0
(*Stouffer's*), 8 oz.	590	20.0	48.0	35.0	55	910	2.0
(*Swanson*), 7 oz.	380	10.0	34.0	22.0	40	750	2.0
no vegetables (*Blake's* Natural), 8 oz.	360	17.0	34.0	15.0	20	380	1.0
roasted, white meat (*Pepperidge Farm*), 1 cup	500	13.0	38.0	33.0	30	890	2.0
roasted:							
(*Lean Cuisine Dinnertime Selects*), 12 oz.	290	19.0	38.0	7.0	30	890	5.0
(*South Beach Living*), 9.5 oz.	240	17.0	27.0	9.0	50	920	4.0

Food and Measure	cal.	prot. (gms)	carbo. (gms)	fat (gms)	chol. (mgs)	sod. (mgs)	fiber (gms)
breast (*Healthy Choice*), 8.5 oz. .	200	14.0	27.0	3.5	20	600	5.0
w/gravy, potato (*Michelina's Lean Gourmet*), 8 oz. .	170	13.0	20.0	6.0	30	830	2.0
w/gravy, potato (*Stouffer's*), 9.63 oz.	290	16.0	30.0	12.0	45	970	2.0
slow, breast (*Smart Ones*), 10 oz.	210	18.0	18.0	7.0	45	770	2.0
slow, breast, mashed potato (*Healthy Choice*), 8.5 oz. .	200	15.0	24.0	4.0	20	570	5.0
and vegetables (*Lean Cuisine*), 8 oz. . .	150	15.0	12.0	5.0	25	650	3.0
stuffed (*Smart Ones*), 10 oz.	290	17.0	42.0	6.0	25	870	4.0
teriyaki (*Empire Kosher*), 11 oz.	250	27.0	27.0	3.5	65	810	3.0
Turkey entree, microwave, 10-oz. cont.:							
and dressing w/gravy (*Hormel Compleats*)	280	20.0	31.0	8.0	45	1120	3.0
and vegetables, hearty (*Hormel Compleats*)	180	14.0	24.0	3.5	25	1200	1.4
Turkey fat, 1 tbsp.	115	0	0	12.8	13	0	0
Turkey franks, see "Frankfurter"							
Turkey giblets:							
simmered, 4 oz.	189	30.1	2.4	5.8	474	67	0
simmered, diced, 1 cup	243	38.5	3.0	7.4	606	85	0
Turkey gravy, can or jar, ¼ cup:							
(*Campbell's*)	25	1.0	3.0	1.0	0	270	0
(*Campbell's Fat Free*) .	20	1.0	4.0	0	<5	290	0
(*Franco-American Slow Roast*)	25	1.0	4.0	.5	<5	320	0
(*Franco-American Slow Roast Fat Free*)	20	1.0	4.0	0	<5	320	0
(*Pacific Natural*)	25	1.0	4.0	.5	0	270	0
roasted (*Heinz*)	25	1.0	3.0	1.0	<5	290	0
Turkey gravy mix, ¼ cup*:							
(*Lawry's*)	25	<1.0	4.0	1.0	0	320	0
(*McCormick*)	20	0	3.0	0	0	350	0

Food and Measure	cal.	prot. (gms)	carbo. (gms)	fat (gms)	chol. (mgs)	sod. (mgs)	fiber (gms)
Turkey ham, 2 oz., except as noted:							
(*Farmland* Deli Style), 1 oz.	30	5.0	1.0	1.0	20	330	0
(*Foster Farms*)	70	10.0	0	3.0	35	590	0
(*Healthy Deli*)	80	10.0	2.0	2.5	30	470	0
(*Jennie-O*)	80	8.0	1.0	4.0	30	510	0
(*Jennie-O* Extra Lean)	50	10.0	1.0	1.0	20	400	0
(*Louis Rich/Oscar Mayer* 50% Less Fat), 1 oz.	35	5.0	1.0	1.5	20	350	0
honey cured (*Jennie-O*)	70	9.0	3.0	3.0	35	660	0
smoked:							
(*Louis Rich/Oscar Mayer* 50% Less Fat), 1 oz.	35	5.0	1.0	1.5	20	350	0
hickory (*Shady Brook Farms*) . . .	60	9.0	2.0	2.0	25	590	0
Turkey ham salad (*Wampler*), ⅓ cup .	150	7.0	9.0	10.0	30	500	1.0
Turkey kielbasa, see "Kielbasa"							
Turkey lunch meat (see also "Turkey ham," etc.), breast, 2 oz., except as noted:							
(*Alpine Lace* Fat Free)	50	11.0	1.0	0	25	500	0
(*Applegate Farms* No Salt)	60	14.0	0	0	35	25	0
(*Black Bear* Golden Brown/Original) . . .	60	11.0	1.0	.5	20	430	0
(*Black Bear* Homestyle)	60	11.0	1.0	1.0	20	430	0
(*Boar's Head* Premium 50% Lower Sodium Skin On)	60	12.0	0	1.5	25	320	0
(*Boar's Head* Premium 47% Lower Sodium Skinless)	60	12.0	0	.5	20	340	0
(*Carando*)	60	11.0	0	1.0	30	680	0
(*Di Lusso* Golden Brown)	50	11.0	0	1.0	25	470	0
(*Di Lusso* Reduced Sodium)	60	13.0	0	1.0	25	280	0

Food and Measure	cal.	prot. (gms)	carbo. (gms)	fat (gms)	chol. (mgs)	sod. (mgs)	fiber (gms)
(*Dietz & Watson* Banquet)	70	12.0	1.0	1.0	30	320	0
(*Dietz & Watson* Golden Brown/ Original)	70	11.0	1.0	1.0	20	430	0
(*Dietz & Watson* Gourmet Lite)	70	12.0	1.0	1.0	30	240	0
(*Dietz & Watson* Gourmet Lite No Salt)	70	14.0	2.0	.5	30	50	0
(*Dietz & Watson* Homestyle)	70	12.0	1.0	1.0	30	420	0
(*Dietz & Watson* Santa Fe)	60	12.0	1.0	.5	30	420	0
(*Empire Kosher*)	60	15.0	0	1.0	35	570	0
(*Foster Farms*)	60	11.0	1.0	1.0	20	510	0
(*Hansel 'n Gretel*) ...	50	7.0	3.0	1.0	15	550	0
(*Hatfield Deli Choice* Premium), 3 oz. ...	90	18.0	1.0	.5	55	530	0
(*Jennie-O* Golden Classic)	60	14.0	0	1.0	25	340	0
(*Jennie-O VIP*)	80	15.0	0	2.0	30	310	0
bacon flavor (*Dietz & Watson* Bacon Lovers*)	70	12.0	2.0	2.0	30	370	0
Black Forest:							
(*Dietz & Watson*) ..	70	11.0	0	.5	30	400	0
(*Wampler Deli Roast Collection*)	60	10.0	2.0	1.5	25	650	0
hickory smoked (*Boar's Head*) ..	60	13.0	0	.5	25	360	0
braised (*Dietz & Watson* Homestyle)	70	12.0	1.0	1.0	30	430	0
browned:							
(*Jennie-O* Grand Champion)	50	12.0	0	1.0	25	460	0
(*Jennie-O* Natural Choice)	60	13.0	0	1.0	25	440	0
Buffalo (*Jennie-O*) ...	60	12.0	1.0	1.0	25	600	0
Cajun style:							
(*Di Lusso*)	60	11.0	1.0	1.0	25	630	0
(*Jennie-O*)	50	12.0	1.0	0	25	530	0
(*Jennie-O* Premium Portions)	50	12.0	1.0	0	20	460	0

Food and Measure	cal.	prot. (gms)	carbo. (gms)	fat (gms)	chol. (mgs)	sod. (mgs)	fiber (gms)
Turkey lunch meat, Cajun style *(cont.)*							
fried (*Jennie-O* Grand Champion)	60	12.0	1.0	1.0	25	430	0
oven roasted, smoked (*Boar's Head*) ..	60	13.0	1.0	.5	25	750	0
garlic herb (*Jennie-O Natural Choice*) ...	60	14.0	1.0	1.0	25	450	0
garlic pepper (*Jennie-O Mediterranean*)	60	12.0	1.0	0	25	570	0
herb:							
(*Applegate Farms*) .	50	12.0	0	0	30	360	0
(*Applegate Farms Organic*)	50	11.0	0	.5	30	420	0
honey/honey cured:							
(*Black Bear*)	70	11.0	3.0	1.0	20	400	0
(*Di Lusso*)	70	11.0	3.0	1.0	20	480	0
(*Dietz & Watson*) ..	70	11.0	2.0	1.0	25	420	0
(*Farmland* Deli Style), 1 oz.	25	5.0	1.0	.5	15	400	0
(*Healthy Deli*)	60	10.0	3.0	.5	20	480	0
(*Hormel Natural Choice* Sliced) ..	60	10.0	2.0	1.0	25	470	0
(*Jennie-O*)	70	11.0	2.0	2.0	30	480	0
(*Jennie-O* Presliced)	60	11.0	2.0	1.0	20	500	0
(*Jennie-O Grand Champion*)	50	11.0	2.0	0	25	530	0
honey maple:							
(*Applegate Farms*) .	50	12.0	0	0	30	360	0
(*Dietz & Watson*) ..	70	11.0	2.0	1.0	25	400	0
honey mesquite:							
(*Di Lusso*)	70	11.0	3.0	1.0	20	480	0
(*Jennie-O* Deli for Shaving)	50	10.0	1.0	0	20	400	0
(*Jennie-O* Deli for Slicing)	50	11.0	2.0	0	25	530	0
(*Jennie-O* Original for Shaving)	50	10.0	2.0	0	20	500	0
honey roasted:							
(*Foster Farms*), 1-oz. slice	25	6.0	1.0	0	10	240	0
(*Hatfield Deli Choice*), 3 oz.	120	18.0	5.0	3.0	45	890	0
(*Jennie-O Natural Choice*)	60	14.0	1.0	0	25	450	0

Food and Measure	cal.	prot. (gms)	carbo. (gms)	fat (gms)	chol. (mgs)	sod. (mgs)	fiber (gms)
(*Perdue Sandwich Builders*)	60	10.0	4.0	1.5	25	450	0
shaved (*Tyson*) ...	60	10.0	2.0	1.0	20	640	0
hot pepper (*Jennie-O Rio Grande*)	50	12.0	1.0	0	20	550	0
Italian style:							
(*Black Bear*)	60	11.0	1.0	1.0	20	430	0
(*Dietz & Watson*) ..	60	11.0	1.0	1.0	25	430	0
London broil:							
(*Black Bear*)	60	11.0	0	1.0	20	460	0
(*Dietz & Watson*) ..	70	11.0	0	1.0	30	430	0
maple glazed (*Boar's Head Honey Coat*) .	70	14.0	2.0	.5	30	440	0
oven prepared:							
(*Empire Kosher Skinless/Mini*) ..	45	11.0	2.0	0	25	440	0
(*Empire Kosher* Presliced), 3 pcs., 2 oz.	50	11.0	1.0	0	30	300	0
oven-roasted:							
(*Applegate Farms*) .	50	12.0	0	0	30	360	0
(*Applegate Farms* Deli Counter) ...	50	12.0	0	0	30	400	0
(*Black Bear*)	60	11.0	1.0	1.0	20	320	0
(*Boar's Head* Golden Catering Style) ..	60	13.0	0	1.0	25	340	0
(*Boar's Head* Ovengold Skin On) ...	60	12.0	1.0	1.5	35	360	0
(*Boar's Head* Ovengold Skinless) ..	60	13.0	0	1.0	20	350	0
(*Dietz & Watson* Oven Classic) ...	60	12.0	1.0	.5	30	400	0
(*Farmland* Special Select)	50	9.0	1.0	1.0	25	610	0
(*Foster Farms*)	60	9.0	1.0	2.0	15	440	0
(*Healthy Choice* Hearty Slices), 1 oz.	30	5.0	1.0	1.0	15	240	0
(*Healthy Choice* Tub), 5 slices, 1.8 oz. ..	60	9.0	2.0	1.5	25	450	0
(*Healthy Choice* Deli Thin), 4 slices, 1.8 oz.	60	9.0	2.0	1.5	25	450	0
(*Hormel Natural Choice* Sliced) ..	50	10.0	1.0	1.0	25	490	0
(*Jennie-O* Homestyle)	60	12.0	0	1.0	25	390	0

Food and Measure	cal.	prot. (gms)	carbo. (gms)	fat (gms)	chol. (mgs)	sod. (mgs)	fiber (gms)
Turkey lunch meat, oven-roasted *(cont.)*							
(*Jennie-O* Premium Portions)	70	14.0	1.0	0	20	480	0
(*Jennie-O* Presliced)	60	11.0	0	1.0	25	510	0
(*Jennie-O* Blue Ribbon)	50	9.0	2.0	1.0	20	470	0
(*Jennie-O* Grand Champion)	50	11.0	1.0	0	20	540	0
(*Jennie-O* Grand Champion Reduced Sodium) .	50	13.0	0	0	25	260	0
(*Jennie-O* Grand Champion Skin On)	50	11.0	1.0	1.0	20	490	0
(*Louis Rich/Oscar Mayer*), 1 oz. . . .	25	6.0	0	0	10	340	0
(*Oscar Mayer* Deli Fresh Thin Sliced)	60	9.0	2.0	1.0	20	630	0
(*Oscar Mayer* Deli Fresh 98% Fat Free), 1 oz.	30	4.0	1.0	.5	10	310	0
(*Tyson*), 2 slices, 1.6 oz.	40	8.0	1.0	.5	15	560	0
shaved (*Tyson*) . . .	60	10.0	2.0	1.0	20	640	0
white (*Oscar Mayer*), 1 oz.	30	4.0	1.0	1.0	10	300	0
pan-roasted:							
(*Wampler Deli Roast Collection*)	50	12.0	1.0	0	20	400	0
(*Wampler Deli Roast Collection* All Natural)	50	12.0	0	1.0	25	250	0
pepper and garlic:							
(*Black Bear*)	60	11.0	1.0	.5	20	460	0
(*Dietz & Watson*) . .	70	12.0	1.0	.5	25	400	0
pepper/peppered:							
(*Applegate Farms*) .	50	12.0	0	0	30	360	0
(*Jennie-O* Natural Choice)	50	12.0	0	0	25	450	0
(*Wampler Deli Roast Collection*)	40	8.0	1.0	0	20	520	0
black (*Black Bear* Homestyle)	60	11.0	1.0	1.0	20	430	0
black (*Hatfield Deli Choice*), 3 oz.	90	16.0	1.0	2.0	45	350	0

Food and Measure	cal.	prot. (gms)	carbo. (gms)	fat (gms)	chol. (mgs)	sod. (mgs)	fiber (gms)
cracked (*Di Lusso*) .	60	12.0	0	1.0	25	460	0
cracked (*Jennie-O*) .	50	12.0	0	0	25	450	0
cracked (*Jennie-O* Presliced)	50	12.0	0	0	25	450	0
cracked, black (*Dietz & Watson*)	70	12.0	1.0	1.0	30	420	0
roast/roasted:							
(*Applegate Farms* Organic)	50	12.0	0	0	30	360	0
(*Boar's Head Salsalito*)	60	13.0	1.0	.5	25	480	0
(*Farmland* Deli Style), 4 slices, 1.8 oz. .	50	10.0	1.0	.5	25	400	0
(*Hormel*)	50	10.0	0	1.0	20	480	0
(*Jennie-O* Golden Roast), 3 oz. . . .	100	19.0	1.0	2.0	45	620	0
(*Organic Prairie*) . .	70	15.0	0	0	40	390	0
(*Perdue Sandwich Builders*)	60	10.0	2.0	1.5	25	340	0
rotisserie (*Wampler Deli Roast Collection*)	50	9.0	1.0	1.5	25	500	0
smoked:							
(*Applegate Farms*) .	50	12.0	0	0	30	360	0
(*Black Bear*)	60	11.0	1.0	1.0	20	400	0
(*Boar's Head Cracked Pepper Mill*)	60	13.0	0	.5	30	460	0
(*Carando*), 1 oz. . . .	60	11.0	0	1.5	30	430	0
(*Di Lusso*)	60	11.0	1.0	1.0	25	620	0
(*Empire Kosher*) . .	45	9.0	0	0	20	490	0
(*Farmland* Deli Style), 4 slices, 1.8 oz. .	50	10.0	1.0	.5	25	400	0
(*Farmland* Deli Style Fat Free), 1 oz. . .	25	5.0	0	0	15	430	0
(*Farmland* Special Select), 1.1 oz. . .	25	5.0	0	0	15	350	0
(*Hatfield Deli Choice*), 3 oz.	90	18.0	2.0	.5	45	790	0
(*Healthy Choice Deli Thin* 6 oz.), 4 slices, 1.8 oz. .	60	9.0	2.0	1.5	25	450	0
(*Healthy Deli Zero Carb Brick Oven*)	50	11.0	0	.5	20	470	0
(*Hormel*)	50	10.0	0	1.0	20	480	0
(*Hormel Natural Choice* Sliced) . .	50	10.0	1.0	1.0	25	450	0

Food and Measure	cal.	prot. (gms)	carbo. (gms)	fat (gms)	chol. (mgs)	sod. (mgs)	fiber (gms)
Turkey lunch meat, smoked *(cont.)*							
(*Organic Prairie*)	70	16.0	0	0	45	420	0
(*Oscar Mayer* Deli Fresh), 2.2 oz.	60	13.0	0	.5	25	760	0
(*Oscar Mayer* Deli Fresh Thin Sliced)	60	9.0	2.0	1.0	20	630	0
(*Oscar Mayer* 97% Fat Free), 1 oz.	30	5.0	1.0	.5	10	310	0
applewood (*Jennie-O Natural Choice*)	60	13.0	1.0	1.0	25	440	0
cracked pepper (*Jennie-O* Smoky Mountain)	60	11.0	1.0	0	20	430	0
peppercorn (*Dietz & Watson*)	50	12.0	0	.5	25	320	0
peppercorn ranch (*Jennie-O* Deli Thin)	50	9.0	3.0	1.0	20	520	0
shaved (*Oscar Mayer* Deli Fresh), 1/5 of 9-oz. pkg.	50	8.0	2.0	1.0	20	570	0
sun-dried tomato (*Jennie-O* Deli Thin)	50	9.0	2.0	1.0	15	410	0
white (*Louis Rich/ Oscar Mayer*), 1 oz.	30	4.0	1.0	1.0	10	320	0
smoked, hickory:							
(*Foster Farms*)	60	13.0	0	.5	25	340	0
(*Jennie-O*)	60	12.0	0	1.0	25	380	0
(*Jennie-O* Deli Thin)	50	9.0	1.0	1.0	20	410	0
(*Jennie-O* Homestyle)	60	12.0	0	1.0	25	390	0
(*Jennie-O* Presliced)	60	11.0	1.0	1.0	20	560	0
(*Louis Rich/Oscar Mayer* 95% Fat Free), 1 oz.	30	4.0	1.0	1.0	10	320	0
(*Louis Rich/Oscar Mayer* 98% Fat Free), 1 oz.	30	5.0	1.0	.5	10	260	0
smoked, hickory or mesquite (*Jennie-O Grand Champion*)	50	12.0	1.0	0	25	590	0
smoked, honey:							
(*Empire Kosher*)	45	11.0	0	0	25	390	0
(*Healthy Choice Deli Thin*), 4 slices, 1.8 oz.	60	9.0	4.0	1.5	25	450	0

Food and Measure	cal.	prot. (gms)	carbo. (gms)	fat (gms)	chol. (mgs)	sod. (mgs)	fiber (gms)
(*Hormel*)	60	10.0	2.0	1.0	20	480	0
(*Jennie-O* Deli Thin)	50	9.0	4.0	1.0	15	470	0
(*Oscar Mayer* Deli Fresh Thin Sliced)	60	10.0	2.0	1.0	25	610	0
lean (*Oscar Mayer*), 1 oz.	35	3.0	2.0	1.5	10	320	0
shaved (*Oscar Mayer* Deli Fresh), ⅕ of 9-oz. pkg.	60	9.0	1.0	1.0	20	480	0
smoked, mesquite:							
(*Black Bear*)	50	11.0	0	.5	20	390	0
(*Boar's Head Wood Smoked*)	60	13.0	1.0	.5	25	440	0
(*Dietz & Watson*) ..	70	12.0	1.0	.5	30	430	0
(*Foster Farms*)	60	9.0	2.0	1.5	10	520	0
(*Healthy Choice Deli Thin*), 4 slices, 1.8 oz.	60	9.0	2.0	1.5	25	450	0
(*Jennie-O* Home-style)	50	12.0	1.0	0	25	590	0
(*Oscar Mayer* Deli Fresh Thin Sliced)	60	10.0	2.0	1.0	25	690	0
honey (*Wampler 4 Diamond*)	50	9.0	4.0	0	25	380	0
shaved (*Oscar Mayer* Deli Fresh), ⅕ of 9-oz. pkg.	50	9.0	2.0	1.0	20	610	0
Southwestern (*Applegate Farms*) .	50	12.0	1.0	1.0	30	400	0
spiced (*Wampler Deli Roast Collection*) ..	70	16.0	1.0	.5	25	380	0
sun-dried tomato:							
(*Di Lusso*)	60	12.0	0	1.0	25	460	0
(*Jennie-O*)	50	12.0	1.0	0	25	460	0
Tex-Mex (*Black Bear*)	60	12.0	1.0	.5	20	460	0
Turkey pastrami, 2 oz.:							
(*Applegate Farms*) ...	50	12.0	0	0	30	360	0
(*Boar's Head*)	60	13.0	1.0	.5	25	440	0
(*Empire Kosher*)	70	9.0	0	3.5	30	450	0
(*Empire Kosher* Presliced)	60	9.0	0	3.0	40	460	0
(*Foster Farms*)	70	11.0	0	2.5	40	450	0
(*Jennie-O*)	70	10.0	1.0	3.0	40	640	0

Food and Measure	cal.	prot. (gms)	carbo. (gms)	fat (gms)	chol. (mgs)	sod. (mgs)	fiber (gms)
Turkey pepperoni							
(*Hormel Pillow Pack*),							
17 slices, 1.1 oz. ...	70	9.0	0	4.0	40	640	0
Turkey pie, see "Turkey							
entree"							
Turkey salami:							
(*Applegate Farms*), 2 oz.	70	11.0	0	2.0	30	360	0
(*Empire Kosher* Pre-							
sliced), 3 pcs., 2.25 oz.	90	12.0	0	4.5	35	500	0
(*Jennie-O*), 2 oz.	90	8.0	2.0	5.0	40	650	0
cooked, 1 oz.	56	4.6	.2	3.9	23	285	0
cotto (*Louis Rich/Oscar							
Mayer*), 1 oz.	45	4.0	0	3.0	20	310	0
Turkey sandwich (see							
also "Panini" and							
"Wraps, filled"):							
and cheddar Dijon							
(*Oscar Mayer Deli							
Creations*), 6.8 oz. .	430	26.0	48.0	15.0	50	1410	5.0
Monterey (*Oscar Mayer							
Deli Creations*),							
7.2 oz.	450	26.0	51.0	17.0	60	1440	3.0
Turkey sausage, see							
"Sausage"							
Turmeric:							
in brine (*Fanci Food*),							
1 tbsp.	10	0	<1.0	0	0	105	<1.0
ground, 1 tsp.	8	.2	1.4	.2	0	1	.5
Turnip:							
raw:							
1 large 6.5 oz.	49	1.7	11.4	.2	0	123	11.4
cubed (*Glory*), ½ cup	20	1.0	4.0	0	0	45	1.0
cubed, ½ cup	18	.6	4.1	.1	0	44	1.2
boiled, drained:							
cubed, ½ cup	16	.6	3.8	.6	0	39	1.6
mashed, ½ cup ...	24	.8	5.6	.9	0	58	2.3
Turnip, frozen, boiled,							
drained, ½ cup ...	18	1.2	3.4	.2	0	28	1.6
Turnip greens, fresh:							
raw, untrimmed, 1 lb.	85	4.8	18.2	1.0	0	126	7.6
raw, chopped:							
(*Del Monte*), 2 cups	25	1.0	5.0	0	0	30	1.0
chopped, ½ cup ...	7	.4	1.6	.1	0	11	.7
boiled, chopped, ½ cup	15	.8	3.1	.2	0	21	2.2

Food and Measure	cal.	prot. (gms)	carbo. (gms)	fat (gms)	chol. (mgs)	sod. (mgs)	fiber (gms)
Turnip greens, canned, ½ cup:							
chopped (*Bush's*)	25	2.0	3.0	0	0	300	2.0
w/diced turnip:							
(*Bush's*)	30	1.0	5.0	0	0	380	2.0
seasoned (*Sunshine*)	35	4.0	5.0	.5	0	860	2.0
seasoned (*Glory*) ..	35	2.0	3.0	0	0	490	1.0
seasoned:							
(*Sunshine*)	35	4.0	5.0	.5	0	860	2.0
(*Glory*)	35	1.0	4.0	0	0	490	2.0
(*Glory* Sensibly) ...	20	1.0	4.0	0	0	240	2.0
turkey flavor (*Glory*) .	25	1.0	5.0	0	0	590	2.0
Turnip greens, frozen boiled, drained, 1 cup	28	3.4	4.7	.3	0	24	2.9
Turnover, frozen or refrigerated, 1 pc., except as noted:							
apple:							
(*The Fillo Factory* Organic), 3 pcs., 3 oz.	180	2.0	30.0	6.0	0	90	1.0
(*Pepperidge Farm*) .	290	4.0	36.0	15.0	0	230	2.0
(*Pillsbury*)	180	2.0	24.0	8.0	0	260	0
blueberry (*Pepperidge Farm*)	280	4.0	33.0	15.0	0	230	1.0
cherry:							
(*Pepperidge Farm*) .	280	4.0	34.0	15.0	0	250	1.0
(*Pillsbury*)	180	2.0	24.0	8.0	0	250	0
peach (*Pepperidge Farm*)	290	4.0	35.0	15.0	0	230	1.0
raspberry (*Pepperidge Farm*)	290	4.0	35.0	15.0	0	230	2.0
Turtle, green, raw, meat only, 4 oz. ...	101	22.5	0	.6	57	68	0
Tzaziki (*Fega* Greek), 2 tbsp.	30	1.0	2.0	2.0	5	120	0

Food and Measure	cal.	prot. (gms)	carbo. (gms)	fat (gms)	chol. (mgs)	sod. (mgs)	fiber (gms)
Umeboshi plum, (*Eden* Organic), .3-oz. pc.	5	0	1.0	0	0	690	0
Umeboshi plum paste (*Eden* Organic), 1 tsp.	5	0	0	0	0	340	0
Uzbek melon (*Frieda's*), 1 cup, 1.4 oz.	35	1.0	9.0	0	0	15	1.0
Vanilla drink mix (*GoLean* Shake), 2 scoops	220	21.0	33.0	.5	0	130	7.0
Vanilla extract, imitation, 1 tbsp.:							
w/alcohol	31	0	.3	0	0	<1	0
w/out alcohol	7	0	1.8	0	0	<1	0
Veal, meat only, 4 oz.:							
cubed, lean only, braised or stewed .	213	39.6	0	4.9	164	105	0
ground, broiled	195	27.6	0	8.6	117	94	0
leg:							
braised, lean w/fat .	239	41.0	0	7.2	152	76	0
braised, lean only . .	230	41.6	0	5.8	159	76	0
roasted, lean w/fat .	181	31.4	0	5.3	117	77	0
roasted, lean only .	170	31.8	0	3.8	117	77	0
loin:							
braised, lean w/fat .	322	34.2	0	19.5	134	91	0
braised, lean only . .	256	38.1	0	10.4	142	95	0
roasted, lean w/fat .	246	28.1	0	14.0	117	105	0
roasted, lean only .	198	29.8	0	7.9	120	109	0
rib:							
braised, lean w/fat .	285	36.8	0	14.2	158	108	0
braised, lean only . .	247	39.1	0	8.9	163	112	0
roasted, lean w/fat .	259	27.2	0	15.8	125	104	0
roasted, lean only .	201	29.2	0	8.4	130	110	0
shank, braised:							
lean w/fat	217	35.8	0	7.0	141	105	0

Food and Measure	cal.	prot. (gms)	carbo. (gms)	fat (gms)	chol. (mgs)	sod. (mgs)	fiber (gms)
lean only	201	35.4	0	4.9	143	107	0
shoulder, whole:							
braised, lean w/fat .	259	36.4	0	11.5	143	108	0
braised, lean only ..	226	38.2	0	6.9	147	110	0
roasted, lean w/fat .	209	28.7	0	9.5	128	109	0
roasted, lean only .	193	29.3	0	7.5	129	110	0
shoulder, arm:							
braised, lean w/fat .	268	38.1	0	11.6	168	99	0
braised, lean only ..	228	40.5	0	6.0	176	102	0
roasted, lean w/fat .	208	28.9	0	9.4	122	102	0
roasted, lean only .	186	29.6	0	6.6	124	103	0
shoulder, blade:							
braised, lean w/fat .	255	35.4	0	11.4	174	111	0
braised, lean only ..	224	37.0	0	7.3	179	115	0
roasted, lean w/fat .	211	28.5	0	9.8	133	113	0
roasted, lean only .	194	29.1	0	7.8	135	116	0
sirloin:							
braised, lean w/fat .	286	35.4	0	14.9	122	90	0
braised, lean only ..	231	38.5	0	7.4	128	92	0
roasted, lean w/fat .	229	28.5	0	11.9	116	94	0
roasted, lean only .	191	29.8	0	7.1	118	96	0
Veal entree, frozen, parmigiana, w/spaghetti (*Stouffer's*), 11.63-oz. pkg.	430	20.0	46.0	18.0	60	970	5.0
Vegetable burger, see "Burger, vegetarian" and "Burger patty, vegetarian"							
Vegetable cake (see also "Burger patty, vegetarian"), frozen, 2.4 oz.:							
ginger teriyaki (*Morningstar Farms*)	110	5.0	19.0	1.5	0	320	2.0
Southwest style (*Morningstar Farms*)	130	6.0	21.0	3.0	5	340	2.0
Vegetable chips/crisps (see also specific listings), 1 oz., except as noted:							
(*Eatsmart* Veggie Crisps), 1.1 oz. ...	140	1.0	18.0	7.0	0	290	2.0

Food and Measure	cal.	prot. (gms)	carbo. (gms)	fat (gms)	chol. (mgs)	sod. (mgs)	fiber (gms)
Vegetable chips/crisps *(cont.)*							
(*Eden/Eden* Organic Wasabi Chips), 1.1 oz.	130	<1.0	24.0	4.0	0	260	0
(*Terra Exotic Vegetable Chips*)	150	1.0	16.0	9.0	0	50	3.0
(*Terra Exotic Vegetable Chips* Mediterranean)	150	1.0	16.0	9.0	0	150	3.0
(*Terra Stix*)	150	1.0	16.0	9.0	0	110	3.0
cheddar or garlic herb (*Flat Earth* Baked) .	130	2.0	19.0	5.0	0	190	2.0
cheddar jalapeño (*Eatsmart* Veggie Crisps), 1.1 oz. ...	130	1.0	18.0	7.0	0	430	2.0
sun-dried tomato/pesto (*Eatsmart* Veggie Crisps), 1.1 oz. ...	140	1.0	19.0	7.0	0	390	3.0
tomato, zesty (*Terra Exotic Vegetable Chips*)	150	1.0	16.0	9.0	0	190	3.0
tomato ranch (*Flat Earth* Baked)	130	2.0	19.0	5.0	0	210	2.0
Vegetable dip mix (*McCormick*), ½ tsp.	5	0	0	0	0	130	0
Vegetable dish, frozen (see also "Vegetable entree, frozen" and specific listings):							
balls (*Dr. Praeger's*), 2 pcs., 2 oz.	80	4.0	10.0	2.5	0	190	3.0
crepes (*Kineret*), 2.2-oz. pc.	100	2.0	13.0	5.0	45	440	1.0
pancake:							
(*Golden*), 1.3-oz. pc.	70	2.0	10.0	3.0	<5	210	<1.0
(*Old Fashioned Kitchen*), 4 pcs., 3 oz.	160	4.0	22.0	7.0	10	470	<1.0
Southern casserole (*Glory Savory Accents*), ½ cup ..	140	2.0	20.0	5.0	15	480	2.0
Vegetable entree, frozen (see also "Vegetarian entree,							

Food and Measure	cal.	prot. (gms)	carbo. (gms)	fat (gms)	chol. (mgs)	sod. (mgs)	fiber (gms)
frozen" and specific listings), 1 pkg., except as noted:							
curry, w/rice:							
(*Ethnic Gourmet* Gujarati), 10 oz.	380	8.0	63.0	11.0	0	540	4.0
coconut, creamy (*Patak's*), 10.5 oz.	400	6.0	54.0	18.0	10	990	5.0
korma (*Amy's Meal*), 9.5 oz.	300	9.0	41.0	12.0	0	680	6.0
korma (*Ethnic Gourmet*), 11 oz.	300	8.0	52.0	6.0	0	680	4.0
lemon and cilantro (*Patak's*), 10.5 oz.	300	5.0	54.0	7.0	0	1020	5.0
tomato and onion (*Patak's*), 10.5 oz.	290	6.0	53.0	6.0	0	900	5.0
pie/pot pie, 7.5 oz.:							
(*Amy's*)	420	9.0	54.0	19.0	50	590	4.0
(*Amy's* Country)	370	12.0	47.0	16.0	40	580	4.0
(*Amy's* Nondairy)	360	10.0	50.0	13.0	0	640	4.0
wraps, see "Wraps, filled"							
Vegetable entree, microwave or pkg., ½ of 10-oz. pkg., except as noted:							
w/cheese:							
(*Tamarind Tree* Navratan Korma), 9.25-oz. pkg.	430	12.0	60.0	16.0	5	700	7.0
(*Tasty Bite* Jaipur)	169	7.0	10.0	11.0	3	372	4.0
curry:							
red (*Tasty Bite*)	100	2.0	11.0	6.0	0	305	1.5
yellow (*Tasty Bite*)	130	2.0	14.0	8.0	0	355	1.5
w/jasmine rice (*Tasty Bite*)	380	7.0	61.0	13.0	0	440	3.0
in peanut sauce:							
(*Tasty Bite* Massaman)	140	3.0	16.0	7.0	0	370	2.0
(*Tasty Bite* Satay)	200	4.0	31.0	11.0	0	450	3.0
spicy (*Tamarind Tree* Vegetable Jalfrazi), 9.25-oz. pkg.	310	8.0	57.0	6.0	0	600	7.0

Food and Measure	cal.	prot. (gms)	carbo. (gms)	fat (gms)	chol. (mgs)	sod. (mgs)	fiber (gms)
Vegetable entree, microwave or pkg. *(cont.)*							
stew:							
w/meatballs (*Dinty Moore* Big Bowl), 1 cup	190	39.0	25.0	6.0	20	660	0
spicy coconut (*Tasty Bite* Kerala)	140	2.0	15.0	4.0	0	430	2.0
Thai (*Tasty Bite* Rendang)	120	2.0	16.0	7.0	0	360	2.0
Vegetable entree mix, frozen (*Green Giant Create a Meal!*), stir-fry, w/out meat, frozen:							
lo mein, 2 cups	140	5.0	28.0	1.0	0	740	2.0
sesame, 2 cups	100	4.0	12.0	5.0	0	1100	4.0
sweet and sour, 1¼ cups	150	2.0	36.0	0	0	490	3.0
Szechuan, 1⅓ cups ..	50	3.0	10.0	0	0	860	3.0
teriyaki, 1½ cups	50	3.0	11.0	0	0	650	3.0
teriyaki, spicy, 1½ cups	80	3.0	16.0	.5	0	810	3.0
Vegetable juice, 8 fl. oz.:							
(*Bolthouse Farms Vedge*)	67	2.0	14.0	0	0	458	2.0
(*R.W. Knudsen Very Veggie* Low Sodium)	50	2.0	11.0	0	0	35	2.0
(*R.W. Knudsen Very Veggie* Organic Low Sodium)	70	2.0	14.0	0	0	35	2.0
(*R.W. Knudsen Very Veggie* Original/ Organic)	50	2.0	11.0	0	0	580	2.0
(*R.W. Knudsen Very Veggie* Untomato) .	70	<1.0	16.0	0	0	130	2.0
(*V8* Calcium Enriched)	50	2.0	11.0	0	0	460	2.0
(*V8* Essential Anti- oxidants)	50	2.0	11.0	0	0	480	2.0
(*V8* Low Sodium)	50	2.0	10.0	0	0	140	2.0
(*V8/V8* Organic)	50	2.0	10.0	0	0	480	2.0
lemon twist (*V8*)	50	2.0	10.0	0	0	590	2.0
spicy (*R.W. Knudsen Very Veggie*)	50	2.0	11.0	0	0	590	2.0
spicy hot (*V8*)	50	2.0	10.0	0	0	620	2.0

Food and Measure	cal.	prot. (gms)	carbo. (gms)	fat (gms)	chol. (mgs)	sod. (mgs)	fiber (gms)
Vegetable juice blends, (*V8 V.Fusion*), 8 fl. oz.:							
peach mango	120	1.0	28.0	0	0	70	0
peach mango, light ...	50	0	13.0	0	0	40	0
pomegranate blueberry	100	0	25.0	0	0	60	0
strawberry banana ...	120	1.0	28.0	0	0	70	0
strawberry banana, light	50	0	13.0	0	0	40	0
tropical orange	120	1.0	28.0	0	0	80	0
Vegetable oyster, see "Salsify"							
Vegetable pancake, see "Vegetable dish, frozen"							
Vegetable pie, see "Vegetable entree, frozen"							
Vegetable pocket sandwich (see also specific listings), 1 pc.:							
(*Amy's Pie Pocket*) ...	300	8.0	45.0	9.0	0	490	3.0
Asian (*Aunt Trudy's Organic*)	240	5.0	34.0	10.0	0	390	3.0
Mexicali (*Aunt Trudy's Organic*)	230	6.0	38.0	7.0	0	350	3.0
olives and (*Aunt Trudy's Mediterranean*)	270	6.0	41.0	10.0	0	550	2.0
roasted:							
(*Amy's Pocket*)	230	6.0	35.0	8.0	0	480	4.0
(*Aunt Trudy's Organic*)	240	5.0	33.0	11.0	0	280	3.0
samosa (*Aunt Trudy's Organic*)	280	6.0	43.0	10.0	0	350	3.0
Vegetable protein, minced (*Tree of Life*), 2.8 oz.	216	41.0	24.0	1.0	0	8	14.0
Vegetable seasoning:							
(*McCormick Vegetable Supreme*), ¼ tsp. ...	0	0	0	0	0	180	0
cheddar (*McCormick Veggie Steamers*), 1 tbsp.	25	1.0	2.0	1.0	5	350	0

Food and Measure	cal.	prot. (gms)	carbo. (gms)	fat (gms)	chol. (mgs)	sod. (mgs)	fiber (gms)
Vegetable seasoning *(cont.)*							
garlic basil (*McCormick Veggie Steamers*), 2 tsp.	15	0	2.0	.5	0	270	0
Vegetable spread, roasted (*Va Va Pindjur*), 1 oz.	55	2.3	3.2	4.5	0	300	<1.0
Vegetables, see specific listings							
Vegetables, mixed, canned, ½ cup:							
(*Del Monte*)	40	2.0	8.0	0	0	360	2.0
(*Del Monte Savory Sides* Homestyle Medley)	70	1.0	11.0	2.5	0	380	2.0
(*Freshlike*)	45	1.0	8.0	.5	0	410	2.0
(*S&W*)	45	2.0	10.0	0	0	360	2.0
(*Veg-All* Homestyle Large Cut)	40	1.0	8.0	0	0	350	2.0
(*Veg-All* Original)	40	1.0	8.0	0	0	290	2.0
Cajun (*Veg-All*)	50	2.0	10.0	0	0	410	3.0
Chinese (*La Choy*)	15	1.0	3.0	0	0	60	1.0
chop suey (*La Choy*)	15	1.0	3.0	0	0	640	<1.0
w/potato (*Del Monte*)	45	2.0	10.0	0	0	360	2.0
spiced (*Veg-All* Hot 'n Spicy)	40	1.0	8.0	0	0	370	2.0
stir-fry (*La Choy*)	15	<1.0	3.0	0	0	180	2.0
Vegetables, mixed, frozen (see also "Vegetable dish, frozen" and specific listings):							
(*Birds Eye* Classic/ *Birds Eye Steamfresh*), ⅔ cup	60	2.0	12.0	0	0	20	2.0
(*Cascadian Farm Organic*), ⅔ cup	60	2.0	12.0	0	0	20	2.0
(*Cascadian Farm Organic Gardener's Blend*), ¾ cup	60	2.0	12.0	0	0	35	2.0
(*Cascadian Farm Purely Steam* Organic Garden Medley), 1 cup	60	2.0	12.0	1.0	0	270	1.0

Food and Measure	cal.	prot. (gms)	carbo. (gms)	fat (gms)	chol. (mgs)	sod. (mgs)	fiber (gms)
(C&W Organic Fancy), ¾ cup	60	2.0	12.0	0	0	15	2.0
(C&W Farmer's Harvest Fancy), ¾ cup	50	2.0	10.0	0	0	70	2.0
(C&W Farmer's Harvest Healthy Garden), 1 cup	25	1.0	4.0	0	0	30	2.0
(C&W The Ultimate Asian Blend), ½ cup	60	3.0	9.0	1.0	0	180	2.0
(C&W The Ultimate Early Harvest Blend), ½ cup	60	3.0	9.0	2.0	0	190	2.0
(C&W The Ultimate Petite Mixed Vegetables), ⅔ cup	50	2.0	10.0	0	0	70	2.0
(C&W The Ultimate Southwest Blend), ⅔ cup	90	5.0	16.0	1.0	0	80	6.0
(C&W The Ultimate Stir Fry), ¾ cup	30	1.0	5.0	0	0	15	1.0
(C&W The Ultimate Tuscan Blend), ⅔ cup	45	3.0	6.0	1.0	0	200	2.0
(Green Giant Garden Medley), ½ cup cooked	70	2.0	14.0	.5	0	220	2.0
(Green Giant Simply Steam Garden Medley), ½ cup cooked	50	2.0	11.0	.5	0	280	1.0
(Tree of Life Organic), ½ cup	65	3.0	13.0	0	0	60	3.0
(Tree of Life Organic Garden Blend), ⅔ cup	60	4.0	10.0	.5	0	20	2.0
Alfredo sauce:							
(Green Giant Bag), 1 cup	60	3.0	9.0	1.5	0	360	2.0
(Green Giant Box), ¾ cup	60	3.0	10.0	2.0	5	420	3.0
Asian, 1 cup:							
seasoned (Birds Eye Steamfresh Medley)	50	2.0	6.0	2.0	0	310	2.0
sesame ginger sauce (Birds Eye)	60	2.0	12.0	1.0	0	630	2.0

Food and Measure	cal.	prot. (gms)	carbo. (gms)	fat (gms)	chol. (mgs)	sod. (mgs)	fiber (gms)
Vegetables, mixed, frozen *(cont.)*							
baby, seasoned (*Green Giant* Medley), ¾ cup	40	1.0	9.0	1.0	<5	250	2.0
California blend:							
(*Cascadian Farm* Organic), ⅔ cup	25	1.0	5.0	0	0	25	2.0
(*Tree of Life* Organic), ¾ cup	30	2.0	5.0	0	0	25	2.0
in cheddar sauce (*Birds Eye* California Blend), ½ cup	80	2.0	8.0	4.0	5	390	1.0
Chinese stir-fry (*Cascadian Farm* Organic), 1 cup ...	25	1.0	5.0	0	0	15	2.0
edamame blends:							
(*Seapoint Farms* Eat Your Greens), 3 oz.	60	5.0	7.0	1.5	0	30	3.0
garden blend (*Seapoint Farms*), ¾ cup	60	4.0	7.0	1.5	0	25	3.0
oriental blend (*Seapoint Farms*), ¾ cup	60	4.0	8.0	1.0	0	20	3.0
gumbo mix (*McKenzie's*), ⅔ cup	35	1.0	8.0	0	0	30	2.0
Italian blend (*Birds Eye*), ¾ cup	30	1.0	5.0	0	0	35	2.0
Parmesan asiago sauce (*Green Giant Select*), 1 cup	50	3.0	8.0	1.5	<5	240	2.0
soup mix, ⅔ cup:							
(*Birds Eye*)	50	1.0	9.0	0	0	60	2.0
(*McKenzie's*)	40	2.0	9.0	0	0	40	2.0
Szechuan, in sauce:							
(*Green Giant*), ½ cup cooked	50	2.0	9.0	.5	0	410	2.0
sesame sauce (*Birds Eye*), 1 cup	60	1.0	9.0	2.0	0	460	2.0
teriyaki (*Green Giant*), 1¼ cups	70	2.0	7.0	4.5	0	490	2.0
Thai stir-fry (*Cascadian Farm* Organic), ¾ cup	25	1.0	5.0	0	0	15	2.0

Food and Measure	cal.	prot. (gms)	carbo. (gms)	fat (gms)	chol. (mgs)	sod. (mgs)	fiber (gms)
Tuscan herb sauce:							
(*Green Giant Select*), 1¼ cups	50	2.0	7.0	1.5	<5	270	2.0
tomato (*Birds Eye*), 1 cup	50	1.0	7.0	2.0	0	180	2.0
Vegetables, mixed, pickled:							
(*B&G* Giardiniera), 2 pcs., 1 oz.	7	0	1.0	0	0	420	0
(*Seres*), 1.4 oz.	10	0	1.0	0	0	625	1.0
Vegetarian dish (see also "Vegetarian entree" and specific listings):							
canned:							
(*Loma Linda* Dinner Cuts), 2 pcs., 3.3 oz.	90	18.0	4.0	1.0	0	500	2.0
(*Loma Linda* Tender Bits), 6 pcs., 3 oz.	120	13.0	7.0	4.0	0	440	3.0
(*Worthington Choplets*), 2 slices, 3.3 oz.	90	18.0	4.0	1.0	0	500	2.0
(*Worthington Multi-Grain Cutlets*), 2 slices, 3.2 oz. .	100	17.0	5.0	1.0	0	290	3.0
frozen:							
(*Worthington* Dinner Roast), ¾" slice, 3 oz.	180	14.0	6.0	11.0	0	580	3.0
schnitzels (*Garden Gourmet*), 2.9-oz. pc.	100	10.0	5.0	4.0	0	500	6.0
Vegetarian entree, frozen (see also specific listings), 1 pkg.:							
black bean mango (*Kashi*), 10 oz.	340	8.0	58.0	8.0	0	430	7.0
nuggets, Hawaiian (*Hain Vegetarian Classics*), 10 oz.	310	13.0	55.0	5.0	0	495	6.0
"osso bucco" w/fettuccine (*Ethnic Gourmet*), 10 oz.	340	15.0	43.0	11.0	0	1040	3.0

Food and Measure	cal.	prot. (gms)	carbo. (gms)	fat (gms)	chol. (mgs)	sod. (mgs)	fiber (gms)
Vegetarian entree, frozen *(cont.)*							
Southern entree (*Amy's* Whole Meal), 10 oz.	340	12.0	53.0	10.0	.25	780	8.0
Venison, meat only, 4 oz.:							
roasted	179	34.3	0	3.6	127	61	0
ground, pan-broiled . .	212	30.0	0	9.3	111	88	0
Vermicelli entree mix, garlic/olive oil:							
(*Near East*), 2.5 oz. . .	240	9.0	48.0	2.5	5	510	2.0
(*Near East*), 1 cup* . .	300	9.0	48.0	9.0	<5	510	2.0
(*Pasta Roni*), 1 cup* .	350	9.0	47.0	15.0	0	1020	2.0
Vine spinach, raw, untrimmed, 1 lb. . .	86	8.2	15.4	1.4	0	109	4.0
Vinegar, 1 tbsp., except as noted:							
apple cider:							
(*Musselman's*)	6	0	0	0	0	4	0
(*Roland*)	0	0	0	0	0	0	0
(*Spectrum* Organic)	5	0	0	0	0	0	0
or red wine (*Eden*) .	0	0	0	0	0	0	0
balsamic:							
(*Carapelli*)	15	0	4.0	0	0	0	0
(*Holland House*) . . .	15	0	4.0	0	0	0	0
(*Progresso*)	10	0	2.0	0	0	0	0
all varieties (*Consul/ Roland*)	10	0	3.0	0	0	0	0
red (*Vigo*)	15	0	3.0	0	0	0	0
red or fig infused (*Alessi*)	15	0	3.0	0	0	0	0
white (*Vigo*)	10	0	3.0	0	0	0	0
white, pear, or raspberry (*Alessi*)	10	0	3.0	0	0	0	0
fish and chips (*Crosse & Blackwell*)	0	0	0	0	0	0	0
malt or sherry wine (*Don Brune*)	0	0	0	0	0	0	0
malt or tarragon (*Fanci Food*)	0	0	0	0	0	0	0
red or white wine:							
(*Carapelli*)	5	0	0	0	0	0	0
(*Fanci Food*)	0	0	0	0	0	0	0
all varieties (*Roland*)	0	0	0	0	0	0	0

Food and Measure	cal.	prot. (gms)	carbo. (gms)	fat (gms)	chol. (mgs)	sod. (mgs)	fiber (gms)
rice:							
(*Nakano*)	0	0	0	0	0	0	0
(*Roland*)	0	0	0	0	0	30	0
balsamic blend (*Nakano*)	15	0	4.0	0	0	190	0
brown (*Eden* Organic)	2	0	0	0	0	0	0
brown (*Spectrum* Organic)	10	0	2.0	0	0	0	0
seasoned (*Roland*)	5	0	2.0	0	0	150	0
seasoned, all varieties (*Nakano*)	20	0	5.0	0	0	240	0
ume plum (*Eden*), 1 tsp.	2	0	0	0	0	1050	0
wine, red or white (*Alessi/Vigo*)	0	0	0	0	0	0	0
white wine, raspberry (*Fanci Food*)	6	0	2.0	0	0	0	0

W

Food and Measure	cal.	prot. (gms)	carbo. (gms)	fat (gms)	chol. (mgs)	sod. (mgs)	fiber (gms)
Waffle, frozen, 2 pcs., except as noted:							
(*Aunt Jemima* Homestyle)	190	4.0	31.0	6.0	<5	530	1.0
(*Aunt Jemima* Low Fat)	160	4.0	31.0	3.0	<5	540	1.0
(*Eggo* Homestyle) . . .	180	5.0	27.0	6.0	20	440	1.0
(*Eggo* Homestyle Minis), 3 sets of 4	250	6.0	38.0	8.0	30	620	1.0
(*GoLean* Original)	170	8.0	33.0	3.0	0	330	6.0
(*Heart to Heart*)	160	6.0	31.0	3.0	0	370	3.0
(*Special K*)	160	5.0	30.0	2.5	20	440	<1.0
(*Van's* Belgian)	172	5.0	30.0	3.5	0	196	2.0
(*Van's* Gourmet)	145	4.5	24.0	3.5	0	152	2.0
(*Van's* Gourmet 97% Fat Free)	180	5.0	30.0	2.0	0	306	5.0
(*Van's* Homestyle), 2 sets of 4	116	3.0	18.0	3.5	0	114	2.0
(*Van's* Organic)	190	6.0	30.0	4.5	0	230	6.0
(*Van's* Wheat Free) . . .	189	4.0	32.0	5.0	0	390	5.0
(*Van's* Wheat Free Minis), 2 sets of 4 .	160	1.0	30.0	4.5	0	290	<1.0
apple cinnamon:							
(*Eggo*)	190	4.0	30.0	6.0	15	370	1.0
(*Van's* Wheat Free) .	189	4.0	32.0	5.0	0	390	5.0
banana bread (*Eggo*) .	190	4.0	29.0	6.0	0	280	1.0
berries, red (*Special K*)	160	4.0	31.0	2.5	15	440	<1.0
blueberry:							
(*Aunt Jemima*)	190	4.0	33.0	6.0	<5	510	1.0
(*Eggo*)	190	4.0	30.0	6.0	15	370	1.0
(*Eggo* Nutri-Grain) .	180	4.0	31.0	4.5	0	380	3.0
(*GoLean*)	170	8.0	33.0	3.0	0	300	6.0
(*Van's* Belgian)	184	5.0	33.0	3.5	0	196	2.0
(*Van's* Gourmet) . . .	157	4.5	24.0	3.5	0	152	2.0

Food and Measure	cal.	prot. (gms)	carbo. (gms)	fat (gms)	chol. (mgs)	sod. (mgs)	fiber (gms)
(Van's Mini), 2 sets of 4	119	3.0	21.0	3.5	0	114	2.0
(Van's Organic) ...	240	5.0	29.0	10.0	0	320	4.0
(Van's Wheat Free) .	201	4.0	35.0	5.0	0	390	5.0
brown sugar cinnamon (Eggo Flip Flop) ...	190	4.0	31.0	6.0	15	390	1.0
buckwheat:							
(Van's Wheat Free) .	230	4.0	37.0	8.0	0	410	4.0
wildberry (Life- stream Organic) .	220	1.0	38.0	7.0	0	430	1.0
buttermilk:							
(Aunt Jemima)	200	5.0	33.0	6.0	<5	550	1.0
(Eggo)	180	5.0	26.0	6.0	15	420	1.0
buttery maple syrup (Eggo), 3 sets of 4 .	250	5.0	39.0	8.0	20	440	1.0
chocolate chip:							
(Eggo)	210	4.0	32.0	7.0	15	380	1.0
(Van's Mini), 2 sets of 4	119	3.0	18.0	4.0	0	114	2.0
chocolate vanilla (Eggo Flip Flop)	190	4.0	28.0	7.0	15	360	<1.0
cinnamon:							
(Eggo Nutri-Grain) .	170	4.0	27.0	4.5	0	280	3.0
toast (Eggo), 3 sets of 4	290	5.0	46.0	10.0	20	500	1.0
fig plus flax (Life- stream Organic) ...	210	5.0	29.0	10.0	0	410	6.0
flax:							
(Lifesteam Flax Plus Organic)	200	5.0	29.0	8.0	0	430	6.0
(Van's Gourmet) ...	260	6.0	34.0	11.0	0	340	6.0
(Van's Organic) ...	230	6.0	26.0	11.0	0	290	6.0
(Van's Wheat Free) .	230	3.0	42.0	6.0	0	390	5.0
French toast (Eggo), 1 pc.	140	3.0	20.0	5.0	10	250	<1.0
w/hemp (Lifestream Hemp Plus Organic)	210	6.0	28.0	9.0	0	400	5.0
maple cinnamon (Lifestream Organic)	200	4.0	30.0	7.0	0	410	4.0
multigrain:							
(Lifestream Mesa Sunrise Organic Gluten Free)	220	2.0	36.0	8.0	0	480	1.0

Food and Measure	cal.	prot. (gms)	carbo. (gms)	fat (gms)	chol. (mgs)	sod. (mgs)	fiber (gms)
Waffle, frozen, multigrain *(cont.)*							
(*Lifestream Synergy* Organic)	200	5.0	32.0	8.0	0	460	5.0
(*Van's* Gourmet) . . .	190	5.0	30.0	6.0	0	306	5.0
seven (*Van's* Belgian)	230	7.0	42.0	4.0	0	290	7.0
oat:							
berry (*Van's* Hearty Oats Berry Boost)	200	4.0	31.0	8.0	0	280	4.0
and honey (*Van's* Hearty Oats)	200	4.0	30.0	8.0	0	290	4.0
maple (*Van's* Hearty Oats Fusion)	210	4.0	31.0	9.0	0	280	4.0
pomegranate (*Lifestream Pomagran Plus* Organic)	190	5.0	31.0	5.0	0	370	5.0
strawberry (*Eggo*) . . .	190	4.0	30.0	6.0	15	370	1.0
strawberry filled (*Eggo Waf-Fulls*), 1 pc. . .	170	3.0	27.0	5.0	10	300	<1.0
vanilla, French (*Eggo*)	200	4.0	27.0	8.0	20	380	<1.0
whole wheat:							
(*Eggo Nutri-Grain*) .	180	5.0	28.0	6.0	0	420	3.0
(*Eggo Nutri-Grain Low Fat*)	140	5.0	28.0	2.5	0	430	3.0
Waffle mix (see also "Pancake mix"), Belgian (*Krusteaz*), 7"-round pc.*	450	12.0	58.0	19.0	85	880	2.0
Walnut, dried:							
(*Fisher*), 1 oz.	200	5.0	3.0	20.0	0	0	3.0
(*Planters*), 1.2 oz. . . .	210	5.0	6.0	20.0	0	0	2.0
(*SunRidge Farms* Organic), 1.1 oz. . .	200	5.0	4.0	20.0	0	0	2.0
black:							
(*Planters*), 2-oz. pkg.	340	14.0	8.0	31.0	0	0	3.0
shelled (*Diamond*), ¼ cup, 1.1 oz. . .	190	7.0	3.0	18.0	0	0	2.0
shelled, 1 oz.	172	6.9	3.4	16.1	0	<1	1.4
chopped, 1 cup . . .	759	30.4	15.1	70.7	0	2	6.3
English or Persian:							
all varieties (*Diamond*), 1.1 oz. . . .	200	5.0	4.0	10.0	0	0	2.0
shelled, 1 oz.	182	4.1	5.2	17.6	0	3	1.4
pieces., 1 cup	770	17.2	22.0	74.2	0	12	5.8

Food and Measure	cal.	prot. (gms)	carbo. (gms)	fat (gms)	chol. (mgs)	sod. (mgs)	fiber (gms)
halves, 1 cup	642	14.3	18.3	61.9	0	10	4.8
pieces (*Planters*), 1 oz.	190	4.0	5.0	18.0	0	0	1.0
Walnut topping, in syrup (*Smucker's*), 2 tbsp.	150	2.0	20.0	7.0	0	0	1.0
Wasabi, root, fresh, sliced, ½ cup	71	3.1	15.3	.4	0	11	5.0
Wasabi peas, see "Peas, green, snack"							
Wasabi paste (*Roland*), 1 tsp.	15	0	2.0	.5	0	95	0
Wasabi powder:							
(*Eden* Organic), 1 tsp.	10	0	1.0	0	0	0	.5
(*Roland*), ¼ tsp.	0	0	0	0	0	0	0
Wasabi sauce, 1 tsp.:							
(*S&B* Tube)	15	0	3.0	.5	0	100	0
w/ginger (*Gold's*)	15	0	1.0	1.5	5	15	0
Water chestnut, fresh:							
(*Frieda's*), 1.1 oz.	30	0	7.0	0	0	0	1.0
4 medium, 1.3 oz. ...	35	.5	8.6	<.1	0	5	1.1
sliced, ½ cup	60	.9	14.8	.1	0	9	1.9
Water chestnut, can/jar:							
whole:							
(*La Choy*), ½ cup .	40	<1.0	9.0	0	0	15	1.0
4 pcs., 1 oz.	14	.3	3.5	<.1	0	2	.7
whole or sliced (*Roland*), ½ cup ..	40	1.0	9.0	0	0	20	1.0
sliced, ½ cup:							
(*La Choy*)	25	1.0	5.0	0	0	10	1.0
w/liquid	35	.5	8.7	<.1	0	6	1.8
Watercress:							
(*Frieda's*), 1 cup, 3 oz.	10	2.0	1.0	0	0	35	2.0
10 sprigs, 11¼"	3	.6	.3	<.1	0	10	.6
chopped, ½ cup	2	.4	.2	<.1	0	7	.4
Watermelon, fresh:							
(*Del Monte*), 1/18 medium, 9.9 oz.	80	1.0	27.0	0	0	10	2.0
1" slice, 10" diam. ...	152	3.0	34.6	2.0	0	10	2.4
diced, ½ cup	25	.5	5.7	.3	0	2	.4
yellow seedless (*Frieda's*), 3 oz. ...	25	1.0	6.0	0	0	0	0
Watermelon drink blend, 8 fl. oz.:							
(*AriZona*)	110	0	27.0	0	0	25	0

Food and Measure	cal.	prot. (gms)	carbo. (gms)	fat (gms)	chol. (mgs)	sod. (mgs)	fiber (gms)
Watermelon drink blend *(cont.)*							
strawberry (*Nantucket Nectars*)	120	0	28.0	0	0	25	0
Watermelon rind, pickled, sweet (*Fanci Food*), 2 tbsp.	70	0	17.0	0	0	0	0
Watermelon seeds, dried, 1 oz.	158	8.1	4.4	13.5	0	28	n.a.
Wax beans, fresh, see "Green bean"							
Wax beans, canned, ½ cup:							
(*Del Monte* Golden) . .	20	1.0	4.0	0	0	360	2.0
cut (*S&W*)	20	1.0	4.0	0	0	360	2.0
Wax gourd, 1 cup:							
raw, cubed	17	.5	4.0	.3	0	147	3.8
boiled, drained, cubed	23	.7	5.3	.4	0	187	1.8
Welsh rarebit, frozen (*Stouffer's*), ¼ of 10-oz. pkg.	140	6.0	6.0	10.0	20	270	1.0
Wendy's, 1 serving:							
burgers:							
Baconator	840	56.0	38.0	51.0	195	1880	1.0
cheeseburger, Jr. . .	270	15.0	27.0	11.0	40	690	1.0
w/bacon	320	17.0	26.0	16.0	50	670	1.0
deluxe	300	15.0	29.0	14.0	45	730	2.0
hamburger, Jr.	230	13.0	27.0	8.0	30	490	1.0
w/everything:							
single	430	25.0	39.0	20.0	75	870	2.0
double w/cheese	710	47.0	41.0	40.0	160	1440	2.0
triple w/cheese . .	980	69.0	43.0	60.0	245	2010	2.0
Stack Attack	380	23.0	27.0	20.0	75	750	1.0
chicken sandwiches:							
club	540	34.0	48.0	25.0	75	1360	2.0
crispy	330	16.0	34.0	14.0	35	680	1.0
fillet, homestyle . . .	430	25.0	48.0	16.0	45	1120	2.0
fillet, spicy	440	28.0	46.0	16.0	60	1300	3.0
grill, ultimate	320	28.0	36.0	7.0	70	950	2.0
chicken go wraps:							
grilled	260	17.0	23.0	11.0	45	760	1.0
homestyle	320	15.0	29.0	16.0	35	860	1.0
spicy	320	17.0	28.0	16.0	40	960	2.0

Food and Measure	cal.	prot. (gms)	carbo. (gms)	fat (gms)	chol. (mgs)	sod. (mgs)	fiber (gms)
chicken nuggets:							
4 pcs.	190	10.0	10.0	12.0	30	420	0
5 pcs.	230	12.0	12.0	15.0	35	520	0
10 pcs.	460	24.0	24.0	30.0	70	1040	0
chicken nugget sauce:							
barbecue	45	1.0	11.0	0	0	160	0
honey mustard	130	0	6.0	12.0	10	220	0
ranch, heartland	160	0	1.0	17.0	15	220	0
sweet and sour	50	0	13.0	0	0	120	0
fish fillet sandwich	450	16.0	47.0	22.0	10	1020	1.0
salad, *Garden Sensations:*							
chicken BLT	340	34.0	10.0	19.0	105	990	4.0
garlic croutons	70	2.0	9.0	2.5	0	125	0
honey mustard dressing	250	1.0	9.0	23.0	20	300	0
chicken Caesar	170	24.0	8.0	4.5	70	570	3.0
garlic croutons	70	2.0	9.0	2.5	0	125	0
Caesar dressing	120	1.0	1.0	13.0	20	200	0
Mandarin Chicken	170	21.0	16.0	2.5	60	520	3.0
almonds	130	5.0	4.0	11.0	0	70	2.0
crispy noodles	70	1.0	10.0	2.5	0	190	0
sesame dressing	170	1.0	19.0	9.0	0	340	0
taco, Southwest	430	30.0	30.0	22.0	80	1090	8.0
sour cream	45	1.0	2.0	3.5	10	25	0
tortilla strips	110	2.0	13.0	5.0	0	160	1.0
ancho chipotle ranch dressing	90	1.0	3.0	8.0	10	240	0
salad dressing:							
blue cheese	230	2.0	2.0	24.0	35	370	0
Caesar	120	1.0	1.0	13.0	20	200	0
French, fat free	70	0	17.0	0	0	170	1.0
honey mustard, low fat	100	0	19.0	2.5	0	270	0
Italian vinaigrette	130	0	8.0	11.0	0	320	0
ranch, creamy	200	1.0	4.0	20.0	15	360	0
ranch, reduced fat	90	1.0	6.0	7.0	10	360	1.0
Thousand Island	230	1.0	7.0	22.0	20	350	0
sides:							
chili, large	330	25.0	35.0	9.0	55	1170	8.0
chili, small	220	17.0	23.0	6.0	35	780	5.0
cheddar	70	4.0	1.0	6.0	15	110	0
hot seasoning	5	0	1.0	0	0	270	0
saltines, 2	25	0	4.0	.5	0	95	0

Food and Measure	cal.	prot. (gms)	carbo. (gms)	fat (gms)	chol. (mgs)	sod. (mgs)	fiber (gms)
***Wendy's* sides** *(cont.)*							
fries:							
large	550	7.0	72.0	26.0	0	480	7.0
medium	430	6.0	56.0	20.0	0	370	5.0
small	340	4.0	45.0	16.0	0	290	4.0
mandarin orange cup	80	1.0	19.0	0	0	15	1.0
potato, baked:							
bacon/cheese . . .	450	19.0	67.0	13.0	30	950	7.0
broccoli/cheese .	320	10.0	69.0	2.0	5	450	8.0
sour cream/chive	320	8.0	63.0	4.0	10	50	7.0
side salad	35	1.0	8.0	0	0	25	2.0
side salad, Caesar .	70	6.0	4.0	4.0	10	170	2.0
garlic croutons . .	70	2.0	9.0	2.5	0	125	0
Frosty, medium:							
chocolate, 16 oz. . .	410	11.0	68.0	7.0	45	200	0
vanilla, 16 oz.	410	11.0	68.0	6.0	45	240	0
Wheat, whole grain:							
(*Arrowhead Mills*							
Organic), ¼ cup . . .	150	7.0	31.0	1.0	0	0	5.0
durum, 1 cup	651	26.3	136.6	4.7	0	3	n.a.
hard red:							
spring, 1 cup	632	29.6	130.6	3.7	0	4	24.2
winter (*Shiloh*							
Farms Organic),							
¼ cup	160	6.0	34.0	1.0	0	0	7.0
winter, 1 cup	628	24.2	136.7	3.0	0	4	24.2
hard white:							
1 cup	657	21.7	145.7	3.3	0	4	n.a.
spring (*Shiloh*							
Farms Organic),							
¼ cup	164	5.0	36.0	1.0	0	4	6.0
soft red winter, 1 cup .	556	17.4	124.7	2.6	0	4	21.0
soft white, 1 cup	571	18.0	126.6	3.3	0	3	21.3
Wheat, parboiled, see							
"Bulgur"							
Wheat, sprouted, 1 cup	214	8.1	45.9	1.4	0	18	1.2
Wheat berries, see							
"Wheat kernels"							
Wheat bran (see also							
"Cereal"):							
(*Arrowhead Mills*							
Organic), ⅓ cup . . .	60	3.0	10.0	1.0	0	0	6.0
coarse (*Shiloh Farms*							
Organic), ¼ cup . . .	30	2.0	10.0	0	0	<1	6.0

Food and Measure	cal.	prot. (gms)	carbo. (gms)	fat (gms)	chol. (mgs)	sod. (mgs)	fiber (gms)
crude:							
(*Hodgson Mill* Unprocessed), ¼ cup	30	2.0	10.0	0	0	0	7.0
2 tbsp.	15	1.1	4.5	.3	0	<1	3.0
fine (*Shiloh Farms* Organic), ¼ cup . . .	30	3.0	7.0	.5	0	5	6.0
Wheat flakes (see also "Cereal") (*Shiloh Farms* Organic), ⅓ cup	110	4.0	24.0	.5	0	0	5.0
Wheat flour (see also specific flour listings), ¼ cup, except as noted:							
all purpose, see "white," below							
bread:							
(*Hodgson Mill* Best for Bread)	100	4.0	22.0	0	0	5	1.0
(*Pillsbury Best*) . . .	110	4.0	22.0	0	0	0	<1.0
cake:							
(*Pillsbury Softasilk*), 1 oz.	100	2.0	23.0	0	0	0	<1.0
(*Swans Down*)	100	2.0	22.0	0	0	0	0
self-rising (*Presto*) .	90	3.0	20.0	0	0	310	1.0
gluten, see "Wheat gluten"							
graham, whole wheat:							
(*Hodgson Mill*), <¼ cup	100	3.0	22.0	.5	0	0	4.0
(*Hodgson Mill* Organic), <¼ cup	100	3.0	22.0	1.0	0	0	3.0
pasta, see "Semolina flour"							
pastry:							
(*Arrowhead Mills* Organic)	120	3.0	26.0	.5	0	0	<1.0
whole wheat (*Hodgson Mill* Regular/ Organic), <¼ cup	100	3.0	22.0	.5	0	0	4.0
presifted (*Pillsbury Best* Shake & Blend) . . .	110	4.0	23.0	0	0	0	<1.0
seasoned (*Kentucky Kernel*), 4 tsp.	36	1.0	8.0	0	0	544	0

Food and Measure	cal.	prot. (gms)	carbo. (gms)	fat (gms)	chol. (mgs)	sod. (mgs)	fiber (gms)
Wheat flour *(cont.)*							
self-rising:							
(*Gold Medal*)	100	3.0	23.0	0	0	400	<1.0
(*Martha White*)	110	3.0	23.0	0	0	380	<1.0
(*Pillsbury Best*) . . .	100	0	16.0	0	0	370	7.0
sprouted (*Shiloh Farms* Organic)	90	4.0	22.0	.5	0	5	6.0
tortilla mix, 1 cup	449	10.7	74.5	11.8	0	751	n.a.
white, all-purpose:							
(*Gold Medal/Gold Medal* Organic/ Unbleached)	100	3.0	22.0	0	0	0	<1.0
(*Pillsbury Best*) . . .	110	3.0	23.0	0	0	0	<1.0
white, quick mixing (*Wondra*)	100	3.0	23.0	0	0	0	<1.0
white, unbleached:							
(*Arrowhead Mills* Organic)	120	3.0	26.0	.5	0	0	<1.0
(*Hodgson Mill* All Purpose), <¼ cup	100	3.0	23.0	0	0	0	1.0
(*Hodgson Mill* Organic)	100	3.0	23.0	0	0	0	1.0
(*Pillsbury Best*) . . .	110	3.0	23.0	0	0	0	<1.0
white, whole wheat (*Hodgson Mill*) . . .	100	4.0	21.0	.5	0	0	3.0
whole-grain, 1 cup . . .	407	16.4	87.1	2.2	0	1	15.1
whole wheat:							
(*Arrowhead Mills* Organic Stone Ground)	130	5.0	26.0	1.0	0	0	4.0
(*Gold Medal* Stone Ground)	100	4.0	21.0	.5	0	0	3.0
(*Pillsbury Best*) . . .	100	4.0	21.0	0	0	0	<1.0
(*Shiloh Farms* Organic)	100	4.0	20.0	0	0	0	2.0
whole wheat and white (*Hodgson Mill* 50/50), <¼ cup	100	4.0	21.0	1.0	0	0	2.0
Wheat germ:							
(*Hodgson Mill* Un-toasted), 2 tbsp. . . .	55	4.0	7.0	1.0	0	0	4.0
w/cinnamon and flax seed (*Hodgson Mill*), 2 tbsp.	65	4.0	7.0	2.0	0	0	3.0

Food and Measure	cal.	prot. (gms)	carbo. (gms)	fat (gms)	chol. (mgs)	sod. (mgs)	fiber (gms)
crude, 1 oz.	102	6.6	14.7	2.8	0	3	3.7
raw (*Arrowhead Mills*), 3 tbsp.	60	4.0	7.0	1.5	0	0	2.0
toasted:							
(*Tree of Life*), 3 tbsp.	100	9.0	12.0	3.0	0	0	3.0
1 oz.	108	8.3	14.1	3.0	0	1	3.7
Wheat gluten, vital:							
(*Arrowhead Mills*), 1 tbsp.	35	5	3.0	0	0	0	0
(*Hodgson Mill*), 4 tsp.	40	8.0	3.0	0	0	0	1.0
Wheat kernels, ¼ cup:							
(*Shiloh Farms* Organic Soft Wheat Berries)	160	6.0	34.0	.5	0	0	7.0
(*Vita-Spelt* Organic Wheat Berries)	160	6.0	34.0	1.0	0	0	7.0
Wheat malt syrup, see "Malt syrup"							
Whelk, meat only:							
raw, 4 oz.	156	27.0	8.8	.5	74	234	0
boiled, steamed, or poached, 4 oz.	312	54.1	17.6	.9	147	467	0
Whey, fluid:							
acid, 1 cup	59	1.9	12.6	.2	0	118	0
sweet, 1 cup	66	2.1	12.6	.9	5	132	0
Whey, protein, dry (*Designer Whey*), 1 level scoop:							
chocolate	100	18.0	2.0	2.0	45	80	0
chocolate, double	100	18.0	3.0	2.0	45	80	0
chocolate peanut caramel	90	18.0	2.0	1.5	45	80	0
natural	90	19.0	2.0	1.0	45	50	0
strawberry	90	18.0	2.0	1.0	45	60	0
vanilla, French	90	18.0	2.0	1.5	45	60	0
vanilla praline	90	18.0	2.0	2.0	45	80	0
Whipped topping, see "Cream topping"							
Whiskey sour mix, see "Sour drink mixer"							
White bean, canned:							
(*S&W*), ½ cup	80	7.0	19.0	.5	0	440	6.0
w/liquid, ½ cup	153	9.5	28.7	.4	0	595	6.3
White bean, mature:							
boiled, ½ cup	125	8.6	22.6	.3	0	6	5.7
small, boiled, ½ cup .	124	8.7	22.5	.3	0	5	5.6

Food and Measure	cal.	prot. (gms)	carbo. (gms)	fat (gms)	chol. (mgs)	sod. (mgs)	fiber (gms)
White bean seasoning							
(*Zatarain's*), 1 tsp. . .	15	0	3.0	0	0	420	0
Whitefish, meat only:							
raw, 4 oz.	153	21.7	0	6.7	68	58	0
baked or broiled, 4 oz.	195	27.7	0	8.5	87	74	0
Whitefish, smoked:							
(*Acme*), 2 oz.	120	10.0	0	9.0	30	340	0
(*Acme* Chubs), 2 oz. .	80	9.0	0	4.5	25	380	0
(*Ducktrap River*), 2 oz.	70	12.0	0	2.0	5	730	0
4 oz.	122	26.5	0	1.1	37	1156	0
Whiting, meat only:							
raw, 4 oz.	102	20.8	0	1.5	76	82	0
baked or broiled, 4 oz.	130	26.6	0	1.9	95	150	0
Whiting entree, frozen,							
breaded (*Schooner*),							
3.5-oz. fillet	160	9.0	20.0	5.0	25	160	1.0
Wiener, see "Frankfurter"							
Wild rice:							
raw, ¼ cup:							
(*Lundberg* Organic)	150	6.0	33.0	1.0	0	0	2.0
(*Lundberg* Organic							
Quick)	150	6.0	33.0	.5	0	0	2.0
(*Roland*)	170	6.0	35.0	.5	0	0	2.0
(*Shiloh Farms*							
Organic California)	160	7.0	34.0	0	0	0	3.0
cooked, 1 cup	166	6.5	35.0	.6	0	6	1.5
Wild rice blends, see							
"Rice"							
Wild rice dish, see							
"Rice dish"							
Wine, 3.5 fl. oz., except							
as noted:							
dessert or apertif[1] . . .	158	.2	12.2	0	0	9	0
dry or table:[2]							
red	74	.2	1.8	0	0	5	0
rose	73	.2	1.4	0	0	5	0
white	70	.1	.8	0	0	5	0
sake, 1 fl. oz.	39	.1	.1	0	0	<1	0

[1] Includes fortified wines containing more than 15% alcohol, such as port, sherry, vermouth, etc.

[2] Includes wines containing less than 15% alcohol, such as burgundy, Chablis, champagne, etc.

Food and Measure	cal.	prot. (gms)	carbo. (gms)	fat (gms)	chol. (mgs)	sod. (mgs)	fiber (gms)
Wine, cooking, 2 tbsp., except as noted:							
Burgundy:							
(*Roland*)	10	0	3.0	0	0	230	0
or Chablis (*Fanci Food*)	20	0	0	0	0	150	0
Marsala:							
(*Holland House*) ...	45	0	4.0	0	0	190	0
(*Roland*)	15	5	4.0	0	0	190	0
red (*Holland House*) ..	20	0	1.0	0	0	190	0
rice, 1 tbsp.:							
(*Eden* Organic Mirin)	25	0	7.0	0	0	130	0
(*Mitsukan* Honteri Sweet Mirin) ...	35	0	8.0	0	0	15	0
(*Sun Luck* Mirin) ..	20	0	5.0	0	0	55	0
Sauterne or white Chablis (*Roland*) ..	10	0	3.0	0	0	190	0
sherry:							
(*Fanci Food*)	40	0	2.0	0	0	160	0
(*Holland House*) ...	45	0	2.0	0	0	190	0
(*Roland*)	15	0	4.0	0	0	180	0
vermouth (*Holland House*)	35	0	2.0	0	0	190	0
white, plain or lemon flavor (*Holland House*)	20	0	0	0	0	190	0
Wing sauce (see also "Hot sauce"), (*Ken's* Buffalo), 1 tbsp.	15	0	1.0	1.5	0	490	0
(*World Harbors* After Glow Hot Wings), 2 tbsp.	30	0	7.0	0	0	390	0
spicy (*Fiesta*), 2 tbsp.	30	0	4.0	1.5	0	20	0
Winged bean, fresh:							
raw, sliced, ½ cup ...	11	1.5	1.0	.2	0	1	n.a.
boiled, drained, ½ cup	12	1.6	1.0	.2	0	1	n.a.
Winged bean, mature:							
dry, ½ cup	372	27.0	38.0	14.9	0	35	14.1
boiled, ½ cup	126	9.1	12.8	5.0	0	11	n.a.
Winged bean leaves, trimmed, 1 oz.	21	1.7	4.0	.3	0	3	n.a.
Winged bean tuber, trimmed, 1 oz.	45	3.3	8.0	.3	0	10	n.a.

Food and Measure	cal.	prot. (gms)	carbo. (gms)	fat (gms)	chol. (mgs)	sod. (mgs)	fib (gm
Winter squash (see also specific listings), all varieties, 1 cup:							
raw, cubed	43	1.7	10.2	.3	0	5	1.
boiled, drained, cubed	80	1.8	17.9	1.3	0	2	5.
Winter squash, frozen, ½ cup:							
(*Cascadian Farm Organic*)	70	2.0	19.0	0	0	0	2.
cooked (*Birds Eye*)	45	0	11.0	0	0	0	2.
Witloof, see "Chicory, witloof"							
Wolf fish, Atlantic, meat only:							
raw, 4 oz.	109	19.9	0	2.7	52	97	
baked or broiled, 4 oz.	139	25.4	0	3.5	67	124	
Wonton wrapper (see also "Wrappers"):							
(*Frieda's Fiesta*), 4 pcs., 1 oz.	80	3.0	17.0	0	0	160	1.
(*Nasoya*), 8 pcs.	160	6.0	31.0	.5	10	370	1.
Wontons, filled, see specific listings							
Worcestershire sauce:							
(*Annie's Naturals Organic*), 2 tbsp.	20	<1.0	5.0	0	0	460	
(*Lea & Perrins*), 1 tsp.	5	0	1.0	0	0	65	
(*World Harbors Angostura*), 1 tsp.	5	0	1.0	0	0	20	
Wrappers (see also specific listings):							
round (*Azumaya/ Nasoya*), 10 pcs.	160	6.0	31.0	.5	10	370	1.0
square:							
(*Azumaya*), 8 pcs.	160	6.0	31.0	.5	10	370	1.0
large (*Azumaya*), 3 pcs.	170	7.0	35.0	.5	10	410	1.0
Wraps (see also "Tortilla"), unfilled, 2.5-oz. pc.:							
(*Cedar's Low Carb*)	70	6.0	14.0	1.5	0	320	9.0
spinach (*Cedar's*)	180	6.0	34.0	3.0	0	380	3.0
wheat (*Cedar's*)	220	6.0	38.0	4.5	0	430	3.0
white (*Cedar's*)	160	6.0	27.0	3.0	0	380	1.0

Food and Measure	cal.	prot. (gms)	carbo. (gms)	fat (gms)	chol. (mgs)	sod. (mgs)	fiber (gms)
Wraps, filled (see also "Breakfast sandwich/ pastry" and "Flat-bread melts"), 1 pc.:							
black bean chipotle:							
(*Gardenburger*), 4.8 oz.	240	13.0	32.0	8.0	10	600	6.0
(*Guiltless Gourmet*), 5.75 oz.	270	9.0	51.0	3.0	0	570	7.0
chicken:							
grilled, Caesar (*South Beach Living*), 6.45 oz. .	230	24.0	22.0	11.0	55	820	14.0
sesame (*South Beach Living*), 6.45 oz.	220	21.0	28.0	9.0	40	710	15.0
Southwestern (*South Beach Living*), 7.85 oz. .	240	25.0	26.0	11.0	55	810	15.0
chicken sausage:							
(*Hans' All Natural Hell's Kitchen*), 5.5 oz.	300	19.0	40.0	6.0	45	640	2.0
(*Hans' All Natural Santorini*), 5.5 oz.	320	21.0	40.0	8.0	45	640	2.0
(*Hans' All Natural Sonoma*), 5.5 oz.	330	21.0	44.0	6.0	45	790	3.0
chili, four bean (*Guiltless Gourmet*), 5.75 oz.	300	10.0	53.0	5.0	0	260	6.0
couscous vegetable (*Cedarlane* Low Fat Veggie), 6 oz.	220	14.0	36.0	3.0	0	580	3.0
ham and turkey, deli (*South Beach Living*), 6.85 oz.	220	22.0	23.0	10.0	40	960	15.0
Indian:							
samosa (*Amy's*), 5 oz.	260	8.0	38.0	8.0	0	680	4.0
spinach tofu (*Amy's*), 5.5 oz.	310	11.0	35.0	14.0	0	690	7.0
pizza:							
(*Cedarlane* Low Fat Veggie), 6 oz. . . .	220	17.0	32.0	3.0	0	520	2.0

Food and Measure	cal.	prot. (gms)	carbo. (gms)	fat (gms)	chol. (mgs)	sod. (mgs)	fiber (gms)
Wraps, filled, pizza *(cont.)*							
Margherita *(Garden-burger)*, 4.8 oz. .	240	12.0	34.0	8.0	10	590	5.0
spinach *(Guiltless Gourmet Mediterranean)*, 5.75 oz.	270	10.0	45.0	5.0	<5	270	4.0
turkey, 6 oz.:							
w/cranberry sauce *(Empire Kosher)*	380	13.0	57.0	11.0	30	570	3.0
w/cranberry chipotle sauce *(Empire Kosher)*	370	11.0	62.0	8.0	20	460	3.0
turkey bacon club *(South Beach Living)*, 7.05 oz. . . .	240	24.0	24.0	12.0	40	930	14.0
vegetable *(Guiltless Gourmet California)*, 5.75 oz.	270	9.0	47.0	5.0	0	290	4.0
veggie "ham" and cheese *(Cedarlane Veggie)*, 6 oz.	350	29.0	36.0	10.0	15	660	1.0
Wrap kit, refrigerated *(Hillshire Farms Deli Wrap)*, ½ pkg.:							
chicken, Caesar	310	17.0	21.0	18.0	45	1090	1.0
w/out dressing	200	16.0	20.0	6.0	30	870	1.0
chicken, Southwest . .	260	14.0	21.0	14.0	40	870	2.0
w/out dressing	190	14.0	20.0	6.0	30	790	2.0
ham and Swiss	260	14.0	25.0	11.0	40	960	3.0
w/out dressing	200	13.0	19.0	7.0	30	810	3.0
turkey bacon club . . .	300	16.0	21.0	16.0	40	1160	1.0
w/out dressing	220	16.0	20.0	8.0	30	1040	1.0

Y

Food and Measure	cal.	prot. (gms)	carbo. (gms)	fat (gms)	chol. (mgs)	sod. (mgs)	fiber (gms)
Yachtwurst, w/pistachios, cooked, 2 oz.	150	8.3	.8	12.7	36	524	0
Yam (see also "Name yam"), cubed:							
raw, ½ cup	89	1.2	20.9	.1	0	7	3.1
baked or boiled, ½ cup	79	1.0	18.8	.1	0	6	2.7
Yam, canned/frozen, see "Sweet potato"							
Yam, mountain, Hawaiian, cubed, steamed, ½ cup . . .	59	1.2	14.4	.1	0	9	n.a.
Yam bean, tuber:							
raw:							
(*Frieda's* Jicama), ¾ cup, 3 oz.	35	1.0	7.0	0	0	5	1.0
sliced, ½ cup	23	.4	5.3	.1	0	3	2.9
boiled, drained, 4 oz. .	43	.8	10.0	.1	0	5	n.a.
Yard-long bean, fresh:							
raw (*Frieda's* Dow Gok), ¾ cup, 3 oz. .	40	2.0	7.0	0	0	0	0
boiled, drained, sliced, ½ cup	25	1.3	4.8	.1	0	2	n.a.
Yard-long bean, mature, boiled, ½ cup	102	7.1	18.1	.4	0	4	1.4
Yeast, baker's:							
active, dry:							
(*Hodgson Mill*), ⁵⁄₁₆-oz. pkg.	30	4.0	3.0	0	0	0	1.0
1 tbsp.	35	3.4	4.6	.6	0	6	.3
compressed, .6-oz. . .	6	<.1	1.1	0	0	2	<.1
fast rise (*Hodgson Mill*), ⁵⁄₁₆-oz. pkg.	25	3.0	4.0	0	0	0	1.0

Food and Measure	cal.	prot. (gms)	carbo. (gms)	fat (gms)	chol. (mgs)	sod. (mgs)	fiber (gms)
Yellow beans, dried, boiled, ½ cup	127	8.1	22.2	1.0	0	4	9.2
Yellow squash, fresh (see also "Crookneck squash"), sliced, ¾ cup:							
(*Glory*)	20	1.0	3.0	0	0	20	1.0
and zucchini (*Glory*) .	25	2.0	6.0	0	0	0	3.0
Yellow squash, canned sliced (*Sunshine*), ½ cup	25	0	5.0	0	0	160	2.0
Yellowtail, meat only:							
raw, 4 oz.	166	26.3	0	6.0	62	44	0
baked or broiled, 4 oz.	212	33.6	0	7.6	81	57	0
Yogurt, 8 oz., except as noted:							
plain:							
(*Colombo* Low Fat)	130	10.0	16.0	2.5	15	125	0
(*Colombo* Nonfat) .	100	10.0	16.0	0	10	160	0
(*Dannon*)	160	9.0	12.0	8.0	20	120	0
(*Dannon* Low Fat), 6 oz.	100	8.0	12.0	2.5	10	115	0
(*Dannon* Nonfat), 6 oz.	80	9.0	12.0	0	5	120	0
(*Fage* Total Greek 2%)	150	19.0	9.0	4.5	15	75	0
(*Fage* Total Greek Nonfat)	120	20.0	9.0	0	0	85	0
(*Stonyfield* Organic)	180	9.0	16.0	9.0	35	130	3.0
(*Stonyfield* Organic Low Fat)	120	10.0	15.0	2.0	10	150	0
(*Stonyfield* Organic Nonfat)	110	11.0	16.0	0	0	160	0
(*Yoplait* Grande! Nonfat)	130	15.0	19.0	0	5	220	0
(*Yoplait* Original Nonfat), 6 oz.	100	11.0	14.0	0	5	170	0
all flavors:							
(*Colombo* Light) ...	120	7.0	21.0	0	5	110	0
(*Dannon* All Natural), 6 oz.	150	7.0	25.0	2.5	10	100	0
(*Dannon la Crème*), 4 oz.	140	5.0	19.0	5.0	15	65	0

Food and Measure	cal.	prot. (gms)	carbo. (gms)	fat (gms)	chol. (mgs)	sod. (mgs)	fiber (gms)
(*Dannon Light & Fit Carb & Sugar Control*), 4 oz. . .	60	5.0	3.0	3.0	10	25	0
(*Yoplait* Fridge Pack), 6 oz.	170	5.0	33.0	1.5	10	80	0
(*Yoplait* Fridge Pack Light), 6 oz.	100	5.0	19.0	0	<5	85	0
(*Yoplait* Fridge Pack Thick & Creamy), 6 oz.	190	7.0	32.0	3.5	15	100	0
(*Yoplait* Grande!) . .	220	8.0	42.0	2.5	15	130	0
(*Yoplait* Grande! Light)	140	7.0	27.0	0	5	115	0
(*Yoplait* Thick & Creamy Custard Style*), 6 oz.	190	7.0	32.0	3.5	15	100	0
(*Yoplait* Thick & Creamy Custard Style* Light), 6 oz.	100	5.0	20.0	0	<5	90	0
except banana crème, coconut crème pie, lemon, and piña colada (*Yoplait*), 6 oz.	170	5.0	33.0	1.5	10	80	0
except banana/ Boston/lemon cream pie, and vanilla (*Yoplait* Light), 6 oz.	100	5.0	19.0	0	<5	85	0
except banana strawberry and vanilla (*Colombo Classic* Fruit on Bottom)	220	7.0	42.0	2.0	15	115	0
all fruit flavors, 4 oz.:							
(*Yoplait* 6-Pack) . . .	110	4.0	22.0	1.0	5	55	0
(*Yoplait* Light 6-Pack)	70	4.0	13.0	0	0	60	0
(*Yoplait* Whips) . . .	140	5.0	25.0	2.5	10	75	0
(*Yoplait* Yo-Plus) . .	110	4.0	21.0	1.5	10	70	3.0
all fruit flavors, except raspberries (*Breyers Creme Savers*), 6 oz.	180	6.0	34.0	2.0	15	180	0
apple cinnamon (*Dannon* Fruit on the Bottom), 6 oz.	150	6.0	28.0	1.5	5	130	<1.0

Food and Measure	cal.	prot. (gms)	carbo. (gms)	fat (gms)	chol. (mgs)	sod. (mgs)	fiber (gms)
Yogurt *(cont.)*							
apricot-mango *(Stony-field* YoCalcium Organic Nonfat), 6 oz.	120	7.0	22.0	0	0	120	<1.0
banana crème, 6 oz.:							
(Yoplait Original) ..	100	5.0	20.0	0	<5	90	0
pie *(Yoplait* Light) .	110	6.0	20.0	0	<5	90	0
banana strawberry *(Colombo* Classic) .	230	7.0	47.0	2.0	15	90	0
banana vanilla *(Stony-field* Organic Low Fat Banilla)	200	9.0	35.0	2.5	10	140	0
berry, mixed:							
(Breyers Smart!), 6 oz.	170	6.0	34.0	1.5	10	95	1.0
(Dannon Fruit on the Bottom), 6 oz. ..	150	6.0	27.0	1.5	5	120	<1.0
(Dannon Activia), 4 oz.	110	5.0	19.0	2.0	10	65	0
berry, wild *(Stonyfield* YoCalcium Organic Nonfat), 6 oz.	120	7.0	22.0	0	0	135	<1.0
blackberry:							
(Dannon Light & Fit), 6 oz.	60	5.0	10.0	0	<5	80	0
(Stonyfield Organic Nonfat), 6 oz.	140	7.0	27.0	0	0	115	0
blueberries/cream *(Breyers* Light!), 6 oz.	80	6.0	12.0	0	5	105	0
blueberry:							
(Breyers Light!), 4 oz.	50	4.0	8.0	0	5	70	0
(Breyers Smart!), 6 oz.	170	6.0	34.0	1.5	10	95	1.0
(Dannon Fruit on Bottom), 6 oz. ..	140	6.0	26.0	1.5	5	130	<1.0
(Dannon Activia), 4 oz.	110	4.0	19.0	2.0	5	61	0
(Dannon Light & Fit), 6 oz.	60	5.0	10.0	0	<5	80	0
(Stonyfield Organic Lowfat), 6 oz.	130	6.0	22.0	1.5	5	110	<1.0
(Stonyfield Organic Nonfat), 6 oz.	120	7.0	23.0	0	0	120	2.0

Food and Measure	cal.	prot. (gms)	carbo. (gms)	fat (gms)	chol. (mgs)	sod. (mgs)	fiber (gms)
wild (*Stonyfield* Organic), 6 oz. . .	160	6.0	21.0	6.0	20	95	<1.0
Boston cream pie (*Yoplait* Light), 6 oz.	110	6.0	20.0	0	<5	90	0
boysenberry (*Dannon* Fruit on Bottom), 6 oz.	150	6.0	27.0	1.5	5	110	<1.0
caramel (*Stonyfield* Organic Low Fat), 6 oz.	180	6.0	35.0	1.5	5	105	0
cherry (*Dannon* Fruit on Bottom), 6 oz. . . .	150	6.0	26.0	1.5	5	120	0
cherry, black, 6 oz.:							
(*Breyers* Light! Jubilee)	80	6.0	12.0	0	5	90	0
(*Breyers* Smart!) . .	170	6.0	35.0	1.5	10	95	1.0
(*Breyers* Smooth & Creamy Parfait) .	170	6.0	33.0	1.5	10	90	0
(*Stonyfield* Organic Nonfat)	120	7.0	24.0	0	0	110	2.0
cherry vanilla (*Dannon* Light & Fit), 6 oz. . .	60	5.0	11.0	0	<5	85	0
chocolate:							
(*Stonyfield* Organic Nonfat), 6 oz. . .	180	7.0	37.0	0	0	110	2.0
all varieties (*Yoplait* Whips!), 4 oz. . .	160	5.0	26.0	4.0	10	105	0
white, raspberry (*Dannon* Light & Fit), 6 oz.	60	5.0	10.0	0	<5	80	0
coconut crème pie (*Yoplait* Original), 6 oz.	190	5.0	34.0	3.0	10	85	0
dulce de leche (*Yoplait* Whips!), 4 oz.	150	4.0	25.0	4.0	15	90	0
honey (*Fage* Total Greek 2%), 5.3 oz.	180	10.0	29.0	2.5	5	40	0
latte, creamy (*Yoplait* Whips!), 4 oz.	150	4.0	24.0	4.0	15	85	0
lemon, 6 oz.:							
(*Stonyfield* Organic Low Fat Luscious)	140	6.0	25.0	1.5	5	140	<1.0
(*Stonyfield* Organic Nonfat Lotsa) . . .	140	7.0	26.0	0	0	120	0
(*Yoplait* Original) . .	180	5.0	36.0	1.5	10	80	0

Food and Measure	cal.	prot. (gms)	carbo. (gms)	fat (gms)	chol. (mgs)	sod. (mgs)	fiber (gms)
Yogurt, lemon *(cont.)*							
chiffon (*Breyers* Light!)	80	6.0	11.0	0	5	120	0
chiffon (*Dannon Light & Fit*)	60	5.0	10.0	0	<5	90	0
cream pie (*Yoplait* Light)	110	6.0	20.0	0	<5	90	0
lime, key, 6 oz.:							
(*Stonyfield* Organic Nonfat)	130	7.0	25.0	0	0	135	0
pie (*Breyers* Light!)	80	6.0	11.0	0	5	170	0
maple vanilla (*Stonyfield* Organic Lowfat), 6 oz.	130	7.0	22.0	1.5	5	105	0
mocha latte (*Stonyfield* Organic Low Fat), 6 oz.	140	7.0	21.0	1.5	5	110	0
orange							
(*Breyers Creme Savers*), 4 oz.	120	4.0	22.0	1.5	10	115	0
mango (*Dannon Light & Fit*), 6 oz.	60	5.0	10.0	0	<5	80	0
peach:							
(*Breyers* Light!), 4 oz.	50	4.0	8.0	0	5	70	0
(*Breyers* Smart!), 6 oz.	170	6.0	34.0	1.5	10	95	1.0
(*Breyers Creme Savers*), 4 oz.	120	4.0	22.0	1.5	10	55	0
(*Dannon* Fruit on the Bottom), 6 oz. ..	150	6.0	28.0	1.5	5	115	<1.0
(*Dannon Activia*), 4 oz.	110	5.0	19.0	2.0	10	70	0
(*Dannon Activia* Light), 4 oz.	70	5.0	13.0	0	<5	70	3.0
(*Dannon Fruit Blends*), 6 oz.	170	6.0	33.0	1.5	10	125	0
(*Dannon Light & Fit*), 6 oz.	60	5.0	11.0	0	<5	85	0
(*Stonyfield* Organic Low Fat), 6 oz. ..	130	6.0	23.0	1.5	5	110	<1.0
(*Stonyfield* Organic Nonfat), 6 oz.	120	7.0	25.0	0	0	120	2.0
peaches/cream, 6 oz.:							
(*Breyers* Light!) ...	80	6.0	12.0	0	5	110	0
(*Breyers* Smooth & Creamy)	170	6.0	34.0	1.5	10	85	0

Food and Measure	cal.	prot. (gms)	carbo. (gms)	fat (gms)	chol. (mgs)	sod. (mgs)	fiber (gms)
piña colada (*Yoplait* Original), 6 oz.	170	5.0	33.0	2.0	10	95	0
pineapple, 6 oz.:							
(*Breyers* Smart!) ..	170	6.0	34.0	1.5	10	95	<1.0
(*Dannon* Fruit on the Bottom)	150	6.0	28.0	1.5	5	125	0
prune (*Dannon Activia*), 4 oz.	110	5.0	19.0	2.0	10	75	0
raspberries/cream, 6 oz.:							
(*Breyers* Light!) ...	80	6.0	12.0	0	5	95	0
(*Breyers* Smooth & Creamy)	170	6.0	34.0	1.5	10	85	0
(*Breyers Creme Savers*)	180	6.0	34.0	2.0	15	190	0
raspberry:							
(*Breyers* Smart!), 6 oz.	170	6.0	35.0	1.5	10	95	1.0
(*Dannon* Fruit on the Bottom), 6 oz. ..	150	6.0	28.0	1.5	5	115	<1.0
(*Dannon Activia* Light), 4 oz.	70	5.0	13.0	0	<5	75	3.0
(*Dannon Fruit Blends*), 6 oz.	170	7.0	32.0	1.5	10	125	<1.0
(*Dannon Light & Fit*), 6 oz.	60	5.0	11.0	0	<5	95	0
(*Stonyfield* Organic Low Fat), 6 oz. ...	130	6.0	22.0	1.5	5	140	<1.0
(*Stonyfield* Organic Nonfat), 6 oz.	120	7.0	23.0	0	0	140	2.0
strawberries/cream (*Stonyfield* Organic), 6 oz.	160	5.0	20.0	6.0	20	110	<1.0
strawberry:							
(*Breyers* Light!), 6 oz.	80	6.0	12.0	0	5	105	0
(*Breyers* Smart!), 6 oz.	170	6.0	34.0	1.5	10	95	1.0
(*Breyers* Smooth & Creamy), 6 oz. ..	170	6.0	34.0	1.5	10	90	0
(*Breyers Creme Savers*), 4 oz.	120	4.0	22.0	1.5	10	115	0
(*Colombo* Low Fat)	220	8.0	42.0	2.5	15	130	0
(*Dannon* Fruit on the Bottom), 6 oz. ..	150	6.0	28.0	1.5	5	110	<1.0
(*Dannon Activia*), 4 oz.	110	4.0	19.0	2.0	5	75	0

Food and Measure	cal.	prot. (gms)	carbo. (gms)	fat (gms)	chol. (mgs)	sod. (mgs)	fiber (gms)
Yogurt, strawberry *(cont.)*							
(*Dannon Activia Light*), 4 oz.	70	5.0	13.0	0	<5	80	3.0
(*Dannon Fruit Blends*), 6 oz. . . .	170	6.0	33.0	1.5	10	125	0
(*Dannon Light & Fit*), 6 oz.	60	5.0	11.0	0	<5	90	0
(*Stonyfield* Organic Low Fat)	200	9.0	35.0	2.5	10	140	0
(*Stonyfield* Organic Low Fat), 6 oz. . .	120	6.0	21.0	1.5	5	125	<1.0
(*Stonyfield* Organic Nonfat), 6 oz. . . .	120	7.0	24.0	0	0	150	3.0
strawberry banana, 6 oz.:							
(*Breyers* Smart!) . .	170	6.0	34.0	1.5	10	95	1.0
(*Breyers* Smooth & Creamy)	170	6.0	33.0	1.5	10	90	0
(*Dannon* Fruit on the Bottom)	150	6.0	26.0	1.5	5	95	<1.0
(*Dannon* Fruit Blends)	160	6.0	30.0	1.5	10	100	0
(*Dannon Light & Fit*)	60	5.0	11.0	0	<5	90	0
strawberry cheesecake:							
(*Breyers* Light!), 6 oz.	80	6.0	12.0	0	5	85	0
(*Breyers* Smooth & Creamy), 6 oz. . .	170	6.0	33.0	1.5	10	95	0
strawberry kiwi (*Dannon Light & Fit*), 6 oz.	60	5.0	11.0	0	<5	85	0
strawberry raspberry (*Stonyfield* YoCalcium Organic Nonfat), 4 oz.	120	7.0	22.0	0	0	105	<1.0
vanilla:							
(*Colombo* Classic) .	190	8.0	33.0	2.5	15	135	0
(*Colombo* Low Fat)	220	8.0	42.0	2.5	15	130	0
(*Colombo* Nonfat) .	160	8.0	32.0	0	5	140	0
(*Dannon Activia*), 4 oz.	110	5.0	19.0	2.0	10	70	0
(*Dannon Activia Light*), 4 oz.	70	5.0	13.0	0	<5	75	3.0
(*Dannon Light & Fit*), 6 oz.	60	5.0	10.0	0	<5	80	0
(*Stonyfield* Organic Low Fat)	180	9.0	30.0	2.0	10	140	0

Food and Measure	cal.	prot. (gms)	carbo. (gms)	fat (gms)	chol. (mgs)	sod. (mgs)	fiber (gms)
(*Yoplait* Light Very), 6 oz.	110	6.0	20.0	0	<5	90	0
truffle (*Stonyfield* Organic), 6 oz. . . .	220	6.0	38.0	5.0	20	95	<1.0
vanilla, French:							
(*Stonyfield* Organic)	230	8.0	31.0	8.0	30	130	0
(*Stonyfield* Organic Nonfat)	180	9.0	36.0	0	0	140	3.0
Yogurt, frozen, ½ cup:							
(*Ben & Jerry's Half Baked* Lighten Up!)	180	4.0	35.0	3.0	20	95	1.0
black cherry vanilla swirl (*Dreyer's/Edy's Slow Churned*) . . .	100	2.0	17.0	3.0	10	35	0
cappuccino chip (*Dreyer's/Edy's Slow Churned*)	110	2.0	18.0	3.5	10	40	0
caramel, nutty (*Turkey Hill* Caribou)	120	3.0	19.0	3.5	5	70	1.0
caramel praline crunch (*Dreyer's/Edy's Slow Churned*)	120	3.0	20.0	3.5	10	45	0
cherry chocolate chip (*Ben & Jerry's Cherry Garcia* Lighten Up!)	160	4.0	31.0	3.0	15	60	1.0
chocolate (*Stonyfield Organic* Nonfat) . . .	100	4.0	20.0	0	<5	60	0
chocolate cherry cordial (*Turkey Hill* Nonfat)	100	3.0	23.0	0	0	55	1.0
chocolate chip cookie dough (*Turkey Hill*)	120	3.0	23.0	2.0	5	95	1.0
chocolate fudge brownie:							
(*Ben & Jerry's* Lighten Up!)	170	5.0	34.0	2.5	15	95	1.0
(*Dreyer's/Edy's Slow Churned*)	120	3.0	19.0	3.5	10	40	1.0
chocolate marshmallow (*Turkey Hill* Nonfat)	110	3.0	24.0	0	0	110	1.0
chocolate vanilla swirl (*Dreyer's/Edy's Slow Churned*)	100	3.0	16.0	3.0	10	35	0

Food and Measure	cal.	prot. (gms)	carbo. (gms)	fat (gms)	chol. (mgs)	sod. (mgs)	fiber (gms)
Yogurt, frozen *(cont.)*							
coffee:							
(*Häagen-Dazs*)	200	8.0	31.0	4.5	65	50	0
(*Stonyfield* Organic Nonfat Java)	100	4.0	21.0	0	<5	65	0
cookie (*Stonyfield* Organic Low Fat Cookies 'n Dream) .	130	5.0	25.0	1.5	0	115	0
crème caramel (*Stonyfield* Organic Lowfat)	130	4.0	26.0	1.5	<5	95	0
fudge ripple (*Turkey Hill* Nonfat)	100	3.0	21.0	0	0	65	0
mint cookies and cream (*Turkey Hill*)	110	3.0	22.0	1.5	0	75	0
minty chocolate chip (*Stonyfield* Organic Low Fat)	140	4.0	24.0	3.0	<5	55	<1.0
Neapolitan (*Turkey Hill* Nonfat)	90	3.0	19.0	0	0	55	1.0
raspberry white chocolate chunk (*Stonyfield* Organic Lowfat)	120	4.0	22.0	1.5	0	70	0
strawberry (*Dreyer's/ Edy's Slow Churned*)	100	2.0	17.0	2.5	10	30	0
vanilla:							
(*Dreyer's/Edy's Slow Churned*)	100	2.0	17.0	3.0	10	35	0
(*Häagen-Dazs*)	200	9.0	31.0	4.5	65	55	0
(*Stonyfield* Organic Nonfat)	100	4.0	21.0	0	<5	70	0
bean (*Turkey Hill* Nonfat)	100	3.0	19.0	0	0	60	0
vanilla fudge swirl (*Stonyfield* Organic Nonfat)	120	4.0	25.0	0	<5	65	0
vanilla raspberry swirl (*Häagen-Dazs*)	170	4.0	32.0	2.5	25	35	0
wildberry (*Häagen-Dazs*)	180	7.0	34.0	2.0	35	40	0
"Yogurt," soy, 6 oz., except as noted:							
plain (*Silk Live!*), 8 oz.	150	6.0	22.0	4.0	0	30	1.0
banana strawberry or blueberry (*Silk Live!*)	150	4.0	29.0	2.0	0	25	1.0

Food and Measure	cal.	prot. (gms)	carbo. (gms)	fat (gms)	chol. (mgs)	sod. (mgs)	fiber (gms)
blueberry:							
(*So Delicious*)	150	6.0	28.0	3.0	0	40	3.0
(*Stoneyfield O'Soy Organic*)	170	7.0	29.0	2.5	0	40	2.0
cherry, black (*Silk Live!*)	150	4.0	29.0	2.0	0	20	1.0
chocolate (*Stoneyfield O'Soy Organic*)	160	8.0	26.0	3.0	0	30	2.0
cinnamon bun (*So Delicious*)	160	6.0	29.0	2.5	0	25	3.0
lime, key (*Silk Live!*) .	150	4.0	30.0	2.0	0	25	1.0
peach:							
(*Silk Live!*)	160	4.0	32.0	2.0	0	25	1.0
(*So Delicious*)	160	6.0	29.0	3.0	0	15	3.0
(*Stonayfield O'Soy Organic*)	170	7.0	30.0	2.5	0	45	2.0
raspberry:							
(*Silk Live!*)	150	4.0	30.0	2.0	0	25	1.0
(*So Delicious*)	150	6.0	29.0	3.0	0	35	3.0
(*Stoneyfield O'Soy Organic*)	170	7.0	29.0	2.5	0	55	2.0
strawberry:							
(*Silk Live!*)	160	4.0	31.0	2.0	0	25	1.0
(*Stoneyfield O'Soy Organic*)	170	7.0	29.0	2.5	0	55	2.0
strawberry and peach (*Stoneyfield O'Soy Organic*), 4 oz.	100	5.0	14.0	2.0	0	25	1.0
vanilla:							
(*Silk Live!*)	150	5.0	25.0	3.0	0	20	1.0
(*So Delicious*)	160	6.0	29.0	3.0	0	10	3.0
(*Stoneyfield Organic*)	150	7.0	24.0	3.0	0	35	1.0
Yogurt drink/smoothie (see also "Kefir"):							
plain (*DanActive*), 3.3 fl. oz.	90	3.0	15.0	1.5	5	40	0
all flavors:							
(*Dannon Light 'n Fit Carb & Sugar Control*), 7 fl. oz.	60	6.0	4.0	2.5	15	35	0
(*Stonyfield Organic*), 6 fl. oz.	140	6.0	23.0	2.0	5	90	0
(*Yoplait*), 8 fl. oz. ..	220	6.0	43.0	3.0	15	160	0
(*Yoplait Light*), 8 fl. oz.	90	6.0	18.0	0	5	120	0

Food and Measure	cal.	prot. (gms)	carbo. (gms)	fat (gms)	chol. (mgs)	sod. (mgs)	fiber (gms)
Yogurt, drink/smoothie *(cont.)*							
banana berry, 10 fl. oz.:							
(*Dannon Frusion*) ..	260	8.0	50.0	3.5	15	105	<1.0
(*Stonyfield* Organic)	230	10.0	40.0	3.0	10	150	<1.0
berry:							
mixed (*Dannon Light*							
'n Fit), 7 fl. oz. ..	70	5.0	13.0	0	<5	85	0
wild (*Dannon Frusion*),							
10 fl. oz.	280	8.0	51.0	3.5	15	130	0
wild (*Stonyfield*							
Organic), 10 fl. oz.	230	10.0	39.0	3.0	10	150	<1.0
blueberry (*DanActive*),							
3.3 fl. oz.	90	3.0	17.0	1.5	5	40	0
cherry berry (*Dannon*							
Frusion), 10 fl. oz. .	260	8.0	50.0	3.5	15	190	<1.0
cranberry raspberry							
(*DanActive*), 3.3 fl. oz.	90	3.0	17.0	1.5	5	45	0
peach (*Stonyfield*							
Organic), 10 fl. oz. .	230	10.0	41.0	3.0	10	140	<1.0
peach passion fruit:							
(*Dannon Frusion*),							
10 fl. oz.	260	8.0	49.0	3.5	15	150	0
(*Dannon Light 'n Fit*),							
7 fl. oz.	70	5.0	13.0	0	<5	70	0
piña colada (*Dannon*							
Frusion), 10 fl. oz. .	260	8.0	50.0	‹3.5	15	135	0
raspberry:							
(*Dannon Light 'n Fit*),							
7 fl. oz.	70	5.0	13.0	0	<5	75	<1.0
(*Stonyfield* Organic),							
10 fl. oz.	230	10.0	39.0	3.0	10	150	<1.0
strawberry:							
(*DanActive*), 3.3 fl. oz.	90	3.0	17.0	1.5	5	45	0
(*Dannon Frusions*),							
10 fl. oz.	260	7.0	50	3.5	15	125	<1.0
or strawberry kiwi							
(*Dannon Light 'n*							
Fit), 7 fl. oz.	70	5.0	13.0	0	<5	70	0
strawberry banana							
(*Dannon Light 'n Fit*),							
7 fl. oz.	70	5.0	13.0	0	<5	65	0
vanilla:							
(*DanActive*), 3.3 fl. oz.	90	3.0	17.0	1.5	5	40	0

Food and Measure	cal.	prot. (gms)	carbo. (gms)	fat (gms)	chol. (mgs)	sod. (mgs)	fiber (gms)
(*Stonyfield* Organic), 10 fl. oz.	240	10.0	40.0	3.0	10	140	<1.0
Yogurt drink mix (*C&W Fruit & Yogurt Smoothie Maker*), frozen, ½ cup:							
berry blend	90	2.0	15.0	2.0	10	65	2.0
peach	80	2.0	15.0	2.0	10	65	1.0
strawberry banana ...	80	1.0	15.0	1.5	5	50	2.0
tropical blend	90	1.0	18.0	1.5	5	55	1.0
Yogurt dip, see "Fruit dip"							
Yogurt seasoning (*Neera's* Raita Mix No Salt), 1 tsp.....	6	0	2.0	0	0	2	0
Youngberry juice, (*Ceres*), 8 fl. oz. ...	120	0	30.0	0	0	10	0
Yu choy sum (*Frieda's*), 1 cup, 3 oz.	20	2.0	3.0	0	0	20	0
Yuca root:							
(*Dole*), 3.5 oz.	120	3.0	27.0	0	0	10	2.0
(*Frieda's*), ⅔ cup, 3 oz.	100	3.0	23.0	0	0	5	1.0

Z

Food and Measure	cal.	prot. (gms)	carbo. (gms)	fat (gms)	chol. (mgs)	sod. (mgs)	fiber (gms)
Ziti pasta entree, frozen, 1 pkg.:							
baked (*Amy's* Bowls), 9.5 oz.	390	9.0	62.0	12.0	0	590	5.0
Parmesan (*Michelina's Budget Gourmet Classics*), 8 oz.	250	10.0	37.0	7.0	10	500	3.0
three cheese marinara (*Smart Ones*), 9 oz.	290	12.0	44.0	7.0	10	530	4.0
Zucchini, fresh, w/skin, ½ cup, except as noted:							
raw:							
chopped	9	.7	1.8	.1	0	2	.7
sliced	8	.7	1.6	.1	0	2	.7
baby (*Frieda's*), ⅔ cup, 3 oz.	20	2.0	3.0	0	0	0	0
baby, 1 large, 3⅛" .	3	.4	.5	<.1	0	tr.	<.1
boiled, drained:							
sliced	14	.6	3.5	<.1	0	2	1.3
mashed	19	.8	4.7	.1	0	3	1.7
Zucchini, canned, Italian style, ½ cup:							
(*Del Monte*)	30	1.0	7.0	0	0	490	1.0
w/tomato juice	33	1.2	7.8	.1	0	424	1.0
Zucchini, frozen:							
w/skin, boiled, drained, 1 cup	38	2.6	7.9	.3	0	5	2.9
yellow and green (*C&W*), ⅔ cup . . .	20	1.0	3.0	0	0	5	<1.0
Zucchini, marinated, sun-dried, in jars (*Antica Italia*), 1 oz.	160	0	2.0	17.0	0	15	1.0

Food and Measure	cal.	prot. (gms)	carbo. (gms)	fat (gms)	chol. (mgs)	sod. (mgs)	fiber (gms)
Zucchini flower (*Sabores Aztecas*), ½ of 7.5-oz. can ..	10	1.0	2.0	0	0	15	0
Zucchini pancake, frozen/refrigerated:							
(*Golden*), 1.3-oz. pc. .	70	2.0	10.0	3.0	<5	210	<1.0
(*Old Fashioned Kitchen*), 2.5-oz. pc.	120	3.0	15.0	5.0	0	300	2.0
Zucchini-tomato pocket, frozen (*Aunt Trudy's* Organic), 5-oz. pc.	230	5.0	37.0	8.0	0	330	2.0